T0383222

Handbook of Assessment in Clinical Gerontology

Handbook of Assessment in Clinical Gerontology

2nd edition

Peter A. Lichtenberg

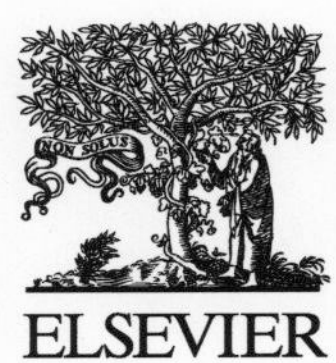

AMSTERDAM • BOSTON • HEIDELBERG • LONDON • NEW YORK • OXFORD
PARIS • SAN DIEGOSAN FRANCISCO • SINGAPORE • SYDNEY • TOKYO

Academic Press is an imprint of Elsevier

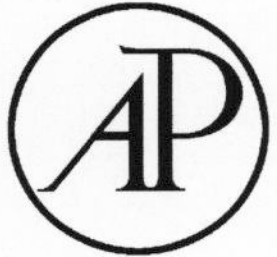

Academic Press is an imprint of Elsevier
32 Jamestown Road, London NW1 7BY, UK
30 Corporate Drive, Suite 400, Burlington, MA 01803, USA
525 B Street, Suite 1800, San Diego, CA 92101-4495, USA

First edition published by John Wiley & Sons, Inc. 1999

Second edition 2010

British Library Cataloguing-in-Publication Data
A catalogue record for this book is available from the British Library

Library of Congress Cataloging-in-Publication Data
A catalog record for this book is available from the Library of Congress

ISBN: 978-0-12-374961-1

For information on all Academic Press publications
visit our website at elsevierdirect.com

Typeset by TNQ Books and Journals Pvt Ltd.
www.tnq.co.in

Printed and bound by CPI Group (UK) Ltd, Croydon, CR0 4YY

Transferred to digital print 2012

Contents

PART II BEHAVIORAL DISORDERS

PART III COGNITION

PART IV EVERYDAY FUNCTIONING

List of Contributors

Michelle S. Ballan
Assistant Professor, Columbia University School of Social Work, New York, NY

Steve Balsis, PhD
Assistant Professor, Department of Psychology, Texas A&M University, College Station, TX

Frederic C. Blow, PhD
Professor, University of Michigan Department of Psychiatry, and Director, Department of Veterans Affairs National Serious Mental Illness Treatment Research and Evaluation Center (SMITREC)

Michelle Braun
Assistant Director, Inpatient Mental Health, Boston VA Healthcare System, Instructor in Psychiatry, Harvard Medical School

Kathryn E. Brogan, PhD, RD K-L
Assistant Professor, Department of Nutrition and Food Science, and Department of Pediatrics, Wayne State University, Detroit, MI

Donna K. Broshek, PhD
Co-Director, Neurocognitive Assessment Lab, University of Virginia School of Medicine, Charlottesville, Virginia

Louis D. Burgio, PhD
Harold R. Johnson Professor of Social Work, Research Professor, Institute of Gerontology, University of Michigan, Ann Arbor, MI

Rebecca P. Cameron, PhD
Associate Professor, Psychology, California State University, Sacramento, CA

Cameron J. Camp
Hearthstone Alzheimer Care, Woburn, MA

Cheryl N. Carmin, PhD
Professor & Director, Department of Psychiatry, University of Illinois at Chicago, Chicago, IL

Brian D. Carpenter, PhD
Associate Professor, Department of Psychology, Washington University, St. Louis, MO

Caroline M. Ciliberti, MS
Department of Psychology, West Virginia University, Morgantown, WV 26506-6010

Colleen Clemency, PhD
Edith Nourse Rogers Memorial Veterans Hospital, Bedford, MA

Jiska Cohen-Mansfield, PhD
George Washington University Medical Center, Washington, DC, USA, Tel Aviv University Herczeg, Institute on Aging and Sackler Faculty of Medicine, Tel-Aviv, Israel

Colin A Depp
Department of Psychiatry, University of California, San Diego, CA

Lisa W. Drozdick, PhD
Research Director II, Clinical Assessment, Pearson, 19500 Bulverde Road, San Antonio, TX 78259

Jamie K. Ducharme
University of Virginia Health System, Department of Neurology, Charlottesville, VA

Barry A. Edelstein
Professor, Department of Psychology, West Virginia University, Morgantown, WV 26506-6040

Erin E. Emery, PhD
Department of Behavioral Sciences, Rush University Medical Center, Chicago, IL

Adam Gerstenecker
University of Louisville

Gali Goldwaser, PhD
PTSD and Stress-related Disorders, Research Service (151), VA San Diego Healthcare System, San Diego, CA

Marcia G. Hunt, PhD
VA Connecticut Healthcare System, Department of Psychiatry, Yale University School of Medicine, New Haven, CT

Alden L. Gross, MHS
Department of Mental Health, Johns Hopkins Bloomberg School of Public Health, Baltimore, MD

Lee Hyer, EdH
Mercer School of Medicine, Macon GA

Renee Hyer
Mercer School of Medicine, Macon GA

Catherine Jen, PhD
Professor and Chair, Department of Nutrition and Food Science, Wayne State University, Detroit, MI

Katherine S. Judge
Department of Psychology, Cleveland State University, Cleveland, OH

Deborah A. King, Ph.D.
University of Rochester Medical Center, Rochester, NY

Jennifer D. Kowalkowski, MS
Doctoral Candidate, Psychology Department, Eastern Michigan University, Ypsilanti, MI

Kristen Lawton Barry, PhD
Research Associate Professor, University of Michigan Department of Psychiatry, and Investigator, Department of Veterans Affairs National Serious Mental Illness Treatment Research and Evaluation Center (SMITREC)

Michelle M. Lee
Department of Behavioral Medicine, Midwestern University, Downers Grove, IL

Larry Lemos, RN MSN MHA GCNS-BC (Chapter 13)
Geriatric Clinical Nurse Specialist, Community Living Center, VA Long Beach Health, Care System; Assistant Professor, Columbia University School of Social Work, New York, NY

Casey Loughran
Department of Psychiatry, University of California, San Diego, CA

Catherine L. Lysack, PhD, OT(C)
Deputy Director, Institute of Gerontology, Professor, Occupational Therapy & Gerontology, Wayne State University, Detroit, MI

Theodore K. Malmstrom, PhD
Department of Neurology & Psychiatry, Saint Louis University School of Medicine

Carol A. Manning
University of Virginia Health System, Department of Neurology, Charlottesville, VA

Bernice A. Marcopulos, PhD
Associate Professor, Psychiatry and Neurobehavioral Sciences, University of Virginia, Charlottesville, VA and Director, Neuropsychology Lab, Western State Hospital, Staunton, VA

Benjamin T. Mast
Associate Professor, Department of Psychological & Brain Sciences, University of Louisville, KT

Aletha R. Miller, PhD
Geropsychology Postdoctoral Fellow, Deer Oaks Mental Health Associates-Behavioral Health Organization, Fort Worth, TX

Victor Molinari, PhD, ABPP
Department of Aging and Mental Health Disparities, College of Behavioral and Community Sciences, Louis de la Parte Florida Mental Health Institute, University of South Florida, Tampa, FL

Linda R. Mona, PhD
Clinical Psychologist, VA, Long Beach Healthcare System, Behavioral Health (06/116-B), Long Beach, CA

Jennifer Moye
Director, Geriatric Mental Health, VA Boston healthcare system, Associate Professor of Psychology, Department of Psychiatry, Harvard Medical School.

Elizabeth A. Mulligan
Department of Psychology, Washington University, St. Louis, MO

Thomas F. Oltmanns, PhD
Edgar James Swift Professor in Arts & Sciences, Professor of Psychology and Psychiatry, Director of Clinical Training, Department of Psychology, Washington University in St. Louis, St. Louis, MO

Raymond L. Ownby, MD, PhD
Professor & Chair, Department of Psychiatry, College of Osteopathic Medicine, Nova Southeastern University, Ft. Lauderdale, FL

Jeanine M. Parisi, PhD
Department of Mental Health, Johns Hopkins Bloomberg School of Public Health, Baltimore, MD

Joseph M. Pellerito, Jr., PhD, OTRL, CDI
Department of Occupatioal Therapy, College of Health and Human Services, Western Michigan University, Kalamazoo, MI

George W. Rebok, PhD
Department of Mental Health, Johns Hopkins Bloomberg School of Public Health, Baltimore, MD

Elizabeth J. Santos, MD
University of Rochester Medical Center, Rochester, NY

Lori Schindel Martin, PhD, RN
Associate Professor, Daphne Cockwell School of Nursing, Ryerson University, Toronto, Ontario

Ciera Scott
Mercer School of Medicine, Macon GA

Michael J. Skrajner
Hearthstone Alzheimer Care, Wiloughby, OH

Adam P. Spira, PhD
Department of Mental Health, Johns Hopkins Bloomberg School of Public Health, Baltimore, MD

Maggie L. Syme, PhD
Geropsychology Postdoctoral Fellow, VA Boston Healthcare System, Psychology Service, Boston, MA

Raymond C. Tait, PhD
Department of Neurology & Psychiatry, Saint Louis University School of Medicine

Tracy Trevorrow
Chaminade University of Honolulu

Chriscelyn M. Tussey, PsyD
Postdoctoral Fellow in Clinical Neuropsychology, Neurocognitive Assessment Lab, University of Virginia School of Medicine, Charlottesville, Virginia and Western State Hospital, Staunton, VA

Ipsit Vahia
Department of Psychiatry, University of California, San Diego, CA

Carey Wexler Sherman, PhD
Research Investigator, Institute for Social Research, University of Michigan, Ann Arbor, MI

Carol J. Whitlatch, PhD
Assistant Director, Margaret Blenkner Research Institute, Benjamin Rose Institute, 11900 Fairhill Rd., Suite 300, Cleveland OH

John L. Woodard
Wayne State University

Erin L. Woodhead, PhD
Department of Behavioral Sciences, Rush University Medical Center, Chicago, IL

Catherine Yeager, PhD
Essex County Hospital Center, Institute of Mental Health Policy, Research, and Treatment, Cedar Grove, NJ

Introduction

Peter A. Lichtenberg, PhD, ABPP

Since I edited the first *Handbook of Assessment in Clinical Gerontology* in 1999, the field has witnessed a continuing explosion of research on clinical issues and a greater availability of assessment instruments. This book is intended primarily for those who use behavioral health (i.e., non-surgical, non-medication) assessments and interventions. The importance of understanding how to assess phenomena like affect, cognition, sleep, nutrition, home safety, driving (and many others) in older age continues to be a key to clinicians having an accurate understanding of change in older individuals. The paradox in clinical gerontology is that with the increase in sophistication and expertise in understanding gerontology syndromes and phenomena, there is a continuing decline in the number of professionals intensively trained to work with older adults, as well as a dearth of training opportunities for those interested in working with older adults. Thus, older adults are being (and will further be) assessed and treated by those practitioners who might only have the barest of training or experience in clinical gerontology.

This version of the *Handbook* is aimed at assisting expert gerontologists, as well as those who have little or no background in gerontology. Each of the book's chapters has the following five common components: (1) assessment instruments thoroughly reviewed; (2) two to four actual instruments embedded into the chapter; (2) case examples to illustrate the strengths and challenges of actual assessments; (4) discussion of the use of reassessment; and (5) addressing multicultural diversity issues in assessment. This introductory chapter reviews and expands upon key basic concepts for clinical gerontologists presented with the first edition of the *Handbook*.

PRINCIPLE 1: AGE AND FUNCTIONING ARE NOT LINEARLY RELATED IN CLINICAL SETTINGS

Clinical gerontologists and those who work with older adults must become familiar with core geriatric medicine concepts. The most common ones are disability, comorbidity, and frailty. Once used synonymously, *disability*, *comorbidity*, and *frailty* are now understood as distinct, although overlapping and related conditions, which have significant implications for gerontologists. Perhaps the most familiar concept is *disability*, defined as "difficulty or dependency in carrying out activities essential to independent living." Impairments affecting lower extremity mobility, for example, may curtail a person's independence in transportation and locomotion. In geriatric rehabilitation, disability increases directly with age (Lichtenberg, 1998). Independence with mobility dropped from 30% for rehabilitation patients in their 60s to 3% for those aged 80–95. Similarly, independence with toileting was 65% in the 60-year-old group, and dropped to 40% in those aged 80–95 (Lichtenberg, 1998).

Frailty describes an aggregate risk of complications for an older patient. Its early definition centered on the presence of more than one system (e.g., heart, lung, kidney, brain) compromised by disease and disability. More recently, frailty has become more clearly defined in its symptoms and effects on rehabilitation outcomes. Fried, Ferrucci, Darer, Williamson, & Anderson (2004) summarized her group's definition as a syndrome with the following elements: decreased appetite and weight loss; gait disturbance and falling; and declining cognition. Some cases also have significant respiratory distress. This constellation of symptoms has an unclear etiology, and, rather, represents multiple system failure. Frailty has been linked to significantly increased rates of nursing home placement and mortality (Ferrucci et al., 2004). In the rehabilitation setting, frailty was related to older age of the patient (Hanks & Lichtenberg, 1996). Discharge from rehabilitation to a dependent situation increased from 35% in those aged 60–79 to near 50% in those aged 80–95. More specifically, discharge to a nursing home increased from 5% of those aged 60–69 to 25% of those aged 80–95. Thus, disability and frailty in clinical settings appeared to have direct relationships to aging, whereas comorbidity and mortality do not.

Comorbidity refers to the presence of two or more medically diagnosed diseases in a given individual. Community-dwelling older adults most commonly suffer from arthritis (48%), hypertension (36%) and heart disease (27%), and the prevalence of these conditions increases with age. This relation often does not hold in rehabilitation settings. That is to say that although there is a clear relation between disability and patient age, there is no clear relation between comorbidity and age. In our studies (Lichtenberg, 1998), those aged 60–69 had 1.4 comorbidities, those aged 70–79 had 1.6 comorbidities, and those aged 80–95 had 1.3 comorbidities. The lack of a relation between age and comorbidity was further supported in a three-year mortality study in which age was not related to mortality, but comorbidity was. In this study (Arfken, Lichtenberg, & Tancer 2000), 36% of the sample died within three years of discharge from rehabilitation, with equal proportions of deaths coming from the 60–69, 70–79, and 80–95 age groups. Crimmins, Kim and Seeman (2009) examined poverty and biological risk, and their findings provide some plausible explanations why age and mortality are not linearly related in clinical settings. Their data were collected from two National Health and Nutrition Examination Survey (NHANES) samples, which they then linked to the national death index. The NHANES data revealed that poor people in each decade of life (20s through 70s) had higher levels of biological risk than people who are not poor in the corresponding ages, thus supporting the notion of premature aging in those who endure poverty.

The overlap between and distinctions among disability, frailty, and comorbidity in older individuals has specific implications for clinical gerontology. Disability is inversely related to strength, coordination, and muscle mass, all characteristics associated with younger versus older ages. Frailty is a specific and extreme expression of the multisystem failures that occur when diseases interact with age-related deficiencies. Thus, in medical rehabilitation, for example, no matter what the primary diagnosis, one finds that younger patients are stronger, suffer less disability, and return more easily to independent living compared with the oldest patients.

Comorbidity issues stand in contrast, however, as younger individuals have amounts of comorbid disease equal to those of the oldest patients. In fact, the finding that mortality does not differ among age groups indicates that perhaps the younger and older sets of geriatric rehabilitation patients represent different populations. The younger group (ages 60–79) present with much more extreme disease and disability than their community-based peers, while the older group more closely resembles their community cohort. It may well be that significant numbers of the young–old cohort never make it to the oldest old-age groups. This last conclusion is critical to minority elders, who have often grown up in and continue to live in poverty.

PRINCIPLE 2: THERE IS NOW A BLURRING OF NORMAL VS. CLINICAL AGING

Whereas 20 years ago the areas of research in normal aging (e.g., cognitive aging, social gerontology) did not intersect with the world of clinical aging (e.g., dementia, depression), these boundaries have blurred over time. Longitudinal data sets which selected healthy older adults created to study "normal aging" are now, because their participants have moved to advanced age and are no longer all healthy, become prime data sets for the study of dementia or late-life depression. There is no longer a clear demarcation between normal aging and clinical aging because gerontologists have recognized that almost every geriatric syndrome (e.g., depression, disability, dementia) has a slow onset to it, and is viewed as a chronic condition. A strategy for effective assessment and treatment of chronic conditions is to identify changes early in the syndrome and intervene. Thus, pathological changes are hypothesized to begin in what would be classified as normal aging. Two examples of this are disability and dementia.

Fried et al. (2004) state that "physical disability in late life is … an outcome of disease and physiologic alterations with aging, with the impact of these underlying causes modified by social, economic, and behavioral factors as well as access to medical care." As such, there are many variables along the pathway toward disability at which intervention and prevention techniques can be aimed to help identify and delay disability onset. In studying pathways toward disability, Fried, Bandeen-Roche, Chaves, & Johnson, (2000) posited that changes in the ability to complete tasks of daily living are preceded by changes in physical functioning. The concept of pre-disability or subclinical disability status, a stage that lies before dependence on the disability spectrum, has been put forth. In this subclinical stage, an older adult is still able to complete a task, but experiences decreased ability and, as a result, has altered the way in which the task is performed. This approach, which is aimed at intervention for high risk groups, now puts a clinical label on a condition without any obvious functional decline. Some people with pre-clinical disability will improve and some will have their conditions worsen and experience disability.

A similar extension of clinical characterization has occurred in issues related to dementia. Viewing Alzheimer's disease as a chronic condition like cancer, diabetes, and hypertension makes early detection and treatment a critical objective. During the past decade there have been several attempts to create new early detection markers. Mild cognitive impairment represents one of the most impacting of these strategies. Mild cognitive impairment was first characterized nearly a decade ago (Petersen et al., 1999). The new category was applied to people who had significantly reduced memory abilities, while retaining strengths in other cognitive and functional areas. Early studies indicated that nearly 60–90% of people suffering from mild cognitive impairment progressed to Alzheimer's disease within five years. Morris and colleagues (2001) concluded that mild cognitive impairment represented early Alzheimer's disease. Morris' study, in which longitudinal data and post mortem examinations were conducted, generated great enthusiasm. Despite these early high hopes, persons meeting mild cognitive impairment criteria have not uniformly progressed to having a dementia. Indeed, a significant number of older adults meeting the criteria for mild cognitive impairment actually demonstrated improved cognition over time (Brooks, Tuerson, & White, 2007). Mild cognitive impairment comes under more criticism than pre-disability because there are no current interventions known to postpone any dementia syndrome.

Pre-disability and mild cognitive impairment provide clinical-like categories for those whose symptoms do not yet meet the criteria for a geriatric syndrome. Clinicians need to be extremely sensitive as to how they use labels like pre-disability and mild cognitive impairment.

PRINCIPLE 3: GERONTOLOGIST MUST WORK TO ACTIVELY REDUCE AGEISM

Ageism, pervasive discrimination against older adults, is widespread in the United States (Palmore, 1990). Allport used his social categorization theory to describe the basic tenants of discrimination (Allport, 1954). The non-dominant group (older adults in this case) is viewed as homogeneous and portrayed as having a variety of negative characteristics. Older adults are viewed stereotypically as: (1) alike; (2) alone and lonely; (3) sick, frail, and dependent; (4) depressed; (5) rigid; and (6) unable to cope (Hinrichsen, 2006). This pervasive view portrays all older adults in a negative light, ignoring the incredible hetereogeneity of aging and the strengths and positive attributes of older adults. Clinical gerontologists, themselves, must be cognizant of their own ageist thoughts and beliefs, and try to minimize these.

Ageism can often be found where age and disability or decline intersect. This can be reflected in interactions whereby gerontologists might direct their comments only to a family caregiver, for example, and ignore the person with dementia who is sitting in the same room. Acting as an expert witness in a conservatorship case, I reviewed the neuropsychological report of a 94-year-old gentleman. The man in question had no cognitive deficits, and performed in the superior range on all cognitive tests. Despite this, the original evaluator, a neuropsychologist with excellent credentials concluded that "all older adults should have a conservator" since on average older people are more susceptible to financial fraud.

Ageism and overly paternalistic conclusions are, in my experience, often found in cases such as the above. In these cases, broad generalizations are applied to individual cases without a close examination of the unique circumstances of the case. General population findings of risk factors and predictive abilities are given too much weight when being applied to an individual. The fact that older adults are more susceptible to financial fraud does not support the notion of the loss of financial freedom for each older individual. Even with good normative (generalized information) data it is paramount for clinical gerontologists to focus on the unique individual being assessed. An individual's assessment must focus on the unique strengths noted in the person, environment or support system, and not simply on whether the assessment supports a diagnosis of a geriatric syndrome. When can a person with dementia make a valid will? What decisions about care can a person with dementia make? These types of questions can only be adequately addressed when details of individual cases are examined objectively and systematically.

PRINCIPLE 4: ALL GERIATRIC CARE OCCURS WITHIN A TEAM CONTEXT AND INTEGRATED CARE IS THE PREFERABLE MODEL

Because older adults are treated by multiple practitioners, whether clinicians realize it or not, a team exists. Often this team of professionals is not activated and contributes to the broken health care system we now have. I had the pleasure of serving on Dr Sharon Brehm's American Psychological Association 2007–08 Presidential task force Integrated Care for an Aging Population. During our background research it became clear how the older adults' experiences of fragmented care contribute to poor assessment and treatment. Older adults are often treated by multiple practitioners, and rarely is any of that care coordinated. This despite evidence which has found geriatric teams lead to better clinical outcomes and for healthier teams to have positive, supportive, and frequent communication among their members (Lemieux-Charles & McGuire, 2006; Sheehan, Robertson, & Ormond, 2007). Integrated care, a team approach that emphasizes a high level of communication and coordination, should be the standard for gerontological assessment and treatment. Most practitioners are not trained in team environments and the following are some core traits that clinicians working with older adults should understand to improve their functioning within teams:

1. Clinical gerontologists should become familiar with the roles of other team members, identifying areas of overlap and areas of non-overlap.
2. Models of health delivery may differ among team members. Some clinicians may be most comfortable adhering to a traditional medical model: acting in more of a paternalistic mode and not including the emotional experiences of the patient. Other clinicians are trained in a more

collaborative approach in which the patient is seen as an equal partner, and the patient's emotional experiences are viewed as highly germane to treatment.

3. Conflict among team members is common and can lead to either a strengthening or weakening of the team. Increased communication brings out differences between different professional beliefs, different personalities, etc. Finding ways to resolve these conflicts in a productive manner is key to effective care.
4. Clinical gerontologists are often aware of and can be useful in applying conflict resolution skills. Since many trained in gerontology have experience in working with teams, clinical gerontologists may be in a good position to assist the team with conflict resolution.
5. Health care teams are communicating in increasingly diverse ways, ranging from team rounds face to face and the use of telemedicine to electronic medical records. Team functioning need not be thought of only as permanent teams; sometimes the coordination of care enables smooth entrance and exits by some members delivering varied or time-limited clinical service.

PRINCIPLE 5: A MAJOR TASK IN ASSESSMENT CONTINUES TO BE THE IDENTIFICATION OF PATHOLOGICAL FROM NORMAL PROCESSES

There are two fundamental needs clinical gerontologists have: (1) the need for ever-increasing specificity of syndromes and familiarity with these syndromes; and (2) the need for good normative data across multiple health domains and assessment tools. Both of these continue to evolve. In my clinical consultation I am often surprised, and indeed alarmed, at the misapplication of symptoms to a diagnosis: delirium confused as dementia; dementia unrecognized in the context of disability or life-long psychiatric conditions; end of life conditions of frailty going unrecognized; and aging equating with incapacity. These common errors originate in the lack of familiarity with geriatric syndromes and also the lack of good normative data to understand the normal range of functioning.

What is the normal range of scores for older adults in domains such as sleep, pain, anxiety, and gait speed, for instance? How much daily variability is there in scores on assessments of depression, cognition, and nutrition, for example? Normative data is so often influenced by age, education, and historical/cultural factors. In fact, one key to improving assessment of under-represented minority elders is the ongoing effort to improve the normative database. Cognitive and affective assessments have been the two areas to receive extensive attention to normative data. Cognitive test interpretations are dependent upon norms, which then can be matched to an individual's age, education, and often quality of education. The Logical Memory subtest, from the Wechsler Memory Scales, has consistently been related to reading ability, whereas the Fuld Object Memory Exam has not. Thus, over-reliance on norms for White elders on tests of logical memory overestimated memory decline in Black elders. Depression scales have been compared across diverse populations, with some studies finding differential item validity for different groups, and some not finding any differences. These studies have demonstrated that reading ability impacts instruments more than we expected. The Beck Depression Inventory, for example, was found to be less accurate for less educated older adults than the Geriatric Depression Scale (see Lichtenberg, 1998) because the Beck test contained questions that were more difficult to understand. How much of a sleep inventory, a treatment adherence questionnaire, or a nutrition questionnaire related to age and education?

Improving our normative base across all instruments is important for adults in general, but is especially important for members of diverse populations. Without a good normative database, assessment tools will likely overestimate pathology in older adults from minority groups. This has clearly been the case for cognitive assessment (see Lucas et al., 2005). As our nation's older population becomes more and more diverse the importance of having adequate norms becomes ever more important. We will need normative data on Spanish versions of assessment tools, as well as many other languages.

PRINCIPLE 6: CLINICAL GERONTOLOGISTS SHOULD USE MULTIPLE METHODS OF ASSESSMENT AND BRIEF ASSESSMENTS

Assessments of domains of interest may be best accomplished by incorporating self-report of abilities, a performance-based test of abilities, a collateral report of abilities (where it makes sense), and an analysis of the consistency or discrepancy between the reports. Accurately estimating one's own abilities or habits (meta-cognition) not only strengthens one's assessment of cognitive abilities, but also allows for the examination of awareness of deficit issues. Self-report measures alone are often not enough for the assessment process. The evaluator looks for converging evidence across these multiple methods of assessment and attempts to integrate these into the assessment.

Conceptual and practical issues continue to support the use of brief assessments. Depending on the setting and purpose of the assessment, a two-tiered approach may be most useful. The first tier would be at the screening level. Most of the assessment instruments embedded in this *Handbook* would qualify as screening tools. Screening instruments are designed for use with high risk populations to call attention to a high likelihood of a problem in a specific behavioral domain. The short version of the MAST-G, for instance, is designed to be sensitive to alcohol problems but only takes a few minutes to administer. The second tier of assessment, triggered by a positive finding on a screening, or other suggestive evidence, consists of a more thorough assessment in which performance and collateral report may also accompany a more robust set of assessment measures. For behavioral health treatments, i.e., alcohol, pain, nutrition, treatment adherence, the assessment process is often intertwined with a brief educational component, assessment of patient beliefs, and even a brief motivational interviewing intervention.

One-third of this second edition of the *Handbook* covers topics not covered in the previous edition. Many of these assessment areas were relatively neglected a decade ago, but are receiving ever-increasing attention. These include personality disorders, elder abuse and financial fraud, family functioning and its role in supporting the older adult, nutrition, treatment adherence for chronic disease, neighborhood and home safety, personal choice in those with dementia, and assessment of cognitive training. The chapters are divided into three sections: psychopathology; behavioral disorders; and cognition. Accurate assessment and the use of assessment data in treatment remain at the cornerstone of excellent clinical care for older adults. This *Handbook* was created to provide clinicians more access to a wide variety of assessment tools in order that older adults receive more accurate assessments which will then guide clinical care and treatment planning.

REFERENCES

Allport, G. W. (1979). *The nature of prejudice*. Cambridge, MA: Perseus Books (Original work published in 1954).

Arfken, C. L., Lichtenberg, P. A., & Tancer, M. (1999). Cognitive impairment and depression predict mortality in medically ill older adults. *Journal of Gerontology: Medical Sciences*, *54A*, M152–M156.

Brooks, B. L., Iverson, G. L., & White, T. (2007). Substantial risk of "Accidental MCI" in healthy older adults: Base rates of low memory scores in neuropsychological assessment. *Journal of the International Neuropsychological Society*, *13*, 490–500.

Crimmins, E. M., Kim, J. K., & Seeman, T. E. (2009). Poverty and biological risk: The earlier "aging" of the poor. *Journal of Gerontology: Medical Sciences*, *64A*, 286–292.

Ferrucci, L., Guralnik, J. M., Studenski, S., Fried, L. P., Cutler, G. B., & Walston, J. D. (2004). Designing randomized, controlled trials aimed at preventing or delaying functional decline and disability in frail, older persons: A consensus report. *Journal of the American Geriatrics Society*, *52*, 625–634.

Fried, L. P., Bandeen-Roche, K., Chaves, P. M., & Johnson, B. (2000). Preclinical mobility disability predicts incident mobility disability in older women. *Journal of Gerontology, Medical Sciences*, *55*, M43–52.

Fried, L., Ferrucci, L., Darer, J., Williamson, J. D., & Anderson, G. (2004). Untangling the concepts of disability, frailty, and comorbidity: Implications for improved targeting and care. *Journal of Gerontology: Medical Sciences*, *59*, 255–263.

Hanks, R. A., & Lichtenberg, P. A. (1996). Physical, psychological and social outcomes in geriatric rehabilitation patients. *Archives of Physical Medicine and Rehabilitation*, *77*, 783–792.

Hinrichsen, G. (2006). Why multicultural issues matter to practitioners working with older adults. *Professional Psychology, Research and Practice*, *37*, 29–35.

Lemieux-Charles, L., & McGuire, W. L. (2006). What do we know about health care team effectiveness: A review of the literature. *Medical Care Research and Review*, *63*, 263–300.

Lichtenberg, P. A. (1998). *Mental Health Practice in Geriatric Health Care Settings*, New York, NY: Haworth Press.

Lucas, J. A., Ivnik, R. J., Smith, G. E., Ferman, T. J., Smith, G. E., Parfitt, F. C., et al. (2005). Mayo's older African Americans normative studies: Normative data for commonly used clinical neuropsychology measures. *The Clinical Neuropsychologist*, *19*, 162–183.

Morris, J. M., Sorandt, M., Miller, J. P., McKeel, D. W., Price, J. L., Rubin, E. H., & Berg, L. (2001). Mild cognitive impairment represents early-stage Alzheimer's disease. *Archives of Neurology*, *58*, 397–405.

Palmore, E. (1990). *Ageism: Negative and Positive*. New York, NY: Springer.

Petersen, R. C., Smith, G. E., Waring, S. C., Ivnik, R. J., Tangalos, E. G., & Kokmen, E. (1999). Mild cognitive impairment: Clinical characterization and outcome. *Archives of Neurology*, *56*(3), 303–308.

Sheehan, D., Robertson, L., & Ormond, T. (2007). Comparison of language used and patterns of communication in interprofessional and multidisciplinary teams. *Journal of Interprofessional Care*, *21*, 17–30.

PART

Psychopathology later in life

1

CHAPTER

1

Assessment of Depression and Bereavement in Older Adults

Barry A. Edelstein[1], Lisa W. Drozdick[2], Caroline M. Ciliberti[1]

[1] *Department of Psychology, West Virginia University Morgantown, WV, USA,*
[2] *Clinical Assessment, Pearson, San Antonio, TX, USA*

This chapter addresses the assessment of older adult depression and bereavement. The assessment of depression in older adults can be complicated due to age-related differences in the presentation of depression, comorbid medical and mental health problems, and age-related changes in cognitive functioning. Moreover, available assessment instruments may have less utility with older adults, either because they were developed with younger adults, or because they were developed to meet diagnostic criteria that may not be appropriate for older adults (see Jeste, Blazer, & First, 2005). Consequently, clinicians may be failing to identify depression adequately in older adults and to identify and treat older adults with subsyndromal or minor depression, which involves considerable disability but is not formally recognized as a clinical disorder.

This chapter addresses both depression and bereavement because loss is often a significant contributor to and risk factor for depression, and adults face increasing losses as they move through older adulthood. Depression is a normal response to a significant loss. The depression can last for a considerable amount of time and be functionally debilitating. Bereavement is one of the more significant risk factors for the first onset of depression and recurrent depression in older adults (Bruce, 2002). In light of the clinical significance of bereavement, its increasing likelihood over the lifespan, and the paucity of assessment literature addressing the topic, we have included the assessment of bereavement in this discussion of late-life depression assessment.

EPIDEMIOLOGY OF LATE-LIFE DEPRESSION

Symptoms of depression tend to be approximately as prevalent in late life as in mid-life (Blazer, 2003). The frequency of depressive symptoms among the oldest old appears higher than among younger adults, although factors other than age (e.g., greater proportion of women, increased cognitive impairment, lower socioeconomic status, greater physical disability) may account for the difference (Blazer, 2003). The prevalence of clinically significant symptoms of depression ranges from 8–16% among community-dwelling older adults (Blazer, 2003). The prevalence of major depression in community-dwelling older adults ranges from approximately 1–4% (Beekman, Copeland, & Prince, 1999). Prevalence estimates for minor depression among community-dwelling older adults range from approximately 4–13%, with the highest estimate found in the Netherlands (Beekman et al., 1995). With minor and major depression combined, Steffens, Fisher, Langa, Potter, and Plassman (2009) found an overall prevalence of 11.19%, with the prevalence being similar for community-dwelling older men and women.

Handbook of Assessment in Clinical Gerontology. DOI: 10.1016/B978-0-12-374961-1.10001-6

Prevalence estimates of major depression vary across settings, with increases in prevalence as one moves from outpatient to inpatient settings. The prevalence of major depression among older adults seen in primary care settings ranges from 5–10% (Lyness et al., 2002; Schulberg et al., 1998). Among hospitalized older adults, prevalence rates of major depression range from 10–12% (Blazer, 1994; Koenig, Meador, Cohen, & Blazer, 1988). Prevalence estimates for major depression among long-term care residents are even higher, ranging from 12.4% to 14.4% (Parmalee, Katz, & Lawton, 1989; Teresi, Abrams, Holmes, Ramirez, & Eimicke, 2001).

These epidemiological findings must be tempered by the questionable adequacy of our current diagnostic system for older adults (see discussion below) and the finding of different relations between age and depression across studies. Researchers have noted varied relations between age and depression, including negative linear, curvilinear, and positive linear relations (Nguyen & Zonderman, 2006). Nguyen and Zonderman suggest that the differences in relations can be attributed, in part, to the nature of the assessment measures employed. Measures of *depressive symptoms* reveal a negative linear relation or positive curvilinear relation. Such relations suggest fewer symptoms of depression as one ages, or increased symptoms among younger and older adults when compared with an intermediate age group. The authors note that when *diagnostic measures of major depression* are used, there tends to be a positive linear or negative curvilinear relation between age and depression. Thus, major depression increases with age, or is lower among younger and older groups when compared with an intermediate age group.

CONCEPTUAL APPROACHES TO ASSESSMENT

The assessment paradigm employed by the clinician determines the assessment methods and instruments employed, the questions addressed, and the integration and use of the assessment results (Edelstein, Martin, & Koven, 2003; Edelstein & Koven, in press). Haynes and O'Brien (2000) have defined an assessment paradigm as "a set of principles, beliefs, values, hypotheses, and methods advocated in an assessment discipline or by its adherents" (p. 10). Two conceptually distinct paradigms are the traditional (e.g., trait-oriented, psychodynamic) and the behavioral (e.g., behavior–analytic, cognitive–behavioral). One can distinguish between traditional and behavioral paradigms through an examination of how each explains or accounts for behavior. More traditional approaches tend to emphasize an individual's dispositional characteristics (see Mischel, 1968) or hypothetical constructs (e.g., anxiety, depression), which are inferred from the individual's self-reports and observed behavior (Edelstein, Woodhead, Bower, & Lowery, 2006). Such approaches to psychopathology often include exploration of an individual's feelings or affective states.

Behavioral approaches tend to be more contextual and emphasize descriptions of environmental conditions under which the behavior of interest is more or less likely to occur. A behavioral account of an individual's behavior involves a description of the conditions under which the behavior occurs (see Edelstein & Koven, in press). More emphasis is placed on the variables controlling the behavior of interest, and less emphasis is placed on characteristics of the individual. It is important to note that behavioral approaches do not discount the role of cognitions or private events; however, they do not consider cognitions to have causal efficacy. Cognitions are treated as any other behavior, whether observable or not. For the purposes of the present discussion, emphasis is placed on behavioral assessment that relies primarily on direct observation of overt behaviors.

One might also distinguish between traditional and behavioral approaches by considering the distinction between nomothetic and idiographic approaches to personality assessment (see Allport, 1936). Traditional approaches are more closely aligned with a nomothetic approach, which involves an examination of the commonalities among individuals. This approach underlies classification systems such as the *Diagnostic and Statistical Manual—Fourth Edition* (DSM-IV) (American Psychiatric Association, 1994). In contrast, behavioral approaches are more similar to the idiographic approach, which is used to ascertain the uniqueness of an individual.

Traditional and behavioral approaches and instruments are often combined. For example, one might administer a self-report depression inventory and examine the individual item responses to gain an individualized understanding of the individual's mood. The total score on the instrument may also be compared with that of a normative sample to enable one to make a judgment about whether the individual's score is below or above a cutoff score that signals a clinical level of depression. Each approach has its strengths and weaknesses.

As one moves from cognitively intact to cognitively impaired older adults, one must rely more on the direct observation of behavior, because the self-reported experiences of depression become unreliable and/or invalid, and eventually unavailable as cognitive skills diminish. Nomothetic assessment instruments must now depend upon the inferences of clinicians based on direct observations of the older adult. Mood and other symptoms must now be inferred from overt behavior. The question of why an individual is reporting particular experiences and engaging in particular behaviors can no longer be answered by questioning that individual. The nomothetic and idiographic assessment methods tend to converge on the observation of behavior.

DEFINITION AND DIAGNOSTIC ISSUES

Jeste et al. (2005) cogently argued that age-appropriate diagnostic criteria are needed for the major DSM psychiatric diagnoses. This issue is particularly salient for the diagnosis of late-life depression, as older adults often present a different array or profile of symptoms than younger adults (Caine, Lyness, King, & Connors, 1994; Fiske & O'Riley, 2008). For example, older adults are less likely than younger adults to report suicidal ideation (Blazer, Bachar, & Hughes, 1987), guilt (Gallo, Rabins, & Anthony, 1999; Musetti et al., 1989; Wallace & Pfohl, 1995), and dysphoria (Gallo, Anthony, & Muthen, 1994; Gallo et al., 1999). In contrast, older adults are more likely than younger adults to report hopelessness and helplessness (Christensen et al., 1999), somatic symptoms (Gallo et al., 1994), psychomotor retardation (Gallo et al., 1994), weight loss (Blazer et al., 1987), and loss of appetite (Blazer et al., 1987).

The issue of whether somatic symptoms should be considered among the diagnostic criteria for depression among older adults has been somewhat controversial (see Norris, Snow-Turek, & Blankenship, 1995), in part because of the overlap of symptoms of physical disease and somatic symptoms of depression (e.g., low energy, sleep disturbance, diminished appetite and sexual drive). The frequency and severity of medical conditions increase with age and can lead to many of the somatic symptoms included in the diagnosis of depression (e.g., weight loss or gain, insomnia, fatigue). Moreover, depression is frequently comorbid with physical illness and cognitive dysfunction, both of which increase with age.

Several studies reported increased endorsement of somatic symptoms of depression with increasing age and suggest removing somatic symptoms from self-report measures of depression (e.g., Barefoot, Mortensen, Helms, Avlund, & Schroll, 2001; Berry, Storandt, & Coyne, 1984; Bolla-Wilson & Bleecker, 1989; Goldberg, Breckenridge, & Sheikh, 2003; Mahurin & Gatz, 1983). However, many studies suggest that removing somatic items from assessment instruments may result in decreased sensitivity to depression in older adults (Drayer et al., 2005; Kirmayer, 2001; Norris, Arnau, Bramson, & Meagher, 2004). Moreover, somatic symptoms cannot always be attributed to physical disease (Gatz & Hurwicz, 1990; Olin, Schneider, Eaton, Zemansky, & Pollock, 1992; Wagle, Ho, Wagle, & Berrios, 2000). There is evidence to suggest that while changes in appetite and sexual drive may not be indicative of depression among older adults, the remaining somatic symptoms are indicative (Nguyen & Zonderman, 2006; Norris et al., 2004). Clinicians should consider assessing somatic symptoms of depression, although caution should be used when interpreting results obtained in individuals for whom medical issues may be contributing to results.

Several other factors can complicate the assessment of late-life depression, including the onset of symptoms. The time of onset of the first depressive episode of major depression may be related to the nature of depression symptoms (Jeste et al., 2005). The symptoms of first-onset, late-life depression (after age 60) may be different from depression that occurs early in life (before age 60) and recurs in late life (Brodaty et al., 2001).

Older adults can experience symptoms of depression that do not meet criteria for a depression diagnosis, yet are associated with psychosocial and functional impairment similar to that associated with major depression (Beekman et al., 1995; Hybels, Blazer, & Pieper, 2001; Lavretsky, Kurbanyan, & Kumar, 2004). Various authors have argued that depression should be conceptualized along a continuum of severity (e.g., Rapaport et al., 2002), with major depressive disorder at one end, subsyndromal depression at the other end, and minor depression in the middle (e.g., Hybels et al., 2001; Lavretksy et al., 2004). Although subsyndromal depression is not currently classified, minor depression appears in the appendix of DSM-IV. Subthreshold depressions are of particular importance for older adults, as their prevalence increases with age (Judd, Schettler, & Akiskal, 2002). Moreover, in an examination of older primary care patients, Lyness, King, Cox, Yoediono, and Caine (1999) found that the prevalence of subsyndromal depression exceeded that of major depression, minor depression, and dysthymia.

There are two additional presentations of depression that do not meet criteria for major depression, dysthymia, or minor depression, and are thought to be more common in older adults. The first is termed "depression without sadness," (Gallo, Rabins, Lyketsos, Tien, & Anthony, 1997) in which individuals present with symptoms of depression (e.g., hopelessness, worthlessness, thoughts of death or suicide) but do not report sadness or loss of interest or pleasure in formerly enjoyed activities. Even though these individuals fail to meet DSM-IV criteria for depression, they are at risk for functional disability, psychological distress, cognitive impairment, and death (Gallo & Rabins, 1999). Similarly, Newmann, Engel, and Jensen (1991) characterized a "depletion syndrome" with symptoms of loss of appetite, lack of interest, thoughts of dying, and hopelessness (see also Adams, 2001).

Olin, Katz, Meyers, Schneider, and Lebowitz (2002) have argued that the depression that occurs with Alzheimer's disease is different from other depressive disorders and have proposed provisional criteria for "depression of Alzheimer's disease." They suggest that the depression observed with Alzheimer's patients is different from "depression due to a general medical condition." The outcome of the authors' proposal remains to be seen. Mayer et al. (2006) compared three rating scales for use as outcome measures in treatment trials of "depression of Alzheimer's disease." The Cornell Scale for Depression in Dementia (CSDD) (Alexopoulos, Abrams, Young, & Shamoian, 1988), particularly the mood subscale, appeared to be the best choice for measuring the effects of treatment. The CSDD is discussed later in this chapter.

Multicultural Issues

The racial and ethnic diversity of older adults in the United States is expected to increase with the growing population (U.S. Census Bureau, 2008a), with minority populations expected to become the majority in 2042. This is particularly important to appreciate, as prevalence estimates of depression vary across racial and ethnic groups. Some authors (e.g., Mui, Burnette, & Chen, 2002) have argued that the prevalence data for some racial and ethnic groups are biased due to the low acceptability of measures used to report symptoms in minority populations, and various socio–cultural factors (e.g., tolerance of symptoms). Moreover, norms are often not available for racial and ethnic groups, and psychometric properties are often not available for racial and ethnic groups on assessment instruments that were developed with Caucasian samples. Moreover, there appear to be cross-cultural differences in the expression of depression symptoms (Futterman, Thompson, Gallagher-Thompson, & Ferris, 1997). For example, Japanese individuals tend to report interpersonal complaints, whereas Chinese individuals tend to present somatic symptoms (Krause & Liang, 1992). However, whether these cultural differences are exhibited through old age is unclear at this time. Readers are cautioned to carefully consider the available normative data for racially or ethnically diverse clients, to avoid stereotypes when considering culturally specific information in the assessment process. Interested readers are referred to Sue and Sue (2007), who provide helpful information on working with racially and ethnically diverse populations. Many of their suggestions are particularly useful for understanding perspectives on mental health care by first generation immigrants, and those who maintain a strong cultural identity.

Symptoms of depression vary between community-dwelling African American and non-African American individuals, including endorsement rates for “less hope about the future, poor appetite, difficulty concentrating, requiring more effort for usual activities, less talking, feeling people were unfriendly, feeling disliked by others, and being more ‘bothered’ than usual” (Blazer, Landerman, Hays, Simonsick, & Saunders, 1998). However, these authors found when such factors as education, income, cognitive impairment, chronic health problems, and disability were controlled, the differences across race/ethnic groups in somatic complaints and satisfaction were minimal. Rates of depression among older adult African American individuals tend to be lower than the rates for Caucasian older adults (Blazer, 2003). Results of the recent *Aging, Demographics, and Memory Study* (Steffens et al., 2009) revealed a prevalence of depression (minor and major combined) among African Americans that was one-third of the prevalence for Whites and Hispanics. With the exception of a greater number of somatic complaints by African American women, there appear to be no significant differences in the symptoms of depression as expressed by African American and Caucasian older adults (Myers et al., 2002).

The population of Hispanic individuals in the United States is large and diverse, suggesting that any attempt to generalize across Hispanic subgroups would be unwise. The largest Hispanic groups of older adults (65+), according to the U.S. Census Bureau (2006), are Mexican Americans (64%), Central and South Americans (13.1%), Puerto Rican Americans (9.0%), Cuban Americans (3.4%), Dominican Americans (2.8%), and other Hispanics (7.7%). The prevalence of depression among Hispanic Americans is relatively high. A study of depression among older Mexican Americans in the Sacramento area (Gonzalez, Haan, & Hinton, 2001) revealed a prevalence of 24.5% using a CES–D cutoff of 16 or more. The prevalence was higher among immigrants (30.4%) and less acculturated participants (36.1%). In comparison, the prevalence rate for U.S. born participants was 20.5%. In a recent examination of the *Health and Retirement Study*, Yang, Cazorla-Lancaster, and Jones (2008) found that Puerto Rican American older adults have a higher prevalence rate for major depression (19.3%) than other Hispanic individuals living in the United States; Cuban Americans had the next highest rate (11.7%), followed by Mexican Americans (8.2%).

The population of Asian individuals in the United States is also quite diverse, with level of acculturation playing a role in the prevalence of depression. In a study of acculturation stress and depression among Asian (i.e., Chinese, Korean, Indian, Filipino, Vietnamese, and Japanese) immigrant older adults, Mui and Kang (2006) found that higher acculturation stress was associated with higher depression levels. Similarly, a review by Kuo, Chong, and Joseph (2008) found that depression is prevalent among older adult Asian immigrants, and is linked to a variety of variables (e.g., gender, how long they have been an immigrant, English proficiency, acculturation, health status, social support).

A recent study of 2611 community-dwelling Chinese adults (Niti, Ng, Kua, Ho, & Tan, 2007) in Singapore, aged 55 and older, revealed a 13.3% prevalence of depressive symptoms based upon scores on a Chinese version of the Geriatric Depression Scale (Yesavage, Brink, & Rose, 1983). This rate is similar to the 12.5% rate reported in Hong Kong (Chi et al., 2005) and the 20.1% rate reported in Taiwan (Chiu, Chen, Huang, & Mau, 2005) using the Geriatric Depression Scale. Asian individuals are likely to hold a holistic view of the mind and body (Sue & Sue, 2007). A physical complaint is a culturally acceptable means of expressing an emotional disorder (Sue & Sue, 2007). This is consistent with the finding that somatic complaints are common among depressed Asian individuals (Parker, Cheah, & Roy, 2001).

Depression is a major concern among American Indian older adults (Greer, 2004). However, until recently, information regarding the prevalence of depression among American Indians remained insufficient because few studies had sufficient sample sizes, and some were conducted with nonrandom samples (Beals et al., 2005). Unfortunately, the most recent and carefully conducted epidemiological study of American Indians, the American Indian Service Utilization, Psychiatric Epidemiology, Risk and Protective Factors Project (AI-SUPERPFP; Beals et al., 2005) failed to include individuals over the age of 54. Thus, adequate prevalence estimates for older adult American Indians remain unknown.

One must remember that there are considerable within-group and between-group cultural differences among racial and ethnic groups, and that degree of assimilation, educational experience, and acculturation can yield very different individual clinical presentations. One must be careful not to overgeneralize with regard to behavioral characteristics, cultural values, and the presentations of symptoms when working with an individual client.

Multi-method Assessment

No single method of assessment is consistently superior to any other. Each method (e.g., interviews, direct observation, self-reports, reports by others, psychophysiological recordings) has its strengths and shortcomings. Because of that, using multiple methods and sources of information has been strongly recommended in the assessment literature (e.g., Eid & Diener, 2006; Haynes & O'Brien, 2000) to ensure accurate, reliable, and valid information. This is particularly true when assessing individuals with cognitive impairment. One can avoid, to some degree, the shortcomings of any one method, and capture information unique to any one method, by employing multiple methods. For the sake of simplicity, we have focused on three general methods. The interested reader is referred to Eid and Diener (2006) for a more comprehensive treatment of multiple method measurement.

Self-Report

Self-report is arguably the most popular assessment method. The most commonly used assessment instrument, the clinical interview, employs self-report. It is also the method used for the multitude of questionnaires and inventories designed to examine various forms of psychopathology and cognitive functioning. Clinicians should be sensitive to the specific wording of the questions, question format, and question context, as these can influence self-reports of older adults (Schwarz, 1999; 2003). Older adults are more likely than younger adults to be cautious when responding, give more acquiescent responses, refuse to answer certain types of questions, and respond "don't know" (Edelstein, Woodhead, Bower & Lowery, 2006). Older adults may also minimize or deny symptoms (Blazer, 2009; Wong & Baden, 2001). The accuracy, reliability, and validity of older adult self-reports is mixed, suggesting that one should be cautious when using the self-report method and, when possible, utilize multiple methods.

There are limited findings which shed light on the adequacy of self-reported information that relates specifically to depression assessment. Older adult self-reports of insomnia, when compared with the results of polysomnography, have been good (e.g., Reite, Buysse, Reynolds, & Mendelson,

1995). In addition, self-reports of activities of daily living by older adults in outpatient settings are strongly related to performance measures (Sager et al., 1992); although the accuracy of estimates of functional ability are mixed (e.g., Rubenstein, Schairer, Wieland, & Kane, 1984; Sager et al., 1992). Among the factors that contribute to the adequacy of older adult self-reports are physical health and acute or chronic cognitive impairment. As one might expect, cognitively impaired older adults often have impaired memory, and are less likely to comprehend questions or the nature of information requested. Moreover, older adults in the earlier stages of dementia often deny memory impairment, and may also deny other symptoms (e.g., Larrabee & Crook, 1989). In contrast, older adults with mild to moderate dementia may offer reliable and valid self-reports when only recent memory is required (see Feher, Larrabee, & Crook, 1992).

Finally, when using self-report measures, it is important to determine the quality of their psychometric support. There are an increasing number of self-report instruments being developed with, and for use with, older adults (e.g., assertiveness, Northrop & Edelstein, 1998; worry, Wisocki, Handen, & Morse,1986; fear, Kogan & Edelstein, 2004; depression, Yesavage et al., 1983; anxiety, Pachana et al., 2007; suicide risk, Edelstein et al., in press). However, clinicians too often adopt self-report measures that were developed with younger adults, and utilize them with older adults without considering their psychometric properties and whether suitable normative data are available.

Report-By-Others

The report-by-other (e.g., spouse, caregiver, adult child) assessment method has many of the strengths and weaknesses of the self-report method. The principal shortcoming is that those reporting on an individual rarely have continuous access to the individual's behavior, both covert and overt. An advantage of including reports-by-other is that they often provide unique and converging information. Information obtained from multiple sources can provide a rich array of information across contexts and time. Reports-by-others become invaluable when assessing cognitively impaired individuals. As one gathers information from various individuals, it is important to remember that these reports are subject to the same potential problems of unreliability, invalidity, and inaccuracy as self-report and other assessment methods. The characteristics of the individual providing the report can influence the accuracy of the information obtained. For example, when Zanetti, Geroldi, Frisoni, Bianchetti, and Trabucchi (1999) compared caregiver reports of patients' ADLs against direct measurement of the patients' ADLs, they found that the accuracy of the caregiver reports varied as a function of the caregiver's depressive symptoms and burden level.

Direct Observation

Direct observation is an important source of information, regardless of the patient's level of physical, medical, and psychosocial functioning. One can begin to formulate hypotheses about an individual's functioning by merely watching that individual walk down a hallway, rise from a bed, or formulate a greeting as he or she is met for the first time. The psychomotor speed, characteristics of speech, frequency and duration of eye contact, quality of grooming, and many other characteristics can provide clues as to psychological functioning before the first words are spoken. Does the individual leave his or her bedroom or house? Does he or she continue to engage in once pleasurable activities? Does the individual remain in bed for long periods of time? The number of potentially relevant, observable behaviors is considerable. Direct observation is a source of convergent information that can be incorporated into a multi-method assessment.

Direct observation can be particularly useful when assessing cognitively impaired older adults, and those who are uncooperative with interviews. As with the other assessment methods, direct observation of behavior must be reliable, valid, and accurate. Discrepancies among reports of direct observations should be explored, and training to avoid such discrepancies should be provided if the setting permits (e.g., inpatient medical facilities, long-term care facilities). Techniques for systematically sampling and recording behaviors can easily be taught to hospital or nursing home staff, as well as family members. Observational methods can be tailored to the behavior of the individual and the demands of the caregivers and staff members. Ideally, a list of specific behaviors and symptoms can be provided, rather than asking staff or family members to "watch out for symptoms of depression."

Multidimensional Assessment

Late-life depression is a multidimensional problem for older adults, whose health and cognitive, social, adaptive and psychological functioning collectively yield a complex assessment challenge that often requires the expertise of multiple disciplines (see Zeiss & Steffen, 1996). Such an approach to assessment is often termed "comprehensive geriatric assessment" (Rubenstein, 1995). Support for the assessment of these domains is found in the DSM-IV and in the nursing home assessment recommendation of the Omnibus Budget Reconciliation Act (1987). Multidimensional assessment can lead to improved diagnostic accuracy, more appropriate placement, improved functional status, more appropriate use of medications, improved coordination of services, and improved emotional status (Edelstein et al., 2003). A recent review of the comprehensive geriatric assessment literature (Ellis & Langhorne, 2005) also revealed that such assessments increase the chances of patients remaining at home and avoiding hospitalization.

We have confined our brief discussion of multidimensional assessment to a discussion of functioning in the following domains: adaptive functioning, health, cognitive functioning, and social support. The focus of this chapter is depression, which would fall under the domain of psychological functioning. A broader discussion is beyond the scope of this chapter.

Assessment of Adaptive Functioning

Adaptive functioning is usually defined by an individual's ability to perform activities of daily living (ADLs) (e.g., eating, dressing, bathing) and instrumental activities of daily living (IADLs) (e.g., meal preparation, money management). Numerous medical and psychological disorders, and physical disabilities, can diminish one's adaptive functioning (e.g., depression, dementia, diabetes, Parkinson's disease, chronic obstructive pulmonary disease). Depression can be particularly devastating on the ability to perform activities of daily living (e.g., Penninx, Leveille, Ferrucci, Van Eijk, & Guralnik, 1999). In addition, individuals whose daily activities are already compromised by disease or disability prior to experiencing depression are at increased risk of experiencing diminished adaptive behaviors with the presence of depression. This is particularly a problem for older adults as they transition from community residences or residential facilities to long-term care facilities (Achterberg, Pot, Kerkstra, & Ribbe, 2006).

The relation between depression and adaptive functioning can be reciprocal, as diminished adaptive behaviors can lead to depression (Blazer, Steffens, & Koenig, 2009). Several ADL and IADL assessment instruments are available, including the Katz Activities of Daily Living Scale (Katz, Downs, Cash, & Grotz, 1970), the Adult Functional Adaptive Behavior Scale (Spirrison & Pierce, 1992), the Texas Functional Living Scale (Cullum, Weiner, & Saine, 2009), and the Independent Living Scales (Loeb, 1996).

Assessment of Physical Health

Approximately 80% of older adults experience at least one chronic health problem, with 50% having two or more chronic conditions (He, Sengupta, Velkoff, & DeBarros, 2005). Moreover, approximately

20% of older adults suffer from at least one disability (He et al., 2005). The prevalence of major depression in primary care patients is 5–10%, and 11% for medical inpatients (Alexopoulos et al., 2002). The assessment of depression is complicated by the comorbidity of health problems: physical diseases can both accompany and present as depression. For example, hypothyroidism can initially present as depression (Fountoulakis, Iacovides, Grammaticos, St. Kaprinis, & Bech, 2004). Moreover, hypothyroidism and cerebrovascular disease can precede the diagnosis of late-life depression (Alexopoulos, 2005; Alexopoulos et al., 2002; Fountoulakis et al., 2004). Depression also can follow or result from other medical conditions, e.g., Alzheimer's disease, stroke, Parkinson's disease, myocardial infarctions, chronic obstructive pulmonary disease (Cummings & Victoroff, 1990; Rodin, Craven, & Littlefield, 1991; van Manen et al., 2002). One of the more challenging tasks in the assessment of late-life depression is deciphering the contributions of physical disease to the presentation of depression.

To further complicate the assessment, one must consider the potential contributions of medications taken by older adults. Older adults consume 34% of all prescription medications, and 30% of all over-the-counter medications, although they constitute only 12% of the U.S. population (Centers for Disease Control and Prevention, 2004; Hajjar, Cafiero, & Hanlon, 2007). Older adults take an average of two to five medications, and 20–40% of older adults take five or more medications (McLean & Le Couteur, 2004).

As one ages, one's body undergoes anatomical and physiological changes that affect drug pharmacokinetics (e.g., absorption, distribution, metabolism, excretion) and pharmacodynamics (e.g., effect of drug on its target site; Mangoni & Jackson, 2004). These changes often increase the sensitivity of the older adult to medications and the potential for adverse effects. In light of the number of medications taken by older adults, the task of sorting out potential drug interactions and adverse medication effects can be challenging. Perhaps more directly relevant to the assessment of depression are drugs that can produce depressive symptoms as side effects (see Patten & Love, 1994); for example, corticosterioids, sedatives, and drugs used to treat hypertension, elevated cholesterol, and asthma.

Assessment of Cognitive Functioning

The difficulty of distinguishing dementia from depression has long been recognized, and represents yet another assessment challenge (see Storandt & VandenBos, 1994). The difficulty stems from the overlapping symptoms of depression and dementia, and the fact that the two can coexist. An individual with depression can exhibit deficits in attention and concentration, which interfere with the learning of new information. Difficulty in retrieving information may also be impaired. Depressed individuals may also appear apathetic and withdrawn. The interested reader is referred to Kaszniak and Christensen (1994) for a discussion regarding the differentiation of dementia and depression. Moreover, there is increasing evidence of deficits in executive function in late-life depression (Alexopoulos, 2003; Elderkin-Thompson, Mintz, Haroon, Lavretsky, & Kumar, 2007). Some of these symptoms may improve once depressive symptoms abate (Butters et al., 2000). However, even if symptoms of cognitive impairment improve or remit, those who experience symptoms of cognitive impairment during a depressive episode are more likely to develop dementia in the future (Alexopoulos, Meyers, Young, & Mattis (1993).

The initial evaluation of an older adult whom one suspects is depressed or cognitively impaired should at least include screening for cognitive impairment. Several cognitive screening instruments are available, each with its strengths and weaknesses (see Cullen, O'Neill, Evans, Coen, & Lawlor, 2007, and Edelstein et al., 2008). Though the Mini-Mental State Examination (MMSE; Folstein, Folstein, & McHugh, 1975) is probably the most popular of the available screening instruments, there are several alternatives, some of which may be more sensitive to mild cognitive impairment than the MMSE; for example, the St. Louis University Mental Status Examination (SLUMS; Tariq, Tumosa, Chibnall, Perry, & Morley, 2006), and the Montreal Cognitive Assessment (MoCA; Nasreddine et al., 2005), which is available in more than 10 languages. If impairment is suggested by performance on a cognitive screening instrument, additional cognitive or neuropsychological assessment can be performed. The interested reader is referred to Woodford and George (2007) for a review of cognitive assessment methods.

Assessment of Social Support

A relation between social support and depression is well established in the literature (Barnett & Gotlib, 1988), although the direction of that relation has been questioned (Krause, Liang, & Yatomi, 1989). Although social support has the potential for buffering stress, consideration of both positive and negative social support is important. One should not presume that because someone has a relationship with another individual, that the sum of their social interactions is positive for that individual. Negative social support (see Rook, 1994) is positively related to depression among older adults (e.g., Pagel, Erdly, & Becker, 1987). When exploring social support, the number of individuals providing social support should be considered separately from the individual's satisfaction with support.

DEPRESSION ASSESSMENT INSTRUMENTS

Many depression assessment instruments have been validated for use with older adults. When selecting instruments, appropriate normative data and adequate indications of reliability and validity are required; however, reliability estimates and diagnostic statistics (e.g., sensitivity) are highly dependent on sample characteristics. Larger samples, lengthier assessment instruments, greater score variability, and larger score ranges produce higher estimates of reliability. It is important to consider these factors when interpreting the results of studies and selecting a particular instrument to use with an individual.

Here we review only the depression assessment instruments most commonly used with older adults. While other instruments show promise, such as the Quick Inventory of Depressive Symptomatology (QIDS; Rush et al., 2003), there is limited research on their use in older adults and they are not discussed further in this chapter. Each of the following instruments is considered in terms of its psychometric properties and overall strengths and weaknesses. For a review of the validity of using depression instruments in older adults for diagnostic purposes, monitoring change, or rating severity, see Fiske and O'Riley (2008).

Self-Report Instruments

We have found self-report assessment instruments to be the most valuable objective assessment instruments, as they are often easy and quick to administer. However, it is important to note examinee characteristics (e.g., low educational attainment or compromised cognition may relate to difficulty comprehending and completing self-report measures) and the potential for response bias when interpreting results. For example, Burke, Houston, Boust, and Roccaforte (1989) found elevated rates of false-negative errors on the Geriatric Depression Scale (GDS) (Yesavage et al., 1983) in Alzheimer's patients. It is important to note that many of the instruments were administered orally to examinees, particularly to individuals with suspected cognitive impairment, difficulty completing the forms, or residing in nursing homes. In most cases the psychometric data obtained was similar to that obtained with individuals who self-completed the forms.

Beck Depression Inventory

Several versions of the Beck Depression Inventory are available. The Beck Depression Inventory (BDI; Beck, Ward, Mendelson, Mock, & Erbaugh, 1961) is the most well-researched depression self-report inventory with older adults. It is a 21-item, multiple-choice inventory employing Guttman scaling designed to assess the level of depression in adults. Each item is scored 0 to 3 points for a total score range of 0 to 63. The scale was developed as a quantitative measure of depression and was not originally intended as a diagnostic instrument (Kendall, Hollon, Beck, Hammen, & Ingram, 1987). Suggested score ranges for mild depression, moderate to severe depression, and severe depression are 10–19, 20–30, and 31 or higher, respectively (Kendall et al., 1987). A 13-item short form (Beck & Beck, 1972) is also available with score ranges of 5–7 for mild depression, 8–15 for moderate depression, and 16 or higher for severe depression. The full-scale BDI requires approximately 5–10 minutes to administer, whereas the short form requires approximately 5 minutes. Estimates of internal consistency for the full-scale and short-form BDI have been acceptable (0.82–0.91; Gallagher, 1986; Gallagher, Nies, & Thompson, 1982; Kim, Pilkonis, Frank, Thase, & Reynolds, 2002; Scogin, Beutler, Corbishley, & Hamblin, 1988) in both normal and depressed older adults. Estimates of test–retest reliability and concurrent validity have also been acceptable (0.77–0.90; Gallagher et al., 1982; Giordano et al., 2007; Scogin, 1994).

Using a cutoff of 10, the full-scale BDI demonstrated good sensitivity and specificity with older adult depressed outpatients (sensitivity = 100%, specificity = 96%; Olin et al., 1992), medical outpatients (sensitivity = 89%, specificity = 82%; Norris, Gallagher, Wilson, & Winograd, 1987), and medical inpatients (sensitivity = 83%, specificity = 65%; Rapp, Parisi, Walsh, & Wallace, 1988). A cutoff score of 17 yielded a sensitivity of 50% and specificity of 92%, suggesting that a cutoff of 10 would be the best score if one is screening for depression. Using discriminant function analysis to examine the classification accuracy of the BDI, Bentz and Hall (2008) obtained adequate sensitivity of 72.5% and specificity of 80.9% in an inpatient, mostly cognitively impaired, geriatric sample. The 13-item short form demonstrated good sensitivity (97%) and adequate specificity (77%) at a cutoff score of 5 (Scogin et al., 1988).

The BDI can be divided into psychological (1–0.4) and somatic items (15–21). Rapp and coauthors (1988) also found that using a cutoff score of 5 for the psychological items yielded better indices of sensitivity (75%) and specificity (92%) than when combined with the somatic items in medical inpatients. Scogin and associates (1988) obtained sensitivity and specificity estimates of 77% and 97%, respectively, using the cutoff score of 5 with non-patient older adults and a group diagnosed with major depression. These results reinforce the need to consider the influence of older adults' somatic complaints when assessing depression, particularly among medical patients.

The BDI correlates moderately to highly with the Geriatric Depression Scale in various inpatient and community-dwelling older adult populations (Allen-Burge, Storandt, Kinscherf, & Rubin, 1994; Giordano et al., 2007; Snyder, Stanley, Novy, Averill, & Beck, 2000). Gallagher et al. (1982) found moderately high test–retest stability in older adult community volunteers and outpatients diagnosed with depression. However, Kendall and colleagues (1987) argue cogently for the use of multiple assessment periods, noting that in spite of the relatively high test–retest coefficients obtained with the BDI, over 50% of individuals scored above a defined cutoff change classification following retesting within hours, days, or one to four weeks. They argue that the overall stability of the measurement appears primarily due to scores from non-depressed subjects.

Among the positive features of the BDI are the fact that it has been evaluated frequently with generally positive outcomes and is brief, easily scored, and easily administered (Scogin, 1994). On the negative side, individuals with cognitive impairment may have difficulty completing the BDI, particularly the Guttman response scale (Edelstein et al., 2008). This difficulty is reflected by higher false positive rates in Alzheimer's patients (Wagle et al., 2000). Interestingly, these differences cannot be attributed to somatic symptoms. However, the somatic content of some items may complicate interpretation of scores, as the complaints can result from depression, physical disorders, or both. Olin et al. (1992) reported a high rate of difficulty by older adults in completing the BDI. Forty-six percent of community-dwelling older adults endorsed multiple responses on at least one item and 12% failed to complete at least one item. Depressed individuals were more likely to fail to complete at least one item correctly. Finally, Allen-Burge et al. (1994) reported gender differences in the BDI, with lower detection of depressive symptoms in men. Moreover, Jefferson, Powers, and Pope (2001) found that older women may be more hesitant to complete the BDI than other measures of depression. Overall, the BDI is a useful screening instrument for depression.

A second version of the Beck Depression Inventory (BDI—II; Beck, Steer, & Brown, 1996) included older adults in the normative sample and addressed many of the problems noted in the BDI. Although the number of items and response style remains the same as with the original version, the item content was modified to address all DSM-IV criteria for Major Depressive Disorder and rates behavior over the past two weeks. Senior et al. (2007) administered the BDI—II via telephone and obtained good reliability and validity with older adults diagnosed with generalized anxiety disorder. The BDI—II has good internal consistency in community-dwelling older adults (Norris et al., 2004; Segal, Coolidge, Cahill, & O'Riley, 2008), older cardiac patients (Low & Hubley, 2007), and women residing in retirement communities (Jefferson et al., 2001). The BDI—II has growing support in the research literature for use with older adults and is a useful update of the BDI for use with older adults.

In addition, the Beck Depression Inventory—Fast Screen for Medical Patients (BDI—FS; Beck, Steer, & Brown, 2000), previously known as the Beck Depression Inventory for Primary Care, is a 7-item scale that omits somatic items. It maintains the item structure from the BDI—II and rates items occurrence over the past two weeks. The BDI—FS demonstrated high sensitivity and specificity in older adults with health problems (Scheinthal, Steer, Giffen, & Beck, 2001), and adequate reliability in older adult post-stroke patients (0.75; Healey, Kneebone, Carroll, & Anderson, 2008) and geriatric outpatients (0.83; Scheinthal et al., 2001). A cutoff score of 4 produced a sensitivity of 100% and a specificity of 84% in an older adult outpatient population. The BDI—FS is a quick alternative to the full BDI or BDI—II. It shows potential for use with older adults, particularly those with medical conditions. However, further research is needed to fully recommend its use as a standard assessment of depression in older adults.

Geriatric Depression Scale

The Geriatric Depression Scale (see Appendix A) was developed specifically for use with older adults and contains 30 items. Each item is scored 0 to 1 for a total score range of 0 to 30. The GDS utilizes a simple "yes—no" item format, omits somatic items, and demonstrated utility when used over the telephone (Burke, Roccaforte, Wengel, Conley, & Potter, 1995). Recommended cutoffs for the full-scale version range from 10—16, with sensitivity and specificity varying in different subject populations (Fiske, Kasl-Godley, & Gatz, 1998; Harper, Kotik-Harper, & Kirby, 1990; Watson, Lewis, Kistler, Amick, & Boustani, 2004). Lower accuracy was found in healthy, highly-educated community-dwelling older adults (Watson et al., 2004). Reliability and validity evidence has been established for older, medically ill outpatients (Norris et al., 1987), non-cognitively impaired nursing home residents (Lesher, 1986; Smalbrugge, Jongenelis, Pot, Beekman, & Eefsting, 2008), older adults diagnosed with GAD (Snyder et al., 2000), and hospitalized older adults (Rapp et al., 1988). Kieffer and Reese (2002) analyzed reliability across 338 studies using the GDS and found a mean reliability of 0.85.

Evidence supporting the use of the GDS with cognitively impaired individuals is mixed, with Feher et al. (1992) finding it a valid measure of mild to moderate depressive symptoms in Alzheimer's patients with mild to moderate dementia; although some dementia patients disavow memory loss and tend to deny depressive symptoms on the GDS. This response bias could account for the less than desirable findings in some studies employing the GDS with dementia patients. Hyer and Blount (1984) found that the GDS discriminated between depressed and non-depressed older adult psychiatric patients, and had better sensitivity and specificity than the Zung Self-Rating Depression Scale (SDC) (Zung, 1965) and the Hamilton Rating Scale for Depression (HRSD) (Hamilton, 1960; 1967). Lichtenberg, Steiner, Marcopulos, and Tabscott (1992) found moderate sensitivity (82%) and specificity (86%) with dementia patients in a long-term care facility using the diagnosis of a psychiatrist as the criterion measure. Using discriminant function analysis to examine the classification accuracy of the GDS, Bentz and Hall (2008) obtained sensitivity of 82.6% and specificity of 81.3% in an inpatient, mostly cognitively impaired, geriatric sample.

Allen-Burge et al. (1994) reported gender effects on the GDS, with poorer detection of depression in males. In addition, Olin et al. (1992) reported a mild level of difficulty by older adults in completing the GDS. Eight percent of community-dwelling older adults endorsed both responses (yes and no) on at least one item and 14% failed to complete at least one item. Depressed individuals were more likely to fail to complete at least one item correctly.

Ott and Fogel (1992) found a moderately strong correlation ($r = 0.77$) between the GDS and the Cornell Scale for Depression in Dementia (CS; Alexopoulos et al., 1988) in patients with mild dementia (Mini-Mental State Exam [MMSE; Folstein et al., 1975] of 22 or less), but a weaker relationship between the two with increased cognitive impairment. Stiles and McGarrahan (1998), in their review of the GDS literature, present the cutoff scores associated with levels of sensitivity and specificity for virtually all GDS studies with older adults. Various cutoff scores have been suggested, varying to some extent by the sample population characteristics. Stiles and McGarrahan recommend cutoff scores of 11 for maximal sensitivity and 14 for higher specificity.

A 15-item short form of the GDS is also available (Lesher & Berryhill, 1994) with high internal consistency ($r = 0.88$). Lesher and Berryhill found a strong relation between scores on the long and short forms of the GDS ($r = 0.89$) and similar sensitivity and specificity with heterogeneous diagnostic groups. (See also Cwikel & Ritchie, 1988.) Baker and Miller (1991) found support for its sensitivity and specificity when used with medically ill skilled nursing home residents, whereas Burke, Roccaforte, and Wengel (1991) found less support when used with cognitively impaired individuals. Recommended cutoff scores vary from 5–7 (Almeida & Almeida, 1999; Haworth, Moniz-Cook, Clark, Wang, & Cleland, 2007; Lesher & Berryhill, 1994) in various older adult populations. Brown, Woods, and Storandt (2007) examined the factor structure of the GDS–15 in samples of non-demented, demented, and depressed older adults. A 2-factor model, including Life Satisfaction and General Depressive Affect factors, was stable across the non-demented and demented samples but only 1-factor was evident in the depressed older adults, suggesting that poor life satisfaction impacts scores on the GDS–15. Overall, the utility of the GDS appears to diminish with increases in cognitive impairment. Although the short form may be useful when time constraints or fatigue are issues, the longer form appears to be more reliable and valid (Stiles & McGarrahan, 1998).

The GDS appears to be a useful screening instrument for depression in older adults. It was developed for use with older adults, employs a yes–no format that is relatively easy to use with cognitively impaired older adults, and has been validated with a wide range of populations. On the less positive side, results with cognitively impaired populations have been mixed (Korner et al., 2006). As a practical measure, Stiles and McGarrahan (1998) offer the following approach to the use of the GDS in individuals suspected of cognitive impairment. Initially screen the older adult for cognitive impairment using the MMSE. If the MMSE score is less than 15, the GDS score is suspect and can be disregarded as unreliable. However, if the MMSE score is below 24, the GDS cutoff of 14 is suggested.

Center for Epidemiological Studies—Depression Scale

The Center for Epidemiological Studies—Depression Scale (CES—D; Radloff, 1977), designed for large-scale epidemiological studies in the general population, is a 20-item self-report inventory that can be completed in approximately 5 minutes. Each item is scored 0 to 3 on a Likert-type scale for frequency of symptoms in the last week, for a total score range of 0 to 60. It consistently demonstrates four factors: depressive affect, well-being, somatic symptoms, and interpersonal relations across multiple older adult samples (Hertzog, Van Alstine, Usala, Hultsch, & Dixon, 1990; O'Rourke, 2005; Williams et al., 2007), although some items cross factors across studies. The suggested cutoff for depression is a score of 16 or more. However, as seen in cutoff scores for all the measures, some studies suggest this may be too low for some older adult populations, producing too many false positives (Haringsma, Engels, Beekman, & Spinhoven, 2004; Himmelfarb & Murrell, 1983), and too high for detecting depression in healthy populations (Watson et al., 2004).

Split-half and coefficient alpha estimates of internal consistency (0.85 to 0.92) reported by Radloff were high across age, sex, geographic, and racial and ethnic subgroups. High reliabilities were also reported in community-dwelling older adults (0.82; Lewinsohn, Seeley, Roberts, & Allen, 1997), older medical inpatients (0.86; Schein & Koenig, 1997), and older adult caregivers (0.88; O'Rourke, 2005). High rates of false positives with the suggested cutoff score of 16 were reported by Schein and Koenig (1997) in medical patients. They suggest a two-stage approach to the use of the CES—D in this population to improve the diagnostic efficiency of the instrument. First, examinees must meet the minimum cutoff total score of 16. Second, the examinee must obtain a score of at least 4 on the depressed affect subscale.

A 10-item short form of the CES—D also has been used with a cutoff score of 10 or more (Andresen, Malmgren, Carter, & Patrick, 1994). Test—retest reliability was reasonably good ($r = 0.71$). Comparison of the CES—D—10 with the 20-item CES—D was quite favorable, resulting in only one misclassification using the CES—D—10. The strengths of the CES—D include its widespread use in epidemiological studies, the availability of norms based on a large representative sample (Himmelfarb & Murrell, 1983), its factor invariance across age groups, and its demonstrated reliability and sensitivity in older adults. A revision of the CES—D (Eaton, Smith, Ybarra, Muntaner, & Tein, 2004) has been developed to reflect changes in diagnostic criteria from the original version, but has not yet been validated in older adults.

Overall, the CES—D appears to be a good instrument for screening community-dwelling older adults. On the less positive side are its response format and low specificity in several studies (see Radloff & Teri, 1986). The response format requires frequency ratings of how often one experienced symptoms over the past week, which may be difficult and somewhat less reliable among individuals with cognitive impairments. Boutin-Foster (2008) reported differential responding patterns in different ethnic groups. Latinos obtained higher scores than African Americans and Caucasians in all domains, and were three times more likely to obtain scores at or above the cutoff score. Moreover, Kohout, Berkman, Evans, and Cornoni-Huntley (1993) reported that 10% of the older adults completing the CES—D failed to complete at least one item. Its low specificity at the cutoff of 16 (Boyd, Weissman, Thompson, & Myers, 1982; Myers & Weissman, 1980; Roberts & Vernon, 1983), using a diagnosis of major depression as a criterion, suggests that it is better suited as a screening than a diagnostic instrument.

Hospital Anxiety and Depression Scale

The Hospital Anxiety and Depression Scale (HADS) (Zigmond & Snaith, 1983) is a 14-item measure designed to assess anxiety and depression symptoms in medical patients, with emphasis on reducing the impact of physical illness on the total score. The depression items tend to focus on the anhedonic symptoms of depression. Items are rated on a 4-point severity scale. The HADS produces two scales, one for anxiety (HADS–A) and one for depression (HADS–D), differentiating the two states. Scores of greater than or equal to 11 on either scale indicate a definitive case. Kenn, Wood, Kucyj, Wattis, and Cunane (1987) reported good differentiation of depressed and non-depressed older adults, and Haworth et al. (2007) found similar results in cardiac patients, although a lower cutoff score was used to minimize false negatives. The HADS–D correlates 0.72 with the GDS and 0.61 with the HRSD in Parkinson's patients (Mondolo et al., 2006), and 0.82 with the GDS–15 in older cardiac patients (Haworth et al., 2007). Mondolo et al. reported sensitivity and specificity with Parkinson's patients to be 100% and 95%, respectively.

Although initial studies suggest the HADS–D is a useful instrument to assess depression in older adults, Davies, Burn, McKenzie, Brothwell, and Wattis (1993) reported a high degree of false positives, with over a quarter of medical inpatients misclassified by the HADS–D. Moreover, Haworth et al. (2007) suggest the use of the GDS over the HADS–D due to the lower sensitivity and specificity of the HADS–D. Alternatively, Mondolo et al. (2006) found the HADS–D better at diagnosing depression than the GDS in Parkinson's patients. Overall, in light of the mixed psychometric evidence, the HADS–D is probably not the best choice for depression assessment instruments for older adults at this time. Further research may yield more support for the use of this scale in older adults.

Zung Self-Rating Depression Scale

The Zung Self-Rating Depression Scale (SDS) is a 20-item measure, with each item rated on a 4-point scale. It requires approximately 5–10 minutes to complete. Ranges for mild to moderate depression, moderate to severe depression, and severe depression are 50–59, 60–69, and over 70, respectively (Zung, 1967). Reliability with older adults appears to be low to moderate, which is most apparent among the oldest old (Kivela & Pahkala, 1986; McGarvey, Gallagher, Thompson, & Zelinski, 1982—cited in Fiske et al., 1998). Older adults tend to score higher than younger adults, possibly due to the somatic items on the scale (Berry et al., 1984). Kitchell, Barnes, Veith, Okimoto, and Raskind (1982) estimated the sensitivity and specificity with medically ill inpatients to be 58% and 87%, respectively. Somewhat better efficiency has been demonstrated with medical outpatients (sensitivity = 82%, specificity = 87%; Okimoto et al., 1982). Finally, age and sex differences have been suggested in the SDC factor structure (Kivela & Pahkala, 1986). Overall, in light of the evidence of its psychometric characteristics, the SDC is probably not the best choice for a depression assessment instrument for older adults at this time. Further research on its psychometric properties and norms may yield a more positive impression of this instrument.

Clinician Rating Scales

Clinician rating scales often require somewhat more time to complete than self-report instruments, but they offer the advantages of providing an "objective" perspective on the depressive symptoms and are particularly useful with older adults experiencing moderate to severe cognitive impairment. They are commonly used in clinical research. As with the self-report instruments, each of the instruments we review has its strengths and weaknesses.

Hamilton Rating Scale for Depression

The Hamilton Rating Scale for Depression (HRSD) has been considered the gold standard for assessing severity of depression and is widely used in research. The HRSD has several versions, with the number of items employed ranging from 17 to 28. The 17-item version is the most commonly used and contains somatic and suicidal ideation items, although it does not include all of the items that would be necessary for the diagnosis of a major depressive episode (e.g., sleep difficulties, weight gain). Each of the behaviorally anchored items is rated on either a 3- or 5-point scale and summed to obtain the total score. Scores greater than 24 are indicative of severe depression, and scores less than 7 are indicative of the absence of depression. It correlates moderately with the BDI (0.68) in community-dwelling older adults and more strongly with the GDS (0.84) in a mixed Danish geriatric sample (Korner et al., 2006).

Williams (1988) developed the Structured Interview Guide for the HRSD (SIGH—D) to address the problem of variability in inter-rater reliability resulting from the relatively unstructured nature of the original 17-item scale. The structured interview can be completed with the patient or a collateral source. Gilley et al. (1995) found low rates of symptom endorsement in Alzheimer's patients, suggesting that the use of collateral sources may be a more valid approach in this population. Even with the increased structure, reliability remained fair to poor for half of the items (Pachana, Gallagher-Thompson, & Thompson, 1994). Gallagher (1986) noted that approximately 20 training interviews were required to achieve acceptable reliability. In addition, Hammond (1998) found low internal reliability in geriatric medical inpatients and suggested that anxiety symptoms may confound results on the scale.

On a more positive note, Korner et al. (2006) reported an inter-rater reliability of 0.90 in a geriatric sample. In addition, Rapp, Smith, and Britt (1990) found the 17-item version of the HRSD to have good psychometric properties with older medical patients and Leentjens, Verhey, Lousberg, Spitsbergen, and Wilmink (2000) and Olden, Rosenfeld, Pessin, and Breitbart (2009) established good concurrent validity with DSM-IV criteria. The HRSD may be a good alternative for older adults who have difficulty completing self-report inventories. A new version of the HRSD was presented in Williams et al. (2008) with good psychometric support in an adult sample. More research is needed on its use in older adults before it can be recommended.

Geriatric Depression Rating Scale

The Geriatric Depression Rating Scale (GDRS) (Jamison & Scogin, 1992) is a 35-item clinician rating scale that contains 29 of the 30 GDS items plus six items with somatic content. The scale combines the format of the HRSD, for the purpose of obtaining severity ratings, with the content of the GDS, which de-emphasizes somatic content. Preliminary evidence of internal consistency is good (alpha = 0.92). Preliminary estimates of concurrent validity with hospitalized, outpatient, and community-dwelling older adults are also good, with moderate to strong correlations obtained between the GDRS and the HRSD (r = 0.83), BDI (r = 0.69), and GDS (r = 0.84). A cutoff score of 20 yielded 88% sensitivity and 82% specificity. The GDRS requires a trained interviewer and approximately 35 minutes to administer. An advantage of the GDRS over the HRSD is that it probably requires less experience and training to administer reliably (Scogin, 1994).

Geriatric Mental State Schedule—Depression Scale

The Geriatric Mental State Schedule—Depression Scale (GMSS—DS) (Ravindran, Welburn, & Copeland, 1994) is a 33-item, semi-structured interview that employs a 3-point rating scale for most items. The items were drawn from the Geriatric Mental State Schedule on the basis of their ability to discriminate between depressed and non-depressed older adults, and their sensitivity to change following pharmacological treatment. The scale is intended for rating symptomatological changes of depression. The authors have presented sound evidence of its internal consistency (alpha = 0.95; Spearman-Brown split half = 0.92). Moreover, strong correlations were demonstrated between

GMSS–DS scores and scores on the BDI, HRSD, and clinician ratings of severity (r = 0.86, 0.91, and 0.84). A cutoff score of 18 yielded a sensitivity estimate of 97% and specificity estimate of 90% with regard to improvement following treatment (improved versus not improved).

In constructing the instrument, the authors included a large number of items because the frequency of different depressive symptoms appears to be more variable in older than younger adults. The large number of items could make this a particularly sensitive instrument for monitoring symptom change, although the large number of items may make it too cumbersome for use with medical populations (Davies et al., 1993). Some symptoms (e.g., guilt, pessimism, dissatisfaction) that have been shown to be sensitive to change in younger adults were not included because the symptoms appear to continue as residual symptoms in older adults following clinical improvement in depressive symptoms. While the initial psychometric characteristics appear very promising for the GMSS–DS as an index of change in depressive symptoms, the instrument could benefit from cross validation with different older populations.

Structured Interviews

Structured and semi-structured diagnostic interviews can be quite helpful to ensure reliable diagnoses for researchers. However, their utility for the practicing clinician is often limited because of the time and skills required to administer them reliably.

Structured Clinical Interview

The Structured Clinical Interview (SCID) (First, Spitzer, Gibbon, & Williams, 1997) for DSM-IV has not been evaluated in older adults, but is one of the best-known and best-accepted structured interviews. There is, however, little evidence that it is used frequently in clinical practice although it is widely used in research on depression in various populations (e.g., Haworth et al., 2007). Segal, Kabacoff, Hersen, VanHasslet, and Ryan (1995) found good inter-rater reliability for major depression in older adults with the DSM-III-R version of the SCID. In their discussion of the previous edition of the SCID for the DSM-III-R, Pachana and coauthors (1994) stated that they did not find it very useful as a diagnostic standard for depression among older adults, as it appears less sensitive than they had anticipated for identifying depressive disorders. In light of the apparent limited use, lengthy administration time, and limited information on the validity and utility of the SCID with older adults, at this time we cannot recommend it for standard use with older adults.

Measures of Depression with Coexistent Dementia

The assessment of depression among individuals with dementia can be a particularly challenging task due to both the overlapping symptoms of dementia and depression, and the effects of cognitive deficits in general. (For more thorough treatments of this topic see: Katz & Parmelee, 1997; Shue, Beck, & Lawton, 1997; and Storandt & VandenBos, 1994.) There is a significant need for instruments that work well in patients with dementia, considering that estimates of depressed mood among individuals with Alzheimer's disease range from 0–87% (median = 41%), and depressive disorders among this population range from 30–50% (Olin et al., 2002). When possible, information obtained from caregivers can be quite helpful in the assessment of depression, particularly in an individual with cognitive deficits (Logsdon & Teri, 1995; Stone, 1995). A few instruments have been designed specifically to be used with individuals experiencing dementia, the two most notable being the Cornell Scale for Depression in Dementia (CSDD) (Alexopoulus et al., 1988) and the Dementia Mood Assessment Scale (DMAS) (Sunderland et al., 1988).

Cornell Scale for Depression in Dementia

The CSDD is a 19-item instrument whose items were constructed so they could be completed primarily on the basis of direct observation and interviews with the client and caregiver. Each item is rated on a severity scale of 0 to 2 with a total score range of 0 to 38. It is similar in item content to the Hamilton Rating Scale for Depression. Administration requires two steps, and requires approximately 30 minutes for completion. The first step is a semi-structured interview of the patient's caregiver using the CSDD items to evaluate the patient's behaviors over the past week. The second step involves an interview of the patient using the same items.

The CSDD was designed to provide a severity rating once depression has been established, rather than determining whether a diagnosis is present. Nevertheless, the CSDD has been shown to differentiate between Research Diagnostic Criteria categories for depression among nursing home residents, although it failed to adequately discriminate between residents with no depression and residents with minor depression (Alexopoulus et al., 1988). Indices of internal consistency and inter-rater reliability are quite good when the scale is used with patients with dementia (alpha = 0.84, kappa = 0.67). Korner et al. (2006) reported high inter-rater reliability (0.84), high correlations with the GDS (0.82) and HDRS (0.91), and excellent sensitivity (0.93) and specificity (0.97) at a cutoff of 6 in a mixed dementia and normal older adult population. Overall, the CSDD may be a reasonable choice of screening instruments when assessing cognitively impaired older adults for major depression.

Dementia Mood Assessment Scale

The DMAS is a 17-item rating scale and semi-structured interview, with most items scaled from 0 (within normal limits) to 6 (most severe). It was developed as a brief measure of mood in dementia patients, requiring an interview of the client and direct observation of the client over time. Approximately 20–30 minutes are required to complete the test. The scale is designed for use by trained raters, requiring skills and knowledge similar to those required for administration of the HRSD, from which part of the DMAS was derived. Symptom severity is rated on the basis of clinical observation and a semi-structured interview. Sunderland et al. (1988) found only a modest relation between DMAS and HRSD scores (r = 0.47), which is rather weak concurrent validity evidence. Inter-rater reliability estimates were also modest (r = 0.74 for core raters and r = 0.69 for other raters). Overall, there has been limited evaluation of the DMAS. Its principal advantage is that it incorporates data from interviews and direct observation.

In spite of the advantages of using these instruments designed for individuals with dementia, Katz and Parmalee (1997) concluded in their review that "of non-diagnostic methods, the Geriatric Depression Scale (GDS) seems to offer the best available assessment approach. Self-ratings of depression with the GDS appear to be reliable and valid in mild to moderate dementia" (p. 98). Their argument is that while measures obtained via the non-self-reports can be reliable and valid, even with moderately to severely impaired older adults, the attainment of adequate levels of reliability and validity requires standardization and formalization of administration.

EPIDEMIOLOGY OF BEREAVEMENT

Older adults are more likely to experience the death of friends, family, and loved ones than younger adults. For many, learning to cope with death and loss is simply part of aging. The death of a spouse is considered to be one of life's greatest stressors (Holmes & Rahe, 1967). According to the U.S. Census Bureau (2008b), an estimated 14% of men, and 42% of women, over the age 65 and older are widowed. Among those aged 85 and older, 38% of men and 76% of women are widowed.

Grief is a part of the human experience. However, even the normal grief process can be incredibly stressful. In addition to coping with feelings of loss and loneliness, older adults who have lost a spouse or partner may need to learn new skills and take over new responsibilities (Anderson & Dimond, 1995). Spousal bereavement is associated with poorer physical health (Charlton, Sheahan, Smith, & Campbell, 2001; Christakis & Allison, 2006; Kowalski & Bondmass, 2008), and lower levels of psychological well-being (Thuen, Reime, & Skrautvoll, 1997). Despite the fact that loss is common among older adults, the grief response varies widely. For the majority of older adults, grief diminishes over time (Ott, Lueger, Kelber, & Prigerson, 2007). However, a subset of older adults experience complicated grief, also known as traumatic grief, or prolonged grief (Ott et al., 2007; Zisook & Shear, 2009). The following section discusses grief responses among older adults, and assessment of grief and bereavement.

DEFINITION AND DIAGNOSTIC ISSUES

To clarify the terminology used to refer to the loss of a loved one, Zisook and Shear (2009) noted the differences between the terms "bereavement," "grief," and "mourning." Researchers refer to bereavement as the state of having suffered a loss, while grief refers to a person's response to a loss, including emotional, functional, cognitive, and behavioral reactions. Mourning refers to the cultural and social behavioral manifestations of grief, including funerals and burial rituals. However, the *Diagnostic and Statistical Manual of Mental Disorders*, Fourth Edition, Text Revised (DSM-IV-TR; American Psychiatric Association, 2000) uses the term "bereavement" rather than "grief" to describe the reaction to the loss of a loved one. Complicated grief is the term used to refer to intense and prolonged grief that is associated with an array of negative outcomes (Zisook & Shear, 2009). However, there are still no official or formal diagnostic criteria for complicated grief, and even the terminology used to describe the phenomenon varies throughout the literature. Some describe "complicated grief," others use the term "traumatic grief," and others use the term "prolonged grief disorder." For the sake of simplicity, we will refer to the set of symptoms described above as "complicated grief" in this chapter.

Normal Bereavement

Before discussing complicated grief, we will discuss a typical, or uncomplicated, grief response. Please note, however, that the grief response varies widely according to individual, circumstantial, and cultural factors. Characterization of a universal "normal" grief response is difficult, if not impossible. However, some of the pieces of the grieving process seem to be common. Older adults who are grieving endorse feelings of stress, difficulty dealing with everyday tasks, and loneliness, but also endorse positive feelings about their loved one (Lund, 1998). In a longitudinal study of bereavement in older adults, depressed mood, tearfulness, and loneliness were found to be fundamental symptoms of grief (Grimby, 1993).

The grief response is sometimes described in stages. According to stage theories of grief, people who are bereaved first experience an initial phase of shock and disbelief, then a phase of depression and mourning, followed by a period of resolution, in which the individual recovers and is able to move forward in life (Shuchter & Zisook, 1993; Zisook & Shuchter, 1996). However, more recent research suggests that stage theories of grief cannot account for the variability in the way that people experience loss (Zisook & Shear, 2009).

Although some studies have shown that grief usually lasts for one year (Norris & Murrell, 1990), others indicate that it is not unusual for people to experience symptoms of grief for a significantly longer period of time (Kowalski & Bondmass, 2008; Pasternak et al., 1991). A longitudinal study of spousal bereavement among older adults showed that most bereaved older adults improved over the course of 18 months (Ott et al., 2007). Specifically, Ott and colleagues found that most older adults experienced an increase in symptoms of grief alone, or symptoms of grief and depression, that mitigated with time. The majority of the remaining participants met the proposed criteria for complicated grief.

Factors That Affect Grief Response

Certain factors, both personal and situational, can have an impact on the bereavement process. Studies of the effects of gender on grief have yielded varied results. In their chapter discussing gender and cultural variations of grief, Wisocki and Skowron (2000) reported that some studies found that men have poorer outcomes than women following the death of a spouse, whereas other studies found that women have poorer outcomes than men. There is also evidence that men and women experience bereavement similarly (Lund, Caserta, & Dimond, 1986). Wisocki and Skowron (2000) discuss possible reasons for this discrepancy, including differences in the outcome variables examined and study designs.

The presence of depression before the death of a loved one is a predictor of depression after the death (Gilewski, Farberow, Gallagher, & Thompson, 1991; Norris & Murrel, 1990). Higher levels of pre-existing depression are associated with higher levels of depression after the loss. Further, existential factors affect the grieving process. Those with higher levels of religiosity, spirituality, and personal meaning had a greater sense of personal well-being after the loss of a spouse (Fry, 2001). Moreover, a study of widowed men and women age 50 and older showed that experiencing happiness, laughter, and humor in daily life after a loss is associated with lower levels of grief and depression (Lund, Utz, Caserta, & de Vries, 2008).

In addition to individual characteristics, certain relationship and situational factors have been found to affect the grieving process. The nature of the marital relationship has been shown to affect outcomes. Widows and widowers who reported being more dependent on their spouse were more likely to experience chronic grief (Ott et al., 2007). The Changing Lives of Older Couples (or CLOC) study examined other factors that affected grief outcomes (see review by Carr & Utz, 2001). Those who had a close marriage reported more symptoms of yearning for their spouse after death than those who reported having a troubled marriage (Carr et al., 2000).

Beyond the quality of the marriage, the CLOC study found that circumstances surrounding the death of a spouse affected grief outcomes. When widowed persons reported that their spouse had experienced significant pain at the time of death, they were more likely to endorse higher levels of anxiety, anger, and yearning for their spouse (Carr, 2003). Carr (2001) also found that widowed persons who reported that their spouse had died as a result of health care provider negligence reported higher levels of anger. Interestingly, widowed persons who had placed their spouse in a nursing home facility reported better outcomes than those whose spouse lived at home at the time of death (Carr et al., 2000). Ott and colleagues (2007) examined other factors surrounding the nature of the death. A sudden death was associated with chronic grief. Similarly, chronic grief was associated with feeling less prepared for the death. When a spouse died by suicide, or a form of stigmatized death (i.e., AIDS), the bereavement period was especially difficult, particularly for widowers (Gilewski et al., 1991). The poorer outcomes may have resulted from diminished social support.

Bereavement and Depression

The DSM-IV-TR recognizes that people often experience depressive symptoms following the death of a loved one, including depressed mood, insomnia, loss of appetite, and weight loss. However, it specifies that major depressive disorder should be diagnosed only if symptoms persist for more than two months after the death (American Psychiatric Association, 2000). Bereavement can be recorded as a V-Code, indicating a possibly clinically relevant condition. Moreover, the DSM-IV-TR outlines certain symptoms that can help to differentiate a normal grief reaction from major depressive disorder, including:

1) Guilt about things other than actions taken or not taken at the time of the death;
2) Thoughts of death other than the survivor feeling that he or she would be better off dead, or should have died with the deceased person;
3) Morbid preoccupation with worthlessness;
4) Marked psychomotor retardation;
5) Prolonged and marked functional impairment; and
6) Hallucinatory experiences other than thinking that he or she hears the voice of, or transiently sees the image of, the deceased person (pp. 740—741).

Zisook, Paulus, Shuchter, & Judd (1997) conducted a longitudinal study that examined the prevalence of depressive disorders after the loss of a loved one. At two months after the loss, 20% of bereaved individuals met criteria for major depressive disorder. Another 20% met criteria for minor depression, and 11% met criteria for subsyndromal depression. Nearly half (49%) did not meet criteria for any type of depressive disorder (Zisook et al., 1997). Thirteen months after the loss, the percentage meeting full criteria for major depressive disorder dropped to 12%. Of the remaining, 17% met criteria for minor depression, 10% met criteria for subsyndromal depression, and 62% met criteria for no depressive disorder (Zisook et al., 1997). The rates of depression dropped even lower at 25 months after the loss. At that time, only 6% met criteria for major depressive disorder, 13% met criteria for minor depression, and 11% reported subsyndromal depression. A full 70% did not meet criteria for any depressive disorder (Zisook et al., 1997).

Though many people who are experiencing grief endorse feelings of profound sadness, a minority meet full criteria for major depressive disorder, and the prevalence of major depressive disorder declines with time. Differentiating between an episode of major depressive disorder and grief can be challenging, given the often similar presentations (e.g., depressed mood and tearfulness). Further complicating the issue, the loss of a loved one is a major stressor that can sometimes trigger a depressive episode. However, differences can distinguish grief from major depressive disorder. People who are grieving generally experience both positive and negative emotions, in contrast to the pervasive depressed mood that characterizes major depressive disorder (Zisook & Shear, 2009). Further, depressed mood among those who are bereaved tends to be tied to reminders of the deceased, in contrast to the pervasive depressed mood of major depressive disorder (Zisook & Shear, 2009). Many argue that the DSM-IV-TR lacks a clear set of criteria that differentiates normal grief from depression, and normal grief from complicated grief.

Complicated Grief

To adequately capture the experience of abnormal grief, many researchers have advocated for the addition of a diagnosis of complicated grief to the DSM. Several sets of similar criteria have been proposed. One set of criteria, developed by Horowitz and colleagues (2003), includes a current experience, lasting at least 14 months after a loss, of anhedonia, intrusive thoughts of the deceased, yearnings, feelings of loneliness, and disrupted sleep patterns. Jacobs, Mazure, and Prigerson (2000) suggest an alternate set of criteria, including a current disturbance lasting at least two months after a loss, of separation distress (e.g., yearning for or preoccupation with the deceased) and symptoms of trauma (e.g., avoidance, feelings of numbness, or feelings of emptiness).

In an attempt to clarify the concept of complicated grief, a panel of grief and trauma experts met for a consensus conference to develop criteria for complicated grief (Prigerson & Jacobs, 2001). The consensus criteria include daily or marked separation distress (e.g., yearning, intrusive thoughts about the loss, searching for the deceased, or loneliness) and daily or marked symptoms of trauma (e.g., a sense of hopelessness about the future, disbelief about the death, or feelings of numbness), lasting at least six months, and causing significant impairment (Prigerson et al., 1999).

Many advocate for the addition of complicated grief to the DSM-V. Studies have shown that symptoms of complicated grief are distinctly different from normal, or uncomplicated, grief (Boelen & van den Bout, 2008; Dillen, Fontaine, & Verhofstadt-Deneve, 2008). Further, the symptoms of separation distress and trauma associated with complicated grief are distinctly different from bereavement-related depression and anxiety, and are predictive of worse outcomes (Prigerson et al., 1995a; Prigerson et al., 1996). Research shows conflicting evidence as to whether symptoms of complicated grief are resistant to traditional treatments for depression (Reynolds et al., 1999; Zisook, Shuchter, Pedrilli, Sable, & Deaciuc, 2001).

An estimated 10% of bereaved individuals meet the proposed criteria for complicated grief (Shear & Shair, 2005). Among psychiatric outpatients who have experienced a significant loss, the prevalence of complicated grief jumps to almost one-third (Piper, Ogrodniczuk, Azim, & Weideman, 2001). Complicated grief is associated with poorer physical and mental health (Ott, 2003; Gallagher-Thompson, Futterman, Farberow, Thompson, & Peterson, 1993). People who experience symptoms of complicated grief six months after the loss of a spouse are at greater risk for cancer, heart disease, and changes in eating pattern at 13 and 25 months after the loss (Prigerson et al., 1997). Moreover, complicated grief substantially increases risk of suicide (Latham & Prigerson, 2004; Szanto et al., 2002). For these reasons, it is important to identify pathological grief.

Multicultural Issues

Recognizing the importance of correctly identifying abnormal grief responses, clinical assessment should consider cultural variations in grief. This section discusses the considerable heterogeneity in grief responses and mourning rituals across different ethnic populations. Wisocki and Skowron (2000) discuss cultural variations in the expression of emotions following a loss, conceptualizations of the presence of the dead, in body or in spirit, after death, community and family involvement in mourning rituals, and the manner in which people deal with memories of the dead. In some cultures, elaborate mourning rituals are believed to be necessary to assist the dead to an afterworld. For example, in the Hmong culture, a 13-day ritual is completed to allow the soul of the dead to pass to the afterlife (Bliatout, 1993). In contrast, other cultures believe that the soul of the dead remains on earth. Many homes in the Japanese culture maintain altars and individuals make offerings to their deceased ancestors throughout their lives (Wiscocki and Skowron, 2000). The expression of grief can vary greatly from culture to culture as well. In Egyptian culture, the death of a close loved one is often associated with an extended period of depression (Irish, Lundquist, & Nelsen, 1993). However, other cultures do not display typical grief reactions.

Several recent studies have examined differences in grief reactions among African American and Caucasian individuals. Some have found no differences in either the clinical presentation of grief, or treatment outcomes (Cruz et al., 2007). One study of race and grief in widowed older adults showed no differences in overall severity of grief symptoms (including yearning, symptoms of depression and anxiety, and shock), but lower levels of despair and anger were found among African American widows and widowers (Carr, 2004). In addition, African American widows and widowers reported higher levels of support from children, more religious participation, and higher levels of marital conflict before the loss (Carr, 2004).

BEREAVEMENT ASSESSMENT INSTRUMENTS

In the following section, we discuss several measures used to assess grief. However, few of the available measures have been validated for use with older adults. We discuss several widely used bereavement assessment instruments, but, since there is little psychometric data, we encourage caution when using these instruments with older adults.

Texas Revised Inventory of Grief

The Texas Revised Inventory of Grief (TRIG) (Faschingbauer, Zisook, & DeVaul, 1987) is a 21- item instrument used to assess symptoms of grief. Clinically, the scale is used to measure adjustment and to track change following a loss. Scores can range from 0 to 65 with higher scores indicating increased grief. The items reflect common symptoms of grief and are rated on a 5-point Likert-type scale, where responses range from "completely true" to "completely false."

The TRIG has two subscales: one that assesses current feelings about the death and one retrospective subscale that assesses feelings at the time of the death. Both subscales demonstrated good test–retest reliability (0.86 for the present feelings and 0.77 for the retrospective account). Further, the TRIG demonstrated good predictive validity in a sample of older adults in a study conducted by Gallagher, Breckenridge, Thompson, and Peterson (1983), and has been used extensively with adults over age 55 (Thompson, Gallagher-Thompson, Futterman, Gilewski, & Peterson, 1991). The TRIG has been translated into both French and Spanish (Garcia, Landa, Trigueros, & Gaminde, 2005; Paulhan & Bourgeois, 1995). The Spanish version has been validated for use in a sample of Latino older adults (Wilson, 2007).

The TRIG has been criticized for containing repetitive items and for containing items that may characterize typical grief reactions (e.g., "No one will ever take the place in my life of the person who died."). Further, it may be difficult for older adults to retrospectively recall past feelings.

The Grief Experience Inventory

The Grief Experience Inventory (GEI) (Sanders, Mauger, & Strong, 1985) is a 135-item scale used to measure grief reactions. Individuals are asked to respond with a "yes" or "no" to each of the items. It is organized across nine subscales (despair, guilt, anger, social isolation, loss of control, depersonalization, somatization, rumination, and death anxiety). Cronbach's α ranges from 0.52–81, indicating moderate support for internal consistency (Hansson, Carpenter, & Fairchild, 1993; Tomita & Kitamura, 2002). The GEI has received criticism because it is a lengthy measure. Older adults may be especially susceptible to measure fatigue. Further, it has been criticized for only allowing a dichotomous "yes" or "no" response.

A shortened version of the GEI was developed by Lev, Munro, and McCorkle (1993). This 22-item version utilizes a six-point Likert-type scale to assess severity of grief symptoms. Lev and colleagues (1993) reported good internal consistency ($\alpha = 0.93$) and sensitivity to grief. Although the more complicated response mode may be confusing to older adults, the abbreviated scale reduces fatigue, and appears to be a more efficient scale for assessing grief. However, there are no studies examining its use specifically among older adults.

Inventory of complicated grief

Prigerson and colleagues developed the Inventory of Complicated Grief (ICG) (Prigerson et al., 1995b) to assess the symptoms of complicated grief (see Appendix B). The scale contains 19 items that are rated on a scale from 0 to 4, where 0 indicates "not at all" and 4 indicates "severe." Total scores range from 0–76 with higher scores indicating more distress. A score of 25 or greater defines complicated grief. When tested in a sample of older adults who had lost a spouse, the ICG demonstrated high internal consistency (Cronbach's $\alpha = 0.94$) and good test–retest reliability (0.80). Further, the ICG correlated highly with both the TRIG scores ($r = 0.87$) and Beck Depression Inventory scores ($r = 0.67$) indicating convergent validity. Further, bereaved older adults with higher ICG scores were significantly more impaired (mentally, physically, and socially) than those with lower ICG scores.

Case Study 1

You are a consulting psychologist for a nursing home. Susan, a 75-year-old resident, is referred to you by the Director of Nursing, who is concerned about Susan's apathy, irritability, crying spells, and withdrawal from social activities. Susan complains of difficulties with concentration and memory, and has experienced difficulty remembering the topic of recent conversations. She occasionally becomes disoriented and is frustrated and angry when this occurs.

You peruse Susan's chart and find that she has a family history of Alzheimer's disease, but no known history of other mental disorders. She is currently being treated for hypothyroidism, gastrointestinal reflux disease, and hyperlipidemia. Her medications include levothyroxine sodium, omeprazole, and atorvastatin, respectively. A discussion with the unit nurse reveals that Susan's hypothyroidism is apparently well controlled in light of her thyroid stimulating hormone levels, which suggests that the possible depression symptoms are unlikely due to her hypothyroidism. None of the common adverse effects of omeprazole and atorvastatin include symptoms consistent with those of which Susan complains. Susan has had no medication changes in the past four weeks. She has lost eight pounds in the past three weeks, placing her just under her ideal weight range. Susan was admitted to the nursing home two months ago following surgery to repair a hip fracture resulting from a fall in her home. Because Susan lived alone, she was unable to care for herself following the initial rehabilitation following surgery.

When you approach Susan in her room, you find her lying in her bed and crying in the middle of the day. She reports that she does not want to talk for very long but agrees to do so the following day. You obtain informed consent from Susan to speak with her daughter, who lives in another state and is Susan's agent under a medical power of attorney. Susan's daughter expresses concern about her mother and reports that she had never seen her mother like this before the hip fracture. Her mother was characterized as energetic, cheerful, and involved in several social activities. You learn from her daughter that Susan's memory complaints and disorientation began soon after her hip surgery, as did her symptoms of depression.

When you approach Susan for the interview the next day, she seems surprised to see you and apologizes for forgetting the appointment. You noticed that as she moved very slowly with a walker down the hall, she appeared unsteady at times. She seemed to hesitate and look around between steps as she proceeded into the conference room that you are using for the interview. She is still wearing her bedclothes, apparently from the night before, and her hair is uncombed, even though it is 3:00 p.m. She has forgotten her glasses even though the nurse reminded her to bring them just before she left her room. Susan sits in a comfortable chair at a table and you inform her of the reason for the interview. As you interview her, she is polite but tearful. She reports that she is not interested in activities that she formerly enjoyed, has difficulty sleeping (awaking early in the morning), her appetite is poor, her memory and concentration are markedly impaired (a source of great distress for her), and she reports feeling worthless and unhappy. Susan denies suicidal ideation and describes several reasons for not taking her life. You find that she frequently needs to be prompted to complete sentences because her sentences trail off or she stares out the window. On several occasions, she asks you to repeat questions, and reports that she has forgotten them.

In light of the information you have gathered, you are uncertain whether Susan is experiencing dementia, depression, or both. You decide to: (a) further observe Susan's behavior; (b) administer a depression screening instrument (GDS rather than BDI due to possible cognitive deficits); (c) administer the Mini-Mental State Examination (MMSE) to screen for cognitive deficits; and (e) discuss the temporal sequence of Susan's symptoms with Susan and her daughter.

Susan obtains a score of 19/30 on the MMSE, suggesting possible cognitive deficits. The items missed pertain to orientation, attention, and memory. You recall that depression can affect performance on these items. You observe Susan at various times of the day and find that she leaves her room only for meals. When other residents approach her, she either complains or does not respond. They quickly leave her alone.

Results of the GDS administration suggest that Susan is experiencing moderate to severe depression, with symptoms of fatigue, insomnia, decreased activities, depressed mood, poor concentration, tearfulness, weight loss, and psychomotor retardation. Based on her memory complaints and possible deficits, disorientation, possible gait disturbance, and low MMSE total score, you refer Susan to a neuropsychologist to explore these deficits and determine to what extent they may be transient, and whether they are more likely due to depression or dementia. Results of the neuropsychological evaluation indicate that cognitive deficits, specifically memory deficits and disorientation, are due primarily to extreme distractibility. Thus, the deficits revealed on the MMSE are likely due to her distractibility arising from her depressed mood. You recall that depression is both a risk factor for hip fracture, particularly among women, often follows hip fractures, and is associated with longer recovery.

Based on your interview and observation of Susan, review of her medical records, psychological testing, information gained from Susan's daughter, and results of the neuropsychological evaluation, you conclude that Susan is experiencing a Major Depressive Disorder secondary to her hip fracture. These results should provide treating professionals with sufficient information to begin a treatment regime.

You recommend to the staff that they continue to monitor Susan's mood and cognitive status, and assure her that her symptoms will likely improve with treatment.

Case Study 2—Bereavement

You are the consulting psychologist for a primary care practice. Jean, a 65-year-old widowed woman, is referred to you by her primary care doctor. Jean's husband died suddenly of a heart attack in the home two years ago. Jean became very depressed after his death. She was very tearful, and found it hard to make it through her typical daily routine. Jean's primary care doctor prescribed an antidepressant for her, which she has been taking for about one year. Jean has noticed some improvements but she is still very tearful, and is still "consumed" by her grief. Her husband had been in charge of the family's finances, but since his death the responsibility has fallen to Jean. She is very behind on paying her bills, because she finds it difficult to remember to pay them. When she is able to remember to pay them, she has trouble concentrating on the paperwork.

Looking over her chart, you note that she has no family or personal history of mental illness. Her doctor increased her dose of antidepressant several weeks ago, but otherwise, she has had no changes in her medications.

During your first visit with Jean, you talk to her about the death of her husband. She is tearful throughout the interview. She tells you that she had always been an active person. However, since her husband died she has had trouble maintaining her home, and caring for her pets. She rarely cooks for herself, because making meals reminds her of her husband. As a result, she now weighs 115 pounds, down from 145 pounds at the time of her husband's death. Jean reports nightly initial and middle insomnia. It takes her about 40 minutes to fall asleep each night, and she wakens frequently throughout the night. She also reports daily loss of appetite, fatigue, and anhedonia. She feels depressed nearly every day of the week, for most of the day, However, she notes that she feels especially down at dinnertime and other times when she is reminded of her husband's absence. When you ask her about feelings of guilt, she begins to sob. She goes on to tell you that she feels guilty that she could not save her husband when he collapsed and died at her feet. Jean describes the day of his death in vivid detail. She tells you that she has rearranged the furniture in her home so she does not have to walk by the spot where he died.

Considering her report, you are uncertain whether Jean is experiencing depression or complicated grief. In light of her forgetfulness with bills, you would also like to rule out the beginnings of cognitive decline. You decide to: (a) ask her to track her activities and her mood over the course of the week; (b) administer a depression measure (the BDI–II); (c) administer a bereavement measure (the ICG); (d) administer the Montreal Cognitive Assessment—a brief screen for cognitive status; (e) assess for suicidality using the Geriatric Suicide Ideation Scale (GSIS) (Heisel and Flett, 2006); and (f) continue to discuss Jean's feelings of loss. Jean scores a 29 out of 30 on the Montreal Cognitive Assessment, placing her well in the normal range. She missed one point on the delayed recall task.

Her scores on the BDI–II indicate a moderate to severe level of depression. She adamantly denies all active or passive suicidal ideation, and her score on the GSIS reflects low levels of suicide risk. Her scores on the ICG indicate a severe level of complicated grief. She endorses both symptoms of separation distress, including yearning for her husband and intense loneliness, and symptoms of trauma, including numbness and disbelief about the death. When examining her activity log, you note that her mood is low for most of the day, but that she has periods of time when she feels normal. However, her mood is always low around dinner time. Jean reiterates that dinner time is especially difficult for her, because she used to enjoy cooking for her husband and sharing a meal with him.

When considering a diagnosis, you recommend that she is evaluated by a physician to rule out any organic causes of her symptoms. Because this episode has lasted for over two years, you rule out acute stress disorder. You also rule out Post-traumatic Stress Disorder (PTSD), because Jean is primarily experiencing feelings of sadness, rather than the feelings of fear that typically characterize PTSD. (See Shear, Frank, Houck, and Reynolds, 2005 for a discussion of the differences between PTSD and complicated grief.) You rule out a diagnosis of dysthymia because Jean reports depressed mood for most of the day, nearly every day, indicating that you should consider a diagnosis of major depressive disorder.

Based on the findings of your interview, the measures administered, and her chart, you determine that Jean is experiencing the symptoms of complicated grief and also meets DSM-IV criteria for Major Depressive Disorder. The results of the assessment will guide you in making treatment recommendations.

CONCLUSION

This chapter provides an overview of conceptual, diagnostic, and practical issues associated with the assessment of late-life depression and bereavement. Commonly used assessment instruments are reviewed, followed by case studies illustrating the complexity of assessing older adults who present with symptoms of depression, complicated bereavement, or both. The empirical support for several assessment instruments has improved since the first edition of this book was published in 1999, and new instruments have appeared that show considerable promise. Nevertheless, the definitional and diagnostic issues continue to contribute to the difficulty of identifying older adults who are distressed by their symptoms but who do not meet criteria for the current DSM diagnoses.

The need for multidimensional and multi-method assessment cannot be overemphasized, particularly in light of the multiple factors that can contribute to the presentation of depression and bereavement. The mounting evidence of the importance of cultural factors in the presentation and epidemiology of depression should not be ignored.

Finally, there is a continuing need for assessment instrument development and refinement, particularly as we come to better understand the unique experience and presentations of older adults, and the need to address subsyndromal symptoms that can curtail daily activities and diminish quality of life.

APPENDIX A: GERIATRIC DEPRESSION SCALE (GDS)

Choose the best answer for how you felt this past week circle one

*1.	Are you basically satisfied with your life?	Yes	No
2.	Have you dropped many of your activities and interests?	Yes	No
3.	Do you feel that your life is empty?	Yes	No
4.	Do you often get bored?	Yes	No
*5.	Are you hopeful about the future?	Yes	No
6.	Are you bothered by thoughts you can't get out of your head?	Yes	No
*7.	Are you in good spirits most of the time?	Yes	No
8.	Are you afraid that something bad is going to happen to you?	Yes	No
*9.	Do you feel happy most of the time?	Yes	No
10.	Do you often feel helpless?	Yes	No
11.	Do you often get restless and fidgety?	Yes	No
12.	Do you prefer to stay at home, rather than going out and doing new things?	Yes	No
13.	Do you frequently worry about the future?	Yes	No
14.	Do you feel you have more problems with memory than most?	Yes	No
*15.	Do you think it is wonderful to be alive now?	Yes	No
16.	Do you often feel downhearted and blue?	Yes	No
17.	Do you feel pretty worthless the way you are now?	Yes	No
18.	Do you worry a lot about the past?	Yes	No
*19.	Do you find life very exciting?	Yes	No
20.	Is it hard for you to get started on new projects?	Yes	No
*21.	Do you feel full of energy?	Yes	No
22.	Do you feel that your situation is hopeless?	Yes	No
23.	Do you think that most people are better off than you are?	Yes	No
24.	Do you frequently get upset over little things?	Yes	No
25.	Do you frequently feel like crying?	Yes	No
26.	Do you have trouble concentrating?	Yes	No
*27.	Do you enjoy getting up in the morning?	Yes	No
28.	Do you prefer to avoid social gatherings?	Yes	No
*29.	Is it easy for you to make decisions?	Yes	No
*30.	Is your mind as clear as it used to be?	Yes	No

**Appropriate (nondepressed) answers = yes, all others= no or count number of CAPITALIZED (depressed) answers*

Score: _____ (Number of "depressed" answers)

Norms

Normal 5 ± 4

Mildly depressed 15 ± 6

Very depressed 23 ± 5

The Geriatric Depression Scale may be used freely for patient assessment according to the authors.

APPENDIX B: INVENTORY OF COMPLICATED GRIEF (ICG)

PLEASE fill in the circle next to the answer which best describes how you feel right now:

1. I think about this person so much that it's hard for me to do the things I normally do…
☐ never ☐ rarely ☐ sometimes ☐ often ☐ always
2. Memories of the person who died upset me…
☐ never ☐ rarely ☐ sometimes ☐ often ☐ always
3. I feel I cannot accept the death of the person who died…
☐ never ☐ rarely ☐ sometimes ☐ often ☐ always
4. I feel myself longing for the person who died…
☐ never ☐ rarely ☐ sometimes ☐ often ☐ always
5. I feel drawn to places and things associated with the person who died…
☐ never ☐ rarely ☐ sometimes ☐ often ☐ always
6. I can't help feeling angry about his/her death…
☐ never ☐ rarely ☐ sometimes ☐ often ☐ always
7. I feel disbelief over what happened…
☐ never ☐ rarely ☐ sometimes ☐ often ☐ always
8. I feel stunned or dazed over what happened…
☐ never ☐ rarely ☐ sometimes ☐ often ☐ always
9. Ever since s/he died it is hard for me to trust people…
☐ never ☐ rarely ☐ sometimes ☐ often ☐ always
10. Ever since s/he died I feel like I have lost the ability to care about other people or I feel distant from people I care about…
☐ never ☐ rarely ☐ sometimes ☐ often ☐ always
11. I have pain in the same area of my body or have some of the same symptoms as the person who died…
☐ never ☐ rarely ☐ sometimes ☐ often ☐ always
12. I go out of my way to avoid reminders of the person who died…
☐ never ☐ rarely ☐ sometimes ☐ often ☐ always
13. I feel that life is empty without the person who died…
☐ never ☐ rarely ☐ sometimes ☐ often ☐ always
14. I hear the voice of the person who died speak to me…
☐ never ☐ rarely ☐ sometimes ☐ often ☐ always
15. I see the person who died stand before me…
☐ never ☐ rarely ☐ sometimes ☐ often ☐ always
16. I feel that it is unfair that I should live when this person died…
☐ never ☐ rarely ☐ sometimes ☐ often ☐ always
17. I feel bitter over this person's death…
☐ never ☐ rarely ☐ sometimes ☐ often ☐ always
18. I feel envious of others who have not lost someone close…
☐ never ☐ rarely ☐ sometimes ☐ often ☐ always
19. I feel lonely a great deal of the time ever since s/he died…
☐ never ☐ rarely ☐ sometimes ☐ often ☐ always

References

Achterberg, W., Pot, A. M., Kerkstra, A., & Ribbe, M. (2006). Depressive symptoms in newly admitted nursing home residents. *International Journal of Geriatric Psychiatry, 21*, 1156–1162.

Adams, K. B. (2001). Depressive symptoms, depletion, or developmental change? Withdrawal, apathy, and lack of vigor in the Geriatric Depression Scale. *The Gerontologist, 41*, 768–777.

Alexopoulos, G. S. (2003). The role of executive function in late-life depression. *Journal of Clinical Psychiatry, 64*(Suppl. 14), 18–23.

Alexopoulos, G. S. (2005). Depression in the elderly. *The Lancet, 365*, 1961–1970.

Alexopoulos, G. S., Abrams, R. C., Young, R. C., & Shamoian, C. A. (1988). Cornell Scale for Depression in Dementia. *Biological Psychiatry, 23*, 271–284.

Alexopoulos, G. S., Borson, S., Cuthbert, B. N., Devanand, D. P., Mulsant, B. H., Olin, J. T., et al. (2002). Assessment of late life depression. *Biological Psychiatry, 52*, 164–174.

Alexopoulos, G. S, Meyers, S. B., Young, R. C., Mattis, S., & Kakuma, T. (1993). The course of geriatric depression with " reversiable dementia." A controlled study. *American Journal of Geriatric Psychiatry, 150*, 1693–1699.

Allen-Burge, R., Storandt, M., Kinscherf, D. A., & Rubin, E. H. (1994). Sex differences in the sensitivty of two self-report depression scales in older depressed inpatients. *Psychology and Aging, 9*, 443–445.

Allport, G. W. (1937). *Persionality: A psychological interpretation*. New York, NY: Henry Holt.

Almeida, O. P., & Almeida, S. A. (1999). Short versions of the Geriatric Depression Scale: A study of their validity for the diagnosis of a major depressive episode according to ICD–10 and DSM-IV. *International Journal of Geriatric Psychiatry, 14*, 858–865.

American Psychiatric Association. (1994). *Diagnostic and Statistical Manual—Fourth Edition*. Washington, DC: Author.

American Psychiatric Association. (2000). *Diagnostic and Statistical Manual of Mental Disorders—Fourth Edition*—Text Revision. Washington, DC: Author.

Anderson, K. L., & Dimond, M. F. (1995). The experience of bereavement in older adults. *Journal of Advanced Nursing, 22*, 308–315.

Andresen, E. M., Malmgren, J. A., Carter, W. B., & Patrick, D. L. (1994). Screening for depression in well older adults: Evaluation of a short-form of the CES–D. *American Journal of Preventive Medicine, 10*, 77–84.

Baker, F. M., & Miller, C. L. (1991). Screening a skilled nursing home population for depression. *Journal of Geriatric Psychiatry and Neurology, 4*, 218–221.

Barefoot, J. C., Mortensen, E. L., Helms, M. J., Avlund, K., & Schroll, M. (2001). A longitudinal study of gender differences in depressive symptoms from age 50 to 80. *Psychology and Aging, 16*, 342–345.

Barnett, P. A., & Gotlib, I. H. (1988). Psychosocial functioning and depression: Distinguishing among antecedents, concomitants, and consequences. *Psychological Bulletin, 104*, 97–126.

Beals, J., Manson, S. M., Whitesell, N. R., Mitchell, C. M., Novins, D. K., Simpson, S., et al. (2005). Prevalence of major depressive episode in two American Indian reservation populations: Unexpected findings with a structured interview. *American Journal of Psychiatry, 162*, 1713–1722.

Beck, A. T., & Beck, R. W. (1972). Screening depressed patients in family practice: A rapid technique. *Postgraduate Medicine,* 81–85.

Beck, A. T., Steer, R. A., & Brown, G. K. (1996). *Manual for the Beck Depression Inventory* (2nd ed.). San Antonio, TX: The Psychological Corporation.

Beck, A. T., Steer, R. A., & Brown, G. K. (2000). *Beck Depression Inventory—Fast Screen for Medical Patients*. San Antonio, TX: The Psychological Corporation.

Beck, A. T., Ward, C. H., Mendelson, M., Mock, J., & Erbaugh, J. (1961). An inventory for measuring depression. *Archives of General Psychiatry, 44*, 53–62.

Beekman, A. T., Copeland, J. R., & Prince, M. J. (1999). Review of community prevalence of depression in later life. *British Journal of Psychiatry, 174*, 307–311.

Beekman, A. T. F., Deeg, D. J. H., van Tilburg, T., Smit, J. H., Hooijer, C., & van Tilburg, W. (1995). Major and minor depression in later life: A study of prevalence and risk factors. *Journal of Affective Disorders, 36*, 65–75.

Bentz, B. G., & Hall, J. R. (2008). Assessment of depression in a geriatric inpatient cohort: A comparison of the BDI and GDS. *International Journal of Clinical and Health Psychology, 8*, 93–104.

Berry, J. M., Storandt, M., & Coyne, A. (1984). Age and sex differences in somatic complaints associated with depression. *Journal of Gerontology, 39*, 465–467.

Blazer, D. G. (1994). Epidemiology of late-life depression. In L. S. Schneider, C. F. Reynolds, B. D. Lebowitz, & A. J. Freidhoff (Eds.), *Diagnosis and treatment of depression in late life: Results of the NIH consensus development conference* (pp. 9–19). Washington, D.C.: American Psychiatric Press.

Blazer, D. G. (2003). Depression in late life: Review and commentary. *Journal of Gerontology: Medical Sciences, 58A*, 249–265.

Blazer, D. G. (2009). The psychiatric interview of older adults. In D. G. Blazer, & D. C. Steffens (Eds.), *The American Psychiatric Publishing Textbook of Geriatric Psychiatry* (4th ed.). (pp. 187–200) Arlington, VA: American Psychiatric Publishing.

Blazer, D., Bachar, J. R., & Hughes, D. C. (1987). Major depression with melancholia: A comparison of middle-aged and elderly adults. *Journal of the American Geriatrics Society, 35*, 927–932.

Blazer, D. G., Steffens, D. C., & Koenig, H. G. (2009). Mood disorders. In D. G. Blazer, & D. C. Steffens (Eds.), *The American Psychiatric Publishing Textbook of Geriatric Psychiatry* (4th ed.). (pp. 275–299) Arlington, VA: American Psychiatric Publishing.

Blazer, D. G., Landerman, L. R., Hays, J. C., Simonsick, E. M., & Saunders, W. B. (1998). Symptoms of depression among community-dwelling elderly African American and White older adults. *Psychological Medicine, 28*, 1311–1320.

Bliatout, B. T. (1993). Hmong death customs: Traditional and acculturated. In D. P. Irish, K. F. Lundquist, & V. J. Nelsen (Eds.), *Ethnic Variations in Dying, Death, and Grief: Diversity in Universality* (pp. 79–100). Philadelphia, PA: Taylor and Francis.

Boelen, P. A., & van den Bout, J. (2008). Complicated grief and uncomplicated grief are distinguishable constructs. *Psychiatry Research, 157*, 311–314.

Bolla-Wilson, K., & Bleecker, M. L. (1989). Absence of depression in elderly adults. *Journals of Gerontology, 44*, 53–55.

Boutin-Foster, C. (2008). An item-level analysis of the Center for Epidemiologic Studies Depression Scale (CES–D) by race and ethnicity in patients with coronary artery disease. *International Journal of Geriatric Psychiatry, 23*, 1034–1039.

Boyd, J. H., Weissman, M. M., Thompson, W. D., & Myers, J. K. (1982). Screening depression in a community sample: Understanding the discrepancies between depression symptoms and diagnostic scales. *Archives of General Psychiatry, 39*, 1195–2000.

Brodaty, H., Luscombe, G., Parker, G., Wilhelm, K., Hickie, I., Austin, M.-P., et al. (2001). Early and late onset depression in old age: Different aetiologies, same phenomenology. *Journal of Affective Disorders, 66*, 225–236.

Brown, P. J., Woods, C. M., & Storandt, M. (2007). Model stability of the 15-item Geriatric Depression Scale across cognitive impairment and severe depression. *Psychology and Aging, 22*, 372–379.

Bruce, M. L. (2002). Psychosocial risk factors for depressive disorders in late life. *Biological Psychiatry, 52*, 175–184.

Burke, W. J., Roccaforte, W. H., & Wengel, S. P. (1991). The short form of the Geriatric Depression Scale: A comparison with the 30-item form. *Journal of Geriatric Psychiatry and Neurology, 4*, 173–178.

Burke, W. J., Houston, M. J., Boust, S. J., & Roccaforte, W. H. (1989). Use of the Geriatric Depression Scale in dementia of the Alzheimer's type. *Journal of the American Geriatrics Society, 37*, 856–860.

Burke, W. J., Roccaforte, W. H., Wengel, S. P., Conley, D. M., & Potter, J. F. (1995). The reliability and validity of the Geriatric Depression Scale administered by telephone. *Journal of the American Geriatrics Society, 43*, 674–679.

Butters, M. A., Becker, J. T., Nebes, R. D., Zmuda, M. D., Mulsant, B. H., Pollock, B. G., et al. (2000). Changes in cognitive functioning following treatment of late-life depression. *American Journal of Psychiatry, 157*, 1949–1954.

Caine, E. D., Lyness, J. M., King, D. A., & Connors, L. (1994). Clinical and etiological heterogeneity of mood disorders in elderly patients. In L. S. Scneider, C. F. Reynolds, B. D. Lebowitz, & A. J. Friedhoff (Eds.),

Diagnosis and treatment of depression in late life: Results of the NIH Consensus Development Conference (pp. 21–53). Washington, D.C.: American Psychiatric Press.

Carr, D. (2003). A "good death" for whom? Quality of spouse's death and psychological distress among older widowed persons. *Journal of Health and Social Behavior, 44*, 215–232.

Carr, D. S. (2004). Black/white differences in psychological adjustment to spousal loss among older adults. *Research on Aging, 26*, 591–622.

Carr, D., & Utz, R. (2001). Late-life widowhood in the United States: New directions in research and theory. *Ageing International, 27*, 65–88.

Carr, D., House, J. S., Kessler, R. C., Nesse, R. M., Sonnega, J., & Wortman, C. (2000). Marital quality and psychological adjustment to widowhood among older adults: A longitudinal analysis. *Journal of Gerontology: Psychological Sciences and Social Sciences, 55*, S197–S207.

Centers for Disease Control and Prevention. (2004). *The State of Aging and Health in America*. Retrieved March 2, 2009. http://www.cdc.gov/aging/pdf/State_of_Aging_and_Health_in_America_2004.pdf

Charlton, R., Sheahan, K., Smith, G., & Campbell, I. (2001). Spousal bereavement—implications for health. *Family Practice, 18*, 614–618.

Chi, I., Yip, P. S., Chiu, H. F., Chou, K. L., Chan, K. S., Kwan, C. W., et al. (2005). Prevalence of depression and its correlates in Hong Kong's Chinese older adults. *American Journal of Geriatric Psychiatry, 13*, 409–416.

Chiu, H. C., Chen, C. M., Huang, C. J., & Mau, L. W. (2005). Depressive symptoms, chronic medical conditions and functional status: A comparison of urban and rural elders in Taiwan. *International Journal of Geriatric Psychiatry, 20*, 635–644.

Christakis, N. A., & Allison, P. D. (2006). Mortality after the hospitalization of a spouse. *New England Journal of Medicine, 354*, 719–730.

Christensen, H., Jorm, A. F., MacKinnon, A. J., Korten, A. E., Jacomb, P. A., Henderson, A. S., et al. (1999). Age differences in depression and anxiety symptoms: A structural equation modeling analysis of data from a general population sample. *Psychological Medicine, 29*, 325–339.

Cruz, M., Scott, J., Houck, P., Reynolds, C. F., Frank, E., & Shear, M. K. (2007). Clinical presentation and treatment outcome of African Americans with complicated grief. *Psychiatric Services, 58*, 700–702.

Cullen, B., O'Neill, B., Evans, J. J., Coen, R. F., & Lawlor, B. A. (2007). A review of screening tests for cognitive impairment. *Journal of Neurology and Neurosurgery, and Psychiatry, 78*, 790–799.

Cullum, C. M., Weiner, M. F., & Saine, K. C. (2009). *The Texas Functional Living Scale.* San Antonio, TX: Pearson NCS.

Cummings, J. L., & Victoroff, J. I. (1990). Noncognitive neuropsychiatric syndromes in Alzheimer's disease. *Cognitive and Behavioral Neurology, 3*, 140–158.

Cwikel, J., & Ritchie, K. (1988). The short GDS: Evaluation in a heterogeneous, multilingual population. *Clinical Gerontologist, 8*, 63–83.

Davies, K. N., Burn, W. K., McKenzie, F. R., Brothwell, J. A., & Wattis, J. P. (1993). Evaluation of the Hospital Anxiety and Depression Scale as a screening instrument in geriatric medical inpatients. *International Journal of Geriatric Psychiatry, 8*, 165–169.

Dillen, L., Fontaine, J. R., & Verhofstadt-Deneve, L. (2008). Are normal and complicated grief different constructs? A confirmatory factor analytic test. *Clinical Psychology and Psychotherapy, 15*, 386–395.

Drayer, R. A., Mulsant, B. H., Lenze, E. J., Rollman, B. L., Dew, M. A., Kelleher, K., et al. (2005). Somatic symptoms of depression in elderly patients with medical comorbidities. *International Journal of Geriatric Psychiatry, 20*, 973–982.

Eaton, W. W., Smith, C., Ybarra, M., Muntaner, C., & Tien, A. (2004). Center for Epidemiological Studies Depression Scale: Review and revision (CESD and CESD-R). In M. E. Maruish (Ed.), *The use of psychological testing for treatment planning and outcomes assessment—Third Edition: Volume 3: Instruments for adults* (pp. 363–377). Mahwah, NJ: Lawrence Erlbaum Associates.

Edelstein, B.A., & Koven. L.P. (in press). Older adult assessment issues and strategies. In V. Molinari (Ed.), *Competencies in gerontological psychology.* New York: Oxford University Press.

Edelstein, B. A., Martin, R. R., & Koven, L. P. (2003). Psychological assessment in geriatric settings. In J. R. Graham, & J. A. Naglieri (Eds.), *Handbook of Psychology: Volume 10: Assessment Psychology.* Hoboken, NJ: John Wiley & Sons, Inc.

Edelstein, B. A., Woodhead, E. L., Bower, E. H., & Lowery, A. J. (2006). Evaluating older adults. In M. Hersen (Ed.), *Clinician's handbook of adult behavioral assessment* (pp. 497–528). New York: Academic Press.

Edelstein, B. A., Heisel, M. J., McKee, D. R., Martin, R. P., Koven, L. P., Duberstein, P. R., et al. (in press). Development and psychometric evaluation of the Reasons for Living–Older Adults Scale: A suicide risk assessment inventory. *The Gerontologist*.

Edelstein, B. A., Woodhead, E. L., Segal, D. L., Heisel, M. J., Bower, E. H., Lowery, A. J., et al. (2008). Older adult psychological assessment: Current instrument status and related considerations. *Clinical Gerontologist*, *31*, 1–35.

Eid, M., & Diener, E. (2006). *Handbook of multimethod measurement in psychology*. Washington, DC: American Psychological Association.

Elderkin-Thompson, V., Mintz, J., Haroon, E., Lavretsky, H., & Kumar, A. (2007). Executive dysfunction and memory in older patients with major and minor depression. *Archives of Clinical Neuropsychology*, *22*, 261–270.

Ellis, G., & Langhorne, P. (2005). Comprehensive geriatric assessment for older hospital patients. *British Medical Bulletin*, *71*, 45–59.

Faschingbauer, T., Zisook, S., & DeVaul, R. (1987). The Texas revised inventory of grief. In S. Zisook (Ed.), *Biopsychosocial Aspects of Bereavement* (pp. 111–124). Washington, D.C: American Psychiatric Press, Inc.

Feher, E. P., Larrabee, G. J., & Crook, T. J. (1992). Factors attenuating the validity of the geriatric depression scale in a dementia population. *Journal of the American Geriatrics Society*, *40*, 906–909.

First, M. B., Spitzer, R. L., Gibbon, M., & Williams, J. B. W. (1997). *User's Guide for the Structured Clinical Interview for DSM-IV Axis I Disorders Clinician's Version (SCID–CV)*. Washington, D.C.: American Psychiatric Press Inc.

Fiske, A., & O'Riley. (2008). Depression in late life. In J. Hunsley, & E. J. Marsh (Eds.), *A Guide to Assessments that Work*. New York: Oxford University Press.

Fiske, A., Kasl-Godley, J. E., & Gatz, M. (1998). Mood disorders in late life. In B. Edelstein (Ed.), *Clinical geropsychology* (pp. 193–230). Oxford: Elsevier Science.

Folstein, M. F., Folstein, S. E., & McHugh, P. R. (1975). Mini-Mental State: A practical method for grading the cognitive state of patients for the clinician. *Journal of Psychiatric Research*, *12*, 189–198.

Fountoulakis, K. N., Iacovides, A., Grammaticos, P., St. Kaprinis, G., & Bech, P. (2004). Thyroid function in clinical subtypes of major depression: An exploratory study. *BMC Psychiatry*, *4*, 1–9.

Fry, P. S. (2001). The unique contribution of key existential factors to the prediction of psychological well-being of older adults following spousal loss. *The Gerontologist*, *41*, 69–81.

Futterman, A., Thompson, L., Gallagher-Thompson, D., & Ferris, R. (1997). Depression in later life: Epidemiology, assessment, etiology, and treatment. In E. E. Beckham, & W. R. Leber (Eds.), *Handbook of depression* (2nd ed.). (pp. 494–525) New York: Guildford.

Gallagher, D. (1986). The Beck Depression Inventory and older adults: Review of its development and utility. *Clinical Gerontologist*, *5*, 149–163.

Gallagher, D., Nies, G., & Thompson, L. W. (1982). Reliability of the Beck Depression Inventory with older adults. *Journal of Consulting and Clinical Psychology*, *50*, 152–153.

Gallagher, D. E., Breckenridge, J. N., Thompson, L. W., & Peterson, J. A. (1983). Effects of bereavement on indicators of mental health in elderly widows and widowers. *Journal of Gerontology*, *38*, 565–571.

Gallagher-Thomspon, D., Futterman, A., Farberow, N., Thompson, L. W., & Peterson, J. (1993). The impact of spousal bereavement on older widows and widowers. In M. S. Stroebe, W. Stroebe, & R. Hansson (Eds.), *Handbook of Bereavement: Theory, Research, and Intervention* (pp. 227–239). Cambridge, United Kingdom: Cambridge University Press.

Gallo, J. J., & Rabins, P. V. (1999). Depression without sadness: Alternative presentations of depression in late life. *American Family Physician*, *60*, 820–826.

Gallo, J. J., Anthony, J. C., & Muthen, B. O. (1994). Age differences in the symptoms of depression: A latent trait analysis. *Journal of Gerontology: Psychological Sciences*, *49*, P251–P264.

Gallo, J. J., Rabins, P. V., & Anthony, J. C. (1999). Sadness in older persons: 13-year follow-up of a community sample in Baltimore, Maryland. *Psychological Medicine*, *29*, 341–350.

Gallo, J. J., Rabins, P. V., Lyketsos, C. G., Tien, A. Y., & Anthony, J. C. (1997). Depression without sadness: Functional outcomes of nondysphoric depression in later life. *Journal of the American Geriatrics Society, 45*, 570–578.

Garcia, G. J. A., Landa, P. V., Trigueros, M. M. C., & Gaminde, I. I. (2005). Texas Revised Inventory of Grief: Adaptation to Spanish, reliability and validity. *Atencion Primaria, 35*, 353–358.

Gatz, M., & Hurwicz, M.-L. (1990). Are old people more depressed? Cross-sectional data on Center for Epidemiological Studies Depression Scale factors. *Psychology and Aging, 2*, 284–290.

Gilewski, M. J., Farberow, N. L., Gallagher, D. E., & Thompson, L. W. (1991). Interaction of depression and bereavement on mental health in the elderly. *Psychology and Aging, 6*, 67–75.

Gilley, D. W., Wilson, R. S., Fleischman, D. A., Harrison, D. W., Goetz, C. G., & Tanner, C. M. (1995). Impact of Alzheimer's-type dementia and information source on the assessment of depression. *Psychological Assessment, 7*, 42–48.

Giordano, M., Tirelli, P., Ciarambino, T., Gambardella, A., Ferrara, N., Signoriello, G., et al. (2007). Screening of depressive symptoms in young–old hemodialysis patients: Relationship between Beck Depression Inventory and 15-item Geriatric Depression Scale. *Nephron Clinical Practice, 106*, 187–192.

Goldberg, J. H., Breckenridge, J. N., & Sheikh, J. I. (2003). Age difference in symptoms of depression and anxiety: Examining behavioral medicine outpatients. *Journal of Behavioral Medicine, 26*, 119–132.

Gonzalez, H. M., Haan, M. N., & Hinton, L. (2001). Acculturation and the prevalence of depression in older Mexican Americans: Baseline results of the Sacramento Area Latino Study on Aging. *Journal of the American Geriatrics Society, 49*, 948–953.

Greer, M. (2004). Statistics show mental health services still needed for native populations. *Monitor on Psychology, 35*, 23.

Grimby, A. (1993). Bereavement among elderly people: Grief reactions, post-bereavement hallucinations, and quality of life. *Acta Psychiatrica Scandinavica, 87*, 72–80.

Hajjar, E. R., Cafiero, A. C., & Hanlon, J. T. (2007). Polypharmacy in elderly patients. *American Journal of Pharmacotherapy, 5*, 345–351.

Hamilton, M. (1960). A rating scale for depression. *Journal of Neurology, Neurosurgery, and Psychiatry, 23*, 56–62.

Hamilton, M. (1967). Development of a rating scale for primary depressive illness. *British Journal of Social and Clinical Psychology, 6*, 278–296.

Hammond, M. F. (1998). Rating depression severity in the elderly physically ill patient: Reliability and factor structure of the Hamilton and the Montgomery-Asberg Depression Rating Scales. *International Journal of Geriatric Psychiatry, 13*, 257–261.

Hansson, R. O., Carpenter, B. N., & Fairchild, S. K. (1993). Measurement issues in bereavement. In M. S. Stroebe, W. Stroebe, & R. Hansson (Eds.), *Handbook of Bereavement: Theory, Research, and Intervention* (pp. 62–74). Cambridge, United Kingdom: Cambridge University Press.

Haringsma, R., Engels, G. I., Beekman, A. T. F., & Spinhoven, P. (2004). The criterion validity of the Center for Epidemiological Studies–Depression Scale (CES–D) in a sample of self-referred elders with depressive symptomatology. *International Journal of Geriatric Psychiatry, 19*, 558–563.

Harper, R. G., Kotik-Harper, D., & Kirby, H. (1990). Psychometric assessment of depression in an elderly general medical population over- or underassessment? *The Journal of Nervous and Mental Disease, 178*, 113–111.

Haworth, J. E., Moniz-Cook, E., Clark, A. L., Wang, M., & Cleland, J. G. F. (2007). An evaluation of two self-report screening measures for mood in an out-patient chronic heart failure population. *International Journal of Geriatric Psychiatry, 22*, 1147–1153.

Haynes, S. N., & O'Brien, W. H. (2000). *Principles and practice of behavioral assessment*. New York: Plenum/Kluwer.

He, W., Sengupta, M., Velkoff, V. A., & DeBarros, K. A. (2005). U.S. Census Bureau. *Current Population Reports, P23–209, 65+ in the United States: 2005*. Washington, DC.

Healey, A. K., Kneebone, I. I., Carroll, M., & Anderson, S. J. (2008). A preliminary investigation of the reliability and validity of the Brief Assessment Schedule Cards and the Beck Depression Inventory–Fast Screen to screen for depression in older stoke survivors. *International Journal of Geriatric Psychiatry, 23*, 531–536.

Heisel, M. J., & Flett, G. L. (2006). The development and initial validation of the Geriatric Suicide Ideation Scale. *The American Journal of Geriatric Psychiatry*, *14*, 742–751.

Hertzog, C., Van Alstine, J., Usala, P. D., Hultsch, D. F., & Dixon, R. (1990). Measurement properties of the Center for Epidemiological Studies–Depression Scale (CES–D) in older populations. *Psychological Assessment: A Journal of Consulting and Clinical Psychology*, *2*, 64–72.

Himmelfarb, S., & Murrell, S. A. (1983). Reliability and validity of five mental health scales in older persons. *Journal of Gerontology*, *3*, 333–339.

Holmes, T. H., & Rahe, R. H. (1967). The social readjustment rating scale. *Journal of Psychosomatic Research*, *11*, 213–218.

Horowitz, M. J., Siegel, B., Holen, A., Bonanno, G. A., Milbrath, C., & Stinson, C. H. (2003). Diagnostic criteria for complicated grief disorder. *Focus*, *1*, 290–298.

Hybels., C. F., Blazer, D. G., & Pieper, C. F. (2001). Toward a threshold for subthreshold depression: An analysis of correlates of depression by severity of symptoms using data from an elderly community sample. *The Gerontologist*, *41*, 357–365.

Hyer, L., & Blount, J. (1984). Concurrent and discriminant validation of the Geriatric Depression Scale with older psychiatric inpatients. *Psychological Reports*, *54*, 611–616.

Irish, D. P., Lundquist, K. F., & Nelsen, V. J. (1993). *Ethnic variations in dying, death, and grief: Diversity in universality.* Philadelphia, PA: Taylor and Francis.

Jacobs, S., Mazure, C., & Prigerson, H. (2000). Diagnostic criteria for traumatic grief. *Death Studies*, *24*, 185–199.

Jamison, C., & Scogin, F. (1992). Development of an interview-based geriatric depression rating scale. *International Journal of Aging and Human Development*, *35*, 193–204.

Jefferson, A. L., Powers, D. V., & Pope, M. (2001). Beck Depression Inventory–II (BDI–II) and the Geriatric Depression Scale (GDS) in older women. *Clinical Gerontologist*, *22*, 3–12.

Jeste, D. V., Blazer, D. G., & First, M. (2005). Aging-related diagnostic variations: Need for diagnostic criteria appropriate for elderly psychiatric patients. *Biological Psychiatry*, *58*, 265–271.

Judd, L. L., Schettler, P. J., & Akiskal, H. S. (2002). The prevalence, clinical relevance, and public health significance of substhreshold depressions. *Psychiatric Clinics of North America*, *25*, 685–698.

Kaszniak, A. W., & Christensen, G. D. (1994). Differential diagnosis of dementia and depression. In M. Storandt, & G. R. VandenBos (Eds.), *Neuropsychological assessment of dementia and depression in older adults: A clinician's guide* (pp. 81–118). Washington, DC: American Psychological Association.

Katz, I. A., & Parmelee, P. (1997). Assessment of depression in patients with dementia. In J. A. Teresi, M. P. Lawton, D. Holmes, & M. Ory (Eds.), *Measurement in elderly chronic care populations* (pp. 90–103). New York: Springer.

Katz, S., Downs, T. D., Cash, H. R., & Grotz, R. C. (1970). Progress in development of the index of ADL. *The Gerontologist*, *10*, 20–30.

Kendall, P. C., Hollon, S. D., Beck, A. T., Hammen, C. L., & Ingram, R. E. (1987). Issues and recommendations regarding use of the Beck Depression Inventory. *Cognitive Therapy and Research*, *11*, 289–299.

Kenn, C., Wood, H., Kucyj, M., Wattis, J., & Cunane, J. (1987). Validation of the Hospital Anxiety and Depression Scale (HADS) in an elderly psychiatric population. *International Journal of Geriatric Psychiatry*, *2*, 189–193.

Kieffer, K. M., & Reese, R. J. (2002). A reliability generalization study of the Geriatric Depression Scale. *Educational and Psychological Measurement*, *62*, 969–994.

Kim, Y., Pilkonis, P. A., Frank, E., Thase, M. E., & Reynolds, C. F. (2002). Differential functioning of the Beck Depression Inventory in late-life patients: Use of item response theory. *Psychology and Aging*, *17*, 379–391.

Kirmayer, L. J. (2001). Cultural variations in the clinical presentation of depression and anxiety: Implications for diagnosis and treatment. *Journal of Clinical Psychiatry*, *62*(Suppl. 13), 22–28.

Kitchell, M. A., Barnes, R. F., Veith, R. C., Okimoto, J. T., & Raskind, M. A. (1982). Screening for depression in hospitalized geriatric medical patients. *Journal of the American Geriatrics Society*, *30*, 174–177.

Kivela, S., & Pahkala, K. (1986). Sex and age differences of factor pattern and reliability of the Zung Self-Rating Depression Scale in a Finnish elderly population. *Psychological Reports*, *59*, 587–597.

Koenig, H. G., Meador, K. G., Cohen, H. J., & Blazer, D. G. (1988). Depression in elderly hospitalized patients with medical illness. *Archives of Internal Medicine*, *148*, 1929–1936.

Kogan, J. N., & Edelstein, B. A. (2004). Modification and psychometric examination of a self-report measure of fear in older adults. *Journal of Anxiety Disorders*, *18*, 397–409.

Kohout, F. J., Berkman, L. F., Evans, D. A., & Cornoni-Huntley, J. (1993). Two shorter forms of the CES–D Depression Symptoms Index. *Journal of Aging and Health*, *5*, 179–193.

Korner, A., Lauritzen, L., Abelskov, K., Gulmann, N., Brodersen, A. M., Wedervang-Jensen, T., et al. (2006). The Geriatric Depression Scale and the Cornell Scale for Depression in Dementia. A validity study. *Nordic Journal of Psychiatry*, *60*, 360–364.

Kowalski, S. D., & Bondmass, M. D. (2008). Physiological and psychological symptoms of grief in widows. *Research in Nursing & Health*, *31*, 23–30.

Krause, N., & Liang, J. (1992). Cross-cultural variations in depressive symptoms in later life. *International Psychogeriatrics*, *4*, 185–202.

Krause, N., Liang, J., & Yatomi, N. (1989). Satisfaction with social support and depressive symptoms: A panel analysis. *Psychology and Aging*, *4*, 88–97.

Kuo, B. C., Chong, V., & Joseph, J. (2008). Depression and its psychosocial correlates among older Asian immigrants in North America. *Journal of Aging and Health*, *20*, 615–652.

Larrabee, G. J., & Crook, T. H. (1989). Dimensions of everyday memory in age-associated memory impairment. *Psychological Assessment: A Journal of Consulting and Clinical Psychology*, *1*, 92–97.

Latham, A. E., & Prigerson, H. G. (2004). Suicidality and bereavement; Complicated grief as a psychiatric disorder presenting greatest risk for suicidality. *Suicide and Life-Threatening Behavior*, *34*, 350–362.

Lavretsky, H., Kurbanyan, K., & Kumar, A. (2004). The significance of subsyndromal depression in geriatrics. *Current Psychiatry Reports*, *6*, 25–31.

Leentjens, A. F. G., Verhey, F. R. J., Lousberg, R., Spitsbergen, H., & Wilmink, F. W. (2000). The validity of the Hamilton and Montgomery-Asberg Depression Rating Scales as screening and diagnostic tools in Parkinson's disease. *International Journal of Geriatric Psychiatry*, *15*, 644–649.

Lesher, E. L. (1986). Validation of the Geriatric Depression Scale among nursing home residents. *Clinical Gerontologist*, *4*, 21–28.

Lesher, E. L., & Berryhill, J. S. (1994). Validation of the Geriatric Depression Scale-Short Form among inpatients. *Journal of Clinical Psychology*, *50*, 256–260.

Lev, E., Munro, B. H., & McCorkle, R. (1993). A shortened version of an instrument measuring bereavement. *International Journal of Nursing Studies*, *30*, 213–226.

Lewinsohn, P. M., Seeley, J. R., Roberts, R. E., & Allen, N. B. (1997). Center for Epidemiologic Studies Depression Scale (CES–D) as a screening instrument for depression among community-residing older adults. *Psychology and Aging*, *12*, 277–287.

Lichtenberg, P. A., Steiner, D. A., Marcopulos, B. A., & Tabscott, J. A. (1992). Comparison of the Hamilton Depression Rating Scale and the Geriatric Depression Scale: Detection of depression in dementia patients. *Psychological Reports*, *70*, 515–521.

Loeb., P. A. (1996). *The Independent Living Scales*. San Antonio, TX: Psychological Corporation.

Logsdon, G. R., & Teri, L. (1995). Depression in Alzheimer's disease patients: Caregivers as surrogate reporters. *Journal of the American Geriatrics Society*, *43*, 150–155.

Low, G. D., & Hubley, A. M. (2007). Screening for depression after cardiac events using the Beck Depression Inventory–II and the Geriatric Depression Scale. *Social Indicators Research*, *82*, 527–543.

Lund, D. A. (1998). Bereavement. In B. Edelstein (Ed.), *Clinical Geropsychology* (pp. 95–112). Oxford: Elsevier Science.

Lund, D. A., Caserta, M. S., & Dimond, M. F. (1986). Gender differences through two years of bereavement among the elderly. *The Gerontologist*, *26*, 314–320.

Lund, D. A., Utz, R., Caserta, M. S., & de Vries, B. (2008). Humor, laughter, and happiness in the daily lives of recently bereaved spouses. *Omega: Journal of Death and Dying*, *58*, 87–105.

Lyness, J. M., King, D. A., Cox, C., Yoediono, Z., & Caine, E. D. (1999). The importance of subsyndromal depression in older primary care patients: Prevalence and associated functional disability. *Journal of the American Geriatrics Society*, *47*, 647–652.

Lyness, J. M., Caine, E. D., King, D. A., Conwell, Y., Duberstein, P. R., & Cox, C. (2002). Depressive disorders and symptoms in older primary care patients: one-year outcomes. *American Journal of Geriatric Psychiatry, 10*, 275–282.

McGarvey, B., Gallagher, D., Thompson, L., & Zelinski, E. (1982). Reliablity and factor structure of the Zung Self-Rating Depression Scale in three age groups. *Essence, 5*, 141–151.

McLean, A. J., & Le Couteur, D. G. (2004). Aging biology and geriatric clinical pharmacology. *Pharmacological Reviews, 56*, 163–184.

Mahurin, K. A., & Gatz, M. (1983). *Depression, health, and somatic complaints in older adults*. Paper presented at the 91st annual convention of the American Psychological Association (August), Anaheim, CA.

Mangoni, A. A., & Jackson, S. H. D. (2004). Age-related changes in pharmacokinetics and pharmacodynamics: Basic principles and practical applications. *British Journal of Clinical Pharmacology, 57*, 6–14.

Mayer, L. S., Bay, R. C., Politis, A., Steinberg, M., Steele, C., Baker, A. S., et al. (2006). Comparison of three rating scales as outcome measures for treatment trials of depression in Alzheimer disease: Findings from DIADS. *International Journal of Geriatric Psychiatry, 21*, 930–936.

Mischel, W. (1968). *Personality and assessment.* New York: Wiley.

Mondolo, F. Jahanshahi, M., Grana, A., Biasutti, E., Cacciatori, E., & Di Benedetto, P. (2006). The validity of the hospital anxiety and depression scale in Parkinson's disease. *Behavioral Neurology, 17*, 109–115.

Mui, A. C., & Kang, S.-Y. (2006). Acculturation stress and depression among Asian immigrant elders. *Social Work, 51*, 243–255.

Mui, A. C., Burnette, D., & Chen, L. M. (2002). Cross-cultural assessment of geriatric depression: A review of the CES–D and the GDS. *Journal of Mental Health and Aging, 7*, 137–164.

Musetti, L., Perugi, G., Soriani, A., Rossi, V. M., Cassano, G. B., & Akiskal, H. S. (1989). Depression before and after age 65. A reexamination. *British Journal of Psychiatry, 155*, 330–336.

Myers, H. F., Lesser, I., Rodriquez, N., Mira, C. B., Hwan, W.-C., Camp, C., et al. (2002). Ethnic differences in clinical presentation of depression in adult women. *Cultural Diversity and Ethnic Minority Psychology, 8*, 138–156.

Myers, J. K., & Weissman, M. M. (1980). Use of a self-report symptom scale to detect depression in a community sample. *American Journal of Psychiatry, 137*, 1081–1084.

Nasreddine, Z. S., Phillips, N. A., Bédirian, V., Charbonneau, S., Whitehead, V., Collin, I., et al. (2005). The Montreal Cognitive Assessment, MoCA: A brief screening tool for mild cognitive impairment. *Journal of the American Geriatrics Society, 53*, 695–699.

Newmann, J. P., Engel, R. J., & Jensen, J. E. (1991). Age differences in depressive symptom experiences. *Journal of Gerontology, 46*, 224–235.

Nguyen, H. T., & Zonderman, A. B. (2006). Relationship between age and aspects of depression: Consistency and reliability across two longitudinal studies. *Psychology and Aging, 21*, 119–126.

Niti, M., Ng, T.-P., Kua, E. H., Ho, R. C. M., & Tan, C. H. (2007). Depression and chronic medical illnesses in Asian older adults: The role of subjective health and functional status. *International Journal of Geriatric Psychiatry, 22*, 1087–1094.

Norris, F. H., & Murrell, S. A. (1990). Social support, life events, and stress as modifiers of adjustment to bereavement by older adults. *Psychology and Aging, 5*, 429–436.

Norris, J. T., Gallagher, D., Wilson, A., & Winograd, C. H. (1987). Assessment of depression in geriatric medical outpatients: The validity of two screening measures. *Journal of the American Geriatrics Society, 35*, 989–995.

Norris, M. P., Snow-Turek, A. L., & Blankenship, L. (1995). Somatic depressive symptoms in the elderly: Contribution or confound? *Journal of Clinical Geropsychology, 1*, 5–17.

Norris, M. P., Arnau, R. C., Bramson, R., & Meagher, M. W. (2004). The efficacy of somatic symptoms in assessing depression in older primary care patients. *Clinical Gerontologist, 27*, 43–57.

Northrop, L. M., & Edelstein, B. A. (1998). An assertive-behavior competence inventory for older adults. *Journal of Clinical Geropsychology, 4*, 315–332.

Okimoto, J. T., Barnes, R. F., Veith, R. C., Raskind, M. A., Inui, T. S., & Carter, W. B. (1982). Screening for depression in geriatric medical patients. *American Journal of Psychiatry, 139*, 799–802.

Olden, M., Rosenfeld, B., Pessin, H., & Breitbart, W. (2009). Measuring depression at the end of life: Is the Hamilton Depression Rating Scale a valid instrument? *Assessment*, *16*, 43–54.

Olin, J. T., Katz, I. R., Meyers, B. S., Schneider, L. S., & Lebowitz, B. D. (2002). Provisional diagnostic criteria for Depression of Alzheimer Disease: Rationale and background. *American Journal of Geriatric Psychiatry*, *10*, 129–141.

Olin, J. T., Schneider, L. S., Eaton, E. M., Zemansky, M. F., & Pollock, V. E. (1992). The Geriatric Depression Scale and the Beck Depression Inventory as screeining instruments in an older adult outpatient population. *Psychological Assessment*, *4*, 190–192.

Omnibus Budget Reconciliation Act of 1987, Public Law No. 100–203, Subtitle C: Nursing Home Reform.

O'Rourke, N. (2005). Factor structure of the Center for Epidemiologic Studies–Depression Scale (CES–D) among older men and women who provide care to persons with dementia. *International Journal of Testing*, *5* (3), 265–277.

Ott, B. R., & Fogel, B. S. (1992). Measurement of depression in dementia: Self vs. clinician rating. *International Journal of Geriatric Psychiatry*, *7*, 899–904.

Ott, C. H. (2003). The impact of complicated grief on mental and physical health at various points in the bereavement process. *Death Studies*, *27*, 249–272.

Ott, C. H., Lueger, R. J., Kelber, S. T., & Prigerson, H. G. (2007). Spousal bereavement in older adults: Common, resilient, and chronic grief with defining characteristics. *The Journal of Nervous and Mental Disease*, *195*, 332–341.

Pachana, N., Gallagher-Thompson, D., & Thompson, L. W. (1994). Assessment of depression. In M. P. Lawton, & J. A. Teresi (Eds.), *Annual review of gerontology and geriatrics: Focus on assessment techniques* (pp. 234–256). New York: Springer.

Pachana, N. A., Byrne, G. J., Siddle, H., Koloski, N., Harley, E., & Arnold, E. (2007). Development and validation of the Geriatric Anxiety Inventory. *International Psychogeriatrics*, *19*, 103–114.

Pagel, M. D., Erdly, W. W., & Becker, J. (1987). Social networks: We get by with (and in spite of) a little help from our friends. *Journal of Personality and Social Psychology*, *53*, 793–804.

Parker, G., Cheah, Y.-C., & Roy, K. (2001). Do the Chinese somatize depression? A cross-cultural study. *Social Psychiatry and Psychiatric Epidemiology*, *36*, 287–293.

Parmalee, P., Katz, I., & Lawton, M. (1989). Depression among institutionalized aged: Assessment and prevalence estimation. *Journal of Gerontology: Medical Science*, *44*, M22–M29.

Pasternak, R. E., Reynolds, C. F., Schlernitzauer, M., Hoch, C. C., Buysse, D. J., Houck, P. R., et al. (1991). Acute open-trial nortriptyline therapy of bereavement-related depression in late life. *Journal of Clinical Psychiatry*, *52*, 307–310.

Patten, S. B., & Love, E. J. (1994). Drug-induced depression. Incidence, avoidance, and management. *Drug Safety*, *10*, 203–219.

Paulhan, I., & Bourgeois, M. (1995). The TRIG (Texas Revised Inventory of Grief): French translation and validation. *Encephale*, *21*, 257–262.

Penninx, B. W., Leveille, S., Ferrucci, L., Van Eijk, J. Th. M., & Guralnik, J. M. (1999). Exploring the effect of depression on physical disability: Longitudinal evidence from the Established Populations for Epidemiologic Studies of the Elderly. *American Journal of Public Health*, *89*, 1346–1352.

Piper, W. E., Ogrodniczuk, J. S., Azim, H. F., & Weideman, R. (2001). Prevalence of loss and complicated grief among psychiatric outpatients. *Psychiatric Services*, *52*, 1069–1074.

Prigerson, H. G., & Jacobs, S. C. (2001). Caring for bereaved patients: "All the doctors just suddenly go." *Journal of the American Medical Association*, *286*, 1369–1376.

Prigerson, H. G., Frank, E., Kasl, S. V., Reynolds, C. F., Anderson, B., Zubenko, G. S., et al. (1995a). Complicated grief and bereavement-related depression as distinct disorders: Preliminary empirical validation in elderly bereaved spouses. *American Journal of Psychiatry*, *152*, 22–30.

Prigerson, H. G., Maciejewski, P. K., Reynolds, C. F., Bierhals, A. J., Newsom, J. T., Fasiczka, A., et al. (1995b). The inventory of complicated grief: A scale to measure maladaptive symptoms of loss. *Psychiatry Research*, *59*, 65–79.

Prigerson, H. G., Bierhals, A. J., Kasl, S. V., Reynolds, C. F., Shear, M. K., Day, N., et al. (1997). Traumatic grief as a risk factor for mental and physical morbidity. *American Journal of Psychiatry*, *154*, 616–623.

Prigerson, H. G., Bierhals, A. J., Kasl, S. V., Reynolds, C. F., Shear, M. K., Newsom, J. T., et al. (1996). Complicated grief as a disorder distinct from bereavement-related depression and anxiety: A replication study. *American Journal of Psychiatry, 153*, 1484–1486.

Prigerson, H. G., Shear, M. K., Jacobs, S. C., Reynolds, C. F., Maciejewski, P. K., Davidson, J. R., et al. (1999). Consensus criteria for traumatic grief. A preliminary empirical test. *The British Journal of Psychiatry, 174*, 67–73.

Radloff, L. S. (1977). The CES–D Scale: A self-report depression scale for research in the general population. *Applied Psychological Measurement, 1*, 385–401.

Radloff, L. S., & Teri, L. (1986). Use of the Center for Epidemiologic Studies–Depression Scale with older adults. *Clinical Gerontologist, 5*, 119–136.

Rapaport, M. H., Judd, L. L., Schettler, P. J., Yonkers, K. A., Thase, M. E., Kupfer, D. J., et al. (2002). A descriptive analysis of minor depression. *American Journal of Psychiatry, 159*, 637–643.

Rapp, S. R., Smith, S. S., & Britt, M. (1990). Identifying comorbid depression in elderly medical patients: Use of the extracted Hamilton Depression Rating Scale. *Psychological Assessment: A Journal of Consulting and Clinical Psychology, 2*, 243–247.

Rapp, S. R., Parisi, S. A., Walsh, D. A., & Wallace, C. E. (1988). Detecting depression in elderly medical inpatients. *Journal of Consulting and Clinical Psychology, 56*, 509–513.

Ravindran, A. V., Welburn, K., & Copeland, J. R. M. (1994). Semi-structured depression scale sensitive to change with treatment for use in the elderly. *British Journal of Psychiatry, 164*, 522–527.

Reite, M., Buysse, D., Reynolds, C., & Mendelson, W. (1995). The use of polysomnography in the evaluation of insomnia. *Sleep, 18*, 58–70.

Reynolds, C. F., Miller, M. D., Pasternak, R. E., Frank, E., Perel, J. M., Cornes, C., et al. (1999). Treatment of bereavement-related major depressive episodes in later life: A controlled study of acute and continuation treatment with nortriptyline and interpersonal psychotherapy. *American Journal of Psychiatry, 156*, 202–208.

Roberts, R. W., & Vernon, S. W. (1983). The Center for Epidemiologic Studies Depression Scale: Its use in a common sample. *American Journal of Psychiatry, 140*, 41–46.

Rodin, G., Craven, J., & Littlefield, C. (1991). *Depression in the Medically Ill: An Integrated Approach.* New York: Brunner/Mazel.

Rook, K. S. (1994). Assessing the health-related dimensions of older adults' social relationships. In M. P. Lawton, & J. A. Teresi (Eds.), *Annual review of gerontology and geriatrics: Focus on assessment techniques, Vol. 14* (pp. 142–181). New York: Springer.

Rubenstein, L. Z. (1995). An overview of comprehensive geriatric assessment: Rationale, history, program models, basic components. In L. Z. Rubenstein, D. Wieland, & R. Bernabei (Eds.), *Geriatric assessment technology: The state of the art* (pp. 11–26). Milan, Italy: Kurtis.

Rubenstein, L. Z., Schairer, C., Wieland, G. D., & Kane, R. (1984). Systematic biases in functional status assessment of elderly adults: Effects of different data sources. *Journal of Gerontology, 39*, 686–691.

Rush, A. J., Trivedi, M. H., Ibrahim., H. M., Carmody, T. J., Arnow, B., Klein, D. N., et al. (2003). The 16-item Quick Inventory of Depressive Symptomatology (QIDS), Clinician Rating (QIDS–C), and Self-report (QIDS–SR): A psychometric evaluation in patients with chronic major depression. *Biological Psychiatry, 54*, 573–583.

Sager, M. A., Dunham, N. C., Schwantes, A., Mecum, L., Halverson, K., & Harlowe, D. (1992). Measurement of activities of daily living in hospitalized elderly: A comparison of self-report and performance-based methods. *Journal of the American Geriatrics Society, 40*, 457–462.

Sanders, C. M., Mauger, P. A., & Strong, P. N. (1985). *A manual for the Grief Experience Inventory.* Palo Alto, CA: Consulting Psychologists Press.

Schein, R. L., & Koenig, H. G. (1997). The Center for Epidemiological Studies–Depression (CES–D) Scale: Assessment of depression in the medically ill elderly. *International Journal of Geriatric Psychiatry, 12*, 436–446.

Scheinthal, S. M., Steer, R. A., Giffen, L., & Beck, A. T. (2001). Evaluating geriatric medical outpatients with the Beck Depression Inventory–Fast Screen for Medical Patients. *Aging and Mental Health, 5*, 143–148.

Schulberg, H. C., Mulsant, B., Schulz, R., Rollman, B. L., Houck, P. R., & Reynolds, C. F. (1998). Characteristics and course of major depression in older primary care patients. *International Journal of Psychiatry in Medicine*, *28*, 421–436.

Schwarz, N. (1999). Self-reports: How the questions shape the answers. *American Psychologist*, *54*, 93–105.

Schwarz, N. (2003). Self-reports in consumer research: The challenge of comparing cohorts and cultures. *Journal of Consumer Research*, *29*, 588–594.

Scogin, F. R. (1994). Assessment of depression in older adults: A guide for practitioners. In M. Storandt, & G. R. VandenBos (Eds.), *Neuropsychological assessment of dementia and depression in older adults: A clinician's guide* (pp. 61–80). Washington, DC: American Psychological Association.

Scogin, F., Beutler, L., Corbishley, A., & Hamblin, D. (1988). Reliability and validity of the short-form Beck Depression Inventory with older adults. *Journal of Clinical Psychology*, *44*, 853–857.

Segal, D. L., Coolidge, F. L., Cahill, B. S., & O'Riley, A. A. (2008). Psychometric properties of the Beck Depression Inventory–II (BDI–II) among community-dwelling older adults. *Behavior Modification*, *32*, 3–20.

Segal, D. L., Kabacoff, R. I., Hersen, M., VanHasslet, V. B., & Ryan, C. F. (1995). Update on the reliability of diagnosis in older psychiatric outpatients using the Structured Clinical Interview for DSM-III-R. *Journal of Clinical Geropsychology*, *1*, 313–321.

Senior, A. C., Kunik, M. E., Rhoades, H. M., Novy, D. M., Wilson, N. L., & Stanley, M. A. (2007). Utility of telephone assessments in an older adult population. *Psychology and Aging*, *22*, 392–397.

Shear, K., & Shair, H. (2005). Attachment, loss, and complicated grief. *Developmental Psychobiology*, *47*, 253–267.

Shear, K., Frank, E., Houck, P. R., & Reynolds, C. F. (2005). Treatment of complicated grief: A randomized controlled trial. *Journal of the American Medical Association*, *293*, 2601–2608.

Shuchter, S. R., & Zisook, S. (1993). The course of normal grief. In M. S. Stroebe, W. Stroebe, & R. Hansson (Eds.), *Handbook of Bereavement* (pp. 23–43). Cambridge, United Kingdom: Cambridge University Press.

Shue, V., Beck, C., & Lawton, M. (1997). Measuring affect in frail and cognitively impaired elderly. In J. Teresi, M. P. Lawton, D. Holmes, & M. Ory (Eds.), *Measurement in elderly chronic care populations* (pp. 104–116). New York: Springer.

Smalbrugge, M., Jongenelis, L., Pot, A. M., Beekman, A. T. F., & Eefsting, J. A. (2008). Screening for depression and assessing change in severity of depression. Is the Geriatric Depression Scale (30-, 15- and 8-item versions) useful for both purposes in nursing home patients? *Aging and Mental Health*, *12*, 244–248.

Snyder, A. G., Stanley, M. A., Novy, D. M., Averill, P. M., & Beck, J. G. (2000). Measures of depression in older adults with generalized anxiety disorder: A psychometric evaluation. *Depression and Anxiety*, *11*, 114–120.

Spirrison, C. L., & Pierce, P. S. (1992). Psychometric characteristics of the Adult Functional Adaptive Behavior Scale (AFABS). *The Gerontologist*, *32*, 234–239.

Steffens, D. C., Fisher, G. G., Langa, K. M., Potter, G. G., & Plassman, B. L. (2009). Prevalence of depression among older Americans: The Aging, Demographics, and Memory Study. *International Psychogeriatrics*. On Line. June 12, 2009.

Stiles, P. G., & McGarrahan, J. F. (1998). The Geriatric Depression Scale: A comprehensive review. *Journal of Clinical Geropsychology*, *4*, 89–110.

Stone, A. A. (1995). Measurement of affective response. In S. Cohen, R. C. Kessler, & G. L. Underwood (Eds.), *Measuring stress: A guide for health and social scientists* (pp. 148–171). New York: John Wiley & Sons.

Storandt, M., & VandenBos, G. (1994). *Neuropsychological Assessment of Dementia and Depression in Older Adults: A Clinician's Guide*. Washington, D.C.: American Psychological Association.

Sue, D. W., & Sue, D. (2007). *Counseling the culturally diverse: Theory and practice*. New York: Wiley.

Sunderland, T., Alterman, I. S., Yount, D., Hill, J. L., Tariot, P. N., Newhouse, P. A., et al. (1988). A new scale for the assessment of depressed mood in demented patients. *American Journal of Psychiatry*, *145*, 955–959.

Szanto, K., Gildengers, A., Mulsant, B. H., Brown, G., Alexopoulos, G. S., & Reynolds, C. F. (2002). Identification of suicidal ideation and prevention of suicidal behavior in the elderly. *Drugs & Aging*, *19*, 11–24.

Tariq, S. H., Tumosa, N., Chibnall, J. T., Perry, M. H., & Morley, J. E. (2006). Comparison of the Saint Louis University Mental Status Examination and the Mini-Mental State Examination for detecting dementia and mild neurocognitive disorder—A pilot study. *American Journal of Geriatric Psychiatry*, *14*, 900–910.

Teresi, J., Abrams, R., Holmes, D., Ramirez, M., & Eimicke, J. (2001). Prevalence of depression and depression recognition in nursing homes. *Social Psychiatry and Psychiatric Epidemiology*, *36*, 613–620.

Thompson, L. W., Gallagher-Thompson, D., Futterman, A., Gilewski, M. J., & Peterson, J. (1991). The effects of late-life spousal bereavement over a 30-month interval. *Psychology and Aging*, *6*, 434–441.

Thuen, F., Reime, M. H., & Skrautvoll, K. (1997). The effect of widowhood on psychological wellbeing and social support in the oldest groups of the elderly. *Journal of Mental Health*, *6*, 265–274.

Tomita, T., & Kitamura, T. (2002). Clinical and research measures of grief: A reconsideration. *Comprehensive Psychiatry*, *43*, 95–102.

U.S. Census Bureau. (2006). *American Community Sample*. Retrieved 7/1/09 from. http://www.census.gov/population/www/socdemo/hispanic/files/Internet_Hispanic_in_US_2006.pdf

U.S. Census Bureau. (2008a). *An older more diverse nation by midcentury*. Retrieved 7/1/09 from. http://www.census.gov/Press-Release/www/releases/archives/population/012496.html

U.S. Census Bureau. (2008b). *Marital Status of the population 55 years and over by sex and age*. Available online at <http://www.census.gov/population/socdemo/age/2008_older_table10.xls>

van Manen, J. G., Bindels, P. J. E., Dekker, F. W., Jzermans, C. J. I., van der Zee, J. S., & Schadé, E. (2002). Risk of depression in patients with chronic obstructive pulmonary disease and its determinants. *Thorax*, *57*, 412–416.

Wagle, A. C., Ho, L. W., Wagle, S. A., & Berrios, G. E. (2000). Psychometric behaviour of BDI in Alzheimer's disease patients with depression. *International Journal of Geriatric Psychiatry*, *15*, 63–69.

Wallace, J., & Pfohl, B. (1995). Age-related differences in the symptomatic expression of major depression. *Journal of Nervous and Mental Disease*, *183*, 99–102.

Watson, L. C., Lewis, C. L., Kistler, C. E., Amick, H. R., & Boustani, M. (2004). Can we trust depression screening instruments in healthy "old-old" adults? *International Journal of Geriatric Psychiatry*, *19*, 278–285.

Williams, C. D., Taylor, T. R., Makambi, K., Harrell, J., Palmer, J. R., Rosenberg, L., et al. (2007). CES–D four-factor structure is confirmed, but not invariant, in a large cohort of African American women. *Psychiatry Research*, *150*, 173–180.

Williams, J. B. (1988). A structured interview guide for the Hamilton Depression Rating Scale. *Archives of General Psychiatry*, *45*, 742–747.

Williams, J. B. W., Kobak, K. A., Bech, P., Engelhardt, N., Evans, K., Lipsitz, J., et al. (2008). The GRID–HAMD: Standardization of the Hamilton Depression Rating Scale. *International Clinical Psychopharmacology*, *23*, 120–129.

Wilson, S. (2007). The validation of the Texas Revised Inventory of Grief on an older Latino sample. *Journal of Social Work in End-of-Life and Palliative Care*, *2*, 33–60.

Wisocki, P. A., & Skowron, J. (2000). The effects of gender and culture on adjustment to widowhood. In R. M. Eisler, & M. Hersen (Eds.), *Handbook of Gender, Culture, and Health* (pp. 417–436). Mahwah, NJ: Erlbaum Associates.

Wisocki, P. A., Handen, B., & Morse, C. K. (1986). The Worry Scale as a measure of anxiety among homebound and community active elderly. *The Behavior Therapist*, *5*, 91–95.

Wong, G., & Baden, A. L. (2001). Multiculturally Sensitive Assessment with Older Adults: Recommendations and Areas for Additional Study. In L. A. Suzuki, P. G. Ponterotto, & J. Meller (Eds.), *Handbook of Multicultural Assessment: Clinical, Psychological, and Educational Applications* (2nd Ed.). (pp. 497–522) San Francisco, CA: Jossey-Bass Publishers.

Woodford, H. J., & George, J. (2007). Cognitive assessment in the elderly: A review of clinical methods. *QJM*, *100*, 469–484.

Yang, F. M., Cazorla-Lancaster, Y., & Jones, R. N. (2008). Within-group differences in depression among older Hispanics living in the United States. *Journals of Gerontology Series B: Psychological Sciences and Social Sciences*, *63B*, 27–32.

Yesavage, J. A., Brink, T. L., & Rose, T. L. (1983). Development and validation of a geriatric depression scale: A preliminary report. *Journal of Psychiatric Residents*, *17*, 37–49.

Zanetti, O., Geroldi, C., Frisoni, G. B., Bianchetti, A., & Trabucchi, M. (1999). Contrasting results between caregiver's report and direct assessment of activities of daily living in patients affected by mild and very mild dementia: The contribution of the caregiver's personal characteristics. *Journal of the American Geriatrics Society*, *47*, 196–202.

Zeiss, A. M., & Steffen, A. M. (1996). Interdisciplinary health care teams: The basic unit of geriatric care. In L. L. Carstensen, B. A. Edelstein, & L. Dornbrand (Eds.), *The Practical Handbook of Clinical Gerontology* (pp. 423–450). Thousand Oaks, CA: Sage Publications, Inc.

Zigmond, A. S., & Snaith, R. P. (1983). The Hospital Anxiety and Depression Scale. *Acta Psychiatrica Scandinavica*, *67*, 361–370.

Zisook, S., & Shear, K. (2009). Grief and bereavement: What psychiatrists need to know. *World Psychiatry*, *8*, 67–74.

Zisook, S., & Shuchter, S. R. (1996). Grief and bereavement. In J. Sadavoy, L. W. Lazarus, L. F. Jarvik, & G. T. Grossberg (Eds.), *Comprehensive review of Geriatric Psychiatry* (2nd ed.). (pp. 529–562) Washington, DC: American Psychiatric Press.

Zisook, S., Paulus, M., Shuchter, S. R., & Judd, L. L. (1997). The many faces of depression following spousal bereavement. *Journal of Affective Disorders*, *45*, 85–95.

Zisook, S., Shuchter, S. R., Pedrilli, P., Sable, J., & Deaciuc, S. C. (2001). Bupropion sustained release for bereavement: Results of an open trial. *Journal of Clinical Psychiatry*, *62*, 227–230.

Zung, W. K. (1965). A self-rating scale. *Archives of General Psychiatry*, *12*, 63–70.

Zung, W. K. (1967). Depression in the normal aged. *Psychosomatics*, *8*, 289–292.

CHAPTER

2 Assessment of Anxiety in Older Adults

Cheryl Carmin[1], Raymond L. Ownby[2]

[1]*Department of Psychiatry, University of Illinois at Chicago, Chicago, IL, USA,*

[2]*Department of Psychiatry, Nova Southeastern University, Fort Lauderdale, FL, USA*

Over the course of a lifetime, anxiety disorders affect more than one in four adults in the United States (Kessler et al., 2005) making these conditions the most prevalent category of psychiatric illness affecting adults. Further, the economic burden of these conditions approximated $42.3 billion annually in 1999 (Greenberg et al., 1999). Given the increase in health care costs, inflation, and taking OCD into consideration, which was excluded in the Greenberg et al. (1999) study, this figure is undoubtedly an underestimate of the burden placed on society, especially in light of the chronic and unremitting nature of these conditions if they are left untreated.

Despite anxiety disorders being more prevalent than mood disorders at any stage of adulthood, surprisingly little attention has been paid to anxiety disorders in older adults (Beck & Stanley, 1997; Kessler et al., 2005) whereas depression has received considerable attention. While there has been a limited increase in research into the treatment of specific anxiety disorders in older adults, there had not been a substantial increase in the investigation of anxiety assessment of adults in their later years since we first reviewed the literature (Carmin, Pollard, & Gillock, 1999). It is the purpose of this chapter to review the current state of knowledge regarding anxiety disorders assessment in older adults.

EPIDEMIOLOGICAL CONSIDERATIONS

The prevalence of anxiety disorders appears to diminish over the course of adulthood. The replication of the National Comorbidity Survey (NCS-R; Kessler et al., 2005) examined prevalence across adult cohorts (i.e., adults aged 18–29, 30–44, 45–59, 60 and older). While the lifetime prevalence of anxiety disorders in adults under 60 years ranged from approximately 30–35%, for those 60 years and older the prevalence dropped to 15.3%. This age-related decline may provide some explanation for the inattention given to geriatric anxiety. Consistent with the NCS-R data, in a recent survey of mental disorders in older African Americans, the National Survey of American Life (NASL; Ford et al., 2007), anxiety disorders were more than twice as prevalent (13.23%) as mood disorders (6.33%) and the most frequently occurring category of psychiatric illness. Notably, Post-traumatic Stress Disorder (6.19%) and Social Phobia (4.49%) were the two most prevalent conditions in the Ford et al. (2007) study, whereas the NCS-R data found that Specific Phobia (7.5%) and Social Phobia (6.4%) were the most prevalent diagnoses. Interestingly, the Longitudinal Aging Study, which was conducted in Amsterdam, found Generalized Anxiety Disorder (7.3%) was the most prevalent condition and the overall prevalence of anxiety disorders was 10.2% (Beekman et al., 1998). However, as noted above,

Handbook of Assessment in Clinical Gerontology. DOI: 10.1016/B978-0-12-374961-1.10002-8

regardless of the prevalence dropping by roughly half, anxiety disorders remain the most frequently occurring diagnoses across all age groups including those aged 60 and above.

The epidemiological data can be both compelling and misleading. The majority of such studies survey community-dwelling individuals. In many instances, older adults may reside in alternative housing such as nursing homes or retirement communities and are not included in such studies (Bland, Newman, & Orn, 1988), thereby resulting in an underestimate of actual prevalence. However, this may have been more the case with early studies, such as the Epidemiologic Catchment Area Survey that found a 1-month anxiety prevalence rate of 5.5% in adults 65 years and older (Regier, Narrow, & Rae, 1990).

SPECIAL CONSIDERATIONS

The assessment of anxiety in older persons may present issues not found when evaluating younger individuals. Perhaps most importantly, the clinician should understand the social, developmental, and medical context in which the client presents in order to understand the extent to which specific symptoms or behaviors represent pathology. This is not always a simple decision, and it is made more complex by the dearth of normative information on older persons. Interestingly, in one study of elderly persons' fears, these differed most from the fears of adults and college students in having less frequent and intense fears of such things as economic problems, the ecology, or political issues (Croake, Myers, & Singh, 1988). Although they reported somewhat more frequent and intense fears of sickness and aging, the differences among age groups in this study were not statistically significant.

Other issues that arise in consideration of anxiety in the elderly include the importance of recognizing clinically significant but subsyndromal patterns of anxiety symptoms, and the possible increased prevalence of mixed anxiety and depression in older persons. Investigators have argued that a combination of anxiety and depression symptoms, referred to as Mixed Anxiety and Depressive Disorder (MADD), may be seen more frequently in elderly persons (Schoevers et al., 2003). Psychometric evidence has accumulated to suggest a considerable overlap between anxiety and depression in the elderly (Koloski, Smith, Pachana, & Dobson, 2008). Although a full discussion of these topics is beyond the scope of this chapter, the clinician evaluating anxiety in an elderly person should be aware that anxiety syndromes in younger and older persons may be different.

When evaluating anxiety symptoms that arise in later life, consideration should be given to the possibility that some symptoms may represent aspects of medical illnesses or common developmental trajectories. For example, older adults may have poorer balance than younger persons. This fact may contribute to older persons' fear of falling, a concern that may seem irrational or exaggerated out of its developmental context. The fear may still be excessive and may affect the older individual's quality of life and functioning, but understanding the physical basis for observed changes in balance (and the potential benefit of balance training) may help in making the assessment process more sensitive to the specific needs of the older person. For example, symptoms such as heart palpitations or shortness of breath can arise from cardiovascular or pulmonary disease but may also be symptoms of anxiety. Further, the anxious patient with chronic obstructive pulmonary disease (COPD) may have worsening of their symptoms of shortness of breath when anxiety is increased.

Case Study

Ms Smith, a 75-year-old woman, was referred for psychiatric evaluation because of her pathological fear of falling. With a Beck Depression Inventory score of 12 and a GAF of 80, however, she appeared to have a single fear of near-phobic level. She had no previous history of psychological disorder. She lived with her husband of 40 years and was a happy mother and grandmother. She was treated for hypertension and hyperlipidemia with a calcium channel blocker and a statin, respectively, but no changes in her medications had been made recently. She had been treated with oral hormone replacement therapy during the peri-menopause but had not taken any HRT for about 20 years.

She arrived in the company of her husband who assisted her in walking down the hall. She leaned on his arm from the waiting area until he assisted her into the office where they were interviewed together. She had particular difficulty in crossing the threshold into the office from the hallway. Examination revealed that she did in fact have lower body weakness that had become progressively worse over the past two years. Referral to a movement disorders specialist revealed that she was suffering from Parkinson's disease. Treatment for that disorder was initiated with considerable improvement in her gait and decreased concerns about falling.

This case study illustrates the importance of understanding the many ways in which physical diseases can be manifested as psychological symptoms. While true in all age groups, the increased frequency of some diseases in older persons makes an awareness of this issue critical. The availability of appropriate specialists for assistance in diagnosis of unusual presentations or uncommon conditions is also essential in some cases.

FACTORS INFLUENCING ANXIETY ASSESSMENT IN THE ELDERLY

Also influencing the outcome of epidemiological investigations and the assessment of anxiety in general is whether the descriptive and diagnostic measures used to assess anxiety in younger adults are applicable to older individuals (Beck & Stanley, 1997a). On the one hand, some studies (e.g., Diefenbach, Stanley, & Beck, 2001; Owens, Hadjistavropoulos, & Asmundson, 2000; Shapiro, Roberts, & Beck, 1999) report age-related differences in anxiety across the lifespan. Other studies have found that anxiety symptoms are relatively invariant across age-based cohorts (e.g., Stanley, Beck, & Zebb, 1996). Thus, it has yet to be determined whether the fundamental nature and experience of anxiety evolves over the lifespan (Lawton, Kleban, & Dean, 1993). Perhaps a more salient consideration than whether individuals meet full diagnostic criteria for an anxiety disorder is whether anxiety is causing a significant disruption in the lives of older adults (Fisher & Noll, 1996).

Finally, and most relevant to this chapter, is the observation that the majority of psychometric instruments used to study anxiety were developed for use with younger populations, and the psychometric properties of these instruments have remained largely uninvestigated with regard to geriatric samples. As Beck and Stanley (2001) note, either measures can be developed that are specific to older adults, or established measures can be evaluated to determine their validity and utility with the elderly, the latter approach being representative of a more economical research effort.

CLINICAL UTILITY OF INSTRUMENTS TO ASSESS ANXIETY IN OLDER ADULTS

Assessment has a variety of purposes and can take several forms. From a clinical standpoint, the purpose of assessment is to aid in the process of diagnosis or to provide descriptive information that can be utilized to gain a perspective on symptoms and/or functioning, or to provide a means of gauging progress in treatment. The form that assessment takes may include a clinician administered interview, self-report, or behavioral observation. Less frequently, assessment may involve psychophysiological measurement.

Diagnostic Assessment

For the purpose of diagnosis, there are two structured diagnostic clinical interviews that are most widely used, namely the Anxiety Disorders Interview Schedule for DSM-IV (ADIS-IV; Brown,

DiNardo, & Barlow, 1994) and the Structured Clinical Interview for DSM-IV Axis I Disorders (SCID; First, Spitzer, Gibbon, & Williams, 1997). Both of these instruments have been found to yield reliable diagnoses with elderly patients (Beck & Stanley, 1997a; Segal, Hersen, Hasselt, Kabacoff, & Roth, 1993; Stanley et al., 1996). While other measures, for example the World Mental Health—Composite International Diagnostic Interview (WMH-CIDI), have been used in large-scale epidemiological studies such as the NCS-R (Kessler et al., 2005) and NSAL (Ford et al., 2007), there has been no systematic investigation of the use of the WMH-CIDI with elderly cohorts, although the prevalence rates reported in the two noted studies are relatively consistent and more in line with expectations than earlier, similar investigations.

The ADIS-IV (Brown et al., 1994) and the SCID (First et al., 1997) classify disorders based on DSM-IV criteria. Each disorder is presented in a discrete section beginning with a few key questions to screen for responses that suggest further in-depth questions are needed to confirm a diagnosis. If the screening questions are answered affirmatively, the balance of the section is administered; if not, the remainder of the section is skipped. All of the adult anxiety disorders and many pre-emptory disorders (i.e., psychosis, substance abuse, depression, dysthymia and somatoform disorders) are included in the ADIS-IV. Unlike the ADIS-IV, the SCID includes all DSM-IV diagnoses.

Both of these clinical interviews are designed to be administered by a highly trained examiner. Because it requires clinical judgment to evaluate responses and determine the direction of questioning, examiners must be familiar with the diagnostic criteria for anxiety or other disorders. Administration time averages one to two hours, but could require more time if the patient endorses a significant number of symptoms indicative of comorbid diagnoses.

Despite their wide use in clinical research, there are only a handful of studies which have examined the properties of either of these diagnostic measures specifically with elderly individuals. Studies using the ADIS-IV with a sample of older patients report excellent inter-rater reliability for the diagnoses of social phobia, specific phobia, and panic disorder, and moderate reliability for major depression (Beck, Stanley, & Zebb, 1996; Stanley et al., 1996). With a small sample of inpatient and outpatient elderly adults (56—84 years), Segal and colleagues (1993) found that the SCID-I (DSM-III-R, Axis I version) had good reliability for the general category of anxiety disorders and an inter-rater agreement of 94%.

There is one other interview measure, the Clinician Administered PTSD Scale (CAPS), that has been developed for the purpose of diagnosis, although its use is limited to Post-traumatic Stress Disorder (PTSD). The CAPS, developed by Blake and colleagues (Blake et al., 1990), is a semi-structured clinical interview. Like SCID and ADIS, the CAPS is designed for administration by a highly trained examiner. This instrument has been used extensively with elderly samples, primarily those involved in wartime events, was found to have good discriminative validity (Hyer, Summers, Boyd, Litaker, & Boudewyns, 1996), and was useful in assessing the presence and severity of current PTSD in veterans (Yehuda et al., 1995). The CAPS has also been used in a number of non-combat-related treatment outcome studies with samples that include older persons. These studies include treatment of PTSD due to motor vehicle accidents (Hickling & Blanchard, 1997) and treatment with brofaromine (Baker et al., 1995). The combined results of these studies suggest that the CAPS is an appropriate scale for use in elderly populations.

In summary, while this work is encouraging, further research using the SCID to diagnose specific anxiety disorders in elderly populations is needed. In fact Kogan, Edelstein, and McKee (2000) suggest that a clear limitation in the use of either the SCID or ADIS is that more representative samples are needed in order to enhance generalizability. It is also noteworthy that all of these clinician-administered instruments require that interviewers receive substantial training, which may limit the utility of these measures in clinical rather than research settings. In addition, the use of a structured clinical interview is further limited in that these diagnostic measures can require considerable stamina on the part of elderly patients, may utilize terminology that is infrequently used or considered stigmatizing by older adults, or the results may be confounded by cognitive deficits (Mohlman, Gainer Sirota, King, Papp, & Gorenstein, in press).

Descriptive Measures of Anxiety—General Measures

A number of scales have been used to either screen for or describe anxiety symptoms and their severity. Some measures are exclusive to anxiety symptoms whereas others include an anxiety subscale among the variety of syndromes or symptoms that are assessed. We have briefly described below measures that are psychometrically sound and designed specifically for use with elderly populations, or have been adopted for use with older adults.

Beck Anxiety Inventory (BAI)

The BAI (Beck, Epstein, Brown, & Steer, 1988) is a self-report questionnaire measuring 21 common somatic and cognitive symptoms of anxiety. In a study of adults age 55 years and older in a community-based outpatient facility, the BAI was found to have good discriminant validity (Kabacoff, Segal, Hersen, & Van Hasselt, 1997). Using the SCID to make a diagnostic determination, the BAI was effective in differentiating between those with and without an anxiety disorder. Two factors (somatic and subjective) best described the elderly sample and discriminated between groups (Kabacoff et al., 1997). In this elderly sample, no single cutoff score proved optimal when used to predict the presence of an anxiety disorder due to considerations regarding sensitivity (the proportion of true cases who score above the cutoff score) versus specificity (the proportion of normals who score below the cutoff point).

Using a community and residential sample of older adults, the BAI demonstrated adequate internal consistency and yielded six factors with a somatic factor accounting for much of the variance (Morin et al., 1999). Morin et al. caution that given the prevalence of somatic concerns in this non-clinical sample, their results suggest a cautious use of the inventory. In a recent study, the BAI performed well on most analyses, demonstrating one of the highest correlations with measures of anxiety severity, good discriminant validity for anxiety, and a good balance between specificity and sensitivity when using the cutoff point of 15/16 (Dennis, Boddington, & Funnell, 2007). The BAI has also been used in a clinical trial comparing cognitive behavior therapy with enhanced usual treatment (Stanley et al., 2009).

Depression Anxiety Stress Scale (DASS)

The DASS (Lovibond & Lovibond, 1995) has been receiving increasing support due to its strong psychometric properties (see Brown, Chorpita, Korotitsch, & Barlow, 1997). Consistent with younger samples, in older adults a 3-factor structure best fit the data. Results also indicated good internal consistency, excellent convergent validity, and good discriminative validity. Receiver operating curve analyses indicated that the DASS-21 predicted the diagnostic presence of generalized anxiety disorder and depression, as well as other commonly used measures. These data suggest that the DASS may be used with older adults in lieu of multiple scales designed to measure similar constructs (Gloster et al., 2008).

Geriatric Anxiety Inventory (GAI)

The GAI (Pachana et al., 2007) is a recent addition to the anxiety assessment literature and was developed specifically for use with older adults. It is a 20-item measure of dimensional anxiety which, during its development, successfully discriminated between those with and without an anxiety disorder, as well as those with and without DSM-IV diagnosed GAD. Pachana et al. (2007) investigated the psychometric properties of the instrument (i.e., internal consistency, test–retest reliability, concurrent and discriminant validity, receiver operating characteristics) with a psychogeriatric sample, as well as with normal older adults. A subsequent study (Boddice & Pachana, 2008) examined the use of the GAI in a residential care setting in order to determine the utility of the instrument with elderly individuals who were experiencing cognitive impairments, and found the classification (i.e., presence or absence) of anxiety symptoms by the GAI was not significantly associated with an individual's cognitive status in either community-dwelling or residential care samples. In addition, data supported the predictive validity of the GAI in residential care settings with respect to diagnosis of anxiety disorders.

Hamilton Anxiety Rating Scale (HAM-A)

The HAM-A (Hamilton, 1959) is a clinician administered rating scale designed to assess anxiety symptom severity. Somatic, cognitive, and affective symptoms are included. A trained examiner rates the severity and intensity of 14 primarily somatic symptoms. The utility of the scale with older adults has received preliminary support (Beck & Stanley, 1997b), with Beck and colleagues (Beck, Stanley, & Zebb, 1996; Beck, Stanley, & Zebb, 1999) concluding that the HAM-A differentiated older adults with GAD from matched normal community participants.

State-Trait Anxiety Inventory (STAI)

The STAI (Speilberger, Gorsuch, Luchene, Vagg, & Jacobs, 1983) is a 40-item self-report scale that assesses separate dimensions of "state" and "trait" anxiety. Examples of what the STAI measures include feelings of apprehension, tension, nervousness, and worry. Norms from the original version (STAI-X) include a small sample of elderly persons aged 50–69 years. An early study found modest construct and discriminant validity using the original version of the STAI (Patterson, O'Sullivan, & Speilberger, 1980) in adults 55–87 years old. A subsequent study supported the use of the Trait but not the State scale of the STAI in anxiety disordered older patients (Kabacoff et al., 1997). A recent study found that compared with the State Scale, the Trait Scale did not fare well in comparison with other measures of anxiety in an elderly sample (Dennis et al., 2007). Thus, despite its widespread use, there is inconsistent data supporting the use of the STAI.

Descriptive Measures of Anxiety—Measures Related to Diagnoses

The instruments described above measure anxiety as a general construct. What is at least as relevant are those measures which have been developed that assess anxiety as it relates to specific diagnoses.

Panic Disorder and Agoraphobia

The primary assessment targets for patients with panic disorder are panic attacks, anticipatory anxiety, and, when agoraphobia is present, phobic avoidance. Frequency and intensity of panic attacks are usually assessed via self-monitoring instruments such as panic diaries.

A few instruments have been studied specifically with elderly patients diagnosed with panic disorder. Researchers used two self-report measures, the Phobia Scale (Marks & Mathews, 1979) and the Sheehan Patient-Rated Anxiety Scale (Sheehan, 1986), to assess 51 elderly patients with panic disorder (Raj, Corvea, & Dagon, 1993). Another study assessed 75 older adults with panic disorder and agoraphobia using the Stanford Agoraphobia Severity Scale (Telch, 1985), a self-report measure requesting respondents to rate their level of anxiety for each of 10 common agoraphobic situations. These studies provide some preliminary normative data on a very small number of instruments. However, a great deal more psychometric research is needed on these and other measures that could be used to assess panic disorder in the elderly.

Generalized Anxiety Disorder Severity Scale (GADSS)

Since we last reviewed anxiety assessment in the elderly, the one area that has received the greatest amount of attention is that of worry, which is a hallmark feature of GAD (Beck & Stanley, 1997). It is not entirely clear why so much attention has been focused on this one dimension and/or disorder, other than the fact that GAD was presumably the most common of the anxiety disorders affecting elderly patients. Recent epidemiological studies may question this emphasis but, the prevalence of worry notwithstanding, it is among the few areas where specific measures have been developed for use with older adults.

As its name suggests, the Generalized Anxiety Disorder Severity Scale (GADSS) (Shear, Belnap, Mazumdar, Houck, & Rollman, 2006) is a 6-item interview that was developed to assess the severity of GAD symptoms. The measure was subsequently validated in a sample of 134 older adults (Andreescu et al., 2008). In this latter study, the authors concluded that the GADSS demonstrated high internal consistency and inter-rater reliabilities, and good convergent and divergent validity. However, Weiss and colleagues (Weiss et al., 2009) note that there is only mixed support for the use of the GADSS with older adults. Of concern is the fact that they found poor diagnostic accuracy, indicating a lack of divergent validity. Interestingly, Weiss at al. (2009) found that using only the three items that assessed impact, rather than frequency/duration of symptoms, provided a more accurate (and parsimonious) measure of symptom severity.

The Worry Scale (WS; Wisocki, Handen, & Morse, 1986) is a 35-item self-report scale developed specifically for use with older adults. The subscales reflect severity of worry-related content concerning financial, health, and social concerns. Mean worry scores from seven studies of the original WS are available (Wisocki, 1994), and there are studies supporting the concurrent validity of the WS (Powers, Wisocki, & Whitbourne, 1992; Wisocki et al., 1986). Comparisons between the WS and anxiety dimensions of the SCL-90 found significant correlations in both community-dwelling and homebound older adults (Wisocki et al., 1986; Wisocki, 1988). With the exception of the health subscale, test–retest reliability in older adults without psychiatric diagnoses is adequate (Beck et al., 1996). To date, in older adults with and without GAD, psychometric data indicate adequate internal consistency, test–retest reliability, and convergent and divergent validity (Beck et al., 1996; Stanley et al., 1996). A recent revision to the Worry Scale expanded the number of items to 88 by including those worries specified by elderly participants in normative studies and contains additional questions about the amount of time spent worrying, the age at which worrying began and was most common, and significant life events associated with worry (Wisocki, 1994).

The Penn State Worry Questionnaire (PSWQ; Meyer, Miller, Metzger, & Borkovec, 1990) is a 16-item measure of trait worry. Unlike many measures that assess worry content, the PSWQ is a content-free measure of the excessiveness, duration, and uncontrollability of worry. Strong psychometric support is available for the use of this measure in both younger and older adults (Beck et al., 1995, 1996; Beck & Stanley, 1997; Brown, Antony, & Barlow, 1992; Molina & Borkovec, 1994). In a descriptive study of GAD in the elderly (55–81 years), community-dwelling participants were diagnosed using the ADIS and compared with matched controls (Beck et al., 1996). Using self-report measures alone (PSWQ, WS social subscale, Fear Questionnaire social subscale, and the Beck Depression Inventory), near-perfect classification (95%) was achieved. These results suggest that worry, based on the PSWQ and other measures, can be reliably assessed in older adults diagnosed with GAD.

Despite its widespread use, when confirmatory factor models that were developed using younger subjects were applied to an older adult sample, the data were a poor fit with both 1- and 2-factor models (Hopko et al., 2003). When the single factor model was modified by eliminating eight items, the researchers found strong fit indices, high internal consistency, adequate test–retest reliability, and good convergent and divergent validity. The author concluded that further psychometric work is required to assess whether the revised model is a more parsimonious method to assess late-life anxiety, possibly further indicating that the nature of worry differs in older versus younger adults.

Just as in both children and younger adults, among the elderly phobias appear to be common. The Fear Questionnaire (FQ; Marks & Mathews, 1979) is a self-report instrument that provides three main scores for agoraphobia, social phobia, and blood-illness-injury phobia. Items measure the degree to which specific situations are avoided, the extent to which phobic symptoms are disturbing, and the impact of various symptoms. In a study of older community volunteers, internal consistency for the Social Phobia and Blood-Illness-Injury Phobia Scales and test—retest reliability was poor (Stanley et al., 1996). Due to equivocal psychometric performance of two of the three scales in elderly populations, the FQ should be used with care.

The Fear Survey Schedule II (FSS-II; Geer, 1965) was designed primarily for research use and was normed on a college student sample. Unfortunately, it is the only version of this measure that has been used with an elderly sample (Liddell, Locker, & Burman, 1991), and no information regarding its psychometric adequacy with older adults has been provided.

Fear of falling is not an uncommon concern among older adults. In response to this concern, Huang developed the Geriatric Fear of Falling Measure (Huang, 2006) based on preliminary, qualitative research with community-dwelling Taiwanese subjects. The 15-item measure has four subscales: psychosomatic symptoms (PS); adopting an attitude of risk prevention (RP); paying attention to environmental safety (ES); and modifying behavior (MB); and additional research into the psychometric properties of this measure is needed.

Social Anxiety Disorder

Until recent epidemiological studies highlighted that Social Anxiety Disorder (SAD) persists into late life, conventional wisdom had dictated otherwise. As a result, there are no measures of social fears, fear of embarrassment, or constructs related to this condition that have been developed for use with socially anxious older adults. The best currently available alternative may be subscales of more general instruments that have been studied with older samples, such as the WS Social scale (Wisocki et al., 1986).

Obsessive—Compulsive Disorder (OCD)

There are several treatment outcome studies of older adults diagnosed with OCD (e.g., Calamari, Faber, Hitsman, & Poppe, 1994; Carmin & Wiegartz, 2000; Carmin, Pollard, & Ownby, 1999). However, while using widely accepted measures of OCD symptoms, there are no established norms or other psychometric data available for the measures used. One study (Stanley et al., 1996) compared responses of normal elder controls and elders with GAD on the Padua Inventory (PI; Sanavio, 1988).

The PI is a 60-item questionnaire designed to evaluate obsessive compulsive symptoms. Four scales measure severity of contamination and checking rituals, and fear of losing control over mental activities and motor behaviors. Results indicated that for the normal controls, there was adequate internal consistency for the PI overall and for three of the four scales, with the Behavior Control Scale the notable exception. In the GAD group, there was evidence of convergent validity with other measures of anxiety and worry, and good test—retest reliability. While this is the first study to use the PI with an elderly clinical sample, subjects were not diagnosed with OCD. While it could be argued that there is some similarity between the intrusive thoughts related to OCD and worry characteristic of GAD, these are two different constructs. Thus, analyses of the PI with older OCD subjects is still needed.

Post-traumatic Stress Disorder (PTSD)

Much of the research in PTSD with elderly groups has focused on dated events (e.g., WWII, the Holocaust) and less is known about age-related differences in PTSD symptomatology when the trauma occurs during later life (Beck & Stanley, 1997b). A series of studies of PTSD symptoms in Holocaust survivors (Yehuda et al., 1995; Yehuda et al., 1996) utilized a variety of PTSD measures and provide descriptive data for the measures for both elderly trauma survivors and non-exposed age-matched controls.

Global effects of stressful events are measured with the combat or civilian forms of the Mississippi PTSD Scales (MISS; Watson, 1990). Neal and colleagues (Neal, Hill, Hughes, Middleton, & Busuttil, 1995) found the Combat Scale to be the most accurate measure of PTSD severity in a small sample of elderly former prisoners of war (age range = 70–85 years).

MULTICULTURAL ISSUES IN ANXIETY ASSESSMENT IN THE ELDERLY

The potential for different expressions of anxiety across cultural or ethnic groups is largely unexplored. Anxiety in Hispanics has been characterized as similar to that in other groups, although some have argued for a specific syndrome of *ataque de nervios,* a group of symptoms similar to but not the same as panic disorder (Liebowitz et al., 1994; Sadock & Sadock, 2007, p. 523). The frequency and phenomenology of these symptoms in Hispanic elderly have not been widely researched. One study (Tolin, Robison, Gaztambide, Horowitz, & Blank, 2007) showed that 26% of a group of 303 Puerto Rican primary care patients aged 50 years and older reported having had at least one episode. Their reports were closely associated with other disorders, with 84% of those reporting an episode of *ataque* meeting criteria for another disorder, most frequently either a depression or anxiety spectrum disorder.

In an analysis of the Cornell Scale for Depression in Dementia (CSDD; Ownby, Harwood, Acevedo, Barker, & Duara, 2001; Ownby, Acevedo, Harwood, Barker, & Duara, 2008), the factor structure of this instrument was found to be essentially similar between groups of Spanish- and English-speaking elders with Alzheimer's disease. One difference that emerged was the importance of somatic complaints in Hispanic patients, consistent with cultural differences in the manner in which anxiety symptoms are expressed. While the CSDD item "somatic complaints" was most directly related to other symptoms of depression in Anglos, it was more closely related to complaints of sleep and appetite disturbance in Hispanic patients. This finding could be interpreted as a more general tendency to express symptoms somatically among the Hispanic patients.

In an analysis of the same group of patients with AD, Ownby et al. (2008) showed that both Spanish- and English-speaking patients could be grouped into several distinct latent classes. As one of the classes that emerged in this analysis was characterized by prominent anxiety, Ownby et al. (2008) suggest that this might either represent a group with agitated depression or with a specific anxiety disorder. The membership of Spanish- and English-speaking patients across classes, however, was not different, although the number of patients in each group was small.

More substantial data are available on anxiety disorders among older African Americans. Ford et al. (2007) report data on the prevalence of DSM-IV disorders from the National Survey of American Life. They found that 23% of African Americans aged 55–93 years (mean age of 66.6 years) reported a lifetime prevalence of at least one disorder, and 13.2% reported a lifetime history of any anxiety disorder, the most common of which were PTSD (6.2%), social phobia (5.5%), and GAD (3.1%). Twelve-month prevalence of any anxiety disorder was 6.6%, with the most common being PTSD (2.9%) and social phobia (2.1%).

CLINICAL ILLUSTRATIONS

While OCD has been found to occur in 1.3% of older adults (Kessler et al., 2005), the occurence of OCD in late life has been regarded as a rare occurrence (Rasmussen & Eisen, 1992). Further, when the onset is coupled with a neurological problem, such as a stroke, treatment can be complicated and may often take the form of pharmacological interventions due to a perception that psychotherapy will not succeed when there is documented brain damage. Consistent with the general adult literature, reviews of OCD treatment in the elderly (Calamari et al., 1994; Pollard, Carmin, & Ownby, 1997) support the use of cognitive behavior therapy in the form of exposure and response prevention as the treatment of choice. Case Study 2 illustrates a successful combined approach involving intensive, inpatient treatment of a newly diagnosed patient with OCD (see Carmin & Wiegartz, 2000 for a complete discussion).

Case Study 2—Obsessive Compulsive Disorder Treatment and Basal Ganglia Infarct

The patient was a 78-year-old man experiencing a first episode of OCD. Data from the ADIS-IV and the Yale Brown Obsessive Compulsive Scale (YBOCS) (Goodman et al., 1989b; Goodman et al., 1989a) along with a clinical interview revealed that his symptoms, which began 8 months prior to his hospital admission, involved "needing to know" and fears of being unable to correctly remember names and other information. When he could not spontaneously produce an answer or was unsure, he felt compelled to neutralize the anxiety produced by his uncertainty by repeatedly reviewing or checking his accumulated lists of names and references or by engaging in mental rituals. If the information was not in his archive or he could not produce the information by "quizzing" himself, he would call friends, acquaintances, his secretary, libraries, radio stations, etc. all over the world in an effort to find what he needed. He was unsuccessfully treated as an outpatient and came to us for intensive, inpatient treatment.

This patient's medical history was significant. On review of his MRI, recent small basal ganglia infarcts were noted. These infarcts were estimated to have occurred prior to the onset of Mr. X's OCD symptoms and may have etiologic significance. Teachman (Teachman, 2007) suggests that it is not clear whether existing cognitive therapy models apply to older populations due to the changes in older persons' cognitive functioning that accompany normal aging. As a means of ruling out any cognitve deficit, we opted to administer the Dementia Rating Scale (DRS; Mattis, 1976). Our patient's scores (DRS Total Score and scales of Attention, Construction, Initiation/Perseveration, and Memory) fell in the normal range for elderly subjects. He did show a deficit on the Conceptualization scale due to a tendency to respond to questions in a somewhat concrete fashion. We did not believe this would have an effect on his treatment.

Treatment began with psychoeducation. We provided a cognitive behavioral conceptualization of OCD and the rationale for exposure and response prevention (ERP). Obsessive intrusions and rituals were explained to the patient as a "learned pattern of reacting to certain situations or objects" and were likened to "habits" that can be broken or weakened with effort. In order to "break these habits" and learn that anxiety will decrease, even in the absence of rituals, the patient would need to confront the situations, or OCD-producing stimuli that provoke anxiety, and refrain from engaging in rituals. Through repeated exposure, anxiety decreases to a manageable level and it was expected that the patient would learn that rituals were unnecessary, in that they neither prevented nor ended his distress.

ERP was introduced gradually due to both his high levels of anxiety and his difficulty understanding the rationale for treatment. He was seen for individual ERP sessions twice daily, with each session lasting 60–90 minutes. A hierarchy of exposure experiences was developed and situations were presented to the patient in a gradual fashion beginning with the lower anxiety items. In creating the hierarchy, a situation was introduced and the patient was asked to rate his subjective anxiety as low, medium, or high. He was asked to refrain from note writing for a 30-minute period each day. Once he could successfully accomplish this task, the period was lengthened. Within one week he was able to discontinue all note taking, and all of his accumulated lists, both at home and at the hospital, were discarded.

He was then exposed to those situations that typically triggered his note taking, such as reading newspapers or magazines and watching television. While he could successfully abstain from taking notes, his anxiety caused him to ask questions of or seek reassurance from staff, family, and other patients. Response prevention took the form of reducing his telephone calls to elicit answers to no more than two per day, and staff members were instructed to redirect him when he attempted to solicit information from them.

Finally, the complete cessation of information-seeking phone calls and a continued ban on note taking were implemented. With the patient's permission, his wife, coworkers, and staff on the unit were apprised of this goal and worked collaboratively to ensure his compliance with the ritual ban. Within the week, the patient was asking questions only infrequently and receiving virtually no information from the above sources. Discharge planning and relapse prevention strategies were initiated. The patient, as well as his family and coworkers, was instructed in the potential barriers to treatment maintenance and in appropriate responses to difficult or stressful situations.

In addition to ERP, this gentleman also received pharmacological treatment. Over the course of his stay, his prior medications were discontinued and he was placed on Zoloft 200 mg every morning, Ativan 0.5 mg twice a day and Depakote 750 mg daily.

At the outset of treatment, this patient's YBOCS score was in the severe range (YBOCS = 24). While not completely ritual-free, by the time of his discharge (day 21), his score had dropped to 19 and he had dramatically reduced the amount of time he spent ritualizing. He continued to increase his gains after leaving the hospital. At 12 weeks post treatment, his YBOCS had dropped to 2 and, while he reported experiencing mild intrusive thoughts, he was able to resist any impulse to ritualize and return to his pre-OCD level of social functioning.

Case Study 3—Anxiety in Alzheimer's Disease

Mr Jones, an 81-year-old with mild cognitive impairment due to Alzheimer's disease, was referred for treatment of his continuing severe anxiety and worries. He complained of nearly constant dysphoric mood, a feeling of inner tension, and difficulty relaxing.

On initial evaluation the patient's score on the BDI was 23 and his GAF was 60, in part due to his cognitive limitations and in part to his psychological symptoms. His MMSE score was 22 out of 30, considered typical of relatively mild cognitive impairment in a dementing illness. The patient was aware of his surroundings, knew important people around him, remembered treating clinicians from one visit to the next, but could not say the day, date, month, or year, and if not prompted would not have taken medications regularly. Over a period of several years, he had shown very mild evidence of continuing cognitive decline and was treated with a cholinesterase inhibitor (donepezil, 10 mg) for cognitive impairment. The patient was thus cognitively and functionally stable, but had significant impairment in quality of life as a result of his severe anxiety.

Pharmacologic treatments attempted included treatment with antidepressant medications, anticonvulsants, anxiolytics (benzodiazepines), and antipsychotics, all with minimal treatment effects or dose-limiting side effects. Cognitive interventions were difficult due to his anxiety-related short attention span and the patient's uncooperativeness with activity scheduling in spite of the support of his wife of 30 years.

Case Study 4—Post-Traumatic Stress Disorder

Mr W was referred by the fundraising staff of a local hospital to which he was a substantial financial contributor. A mild-mannered and self-effacing man who had retired 10 years earlier, he came for treatment because of his wife's concerns about his agitated behavior during apparent nightmares while asleep. His wife stated that his behavior was so agitated that she feared for her safety when these episodes occurred. Mr W's personal history was significant for having been incarcerated in a concentration camp during World War II. He was still at the camp when it was liberated at the end of the war when he was aged 13. American officers of the liberating force took care of him as he had been orphaned, and assisted his move to the U.S. to complete his education. Mr W had become successful in business and had retired after selling his business to a large corporation about 10 years before he came to my attention.

While Mr W denied feeling depressed, he acknowledged multiple related symptoms including sadness, low energy, lack of interest, and sleep disturbance. Although Mr W denied knowing what occurred during the episodes of sleep disturbance, it was assumed that his nightmares were caused by post-traumatic stress disorder. He was reluctant to discuss his recollections of his time in the camp or other war-related events, and declined other treatment for specific PTSD-related symptoms. He stated that he felt that his memories were better left undisturbed. He readily engaged in treatment, however, and stated that he enjoyed the opportunity to interact with his therapist.

Previous treatment by another psychiatrist had included antidepressant treatment with a serotonergic agent, a second-generation antipsychotic, and benzodiazepines. Mr W complained of feeling tired on these medications and noted that they did not relieve his disturbed sleep.

Treatment for Mr W focused on changes in his medications and cognitive–behavioral treatment. His denial of depression while acknowledging multiple symptoms of depression is commonly encountered in work with older individuals. Little is to be accomplished in trying to persuade the client that they do, in fact, have depression. It is preferable to focus on specific symptoms such as lack of interest or hopelessness and address them as appropriate. In Mr W's case, we focused on increasing physical activity through activity scheduling and developing better social relations with a group of friends. He developed a higher level of physical activity and greater social connectedness, and responded positively to supportive therapy.

References

Andreescu, C., Belnap, B. H., Rollman, B. L., Houck, P., Ciliberti, C., Mazumdar, S., et al. (2008). Generalized anxiety disorder severity scale validation in older adults. *The American Journal of Geriatric Psychiatry: Official Journal of the American Association for Geriatric Psychiatry, 16*(10), 813–818. doi: 10.1097/JGP.0b013e31817c6aab

Baker, D., Diamond, B., Gillette, G., Hamner, M., Katzelnick, D., Keller, T., et al. (1995). A double-blind, randomized, placebo-controlled, multi-center study of brofaromine in the treatment of post-traumatic stress disorder. *Psychopharmacology, 122*(4), 386–389. doi: 10.1007/BF02246271

Beck, A. T., Epstein, N., Brown, G., & Steer, R. A. (1988). An inventory for measuring clinical anxiety: Psychometric properties. *J Consult Clin Psychol, 56*(6), 893–897.

Beck, J. G., & Stanley, M. A. (1997). Anxiety disorders in the elderly: The emerging role of behavior therapy. *Behavior Therapy, 28*(1), 83–100. doi: 10.1016/S0005-7894(97)80035-4

Beck, J. G., Stanley, M. A., & Zebb, B. J. (1995). Psychometric properties of the Penn State Worry Questionnaire in older adults. *Journal of Clinical Geropsychology, 1*, 33–42.

Beck, J. G., Stanley, M. A., & Zebb, B. J. (1996). Characteristics of Generalized Anxiety Disorder in older adults: A descriptive study. *Behaviour Research and Therapy, 34*(3), 225–234. doi: 10.1016/0005-7967(95)00064-X

Beck, J. G., Stanley, M. A., & Zebb, B. (1999). Effectiveness of the Hamilton Anxiety Rating Scale with older Generalized Anxiety Disorder patients. *Journal of Clinical Geropsychology, 5*(4), 281–290. doi: 10.1023/A:1022962907930

Beekman, A. T. F., Bremmer, M. A., Deeg, D. J. H., Van Balkom, A. J. L. M., Smit, J. H., De Beurs, E., et al. (1998). Anxiety disorders in later life: A report from the Longitudinal Aging Study Amsterdam. *International Journal of Geriatric Psychiatry, 13*(10), 717–726. doi: Article

Blake, Weathers, F., Nagy, L., Kaloupek, D., Klauminzer, G., Charney, D., et al. (1990). A clinician rating scale for assessing current and lifetime PTSD: The CAPS-1. *Behavioral Therapist, 13*, 187–188.

Bland, R. C., Newman, S. C., & Orn, H. (1988). Prevalence of psychiatric disorders in the elderly in Edmonton. *Acta Psychiatrica Scandinavica. Supplementum, 338*, 57–63. doi: 3165596

Boddice, G., & Pachana, N. A. (2008). The clinical utility of the geriatric anxiety inventory in older adults with cognitive impairment. *Nursing Older People, 20*(8), 36–39, quiz 40. Retrieved February 5, 2009, from http://www.ncbi.nlm.nih.gov/pubmed/18982897

Brown, T. A., Antony, M. M., & Barlow, D. H. (1992). Psychometric properties of the Penn State Worry Questionnaire in a clinical anxiety disorders sample. *Behaviour Research and Therapy, 30*(1), 33–37. doi: 10.1016/0005-7967(92)90093-V

Brown, T. A., DiNardo, P., & Barlow, D. (1994). *Anxiety Disorders Interview Schedule for DSM-IV.* New York, NY: Oxford University Press.

Brown, T. A., Chorpita, B. F., Korotitsch, W., & Barlow, D. H. (1997). Psychometric properties of the Depression Anxiety Stress Scales (DASS) in clinical samples. *Behaviour Research and Therapy, 35*(1), 79–89, Retrieved August 4, 2009, from http://www.ncbi.nlm.nih.gov/pubmed/9009048

Calamari, J. E., Faber, S. D., Hitsman, B. L., & Poppe, C. J. (1994). Treatment of obsessive compulsive disorder in the elderly: a review and case example. *Journal of Behavior Therapy and Experimental Psychiatry, 25*(2), 95–104. doi: 7983229

Carmin, C. N., & Wiegartz, P. S. (2000). Successful and unsuccessful treatment of Obsessive-Compulsive Disorder in older adults. *Journal of Contemporary Psychotherapy, 30*(2), 181–193. doi: 10.1023/A:1026566729195

Carmin, C. N., Pollard, C., & Gillock, K. L. (1999). Assessment of anxiety disorders in the elderly. In P. Lichtenberg (Ed.), *Handbook of Assessment in Clinical Gerontology.* New York, NY: John Wiley & Sons.

Carmin, C. N., Pollard, C. A., & Ownby, R. L. (1999). Cognitive behavioral treatment of older adults with obsessive-compulsive disorder. *Cognitive and Behavioral Practice*, *6*(2), 110–119. doi: 10.1016/S1077-7229 (99)80019-4

Croake, J. W., Myers, K., & Singh, A. (1988). The fears expressed by elderly men and women: A lifespan approach. *International Journal of Aging and Human Development*, *26*, 139–146.

Dennis, R. E., Boddington, S. J. A., & Funnell, N. J. (2007). Self-report measures of anxiety: Are they suitable for older adults? *Aging & Mental Health*, *11*(6), 668–677. doi: 10.1080/13607860701529916

Diefenbach, G. J., Stanley, M. A., & Beck, J. G. (2001). Worry content reported by older adults with and without generalized anxiety disorder. *Aging & Mental Health*, *5*(3), 269–274. doi: 10.1080/13607860120065069

First, M., Spitzer, R., Gibbon, M., & Williams, J. (1997). *Structured Clinical Interview for DSM-IV Axis I Disorders*. Washington, DC: American Psychiatric Press.

Fisher, J., & Noll, J. (1996). Anxiety disorders. In L. Carstensen, B. Edelstein, & L. Dornbrand (Eds.), *The practical handbook of clinical gerontology* (pp. 304–323). Thousand Oaks, CA: Sage Publications.

Ford, B. C., Bullard, K. M., Taylor, R. J., Toler, A. K., Neighbors, H. W., & Jackson, J. S. (2007). Lifetime and 12-month prevalence of Diagnostic and Statistical Manual of Mental Disorders, Fourth Edition disorders among older African Americans: findings from the National Survey of American Life. *The American Journal of Geriatric Psychiatry: Official Journal of the American Association for Geriatric Psychiatry, 15*(8), 652–659. doi: JGP.0b013e3180437d9e

Geer, J. H. (1965). The development of a scale to measure fear. *Behaviour Research and Therapy, 3*(1), 45–53. doi: 10.1016/0005-7967(65)90040-9

Gloster, A. T., Rhoades, H. M., Novy, D., Klotsche, J., Senior, A., Kunik, M., et al. (2008). Psychometric properties of the Depression Anxiety and Stress Scale-21 in older primary care patients. *Journal of Affective Disorders*, *110*(3), 248–259. doi: 10.1016/j.jad.2008.01.023

Goodman, W. K., Price, L. H., Rasmussen, S. A., Mazure, C., Delgado, P., Heninger, G. R., et al. (1989a). The Yale-Brown Obsessive Compulsive Scale: II. Validity. *Arch Gen Psychiatry, 46*(11), 1012–1016. doi: 10.1001/archpsyc.1989.01810110054008

Goodman, W. K., Price, L. H., Rasmussen, S. A., Mazure, C., Fleischmann, R. L., Hill, C. L., et al. (1989b). The Yale-Brown Obsessive Compulsive Scale. I. Development, use, and reliability. *Archives of General Psychiatry, 46*(11), 1006–1011. Retrieved August 23, 2009, from http://www.ncbi.nlm.nih.gov/pubmed/2684084

Greenberg, P. E., Sisitsky, T., Kessler, R. C., Finkelstein, S. N., Berndt, E. R., Davidson, J. R., et al. (1999). The economic burden of anxiety disorders in the 1990s. *The Journal of Clinical Psychiatry, 60*(7), 427–435. doi: 10453795

Hamilton, M. (1959). The assessment of anxiety states by rating. *British Journal of Medical Psychiatry, 23*, 56–62.

Hickling, E. J., & Blanchard, E. B. (1997). The private practice psychologist and manual-based treatments: Post-traumatic stress disorder secondary to motor vehicle accidents. *Behaviour Research and Therapy, 35*(3), 191–203. doi: 10.1016/S0005-7967(96)00090-3

Hopko, D. R., Stanley, M. A., Reas, D., Wetherell, J. L., Beck, J. G., Novy, D. M., et al. (2003). Assessing worry in older adults: Confirmatory factor analysis of the Penn State Worry Questionnaire and psychometric properties of an abbrieviated model. *Psychological Assessment*, *15*(2), 173–183.

Huang, T. (2006). Geriatric fear of falling measure: development and psychometric testing. *International Journal of Nursing Studies*, *43*(3), 357–365. doi: 10.1016/j.ijnurstu.2005.04.006

Hyer, L., Summers, M. N., Boyd, S., Litaker, M., & Boudewyns, P. (1996). Assessment of older combat veterans with the clinician-administered PTSD Scale. *Journal of Traumatic Stress*, *9*(3), 587–593. doi: Article

Kabacoff, R. I., Segal, D. L., Hersen, M., & Van Hasselt, V. B. (1997). Psychometric properties and diagnostic utility of the Beck Anxiety Inventory and the State-Trait Anxiety Inventory with older adult psychiatric outpatients. *Journal of Anxiety Disorders*, *11*(1), 33–47. Retrieved February 3, 2009, from http://www.ncbi.nlm.nih.gov/pubmed/9131880

Kessler, R., Berglund, P., Demler, O., Jin, R., Merikangas, K. R., & Walters, E. E. (2005). Lifetime prevalence and age-of-onset distributions of DSM-IV disorders in the National Comorbidity Survey Replication. *Archives of General Psychiatry, 62*(6), 593–602. doi: 10.1001/archpsyc.62.6.593

Kogan, J. N., Edelstein, B. A., & McKee, D. R. (2000). Assessment of anxiety in older adults: Current status. *Journal of Anxiety Disorders, 14*(2), 109–132. doi: 10.1016/S0887-6185(99)00044-4

Koloski, N. A., Smith, N., Pachana, N. A., & Dobson, A. (2008). Performance of the Goldberg Anxiety and Depression Scale in older women. *Age and Ageing, 37*(4), 464–467. doi: 10.1093/ageing/afn091

Lawton, M., Kleban, M. H., & Dean, J. (1993). Affect and age: Cross-sectional comparisons of structure and prevalence. *Psychology and Aging, 8*(2), 165–175. Retrieved July 17, 2009, from http://www.sciencedirect.com/science/article/B6WYV-46T99YS-1S/2/6fb8931f60f738ec3ac7a3dda5f785b8

Liddell, A., Locker, D., & Burman, D. (1991). Self-reported fears (FSS-II) of subjects aged 50 years and over. *Behaviour Research and Therapy, 29*(2), 105–112. doi: 10.1016/0005-7967(91)90037-4

Liebowitz, M., Salman, E., Jusino, C., Garfinkel, R., Street, L., Cardenas, D., et al. (1994). Ataque de nervios and panic disorder. *Am J Psychiatry, 151*(6), 871–875. Retrieved from PM:8184996

Lovibond, P. F., & Lovibond, S. H. (1995). The structure of negative emotional states: Comparison of the Depression Anxiety Stress Scales (DASS) with the Beck Depression and Anxiety Inventories. *Behaviour Research and Therapy, 33*(3), 335–343. doi: 10.1016/0005-7967(94)00075-U

Marks, I., & Mathews, A. (1979). Brief standard self-rating for phobic patients. *Behaviour Research and Therapy, 17*(3), 263–267. doi: 10.1016/0005-7967(79)90041-X

Mattis, S. (1976). Mental state examination for organic mental syndrome in the elderly patient. In L. Bellak, & T. Karasu (Eds.), *Geriatric Psychiatry.* New York, NY: Grune & Stratton.

Meyer, T. J., Miller, M. L., Metzger, R. L., & Borkovec, T. D. (1990). Development and validation of the Penn State Worry Questionnaire. *Behaviour Research and Therapy, 28*(6), 487–495. doi: 10.1016/0005-7967(90)90135-6

Mohlman, J., Gainer Sirota, K., King, A., Papp, L., & Gorenstein, E. (in press). Augmenting the SCID and ADIS interviews for use with anxious older adults. *Cognitive and Behavioral Practice.*

Molina, S., & Borkovec, T. (1994). The Penn State Worry Questionnaire: Psychometric properties and associated characteristics. In G. Davey, & F. Tallis (Eds.), *Worrying: Perspectives on theory, assessment and treatment* (pp. 265–283). New York, NY: John Wiley & Sons.

Morin, C., Landreville, P., Colecchi, C., McDonald, K., Stone, J., & Ling, W. (1999). The Beck Anxiety Inventory: Psychometric properties with older adults. *Journal of Clinical Geropsychology, 5*(1), 19–29. doi: 10.1023/A:1022986728576

Neal, L., Hill, N., Hughes, J., Middleton, A., & Busuttil, W. (1995). Convergent validity of measures of PTSD in an elderly population of former prisoners of war. *International Journal of Gerliatric Psychiatry, 10*(7), 617–622.

Owens, K. M. B., Hadjistavropoulos, T., & Asmundson, G. J. G. (2000). Addressing the need for appropriate norms when measuring anxiety in seniors. *Aging & Mental Health, 4*(4), 309–314. doi: 10.1080/13607860020010448

Ownby, R., Acevedo, A., Harwood, D., Barker, W., & Duara, R. (2008). Patterns of depression in Spanish- and English-speaking patients with Alzheimer's disease. *J Geriatr Psychiatry Neurol, 21*(1), 47–55. Retrieved from PM:18287170

Ownby, R., Harwood, D., Acevedo, A., Barker, W., & Duara, R. (2001). Factor structure of the Cornell Scale for Depression in Dementia for Anglo and Hispanic patients with dementia. *Am J Geriatr Psychiatry, 9*(3), 217–224. Retrieved from PM:11481129

Pachana, N. A., Byrne, G. J., Siddle, H., Koloski, N., Harley, E., & Arnold, E. (2007). Development and validation of the Geriatric Anxiety Inventory. *International Psychogeriatrics/IPA, 19*(1), 103–114. doi: 10.1017/S1041610206003504

Patterson, R., O'Sullivan, M., & Speilberger, C. (1980). Measurement of state and trait anxiety in elderly mental health clients. *Journal of Behavioral Assessment, 2*, 89–97.

Pollard, C. A., Carmin, C. N., & Ownby, R. (1997). Obsessive-Compulsive Disorder in later life. In M. Pato, & G. Steketee (Eds.), *Review of Psychiatry, Vol. 16* (pp. III-57–III-72). Washington, DC: American Psychiatric Press.

Powers, C. B., Wisocki, P. A., & Whitbourne, S. K. (1992). Age differences and correlates of worrying in young and elderly adults. *Gerontologist*, *32*(1), 82–88. doi: 10.1093/geront/32.1.82

Raj, B., Corvea, N., & Dagon, E. (1993). The clinical characteristics of panic disorder in the elderly: A retrospective study. *Journal of Clinical Psychiatry*, *54*, 150–155.

Rasmussen, S., & Eisen, J. L. (1992). The epdemiology and clinical features of obsessve compulsive disorder. *Child and Adolescent Psychiatric Clinics of North America*, *15*, 743–758.

Regier, D. A., Narrow, W. E., & Rae, D. S. (1990). The epidemiology of anxiety disorders: The epidemiologic catchment area (ECA) experience. *Journal of Psychiatric Research*, *24*(Suppl. 2), 3–14. doi: 10.1016/0022-3956(90)90031-K

Sadock, B., & Sadock, V. (2007). *Kaplan & Sadock's synopsis of psychiatry* (Vol. 10). Philadelphia, PA: Wolters Kluwer.

Sanavio, E. (1988). Obsessions and compulsions: The Padua inventory. *Behaviour Research and Therapy*, *26*(2), 169–177. doi: 10.1016/0005-7967(88)90116-7

Schoevers, R. A., Beekman, A. T., Deeg, D. J., Hooijer, C., Jonker, C., & van Tilburg, W. (2003). The natural history of late-life depression: results from the Amsterdam Study of the Elderly (AMSTEL). *Journal of Affective Disorders*, *76*, 5–14.

Segal, D. L., Hersen, M., Hasselt, V. B., Kabacoff, R. I., & Roth, L. (1993). Reliability of diagnosis in older psychiatric patients using the structured clinical interview for DSM-III-R. *Journal of Psychopathology and Behavioral Assessment*, *15*(4), 347–356. doi: 10.1007/BF00965037

Shapiro, A., Roberts, J., & Beck, J. G. (1999). Differentiating symptoms of anxiety and depression in older adults: Distinct cognitive and affective profiles? *Cognitive Therapy and Research*, *23*, 53–74.

Shear, K., Belnap, B. H., Mazumdar, S., Houck, P., & Rollman, B. L. (2006). Generalized anxiety disorder severity scale (GADSS): A preliminary validation study. *Depression and Anxiety*, *23*(2), 77–82. doi: 10.1002/da.20149

Sheehan, D. V. (1986). *The anxiety disease*. Des Plaines, IL: Bantam Books.

Speilberger, C., Gorsuch, R., Luchene, R., Vagg, P., & Jacobs, G. (1983). *Manual for the STAI*. Palo Alto, CA: Consulting Psychologists Press.

Stanley, M. A., Beck, J. G., & Zebb, B. J. (1996). Psychometric properties of four anxiety measures in older adults. *Behaviour Research and Therapy*, *34*(10), 827–838. Retrieved February 3, 2009, from http://www.ncbi.nlm.nih.gov/pubmed/8952126

Stanley, M. A., Wilson, N. L., Novy, D. M., Rhoades, H. M., Wagener, P. D., Greisinger, A. J., et al. (2009). Cognitive behavior therapy for generalized anxiety disorder among older adults in primary care: A randomized clinical trial. *JAMA: The Journal of the American Medical Association*, *301*(14), 1460–1467. doi: 10.1001/jama.2009.458

Teachman, B. A. (2007). Linking obsessional beliefs to OCD symptoms in older and younger adults. *Behaviour Research and Therapy*, *45*(7), 1671–1681. doi: 10.1016/j.brat.2006.08.016

Telch, M. (1985). *The Stanford Agoraphobia Scale*. Stanford, CA: Stanford University.

Tolin, D., Robison, J., Gaztambide, S., Horowitz, S., & Blank, K. (2007). Ataques de nervios and psychiatric disorders in older Puerto Rican primary care patients. *Journal of Cross-Cultural Psychology*, *38*, 659–669.

Watson, C. G. (1990). Psychometric posttraumatic stress disorder measurement techniques: A review. *Psychological Assessment: A Journal of Consulting and Clinical Psychology*. Vol. *2*(*4*), 2(4), 460–469.

Weiss, B. J., Calleo, J., Rhoades, H. M., Novy, D. M., Kunik, M. E., Lenze, E. J., et al. (2009). The utility of the Generalized Anxiety Disorder Severity Scale (GADSS) with older adults in primary care. *Depression and Anxiety*, *26*(1), E10–E15. doi: 10.1002/da.20520

Wisocki, P. A. (1988). Worry as a phenomenon relevant to the elderly. *Behavior Therapy*, *19*, 369–379.

Wisocki, P. (1994). The experience of worry among the elderly. In G. Davey, & F. Tallis (Eds.), *Worrying: Perspectives on theory, assessment and treatment*. New York, NY: Wiley.

Wisocki, P., Handen, B., & Morse, C. (1986). The Worry Scale as a measure of anxiety among homebound and community active elderly. *The Behavior Therapist*, *9*, 91–95.

Yehuda, R., Elkin, A., Binder-Brynes, K., Kahana, B., Southwick, S., Schmeidler, J., et al. (1996). Dissociation in aging Holocaust survivors. *Am J Psychiatry, 153*(7), 935–940. Retrieved August 4, 2009, from http://ajp.psychiatryonline.org/cgi/content/abstract/153/7/935

Yehuda, R., Kahana, B., Schmeidler, J., Southwick, S., Wilson, S., & Giller, E. (1995). Impact of cumulative lifetime trauma and recent stress on current posttraumatic stress disorder symptoms in holocaust survivors. *Am J Psychiatry, 152*(12), 1815–1818. Retrieved August 2, 2009, from http://ajp.psychiatryonline.org/cgi/content/abstract/152/12/1815

CHAPTER

3

Psychotherapy with Older Adults: The Importance of Assessment

Lee Hyer[1], Catherine Yeager[2], Renee Hyer[1], Ciera Scott[1]

[1] *Mercer School of Medicine, Macon, GA, USA*

[2] *Essex County Hospital Center, Institute of Mental Health Policy, Research and Treatment, Cedar Grove, NJ, USA*

Assessment is an eminent theoretical process which requires a weighting of this and a disqualifying of that across the idiosyncrasies and commonalities of methods and data sources through multiple iterations of hypothesis generation and testing. The ideal result is a "theory of the client," a theory in which every loose end has been tied up in a logic so compelling that it seems to follow from a logic of the client's own psyche, so convincing that one gets the feeling that things could not be otherwise.

Ted Millon

Ten years ago the chapter in this book on assessment for older adults surveyed the common psychotherapy constructs and softly evaluated the then reasonable universe of outcomes as they apply to psychotherapy. In the past decade there have been several reviews on psychotherapy (e.g., Ayers, Sorrell, Thorp, & Wetherell, 2007; Wetherell, Lenze, & Stanley, 2005), a spate of studies, largely in primary care on anxiety and depression (e.g., Arean, Hegel, Vannoy, Fan, & Unutzer, 2008; Stanley et al., 2009), several cognitive training studies (e.g., Rebok et al., 2008), and a broadening of outcomes to consider, including functioning and quality of life (e.g., Scogin et al., 2005) in various treatment settings. About these and others, Gatz (2007) noted that "the older adult in mental distress can very likely be helped" (p. 52). There is then a lot to say and in this chapter we must truncate and delimit.

In the past two decades there have been major changes in the psychotherapy of older adults. No longer is the stance fixed in which the therapist knows all and the client is ignorant and needs the therapist to tell him or her what to do; no longer is it the case that only techniques or manuals are helpful; no longer is it true that common factors are not important or that we have codified winners in therapy; no longer is it acceptable that measurable outcomes are unimportant; and no longer is it so that medication is superior to the psychotherapies. Our challenge in 2010 is what works in the interface of psychotherapy and medication: are additive, synergistic, or attenuation models viable?

In this chapter we address the core disorders of depression, anxiety, dementia, somatic issues, and caregiving as they relate to psychotherapy for older adults. We intentionally ignore other promising areas of person change at late-life, like disruptive behavior in dementia, sleep, pain, as well as positive aging. Our focus is assessment and we will highlight measures that mark outcomes and process in therapy, both psychosocial and medical. The issue of outcome has a rich tradition in psychotherapy and, in 2010, it has taken on a renewed importance. In this chapter we consider outcomes as they are portrayed in comparative studies and ones that apply to individuals in therapy.

We believe strongly that a focus on the immediate outcome alone is shortsighted and does little to inform about process changes over time. Therefore, we tier our efforts and address the total picture of

Handbook of Assessment in Clinical Gerontology. DOI: 10.1016/B978-0-12-374961-1.10003-X

the older adult in psychotherapy: both the longer view of the importance of psychotherapy, and general as well as more focused outcomes. Context is requisite. Specifically, this chapter addresses assessment in psychotherapy with an emphasis on the research base and rationale for assessment. Then we consider the nuances of testing older adults from the perspective of the therapeutic relationship. We discuss psychometric issues related to older adults. We then present typical measures used in psychotherapy research and in everyday therapy. We also consider the core elements of psychotherapy, such as alliance and readiness for therapy, among others. We end with a discussion of the important role of caregivers and of attention to cultural influences; and we provide a model for thinking about older adults in psychotherapy. An illustrative case is presented as well.

RESEARCH AND PSYCHOTHERAPY

> *Psychologists rely on scientifically and professionally derived knowledge when making scientific or professional judgments or when engaging in scholarly or professional endeavors.*
>
> **(APA Standard 1.06: American Psychological Association, 1992)**

In medicine, the issue of care involves the best interventions/medicines for treating the disease; in psychotherapy, treatment is more complex, involving the relentless complexity of the person. Evidence-based practice (EBP) has mostly taken over from evidence-based treatments (EBTs) and is defined as "the integration of the best available research with clinical expertise in the context of client characteristics, culture and preferences" (APA, 2006, p. 273). The three pillars of EBTs include a research base, clinical expertise, and client characteristics (e.g., culture, and client's preferences) (Institute of Medicine, 2004). The "culture wars" (Messer, 2004) surrounding this topic come honestly to the table of debate with a long past but, more precisely, a short history.

In recent years there has been an explosion in the number of articles that invoke EBT or EBP. Several APA divisions have embraced EBPs to include therapeutic relationships (Norcross, 2002), clinical assessment (Hunsley, Crabb, & Mash, 2004), and principles of change (Castonguay & Beutler, 2006). Moreover, the American Psychiatric Association, especially the American Association of Geriatric Psychiatry (Lyketsos et al., 2006), has published practice guidelines in recent years on a number of psychiatric disorders and more exacting interventions. Wampold (2001), no stranger to the dialog on the efficacy of psychotherapy, highlighted, perhaps as close to a consensus as possible regarding psychotherapies for older adults:

> *... all psychotherapies are instances of the contextual model, and therefore, all treatments should produce equivalent outcomes. That is, all bona fide treatments should possess the proper context and common factors necessary to produce beneficial outcomes...*

Psychotherapy research has done this to itself. As a science, research targets internal validity of the intervention, first and foremost. In that way, we can know that any competing causes of change are ruled out. We eliminate confounds by attempting to hold all constant but the independent variable. We also include randomization, "clean" subjects, a fair placebo or alternative therapy, blinded raters, and multiple perspectives of comparison. Given these restrictions, if we find for statistical significance, we must go the next step and dismantle the intervention to learn what factor(s) could account for the difference (e.g., relaxation, extinction, parasympathetic system, attention processes, different cognitions). And, after all this, if we still have a robust therapy, we perform two more steps: (1) examine cost efficiency (is the clinical effect large enough?); and (2) does the intervention work differently on different types of clients? Finally, we must assure that the treatment is *effective.* In other words, does the particular intervention work in this setting? How about other settings? Clearly, validating a unique psychotherapeutic intervention is a long, effortful, and potentially expensive process. Nonetheless, this kind of research must be undertaken in order to demonstrate the efficacy and effectiveness of psychotherapeutic interventions (ESTs), so that psychotherapy can stand toe-to-toe with psychopharmacology in the treatment of mental health problems (Olfson & Marcus, 2009).

There are changes to be considered, however. When dealing with older adults, we are often doing some application of translational research because few psychotherapy interventions have been designed expressly for elders. The translational component involves focusing on the time span of the problem, nature and scope of hypothesis, dose adjustments, and patient population characteristics. Early on in therapy with older individuals, treatment is titrated. This includes a timeframe that is short, hypotheses that are narrow in scope, small doses of the intervention, close monitoring of suicide potential, and choosing narrow treatment targets. In later phases of treatment, there is the requisite alteration in goals, which are simplified for reality's sake. Psychotherapies are never just pure techniques to be used off-the-shelf. As this process has unfolded over the years, however, efforts to document the applicability of all-purpose psychotherapy research data appears to be relevant to older adults if practiced in an aging-informed manner (Hinrichsen, 2008).

Outcomes then matter, and with older adults outcomes are complex. The issue is never just symptom abatement. Rather, therapy should aim at symptom relief *and* improving overall quality of life (QoL). Moreover, although evaluation questions necessarily focus on the reasons why an elder is seeking treatment, such a narrow focus is not helpful for understanding process changes over time, or other longer-term and broader concerns. In translating ESTs to older adults, and in targeting this to the most researched psychotherapy, Cognitive Behavioral Therapy (CBT), we must concentrate on more general outcomes (e.g., diagnosis), as well as specific markers associated with the identified problem. For the treatment of depression, for example, CBT will involve the alteration of cognitions to reduce depressive symptomatology. With older adults, however, the therapy also demands a scientific attitude, a skillful and flexible delivery of services, quantitative monitoring of the client's progress, and an awareness of the personal, interpersonal, and cultural characteristics of the client, as well as QoL themes.

We suggest here that, for elders, the efficacy of change also resides in the common factor details: the context of therapy. Reality constraints on outcome that cannot be easily captured by research include: the client's readiness to change; acceptability of the treatment and preferences of the client; caregiver acceptance; availability of desired or needed services; probability of third party payer approval; tolerance of incongruous recommendations; prior treatment failures or successes; and side effects. Hence, with older adults, the big three components of therapy—research, clinical experience, and client characteristics—are added to by generic psychotherapy markers for adequate outcome coverage.

Moreover, we believe that psychotherapy outcomes need to be multimodal and comprehensive, both at the broad and specific levels. Perhaps we may reach the point where the line between assessment and therapy becomes artificial and they meld into one. But for now, different outcomes provide very different information, even in long-term care facilities where residents with diabetes, for example, have different end points from those with physical disabilities and depression (Degenholtz, Rosen, Castle, Mittal, & Liu, 2008). We know that the basic psychometrics of any assessment scale are not an integral feature of the measurement instrument; rather it is a product of the context and population in which it was produced. In short, one can argue that all therapy and assessment is both general and local.

WHY ASSESS BASELINE FUNCTIONING AND OUTCOMES?

Psychological assessment has been under siege for sometime by third party payers and others who argue that it lacks sufficient empirical support for improving diagnostic accuracy or treatment outcomes, and is no more informative than those data gleaned from the clinical interview (see Eisman et al., 2000; Kubiszyn et al., 2000). Psychologists themselves have complained that psychological assessment, especially neuropsychological assessment, is too complicated, time-intensive, and expensive (Piotrowski, 1999; Turchik, Karpenko, Hammers & McNamara, 2007), in spite of the fact that a well-constructed multi-method assessment can provide invaluable diagnostic and treatment planning information, as well as shorten treatment time by highlighting issues for targeted intervention (Groth-Marnat, 2003). Only recently, in response to lobbying by APA and its affiliates, have billing codes been altered to permit psychologists to be more fully remunerated for psychological assessment. Meyer et al. (1999) and Kubiszyn and colleagues (2000) present a thorough review of relevant research supporting the empirical validity and clinical utility of psychological assessment.

Psychological assessment is at least as valid as most medical tests (Meyer et al., 2001). As a prelude to and follow-up after psychotherapy, psychological assessment can enhance the therapeutic process in several ways, including:

1) the delineation of clinical symptomatology;
2) hypothesis testing and decision-making regarding differential diagnoses;
3) assisting in case formulation;
4) predicting a client's ability to participate, as well as their degree of participation in psychotherapy;
5) predicting health care utilization;
6) hypothesis testing for therapy impasses or looming therapy failure;
7) monitoring treatment effects over time;
8) the confirmation (or disconfirmation) of perceived psychotherapy outcomes;
9) improving prediction of relapse; and
10) enabling the clinician to respond to managed care and other external pressures.

The most common method that psychologists use for clinical data collection is the unstructured interview, coupled with informal observation (Mash & Foster, 2001; Mash & Hunsley, 1993; Meyer et al., 2001). As we noted early in this chapter, humans are relentlessly complex beings, so these methods, although seemingly time-efficient, can have significant limitations. In fact, Fennig and colleagues (1994) long ago showed that diagnoses derived from clinical interviews alone agreed only about 50% of the time with diagnoses derived from multi-method assessments. In short, our reliance on using one clinician and one source of information (i.e., patient interview) to generate a diagnosis may well create an unreliable and erroneous understanding of the patient.

Indeed, there are a number of shortcomings associated with unstructured, single method approaches to information gathering. First, reliance solely on the unstructured interview can mislead clinicians into overlooking potentially important areas of distress or dysfunction while focusing too much on others (e.g., the chief complaint). A second shortcoming is the clients themselves, who may be poor historians, have issues to hide from the assessor, or have personality characteristics that bias their self-presentation. Third, if the clinician's therapy objectives are at odds with those of the client, or if the client lacks motivation for psychotherapy, the interview will almost invariably be unrevealing. Fourth, certain neuropsychiatric conditions, such as anosognosia, amnesia or confabulation, paranoia, or delusions and other subtle psychotic symptoms, interfere with the accurate reporting of information. This is especially true with regard to elders who may present with occult cognitive problems that cloud or distort the history and clinical picture. On the other hand, using a semi-structured clinical interview alone (e.g., Structured Clinical Interview for DSM-IV Axis I Disorders [SCID; First & Gibbon, 2004]), can mislead the clinician into focusing too much on the yes/no response to the question at hand and ignoring clues that point to less obvious biopsychosocial inputs to the symptom picture. Multi-method assessments, in contrast, enable the clinician to "deconstruct" the client in terms of cognitive/neuropsychological, personality, and behavioral/functional contributions to the chief complaint using standardized, quantifiable, norm-referenced tests coupled with self-report and input from significant others.

There is also the need, however, for care and accuracy when using multiple measures so that one does not miss the forest for the trees. In the main, tests are often sensitive but not very specific, so sound clinical judgment is vital in "reconstructing" the person from multiple sources of data. One must be especially prudent when assessing older adults because there often can be a serious disconnect between raters on target symptoms or behaviors, even when markers are quite specific. For example, when one compares depression ratings on the Geriatric Depression Scale (GDS; Yesavage, et al., 1982) for a client with cognitive decline, clients and caregivers part company on just about every item. Similarly, in dementia, caregivers almost always overrate problems while patients generally underrate them (i.e., anosognosia). Regarding functional assessments, caregivers and clients also are at odds, with the caregiver typically reporting that the client is less functional than what the client perceives to be true.

In late life, constructs interact in ways that are not problematic at younger ages. For example, cross-sectional investigations generally support the hypothesis that the presence and severity of anxiety in an older adult is associated with lower cognitive performance. An older adult who is anxious has a reasonable probability of having cognitive problems as well, especially in processing speed and/or executive functioning. Longitudinal studies that took into account baseline performance levels showed that clinically significant anxiety predicted accelerated cognitive decline (e.g., Sinoff & Werner, 2003). Comorbid depression and generalized anxiety also are special problems to attend to in the assessment of older adults. It now appears that there is reasonable, even probable, likelihood that the brain is involved, either subtly as in working memory dysfunction, or more globally as in an under-active prefrontal cortex and disinhibited amygdala (Beaudreau & O'Hara, 2008). As such, a thorough pre-therapy assessment for the elder who presents with depression and/or anxiety is vital for understanding the full complement of issues that may be playing a role in the chief complaint.

Psychological assessment also can be a rich short-term therapeutic intervention in its own right. Regardless of age, sharing test results with the client has been found to increase hope and motivation to change, increase self-awareness, decrease the sense of aloneness and isolation with one's condition, confirm one's self-efficacy, and enhance the therapeutic alliance (Finn & Butcher, 1991). Caregivers and family members who participate in the assessment process also benefit from testing feedback; they, too, can experience a healthier appreciation of their loved one's strengths and weaknesses, and are empowered to meet their loved one's needs in a more compassionate, competent, and realistic way. Finn and Tonsager (1997; 2002) describe a major goal of the "therapeutic" style of assessment as making it possible for clients to leave the assessor's office having gained new information or experiences about themselves that will increase hope and facilitate change. This point has not escaped the personality-based (Millon & Bloom, 2008) or case-based (Persons, 2006) therapy formulations that depend on buy-in from the older patient. One also cannot discount the placebo effect here.

To make the assessment process therapeutic, the assessor must not only develop an empathic connection with the client, but also create a collaborative environment in which the client (and caregiver) is encouraged to actively participate in answering the questions that brought them to the office in the first place. Testing older adults requires special sensitivity toward this cohort's suspicion of mental health providers in general and toward the strangeness of undergoing performance and personality testing specifically (Karlin & Duffy, 2004). When used therapeutically, the tests serve to stimulate discussion about the client's self-perceived strengths and weaknesses, as well as their response patterns to novel or problematic situations.

Although the need for standard administration is respected, older adults are often confused by the assessment process, test instructions, or test items. Furthermore, elders, who may be anxious and who may feel disrespected by an "all business" professional stance, will indeed be put off by a strictly standard administration that doesn't allow for interjections by the client or caregiver, or explanation and encouragement by the assessor. As such, nonstandard test administration is often necessary to draw out the client's best performance, as well as gain an accurate understanding of the ways in which symptoms or deficits get in the way of day-to-day functioning.

There are, additionally, benefits for the psychologist who uses the assessment process as a therapeutic intervention. Test results are no longer a composite of scores reflecting performance in light of age-based norms. Rather, you now *know* your client, and can make a difference in their experience of the world and of the self (see Hyer, Molinari, Mills, & Yeager, 2008).

PSYCHOTHERAPY MEASURES

All models are wrong; some are useful.

John Tukey

The criteria for change in psychotherapy have been variously defined. We have alluded to the traditional method: it evaluates the null hypothesis on therapy groups adjusted for power. In the past two decades, however, other methods have been put to use, such as that of Jacobson and Truax (1991), and Borkovec and Costello (1993), who require more change for successful end-state functioning. This latter method requires the post-treatment score to be within one standard deviation of the normalized mean on each outcome measure. This would be done pre- and post-therapy. In addition, Hamadi et al. (2007) recommend that the person show a decrease from pretest scores on at least three-quarters of standard outcome measures (e.g., Beck Depression Inventory—BDI-II) to demonstrate clinically significant change, and have a remission of the DSM (American Psychiatric Association, 2000) diagnoses established at entry into therapy.

Recently, a "movement" has begun that attempts to optimize the tripartite model of psychopathology: negative affect, positive affect, and physiological reaction (Mineka, Watson, & Clark, 1998). This model is tied to a dimensional approach to patient classification in lieu of the DSM system in which core components of the tripartite variables share factors across disorders. Brown, Antony, and Barlow (1995) found, for example, that patients who receive CBT for panic disorder also experience a decline in comorbidities over the course of treatment. The general trend in the past two decades of excessive comorbidities, frequent NOS diagnoses, and problems with subsyndromal domains have presented the DSM-V committees with the challenge to be more dimensional in the diagnostic and more encompassing in their approach. The tripartite model (Watson, Wiese, Vaidya, & Tellegen, 1999) explicates this process, holding that many psychiatric disorders are attached to negative affect, positive affect, and physiological reactions to varying degrees. In effect, these three dimensions can account for pathology better than diagnoses.

The transdiagnostic model addresses this. Brown and Barlow (2005) held that all emotional disorders have a similar underlying structure and there is a unified approach to treating depression/anxiety. Patients with depression and anxiety especially are served well by this model. This model holds that a single negative affective (NA) vulnerability factor influences the development of an anxiety disorder and depression. Individuals high in NA increase the likelihood of negative life events, have high levels of physical and mental health problems, are prone to multiple Axis I and Axis II disorders, and have multiple negative lifestyle habits (Lahey, 2009). NA individuals undergo multiple learning experiences that promote problems (fears and depression) that eventuate in comorbidity. Day-to-day, these individuals are excessively irritable, sad, anxious, self-consciousness, and vulnerable—out of proportion to circumstances. A good intervention protocol would therefore indicate a multimodal approach, including psychoeducation, cognitive restructuring, breathing retraining, exposure, and self-monitoring, regardless of the presenting DSM diagnosis. Procedurally, a case-driven formulation under the umbrella of the transdiagnostic model is given to patients using parallel care strategies (not serial) and a holistic understanding of the person.

Obviously, mental disorders are not discrete events. Most psychological phenomena can be better described and understood according to a dimensional model. Older patients especially experience a high rate of comorbid symptoms. The presence of subsyndromal conditions also is robust and produces uncommonly poor outcomes for older adults (Chopra, et al., 2005). This is especially apt for the rather common presentation in late-life of depression and anxiety mixed with somatic concerns. The effort of including an Axis II presence in this taxonomy has yet to be adequately evaluated. The question also arises: What should assessment in psychotherapy really measure? Is it more theoretically oriented (e.g., CBT and attributions) or general symptom-based (e.g., functional outcomes) (Lambert & Lambert, 1999)?

So, the assessment of psychotherapy outcomes is tiered, global, symptom-based, and target-specific. In cognitive behavioral therapy (CBT), for example, evidence suggests that adjustment can be measured by quality of life (QoL) or overall adjustment scales; depression by a focused psychological measure like the BDI-II; and target-specific in the form of scales unique to cognitive change. In CBT, cognitive change is associated with changes in depressive symptomatology, for the prevention of relapse, and for quality of life. This unique therapy then requires specific assessments if it is applied.

Measurement of psychotherapy outcomes must have acceptable psychometric properties. Table 3.1 presents common assessment measures used in psychotherapy. We begin with recommended measures for depression and general anxiety for older adults. Fortunately, where older adults are concerned, most of the

Table 3.1 Model Tests Applied in Clinic Settings*

Session	Depression: Recommended Instruments	Anxiety: Recommended Instruments
Initial session	HAM-D MINI MADRS BDI-II/GDS Beck Hopelessness Scale GSIS MBMD MoCA and/or RBANS Stroop Color Word Test ADCS-ADL, FAQ QoL	ADIS-IV-L MINI Penn State Worry Scale MBMD MoCA and/or RBANS Stroop Color Word Test ADCS/FAQ QoL
Each Session	BDI-II, GDS QoL	Penn State Worry Scale QoL
Discharge Session	HAM-D MADRS BDI-II/GDS MINI QoL	Penn State Worry Scale HAM-A/HARS ADIS-IV-L MINI QoL
Follow-up assessment	MINI MADRS BDI-II HAM-D	MINI HAM-A/HARS Penn State Worry Scale

**Hamilton Depression Scale (HAMD), MINI International Neurospsychiatric Interview (MINI), Montgomery Asberg Depression Rating Scale (MADRS), Beck Depression Inventory-II (BDI-II), Geriatric Depression Scale (GDS), Millon Behavioral Medical Diagnostic (MBMD), Montreal Cognitive Assessment (MoCA), RBANS-Repeated Battery for the Assessment of Neurological Status (RBANS), Quality of Life (QoL), Anxiety Disorder Interview Scale-Lifetime (ADIS–L), Hamilton Anxiety Scale (HAMA), Hamilton Anxiety Rating Scale (HARS), General Suicide Index Scale (GSIS), Alzheimer's Disease Cooperative Studies Scale–Activities of Daily Living (ADCS–ADL), Functional Assessment Questionnaire (FAQ)* measures that apply to younger adults have applicability to them. Differences have to do with norms or with constructs that require an aging emphasis. As for the former, we do not yet have adequate norms on symptom-based measures to assert that clinical significance represents some measure of change. As for the latter, the constructs relevant to aging are many and change even as a function of young old to oldest old.

The measurement and treatment of specific anxiety disorders (e.g., panic, agoraphobia, PTSD, OCD, and phobias) in older adults is not very different from that applied to younger adults. Regarding depression and generalized anxiety, however, the measures of older adults demand more consideration. While the factor structure of both constructs remains similar across ages (Blazer, 2003), there are differing cutoff points and different features unique to each. Depressed older adults, for example, have less irritability and negative cognitions, but show more sleep and health problems. In Table 3.1 we provide a listing of measures that can serve for the initial session and diagnoses, as well as markers for change. In the initial session we establish the diagnoses, its severity, and possible related problems, such as treatment issues (e.g., MBMD), suicidal thinking (GSIS), and function (IADLs). We also establish the possible existence of cognitive problems with a short battery that subserves multiple domains. Each session then can apply short forms of these scales that are sensitive to change. Monthly measures also can be applied to assure the status of the diagnosis and symptom severity. Discharge and follow-up sessions largely do the same. The hope is that the patient will be diagnosis-free and have a substantial reduction in symptom severity (Hamadi et al., 2007).

Table 3.2 outlines more general and specific psychotherapy goals, as well as measures for typical depressive or anxious older patients. This table is worth paying attention to because it targets specific sub-goals and measures for change that would apply to a given case formulation. Outcomes then would be very different given general and specific goals. These have special merit to older adults.

Practically speaking, effective therapy for older adults does not involve a strict interpretation of a manualized program, even if that program is empirically supported. The therapist shall not rely on one treatment approach for a given set of symptoms, but, rather, reviews the range of possible strategies and tactics and applies them to a given client. A goal attainment map can be formulated for the individual that includes potential intervention strategies, treatment targets, and ultimate outcomes. What is most important here is that for each goal there is a goal-specific assessment tool (e.g., PES for the target of increasing positive reinforcement) and goal-specific potential interventions (e.g., behavior activation) that is focused, monitored, and collaborative. Here, empirical research gives way to real world practice in the actual foxhole of the clinical situation. Whereas researchers can respond to uncertainty with abstraction and curiosity, practitioners must resolve uncertainty through action.

Several omnibus measures are often applied in research related to older adults both as a screen and as an outcome measure (see Table 3.3). These relate to general functioning, psychiatric problems, QoL, health, and coping. Importantly, these measures can be summed or disaggregated and applied for general or specific purposes. These measures also provide reasonable reliability as the structure of the interview or self-report allows for feedback and checking. The cost of in-depth information is always an issue with these shorter general measures (bandwidth versus fidelity). Again, any measurement instrument is a product of the context in which it was produced, and these scales were not originally developed on older adults. Also, it is worth mentioning that these and most other measures suffer when we are interested in retrospective events related to the psychopathology.

We note too that several other measures have been consistently applied to outcome studies related to older adults. These include the Montgomery-Asberg Depression Rating Scale (MADRS); the Generalized Anxiety Disorder Symptoms Scale (GADSS); Clinician Administered PTSD Scale (CAPS); Psychiatric Diagnostic Screening Questionnaire (PDSQ); and Personal Health Questionnaire (PHQ-9), among many others. Finally, we note that there are several other structured or semi-structured measures that address the DSM for Axis I diagnoses (e.g., ADIS, DIS, SADS, SCID), which have high kappa coefficients for the general population.

Table 3.2 Psychotherapy Goals and Assessment Interventions*

Depression

1. Decrease dysfunctional thinking
   Goal-specific assessment tools (ATQ, DAS)
   Goal-specific interventions (PST)
2. Improve problem solving
   Goal-specific assessment tools (PSI)
   Goal-specific interventions (PST)
3. Improve self-control skills
   Goal-specific assessment tools (SCQ)**
   Goal-specific potential interventions (PST, SCT)
4. Improve rates of positive reinforcement
   Goal-specific assessment tools (PES)
   Goal-specific potential interventions (Behavioral Activation)
5. Enhance social and interpersonal skills
   Goal-specific assessment tools (Inter Events Schedule)
   Goal-specific potential interventions (social skills training, assertiveness)

Also decrease suicidal ideation, reduce stress, improve marital relationships, improve physical health, decrease relapse

Generalized Anxiety Disorder (GAD)

1. Alter maladaptive metacognitions
   Goal-specific assessment tools (ATI, Why Worry Scale)
   Goal-specific interventions (Cognitive restructuring, PST, Mindfulness)
2. Decrease intolerance of uncertainty
   Goal-specific assessment tools (Intolerance of Uncertainty Scale)
   Goal-specific interventions (PST, self-monitoring, stimulus control)
3. Decrease avoidant behavior
   Goal-specific assessment tools (SUDS, BAT)
   Goal-specific potential interventions (Exposure, Behavioral experiments, Interpersonal strategies)
4. Decrease physical symptoms of anxiety
   Goal-specific assessment tools (Relaxation measures)
   Goal-specific potential interventions (Relaxation, self-control desensitization, sleep hygiene)
5. Enhance time management skills
   Goal-specific assessment tools (Calendar monitoring)
   Goal-specific potential interventions (Assertiveness)

Other goals include decrease stress, increase self-efficacy, decrease need for medications

**Extrapolated from Nezu, Nezu, and Lombardo, 2004: Automatic Thought Questionnaire (ATQ), Dysfunctional Attitude Scale (DAS), Problem Solving Inventory (PSI), Problem Solving Therapy (PST), Self-Control Questionnaire (SCQ), Self-Control Therapy (SCT), Pleasant Events Schedule (PES), Anxious Thoughts Inventory (ATI), Subjective Units of Distress Scale (SUDS), Behavioral Avoidance Test (BAT)*

***Self-Control Questionnaire (SCQ) is in Appendix A*

Finally, we focus our attention on constructs of psychotherapy research that are directly applicable to the phenomenon of therapy. Constructs integral to psychotherapy are now more refined and operationalized with improved psychometric properties. Psychotherapy variables have blossomed beyond initial therapy notions of transference and counter-transference. They now include the working alliance, readiness for treatment, therapist allegiance and skills, common factors, therapeutic bond, patient enactment and reception, treatment fidelity, and cognitive skills, among others. Aging-related alterations involve the nuancing of these variables. To this are added other mediators of therapy such as problem complexity, readiness to change/motivation, potential to resist therapeutic intervention, social support,

Table 3.3 Generic Measures in Psychotherapy Outcome Studies

Measure	Content	Reliability	Comment
General Health Questionnaire (GHQ)	60 items for severity of psychiatric symptoms	0.8 test–retest	15 minutes self-report; Problem is under-reporting
Symptom Checklist-90-Revised (SCL-90-R)	90 items for general psychopathology and subscales	0.7–0.85 test–retest	20 minute self-report, not disorder based
Multidimensional Health Profile–Psychosocial Functioning	58 items assessing mental health, social resources, stress, and coping	0.7–0.8 test–retest	20 minute brief screen for primary care
Medical Outcomes Study 36*	36 items for social functioning, body pain, mental health, roles, vitality, general health	0.8 test–retest	10 minutes assess medical (and mental health) outcomes; Likert scale
Behavior and Symptom Identification Scale*	32 items assessing symptoms and functional abilities	0.7–0.8 test–retest	10 minutes with excellent use for inpatient and outpatient settings
Treatment Outcome Package	Depression, anxiety, thought problems, paranoid ideas	0.8 test–retest	20–30 minutes self-report; useful for OPT settings; based on DSM-IV
Mini-International Neuropsychiatric Interview (MINI)	Comprehensive DSM criteria	High inter-rater reliability (kappas)	15–20 minutes; training necessary
Primary Care Evaluation of Mental Disorders	Matched to DSM-IV, generates specific diagnoses	Inter-rater reliability is suspect	10–20 minutes; inadequate provision of accurate diagnoses

**in Appendix A*

coping styles, and patient strengths. Morey (1996) provides a taxonomy of treatment process indices for patients—friendliness, likeability, motivation, psychological mindedness, conscientiousness factors, self-discipline, impulse control, defensive style, internalization, empathy, paternal factors, and social supports.

Table 3.4 provides a partial listing of variables relevant to the phenomenology of psychotherapy, broken down by therapist and client. These constructs have been in the foreground of therapy for many years. Unfortunately, the EST movement relegated them to a less relevant status until very recently. It is estimated that these variables account for approximately 30% of the variance of change in psychotherapy (Norcross, Koocher, & Hogan, 2008). This figure is not known, however, when the psychotherapy of older adults is at issue. Nonetheless, we believe their value is significant (Hyer, Kramer, & Sohnle, 2004). The following factors are also important: (1) the extent to which the therapist is age-informed and motivated; (2) the extent to which the client expects results and is positively attuned to the therapist; (3) the extent to which health literacy and compliance are addressed and supported; and (4) the extent to which the elder is willing to do off-session tasks; to these extents the chance of change is maximized, considerably more so than for younger age groups.

A MODEL OF OLDER ADULTS IN PSYCHOTHERAPY

So far we have discussed the various types of measures applied in psychotherapy. What is central to this effort is the ability to form a case formulation, manage the client, and assess the outcomes. Client-focused research (e.g., Howard, Moras, Brill, Martinovich, & Lutz, 1996; Lambert et al., 2001) aims to

Table 3.4 Psychotherapy Constructs Related to the Therapy Session

Key Client Factors	Key Therapist Factors
Therapeutic alliance*	Empathy
Stages of change*	Positive regard
Expectations	Feedback
Personality disorders	Therapeutic counter-transference
Insight*	
Motivation	
Resistance	

Working Alliance Inventory (for client and therapist), University of Rhode Island Change Assessment and Clinical Insight Rating Scale are in Appendix A

predict the course of individual patients' progress in psychotherapy (i.e., usually by decreases in symptom intensity) on the basis of their initial characteristics or on the basis of change over a brief period in therapy. In regard to the latter point, Lambert et al. (2003) demonstrated beneficial effects of simply providing feedback on patients' progress relative to their baseline and established trajectories. There are also markers of change that focus on sudden gains, positive treatment alliance, and readiness or motivation in therapy, among others (see Hyer & Intrieri, 2006).

In a multidimensional framework of case management, patient-related variables, environmental variables, the temporal dimension, and the functional dimension are core features. Nezu, Nezu, and Lombardo (2004) have developed one model, a *Clinical Pathogenesis Map* that outlines in a path analysis or causal modeling diagram the individual components of a patient's problem state. The elements include distal variables, antecedent variables, organismic variables, response variables, and consequences. This is a hypothesis-testing model of care that is based on the case formulation in which the therapist and client attempt to verify (confirm or disconfirm) the model. Under this model a variety of treatment tactics and strategies can be validated. The operative word is "validated," as this component becomes testable by selected interventions. These can include exposure, guided imagery, covert conditioning, and the like. The efficacy of any of these techniques is dependent on the unique characteristics and responses of the patient. Fortunately, there is a set number of empirically applied tactics that are used for different DSM problem states.

One other therapy model, espoused by Norcross et al. (2008), is the PICO model (Patient, Intervention, Comparison, and Outcome). This model provides a throughput for dialog about the operative issues in the therapy process. Patient variables (background, abilities, desires, etc.) are matched with interventions that are chosen in a sea of options (comparison) with outcomes defined. This model provides a holistic and ongoing approach that incorporates a body of data, multiple problems, failed treatment attempts, and collaborative assessment.

As we've argued in this chapter, assessment is important at all stages of therapy (see Table 3.1), but especially at entry. The PICO model allows for a refined formulation of the case and the necessary follow-up of intervention effects. It also provides feedback for all parties, as well as allowing for a convenient method for patient input and buy-in. Table 3.5 provides data on this model.

CAREGIVERS

The term "caregiving" implies a wide range of activities from overall management of the patient, medication input, appointments, ADL/IADL negotiation, to a focus on surrogate issues of choice at the

Table 3.5 PICO Model of Psychotherapy

	Ask Yourself:	Include in Your Inquiry	Assessment Choices
P (Patient)	Who is the patient? Who is the caregiver? What is the population of interest? Specific concerns?	Patient's primary complaint and background Collateral information Cognition/pain/sleep/ medical issues/QoL, etc.	SCID, ADIS-IV MINI RBANS/Pain scale/ESS/ Charlson Comorbidity Index
I (Intervention)	What are you planning to do?	Assessment and treatment	Monitor change; GDS, BDI, STAI. PSWQ, Other scales (e.g., EF, sleep, pain)
C (Comparison)	Is there an alternative to your Rx?	The alternative treatments, if any	Comparator outcomes
O (Outcome)	What is the planned outcome?	Specific outcomes	Evaluate changes pre- and post-treatment

end of life. This term was barely known 30 years ago. Research over this period has shown that the care process in dementia is critical, and it is both dynamic and challenging (Aneshensel, Pearlin, Mullan, Zarit, & Whilatch, 1995; Max, Webber, & Fox, 1995; Pruchno, Kleban, Michaels, & Dempsey, 1990; Wright, Clipp, & George, 1993). Caregivers of individuals with dementia often experience high levels of stress, and it is not uncommon for them to experience depression and anxiety symptoms as well (Schultz et al., 2008; Yeager, Hyer, Hobbs, & Coyne, 2010). Percentages of common problems can reach as high as 50% for caregivers (Williamson & Schultz, 1993). In fact, in addition to burden, estimates show that 40–70% of caregivers of older adults with various medical conditions experience clinically significant depressive symptoms, with approximately one-quarter to one-half of caregivers meeting criteria for a depressive disorder (Zarit, 2006). There is reasonable evidence, too, that older caregivers, who are mostly female, and spouses with health problems are especially at risk (see Mausbach et al., 2006).

Two core issues come to mind when working with an older adult with a caregiver. The first involves assessment of the caregiver regarding the identified patient. As noted, caregiving is commonly associated with depression and burden, especially when both the carer and care receiver are older adults. The usual measures related to caregiving are caregiver burden, caregiver/care receiver relationship, ADL and IADL ratings of the care receiver, and, increasingly, scales related to the care receiver's executive functioning, such as FAQ and the DAD. In addition, depression and anxiety markers also are highly relevant for caregiver status and should be applied. Norms need to be adjusted for at least age, but also for gender and ethnicity, and perhaps for education. Perhaps local norms are best, as these can easily be developed after assessing approximately 100 cases.

The second issue concerns the caregiver role and what we know as it relates to the carer's health status and therapy with the identified patient. Recent studies demonstrate that if the caregiver is depressed, the identified patient becomes depressed and more impaired (Schulz et al., 2008). The added burden of the care receiver's cognitive deterioration has been attributed to increased problems in caregiving over the course of a day and the degree of assistance needed for basic and complex activities of daily living (Russo & Vitaliano, 1995). In their meta-analysis, Pinquart and Sörenson (2003) found that patient behavior problems were more strongly related to caregiver burden than were patient physical and cognitive impairments, the amount of care provided, or duration of caregiving. Furthermore, Vitalino and colleagues (2009) recently showed that the caregiver who is stressed and

Table 3.6 Overall Assessment of Caregiver

Idiographic Assessment—Goal Attainment Markers for the Care Receiver
Core Problems
Burden—Zarit Caregiver Burden Interview* Depression—CES-D, GDS, POMS Anxiety—STAI, BAI Cognition—MoCA*, Revised Memory and Behavior Checklist, reaction-response
Related Constructs
Social support—Perceived Social Support Scale Caregiver health—General Health Questionnaire (GHQ) Coping—especially avoidance—Revised Ways of Coping Scale Quality of Life Scale (WHOQOL) Cultural specificity—language-specific measures
Center for Epidemiological Scale–Depression (CES-D), Geriatric Depression Scale (GDS), Profile of Mood Scale (POMS), State Trait Anxiety Inventory (STAI), Beck Anxiety Inventory (BAI), Montreal Cognitive Assessment (MoCA), WHO Quality of Life (WHOQOL) **Zarit Caregiver Burden Interview and MoCA are in Appendix A*

depressed is at risk for cognitive decline as well as the patient. Assessment may therefore involve more than just the usual markers of burden in caregiving.

One other issue is relevant here: the lack of concordance between caregiver and care receiver is a concern for the practitioner. Estimates of the patient's problems typically result in the caregiver's seeing a worse situation, whereas the care receiver sees less pathology. Extant measures of self-reported patient insight appear to allow for inflated ratings of current functional status (Hyer, Yeager, Shah, Nizam & Coleman, 2007). Often, too, the caregiver can overstate problems because of the lenses of frustration and burden. So, the practitioner must be wary, obtain data from multiple sources over time, and pay attention to outcomes.

Idiographic assessment is most relevant to caregiving as this allows for measurement in each individual setting. Commonly used scales are outlined in Table 3.6. Most studies assess caregiver burden, depression and anxiety, in addition to cognition (see Gallagher-Thompson & Coon, 2007). We also highlight several related constructs that have been used as outcomes for caregivers. Among caregiver studies, the issue of diversity has been an important consideration. The REACH (Resources for Enhancing Alzheimer's Caregivers Health) project addresses this issue specifically and endorses psychoeducation, counseling and multi-component interventions as effective, but these must be tailored to the cultural mores of the carer (see Gallagher-Thompson & Coon, 2007).

TESTING IN DIFFERENT SETTINGS

The treatment setting in which the assessment takes place matters. Increasingly, the variety of settings, from outpatient primary care and outpatient mental health clinic to inpatient medical treatment (including rehabilitation) or psychiatric care, as well as the continuum of older adult living settings (continuing care retirement communities, assisted living, and nursing homes), each have unique features that influence assessment. The primary variables that are associated with different settings are degree of frailty, types of medical comorbidities, and psychiatric intensity. Most important is what is emphasized in each setting, what is possible for treatment, and what are reasonable outcomes in given treatment settings. Cognition is important in all, followed closely by markers of depression, anxiety, somatic problems, and adjustment (overall and functioning).

We briefly address two settings here: primary care and long-term care. These are the most common venues in which mental health issues present, and in some ways are the least understood. Primary care continues to have high psychiatric comorbidities (17–37% for depression alone), which are frequently missed by primary care physicians (Miller et al., 2009). Missed psychiatric diagnoses (false negatives) can be as high as 50%, while false positives are approximately 75%. Proper diagnosis of dementia and anxiety fare no better in these settings. The integration of psychology into primary care is increasingly recommended and effective, especially when focused case management models are applied (see Arean et al., 2008).

Long-term care, both nursing homes and assisted living facilities (ALFs), provides unique settings for assessment. In recent years ALFs have become more like nursing homes in prevalence rates of psychopathology, including dementia. In comparison, nursing homes have fewer numbers of long stay residents, more frail elders, and increased numbers with psychiatric problems (Hyer & Intrieri, 2006). Measures in this setting are increasingly proscribed by insurance and CMS regulations (e.g., Minimum Data Set). All residents must be evaluated by facility staff at set times during the year and these ratings tend to be relatively accurate (Hawes, Phillips, Holan, Sherman, & Hutchison, 2005). Recent reviews on cognition, depression, anxiety, adjustment, and quality of life in long-term care (see Reichman & Katz, 2008) have fostered the use of common measures with careful attention to purpose of testing and norms. Domains of sleep and pain, as well as behavior disruptions, require attention in these settings, because close to 80% of residents will have these problems (Kim & Rovner, 1996). Any evaluation must account for the unique phenomenology of the long-term care setting where activity and sleep are compromised, as well as the fit between the construct measured and requirements to do tasks in a setting where there is considerable help.

CULTURAL DIVERSITY AND ASSESSMENT

> *The combination of emic and etic perspectives we espouse assumes that while the behaviors targeted by the intervention are exhibited across cultures, how persons understand those behaviors and how willing they are to engage in the process of therapy to change the problematic behavior may differ by cultural groups.*
>
> **Domenech-Rodríguez & Wieling, 2004**

The U.S. is ever more ethnically and culturally diverse. Approximately 34% of the population is currently estimated to self-identify as non-white, and ethnic minorities are projected to comprise over 50% of the U.S. by 2050 (U.S. Census Bureau, 2004). Yet, too few EBTs/ESTs have included representative numbers of racial/ethnic minority groups in their study samples. Indeed, in an examination of 379 NIMH sponsored clinical trials, Mak and colleagues (2007) found that fewer than half provided information on the race or ethnicity of their study populations. Among those studies that provided sample demographics in sufficient detail, Caucasians and African Americans tended to be over-represented and all other U.S. racial/ethnic groups were significantly underrepresented. What is more, even among those clinical trials that had substantial sample sizes, there were too few racial/ethnic minority participants to compare their treatment outcomes against those of the white majority. Lack of racial/ethnic diversity in the development of EBPs, as well as inattention to cultural context or social class, is also problematic. For example, of the four evidence-based individual psychotherapies for older adults identified on the National Registry of Evidence-Based Programs and Practices (CBT for Late Life Depression, IMPACT, PROSPECT, Prolonged Exposure Therapy for PTSD), study populations were predominantly white and female (see www.nrepp.samhsa.gov/index.asp).

These and other psychotherapies are designed, then, on the dominant American (white) culture; as such, the change process is conceptualized as occurring within an individual, with outcome measures focused on the individual. Contrast this with what we know about other American ethnocultural groups (e.g., African American, Hispanic/Latino) in which the change process may be better contextualized by including family and community (LaRoche & Christopher, 2008). It is notable that three cognitive–behavioral interventions have been adapted for depressed and/or anxious Latino/Hispanic adults (Escobar et al., 2007) and Asians (Chen, et al., 2007; Hwang, et al., 2006), but there are no data on the transferability of these therapies to older adults. In sum, given the lack of attention to minority group representation in ESTs/EBTs, and EBPs, the practitioner must exercise great caution and care when drawing on ESTs/EBTs to treat racially/ethnically diverse elders.

In practice, all psychotherapy problems are contextualized by culture. Cultural factors, especially ethnicity, gender, age, religious or spiritual beliefs, and education, significantly influence a person's perception of illness. As such, individuals from different cultures will experience and manifest symptoms of mental illness differently, and psychiatric diagnoses will vary across cultures. Cultural factors also affect an elder's decisions about treatment and compliance, as well as serve as moderators for treatment prognostics. The practitioner must therefore carefully consider a client's cultural history, world view, education, preferences for treatment, and, of special significance to older adults, degree of acculturation, when determining how best to intervene psychotherapeutically. Acculturation, which represents the level at which values, language, and cognitive styles are shared within an ethnic community versus those of the dominant culture, is an especially potent variable when developing an assessment and treatment plan (Manley, 2006).

Furthermore, differences continue to exist among ethnic groups in prevalence rates for many psychiatric disorders, as well as treatment outcomes, and in basic issues such as health utilization (Bernal & Domenech-Rodriguez, 2009). The importance of accounting for ethnocultural factors in the diagnostic assessment is emphasized in the DSM (American Psychiatric Association, 2000). Five areas are recommended for consideration, especially for concerns regarding assessment and treatment: (1) the cultural identity of the person (self-identified); (2) a cultural explanation of the individual's disorder; (3) cultural factors related to psychosocial environment and levels of functioning; (4) cultural elements of the relationship between patient and clinician; and (5) overall assessment of diagnosis and care. Likewise, the application of a culturally informed functional analysis has been raised as an important issue for CBT. This applies to race/ethnicity, socioeconomic status/social class, and gender. Tanaka-Matsumi, Seiden, and Lam (1996) have identified eight steps in this effort:

1) Assess cultural identity and degree of acculturation.
2) Assess and evaluate the presenting problems with reference to the client's cultural norms.
3) Evaluate the client's causal attributions regarding their problems.
4) Conduct a functional analysis.
5) Compare one's case formulation with the client's belief system.
6) Negotiate treatment objectives and methods with the client.
7) Discuss with the client the need for data collection to assess treatment progress.
8) Discuss with the client the anticipated treatment duration, course, and expected outcomes.

Measures of acculturation are available for a number of racial/ethnic groups found in the U.S. Some scales are linear; that is, they measure the extent to which an individual has assimilated into the dominant culture. More preferable are bi-linear or, even better, multidimensional scales, which measure both the degree of assimilation and degree to which an individual retains the culture of origin (see Kim, & Abreu, 2001; Zane & Mak, 2003; Zea, Asner-Self, Birman, & Buki, 2003 for reviews). A well-designed acculturation scale measures aspects of behavior, cultural identity, knowledge, language, and, most importantly, values. Zea and colleagues (2003) suggest that the first four factors reflect a more superficial degree of cultural immersion, whereas values are indicative of a deeper degree of cultural identity with either the traditional or host culture. Understanding the client's, and caregiver's, value systems is essential for successful psychotherapy. Table 3.7 lists examples of bilinear and multidimensional scales that have a reasonable evidence base for younger adults. Data on older adults is wanting, however.

Because of the dearth of data regarding the ecological validity of cognitive, personality, and neuropsychological assessment instruments for racial/ethnic minority older adults, Byrd and Manley (2005) suggest that the clinical interview might be the best way to evaluate a minority elder's premorbid level of functioning, current functional status, and cultural norms for functional behaviors (e.g., gender expectations for ADLs, IADLs). Collateral information from the spouse, children, or siblings can be especially helpful here. We also highlight that ethnic minority groups, especially elders, score significantly lower than whites on cognitive and neuropsychological tests, so every effort must be made to use test norms that have been adjusted for age, sex, ethnicity, and education (Nell, 2000).

Furthermore, Manley and colleagues (Manley et al., 1998; Manley, Jacobs, Touradji, Small, & Stern, 2002), as well as Gasquoine (2001), have pointed out that reading grade level and/or degree of bilingualism have more impact on verbal test performance than does educational attainment. Education quality also is important to consider. This is especially true in the case of African Americans who were schooled before versus after the Brown v. Board of Education decision. In a word, literacy and degree of bilingualism should be assessed prior to the administration of any tests. Additionally, bilingual clients should be given the choice of language to be used for testing. However, when the client has only limited English and the clinician does not speak the client's native language, the use of a professional translator trained in assessment techniques or referring out must be considered. The use of untrained interpreters, such as family members or coworkers, can invalidate the assessment and should be avoided.

This section underscores the necessity of a careful selection of measures when assessing racial/ethnic minority elders. This is especially critical for cognitive evaluations. A cognitive screening measure as seemingly simple as the Mini Mental Status Exam (MMSE; Folstein, Folstein & McHugh, 1975) may not be appropriate for some ethnic minority elders. Fillenbaum, Heyman, Huber, Ganguli, and Unverzagt (2001), for example, showed that the specificity of the MMSE for detecting dementia was significantly lower for African Americans (59%) than for whites (94%). False positives may result. Fortunately, some commonly used neuropsychological tests have normative data on different minority groups gleaned from individual studies (see Mitrumshina, Boone, Razani, & D'Elia, 2005; Strauss, Sherman, & Spreen, 2006), but these data, again, must be used with caution because limitations such as small sample sizes, lack of education information, limited age range, and lack of

Table 3.7 Acculturation Scales for Racial and Ethnocultural Minorities*

Racial/Ethnic Group	Acculturation Scales
Any US minority group	Abbreviated Multidimensional Acculturation Scale (AMAS)
Black/African American	African American Acculturation Scale-Revised (AAAS-R)
Asian	Suinn-Lew Asian Self-Identity Acculturation Scale (SL-ASIAN)
	Asian Values Scale-Revised (AVS-R)
Hispanic/Latino	Bicultural Scale for Puerto Ricans
	Acculturation Rating Scale for Mexican-Americans-II (ARSMA-II)
Native American	Tribe-specific measures are recommended

**AAAS-R (Klonoff & Landrine, 2000); SL-ASIAN (Suinn, Knoo, & Ahuna, 1995); AVS-R (Kim & Hong, 2004); Bicultural Scale for Puerto Ricans (Cortéz, Rogler & Malgady, 1994); ARSMA-II (Cuéllar, Arnold & Maldonado, 1995); Native American measures (see Dana, 1993, pp. 128–130); AMAS (Zea et al., 2003)*

co-normed measures are widespread (Byrd & Manley, 2005). Also, Heaton and colleagues (Heaton, Miller, Taylor, & Grant, 2004) have produced a set of age, gender, and education-corrected norms for many traditional neuropsychological tests appropriate for White and African American individuals. Finally, several groups have adapted existing or developed new neuropsychological batteries specifically for Hispanic/Latino clients. They include: the Spanish language version of the Repeatable Battery for the Assessment of Neuropsychological Status (RBANS; Randolph, Tierney, Mohr, & Chase, 1998); Neuropsychological Screening Battery for Hispanics (NeSBHIS; Ponton et al., 1996); Bateria Neuropsychologica en Espanol (Artiola, Fortuny, Hermosillo-Romo, Heaton, & Pardee, 1999). The RBANS also has recently been adapted for Chinese clients (Zhang et al., 2008).

Case Study

Mrs B is an 86-year-old white female who presents with primary pathogenic components of depression, grief, and cognitive slowness. She has been widowed for just over two years. She is living with her son but also stays with her daughter at least once a week. Mrs B is college educated. In her youth, she had married a minister whose career was in the Air Force. Her husband retired from there and started several churches where he was very popular. She was the dutiful pastor's wife. When it became clear that they could not have children, they adopted a child and, later, a set of twins. She believes that she was an excessively permissive parent, which, she is convinced, led to drug problems for the oldest child and divorces for the twins. Mrs B feels guilty about all this. Currently, her older son, now in his 50s, is in a rehab home and the twins have taken a protective stance toward their mother as the older son has "abused" her financially over the years.

Mrs B has been forlorn for a period predating her husband's death. She expresses this by yearning after her husband, and also by being inactive, not making decisions, and manifesting cognitive confusion. Mrs B also complained of visual hallucinations. She has been dealing with these problems for at least two years. Medically she has arthritis and hypertension, as well as Parkinsonism, but she does not attend any primary care clinic. Worried, the twins brought her into the clinic for an evaluation.

Pre-treatment Assessment

Table 3.8 provides information on Mrs B's pre- and post-assessments. Her diagnoses were set initially by the MINI, as well as clinician ratings and by findings from selected cognitive tests. Her current depression recurred from an earlier period in her life when she was having problems with her children. She had always been a worrier, but recently Mrs B expressed concern about several issues: her health; being a burden to her children; and her son's condition. She does not feel in control of her situation. Scores on the HAMD and HARS as well as the MINI indicate current depression and anxiety. Mrs B also completed several self-report measures that confirmed this. She also reported an overall lower quality of life (QoL) and trouble with sleep, but she denied having pain (to any degree). Mrs B also was mildly suicidal (GSIS [Factor I]—no operative plans). For the most part she handled day-to-day functioning well.

Mrs B was found to suffer mild cognitive impairment. In brief, Mrs B's cognitive profile was set by her score on the Oklahoma Premorbid Intelligence Estimate–Vocabulary (OPIE–V IQ) of 98, placing her in the average area intellectually. Although this has a wide confidence interval (~12 points), this is a reasonable marker with which to gauge her skills at present. Her MoCA was moderately impaired, somewhat lower than what would be suggested by her premorbid intelligence estimate. As such, the screening indicated the necessity for further neuropsychological testing. Mrs B scored an RBANS Index of 80, placing her at the 5th percentile for her age group. RBANS subscale scores were generally in the Below Average/Low Average range; Attention Index = 88 (21st percentile); Visuospatial Index = 89 (19th percentile); Language index = 89 (23rd percentile); Immediate Memory Index = 75 (7th percentile); and Delayed Memory index = 78 (7th percentile). Mrs B's performance on executive function tasks was poor. This included the Stroop, the Trail Making test, semantic fluency, and several working memory tasks on the WAIS-III. There also were mild deficits on the FAQ (see below), a measure of executive functions in relation to activities of daily living. Most concerning of these test findings were Mrs B's memory deficit (lower by a standard deviation on recall) and her impaired executive functioning (EF). This last deficit was viewed to be sufficiently troublesome to warrant EF as a major target for treatment. Importantly, Mrs B showed that she currently possesses adequate skills to handle her day-to-day requirements. Furthermore, she is cognitively competent for all decisions, medical or otherwise.

Mrs B was also given the MBMD to determine personality styles as well as treatment issues (treatment prognostics and stress moderators). Her personality registers as passive, but generally cooperative, and dependent. She is decidedly not assertive and socialization is an issue. There were treatment concerns about her functioning and

Table 3.8 Pre-treatment to Post-treatment Changes on Key Measures

Pre-treatment

Axis I: 296.30 Major Depressive Disorder, Recurrent
300.02 Generalized Anxiety Disorder
294.9 Cognitive Disorder, NOS
Axis II : Deferred
Axis III : CHF, arthritis, "MCI"
Axis IV: Lack of resources: social support, family problem
Axis V : GAF: 60

Post-treatment (2 weeks after Rx)

Axis I : 296.30 Major Depressive Disorder, Recurrent (subsyndromal)
300.02 Generalized Anxiety Disorder (subsyndromal)
294.9 Cognitive Disorder, NOS
Axis II : Deferred
Axis III : CHF, HTN, arthritis, "MCI"
Axis IV: Social support, family problem
Axis V : GAF: 65

Six-Month Follow-Up (MINI interview administered)

Axis I: 296.30 Major Depressive Disorder, Recurrent (subsyndromal)
300.02 Generalized Anxiety Disorder (subsyndromal)
294.9 Cognitive Disorder, NOS
Axis II : Deferred
Axis III : CHF, HTN, arthritis, Parkinsonism, "MCI"
Axis IV: Family problem
Axis V : GAF: 60

Measure	Pre-Score	Post-Score (2 wks)
Cognitive		
RBANS (total)	80 (below average)	88 (low average)
MoCA	23 (below average)	26 (average)
Stroop Color-Word	15 (low average)	42 (average)
Phonemic Fluency (FAS)	24 (low)	48 (average)
Affective		
HAMD	24 (high)	7 (normal)
HARS	28 (high)	9 (normal)
BDI-II	28 (high/moderate)	12 (minor problem)
PSWS	67 (moderate)	42 (normal)
GSIS	22 (moderate)	14 (normal)
SWLS	12 (low)	27 (normal)
Pain Rating	3/10 (low)	2/10 (low)
Sleep (ESS)	12 (high)	6 (average)

Functional		
ADCS-ADL	7 (normal)	8 (normal)
FAQ	8 (problem normal)	9 (high normal)
Charlson Comorbidity Index	6 (problem)	—
Personality and Treatment Issues		
MBMD: Personality styles • Cooperative and Inhibited MBMD: Stress Moderators • Functional deficits • Illness apprehension • Social isolation MBMD: Treatment Prognostics • Interventional fragility • Problematic compliance		

CHF is Congestive Heart Failure; HTN is hypertension; MCI is mild cognitive impairment; GAF is Global Aassessment of Functioning. RBANS-Repeated Battery for the Assessment of Neurological Status-Form A (RBANS); Montreal Cognitive Assessment (MoCA), Beck Depression Inventory-II (BDI-II), Letter Fluency (FAS), Penn State Worry Scale (PSWS), Hamilton Depression Scale (HAMD), Hamilton Anxiety Rating Scale HARS), General Suicide Index Scale (GSIS), Life Satisfaction (SWLS), Epworth Sleep Scale (ESS), Alzheimer's Disease Cooperative Studies Scale-Activities of Daily Living (ADCS-ADL), Functional Assessment Questionnaire (FAQ), and Millon Behavioral Medical Diagnostic (MBMD)

Table 3.9 Therapy Sessions

Session 1:	Discussion of case, transdiagnostic targets, socialize to EF training
	Monitor moods
	Activity scheduling
	Increase PE (three of them)
	MD consult/Med labs (bring in physician)
Session 2:	EF training
	Monitor moods/Activity Scheduling/Increase PE
	Decrease avoidance
	Positive aging image priming
	Call son
	Emotional awareness
	Sleep diary: Sleep hygiene—option of meds
	Belly breathing
Session 3:	EF training
	Monitor moods/Activity Scheduling/Increase PE/Decrease Avoidance
	Positive aging image priming
	Worry schedule
	Sleep diary: Sleep hygiene
	Emotional awareness
	All interpersonal tasks (role play)
	Breathing
Session 4:	EF training
	Monitor moods/Increase PE/Activity Schedule/Avoidance/Worry Schedule
	Positive aging image priming

(Continued)

Table 3.9 Therapy Sessions *Continued*

	Emotional awareness
	Sleep monitoring and hygiene
	Bring in family (all interpersonal issues)
	Breathing
Session 5:	EF training
	Monitor moods/Increase PE/Decrease Avoidance/Act Schedule/Worry Schedule
	Improve problem solving (target family issues)
	Death ideation challenge (monitor GSIS)
	Sleep monitoring and hygiene
	Breathing
Session 6:	EF training
	Monitor moods/Increase PE/Decrease Avoidance/At Schedule/Worry Schedule
	Problem solving
	Death ideation challenge (monitor GSIS)
	Sleep hygiene
	Breathing
Session 7:	EF training
	Monitor moods/Increase PE/Act Schedule/Worry Schedule
	Problem solving
	Death ideation challenge (monitor GSIS)
	Sleep hygiene (resolved)
	Breathing
Session 8:	EF Training
	Monitor moods/Increase PE/Act Schedule/Increase PE/Worry Schedule
	Problem solving
	Breathing
Session 9:	EF training
	Monitor moods/Increase PE/Decrease Avoidance/Worry Schedule/Act Schedule
	Loss of husband (mood monitoring and ritual)
	MD follow-up/Sleep check-up
	Problem solving
Session 10:	EF training
	Monitor moods/Increase PE/Decrease Avoidance/Worry Scheduling
	Loss of husband (mood monitoring and ritual)
	Activity Scheduling (family for last session)
	Call physician
	Problem solving
	Breathing
Session 11:	EF training
	Monitor moods/Increase PE/Decrease Avoidance/Worry Schedule
	Problem solving
	Family issues
	Breathing
Session 12:	Sum up
	Relapse issues

Table 3.10 Stroop CW and BDI Across Sessions

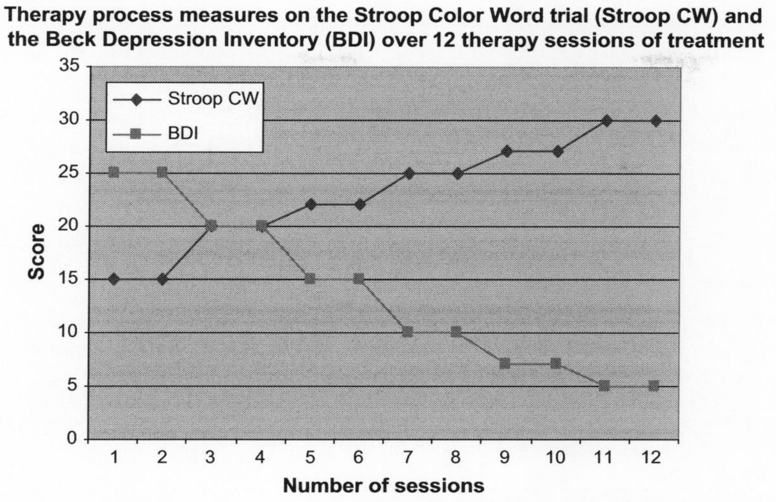

Therapy process measures on the Stroop Color Word trial (Stroop CW) and the Beck Depression Inventory (BDI) over 12 therapy sessions of treatment

Stroop CW
BDI
Score
0
5
10
15
20
25
30
35
1 2 3 4 5 6 7 8 9 10 11 12
Number of sessions

illness apprehension, as well as concerns about interventional fragility and problematic compliance. These descriptors are face valid, given her history, and therefore they can be folded into her treatment. She scored a 6 on the Charlson Comorbidity Index, a high predictor of further morbidity and possible mortality.

There were several targets selected for therapy. These included problems related to: (1) depression, notably to increase behavioral activation and positive events, improve problem solving and emotional awareness, prime her self-image for positive self-assessment, and monitor death ideation; (2) anxiety, to teach relaxation techniques, decrease avoidance (via assertiveness training), reinforce activity scheduling as well as worry scheduling; (3) interpersonal functioning—this would be task based, including talking to her son and daughter; (4) loss of husband, including monitoring mood and scheduling rituals, as well as restricting time devoted to grief tasks; and (5) medical behaviors, specifically to acquire labs and attend a neurology consult for Parkinson's disease. Importantly, in every treatment session Mrs B trained on EF exercises (ACTIVE trial exercises, Stroop CW test, as well as a Memory Group). This training lasted from one-third to half all sessions.

Structure of Therapy

Therapy sessions were constructed directly from the problem list. Initial sessions confirmed diagnoses and socialized Mrs B to the problem list. Collaboratively, priorities for therapy were set. In addition to EF training, these included activity scheduling (as she is excessively passive and unstructured), monitoring moods so that she would better assess her day, and psychological status, relaxation, problem solving (in middle and later sessions), and family needs, followed by health maintenance/physician issues, sleep hygiene, grief, and some interpersonal challenges. These tasks were agreed to within the context of the transdiagnostic model: Mrs B would try the tasks, monitor outcomes and change focus, if necessary. Early sessions stressed the importance of activity scheduling, her ability to control her situation, and her challenge to monitor her own psychological status. Mrs B also was primed with several positive self-identity images. This had a very positive effect on her. Table 3.9 presents these topics. Table 3.10 provides objective data on the two key outcomes of her therapy: depression (BDI-II) and EF training (Stroop CW test).

CONCLUSION

This chapter highlighted the importance of assessment in psychotherapy that now has empirical support behind the various interventions. Assessment is the sine qua non for ESTs or EBTs. However, "there are many roads to Rome." The field of psychology and, for that matter, psychiatry, has rediscovered the value of monitoring and measuring, as they provide perspective, a course for care, and markers for success. In this chapter we have provided input for many levels of evaluation in the therapy process, and made suggestions as to how to foster change. Finally, we have endorsed one method, above all others, to assist in this process: the development of the case formulation using a transdiagnostic model.

Ultimately, an unearthing of the biological and behavioral mechanisms that mediate psychological disturbances will be necessary for a full understanding of the origin, symptomatology, cultural context, maintenance, treatment, and course of a mental disorder. This may yet be a distant vision, but one that is ever nearer on the horizon for older adults. The commitment to using assessments in all our interventions will bring this vision closer.

APPENDIX A: SELF-CONTROL QUESTIONNAIRE

Please read over read over the following statements. For each item, circle a number from 1 (very little) to 5 (very much) that best represents *how much the statement applies to you in general*. There are no right or wrong answers. Do not spend too much time on any statement.

	Item	Very Little	A Little	Some	Much	Very Much
1.	I don't try hard enough at anything I do.	1	2	3	4	5
2.	I am very self-critical.	1	2	3	4	5
3.	When there is some goal I'd like to reach, I find it best to list specifically what I have to do to get there.	1	2	3	4	5
4.	When bad things happen to me, I feel responsible.	1	2	3	4	5
5.	A long-term benefit is more important to me than a short-term payoff.	1	2	3	4	5
6.	I am always noticing the positive things that happen.	1	2	3	4	5
7.	I judge myself based on what others think.	1	2	3	4	5
8.	I don't work hard enough.	1	2	3	4	5
9.	I am always looking for the next bad thing to happen.	1	2	3	4	5
10.	Things beyond my control rule my moods.	1	2	3	4	5
11.	When I fail, it is because of my own inadequacy.	1	2	3	4	5
12.	I don't reward myself for the difficult things I've done.	1	2	3	4	5
13.	Good things happen only because I get lucky.	1	2	3	4	5
14.	I usually succeed in what I try to do.	1	2	3	4	5
15.	I always set specific, concrete goals for myself.	1	2	3	4	5
16.	I often do things I know will be bad for me in the long run.	1	2	3	4	5
17.	Positive things in life do not happen routinely, they are few and far between.	1	2	3	4	5
18.	Other people's approval determines how I feel about myself.	1	2	3	4	5
19.	I spend a lot of time thinking about my faults and failures.	1	2	3	4	5
20.	I have a hard time dismissing the negative thoughts about myself.	1	2	3	4	5
21.	I reward myself for my efforts towards accomplishing a goal.	1	2	3	4	5
22.	Even though I know that doing something now will produce the most positive results for me in the long run, I tend not to do it.	1	2	3	4	5
23.	I feel unhappy about my work unless other people approve.	1	2	3	4	5
24.	I like to reward myself with something special, such as buying something I've been wanting.	1	2	3	4	5
25.	I notice all the little steps I've accomplished as I work toward a goal.	1	2	3	4	5
26.	Often my goals are so distant, they seem impossible to reach.	1	2	3	4	5
27.	My efforts are never enough.	1	2	3	4	5
28.	When I think about the future, I can see many positive things.	1	2	3	4	5

	Item	Very Little	A Little	Some	Much	Very Much
29.	I usually place more weight on the long-term benefits of an action than on the immediate consequences.	1	2	3	4	5
30.	Even when I am doing a good job, I am not happy unless other people like my work.	1	2	3	4	5
31.	If I've done a good job, it doesn't matter what others think.	1	2	3	4	5
32.	I get myself through hard jobs by rewarding myself after I complete them.	1	2	3	4	5
33.	I am good at setting goals for myself.	1	2	3	4	5
34.	When I accomplish something, I reward myself with a pleasant activity.	1	2	3	4	5
35.	If I make a mistake, I judge myself more harshly than anyone else would.	1	2	3	4	5
36.	I can make myself feel better by thinking about something positive.	1	2	3	4	5
37.	I am often hard on myself for no apparent reason.	1	2	3	4	5
38.	When things go wrong, it is usually because of something I did.	1	2	3	4	5
39.	When I do something good, I give myself credit for a job well done.	1	2	3	4	5
40.	There are things I can do to control my mood.	1	2	3	4	5
41.	I reward myself for the little steps I take toward my goal.	1	2	3	4	5
42.	I reward myself if I do a difficult or unpleasant task.	1	2	3	4	5
43.	I tend to set realistic goals.	1	2	3	4	5
44.	When I do something well, I know I can make it happen again.	1	2	3	4	5
45.	If I don't immediately gain from my effort, I'd rather not do it at all.	1	2	3	4	5
46.	I don't feel good about something I've done, unless someone else approves of it.	1	2	3	4	5
47.	Often my goals are vague.	1	2	3	4	5
48.	I always seem to remember the bad things that are upsetting me.	1	2	3	4	5

SCQD Scoring

1, 2, 4, 7–13, 16–20, 22, 23, 26, 27, 30, 35, 37, 38, 45–48 are REVERSE-CODED. Scores for these items are (6-circled number). Sum up scores for 48 items to obtain total score (range: 48–240). Items load onto seven general domains as listed below.

Factor/Category	# of items	Item #s
Monitoring and control of mood	8	6,9,10,19,20,36,40,48
Future orientation	6	5,16,22,28,29,45
Attributional style	7	
For positive events	4	13,14,17,44
For negative events	3	4,11,38
Internal standards	6	7,18,23,30,31,46
Goal setting	7	3,15,25,26,33,43,47
Self-reinforcment	8	12,21,24,32,34,39,41,42
Self-punishment	6	
Criticism of effort	3	1,8,27
Criticism of self	3	2,35,37
Total	**48**	

The Self-Control Questionnaire is a measure that was originally devised to assess self-management behavior that creators of the measure believe to be possible factors involved with depression. This assessment measures the impact of various self-control behaviors and attitudes on a person's overall ability to live productively.

SHORT FORM HEALTH SURVEY (SF-36)

1. In general, would you say your health is:
☐ 1. Excellent ☐ 2. Very good ☐ 3. Good ☐ 4. Fair ☐ 5. Poor

2. Compared with ONE YEAR AGO, how would you rate your health in general NOW?
☐ 1. MUCH BETTER than one year ago.
☐ 2. Somewhat BETTER now than one year ago.
☐ 3. About the SAME as one year ago.
☐ 4. Somewhat WORSE now than one year ago.
☐ 5. MUCH WORSE now than one year ago.

3. The following items are about activities you might do during a typical day. Does your health now limit you in these activities? If so, how much?

Activities			
a) **Vigorous activities,** such as running, lifting heavy objects, participating in strenuous sports?	☐ 1. Yes, limited a lot	☐ 2. Yes, limited a little	☐ 3. No, not limited at all
b) **Moderate activities,** such as moving a table, pushing a vacuum cleaner, bowling, or playing golf?	☐ 1. Yes, limited a lot	☐ 2. Yes, limited a little	☐ 3. No, not limited at all
c) Lifting or carrying groceries?	☐ 1. Yes, limited a lot	☐ 2. Yes, limited a little	☐ 3. No, not limited at all
d) Climbing **several flights** of stairs?	☐ 1. Yes, limited a lot	☐ 2. Yes, limited a little	☐ 3. No, not limited at all
e) Climbing **one** flight of stairs?	☐ 1. Yes, limited a lot	☐ 2. Yes, limited a little	☐ 3. No, not limited at all
f) Bending, kneeling or stooping?	☐ 1. Yes, limited a lot	☐ 2. Yes, limited a little	☐ 3. No, not limited at all
g) Walking **more than a mile**?	☐ 1. Yes, limited a lot	☐ 2. Yes, limited a little	☐ 3. No, not limited at all
h) Walking **several** blocks?	☐ 1. Yes, limited a lot	☐ 2. Yes, limited a little	☐ 3. No, not limited at all
i) Walking **one** block?	☐ 1. Yes, limited a lot	☐ 2. Yes, limited a little	☐ 3. No, not limited at all
j) Bathing or dressing yourself?	☐ 1. Yes, limited a lot	☐ 2. Yes, limited a little	☐ 3. No, not limited at all

4. During the **past four weeks**, have you had any of the following problems with your work or other regular activities as a result of **your physical health**?

	Yes	No
a) Cut down on the **amount of time** you spent on work or other activities?	☐ 1. yes	☐ 2. No
b) **Accomplished less** than you would like?	☐ 1. yes	☐ 2. No
c) Were limited in the **kind** of work or other activities?	☐ 1. yes	☐ 2. No
d) Had **difficulty** performing the work or other activities (for example it took extra effort)?	☐ 1. yes	☐ 2. No

5. During the **past four weeks**, have you had any of the following problems with your work or other regular daily activities as a result of any **emotional problems** (such as feeling depressed or anxious)?

	Yes	No
a) Cut down on the **amount of time** you spent on work or other activities?	☐ 1. yes	☐ 2. No
b) **Accomplished less** than you would like?	☐ 1. yes	☐ 2. No
c) Didn't do work or other activities as **carefully** as usual?	☐ 1. yes	☐ 2. No

6. During the **past four weeks**, to what extent has your physical health, or emotional problems, interfered with your normal social activities with family, friends, neighbors, or groups?
☐ 1. Not at all ☐ 2. Slightly ☐ 3. Moderately ☐ 4. Quite a bit ☐ 5. Extremely

7. How much **bodily** pain have you had during the **past four weeks**?
☐ 1. None ☐ 2. Very mild ☐ 3. Mild ☐ 4. Moderate ☐ 5. Severe ☐ 6. Very severe

8. During the **past four weeks**, how much did **pain** interfere with your normal work (including both work outside the home and housework)?
☐ 1. Not at all ☐ 2. A little bit ☐ 3. Moderately ☐ 4. Quite a bit ☐ 5. Extremely

9. These questions are about how you feel and how things have been with you **during the past four weeks**. For each question, please give the one answer that comes closest to the way you have been feeling. How much of the time during the **past four weeks** …

	1. All of the time	2. Most of the time	3. A good bit of the time	4. Some of the time	5. A little of the time	6. None of the time
a) Did you feel full of pep?	☐ 1. All of the time	☐ 2. Most of the time	☐ 3. A good bit of the time	☐ 4. Some of the time	☐ 5. A little of the time	☐ 6. None of the time
b) Have you been a very nervous person?	☐ 1. All of the time	☐ 2. Most of the time	☐ 3. A good bit of the time	☐ 4. Some of the time	☐ 5. A little of the time	☐ 6. None of the time
c) Have you felt so down in the dumps that nothing could cheer you up?	☐ 1. All of the time	☐ 2. Most of the time	☐ 3. A good bit of the time	☐ 4. Some of the time	☐ 5. A little of the time	☐ 6. None of the time
d) Have you felt calm and peaceful?	☐ 1. All of the time	☐ 2. Most of the time	☐ 3. A good bit of the time	☐ 4. Some of the time	☐ 5. A little of the time	☐ 6. None of the time
e) Did you have a lot of energy?	☐ 1. All of the time	☐ 2. Most of the time	☐ 3. A good bit of the time	☐ 4. Some of the time	☐ 5. A little of the time	☐ 6. None of the time
f) Have you felt downhearted and blue?	☐ 1. All of the time	☐ 2. Most of the time	☐ 3. A good bit of the time	☐ 4. Some of the time	☐ 5. A little of the time	☐ 6. None of the time
g) Do you feel worn out?	☐ 1. All of the time	☐ 2. Most of the time	☐ 3. A good bit of the time	☐ 4. Some of the time	☐ 5. A little of the time	☐ 6. None of the time
h) Have you been a happy person?	☐ 1. All of the time	☐ 2. Most of the time	☐ 3. A good bit of the time	☐ 4. Some of the time	☐ 5. A little of the time	☐ 6. None of the time
i) Did you feel tired?	☐ 1. All of the time	☐ 2. Most of the time	☐ 3. A good bit of the time	☐ 4. Some of the time	☐ 5. A little of the time	☐ 6. None of the time

10. During the **past four weeks**, how much of the time has your **physical health,** or **emotional problems,** interfered with your social activities (like visiting with friends, relatives, etc.)?
☐ 1. All of the time
☐ 2. Most of the time.
☐ 3. Some of the time
☐ 4. A little of the time.
☐ 5. None of the time.

11. How TRUE or FALSE is **each** of the following statements for you?

	1. Definitely true	2. Mostly true	3. Don't know	4. Mostly false	5. Definitely false
a) I seem to get sick a little easier than other people.	☐ 1. Definitely true	☐ 2. Mostly true	☐ 3. Don't know	☐ 4. Mostly false	☐ 5. Definitely false
b) I am as healthy as anybody I know.	☐ 1. Definitely true	☐ 2. Mostly true	☐ 3. Don't know	☐ 4. Mostly false	☐ 5. Definitely false
c) I expect my health to get worse.	☐ 1. Definitely true	☐ 2. Mostly true	☐ 3. Don't know	☐ 4. Mostly false	☐ 5. Definitely false
d) My health is excellent.	☐ 1. Definitely true	☐ 2. Mostly true	☐ 3. Don't know	☐ 4. Mostly false	☐ 5. Definitely false

The Short Form Health Survey (SF-36) is a measure that consists of 36 general questions that assess the overall quality of life for a patient. This measure is widely used by medical organizations and managed care groups worldwide to better understand the overall health of a patient.

UNIVERSITY OF RHODE ISLAND CHANGE ASSESSMENT

This questionnaire is to help us improve services. Each statement describes how a person might feel when starting therapy or approaching problems in their lives. Please indicate the extent to which you tend to agree or disagree with each statement.

In each case, make your choice in terms of how you feel right now, not what you have felt in the past or would like to feel. "Here" refers to the place of treatment or the program.

There are FIVE possible responses to each of the items in the questionnaire:

1 = Strongly Disagree
2 = Disagree
3 = Undecided
4 = Agree
5 = Strongly Agree
[for self-evaluation only]

1. As far as I'm concerned, I don't have any problems that need changing.
2. I think I might be ready for some self-improvement.
3. I am doing something about the problems that had been bothering me.
4. It might be worthwhile to work on my problem.
5. I'm not the problem one. It doesn't make much sense for me to be here.
6. It worries me that I might slip back on a problem I have already changed, so I am here to seek help.
7. I am finally doing some work on my problem.
8. I've been thinking that I might want to change something about myself.
9. I have been successful in working on my problem but I'm not sure I can keep up the effort on my own.
10. At times my problem is difficult, but I'm working on it.
11. Being here is pretty much a waste of time for me because the problem doesn't have to do with me.
12. I'm hoping that this place will help me to better understand myself.
13. I guess I have faults, but there's nothing that I really need to change.
14. I am really working hard to change.
15. I have a problem and I really think I should work at it.
16. I'm not following through with what I had already changed as well as I had hoped, and I'm here to prevent a relapse of the problem.
17. Even though I'm not always successful in changing, I am at least working on my problem.
18. I thought once I had resolved my problem I would be free of it, but sometimes I still find myself struggling with it.
19. I wish I had more ideas on how to solve the problem.
20. I have started working on my problems but I would like help.
21. Maybe this place will be able to help me.
22. I may need a boost right now to help me maintain the changes I've already made.
23. I may be part of the problem, but I don't really think I am.
24. I hope that someone here will have some good advice for me.
25. Anyone can talk about changing; I'm actually doing something about it.
26. All this talk about psychology is boring. Why can't people just forget about their problems?
27. I'm here to prevent myself from having a relapse of my problem.
28. It is frustrating, but I feel I might be having a recurrence of a problem I thought I had resolved.
29. I have worries but so does the next guy. Why spend time thinking about them?
30. I am actively working on my problem.
31. I would rather cope with my faults than try to change them.
32. After all I had done to try to change my problem, every now and again it comes back to haunt me.

The University of Rhode Island Change Assessment is utilized to measure how a patient views their own progress during therapy. This assessment is a 32-item scale that includes a total of four subscales that measure the four stages of change: precontemplation, contemplation, action, and maintenance.

CLINICAL INSIGHT RATING SCALE

Following interviews with patient and primary caregiver and comparing their responses, each of the following four items are assessed on a scale of **0–2**:

0 = Good insight
1 = Relatively impaired insight
2 = Poor insight

Degree of patient's awareness regarding the following aspects:

____1) the reason for the visit to see doctor
____2) his or her cognitive deficits
____3) his or her functional deficits
____4) his or her perception of the progression of the disease
_____TOTAL SCORE (0 = insight fully preserved to 8 = insight totally absent)

Interpretation of total CIR scores:

0 and 1 are associated with good insight
2 to 4 associated with relativity impaired insight
4 or higher associated with poor insight

Assessors rating of insight:

_________Strong evidence of memory problem and insight
_________Mild evidence of memory problem and insight
_________No evidence of memory problem and insight

The Clinical Insight Rating Scale serves as a measure of patient insight pertaining to their main problem and perceived progress with improving their problem.

BASIS-32 (BEHAVIOR AND SYMPTOM IDENTIFICATION SCALE)

Instructions to Respondent: Below is a list of problems and areas of life functioning in which some people experience difficulties. Using the scale below, fill in the box with the answer that best describes how much difficulty you have been having in each area **DURING THE PAST WEEK.**

0 = No Difficulty
1 = A Little Difficulty
2 = Moderate Difficulty
3 = Quite A Bit of Difficulty
4 = Extreme Difficulty

Please answer each item. **Do not leave any blank.**

If there is an area that you consider to be inapplicable, indicate that it is *0=No Difficulty.*

IN THE PAST WEEK, how much difficulty have you been having in the area of:

1. **Managing day-to-day life** (For example, getting places on time, handling money, making everyday decisions)... 1 ☐
2. **Household responsibilities** (For example, shopping, cooking, laundry, cleaning, other chores)... 2 ☐
3. **Work** (For example, completing tasks, performance level, finding/keeping a job)... 3 ☐
4. **School** (For example, academic performance, completing assignments, attendance)... 4 ☐
5. **Leisure time or recreational activities**... 5 ☐
6. **Adjusting to major life stresses** (For example, separation, divorce, moving, new job, new school, a death) 6 ☐
7. **Relationships with family members**... 7 ☐
8. **Getting along with people outside of the family**... 8 ☐
9. **Isolation or feelings of loneliness**... 9 ☐
10. **Being able to feel close to others**... 10 ☐
11. **Being realistic about yourself or others**. 11 ☐
12. **Recognizing and expressing emotions appropriately**. 12 ☐
13. **Developing independence, autonomy**... 13 ☐
14. **Goals or direction in life**. 14 ☐

15. Lack of self-confidence, feeling bad about yourself. 15 ☐
16. Apathy, lack of interest in things. 16 ☐
17. Depression, hopelessness. 17 ☐
18. Suicidal feelings or behavior. 18 ☐
19. Physical symptoms (For example, headaches, aches and pains, sleep disturbance, stomach aches, dizziness) 19 ☐
20. Fear, anxiety, or panic... 20 ☐
21. Confusion, concentration, memory... 21 ☐
22. Disturbing or unreal thoughts or beliefs... 22 ☐
23. Hearing voices, seeing things. 23 ☐
24. Manic, bizarre behavior. 24 ☐
25. Mood swings, unstable moods. 25 ☐
26. Uncontrollable, compulsive behavior (For example, eating disorder, hand-washing, hurting yourself) 26 ☐
27. Sexual activity or preoccupation. 27 ☐
28. Drinking alcoholic beverages. 28 ☐
29. Taking illegal drugs, misusing drugs... 29 ☐
30. Controlling temper, outbursts of anger, violence. 30 ☐
31. Impulsive, illegal, or reckless behavior... 31 ☐
32. Feeling satisfaction with your life... 32 ☐

The BASIS-32 measures the change in self-reported symptoms and problem difficulty over the course of treatment. This measure is supported with strong reliability and validity concerning how patients feel before and after receiving treatment.

WORKING ALLIANCE INVENTORY

Form C (Client)

Instructions

On the following pages there are sentences that describe some of the different ways a person might think or feel about his or her therapist (counselor). As you read the sentences mentally insert the name of your therapist (counselor) in place of _____________ in the text.

Below each statement there is a seven point scale:

1	2	3	4	5	6	7
Never	Rarely	Occasionally	Sometimes	Often	Very Often	Always

If the statement describes the way you ***always*** feel (or think) circle the number 7; if it ***never*** applies to you circle the number 1. Use the numbers in between to describe the variations between these extremes.

This questionnaire is **CONFIDENTIAL**. Neither your therapist nor the agency will see your answers.

Work fast, your first impressions are the ones we would like to see.

(PLEASE DON'T FORGET TO RESPOND TO ***EVERY*** *ITEM.)*

Thank you for your cooperation.

1. I feel comfortable with _______________.

1	2	3	4	5	6	7
Never	Rarely	Occasionally	Sometimes	Often	Very Often	Always

2. _________ and I agree about the things I will need to do in therapy to help improve my situation.

1	2	3	4	5	6	7
Never	Rarely	Occasionally	Sometimes	Often	Very Often	Always

3. I am worried about the outcome of these sessions.

1	2	3	4	5	6	7
Never	Rarely	Occasionally	Sometimes	Often	Very Often	Always

4. What I am doing in therapy gives me new ways of looking at my problem.

1	2	3	4	5	6	7
Never	Rarely	Occasionally	Sometimes	Often	Very Often	Always

5. ________________ and I understand each other.

1	2	3	4	5	6	7
Never	Rarely	Occasionally	Sometimes	Often	Very Often	Always

6. ________________ perceives accurately what my goals are.

1	2	3	4	5	6	7
Never	Rarely	Occasionally	Sometimes	Often	Very Often	Always

7. I find what I am doing in therapy confusing.

1	2	3	4	5	6	7
Never	Rarely	Occasionally	Sometimes	Often	Very Often	Always

8. I believe ______________ likes me.

1	2	3	4	5	6	7
Never	Rarely	Occasionally	Sometimes	Often	Very Often	Always

9. I wish ________________ and I could clarify the purpose of our sessions.

1	2	3	4	5	6	7
Never	Rarely	Occasionally	Sometimes	Often	Very Often	Always

10. I disagree with _____________ about what I ought to get out of therapy.

1	2	3	4	5	6	7
Never	Rarely	Occasionally	Sometimes	Often	Very Often	Always

11. I believe the time ______________ and I spend together is not spent efficiently.

1	2	3	4	5	6	7
Never	Rarely	Occasionally	Sometimes	Often	Very Often	Always

12. ________________ does not understand what I am trying to accomplish in therapy.

1	2	3	4	5	6	7
Never	Rarely	Occasionally	Sometimes	Often	Very Often	Always

13. I am clear on what my responsibilities are in therapy.

1	2	3	4	5	6	7
Never	Rarely	Occasionally	Sometimes	Often	Very Often	Always

14. The goals of these sessions are important for me.

1	2	3	4	5	6	7
Never	Rarely	Occasionally	Sometimes	Often	Very Often	Always

15. I find what ________________ and I are doing in therapy is unrelated to my concerns.

1	2	3	4	5	6	7
Never	Rarely	Occasionally	Sometimes	Often	Very Often	Always

16. I feel that the things I do in therapy will help me to accomplish the changes that I want.

1	2	3	4	5	6	7
Never	Rarely	Occasionally	Sometimes	Often	Very Often	Always

17. I believe _____________ is genuinely concerned for my welfare.

1	2	3	4	5	6	7
Never	Rarely	Occasionally	Sometimes	Often	Very Often	Always

18. I am clear as to what ______________ wants me to do in these sessions.

1	2	3	4	5	6	7
Never	Rarely	Occasionally	Sometimes	Often	Very Often	Always

19. ________________ and I respect each other.

1	2	3	4	5	6	7
Never	Rarely	Occasionally	Sometimes	Often	Very Often	Always

20. I feel that _____________ is not totally honest about his/her feelings towards me.

1	2	3	4	5	6	7
Never	Rarely	Occasionally	Sometimes	Often	Very Often	Always

21. I am confident in _____________'s ability to help me.

1	2	3	4	5	6	7
Never	Rarely	Occasionally	Sometimes	Often	Very Often	Always

22. _____________ and I are working towards mutually agreed upon goals.

1	2	3	4	5	6	7
Never	Rarely	Occasionally	Sometimes	Often	Very Often	Always

23. I feel that _____________ appreciates me.

1	2	3	4	5	6	7
Never	Rarely	Occasionally	Sometimes	Often	Very Often	Always

24. We agree on what is important for me to work on.

1	2	3	4	5	6	7
Never	Rarely	Occasionally	Sometimes	Often	Very Often	Always

25. As a result of these sessions I am clearer as to how I might be able to change.

1	2	3	4	5	6	7
Never	Rarely	Occasionally	Sometimes	Often	Very Often	Always

26. ________________ and I trust one another.

1	2	3	4	5	6	7
Never	Rarely	Occasionally	Sometimes	Often	Very Often	Always

27. ________________ and I have different ideas on what my problems are.

1	2	3	4	5	6	7
Never	Rarely	Occasionally	Sometimes	Often	Very Often	Always

28. My relationship with _______________ is very important to me.

1	2	3	4	5	6	7
Never	Rarely	Occasionally	Sometimes	Often	Very Often	Always

29. I have the feeling that if I say or do the wrong things, _________ will stop working with me.

1	2	3	4	5	6	7
Never	Rarely	Occasionally	Sometimes	Often	Very Often	Always

30. _______________ and I collaborate on setting goals for my therapy.

1	2	3	4	5	6	7
Never	Rarely	Occasionally	Sometimes	Often	Very Often	Always

31. I am frustrated by the things I am doing in therapy.

1	2	3	4	5	6	7
Never	Rarely	Occasionally	Sometimes	Often	Very Often	Always

32. We have established a good understanding of the kind of changes that would be good for me.

1	2	3	4	5	6	7
Never	Rarely	Occasionally	Sometimes	Often	Very Often	Always

33. The things that ____________________ is asking me to do don't make sense.

1	2	3	4	5	6	7
Never	Rarely	Occasionally	Sometimes	Often	Very Often	Always

34. I don't know what to expect as the result of my therapy.

1	2	3	4	5	6	7
Never	Rarely	Occasionally	Sometimes	Often	Very Often	Always

35. I believe the way we are working with my problem is correct.

1	2	3	4	5	6	7
Never	Rarely	Occasionally	Sometimes	Often	Very Often	Always

36. I feel ____________cares about me even when I do things that he/she does not approve of.

1	2	3	4	5	6	7
Never	Rarely	Occasionally	Sometimes	Often	Very Often	Always

Form T (Therapist)

Instructions

On the following pages there are sentences that describe some of the different ways a person might think or feel about his or her client. As you read the sentences mentally insert the name of your client in place of ____________ in the text.

Below each statement there is a seven point scale:

1	2	3	4	5	6	7
Never	Rarely	Occasionally	Sometimes	Often	Very Often	Always

If the statement describes the way you ***always*** feel (or think) circle the number 7; if it ***never*** applies to you circle the number 1. Use the numbers in between to describe the variations between these extremes.

This questionnaire is **CONFIDENTIAL**. Neither your client nor the agency will see your answers.

Work fast, your first impressions are the ones we would like to see.

(PLEASE DON'T FORGET TO RESPOND TO ***EVERY*** *ITEM.)*

Thank you for your cooperation.

1. I feel uncomfortable with ____________.

1	2	3	4	5	6	7
Never	Rarely	Occasionally	Sometimes	Often	Very Often	Always

2. ______________ and I agree about the steps to be taken to improve his/her situation.

1	2	3	4	5	6	7
Never	Rarely	Occasionally	Sometimes	Often	Very Often	Always

3. I have some concerns about the outcome of these sessions.

1	2	3	4	5	6	7
Never	Rarely	Occasionally	Sometimes	Often	Very Often	Always

4. My client and I both feel confident about the usefulness of our current activity in therapy.

1	2	3	4	5	6	7
Never	Rarely	Occasionally	Sometimes	Often	Very Often	Always

5. I feel I really understand ______________.

1	2	3	4	5	6	7
Never	Rarely	Occasionally	Sometimes	Often	Very Often	Always

6. ______________ and I have a common perception of her/his goals.

1	2	3	4	5	6	7
Never	Rarely	Occasionally	Sometimes	Often	Very Often	Always

7. __________ finds what we are doing in therapy confusing.

1	2	3	4	5	6	7
Never	Rarely	Occasionally	Sometimes	Often	Very Often	Always

8. I believe ___________ likes me.

1	2	3	4	5	6	7
Never	Rarely	Occasionally	Sometimes	Often	Very Often	Always

9. I sense a need to clarify the purpose of our session(s) for _____________.

1	2	3	4	5	6	7
Never	Rarely	Occasionally	Sometimes	Often	Very Often	Always

10. I have some disagreements with __________________ about the goals of these sessions.

1	2	3	4	5	6	7
Never	Rarely	Occasionally	Sometimes	Often	Very Often	Always

11. I believe the time __________ and I are spending together is not spent efficiently.

1	2	3	4	5	6	7
Never	Rarely	Occasionally	Sometimes	Often	Very Often	Always

12. I have doubts about what we are trying to accomplish in therapy.

1	2	3	4	5	6	7
Never	Rarely	Occasionally	Sometimes	Often	Very Often	Always

13. I am clear and explicit about what _____________'s responsibilities are in therapy.

1	2	3	4	5	6	7
Never	Rarely	Occasionally	Sometimes	Often	Very Often	Always

14. The current goals of these sessions are important for _____________.

1	2	3	4	5	6	7
Never	Rarely	Occasionally	Sometimes	Often	Very Often	Always

15. I find what ___________ and I are doing in therapy is unrelated to her/his current concerns.

1	2	3	4	5	6	7
Never	Rarely	Occasionally	Sometimes	Often	Very Often	Always

16. I feel confident that the things we do in therapy will help _________ to accomplish the changes that he/she desires.

1	2	3	4	5	6	7
Never	Rarely	Occasionally	Sometimes	Often	Very Often	Always

17. I am genuinely concerned for ______________'s welfare.

1	2	3	4	5	6	7
Never	Rarely	Occasionally	Sometimes	Often	Very Often	Always

18. I am clear as to what I expect ____________ to do in these sessions.

1	2	3	4	5	6	7
Never	Rarely	Occasionally	Sometimes	Often	Very Often	Always

19. _______________ and I respect each other.

1	2	3	4	5	6	7
Never	Rarely	Occasionally	Sometimes	Often	Very Often	Always

20. I feel that I am not totally honest about my feelings toward ________________.

1	2	3	4	5	6	7
Never	Rarely	Occasionally	Sometimes	Often	Very Often	Always

21. I am confident in my ability to help _________________.

1	2	3	4	5	6	7
Never	Rarely	Occasionally	Sometimes	Often	Very Often	Always

22. We are working towards mutually agreed upon goals.

1	2	3	4	5	6	7
Never	Rarely	Occasionally	Sometimes	Often	Very Often	Always

23. I appreciate _______________ as a person.

1	2	3	4	5	6	7
Never	Rarely	Occasionally	Sometimes	Often	Very Often	Always

24. We agree on what is important for ________________ to work on.

1	2	3	4	5	6	7
Never	Rarely	Occasionally	Sometimes	Often	Very Often	Always

25. As a result of these sessions ____________ is clearer as to how she/he might be able to change.

1	2	3	4	5	6	7
Never	Rarely	Occasionally	Sometimes	Often	Very Often	Always

26. _____________ and I have built a mutual trust.

1	2	3	4	5	6	7
Never	Rarely	Occasionally	Sometimes	Often	Very Often	Always

27. _______________ and I have different ideas on what his/her real problems are.

1	2	3	4	5	6	7
Never	Rarely	Occasionally	Sometimes	Often	Very Often	Always

28. Our relationship is important to ___________________.

1	2	3	4	5	6	7
Never	Rarely	Occasionally	Sometimes	Often	Very Often	Always

29. ________________ has some fears that if she/he says or does the wrong things, I will stop working with him/her.

1	2	3	4	5	6	7
Never	Rarely	Occasionally	Sometimes	Often	Very Often	Always

30. __________________ and I have collaborated in setting goals for these session(s).

1	2	3	4	5	6	7
Never	Rarely	Occasionally	Sometimes	Often	Very Often	Always

31. _______________ is frustrated by what I am asking her/him to do in therapy.

1	2	3	4	5	6	7
Never	Rarely	Occasionally	Sometimes	Often	Very Often	Always

32. We have established a good understanding between us of the kind of changes that would be good for _________________.

1	2	3	4	5	6	7
Never	Rarely	Occasionally	Sometimes	Often	Very Often	Always

33. The things that we are doing in therapy don't make much sense to _______________.

1	2	3	4	5	6	7
Never	Rarely	Occasionally	Sometimes	Often	Very Often	Always

34. ___________________ doesn't know what to expect as the result of therapy.

1	2	3	4	5	6	7
Never	Rarely	Occasionally	Sometimes	Often	Very Often	Always

35. ______________ believes the way we are working with her/his problem is correct.

1	2	3	4	5	6	7
Never	Rarely	Occasionally	Sometimes	Often	Very Often	Always

36. I respect ___________________ even when he/she does things that I do not approve of.

1	2	3	4	5	6	7
Never	Rarely	Occasionally	Sometimes	Often	Very Often	Always

For Caregivers

The Zarit Burden Interview

Caregiver Name: ______________________ Date: ________________

Relationship to Patient: ________________

Instructions for caregiver: The questions below reflect how persons sometimes feel when they are taking care of another person. There are no right or wrong answers. Just **circle the response that best describes how you feel.**

	Never	**Rarely**	**Some-times**	**Quite frequently**	**Nearly always**
Do you feel that this person asks for more help than he/she needs?					
Do you feel that because of the time you spend with this person that you don't have enough time for yourself?					
Do you feel stressed between caring for this person and trying to meet other responsibilities for your family or work?					
Do you feel embarrassed over this person's behavior?					
Do you feel angry when you are around this person?					
Do you feel that this person currently affects your relationships with other family members or friends in a negative way?					
Are you afraid what the future holds for this person?					
Do you feel this person is dependent on you?					
Do you feel strained when you are around this person?					
Do you feel your health has suffered because of your involvement with this person?					
Do you feel that you don't have as much privacy as you would like because of this person?					
Do you feel that your social life has suffered because you are caring for this person?					
Do you feel uncomfortable about having friends over because of this person?					
Do you feel that this person seems to expect you to take care of him/her as if you were the only one he/she could depend on?					
Do you feel that you don't have enough money to take care of this person in addition to the rest of your expenses?					
Do you feel that you will be unable to take care of this person much longer?					
Do you feel you have lost control of your life since this person's illness?					
Do you wish you could leave the care of this person to someone else?					
Do you feel uncertain about what to do about this person?					
Do you feel you should be doing more for this person?					
Do you feel you could do a better job in caring for this person?					
Overall, how burdened do you feel in caring for this person?					

References

American Psychological Association. (1992). *Ethical principles of psychologists and code of conduct*. Washington, DC: American Psychological Association.

American Pschological Association (2006). Report of the Presidential Task Force on Evidence-Based Practice. See http://www.apa.org/practice/ebpreport.pdf/

American Psychiatric Association. (2000). *Diagnostic and Statistical Manual of Mental Disorders*, (4th ed.). Text Revision. Washington, DC: American Psychiatric Association.

Anheshensel, C. S., Pearlin, L. I., Mullan, J. T., Zarit, S. H., & Whitlatch, C. J. (1995). *Profiles in caregiving: The unexpected career*. San Diego, CA: Academic Press.

Antony, M. M., & Barlow, D. H. (2002). *Handbook of assessment and treatment planning for psychological disorders*. New York, NY: Guilford Publications, Inc.

APA Task Force on Evidence Based Practice. (2006). Report of the 2005 Presidential Task Force on Evidence-Based Practice. *American Psychologist*, *61*, 271–285.

Arean, P., Hegel, M., Vannoy, S., Fan, M. Y., & Unutzer, J. (2008). Effectiveness of problem-solving therapy for older primary care patients with depression: Results from the IMPACT project. *The Gerontologist*, *48*(3), 311–323.

Artiola, I., Fortuny, L., Hermosillo-Romo, D. H., Heaton, R. K., & Pardee, R. E. (1999). *Manual de normas y procedimientos para la Bateria Neuropsychologica en Espanol*. Tucson, AZ: mPress.

Ayers, C. R., Sorrell, J. T., Thorp, S. R., & Wetherell, J. L. (2007). Evidence-based psychological treatments for late-life anxiety. *Psychology and Aging*, *22*(1), 8–17.

Barlow, D. (2008). The Transdiagnostic Model: Interface Between Depression and Anxiety. Workshop presented at the Annual American Psychological Association Meeting in Boston, August 13, 2008.

Beaudreau, S. A., & O'Hara, R. (2008). Late-life anxiety and cognitive impairment: A review. *The American Journal of Geriatric Psychiatry*, *16*(10), 790–803.

Bernal, G., & Domenech Rodriguez, M. M. (2009). Advances in Latino family research: Cultural adaptations of evidence-based interventions. *Family Process*, *48*, 169–178.

Blazer, D. G. (2003). Depression in late life: Review and commentary. *Journal of Gerontology: Medical Sciences*, *58A*(3), 249–265.

Borkovec, T. D., & Costello, E. (1993). Efficacy of applied relaxation and cognitive–behavioral therapy in the treatment of generalized anxiety disorder. *Journal of Consulting and Clinical Psychology*, *61*(4), 611–619.

Brown, T. A., & Barlow, D. H. (2005). Dimensional versus categorical classification of mental disorders in the fifth edition of the Diagnostic and Statistical Manual of Mental Disorders and beyond: Comment on the special section. *Journal of Abnormal Psychology*, *114*(4), 551–556.

Brown, T. A., Antony, M. M., & Barlow, D. H. (1995). Diagnostic comorbidity in panic disorder: Effect on treatment outcome and course of comorbid diagnoses following treatment. *Journal of Consulting and Clinical Psychology*, *63*(3), 408–418.

Byrd, D. A., & Manley, J. J. (2005). Cultural considerations in the neuropsychological assessment of older adults. In S. S. Bush, & T. A. Martin (Eds.), *Geriatric Neuropsychology: Practice Essentials* (pp. 115–139). Philadelphia, PA: Taylor & Francis.

Castonguay, L. G., & Beutler, L. E. (2006). Principles of therapeutic change: A task force on participants, relationships, and techniques factors. *Journal of Clinical Psychology*, *62*(6), 631–638.

Chen, J., Nakano, Y., Ietzugu, T., Ogawa, S., Funayama, T., Watanabe, N., Noda, Y., & Furukawa, T. A. (2007). *BMC Psychiatry*, *7*, ArtID 69.

Chopra, M. P., Zubritsky, C., Knott, K., Have, T. T., Hadley, T., Coyne, J. C., et al. (2005). Importance of subsyndromal symptoms of depression in elderly patients. *American Journal of Geriatric Psychiatry*, *13*, 597–606.

Cortes, D. E., Rogler, L. H., & Malgady, R. G. (1994). Biculturality among Puerto Rican adults in the United States. *American Journal of Community Psychology*, *22*, 707–721.

Cuellar, I., Arnold, B., & Maldonado, R. (1995). Acculturation Rating Scale for Mexican Americans-II: A revision of the original ARSMA scale. *Hispanic Journal of Behavioral Sciences*, *17*, 275–304.

Dana, R. H. (1993). *Multicultural assessment perspectives for professional psychology.* Needham Heights, MA: Allyn & Bacon.

Degenholtz, H. B., Rosen, J., Castle, N., Mittal, V., & Liu, D. (2008). The association between changes in health status and nursing home resident quality of life. *The Gerontologist*, *48*(5), 584–592.

Domenech-Rodriguez, M., & Weiling, E. (2004). Developing culturally appropriate, evidence-based treatments for interventions with ethnic minority populations. In M. Rastogin & E. Wieling (Eds.), *Voices of color: First person accounts of ethnic minority therapists* (pp. 313–333). Thousand Oaks, CA: Sage.

Eisman, E. J., Dies, R. R., Finn, S. E., Eyde, L. D., Kay, G. G., Kubiszyn, T. W., et al. (2000). Problems and limitations in using psychological assessment in contemporary health care delivery system. *Professional Psychology: Research and Practice*, *31*(2), 131–140.

Escobar, J., Gara, M. A., Diaz-Martinez, A. M., Interian, A., Warman, M., Allen, L. A., et al. (2007). Effectiveness of a time-limited cognitive behavior therapy-type intervention among primary care patients with medically unexplained symptoms. *Annals of Family Medicine*, *5*, 328–335.

Fennig, S., Craig, T. J., Tanenberg-Karant, M., & Bromet, E. J. (1994). Comparison of facility and research diagnoses in first-admission psychotic patients. *The American Journal of Psychiatry*, *151*, 1423–1429.

Fillenbaum, G. G., Heyman, A., Huber, M. S., Ganguli, M., & Unverzagt, F. W. (2001). Performance of elderly African American and white community residents on the CERAD Neuropsychological Battery. *Journal of the International Neuropsychological Society*, *7*, 502–509.

Finn, S. E., & Butcher, J. N. (1991). Clinical objective personality assessment. In M. Hersen, & A. E. Kazdin (Eds.), *The clinical psychology handbook* (2nd ed.). (pp. 362–373) New York, NY: Pergamon Press.

Finn, S. E., & Tonsager, M. E. (1997). Information gathering and therapeutic models of assessment: Complimentary paradigms. *Psychological Assessment*, *9*, 374–385.

Finn, S. E., & Tonsager, M. E. (2002). How therapeutic assessment became humanistic. *The Humanistic Psychologist*, *84*, 19–22.

First, M. B., & Gibbon, M. (2004). The Structured Clinical Interview for DSM-IV Axis I Disorders (SCID-I) and the Structured Clinical Interview for DSM-IV Axis II Disorders(SCID-II). In M. J. Hilsenroth, & D. Segal (Eds.), *Comprehensive handbook of psychological assessment* (pp. 134–143). Hoboken, NJ: John Wiley & Sons.

Folstein, M., Folstein, S., & McHugh, P. (1975). Mini-mental state: A practical method for grading the cognitive state of patients for the clinician. *Journal of Psychiatric Research*, *12*, 189–198.

Gallagher-Thompson, D., & Coon, D. W. (2007). Evidence-based psychological treatments for distress in family caregivers of older adults. *Psychology and Aging*, *22*(1), 37–51.

Gasquoine, P. G. (2001). Research in clinical neuropsychology with Hispanic American participants: A review. *Clinical Neuropsychologist*, *15*, 2–12.

Gatz, M. (2007). Commentary on evidence-based psychological treatments for older adults. *Psychology and Aging*, *22*(1), 52–55.

Groth-Marnat, G. (2003). *Handbook of psychological assessment*. Hoboken, NJ: Wiley, John & Sons, Inc.

Hawes, C., Phillips, C. D., Holan, S., Sherman, M., & Hutchison, L. L. (2005). Assisted living in rural America: Results from a national survey. *Journal of Rural Health*, *21*(2), 131–139.

Heaton, R. K., Miller, S. W., Taylor, M. J., & Grant, I. (2004). *Revised comprehensive norms for an expanded Halstead-Reitan Battery: Demographically adjusted neuropsychological norms for African American and Caucasian adults*. Lutz, FL: Psychological Assessment Resources.

Hinrichsen, G. A. (2008). Interpersonal psychotherapy as a treatment for depression in later life. *Professional Psychology: Research and Practice*, *39*(3), 306–312.

Howard, K. I., Moras, K., Brill, P. L., Martinovich, Z., & Lutz, W. (1996). Evaluation of psychotherapy. Efficacy, effectiveness, and patient progress. *The American Psychologist*, *51*(10), 1059–1064.

Hunsley, J., Crabb, R., & Mash, E. J. (2004). Evidence-based clinical assessment. *Clinical Psychologist*, *57*, 25–32.

Hwang, W., Wood, J. J., Lin, K., & Cheung, F. (2006). Cognitive–behavioral therapy with Chinese Americans: Research, theory, and clinical practice. *Cognitive and Behavioral Practice*, *13*, 293–303.

Hyer, L. A., Molinari, V., Mills, W., & Yeager, C. A. (2008). Older Adults: Personalogic Assessment and Treatment. In T. Millon (Ed.), *Personalized Clinical Assessment: A Practitioner's Guide to The Millon Inventories*. New York, NY: John Wiley & Sons, Inc.

Hyer, L. A., Yeager, C. A., Shah, S., Nizam, Z., & Coleman, J. (2007). *Depression and Insight are medicated by language skills in dementia*. San Francisco, CA: American Psychological Association Annual Convention. August 17, 2007.

Hyer, L., & Intrieri, R. (2006). *Geropsychological interventions in long-term care*. New York, NY: Springer Publishing Company, Inc.

Hyer, L., Kramer, D., & Sohnle, S. (2004). CBT with older people: Alterations and the value of the therapeutic alliance. *Psychotherapy: Theory, Research, Practice, Training*, *41*(3), 276–291.

Institute of Medicine. (2004). *"Forum on Evidence Based Medicine."* Washington, DC: Institute of Medicine.

Jacobson, N. S., & Truax, P. (1991). Clinical significance: A statistical approach to defining meaningful change in psychotherapy research. *Journal of Consulting and Clinical Psychology*, *59*(1), 12–19.

Karlin, B. E., & Duffy, M. (2004). Geriatric mental health policy: Impact on service delivery and directions for effecting change. *Professional Psychology: Research and Practice*, *35*, 509–519.

Kim, B. S. K., & Abreu, J. M. (2001). Acculturation measurement: Theory, current instruments, and future directions. In J. G. Ponterotto, J. M. Casas, L. A. Suzuki, & C. M. Alexander (Eds.), *Handbook of multicultural counseling* (2nd ed). (pp. 394–424). Thousand Oaks, CA: Sage Publications, Inc.

Kim, B. S., & Hong, S. (2004). A psychometric revision of the Asian Values Scale using the Rasch Model. *Measurement and Evaluation in Counseling and Development*, *37*, 15–27.

Klonoff, E. A., & Landrine, H. (2000). Revising and improving the African American Acculturation Scale. *Journal of Black Psychology*, *26*, 235–261.

Kim, E., & Rovner, B. (1996). The nursing home as a psychiatric hospital. In W. E. Reichman, & P. R. Katz (Eds.), *Psychiatric care in the nursing home*. New York, NY: Oxford University Press.

Kubiszyn, T. W., Meyer, G. J., Finn, S. E., Eyde, L. D., Kay, G. G., Moreland, K. L., et al. (2000). Empirical support for psychological assessment in clinical health care settings. *Professional Psychology: Research and Practice*, *31*(2), 119–130.

Lahey, B. B. (2009). Public health significance of neuroticism. *American Psychologist*, *64*(4), 241–256.

Lambert, C. E., & Lambert, V. A. (1999). Psychological hardiness: State of the science. *Holistic Nursing Practice*, *13*(3), 11–19.

Lambert, M. J., Hansen, N. B., & Finch, A. E. (2001). Patient-focused research: Using patient outcome data to enhance treatment effects. *Journal of Consulting and Clinical Psychology*, *69*(2), 159–172.

Lambert, M. J., Whipple, J. L., Hawkins, E. J., Nielsen, S. L., Smart, D. W., & Vermeersch, D. A. (2003). Is it time for clinicians to routinely track patient outcome? A meta-analysis. *Clinical Psychology: Science and Practice*, *10*(3), 288–301.

Langbaum, J., Rebok, G. W., Bandeen-Roche, K., & Carlson, M. C. (2009). Predicting memory training response patterns: Results from ACTIVE. *The Journals of Gerontology: Series B: Psychological Sciences and Social Sciences*, *64*, 14–23.

La Roche, M., & Christopher, S. (2008). Culture and empirically supported treatments: On the road to a collision? *Culture and Psychology*, *14*, 333–356.

Lyketsos, C. G., Colenda, C. C., Beck, C., Blank, K., Doraiswamy, M. P., Kalunian, D. A., et al. (2006). Position statement of the American Association for Geriatric Psychiatry regarding principles of care for patients with dementia resulting from Alzheimer disease. *The American Journal of Geriatric Psychiatry*, *14*(7), 561–572.

Mak, M. W., Law, R. W., Alvidrez, J., & Perez-Stable, E. J. (2007). Gender and ethnic diversity in NUMH-funded trials: Review of a decade of published research. *Administration and Policy in Mental Health and Mental Health Services Research*, *34*, 497–503.

Manley, J. J., Miller, S. W., Heaton, R. K., Byrd, D., Reilly, J., Velasquez, R. J., et al. (1998). The effect of African-American acculturation on neuropsychological test performance in normal and HIV-positive individuals. *Journal of the International Neuropsychological Society*, *4*, 291–302.

Manley, J. J., Jacobs, D. M., Touradji, P., Small, S. A., & Stern, Y. (2002). Reading level attenuates differences in neuropsychological test performance between African American and white elders. *Journal of the International Neuropsychological Society*, *8*, 341–348.

Manley, J. J. (2006). Cultural issues. In D. K. Attix, & K. A. Welsh-Bohmer (Eds.), *Geriatric Neuropsychology: Assessment and Intervention*. New York, NY: The Guilford Press.

Mash, E. J., & Foster, S. L. (2001). Exporting analogue behavioral observation from research to clinical practice: Useful or cost-defective? *Psychological Assessment*, *13*(1), 86–98.

Mash, E. J., & Hunsley, J. (1993). Assessment considerations in the identification of failing psychotherapy: Bringing the negatives out of the darkroom: Treatment implications of psychological assessment. *Psychological Assessment*, *5*(3), 292–301.

Mausbach, B. T., Aschbacher, K., Patterson, T. L., Ancoli-Israel, S., von Känel, R., Mills, P. J., et al. (2006). Avoidant coping partially mediates the relationship between patient problem behaviors and depressive symptoms in spousal Alzheimer caregivers. *The American Journal of Geriatric Psychiatry*, *14*(4), 299–306.

Max, W., Webber, P., & Fox, P. (1995). Alzheimer's disease: The unpaid burden of caring. *Journal of Aging and Health*, *7*(2), 179–199.

Messer, S. B. (2004). Evidence-based practice: Beyond empirically supported treatments. *Professional Psychology: Research and Practice*, *35*, 580–588.

Meyer, G. J., Finn, S. E., Eyde, L. D., Kay, G. G., Moreland, K. L., Dies, R. R., et al. (2001). Psychological testing and psychological assessment: A review of evidence and issues. *The American Psychologist*, *56*(2), 128–165.

Millon, T., & Bloom, C. (2008). *The Millon inventories: A practitioner's guide to personalized clinical assessment* (2nd ed). New York, NY: Guilford Press. 732 pp.

Mineka, S., Watson, D., & Clark, L. A. (1998). Comorbidity of anxiety and unipolar mood disorders. *Annual Review of Psychology*, *49*, 377–412.

Mitchell, A., Vaze, A., & Rao, S. (2009). Clinical diagnosis of depression in primary care: A meta-analysis. *The Lancet*, *374*, 609–619.

Mitrushina, M., Boone, K. B., Razani, J., & D'Elia, L. F. (2005). *Handbook of normative data for neuropsychological assessment,* (2nd ed.). New York, NY: Oxford University Press.

Morey, L. C. (1996). *An interpretive guide to the Personality Assessment Inventory*. Odessa, FL: Psychological Assessment Resources.

Nell, V. (2000). *Cross-cultural neuropsychological assessment: Theory and practice*. Mahwah, NJ: Lawrence Erlbaum Associates.

Nezu, A. M., Nezu, C. M., & Lombardo, E. R. (2001). Cognitive-behavior therapy for medically unexplained symptoms: A critical review of the treatment literature. *Behavior Therapy*, *32*(3), 537–583.

Nezu, A. M., Nezu, C. M., & Lombardo, E. (2004). *Cognitive-behavioral case formulation and treatment design: A problem-solving approach*. New York, NY: Springer Publishing Company, Inc.

Norcross, J. C. (2002). *Psychotherapy relationships that work: Therapist contributions and responsiveness to patients*. New York, NY: Oxford University Press.

Norcross, J. C., Koocher, G. P., & Hogan, T. P. (2008). *Clinician's guide to evidence-based practices: Mental health and the addictions*. New York, NY: Oxford University Press.

Olfson, M., & Marcus, S. C. (2009). National patterns in antidepressant medication treatment. *Archives of General Psychiatry*, *66*, 848–856.

Persons, J. B. (2006). Case formulation-driven psychotherapy. *Clinical Psychology: Science and Practice*, *13*(2), 167–170.

Pinquart, M., & Sörenson, S. (2003). Associations of stressors and uplifts of caregiving with caregiver burden and depressive mood: A meta-analysis. *Journal of Gerontology: Psychological Sciences*, *58B*, 122–128.

Piotrowski, C. (1999). Assessment practices in the era of managed care: Current status and future directions. *Journal of Clinical Psychology*, *55*(7), 787–796.

Ponton, M. O., Satz, P., Herrera, L., Ortiz, F., Urrutia, C. P., et al. (1996). Normative data stratified by age and education for the Neuropsychological Screening Battery for Hispanics (NeSBHIS): Initial report. *Journal of the International Neuropsychological Society*, *2*, 96–104.

Pruchno, R. A., Kleban, M. H., Michaels, J. E., & Dempsey, N. P. (1990). Mental and physical health of caregiving spouses: Development of a causal model. *Journal of Gerontology*, *45*(5), 192–199.

Randolph, C., Tierney, M. C., Mohr, E., & Chase, T. N. (1998). The Repeatable Battery for the Assessment of Neuropsychological Status (RBANS): Preliminary clinical validity. *Journal of Clinical and Experimental Neuropsychology*, *20*, 310–319.

Reichman, W., & Katz, P. (2008). *Psychiatry in long-term care*. New York, NY: Oxford University Press.

Russo, J., & Vitaliano, P. P. (1995). Life events as correlates of burden in spouse caregivers of persons with Alzheimer's disease. *Experimental Aging Research*, *21*(3), 273–294.

Schulz, R., McGinnis, K. A., Zhang, S., Martire, L. M., Hebert, R. S., Beach, S. R., et al. (2008). Dementia patient suffering and caregiver depression. *Alzheimer's Disease and Associated Disorders*, *22*(2), 170–176.

Scogin, F., Morthland, M., Kaufman, A., Burgio, L., Chaplin, W., & Kong, G. (2007). Improving quality of life in diverse rural older adults: A randomized trial of a psychological treatment. *Psychology and Aging*, *22*, 657–665.

Sinoff, G., & Werner, P. (2003). Anxiety disorder and accompanying subjective memory loss in the elderly as a predictor of future cognitive decline. *International Journal of Geriatric Psychiatry*, *18*(10), 951–959.

Stanley, M. A., Wilson, N. L., Novy, D. M., Rhoades, H. M., Wagener, H. M., Greisinger, A. J., et al. (2009). Cognitive behavior therapy for generalized anxiety disorder among older adults in primary care: A randomized clinical trial. *The Journal of the American Medical Association*, *301*(14), 1460–1467.

Strauss, E., Sherman, E., & Spreen, O. (2006). *A compendium of neuropsychological tests: Administration, norms, and commentary* (3rd ed.). New York, NY: Oxford University Press.

Suinn, R. M., Khoo, G., & Ahuna, C. (1995). The Suinn-Lew Asian Self-Identity Acculturation Scale: Cross-cultural information. *Journal of Multicultural Counseling and Development*, *23*, 139–148.

Tanaka-Matsumi, J., Seiden, D. Y., & Lam, K. N. (1996). The Culturally Informed Functional Assessment (CIFA) Interview: A strategy for cross-cultural behavioral practice. *Cognitive and Behavioral Practice*, *3*(2), 215–233.

Turchik, J. A., Karpenko, V., Hammers, D., & McNamara, J. R. (2007). Practical and ethical assessment issues in rural, impoverished, and managed care settings. *Professional Psychology: Research and Practice*, *38*(2), 158–168.

U.S. Census Bureau News. (2004). Census Bureau projects tripling of Hispanic and Asian populations in 50 years: Non-Hispanic whites may drop to half total population. Retrieved August 2009 from http://www.census.gov/press-release/www/releases/archives/population.001720.html

Vitaliano, P. P., Zhang, J., Young, H. M., Caswell, L. W., Scanlan, J. M., & Echeverria, D. (2009). Depressed mood mediates decline in cognitive processing speed in caregivers. *The Gerontologist*, *49*(1), 12–22.

Wampold, B. E. (2001). *Great psychotherapy debate: Models, methods, and findings*. Oxford, United Kingdom: Taylor & Francis, Inc.

Watson, D., Wiese, D., Vaidya, J., & Tellegen, A. (1999). The two general activation systems of affect: Structural findings, evolutionary considerations, and psychobiological evidence: The structure of emotion. *Journal of Personality and Social Psychology*, *76*(5), 820–838.

Wetherell, J. L., Lenze, E. J., & Stanley, M. A. (2005). Evidence-based treatment of geriatric anxiety disorders. *The Psychiatric Clinics of North America*, *28*(4), 871–896.

Williamson, G. M., & Schulz, R. (1993). Coping with specific stressors in Alzheimer's disease caregiving. *The Gerontologist*, *33*(6), 747–755.

Wright, L., Clipp, E., & George, L. (1993). Medical consequences of caregiving. *Medicine, Exercise, Nutrition, and Health*, *2*, 181–195.

Yeager, C. A., Hyer, L. A., Hobbs, B., & Coyne, A. (2010). Alzheimer's disease and vascular dementia: The complex relationship between diagnosis and caregiver burden. *Issues in Mental Health Nursing*, *31*, 1–8.

Yesavage, J. A., Brink, T. L., Rose, T. L., Lum, O., Huang, V., Adey, M., et al. (1982). Development and validation of a geriatric depression screening scale: A preliminary report. *Journal of Psychiatric Research*, *17* (1), 37–49.

Zane, N., & Mak, W. (2003). Major approaches to the measurement of acculturation among ethnic minority populations: A content analysis and an alternative empirical strategy. In K. M. Chun, O. P. Balls Organista, & G. Marin (Eds.), *Acculturation: Advances in theory, measurement, and applied research* (pp. 39–60). Washington, DC: American Psychological Association.

Zarit, S. (2006). The history of caregiving in dementia. In S. Lobo-Prabhu, V. Molinari, & J. Lomax (Eds.), *Supporting the caregiver in dementia: A guide for health care professionals* (pp. 3–22). Baltimore, MD: Johns Hopkins University Press.

Zea, M. C., Asner-Self, K. K., Birman, D., & Buki, L. P. (2003). The Abbreviated Multidimentional Acculturation Scale: Empirical validation with two Latino/Latina samples. *Cultural Diversity and Ethnic Minority Psychology*, *9*, 107–112.

Zhang, B. H., Tan, Y. L., Zhang, W. F., Wang, Z. R., Yang, G. G., et al. (2008). Repeatable battery for the assessment of neuropsychological status as a screening test in Chinese: reliability and validity. *Chinese Mental Health Journal*, *22*, 865–869.

CHAPTER

4 Assessment of Personality Disorders in Older Adults

Thomas F. Oltmanns[1], Steve Balsis[2]

[1] *Department of Psychology, Washington University in St. Louis, St. Louis, MO, USA,*

[2] *Department of Psychology, Texas A&M University, College Station, Texas, TX, USA*

OVERVIEW

If depression is the common cold of psychopathology, then personality disorders are the chronic headache. Common colds come and go. But like chronic headaches, personality disorders can be much more persistent, and they are more difficult to treat. While the common cold or depression may temporarily affect an individual's ability to maintain good work habits and social relationships, a chronic headache or personality disorder can plague a person in those areas for decades or even a lifetime. In this way, a personality disorder can have deleterious effects that become cumulative over time and have reverberating effects well into later life.

When personality disorders are present in later life, they can have unique implications for families, society, and the affected individuals. With advancing age, an individual's changing needs often require a greater reliance on family. Meeting the needs of an older adult with a personality disorder may be particularly difficult. Consider a man with narcissistic personality disorder who has steadily alienated his family members through his egotistical conduct over the course of a lifetime. Now, when his family must decide who (if anyone) will have the responsibility of providing care for their abrasive relative, the family members may be understandably reluctant to volunteer for this unpleasant task. This decision process may, in turn, create new tension within the family that may cause difficulties that extend beyond the death of the difficult family member.

Another area of unique concern is the immense cost of health care that treating older adults with personality disorders may entail. People with personality disorders are more prone to suffer from a variety of medical illnesses, have long hospital stays, and generally experience poor treatment outcomes (Gish et al., 2001; Spiessl, Hubner-Liebermann, Binder, & Cording, 2002; Whiteman, Deary, & Fawkes, 2000). To add to these misfortunes, the very nature of personality disorders makes sufferers more likely to exhibit inappropriate behavior when hospitalized. These inappropriate behaviors are known to affect both hospital staff and other residents. Granted that older adults are already the primary users of the health care system, those older adults with personality disorders will inevitably be especially burdensome for the health care system (Agronin & Maletta, 2000; Rosowsky, 1999; Rosowsky & Gurian, 1992; Rosowsky & Smyer, 1999).

In addition to creating difficulty for their families and the health care system, older adults with personality disorders may themselves experience difficulty adjusting to changes that result from the normal aging process. Psychologically healthy adults usually adjust more or less satisfactorily to their gradually declining physical strength, youthful attractiveness, vitality, health, and cognitive abilities.

Handbook of Assessment in Clinical Gerontology. DOI: 10.1016/B978-0-12-374961-1.10004-1

Older adults with personality disorders, however, may experience unique adjustment challenges. Take for example an older woman with a narcissistic personality disorder whose egotism was satisfied in her younger years by a reasonable belief in her own physical attractiveness. As a young woman she may have devoted much energy to focusing on and maintaining her appearance, potentially at the cost of fostering significant character flaws related to this excessive vanity. With ever-increasing age, the challenges to her ego may become particularly incisive. As her primary source of personal pride rests on superficial beauty, her decreasing muscle tone and increased wrinkling of the skin may become psychologically devastating. With no fallback and no alternative source of self-esteem, as this woman's youth wanes she may be prone to develop a mental disorder such as depression.

Understanding the interaction between personality disorder pathology and the challenges posed by aging is a complicated matter. What makes the situation especially difficult to understand is the absence of adequate measurement instruments. Existing measures of personality disorder pathology were not designed with an older adult population in mind (Agronin & Maletta, 2000; Balsis, Woods, Gleason, & Oltmanns, 2007; Segal, Hersen, Van Hasselt, Silberman, & Roth, 1996). Before we can study the influence of personality disorder pathology in the lives of older adults, therefore, it is necessary to develop measurement instruments that are specifically tailored to address the unique context(s) of older people (Agronin & Maletta, 2000; Clarkin, Spielman, & Klausner, 1999; Mroczek, Hurt, & Berman, 1999). The remaining part of this chapter will address fundamental problems with the assessment of personality disorders and highlight the specific challenges that arise when later life is considered. We begin this discussion with a review of some basic definitional issues.

DEFINITIONAL ISSUES

To qualify for a personality disorder diagnosis in DSM-IV-TR, a person must fit the *general definition* of personality disorder (which applies to all 10 subtypes) and must also meet the *specific criteria* for a particular type of personality disorder. The specific criteria consist of a list of traits and behaviors that characterize the disorder. The general definition emphasizes the duration of the pattern and the social impairment associated with the traits in question. The problems must be part of "an enduring pattern of inner experience and behavior that deviates markedly from the expectations of the individual's culture" (American Psychiatric Association, 2000), which is evident in two or more of the following domains: cognition (such as ways of thinking about the self and other people); emotional responses; interpersonal functioning; or impulse control. Beyond these requirements, the pattern of maladaptive experience and behavior must also be:

- Inflexible and pervasive across a broad range of personal and social situations;
- The source of clinically significant distress or impairment in social, occupational, or other important areas of functioning;
- Stable and of long duration, with an onset that can be traced back at least to adolescence or early adulthood.

The concept of social dysfunction plays an important role in the definition of personality disorders. It provides a large part of the justification for defining these problems as mental disorders. If the personality characteristics identified in the DSM-IV-TR criterion sets typically interfere with the person's ability to get along with other people and perform social roles, they become more than just a collection of eccentric traits or peculiar habits. They can then be viewed as a form of harmful dysfunction (Wakefield, 1999). In fact, most of the clusters of pathological personality traits that are described on Axis II do lead to impaired social functioning or occupational impairment (Oltmanns, Melley, & Turkheimer, 2002; Skodol, Johnson, Cohen, Sneed, & Crawford, 2007).

The DSM-IV-TR treats personality disorders as discrete categories, and assumes that there are distinct boundaries between normal and abnormal personalities. However, there are many people with serious personality problems who do not fit the official DSM-IV-TR subtypes. The categorical approach to diagnosis forces clinicians to use a threshold that has been set to distinguish between normal and abnormal personality types. These thresholds have been called arbitrary by many, because most of them have no empirical support or logical justification. Recent work supports the notion that these thresholds are indeed "arbitrary" because they can correspond to varying levels of latent pathology (Balsis, Cooper, Lowmaster, & Benge, in press).

Another frequent complaint about the definition of personality disorders is that there is considerable overlap among categories. Many patients meet the criteria for more than one type (Grant et al., 2005). It is cumbersome to list multiple diagnoses, especially when the clinician is already asked to list problems on both Axis I and Axis II. For this reason, many clinicians are reluctant to make more than one diagnosis on Axis II; consequently, much information is frequently left out.

Developmental issues create additional challenges for the assessment of personality disorders, particularly with regard to the formal diagnostic categories defined in DSM-IV-TR (Tackett, Balsis, Oltmanns, & Krueger, 2009). One problem is that the DSM-IV-TR allows for a diagnosis of a personality disorder if "its onset can be traced back at least to adolescence or early adulthood." The manual does not allow for the possibility of a late-onset personality disorder (Widiger & Seidlitz, 2002). How is information about adolescence and early adulthood collected for an older adult? After all, that time period might have occurred 50 or 60 years ago. If a 70-year-old person currently exhibits a sufficient number of features to qualify for a specific personality disorder diagnosis, the clinician would need to establish that these symptoms were also evident many years ago. Should we rely on the person's recollections of long past experiences to verify the diagnosis, recognizing that autobiographical memories are often flawed? The most practical solution is to focus on the person's recent experience, recognizing that it is difficult to create a completely accurate portrait of the past.

For these reasons and many others most experts favor the development of an alternative classification system for personality pathology, one that would be based on a dimensional view of current personality pathology that is grounded in extensive research on the basic elements of personality. A dimensional system might provide a more complete description of each person, and it would be more useful with patients who fall on the boundaries between different types of personality disorder. It might also be easier to use than the DSM-IV-TR approach. One proposal is to use the 5-factor model as the basic structure for a comprehensive description of personality problems (Widiger & Trull, 2007). Later in this chapter, we will discuss DSM-based and alternative systems in depth. For now though, it is important for the reader to recognize that there are both DSM-based and trait-based conceptualizations of personality pathology.

EPIDEMIOLOGY OF PERSONALITY DISORDERS

Personality disorders are generally considered to be among the most common forms of psychopathology, when they are considered as a general category. Several epidemiological studies in the United States and in Europe have used semi-structured diagnostic interviews to assess personality disorders in samples of people living in the community.

In studies that have examined community-based samples of adults, the overall lifetime prevalence for having at least one personality disorder (any type) varies between 10–14% (Coid, Yang, Tyrer, Roberts, & Ullrich, 2006; Lenzenweger et al., 2007; Torgersen, Kringlen, & Cramer, 2001). While this figure tends to be relatively consistent from one study to the next, prevalence rates for specific types of personality disorder vary quite a bit from one study to the next. The highest prevalence rates are usually found to be associated with obsessive–compulsive personality disorder, antisocial personality disorder, and avoidant personality disorder, which may affect 3 or 4% of adults.

The most precise information that is available regarding the prevalence of personality disorders in community samples is available for the antisocial type (Moran, 1999). In two large-scale epidemiological studies of mental disorders, structured interviews were conducted with several thousand participants. The overall lifetime prevalence rate for antisocial personality disorder (men and women combined) was 3% in both studies (Kessler, McGonagle, Zhao, & Nelson, 1994; Robins & Regier, 1991).

The prevalence of other specific types of personality disorders tends to be approximately 1 or 2% of the population. The most obvious exception is narcissistic personality disorder, which appears to be the least common form, affecting much less than 1% of the population. Investigators tend to identify very few cases of narcissistic personality disorder when they interview people in community samples (as opposed to clinic settings). The fact that almost no one endorses narcissistic symptoms does not necessarily mean, however, that the disorder does not occur. Rather, it seems possible that people who experience these features do not recognize the nature of their own problems or are unwilling to admit them. Self-report measures, such as questionnaires and interviews, may not be effective instruments for assessing narcissistic personality disorder. More accurate information might be obtained from other people who know the person well and can report examples of grandiosity, exploitation, or lack of empathy (Oltmanns & Turkheimer, 2006).

Another issue regarding prevalence rates involves comorbidity. There is considerable overlap among categories in the personality disorders. At least 50% of people who meet the diagnostic criteria for one personality disorder also meet the criteria for another disorder (Coid et al., 2006). To some extent, this overlap is due to the fact that similar symptoms are used to define more than one disorder. For example, impulsive and reckless behaviors are part of the definition of both antisocial and borderline personality disorders. Social withdrawal is used to define schizoid, schizotypal, and avoidant personality disorder.

There is also extensive overlap between personality disorders and disorders that are diagnosed on Axis I of DSM-IV-TR. Approximately 75% of people who qualify for a diagnosis on Axis II also meet criteria for a syndrome such as major depression, substance dependence, or an anxiety disorder (Dolan-Sewell, Krueger, & Shea, 2001). This overlap may also be viewed from the other direction: many people who are treated for a mental disorder listed on Axis I, such as depression or alcoholism, would also meet the criteria for a personality disorder (Thomas, Melchert, & Banken, 1999). Borderline personality disorder appears to be the most common personality disorder among patients treated at mental health facilities (both inpatient and outpatient settings). Averaged across studies, the evidence suggests that this disorder is found among slightly more than 30% of all patients who are treated for psychological disorders (Mattia & Zimmerman, 2001).

The overall prevalence of personality disorders is approximately equal in men and women (Weissman, 1993). There are, however, consistent gender differences with regard to at least one specific disorder: antisocial personality disorder is unquestionably much more common among men than among women, with rates of approximately 5% reported for men and 1% for women (Kessler et al., 1994). Thus, antisocial personality disorder is actually an alarmingly common problem among adult males in the United States. Epidemiological evidence regarding gender differences for the other types of personality disorder is much more ambiguous. Borderline personality disorder and dependent personality disorder may be somewhat more prevalent among women than men, but the evidence is not strong (Skodol & Bender, 2003). There has been some speculation that paranoid and obsessive–compulsive personality disorders may be somewhat more common among men than women (Coid et al., 2006).

The prevalence of personality disorders in later life is an under-studied phenomenon. Still, of the handful of studies that have been conducted, the general conclusion has been that personality disorders become rarer with age. Using community-dwelling samples, Ames and Molinari (1994) found that just under 18% of the younger adults were diagnosed with a personality disorder compared with only about 13% of the older adults. In an examination of a clinical sample of psychiatric inpatient veterans, while many younger adults were diagnosed with a personality disorder (76%), considerably fewer older adults were given this diagnosis (55%) (Kenan et al., 2000). Data from longitudinal studies also provide evidence that increasing age is associated with reduced susceptibility to personality disorders (e.g., Lenzenweger, Johnson, & Willett, 2004; see Paris, 2003, for a brief review).

The underlying cause of this apparent decrease of personality disorders with age is unclear. One theory is that with the general slowing associated with age, some of the vitality that once fueled personality disorders is lost. A "mellowing" effect therefore takes place that reduces the problematic conduct to subclinical levels (Kenan et al., 2000; Paris, 2003). Some studies, however, suggest that this reduction of personality disorders with age may be somewhat illusory. The idea is that while certain symptoms of personality disorders may disappear with increasing age, this does not eliminate all social and interpersonal problems in the lives of these older individuals (Drake, Adler, & Valliant, 1988; Moffitt, Caspi, Harrington, & Milne, 2002). This notion raises the possibility that although the behavioral expression of personality disorders may change over time, these altered forms of conduct are by no means innocuous. In other words, the older adults may still have the personality disorder from youth, but it may express itself differently in later life. If this is true, then the reported reductions in personality disorders for older adults may be best explained as an artifact of the measurement instrument employed. What may be needed is an adapted measure that will be sensitive to the changing face of personality disorder that appears with advancing age (Agronin & Maletta, 2000; Clarkin et al., 1999; Mroczek et al., 1999; Segal et al., 1996). We return to this possibility later in the chapter.

STABILITY AND CHANGE

Temporal stability is one of the most important assumptions about personality disorders. Evidence for the assumption that personality disorders appear during adolescence and persist into adulthood has, until recently, been limited primarily to antisocial personality disorder. A classic follow-up study by Lee Robins (1966) began with a large set of records describing young children treated for adjustment problems at a clinic during the 1920s. Robins was able to locate and interview almost all of these people, who by then were adults. The best predictor of an adult diagnosis of antisocial personality was conduct disorder in childhood. The people who were most likely to be considered antisocial as adults were boys who had been referred to the clinic on the basis of serious theft or aggressive behavior; who exhibited such behaviors across a variety of situations; and whose antisocial behaviors created conflict with adults outside their own homes. More than half of the boys who exhibited these characteristics were given a diagnosis of antisocial personality disorder as adults.

Another longitudinal study has collected information regarding the prevalence and stability of personality disorders among adolescents (Bernstein, Cohen, Velez, & Schwab-Stone, 1993; Cohen, Crawford, Johnson, & Kasen, 2005). This investigation is particularly important because it did not depend solely on subjects who had been referred for psychological treatment, and because it was concerned with the full range of personality disorders. The rate of personality disorders was relatively high in this sample: seventeen percent of the adolescents received a diagnosis of at least one personality disorder. Categorically defined diagnoses were not particularly stable; fewer than half of the adolescents who originally qualified for a personality disorder diagnosis met the same criteria two years later. Nevertheless, many of the study participants continued to exhibit similar problems over the next eight years. Viewed from a dimensional perspective, the maladaptive traits that represent the core features of the disorders remained relatively stable between adolescence and young adulthood (Crawford, Cohen, & Brook, 2001; Skodel et al., 2007).

Several studies have examined the stability of personality disorders among people who have received professional treatment for their problems, especially those who have been hospitalized for schizotypal or borderline disorders. Many patients who have been treated for these problems are still significantly impaired several years later, but the disorders are not uniformly stable (Grilo et al., 2004; Paris, 2003). Recovery rates are relatively high among patients with a diagnosis of borderline personality disorder. If patients who were initially treated during their early twenties are followed up when they are in their forties and fifties, only about one person in four would still qualify for a diagnosis of borderline personality disorder. The long-term prognosis is less optimistic for schizotypal and schizoid personality disorders. People with these diagnoses are likely to remain socially isolated and occupationally impaired. But even these results must be viewed within the lens of age associated measurement bias and the relevant psychometric concerns.

The extent to which personality disorders dissipate or remain stable over the course of a lifetime has received remarkably little attention. One reason for the lack of research on this topic is that we do not have instruments that are sufficiently tailored to the interests and lifestyles of older adults. Despite the dearth of research on late-life changes in personality disorders, a good deal of focus has been given to the relative stability (or change) of normal personality traits over the lifespan. The issue has been examined using both longitudinal and cross-sectional personality data (e.g., Roberts & DelVecchio, 2000). A common finding has been that change in personality is limited to minor increases in agreeableness and conscientiousness, and minor decreases in neuroticism, extraversion, and openness to experience (e.g., Costa & McCrae, 1988; Terracciano, McCrae, Brant, & Costa, 2005). The interpretation of this body of research is, however, equivocal. The primary dispute centers around whether the degree of change observed in these studies is functionally significant or not. While some researchers dismiss the change as being a rather trival difference, others regard the change as being an important one. The latter contingent points out that many of these differences represent as much as a standard deviation of change (Roberts, Walton, & Viechtbauer, 2005).

PSYCHOMETRIC CONCERNS IN LATER LIFE

When applied to older adults, the weak psychometric properties of standard personality disorder assessments are quite evident. Face validity is severely compromised by the use of items clearly relevant only to the lifestyle of younger adults (Segal, Coolidge, & Rosowsky, 2006). One obvious example is the criterion for avoidant personality disorder, which begins, "Avoids occupational activities . . ." As most older adults are either retired or semi-retired, they are unlikely to endorse this item, regardless of whether they have avoidant personality disorder. This item, therefore, would not adequately assess this latent personality disorder. The criterion for schizoid personality disorder, "Neither enjoys nor experiences sexual relations," is another example of an item that has poor face validity for use with older adults. Older adults may not endorse this item because of physical or contextual factors related to aging, rather than for reasons having anything to do with schizoid pathology. Perhaps physical changes have reduced the quality of their sexual experience or their spouse has passed away, making the item largely irrelevant (see Zweig, 2008). Item face validity, of course, is merely a qualitative interpretation of the relevance of an item to the phenomenon it purports to measure.

Any legitimate problem with face validity, however, becomes quantifiable in terms of its influence on a wide range of psychometric properties, including content validity, criterion validity, internal reliability, utility, and so on (Balsis, Segal, & Donahue, 2009). For example, consider how having poor face validity influences the content validity (defined as the ability of a set of items together to measure all aspects of a particular phenomenon) of the eight items for obsessive–compulsive personality disorder (OCPD). At least three of these items (e.g., miserly pattern of spending; difficulty discarding worn-out things; overly conscientious about morals and ethics) measure behavior that, while relevant to OCPD in young adults, may also happen to be associated with generational differences between younger and older cohorts. Since these three items accordingly cannot be relied upon in the assessment of OCPD in older adults, only five items remain to capture behavior associated with the disorder. As any reduction in the number of items on an assessment means that a lesser range of features relevant to the disorder are covered, the content validity of this assessment has been decidedly impaired by the effective loss of nearly one-half of its items.

Content validity is but one negative consequence of poor face validity. The lack of adequate face validity will also have negative consequences for most types of reliability and validity. When an item measures some aspect of aging rather than personality disorder pathology, measurement error has been introduced into the set. The resulting weakness of the assessment will necessarily mean that only weak correlations can be expected with external measures needed for verifying different types of validity (e.g., convergent, divergent, predictive). Inter-rater reliability between independent assessments will be equally difficult to establish. We have been pursuing many of these statistical shortcomings in our own empirical work (e.g., Balsis, Gleason, Woods, & Oltmanns, 2007).

APPROACHES TO ASSESSMENT OF PERSONALITY DISORDERS

Personality disorders are among the most controversial categories in the diagnostic system for mental disorders (Kendell, 2002; Tyrer et al., 2007). They are difficult to identify reliably, their etiology is poorly understood, and there is relatively less evidence to indicate that they can be treated successfully (compared with mood and anxiety disorders, for example). For all of these reasons, it is important to think critically about the validity of these categories.

Although the DSM conceptualization of personality disorders is flawed, and although personality disorders are difficult to define and measure, they are also crucial concepts in the field of psychopathology. Several observations support this argument. First, personality disorders are associated with significant social and occupational impairment. They disrupt interpersonal relationships, including those involving friends and coworkers. Personality disorders also play an important role in many cases of marital discord and violence (Holtzworth-Munroe, 2000; Whisman, Tolejko, & Chatav, 2007). Second, the presence of pathological personality traits during adolescence is associated with an increased risk for the subsequent development of other mental disorders (Cohen, Chen, Crawford, Brook, & Gordon, 2007; Krueger, 1999). Negative emotionality (high neuroticism) often predicts the later onset of major depression or an anxiety disorder. Impulsivity and antisocial personality increase the person's risk for alcoholism. Third, in some cases, personality disorders actually represent the beginning stages of the onset of a more serious form of psychopathology. Paranoid and schizoid personality disorders, for example, sometimes precede the onset of schizophrenic disorders. Finally, the presence of a comorbid personality disorder can interfere with the treatment of a disorder such as depression (Fournier et al., 2008). All of these findings have been gleaned even though these concepts are difficult to measure. The following case study illustrates how personality pathology can present itself in unique ways in late-life, making it difficult to measure using standard measures designed for a younger adult's life context.

Case Study 1

John is a 78-year-old veteran and retired police officer. Although he is clearly somewhat frail, he has a ruggedness that suggests he was once a legitimately tough guy. He presented for therapy at the request of his new physician, who had noticed scarring and a few small punctures on his chest. During his intake, John explained that these punctures were caused years ago by high heels. Specifically, he stated that during sexual encounters with prostitutes (which were frequent) he would demand that the prostitutes stomp on his chest with their heels. He explained further that when younger he experienced only limited injury from this unusual practice, because at that time he was sufficiently strong that he could ensure some level of caution, suffering only the damage that he permitted. He explained further that these stompings made him feel "whole." In a very real way, this was a type of self-harm. In recent years, John has stopped this behavior for several reasons. His ability to perform sexually has changed and he no longer has the strength to resist injury from the high heels. Indeed, the practice had fully become life threatening.

John also described how in middle age he would exhibit what he called a "righteous indignation" against those who broke rules. He provided an example of how he typically reacted. He explained that he once saw a car run through a red light. John was so angered by this traffic violation that he somehow managed to move his truck in front of the offender's vehicle. He then stopped in the middle of the street and slammed his truck in reverse, smashing into the said unlawful automobile. This type of aggression showed up in other areas of his life as well. John often found himself in bar fights and other physical conflicts. As the years have passed, however, John no longer expresses his anger by directly confronting people. Rather, he gives outlet to his indignation through such relatively benign forms of retaliation as, for example, following a recalcitrant driver back to his home and letting the air out of his tires. Thus, while John still experiences some exaggerated emotional reactions, he now finds alternative ways to express these feelings than by the direct physical confrontations that his greater health and fitness emboldened him to engage in when he was younger.

When he was very young, John's temper often got him into trouble. He was often in detention at school and was considered a class bully. He was able to graduate high school, but had terrible grades because of poor effort. Accordingly, with few other options after graduation, he decided to go into the military. He thought entering the military would give him a chance to develop skills for a career. This possibility began to be undermined by his habit of pulling pranks on his peers. This practice may well have been a factor for his premature discharge under somewhat murky circumstances. Following this dismissal, and after changing jobs several times, he eventually became a police officer. His hope was that this job would offer him an ideal (and legal) opportunity to enact revenge on those rule-breakers that were the object of his intense ire. Unfortunately, he soon found that his usual practice of writing tickets to individuals was not enough to satiate his powerful urges for retaliation. He began to escalate the aggressiveness of his responses to violators of the law. Soon, he became more aggressive in the field than the law would allow and was written up several times for exerting too much physical force.

This led to John being reassigned to desk duty for many years. He was eventually let back into the field, not because of good behavior but instead because he had apparently alienated his fellow officers at the police station. The latter were finally successful in getting him out of the station by getting him back into the field. Once he was at last back in the field, John redirected his anger towards the "establishment," an antagonist that he can only vaguely explain. He no longer expressed anger towards, or directed aggression at, those who committed crimes. Instead, he looked upon them with indifference and allowed them to violate the law. This passivity, he explained, was his way of getting back at "The Man."

John's problems were not limited to self-harm, impulsive outbursts of rage, and occupational difficulties. He also had trouble maintaining relationships with friends and family. He had had three wives, all of whom would eventually divorce him. Nor did any relationship remain between himself and either of his two children, so he found himself generally alone in later life.

Although John clearly met a diagnosis of antisocial and borderline PD when younger, his current therapist had a difficult time applying many of the DSM diagnostic criteria to his present situation. For example, although John once met Antisocial criterion #4 (repeated physical fights or assaults), his aggression now manifested itself in non-violent (though malicious) acts of retaliation, such as the letting of air out of people's tires. Further, whereas in earlier life he would have met criteria #1 (performing acts that are grounds for arrest) in the form of physically violent confrontations, he would later harm society in his role as a police officer when he spitefully allowed violent crimes to occur with impunity. Although in this way John has maintained a standard of exaggerated emotional response consistently throughout his life, the DSM criteria were not sensitive to this stability. The same sort of diagnostic dilemma arose for borderline PD. Whereas in the past he would have met criterion #4 (impulsivity in areas that are self-damaging, such as sex and reckless driving), his behavior no longer met the formal criteria for this diagnosis. Although the underlying tendencies are still present, they are not enacted in a behavioral form recognized by DSM verbiage. For a somewhat different reason, John also no longer meets criterion #2 (unstable interpersonal relationships). This is simply because he no longer has any significant interpersonal relationships left of any kind.

This case study illustrates several additional important features of personality disorders that have direct implications for their valid assessment. Most other forms of mental disorder, such as anxiety disorders and mood disorders, are *ego-dystonic*; that is, people with these disorders are distressed by their symptoms and uncomfortable with their situations. The distress is very much accessible to the person. They can readily report the distress. Personality disorders are usually *ego-syntonic*—the ideas or impulses with which they are associated are acceptable to the person. People with personality disorders frequently do not see themselves as being disturbed. John, for example, saw no problems with enacting revenge on those committing crimes. We might also say that they do not have insight into the nature of their own problems. John, for example, did not believe that his repeated antisocial behavior represented a problem. The other people for whom he created problems were suffering, but he was not. Many forms of personality disorder are defined primarily in terms of the problems that these people create for others rather than in terms of their own subjective distress.

The ego-syntonic nature of many forms of personality disorder raises important questions about the limitations of self-report measures—interviews and questionnaires—for their assessment. Many people with personality disorders are unable to view themselves realistically and are unaware of the effect that their behavior has on others. Therefore, assessments based exclusively on self-report may have limited validity (Klein, 2003; Oltmanns & Turkheimer, 2009). Don't forget that John didn't seek therapy on his own. He was encouraged to attend by his physician who noticed punctures all over his chest. People with personality disorders may underestimate the frequency and severity of certain aspects of personality pathology, particularly those problems associated with narcissism. The development of alternative assessment methods, such as collecting information from peers, family members, or mental health professionals, remains an important challenge for future research studies (Clark, 2007). Thus, all of the information in this next section needs to be considered in light of these comments.

Semi-Structured Interviews

The most widely recognized approach to the assessment of personality disorders, in both research and clinical practice, involves the use of interviews. Many different semi-structured interviews have been developed for the diagnosis of personality disorders (Zimmerman, 1994). Examples include the Structured Interview for DSM-IV Personality (SIDP-IV; Pfohl, Blum, & Zimmerman, 1997) and the Personality Disorders Interview (PDI-IV; Widiger, Mangine, Corbitt, Ellis, & Thomas, 1995). Each of the interview schedules provides a list of opening questions on topics related to the diagnostic features, as well as suggested follow-up probes to be used whenever the person admits problems in a particular area.

Clark and Harrison (2001) have described in detail the advantages and potential weaknesses of these instruments. Most efforts to evaluate empirically the utility of semi-structured interviews have focused on the issue of reliability. Inter-rater reliability estimates in a joint interview format are higher (average kappas above 0.60) than either short-interval test–retest or the long interval test–retest. Reliability increases when personality disorders are computed using dimensional scores rather than categorical scores (Pilkonis et.al., 1995; Zimmerman & Coryell, 1989). Less attention has been paid to the validity of diagnostic interviews in the assessment of personality disorders. Convergent reliability (different interviews compared with each other or an interview compared with a self-report questionnaire) has been shown to be relatively poor (Clark, Livesley, & Morey, 1997). Clinicians should therefore consider the results of diagnostic interviews with some caution. These instruments are considered to be the "gold standard" with regard to the diagnosis of personality disorders, but they depend largely on the ability or willingness of the person to recognize the nature of their problems.

Self-Report

Another popular approach to the assessment of personality disorders involves the administration of self-report questionnaires. Several different instruments are available. Some focus on symptoms of specific personality disorders, others focus on personality traits that are related to personality pathology, and a final option would be to collect information regarding interpersonal difficulties that follow as a consequence of personality disorders.

Rather than focusing on diagnostic scales, with an emphasis on somewhat arbitrary thresholds and a categorical view regarding the presence or absence of specific personality disorders, some self-report instruments place greater emphasis on personality dimensions. Some of these focus exclusively on normal personality traits. One popular alternative of this type is the NEO-PI-R, a questionnaire that provides scores based on the five-factor model of personality (Costa & McCrea, 1992). Using this type of measure for the assessment of traits that are related to personality disorders, one might expect patterns of scores that have been shown to be associated with each of the different disorders (Lynam & Widiger, 2001; Miller, Pilkonis, & Clifton, 2005). For example, a person with antisocial personality disorder would be expected to produce scores that are high on some facets of Neuroticism, such as angry hostility and impulsiveness, high on certain facets of Extraversion, such as excitement seeking, low on certain facets of Agreeableness, such as tendermindedness and straightforwardness, and low on certain facets of Conscientiousness, such as self-discipline and dutifulness. A person who is pathologically dependent would also be expected to produce a high score on Neuroticism (especially anxiousness and self-consciousness), as well as high scores on Agreeableness (especially trust, compliance, and modesty). Many leading investigators favor this approach to the assessment of pathological personality characteristics (Mullins-Sweatt, Smit, Verheul, Oldham, & Widiger, 2009; Samuel & Widiger, 2008).

The Schedule for Nonadaptive and Adaptive Personality (SNAP) is a factor analytically derived, self-report instrument that is designed to measure trait dimensions that are important in the domain of personality disorders (Clark, 1993; Simms & Clark, 2006). The instrument includes both obvious and more subtle items which are intended to tap the high and low ends of all of the trait dimensions. The core of the SNAP is composed of 15 scales, including 12 trait scales associated with relatively specific forms of personality pathology and three more general "temperament" scales (negative temperament, positive temperament, and disinhibition). For example, the specific trait scales most related to paranoia include mistrust, aggression, and detachment.

The SNAP also includes five validity scales that can be used to identify subjects who have responded carelessly or defensively. They are also sensitive to various other response sets that might contribute to an invalid profile. In addition to the 15 trait scales, the SNAP can also be used to derive scores on 13 diagnostic scales, which correspond to each of the specific personality disorder categories included in DSM-IV. The combination of validity scales, trait scales, and diagnostic scales makes the SNAP an especially useful instrument to be used in an assessment aimed at the identification of personality problems related to paranoia. For a self-report measure that maps directly onto the DSM-IV criteria, you may want to use the self-report version of the Multi-source Assessment of Personality Pathology (Oltmanns & Turkheimer, 2006; see also Appendix A).

Informant-Report

The fact that semi-structured interviews and self-report questionnaires have traditionally been used in the assessment of personality disorders should not imply that they are the best sources of information. Because realistic, accurate information about a client's behavior may not be obtained from the clients themselves, it is often useful to collect information from other sources. Family members, friends, and other acquaintances may provide an important perspective. Studies that have examined the relation between self-report data and informant-report data regarding personality pathology have found that the two sources often disagree (Klonsky, Oltmanns & Turkheimer, 2002; Oltmanns & Turkheimer, 2009).

Comparisons between self- and peer-reports reveal an interesting paradox regarding personality disorders. Take paranoia as an example. People who are viewed by their peers as being paranoid do not see themselves as being suspicious or lacking in trust. Rather, they described themselves as being angry and hostile (Clifton, Turkheimer, & Oltmanns, 2004). Research has shown that those who had thought of themselves as being paranoid were often regarded by others as cold and unfeeling. While it has not yet been determined how the two very different types of information should be used, it is fair to state that patient and informant evaluation represent two different assessment approaches to personality that produce two different portrayals of a client's personality disorder. Perhaps utilizing information from both sources may help a clinician gain a more comprehensive picture of a client's personality disorder than if the clinician were to rely solely on one source of information.

Later-Life Assessment Issues

As discussed previously, the DSM criteria were developed without closely considering the context of later life. There are different ways to address this measurement issue. Just recently, two age-specific measures have been created. In one (see Appendix B), which is a categorical measure (van Alphen, Engelen, Kuin, Hoijtink, & Derksen, 2006), there are 16 items scored yes/no. Seven items cover habitual behavior and nine cover biographical information. Strengths of this measure include its usability, length, focus on habitual behaviors, and biographical information. Limitations may include its lack of breadth and its categorical scoring system. Although the phenomena of interest likely exist along several associated dimensions, this measure assesses each feature categorically and doesn't concentrate on gradations of personality.

A second measure that was developed is a hybrid personality disorder scale (Balsis, 2009). The goal during item creation in this measure was to improve upon the current diagnostic criteria, many of which poorly capture personality disorder pathology when applied to older adults. This measure sought to establish better indicators of the personality disorders as they present themselves in later life. One hundred items (10 for each personality disorder) were written specifically for older adults on the basis of clinician experiences. Of these items, results showed that 37 worked better than some of the current diagnostic criteria. On average, three or four new items per personality disorder replaced former items that functioned less than optimally. Overall, clinicians favored certain DSM items over particular novel items in some cases, while favoring certain novel items over particular DSM items in other cases. Replacing some of the psychometrically underperforming items with these new items increased the face validity and, correspondingly, the content validity of the diagnostic sets. This measure is available from the chapter's second author.

Although the measures that were just described may work well to assess personality disorder pathology in older adults, it might be preferable for investigators who want to study personality disorder pathology longitudinally into later life or cross-sectionally among younger and older participants (Balsis et al., 2007) to have a measure that is age neutral. Otherwise, longitudinal studies would require researchers either to switch measures at some point (or apply weighting schemes during data analysis) from the younger adult measure to the older adult measure sometime during the data collection process. This would potentially be a serious confound in the analysis of data across time. Of course, the same problem would arise in cross-sectional studies. Any differences between younger and older groups might be an artifact of using separate measures for different groups.

Developing an age-neutral measurement system that would work equally well across all age groups is one way to help solve these problems (Mroczek et al., 1999). Obviously, the benefit of an age-neutral measure is that one can compare scores across age groups and over time without concern for measurement artifact associated with the two separate measures. An age-neutral measure would enable investigators to study the progression of personality change over the lifespan and construct age-related personality theory. It also would allow clinicians to have confidence in using a measure without concern for whether it is appropriate for the age of a client (Zweig, 2008).

Two prominent personality measures that purport to be age-neutral are already available. One such measure is the NEO (Costa & McCrae, 1992), which has been validated across several forms. Many researchers who study personality in older adults support its use because older adults were closely considered during its development. It also has the advantage of using a dimensional instead of a categorical approach in the assessment of each of the five personality traits that it measures. Still, there are legitimate concerns with simply using the NEO as a replacement for the DSM personality system. First and foremost, this measure was designed to assess "normal" or typical personality. Therefore, it is unknown whether it is sufficiently attuned for the assessment of a specific personality disorder pathology as described in the DSM. Nonetheless some have proposed that the NEO can measure personality disorder pathology (Widiger, Trull, Clarkin, Sanderson, & Costa, 1994). While a growing amount of evidence supports this notion, the majority of this research uses samples of younger adults. Thus, it remains unclear whether the NEO can also flexibly assess personality disorder pathology in later life.

The other measure that was developed with the context of aging in mind is the Personality Assessment Inventory (PAI; Morey, 1991). Like the NEO, the PAI measures several personality traits and includes dimensional subscales for each of these traits. The actual development of the PAI was notably different from that of the NEO, however. During its creation, items that contained measurement bias across two broad age groups were systematically identified and eliminated from the measure. The PAI, however, is not an ideal tool for our purposes because it was not designed to identify each of the personality disorders.

Nonetheless, the NEO and the PAI each offers different examples for how to devise an age-neutral assessment of personality. A researcher who wants to develop an ideal age-neutral system should, similar to the developers of the NEO, consider the later-life context during the item generation and selection phase. At the same time, the researcher should make use of analytic techniques (e.g., item response theory) to empirically select items that are appropriate for all age groups. Fortunately, these techniques are by no means mutually exclusive and would presumably be able to be used sequentially to develop a measure of even greater reliability and validity.

Dementia-Related Issues

As people age, they may experience changes secondary to dementia. In addition to the typical cognitive changes, personality changes also occur with dementia. These changes are often "negative," in the sense that individuals tend to move towards what is usually considered the less adaptive end of each trait's continuum. Namely, they tend to become more neurotic, less extraverted, less agreeable, less open, and less conscientious. These changes, especially the most pronounced change of increased neuroticism, are hallmarks of personality pathology and the personality disorders (Lynam & Widiger, 2001). On the surface, accounting for personality pathology and personality disorders that emerge secondary to dementia should be easy. One should simply be able to assess the onset of dementia and the onset of the personality changes and make a good clinical determination as to whether the dementia underlies the personality.

Unfortunately, untangling dementia-related personality change from non-dementia-related personality change is not such an easy task. The reason this is difficult to do is that dementia-related personality changes may occur years before an individual experiences sufficient cognitive changes necessary to warrant a diagnosis. Indeed, there is both anecdotal evidence and good preliminary data to suggest that personality change may precede measurable cognitive loss in Alzheimer's Disease (AD). For example, when Alzheimer (1907) first described the disease in his patient "… Auguste D, indicating that she showed suspiciousness of her husband as the first noticeable sign of the disease (translated with slight variation in Siegler et al., 1991 and Oppenheim, 1994)."

Only recently has Alzheimer's initial clinical description of personality change received empirical support (Balsis, Carpenter, & Storandt, 2005). Using longitudinal data, the Balsis et al. study showed that personality change is a symptom of AD and that it precedes cognitive changes, such as short-term memory loss and word finding difficulties. These results suggest that personality changes may be early indicators of AD. A difficulty, though, arises for understanding non-dementia personality change in later life. When an older adult presents with new personality disorder symptoms, how is a clinician to know if the symptoms are secondary to an insipient undetected dementia?

Ruling out dementia-related personality change is difficult because the measurement instruments to detect dementia are most effective in the moderate range (not the early range) of disease severity. There are no data that suggest that current personality disorder measures can be used to identify which patients experiencing personality change are experiencing it secondary to dementia. This means that when there is a case of personality change in late-life, it is difficult to determine the cause of that change. The best advice in this regard is for a clinician to continue to monitor the individual's cognitive changes to see if the person eventually develops dementia. If not, he or she can be assured that the personality change is independent of such a dementia process.

Multicultural Issues

In DSM-IV-TR, personality disorders are defined in terms of behavior that "deviates markedly from the expectations of the individual's culture." In setting this guideline, the authors of DSM-IV-TR recognized that judgments regarding appropriate behavior vary considerably from one society to the next. Some cultures encourage restrained or subtle displays of emotion, whereas others promote visible, public displays of anger, grief, and other emotional responses. Behavior that seems highly dramatic or extraverted (histrionic) in the former cultures might create a very different impression in the latter cultures. Cultures also differ in the extent to which they value individualism (the pursuit of personal goals) as opposed to collectivism (sharing and self-sacrifice for the good of the group) (Triandis, 1994). Someone who seems exceedingly self-centered and egotistical in a collectivist society, such as Japan, might appear to be normal in an individualistic society like the United States.

Personality disorders may be more closely tied to cultural expectations than any other kind of mental disorder (Alarcón, 2005). Some studies have compared the prevalence and symptoms of personality disorders in different countries, and the data suggest that similar problems do exist in cultures outside the United States and Western Europe (Pinto, Dhavale, Nair, Patil, & Dewan, 2000; Yang et al., 2000). Nevertheless, much more information is needed before we can be confident that the DSM-IV-TR system for describing personality disorders is valid in other societies. Two questions are particularly important: (1) in other cultures, what are the personality traits that lead to marked interpersonal difficulties and social or occupational impairment? Are they different from those that have been identified for our own culture? (2) are the diagnostic criteria that are used to define personality disorder syndromes in DSM-IV-TR (and ICD-10) meaningful in other cultures?

Currently, these questions remain unanswered, making it important that within a particular society, the experiences of people from cultural and ethnic minorities should be considered carefully before diagnostic decisions are made. Phenomena associated with paranoid personality disorder, including strong feelings of suspicion, alienation, and distrust, illustrate this issue. People who belong to minority groups (and those who are recent immigrants from a different culture) are more likely than members of the majority or dominant culture to hold realistic concerns about potential victimization and exploitation. For example, Black Americans may develop and express mild paranoid tendencies as a way of adapting to ongoing experiences of oppression (Whaley, 2001). Clinicians may erroneously diagnose these conditions as paranoid personality disorder if they do not recognize or understand the cultural experiences in which they are formed. In this particular case, it is obviously important for the clinician to consider the person's attitudes and beliefs regarding members of his or her own family or peer group, as well as the person's feelings about the community as a whole.

SUMMARY AND CONCLUSIONS

Personality disorders in later life can have major personal, familial, and societal implications. Yet, it has been difficult to understand the nature and the prevalence of personality disorders in later life because personality disorders may manifest themselves differently in, say, an 80-year-old than in, say, a 20-year-old. This potentially different presentation in later life raises additional challenges for assessing personality disorders across the lifespan—challenges beyond those for assessing personality disorders in general. Future work is needed to develop measures that are suitable for use with people of all ages and to help characterize the nature of personality disorders across the lifespan and in later life in particular. Only then will we be able to appreciate the changing face of personality disorders in later life, begin to grasp the functional impairment associated with personality disorders in late-life, and more fully understand the developmental nature of personality disorders.

APPENDIX A: MULTI-SOURCE ASSESSMENT OF PERSONALITY PATHOLOGY (MAPP)

(Oltmanns & Turkheimer, 2006)

Abbreviated Personality Disorder Code

SZD—Schizoid Personality Disorder
SZT—Schizotypal Personality Disorder
PND—Paranoid Personality Disorder
BDL—Borderline Personality Disorder
NAR—Narcissistic Personality Disorder
ATS—Antisocial Personality Disorder
HST—Histrionic Personality Disorder
OBC—Obsessive–Compulsive Personality Disorder
AVD—Avoidant Personality Disorder
DEP—Dependent Personality Disorder

DSM Item Number Correspondence (1 = item 1, 2 = item 2, etc.)

Answer Values—Are shown by the number choices 0–4 listed after each question.

0 = I am never like this	0% of the time
1 = I am occasionally like this	25% of the time
2 = I am sometimes like this	50% of the time
3 = I am often like this	75% of the time
4 = I am always like this	100% of the time

Scoring of Assessment—To obtain a continuous score, simply sum the item scores per disorder. For categorical scores, one must create dichotomous variables using a threshold cutoff score per item. Subthreshold item responses (0 or 1) are assigned a value of 0, and responses of 2 or higher are assigned a value of 1. Dichotomous scores should then be summed and compared with DSM-IV criteria to determine whether a personality disorder is present.

Narcissistic personality disorder criterion #8 and criterion #5 have each been split into two MAPP items. When using categorical scores, if EITHER of the two items meets threshold, the criterion should be counted as present.

1. I prefer to do things alone **(SZD2)**	0	1	2	3	4
2. I am superstitious or believe in mind-reading **(SZT2)**	0	1	2	3	4
3. I feel emotionally unfulfilled or that life is meaningless **(BDL7)**	0	1	2	3	4
4. I find myself daydreaming about power, success and/or the perfect relationship that will be mine someday **(NAR2)**	0	1	2	3	4
5. I am reserved or shy when meeting new people because I worry that I might not measure up **(AVD5)**	0	1	2	3	4
6. I depend on other people to take care of me **(DEP2)**	0	1	2	3	4
7. I am a perfectionist and my perfectionism gets in the way of getting things done **(OBC2)**	0	1	2	3	4
8. I am not interested in close relationships **(SZD5)**					
9. I have little interest in having a sexual relationship **(SZD3)**	0	1	2	3	4
10. I act or dress in an eccentric (or odd) manner **(SZT7)**	0	1	2	3	4
11. I can be deceitful when I need to be **(ATS2)**	0	1	2	3	4
12. Compared to others, my opinions and preferences change more frequently **(BDL3)**	0	1	2	3	4
13. I am not afraid to show my emotions, and my emotions can change quickly **(HST3)**	0	1	2	3	4
14. Being noticed and/or admired by others is important to me **(NAR4)**	0	1	2	3	4
15. I worry that other people will criticize or reject me **(AVD4)**	0	1	2	3	4
16. I am afraid of being left alone to care for myself **(DEP8)**	0	1	2	3	4
17. I can be rigid and stubborn **(OBC8)**	0	1	2	3	4
18. I have a hard time trusting other people and I often wonder if I can trust my friends **(PND2)**	0	1	2	3	4
19. Close relationships are not important to me (including being part of a family) **(SZD1)**	0	1	2	3	4
20. When I see other people talking, I begin to think that they may be talking about me **(SZT1)**	0	1	2	3	4
21. I like to do things on the fly without planning ahead **(ATS3)**	0	1	2	3	4
22. I expect to be catered to **(NAR5a)**	0	1	2	3	4
23. I have strong mood swings in response to events; I have frequent periods of intense sadness, irritation or anxiety **(BDL6)**	0	1	2	3	4
24. In conversations with other people (such as about my personal beliefs), I usually emphasize my personal feelings and impressions and am bored by details **(HST5)**	0	1	2	3	4
25. It is important to let other people know when they are incompetent and I don't worry about whether they will like me **(NAR9)**	0	1	2	3	4

(Continued)

26. I am not as much fun or as attractive as other people **(AVD6)**	0	1	2	3	4
27. After I break up with a girlfriend/boyfriend, I am likely to jump into another relationship **(DEP7)**	0	1	2	3	4
28. I am more concerned with saving money than my peers are **(OBC7)**	0	1	2	3	4
29. I do not want to share personal information with other people because I am afraid that it may get into the wrong hands **(PND3)**	0	1	2	3	4
30. I don't enjoy doing anything **(SZD4)**	0	1	2	3	4
31. I find myself laughing or crying when those around me are not laughing or crying **(SZT6)**	0	1	2	3	4
32. I have failed to do what was expected of me, such as completing my work or paying bills. (Not due to circumstances that I could not control) **(ATS6)**	0	1	2	3	4
33. In close relationships (with friends and family members), I often switch back and forth between loving a person and hating him or her **(BDL2)**	0	1	2	3	4
34. I have threatened to hurt, or kill myself **(BDL5)**	0	1	2	3	4
35. My expressions of emotion are stronger than most others **(HST6)**	0	1	2	3	4
36. It is not my job to listen to, or solve, other people's problems **(NAR7)**	0	1	2	3	4
37. I do not like to do or try new things because they might be embarrassing **(AVD7)**	0	1	2	3	4
38. I feel scared or uncomfortable when left alone to care for myself **(DEP6)**	0	1	2	3	4
39. I need to do everything myself because no one else will do them right **(OBC6)**	0	1	2	3	4
40. Rather than taking what people say at face value, I try to read between the lines and figure out what they really mean **(PND4)**	0	1	2	3	4
41. I have no close friends (other than family members) **(SZT8)**	0	1	2	3	4
42. Things make sense to me in a way that they may not for other people **(SZT4)**	0	1	2	3	4
43. I get mad easily and often get in fights **(ATS4)**	0	1	2	3	4
44. I seldom feel sorry or guilty for doing things that may have hurt others because I feel that my actions were justified **(ATS7)**	0	1	2	3	4
45. I have sudden, intense outbursts of anger **(BDL8)**	0	1	2	3	4
46. I am easily influenced by other people (suggestible) **(HST7)**	0	1	2	3	4
47. I think other people are jealous of me **(NAR8a)**	0	1	2	3	4
48. I am very controlled or inhibited with close friends because I am afraid people will make fun of me **(AVD3)**	0	1	2	3	4
49. I don't like to disagree with other people because I fear that they may reject me **(DEP3)**	0	1	2	3	4

50. I can't throw out old things even if they are of no use to me **(OBC5)**	**0**	**1**	**2**	**3**	**4**
51. I am not very good at showing my feelings **(SZD7)**	**0**	**1**	**2**	**3**	**4**
52. I repeatedly get in trouble with the police **(ATS1)**	**0**	**1**	**2**	**3**	**4**
53. I will do almost anything to keep those that I love from leaving me **(BDL1)**	**0**	**1**	**2**	**3**	**4**
54. When I am under stress, I may become paranoid or suspicious of people I usually trust, or have other strange experiences that are hard to explain **(MAPP_BDL9)**	**0**	**1**	**2**	**3**	**4**
55. I have gotten hurt in relationships because I thought that the relationship was closer (more intimate) than the other person did **(HST8)**	**0**	**1**	**2**	**3**	**4**
56. I expect other people to do what I say **(NAR5b)**	**0**	**1**	**2**	**3**	**4**
57. I avoid working in teams because I am afraid someone will criticize or reject me **(AVD1)**	**0**	**1**	**2**	**3**	**4**
58. I find it hard to make a simple decision without lots of advice from other people **(DEP1)**	**0**	**1**	**2**	**3**	**4**
59. I am afraid to start or do things by myself **(DEP4)**	**0**	**1**	**2**	**3**	**4**
60. I am very concerned with details, rules, lists and schedules; I spend a great deal of time getting organized (i.e., making lists, schedules, etc.) **(OBC1)**	**0**	**1**	**2**	**3**	**4**
61. I become angry quickly when I am criticized **(PND6)**	**0**	**1**	**2**	**3**	**4**
62. I don't care whether other people praise or criticize me **(SZD6)**	**0**	**1**	**2**	**3**	**4**
63. I am nervous around other people because I don't trust them **(SZT9)**	**0**	**1**	**2**	**3**	**4**
64. I am adventurous; I like to do things even if it could be dangerous to me or others **(ATS5)**	**0**	**1**	**2**	**3**	**4**
65. I like being the center of attention and feel disappointed when I am not **(HST1)**	**0**	**1**	**2**	**3**	**4**
66. I am unwilling to get involved with other people unless I am certain of being liked **(AVD2)**	**0**	**1**	**2**	**3**	**4**
67. I will do just about anything to get other people to take care of me **(DEP5)**	**0**	**1**	**2**	**3**	**4**
68. My work is more important than spending time with friends and family, and/or having fun **(OBC3)**	**0**	**1**	**2**	**3**	**4**
69. I am constantly on the lookout to make sure that other people are not taking advantage, lying to, or harming me **(PND1)**	**0**	**1**	**2**	**3**	**4**
70. I see, hear, or experience things differently from the way other people do **(SZT3)**	**0**	**1**	**2**	**3**	**4**
71. I am impulsive and have done things that could be dangerous to me **(BDL4)**	**0**	**1**	**2**	**3**	**4**
72. I am more flirtatious than other people **(HST2)**	**0**	**1**	**2**	**3**	**4**
73. I think that I am much better than most other people **(NAR1)**	**0**	**1**	**2**	**3**	**4**
74. Compared to others, I have very high standards when it comes to morals and ethics **(OBC4)**	**0**	**1**	**2**	**3**	**4**

(Continued)

75. I have concerns that my sexual partner is not being faithful to me **(PND7)**	**0**	**1**	**2**	**3**	**4**
76. I use physical appearance to draw attention to myself **(HST4)**	**0**	**1**	**2**	**3**	**4**
77. Because I am so unique, only other special people understand me **(NAR3)**	**0**	**1**	**2**	**3**	**4**
78. I am constantly on edge to make sure that other people don't take advantage of me **(SZT5)**	**0**	**1**	**2**	**3**	**4**
79. I will do just about anything to get what I need or think I deserve even if it means having to "step on a few toes" **(NAR6)**	**0**	**1**	**2**	**3**	**4**
80. I hold grudges for a long time if I am insulted or injured **(PND5)**	**0**	**1**	**2**	**3**	**4**
81. I am jealous of other people **(NAR8b)**	**0**	**1**	**2**	**3**	**4**

APPENDIX B: GERONTOLOGICAL PERSONALITY DISORDERS SCALE (GPS)

(van Alphen, Engelen, Kuin, Hoijtink, & Derksen, 2006)

Habitual behavior

1. I don't like growing older because I become less attractive (Yes or No)
2. I often worry about my health (Yes or No)
3. I'm often concerned about my memory (Yes or No)
4. I hope that others solve my problems (Yes or No)
5. I'm often afraid of losing those who care for me, such as members of the family or my partner (Yes or No)
6. I'm often taken advantage of by others (Yes or No)
7. I find it difficult to fend for myself (Yes or No)

Biographical information

1. In my life I've been to see the doctor for many vague physical complaints (Yes or No)
2. I have sometimes said to my family or friends that I don't want to live any longer (Yes or No)
3. In the past I've been admitted to a psychiatric institution or convalescent home because of nerves (Yes or No)
4. At important times in my life I've had a lot of trouble with nerves, stress or moodiness (Yes or No)
5. In the past I've already had treatment from a psychiatrist or psychologist (Yes or No)
6. I have sometimes tried to end my life (Yes or No)
7. At the most I've only had one acquaintance or friend in my life (Yes or No)
8. In my life I've not been very interested in sexual contact (Yes or No)
9. In the past I've often taken tranquilizers and/or sleeping pills (Yes or No)

References

Agronin, M. E., & Maletta, G. (2000). Personality disorders in late life: Understanding the gap in research. *American Journal of Geriatric Psychiatry*, *8*, 4–18.

Alarcón, R. (2005). Cross-cultural issues. *The American Psychiatric Publishing textbook of personality disorders* (pp. 561–578). Arlington, VA: American Psychiatric Publishing.

Alzheimer, A. (1907). Ueber eine eigenartige Erkrankung der Hirnrinde. *Zeitschrift fuer Psychiatrie*, *64*(146), 3 pages.

American Psychiatric Association. (2000). *Diagnostic and statistical manual of mental disorders* (4th ed., text revision). Washington, DC: Author.

Ames, A., & Molinari, V. (1994). Prevalence of personality disorders in community-living elderly. *Journal of Geriatric Psychiatry and Neurology*, *7*, 189–194.

Balsis, S. (2009). Measuring personality disorders in later life: hybrid criteria. Manuscript submitted for publication.

Balsis, S., Carpenter, B. D., & Storandt, M. (2005). Personality change precedes clinical diagnosis of dementia of the Alzheimer type. *Journal of Gerontology: Psychological Sciences*, *60B*, P98–P101.

Balsis, S., Cooper, L. D., Lowmaster, S., & Benge, J. F. (in press). Personality disorder diagnostic thresholds correspond to different levels of latent pathology. *Journal of Personality Disorders*

Balsis, S., Gleason, M. E. J., Woods, C. M., & Oltmanns, T. F. (2007). An item response theory analysis of DSM-IV personality disorder criteria across younger and older age groups. *Psychology and Aging*, *22*, 171–185.

Balsis, S., Segal, D. L., & Donahue, C. (2009). Revising the personality disorder criteria for the Diagnostic and Statistical Manual of Mental Disorders—Fifth Edition (DSM-V): consider the later life context. *American Journal of Orthopsychiatry*, *79*, 452–460.

Balsis, S., Woods, C. M., Gleason, M. E. J., & Oltmanns, T. F. (2007). The over and under diagnosis of personality disorders in older adults. *American Journal of Geriatric Psychiatry*, *15*, 742–753.

Bernstein, D., Cohen, P., Velez, C., & Schwab-Stone, M. (1993). Prevalence and stability of the DSM-III—R personality disorders in a community-based survey of adolescents. *The American Journal of Psychiatry*, *150*, 1237–1243.

Clark, L. A. (1993). *Manual for the Schedule for Nonadaptive and Adaptive Personality.* Minneapolis, MN: University of Minnesota Press.

Clark, L. (2007). Assessment and diagnosis of personality disorder: Perennial issues and an emerging reconceptualization. *Annual Review of Psychology*, *58*, 227–257.

Clark, L. A., & Harrison, J. A. (2001). Assessment Instruments. In *Handbook of Personality Disorders: Theory, Research and Treatment* (pp. 277–306). New York, NY: Guilford Press.

Clark, L. A., Livesley, W. J., & Morey, L. (1997). Personality disorder assessment: The challenge of construct validity. *Journal of Personality Disorders*, *11*, 205–231.

Clarkin, J. F., Spielman, L. A., & Klausner, E. (1999). Conceptual overview of personality disorders in the elderly. In E. Rosowsky, R. C. Abrams, & R. A. Zweig (Eds.), *Personality disorders in older adults: Emerging issues in diagnosis and treatment* (pp. 3–16). Mahwah, NJ: Erlbaum.

Clifton, A., Turkheimer, E., & Oltmanns, T. F. (2004). Contrasting perspectives on personality problems: Descriptions from the self and others. *Personality and Individual Differences*, *36*, 1499–1514.

Cohen, P., Crawford, T. N., Johnson, J. G., & Kasen, S. (2005). The children in the community study of developmental course of personality disorder. *Journal of Personality Disorders*, *19*, 466–486.

Cohen, P., Chen, H., Crawford, T., Brook, J., & Gordon, K. (2007). Personality disorders in early adolescence and the development of later substance use disorders in the general population. *Drug and Alcohol Dependence*, *88*, S71–S84.

Coid, J., Yang, M., Tyrer, P., Roberts, A., & Ullrich, S. (2006). Prevalence and correlates of personality disorder among adults aged 16 to 74 in Great Britain. *British Journal of Psychiatry*, *188*, 423–431.

Costa, P., & McCrae, R. (1988). Personality in adulthood: A six-year longitudinal study of self-reports and spouse ratings on the NEO Personality Inventory. *Journal of Personality and Social Psychology*, *54*, 853–863.

Costa, P. T., & McCrae, R. R. (1992). *Revised NEO Personality Inventory (NEO PI-R) and NEO Five-Factor Inventory (NEO-FFI) professional manual.* Odessa, FL: Psychological Assessment Resources.

Crawford, T., Cohen, P., & Brook, J. (2001). Dramatic—erratic personality disorder symptoms: I. Continuity from early adolescence into adulthood. *Journal of Personality Disorders*, *15*, 319–335.

Dolan-Sewell, R. T., Krueger, R. F., & Shea, M. T. (2001). Co-occurrence with syndrome disorders. In W. J. Livesley (Ed.), *Handbook of personality disorders: Theory, research, and treatment.* (pp. 84–106). New York, NY: Guilford.

Drake, R., Adler, D., & Vaillant, G. (1988). Antecedents of personality disorders in a community sample of men. *Journal of Personality Disorders*, *2*(1), 60–68.

Fournier, J. C., DeRubeis, R. J., Shelton, R. C., Gallop, R., Amsterdam, J. D., & Hollon, S. D. (2008). Antidepressant medications v. cognitive therapy in people with depression with or without personality disorder. *British Journal of Psychiatry*, *192*, 124–129.

Gish, R. G., Lee, A., Brooks, L., Leung, J., Lau, J. Y., & Moore, D. H. (2001). Long-term follow-up of patients diagnosed with alcohol dependence or alcohol abuse who were evaluated for liver transplantation. *Liver Transplant*, *7*, 581–587.

Grant, B., Stinson, F., Hasin, D., Dawson, D., Chou, S., Ruan, W., et al. (2005). Prevalence, correlates, and comorbidity of Bipolar I Disorder and Axis I and II Disorders: Results from the National Epidemiologic Survey on Alcohol and Related Conditions. *Journal of Clinical Psychiatry*, *66*, 1205–1215.

Grilo, C., Sanislow, C., Gunderson, J., Pagano, M., Yen, S., Zanarini, M., et al. (2004). Two-year stability and change of Schizotypal, borderline, avoidant, and obsessive–Compulsive Personality Disorders. *Journal of Consulting and Clinical Psychology*, *72*, 767–775.

Holtzworth-Munroe, A. (2000). A typology of men who are violent toward their female partners: Making sense of the heterogeneity in husband violence. *Current Directions in Psychological Science*, *9*, 140–143.

Kenan, M. M., Kendjelic, E. M., Molinari, V. A., Williams, W., Norris, M., & Kunik, M. E. (2000). Age-related differences in the frequency of personality disorders among inpatient veterans. *International Journal of Geriatric Psychiatry*, *15*, 831–837.

Kendell, R. E. (2002). The distinction between personality disorder and mental illness. *British Journal of Psychiatry*, *180*, 110–115.

Kessler, R., McGonagle, K., Zhao, S., & Nelson, C. (1994). Lifetime and 12-month prevalence of DSM-III-R psychiatric disorders in the United States: Results from the National Comorbidity Study. *Archives of General Psychiatry*, *51*, 8–19.

Klein, D. N. (2003). Patients' versus informants' reports of personality disorders in predicting 7½ year outcome in outpatients with depressive disorders. *Psychological Assessment*, *15*, 216–222.

Klonsky, E. D., Oltmanns, T. F., & Turkheimer, E. (2002). Informant-reports of personality disorder: Relation to self-reports and future research directions. *Clinical Psychology: Science and Practice*, *9*, 300–311.

Krueger, R. (1999). Personality traits in late adolescence predict mental disorders in early adulthood: A prospective-epidemiological study. *Journal of Personality*, *67*, 39–65.

Lenzenweger, M. F., Johnson, M. D., & Willett, J. B. (2004). Individual growth curve analysis illuminates stability and change in personality disorder features: The longitudinal study of personality disorders. *Archives of General Psychiatry*, *61*, 1015–1024.

Lenzenweger, M., Lane, M. C., Loranger, A. W., & Kessler, R. C. (2007). DSM-IV personality disorders in the national comorbidity survey replication. *Biological Psychiatry*, *62*(6), 553–564.

Lynam, D. R., & Widiger, T. A. (2001). Using the five-factor model to represent DSM-IV personality disorders: An expert consensus approach. *Journal of Abnormal Psychology*, *110*, 401–412.

Mattia, J. I., & Zimmerman, M. (2001). Epidemiology. In W. J. Livesley (Ed.), *Handbook of personality disorders: Theory, research, and treatment* (pp. 107–123). New York, NY: Guilford.

Miller, J. D., Pilkonis, P. A., & Clifton, A. (2005). Self- and other reports of traits from the five-factor model: Relations to personality disorders. *Journal of Personality Disorders*, *19*, 400–419.

Moffitt, T., Caspi, A., Harrington, H., & Milne, B. (2002). Males on the life-course-persistent and adolescence-limited antisocial pathways: Follow-up at age 26 years. *Development and Psychopathology*, *14*, 179–207.

Molinari, V., Ames, A., & Essa, M. (1994). Prevalence of personality disorders in two geropsychatric inpatient units. *Journal of Geriatric Psychiatry & Neurology*, *7*, 209–215.

Moran, P. (1999). The epidemiology of antisocial personality disorder. *Social Psychiatry and Psychiatric Epidemiology*, *34*, 231–242.

Morey, L. C. (1991). *Personality Assessment Inventory*. Odessa, FL: Psychological Assessment Resources, Inc.

Mroczek, D. K., Hurt, S. W., & Berman, W. H. (1999). Conceptual and methodological issues in the assessment of personality disorder in older adults. In E. Rosowsky, R. C. Abrams, & R. A. Zweig (Eds.), *Personality disorders in older adults: Emerging issues in diagnosis and treatment* (pp. 135–152). Mahwah, NJ: Erlbaum.

Mullins-Sweatt, S., Smit, V., Verheul, R., Oldham, J., & Widiger, T. (2009). Dimensions of personality: Clinicians' perspectives. *Canadian Journal of Psychiatry*, *54*, 247–259.

Oltmanns, T. F., & Turkheimer, E. (2006). Perceptions of self and others regarding pathological personality traits. In R. F. Krueger, & J. L. Tackett (Eds.), *Personality and psychopathology: Building bridges* (pp. 71–111). New York, NY: Guilford.

Oltmanns, T. F., & Turkheimer, E. (2009). Person perception and personality pathology. *Current Directions in Psychological Science*, *18*, 32–36.

Oltmanns, T. F., Melley, A. H., & Turkheimer, E. (2002). Impaired social functioning and symptoms of personality disorders in a non-clinical population. *Journal of Personality Disorders*, *16*, 438–453.

Oppenheim, G. (1994). The earliest signs of Alzheimer's disease. *Journal of Geriatric Psychiatry and Neurology*, *7*, 116–120.

Paris, J. (2003). Personality disorders over time: Precursors, course, and outcome. *Journal of Personality Disorders*, *17*, 479–488.

Pfohl, B., Blum, N., & Zimmerman, M. (1997). *Structured Interview for DSM-IV Personality (SIDP-IV)*. Washington, DC: American Psychiatric Association.

Pilkonis, P. A., Heape, C. L., Proietti, J. M., Clark, S. W., McDavid, J. D., & Pitts, T. E. (1995). The reliability and validity of two structured diagnostic interviews for personality disorders. *Archives of General Psychiatry*, *52*, 1025–1033.

Pinto, C., Dhavale, H. S., Nair, S., Patil, B., & Dewan, M. (2000). Borderline personality disorder exists in India. *Journal of Nervous and Mental Disease*, *188*, 386–388.

Roberts, B. W., & DelVecchio, W. F. (2000). The rank-order consistency of personality from childhood to old age: A quantitative review of longitudinal studies. *Psychological Bulletin*, *126*, 3–25.

Roberts, B. W., Walton, K. E., & Viechtbauer, W. (2006). Patterns of mean-level change in personality traits across the life course: A meta-analysis of longitudinal studies. *Psychological Bulletin*, *132*, 1–25.

Robins, L. (1966). Deviant children grown up: A sociological and psychiatric study of sociopathic personality. Oxford, England: Williams & Wilkins.

Robins, L. N., & Regier, D. A. (1991). *Psychiatric disorders in America: The Epidemiologic Catchment Area Study*. New York, NY: Free Press.

Rosowsky, E. (1999). The patient–therapist relationship and the psychotherapy of the older adults with personality disorder. In E. Rosowsky, R. C. Abrams, & R. A. Zweig (Eds.), *Personality disorders in older adults: Emerging issues in diagnosis and treatment* (pp. 153–174). Mahwah, NJ: Erlbaum.

Rosowsky, E., & Gurian, B. (1992). Impact of borderline personality disorder in late life on systems of care. *Hospital & Community Psychiatry*, *43*, 386–389.

Rosowsky, E., & Smyer, M. A. (1999). Personality disorders and the difficult nursing home resident. In E. Rosowsky, R. C. Abrams, & R. A. Zweig (Eds.), *Personality disorders in older adults: Emerging issues in diagnosis and treatment* (pp. 257–274). Mahwah, NJ: Erlbaum.

Samuel, D., & Widiger, T. (2008). A meta-analytic review of the relationships between the five-factor model and DSM-IV-TR personality disorders: A facet level analysis. *Clinical Psychology Review*, *28*, 1326–1342.

Segal, D. L., Coolidge, F. L., & Rosowsky, E. (2006). *Personality disorders and older adults: Diagnosis, assessment, and treatment*. Hoboken, NJ: Wiley.

Segal, D. L., Hersen, M., Van Hasselt, V. B., Silberman, C. S., & Roth, L. (1996). Diagnosis and assessment of personality disorders in older adults: A critical review. *Journal of Personality Disorders*, *10*, 384–399.

Siegler, I. C., Welsh, K. A., Dawson, D. V., Fillenbaum, C. G., Earl, N. L., Kaplan, E. B., et al. (1991). *Alzheimer's Disease and Associated Disorders*, *5*, 240–250.

Simms, L., & Clark, L. (2006). The Schedule for Nonadaptive and Adaptive Personality (SNAP): A dimensional measure of traits relevant to personality and personality pathology. *Differentiating normal and abnormal personality* (2nd ed., pp. 431–450). New York, NY: Springer.

Skodol, A., & Bender, D. (2003). Why are women diagnosed borderline more than men? *Psychiatric Quarterly*, *74*, 349–360.

Skodol, A. E., Johnson, J. G., Cohen, P., Sneed, J. R., & Crawford, T. N. (2007). Personality disorder and impaired functioning from adolescence to adulthood. *British Journal of Psychiatry*, *190*, 415–420.

Spiessl, H., Hubner-Liebermann, B., Binder, H., & Cording, C. (2002). Heavy users in a psychiatric hospital: A cohort study of 1,811 patients over five years. *Psychiatrische Praxis*, *29*, 350–354.

Tackett, J. L., Balsis, S. M., Oltmanns, T. F., & Krueger, R. F. (2009). A unifying perspective of personality pathology across the lifespan: Developmental considerations for DSM-V. *Development and Psychopathology*, *21*, 687–713.

Terracciano, A., McCrae, R. R., Brant, L. J., & Costa, P. T. (2005). Hierarchical linear modeling analyses of the NEO-PI-R scales in the Baltimore longitudinal study of aging. *Psychology and Aging*, *20*, 493–506.

Thomas, V. H., Melchert, T. P., & Banken, J. A. (1999). Substance dependence and personality disorders: Comorbidity and treatment outcome in an inpatient treatment population. *Journal of Studies on Alcohol*, *60*, 271–277.

Torgersen, S., Kringlen, E., & Cramer, V. (2001). The prevalence of personality disorders in a community sample. *Archives of General Psychiatry*, *58*, 590–596.

Triandis, H. (1994). *Culture and social behavior*. New York, NY: McGraw-Hill.

Tyrer, P., Coombs, N., Ibrahimi, F., Mathilakath, A., Bajaj, P., Ranger, M., et al. (2007). Critical developments in the assessment of personality disorder. *British Journal of Psychiatry*, *190*(suppl. 49), s51–s59.

van Alphen, S. P. J., Engelen, G. J. J. A., Kuin, Y., Hoijtink, H. J. A., & Derksen, J. J. L. (2006). A preliminary study of the diagnostic accuracy of the gerontological personality disorders scale (GPS). *International Journal of Geriatric Psychiatry*, *21*, 862–868.

Wakefield, J. C. (1999). The measurement of mental disorder. In A. V. Horowitz & T. L. Shield (Eds.), *A Handbook for the study of Mental Health: Social Contexts, Theories and Systems*. Cambridge, UK: Cambridge University Press.

Weissman, M. M. (1993). The epidemiology of personality disorders: A 1990 update. *Journal of Personality Disorders*, *supplement* 44–62.

Whaley, A. (2001). Cultural mistrust and the clinical diagnosis of paranoid schizophrenia in African American patients. *Journal of Psychopathology and Behavioral Assessment*, *23*, 93–100.

Whisman, M. A., Tolejko, N., & Chatav, Y. (2007). Social consequences of personality disorders: probability and timing of marriage and probability of marital disruption. *Journal of Personality Disorders*, *21*, 690–695.

Whiteman, M. C., Deary, I. J., & Fawkes, F. G. (2000). Personality and social predictors of atherosclerotic progression: Edinburgh artery study. *Psychosomatic Medicine*, *62*, 703–714, American Psychological Association.

Widiger, T. A., & Seidlitz, L. (2002). Personality, psychopathology, and aging. *Journal of Research in Personality*, *36*, 335–362.

Widiger, T. A., & Trull, T. J. (2007). Plate tectonics in the classification of personality disorder: Shifting to a dimensional model. *American Psychologist*, *62*, 71–83.

Widiger, T. A., Mangine, S., Corbitt, E. M., Ellis, C. G., & Thomas, G. V. (1995). *Personality Disorder Interview-IV: A Semistructured Interview for the Assessment of Personality Disorders*. Odessa, FL: Psychological Assessment Resources, Inc.

Widiger, T., Trull, T., Clarkin, J., Sanderson, C., & Costa, P. (1994). A description of the DSM-III-R and DSM-IV personality disorders with the five-factor model of personality. Personality disorders and the five-factor model of personality (pp. 41–56). Washington, DC:

Yang, J., McCrae, R. R., Costa, P. T., Yao, S., Dai, X., & Cai, T. (2000). The cross-cultural generalizability of Axis-II constructs: An evaluation of two personality disorder assessment instruments in the People's Republic of China. *Journal of Personality Disorders*, *14*, 249–263.

Zimmerman, M. (1994). Diagnosing personality disorders: A review of issues and research methods. *Archives of General Psychiatry*, *51*, 225–245.

Zimmerman, M., & Coryell, W. (1989). The reliability of personality disorder diagnoses in a non-patient sample. *Journal of Personality Disorders*, *3*, 53–57.

Zweig, R. A. (2008). Personality disorder in older adults: Assessment challenges and strategies. *Research and Practice*, *39*, 298–305.

CHAPTER

5 Assessing Psychosis in Acute and Chronic Mentally Ill Older Adults

Colin A. Depp[1], Casey Loughran[1], Ipsit Vahia[1], Victor Molinari[2]

[1] *Department of Psychiatry, University of California, San Diego, CA, USA*

[2] *Department of Aging and Mental Health Disparities, University of South Florida, Tampa, FL, USA*

INTRODUCTION

Psychosis is broadly defined as a loss of contact with reality. According to the DSM-IV (APA, 2000), a narrow definition of psychosis encapsulates both delusions and hallucinations. Delusions are persistent beliefs that are not accepted in the context of a person's social and cultural background, whereas hallucinations are false sensory perceptions that cannot be attributed to sensory distortions. A slightly broader definition of psychosis includes disorganized speech or behavior, such as in catatonia. Until recently little data have been available to inform clinicians about the prevalence, risk factors, and course of psychosis in older people. It is now understood that psychosis is quite common in older people; its prevalence, irrespective of its underlying cause, is about 4–10% in community-dwelling older adults (Henderson et al., 1998; Ostling & Skoog, 2002), and higher among those residing in institutional settings and the oldest adults (e.g., those aged older than 95) (Ostling, Borjesson-Hanson, & Skoog, 2007). In addition, the absolute number of older people who exhibit psychotic symptoms will increase with the aging of the population (Jeste et al., 1999).

Psychosis manifests in a variety of conditions in older adults, and it often has devastating effects on individual quality of life and caregiver well-being. Delusions and hallucinations are hallmark features of schizophrenia, but may also be evident in late-life mood disorders with psychotic features. Psychotic symptoms are often present in the dementias; and hallucinations and delusions may occur in the context of delirium due to a medical condition or exposure to a toxin. Therefore, the assessment of psychosis in older adults is often challenging in terms of identifying its underlying etiology, in addition to determining how best to guide treatment planning and services. In this chapter, we describe general considerations in assessing older adults who are suspected of exhibiting psychotic symptoms. We then review the definition, prevalence, and features of common syndromes associated with psychosis; and for each of these syndromes, we provide assessment strategies, illustrative case studies, and well-validated instruments for the practitioner.

GENERAL ASSESSMENT CONSIDERATIONS

Given that medical conditions, medications, and toxins cause psychotic experiences, the first step in assessment is to rule out these causes. Older adults, particularly those with diminished physical resources due to medical illnesses, are more vulnerable to central nervous system effects. They are thus more likely to experience psychotic symptoms secondary to a medical cause than are younger adults.

Handbook of Assessment in Clinical Gerontology. DOI: 10.1016/B978-0-12-374961-1.10005-3

Often the psychotic symptoms associated with medical illnesses signify a serious medical condition, making initial differential diagnosis all the more important.

Medical causes of psychosis include infection, metabolic changes, central nervous system abnormalities, head trauma, deliberate or accidental overdoses, and ingestion of illicit substances. Particularly among older adults in whom the onset of symptoms is recent and there is no history of psychiatric disorder, a complete medical work-up is warranted to rule out these causes. However, it is important to note that older adults with long histories of schizophrenia or other psychotic disorders may have organic causes for exacerbations of psychosis. Therefore it should not be automatically assumed that older adults with long-standing psychotic disorders do not have contributory medical etiologies. Moreover, chronically mentally ill older adults are at risk for poorer medical care, which is likely to exacerbate existing medical conditions (Folsom et al., 2002; Vahia et al., 2008).

Biochemical screening should be conducted. Blood work should include checking blood count, electrolytes, metabolic function, urinalysis and urine toxicology. Additionally, hepatic and thyroid panels may be useful. In patients with new onset psychosis without clear cause, computerized tomography or MRI of the brain may be used to rule out intracranial bleeds or neoplasms. Assessment of motor function, sensory function, reflexes, coordination and gait can aid in determining whether acute brain insults precipitated presenting symptoms (Richards & Gurr, 2000).

A thorough psychiatric and medical history is necessary when new or exacerbated psychotic symptoms are present, which would include obtaining collateral information from medical records and proxy informants, recording all the medications that a person is taking, and having direct communication with primary care providers (Jones, Vahia, Cohen, Hindi, & Nurhussein, 2009). After establishing rapport, patients should be asked if they have been experiencing any unusual sensations, hearing voices that others cannot hear, or seeing things that are not there. They may also be asked whether they have held any beliefs that others might not understand or believe. In many cases, the responses to these questions may be met with denial of symptoms and insistence that the phenomena experienced are real. In particular, cognitively impaired older adults may not be able to verbalize their experiences. The role of proxy informants, such as family members, is thus essential. Family members may want to disclose information about their relative's hallucinations or delusions in private so as not to alter trust with, or to offend, the patient.

In nursing home or other institutional settings, staff observations are particularly valuable in characterizing the nature of psychosis and its contextual influences. In addition to the history of the symptoms, clinicians should also inquire about recent changes in social or occupational behavior, such as withdrawal from usual activities, as well as any changes in personal hygiene and habits.

To aid in identifying whether medical causes contribute to the etiology of psychotic symptoms, specification of the time course of symptoms should be a central goal of the evaluation, establishing whether psychosis emerged in the context of a trial of a new medication or emergent medical conditions. A thorough review of medications and identification of potential drug–drug interactions should be undertaken, as well as an indication of how and when the medication(s) are taken so as to identify potential over/underdoses. History of psychiatric treatment, such as whether previous psychiatric symptoms occurred in the context of medical conditions or treatments, should be gathered. Another factor to consider in regard to identifying contributors to psychosis is the degree of social isolation; particularly among homebound elderly people, isolation is a risk factor for psychosis (Richards & Gurr, 2000). Severe hearing loss may also produce experiences that may be similar to auditory hallucinations (Stein & Thienhaus, 1993).

In addition to the course and context of symptoms, the phenomenology of symptoms can provide clues as to whether psychotic symptoms may derive from medical causes. Key distinctions among hallucinations are the modality (i.e., auditory, visual, tactile, olfactory), frequency, and intensity. Delusions can be sub-divided by their content (e.g., delusions of reference, control, persecutory, paranoid, grandiose, somatic, and jealousy/guilt) as well as the degree to which they are bizarre (could not happen) or non-bizarre (represent extensions of reality). Another factor to assess is insight into the origin of delusions and hallucinations, as well as amenability of delusional beliefs to alternative explanations.

Another common distinction, for which evidence is mixed, is the presence of Schneiderian "first rank" symptoms which are thought to be specific to schizophrenia (i.e., voices heard arguing with each other, commenting on behavior, removal of thoughts or insertion of thoughts). The presence of visual, tactile, and olfactory hallucinations is more suggestive of medical causes, whereas auditory hallucinations are more common in psychiatric illnesses. Delusions that are simple, more transient, and involve misidentification of family members are more suggestive of dementia, whereas long-held delusions with intricate themes are more consistent with schizophrenia. Psychosis co-occurring with cognitive impairment, and in particular a waxing and waning state of consciousness and orientation, is often indicative of delirium.

Another general consideration in assessing people with a long history of psychosis is that, while distressing, hallucinations and delusions can be less debilitating than concurrent symptoms of depression (Diwan et al., 2007) and cognitive impairments. Therefore, it should not be assumed that psychotic symptoms are the primary problem experienced by the patient. For example, there is some evidence to suggest that, because psychotic symptoms tend to "stand out," the presence of comorbid medical problems can be overlooked in patients with schizophrenia (Brown, Barraclough, & Inskip, 2000).

Finally, the patient and their caregivers' approach toward psychotic symptoms is important to assess in order to formulate a treatment plan. Whether or not patients are able to consider alternative explanations of their symptoms, and have insight into their illness, can aid in determining the prognosis for rehabilitation. Older adults with long-standing psychotic symptoms often have developed a number of coping skills to aid in dealing with delusions and hallucinations (e.g., distraction, "talking back" to the voices). How family members react to psychotic symptoms, such as whether they argue with the patient or whether they are embarrassed by their family member's illness, can shed light on ways to reduce the impact of psychosis on the family. Indeed, highly emotionally expressive family members have long been associated with relapse in patients with schizophrenia (Brown, Monck, Carstairs, & Wing, 1962; Butzloff & Hooley, 1998) .

In sum, psychosis is a symptom that occurs in many conditions, and medical causes need to be ruled out prior to the diagnosis of a psychiatric disorder. The phenomenology of hallucinations and delusions differs among illnesses and may provide an indication of whether the underlying cause stems from a medical condition or from the psychiatric disorders. A careful evaluation that integrates multiple sources of information can aid in determining the underlying cause of psychosis and point toward targets for treatment plans.

SCHIZOPHRENIA AND DELUSIONAL DISORDERS

Definition, Prevalence and Course

The disorder most classically associated with psychosis is schizophrenia. The DSM-IV criteria for schizophrenia require at least two of the following: (1) hallucinations; (2) delusions; (3) disorganized speech; (4) grossly disorganized or catatonic behavior; or (5) negative symptoms which include alogia, anhedonia, social withdrawal, or apathy. These symptoms must be continuously present for at least one month, must not be attributable to medical causes, and must also produce social and/or occupational impairment.

Other primary psychotic disorders include delusional disorder, which requires the presence of non-bizarre delusions over the course of at least one month. Delusional disorder is characterized by focal delusions that do not impair functioning outside of that affected by the delusion, with no evidence of hallucinations or negative symptoms. Schizoaffective disorder requires fulfillment of criteria for schizophrenia as well as a mood disorder, with evidence for the existence of the psychotic symptoms in the absence of mood disorder.

Historically, schizophrenia with onset in old age has had many different anecdotal characterizations including "late paraphrenia" and "dementia praecox" (Palmer, McClure, & Jeste, 2001), with little empirical data available to describe this disorder until recently. Even now, only 1% of the literature on schizophrenia focuses on older adults (Vahia et al., 2007). The prevalence of schizophrenia in older persons varies somewhat based on the criteria used, with estimates for current diagnosis as low as 0.2% in the Epidemiological Catchment Area studies (Robins et al., 1984) and 0.06% in a British study (Copeland et al., 1998). However, given that many population-based estimates exclude older adults in supported living environments, the actual prevalence is likely around 0.6 to 1% (Cohen, 2003). Delusional disorder is much less common, with estimated prevalence about 0.03%. Although more men than women are diagnosed with schizophrenia at younger ages, the gender ratio reverses in older age. Approximately 85% of older adults with schizophrenia reside in the community, with the remainder in institutional settings.

Most older adults with schizophrenia experience the onset of the illness in their second or third decade of life, and thus have lived with the illness for many years. Even with the increased mortality experienced by people with schizophrenia, particularly due to suicide or homicide, the absolute number of people living to older age with schizophrenia is expected to increase dramatically because of the aging of the population (Jeste et al., 1999). Onset prior to age 40 is referred to as "early-onset" schizophrenia, which accounts for approximately 80% of patients with schizophrenia. In contrast, the age of onset of delusional disorder is later, on average, than that in schizophrenia—typically occurring in middle age (between ages 40 and 60). Schizophrenia with onset after age 60 is referred to as Very-Late-Onset Schizophrenia-Like Psychosis (Howard, Rabins, Seeman, & Jeste, 2000). The literature includes a case report of schizophrenia with onset at age 100 (Cervantes, Rabins, & Slavney, 2006).

Over the years, researchers have explored the differences in clinical presentation and prognosis between individuals with early- versus late-onset schizophrenia. In these studies, late-onset schizophrenia is traditionally defined as having an onset of schizophrenia after the age of 40. Approximately 23% of patients experience onset after age 40 and 7% of older adults with schizophrenia have experienced the onset of illness after age 50 (Harris & Jeste, 1988). Comparing the presentation between early- and late-onset patients, there appear to be more similarities than differences (Palmer et al., 2001). Nevertheless, late-onset patients present somewhat unique features from their early-onset counterparts and, overall, late-onset patients have a somewhat better prognosis. Those with late-onset schizophrenia are more likely to be of the paranoid type and more likely to be women (Jeste et al., 1995). Late-onset patients may be less likely to display negative symptoms, and the neuropsychological profile is that of less impairment in executive functions and learning compared with early-onset patients. Additionally, because they experienced a longer symptom-free life, late-onset patients often have achieved more functional milestones, with better marriage and employment histories (Howard et al., 2000).

Early characterization of the course of late-life schizophrenia was that of progressive deterioration. The pre-eminent psychiatrist Emil Kraeplin referred to schizophrenia in older age as "dementia praecox" (Kraeplelin, 1919). However, long-term follow-up of early-onset patients suggests that, on average, general psychopathology and functional impairment are stable into later life (Jobe & Harrow, 2005). The first 5 to 10 years after the onset of schizophrenia are associated with the sharpest declines in functioning, with general evidence for stability thereafter. Cross-sectional data from middle-aged and older outpatients with schizophrenia suggests that the severity of positive symptoms tends to lessen with age (Jeste et al., 2003). Cognitive abilities remain stable in older adults with schizophrenia for up to 10 years, with a rate of decline similar to that seen in normal aging (Heaton et al., 2001). Some of these observed improvements are influenced by the "survivor" effect, i.e., mortality rates may be higher for more virulent early-onset cases that are at greater risk for self-inflicted injury or greater mortality from other causes. Nevertheless, the few existing long-term cohort studies suggest that improvements may occur, with some patients even attaining "sustained remission" (Auslander & Jeste, 2004; Jobe & Harrow, 2005).

Examining the predictors of positive or negative mental health trajectories, it does appear that worse prognosis in later life is associated with more severe negative symptoms and longer duration of illness. In addition, certain subsets of patients, particularly long-term institutionalized patients, may experience declines in functioning due to their impoverished living conditions (Harvey et al., 1999).

Culture and Diversity Issues

The core symptoms of schizophrenia appear to be consistent across ethnicities and cultures, but there are some key sociocultural considerations. Older people who are ethnic minorities and who have severe mental illnesses may experience a "triple stigma," facing ageism, racism, and biases against individuals with mental illnesses. In some instances, suspected paranoia regarding persecution may be based on actual racial prejudice experienced by the patient. There is also a well-known tendency for African Americans to be diagnosed with schizophrenia rather than bipolar disorder or other mood disorders: it is unclear if this tendency is due to self-selection, actual ethnic differences, or clinician biases (Minsky, Vega, Miskimen, Gara, & Escobar, 2003). Language barriers among patients whose first language is not English may complicate the clinical process of eliciting the nature and history of suspected psychotic symptoms—obtaining additional information from family members is often needed. Determination of whether the patient's unusual experiences are ethically or religiously sanctioned requires cultural competence of the clinician. In addition, older Latinos with schizophrenia appear less likely to utilize mental health services (Vega & Lopez, 2001). In turn, Latinos with schizophrenia are more likely to live with family members who may be more available to provide support, and prognosis may be improved as a result.

Assessment Measures

The first portion of the assessment of older people with suspected schizophrenia would entail the steps described in the early part of this chapter, with regard to ruling out underlying medical causes and contributors by gathering information from multiple sources. The next step is to confirm the diagnosis of schizophrenia and to measure its severity and its impact. Using structured clinical interviews, such as the Structured Clinical Interview for the DSM-IV Interview (SCID; Spitzer, Gibbon, & Williams, 1995), can aid in increasing the rigor in establishing current and lifetime diagnoses. The SCID can take anywhere from 30 minutes to three hours to administer, depending on which modules are included and the patient's history. A briefer alternative to the SCID for a psychiatric diagnostic interview is the Mini International Neuropsychiatric Interview (MINI; Sheehan et al., 1998), which takes approximately 30 minutes to administer.

Once a diagnosis of late-life schizophrenia and delusional disorder is obtained, domains that need ongoing clinical assessment include: (1) psychopathologic symptoms; (2) cognitive ability; (3) functional capacity/community functioning; and (4) medication side effects and adherence. Below we present useful measures in each of these categories. The most common form of assessment used in older adults with severe mental illness is the clinician-rated instrument, but there are also performance-based, observational, and self-reported measures representing these domains. The use of standardized and validated instruments can aid in gauging the overall severity of symptoms relative to established criteria, in assuring the coverage of all of the symptom clusters experienced by the patient, and in adding prognostic precision to the estimation of treatment effects.

Psychopathologic Symptoms

Positive and Negative Syndrome Scale (PANSS) is among the best-validated instruments for assessing positive, negative, and general psychopathology associated with schizophrenia. The PANSS is a standardized, clinical interview that rates the presence and severity of positive and negative symptoms, as well as general psychopathology for people with schizophrenia within the past week. Of the 30 items, seven are positive symptoms, seven are negative symptoms, and 16 are general psychopathology symptoms. Symptom severity for each item is rated according to which anchoring points in the 7-point scale (1 = absent; 7 = extreme) best describe the presentation of the symptom (Kay, Fiszbein, & Opler, 1987).

The Brief Psychiatric Rating Scale (BPRS) is an older, commonly used clinician-rated measure that is somewhat broader in symptom coverage. The BPRS was initially designed to evaluate pharmacologic treatment response in older adults. There are 18 symptom constructs assessed during this interview, encompassing various symptoms of psychosis, depression, and anxiety. Each symptom question is rated on a 7-point scale (1 = not present; 7 = extremely severe). The scoring criteria for each symptom are highly detailed; and consequently, the assessment has solid inter-rater reliability. The information gathered is based on the clinician's observation and the individuals' self-report of the past two to three days (Overall, 1962).

Cognitive Impairment

In addition to psychotic symptoms, the assessment of cognitive functioning is essential given its role in magnifying functional impairment. The assessment of cognition is discussed in greater depth in this book's section on cognition. There has been much recent work in the realm of neuropsychological assessment in schizophrenia, prominently the U.S. National Institute of Mental Health's Measurement and Treatment Research to Improve Cognition in Schizophrenia (MATRICS) initiative, which has identified a core battery of tests for the measurement of cognitive abilities in schizophrenia (Green & Nuechterlein, 2004). Although a full neuropsychological assessment such as the MATRICS battery will provide a more thorough indication of strengths and weakness in differing cognitive abilities, very often clinicians are called upon to obtain a global estimate of cognitive performance in older adults with psychotic disorders who have suspected cognitive impairment. Two brief measures of cognitive ability that that have been used in late-life schizophrenia are the Mattis Dementia Rating Scale (DRS) and the Repeatable Battery for the Assessment of Neuropsychological Status (RBANS).

The DRS takes approximately 15—20 minutes to administer and yields a total score (0—144) that reflects level of overall cognitive functioning, and five subscale scores that measure attention, initiation/perseveration, construction, conceptualization, and memory (Mattis, 1988).

The RBANS takes an average 30 minutes to administer, measuring five subscales of attention, immediate memory, visuospatial constructional skills, delayed memory, and language. The RBANS is particularly useful for longitudinal assessments because it has alternate forms that diminish learning effects of repeated testing (Randolph, Tierney, Mohr, & Chase, 1998).

Functional Abilities

The assessment of functional abilities is often essential in determining the level of care an individual with schizophrenia may require, as well as how the illness and associated factors impact patients' daily lives. There is no gold standard definition of functional dependence or independence, and no single functional instrument that covers all functional domains. Functional assessment separates what an individual does (actual performance) from what an individual can do (capacity). Different assessment strategies are required for performance and capacity: assessing real world functioning provides an indication of disability, while functional capacity assessment allows the clinician to observe functional abilities under optimized conditions. Because functional ability varies by context, assessment modality, and state-level factors (e.g., pain, fatigue), attaining an accurate estimation of functional status should include self- and informant-ratings, as well as performance-based assessment.

The Social-Adaptive Functioning Evaluation (SAFE) is a clinician-rated measure covering instrumental, social-interpersonal, and life-skills functioning, and was specifically designed and validated among older people with severe mental illness. This assessment is unique in its sensitivity to age-related impairments and is commonly used in inpatient and chronically institutionalized populations. There are 19 items, such as "money management" and "social engagement," that are rated on a scale of 0 (no impairment) to 4 (severe impairment). Ratings are restricted to functioning in the preceding month. Ratings are acquired through patient interaction, observation, and caregiver interviews (Harvey et al., 1997).

The Independent Living Skills Survey (ILSS) is a measure to test basic functional living skills of patients with severe and persistent mental illness. There are two versions: an informant-rated version (ILSS-I) and a self-report version (ILSS-SR). The ILSS-I consists of 103 items that assess 12 areas of basic community living skills. The ILSS-SR consists of 70 items, which cover 10 different domains of functioning: personal hygiene; appearance and care of clothing; care of personal possessions and living space; food preparation; care of personal health and safety; money management; transportation; leisure and recreational activities; job seeking; and job maintenance. Participants are asked to indicate "yes" or "no" to whether or not they had performed a specific task in the past month. The ILSS-SR takes approximately 20—30 minutes to complete (Wallace, Liberman, Tauber, & Wallace, 2000).

The UCSD Performance-Based Skills Assessment (UPSA) assesses functional capacity in five domains: comprehension/planning; finance; transportation; and household management. The UPSA involves role-playing tasks, such as navigating a bus route, balancing a checkbook, or rescheduling an appointment. Each subscale is scored on a scale of 0—20 and a total score (0—100) is provided from the sum of these sub-scores. The UPSA has excellent inter-rater reliability and has been empirically validated (Patterson, Goldman, McKibbin, Hughs, & Jeste, 2001).

Another performance-based measure, the Medication Management Ability Assessment (MMAA), focuses solely on prescription medication management. This role-playing task is modeled on prescription medication regimens, similar in complexity to those an older adult might encounter. The MMAA has excellent test—retest reliability and good construct validity, with scores significantly correlated with two other performance-based measures of functionality (Patterson et al., 2002).

Medication Side Effects and Adherence

Finally, medication side effects need to be assessed in older patients with schizophrenia. Antipsychotics (the mainstay of treatment) have side effects that require routine monitoring—older age is a primary risk factor for these side effects. First generation antipsychotics (e.g., haloperidol) carry a risk of inducing tardive dyskenesia (TD), which involves involuntary movements of the face, trunk, and limbs. The incidence of TD in patients treated with first generation antipsychotics is high; in one prospective study it was 5%, 34%, and 53% after one, two, and three years respectively of cumulative antipsychotic treatment (Woerner, Alvir, Saltz, Lieberman, & Kane, 1998). Second generation antipsychotics are less likely to produce TD, but are associated with significant metabolic changes including diabetes, hypertension, and weight gain (Newcomer, 2007). These side effects are of concern in that they may increase the risk of cerebrovascular disease and cardiovascular mortality. There are clinician-rated scales for assessing TD, which include the AIMS Scale (Lane, Glazer, Hansen, Berman, & Kramer, 1985). The monitoring of metabolic side effects of second generation antipsychotics includes regular assessment of serum metabolic profile, lipid profiles, blood pressure, and body mass index (Marder et al., 2004).

The routine assessment of older people with psychotic disorders should include an assessment of medication adherence as well as side effects. In people with bipolar disorder or schizophrenia, the rate of non-adherence is quite high (approximately 40%), and exacerbations of psychosis can frequently occur after episodes of non-adherence (Lacro, Dunn, Dolder, Leckband, & Jeste, 2002). In older adults, non-adherence is more likely to be unintentional, such as via forgetting. Self-report scales of adherence exist (Dolder et al., 2004), but accuracy of self-report may be diminished in older adults with cognitive impairment. Other measures such as pill counts, blood levels of medications, and pharmacy records can be used to provide a more objective measure of adherence.

Case Study 1

Elsa is a 68-year-old woman who lives with her daughter in an apartment. Elsa's daughter brought her to the emergency department after her mother had become increasingly suspicious of the neighbors living upstairs, believing that these neighbors were putting "mind control gas" in the air vents and attempting to poison Elsa. She believed these neighbors were part of a satanic cult. Her paranoia had increased over the previous week, and she had begun to plug the vents with paper towels, creating concern for a fire hazard. In the previous week, Elsa had eaten only sporadically and had refused to take her medications. The daughter finally decided to bring her mother in to the emergency department for an evaluation after she witnessed her mother shouting into the vents, cursing at her neighbors.

From separate interviews with Elsa and her daughter, it was revealed that Elsa had been diagnosed with schizophrenia at age 34 and had spent several months in different psychiatric hospitals over the subsequent 10 years. From middle age onward, Elsa had lived initially with her husband (her primary caretaker) and, since his death five years before, she had lived with her daughter. Elsa had seen a psychiatrist who prescribed antipsychotic medications and she had not worked regularly since she was first diagnosed. Medically, she had a stroke three years before, which had left her with a slight drop on the left side of her face, some generalized muscle weakness, and some decline in short-term memory. Functionally, Elsa's daughter assisted Elsa in nearly all instrumental activities of daily living, including medication management, and expressed feeling distress and being overwhelmed by her caregiving responsibilities. In addition to a second generation antipsychotic medication, she was prescribed cardiovascular medications.

During evaluation, Elsa was noted to appear anxious (i.e., wringing her hands), and guarded in her attitude. After initially denying any problems, Elsa then endorsed beliefs that her neighbors had been trying to harm her; although she did not admit that she had ever been diagnosed with schizophrenia. She scored a 31 on the PANSS, which revealed that she had severe positive symptoms but mild negative symptoms. Brief assessment of cognitive status with the Dementia Rating Scale revealed that Elsa was generally cognitively intact. Laboratory work-up was indicative of a urinary tract infection (UTI). CT of the head revealed a right-sided lacunar infarction consistent with her stroke five years ago, diffuse white matter changes that were consistent with age-related change, and no new concerning changes.

After a long discussion with her daughter, Elsa was willing to be admitted to a psychiatric hospital for a medication evaluation and treatment of her UTI with antibiotics. After five days in which her antipsychotic medications were restarted, Elsa was less anxious and no longer expressed certainty about her neighbor's ill intentions, although she continued to harbor suspicions. She had better insight into her diagnosis of schizophrenia. No auditory hallucinations were observed during hospitalization. At discharge, her symptoms of UTI had remitted and her PANSS score had dropped to 14. Part of the discharge plan was for Elsa to attend a day treatment group at the community mental health center, aimed at providing social engagement for Elsa and allowing Elsa's daughter respite from care.

BIPOLAR DISORDER AND PSYCHOTIC DEPRESSION

Definition, Prevalence and Course

Mood disorders at times present with psychotic features, and include bipolar disorder and depression with psychotic features. There has been a long held dichotomy between schizophrenia and mood disorders, with Emil Kraeplin differentiating "dementia praecox" from "manic depression" by the presence of psychosis in the former and mood symptoms in the latter. However, more recent conceptualizations, stemming from the evidence of shared genetic vulnerabilities between mood and psychotic disorders, challenge the validity of the dichotomy between mood and psychotic disorders. Psychotic disorders including schizophrenia may thus be best viewed as part of a continuum that includes bipolar disorder and other mood disorders (Craddock & Owen, 2005).

The classification of psychotic disorders is evolving. The current approach, based on DSM-IV, differentiates between diagnoses of schizophrenia, schizoaffective disorder, and mood disorder based on the chronological sequence and duration of symptoms, and overlap of psychosis and mood symptoms. To meet criteria for a mood disorder with psychotic features, the DSM-IV specifies that psychotic symptoms must occur in the presence of a mood disorder—if the patient has delusions or hallucinations for two weeks in the absence of a mood disorder then the diagnosis would be schizoaffective disorder or schizophrenia. Most commonly, psychotic mood disorders include psychotic symptoms that are *mood congruent*. Depressive delusions include themes of guilt, hypochondriasis, nihilism, persecution, or jealousy. In manic episodes, the content may be grandiose. However, psychotic symptoms do not *need* to be mood congruent for a person to meet criteria for a mood disorder with psychotic features, so long as the symptoms occur in the context of a mood episode.

The presence of depression in community-dwelling older adults is approximately 1–4%, with higher rates in primary care and higher still in specialty mental health settings. Among older adults with depression, the exact prevalence of depression with psychotic features in late-life is unknown, but, in the general population, about 20% of people with major depression have psychotic features. Bipolar disorder is less common than major depression in late-life, but may be present in up to 10% of geriatric psychiatric inpatients and outpatients. In a review of the phenomenology of older adults with bipolar disorder, 60% of cases had psychotic symptoms (Depp & Jeste, 2004). Delusions are more common than hallucinations in mood disorders with psychotic features, and, when hallucinations are present, delusions generally are also found (Meyers, 1995).

Psychotic symptoms generally predict a worse prognosis in affective disorders. In mixed-age studies, patients with psychotic depression have more frequent relapses and may be at risk for greater residual impairment in functioning after symptoms remit. There is some evidence that suicide risk may be increased among depressed people with psychotic features, but studies are inconsistent. In older adults, there is consistent evidence that cognitive impairment may accompany depression or bipolar disorder, with or without psychosis. These deficits may not be as severe as those associated with schizophrenia, but they are associated with substantial disability. In mixed-age studies of patients with depression or bipolar disorder, psychotic features are associated with a higher risk for cognitive impairment. A number of studies have suggested that dysregulation in the hypothalamic–pituitary–adrenal (HPA) axis may be more evident in psychotic than non-psychotic depression, leading to speculation of a causal role of HPA in psychotic depression (Keller et al., 2006).

Assessment Measures

The assessment of psychosis in the context of mood disorders would include the same procedures and instruments as described for schizophrenia above, covering psychotic symptoms, cognitive functioning, and functional capacity/community functioning. Additional assessment of mood symptoms, covered in the first chapter in this book, would include depression symptom severity measures (e.g., the Hamilton Depression Rating Scale) and manic symptoms (e.g., the Young Mania Rating Scale).

Given that there is a high risk of suicide in older adults with mood disorders in general, and suicide risk may be increased among those with psychotic features, suicide screening should be routinely undertaken. In older adults with psychosis, asking about the presence of command hallucinations should be included in suicide assessment.

ASSESSMENT OF PSYCHOSIS IN DEMENTIA

Definition, Prevalence, and Course

Psychotic symptoms frequently occur among older adults with Alzheimer's disease (AD) and other dementias. In fact, the dementias account for the largest proportion of older adults' cases of psychosis.

Psychotic symptoms in dementia are generally described as part of a constellation of neuropsychiatric symptoms (i.e., non-cognitive symptoms), which also include emotional disturbances (depression, anxiety, irritability, apathy) and behavioral problems (aggression, withdrawal). Psychosis often increases the risk of other behavioral problems; for example, the presence of a persistent delusion may be associated with aggression, or misidentification of the family home may subsequently lead to wandering. The DSM-IV does not specifically recognize "psychotic features" of Alzheimer's disease or other dementias, lumping psychosis with other neuropsychiatric symptoms under the modifier "with behavioral disturbances." Because so many with AD exhibit such behavioral disturbances, and because the symptoms are quite diffuse, future revisions of the DSM may include greater specification of neuropsychiatric symptoms (Jeste, Meeks, Kim, & Zubenko, 2006).

Psychosis in AD was initially described by Alois Alzheimer in 1907. It is now known that psychosis in AD is biologically distinct from psychosis due to schizophrenia; however, due to the overlap in presentation between these conditions, differential diagnosis can be difficult. Jeste and Finkel (2000) have proposed criteria aimed at identifying whether psychosis is due to dementia rather than schizophrenia, delirium, or other conditions. Table 5.1 displays some heuristic differences between psychosis exhibited in AD and schizophrenia (Jeste & Finkel, 2000).

To meet the proposed criteria for psychosis in AD, patients must meet criteria for AD, and they must have exhibited visual or auditory hallucinations or delusions for one month or longer. These symptoms must not have been present continuously prior to the onset of dementia, and the patient must never have met criteria for a psychotic disorder (e.g., schizophrenia, mood disorder with psychotic features). Neurobiological studies, as well as differences in presentation between dementia with psychosis and schizophrenia, support the distinction between these syndromes.

Most of what is known about the prevalence of psychosis in dementia is via patients with Alzheimer's disease, since AD accounts for the largest proportion of dementias. Approximately 40% of people with dementia exhibit psychotic symptoms, although the range in prevalence varies widely across studies. Delusions appear to be more common that hallucinations in AD. In one review of 55 studies reporting a prevalence of psychosis in AD, 36% of patients had delusions and 18% exhibited hallucinations (Ropacki & Jeste, 2005). The cumulative incidence of psychosis in AD in one study was 20% at 1 year, 36% at 2 years, 50% at 3 years, and 51% at 4 years (Paulson et al., 2000).

Psychosis is also common in Parkinson's disease, with about 15–20% of patients exhibiting hallucinations or delusions (Werner, 2003). Some evidence suggests that hallucinations may be more common than delusions in Parkinson's disease. Visual hallucinations are very common in dementia with

Table 5.1 Psychosis of Alzheimer's Disease versus Late-Life Schizophrenia

	Alzheimer's Disease	Schizophrenia
Prevalence in adults older than age 65	1.5 %	<1%
Bizarre delusions	Rare	Frequent
Misidentifications	Common	Rare
Hallucinations	Mostly visual	Mostly auditory
First rank symptoms	Rare	Common
Suicide	Rare	Frequent
Past history	Rare	Common
Remission	Frequent	Uncommon
Need for maintenance	Rare	Common
Antipsychotic doses	Low	Moderate

Lewy bodies, and often are among the earliest presentations. In contrast, fronto-temporal dementia appears to have a much lower prevalence of psychotic symptoms compared with other types of dementia.

Among people with AD followed over time, psychotic symptoms tend to emerge gradually, last for several months or years, and then diminish in frequency. In AD, the middle stage of the illness is most often associated with psychosis, whereas the earlier stages are more commonly associated with depression. Patients in late stages may still experience psychotic symptoms, but may not be able to verbally describe these experiences; their reactions to psychosis may manifest in agitation or refusal to engage in activities. These symptoms may be intermittent, in some cases disappearing and reappearing months later. Abrupt onset of psychosis is more often indicative of delirium.

The presence of psychosis in AD is associated with greater cognitive impairment and faster cognitive decline, as well as reduced quality of life in both patients and caregivers. There is some evidence that the presence of psychosis also increases risk of mortality. Some studies have found a significant association between psychosis and older age (Mizrahi, Starkstein, Jorge, & Robinson, 2006). In Parkinson's disease, dopaminergic agents used to treat the disorder may produce psychotic symptoms.

There are a number of common delusions that occur in dementia. These include misidentification syndromes, in particular believing that a caregiver or familiar person has been replaced by an imposter (Capgras delusion), and believing that one's home has been replaced or that others are living in the home (the Phantom Boarder syndrome). Some authors do not consider misidentification symptoms as true delusions, since they may represent confusion with reality rather than a more complex reconstruction of reality. Other common delusions include beliefs that a spouse has committed infidelity, or that one is the victim of a theft or abuse. In comparison to the delusions evidenced in schizophrenia, those present in dementia are generally more simple and less likely to be bizarre. Delusions in dementia are also more transitory and may diminish or increase in intensity depending on the context. In regard to hallucinations, visual and auditory hallucinations are more common than hallucinations in other sensory modalities.

Not surprisingly, presence of psychosis is frequently associated with caregiver distress. Psychotic symptoms are a frequent cause for possible premature institutionalization and are a primary reason for the prescription of antipsychotic medications in nursing homes, which appears to be on the rise (Molinari et al., 2010).

Multicultural and Diversity Issues

Risk factors for psychosis in AD include African American ethnicity. Rates of institutionalization are lower in Latino and African American older adults with dementia. Hence, care recipients may reside at home for longer, and thus may have more severe cognitive and functional impairments that are less likely to have been present prior to formal assessment and treatment.

Assessment Procedures

The assessment of psychosis, as well as other neuropsychiatric symptoms, in dementia requires gathering detailed information regarding circumstances, timing, frequency, setting, and severity of symptoms. Identifying the antecedents to psychotic symptoms, (e.g., being in an unfamiliar environment) and their timing (e.g., whether symptoms occur at night) can lead to preventative measures. For instance, changes in the home environment, such as a new visitor, may induce misidentification syndromes. Other antecedents may include physiological states, such as hunger, fatigue, or pain, which may either introduce new symptoms or amplify the intensity of existing psychotic symptoms.

Assessing caregiver's response to psychotic symptoms can also be helpful in determining more adaptive responses. For instance, some caregivers engage in lengthy arguments with the patient trying to convince the patient that they are misperceiving reality—these arguments often leave the caregiver exasperated and do little to change the patient's views. Indeed, assessing the emotional expressivity variable for caregivers of those with dementia may yield high therapeutic value, especially in planning interventions for those care recipients exhibiting psychotic symptoms (Adams, 1997). Alternative strategies, such as distraction, may reduce caregiver burden. Assessing the severity of psychosis can help to identify whether symptoms are dangerous and require immediate pharmacological management, or, if not, whether they can be dealt with through distraction or other behavioral strategies.

There is good reason to conduct a careful behavioral assessment in order to guide non-pharmacological strategies—the pharmacological management of behavioral disturbances, including psychosis, in AD has been the subject of much recent discussion. There are potential risks of antipsychotic medications (e.g., the FDA black box warning regarding increased risk of mortality in AD patients who are placed on antipsychotics), and the findings of the recent Multi-center Clinical Antipsychotic Trials of Intervention Effectiveness study indicate that benefits of antipsychotic medications in reducing neuropsychiatric symptoms were questionable (Schneider et al., 2006). As the pharmacologic treatment of psychosis in AD is still evolving, behavioral and family approaches become all the more important.

There are a number of clinician and caregiver rated scales for measuring the neuropsychiatric symptoms of dementia. These scales include questions on psychosis embedded in subscales measuring other neuropsychiatric syndromes.

The Behavioral Pathology in Alzheimer's Disease Rating Scale (BEHAVE-AD) is a psychometrically validated assessment that assesses the nature and severity of behavioral pathology. BEHAVE-AD consists of a 25-item scale with seven categories: paranoid and delusional ideation; hallucinations; activity disturbances; aggressiveness; diurnal rhythm disturbances; affective disturbances; and anxieties and phobias. Each category is scored on a 4-point scale where 0 = not present, 1 = present, 2 = present with an emotional component, 3 = present with an emotional and physical component. There is also a 4-point global assessment scale of caregiver distress and/or perceived danger to the patient. This assessment reliably measures behavioral disturbances independent of cognitive deficiencies, allowing for more appropriate treatment of behavioral symptoms (Reisberg et al., 1987).

The Caregiver-Administered Neuropsychiatric Inventory (CGA-NPI) determines the presence, frequency, and severity of neuropsychiatric symptoms. The CGA-NPI yields 12 domain scores (corresponding to 12 psychiatric symptoms), as well as a total score, each reflecting the product of frequency and severity of symptoms. Although not part of a formal CGA-NPI domain scores or total, each of the 12 domain sections in the CGA-NPI includes a question in which the caregiver rated, on a scale of 0 (not at all) to 5 (very severely or extremely), the level of emotional distress (to the caregiver) from the patient's neuropsychiatric symptoms in that domain (Kang et al., 2004).

The Behavioral Rating Scale for Dementia (BRSD) is a standardized instrument that rates the frequency and severity of a wide range of psychopathology in patients with probable Alzheimer's disease. There are 51 items, 48 of which are related to specific signs and symptoms, and three are open-ended questions about general psychopathological disturbances. Each of the items is rated by frequency of occurrence. The examiner rates each symptom according to anchored scoring guidelines, and the assessment is administered to caregivers (Tariot et al., 1995).

Case Study 2

Ms G, a 78-year-old female, was referred to an Outpatient Geriatric Psychiatry Clinic by her family care practitioner for a psychiatric evaluation and treatment recommendations. History revealed that the patient was diagnosed with mild Alzheimer's disease when she was 75-years-old by a neurologist at the Alzheimer's Disease Research Center. Among other neuropsychological test scores indicating cognitive decline, Ms G had a score of 121 on the Mattis Dementia Rating Scale (DRS). Around that time, the patient and her family noticed increasing memory problems;

she would frequently forget phone messages, family visits, and where she put her belongings. Although Ms G was not able to do her own finances, she was able to independently manage other instrumental activities of daily living, like cooking and doing her own laundry; with assistance, Ms G continued to live alone for two years. However, when Ms G exhibited some potentially dangerous behaviors (leaving the stove on and letting the bathtub overflow), the family arranged for her to move in with her daughter's family.

After the move, Ms G began to exhibit delusions, peaking within two months. She had been accusing her daughter, with whom she lived, of stealing money from her bank accounts. Ms G also held the belief that she only had one granddaughter, and this granddaughter would change identities to disguise herself and steal Ms G's personal belongings out of her room (the Fregoli delusion). Some items Ms G claimed were stolen never existed.

The patient was seen at the Outpatient Geriatric Psychiatry Clinic for evaluation. A medical evaluation, including a blood test, urine sample, physical exam, and a CT scan were completed. Ms G was generally healthy, although she had non-insulin dependent diabetes. These evaluations did not indicate any underlying medical condition that might have contributed to the onset of the patient's psychotic symptoms. An extensive medical and family history was collected from all available sources, i.e., medical records and family members. Ms G had no previous psychiatric history. The patient also underwent a follow-up neuropsychological screening and was administered the Behavioral Pathology in Alzheimer's Disease Rating Scale (BEHAVE-AD). A repeat DRS score of 110 indicated further decline since the patient's initial diagnosis three years prior. The BEHAVE-AD revealed elevations on symptom clusters representing delusions and agitation, but not on hallucinations or other behavior problems.

Evaluation of the context of delusional statements revealed that they seemed to occur during evenings when the entire family was home. Ms G exhibited no potentially dangerous behaviors associated with the delusions (e.g., aggressiveness), however they were extremely distressing for the patient's family. Her granddaughters went to great lengths to try to prove to Ms G that she was not being stolen from, during which Ms G would often become agitated and tearful. Ms G was sometimes agitated and would wander around the house, sometimes late at night. It was apparent that she was having a hard time adjusting to living in a new environment and with other people.

Based on the evaluation, Ms G's symptoms were judged to be consistent with psychotic symptoms associated with Alzheimer's disease, and also consistent with progression to the middle stages of AD. No medical problems or psychotic disorder were suspected. Moreover, antecedent to the patient's psychosis was moving to a new house where other people lived. Weighing treatment options with Ms G's family led to an agreement to observe Ms G over the period of one month to see if assimilation to the new environment might improve her symptoms. To accelerate this adjustment, steps were taken which included putting familiar objects in Ms G's room that would remind her of her old home. Family members were advised to redirect the patient rather than confront her accusations. Additionally, the family was referred to a support group at the Alzheimer's Disease Research Center. If following these recommendations did not result in substantial benefit within one month, the plan was to prescribe a low dose of antipsychotic medication.

Fortunately, at a follow-up appointment one month after being seen at the Outpatient Geriatric Psychiatry Clinic, it was determined that Ms G's delusions had abated somewhat. Ms G continued to express delusional beliefs about being stolen from, but these were less frequent, and the family was less distressed about them. Repeat BEHAVE-AD scores revealed slight declines in symptom severity. The family was advised to follow up with the clinic if there was a worsening of symptoms.

Issues in ReAssessment

This chapter has thus far focused on the initial assessment of individuals with psychosis. Re-assessment is useful for gauging the effectiveness of treatment effects and monitoring the course of illness. Care should be taken to make repeat assessments as equivalent as possible, particularly in terms of factors such as fatigue or pain that may bias the interpretation of results. By doing so, assessment of change in symptoms enables measurement-based care planning. A 50% reduction in symptoms, as measured by standardized scales, indicates effectiveness of medications in most clinical trials. Additionally, criteria for remission on the PANSS and BPRS have been proposed. Failure to attain remission in a specified time frame might suggest altering the treatment plan.

With the cognitive screening and performance-based measures we have discussed, an additional concern is practice effects. Practice effects can reduce the ability of clinicians to measure declines accurately. The use of reliable change indices or adjustments for practice effects may aid in the interpretation of change. With these principles in mind, rehabilitation strategies can become more measurement based.

CONCLUSION

This chapter has described the general assessment approach to older adults with psychosis, the features of psychiatric conditions in later life associated with psychotic symptoms, and selected measures and assessment strategies for patients with these conditions. The absolute number of older adults with psychotic symptoms from all causes will rise as the population ages. A careful and comprehensive approach to assessment will aid in pinpointing the etiology of psychosis, assessing its impact on the person and support system, and gauging the effectiveness of treatments.

POSITIVE AND NEGATIVE SYNDROME SCALE (PANSS)

Patient Information									
Patient		Date	Day	Mth.	Year	Time	Hour	Min
Personal notes								

Scoring Procedure

Tick appropriate box for each item

POSITIVE SCALE (P)

P1. Delusions Beliefs which are unfounded, unrealistic, and idiosyncratic. Basis for rating thought content expressed in the interview and its influence on social relations and behavior.	
1 Absent - Definition does not apply.	☐
2 Minimal - Questionable pathology; may be at the upper extreme of normal limits.	☐
3 Mild - Presence of one or two delusions which are vague, uncrystallized, and not tenaciously held. Delusions do not interfere with thinking, social relations, or behavior.	☐
4 Moderate - Presence of either a kaleidoscopic array of poorly-formed, unstable delusions or of a few well-formed delusions that occasionally interfere with thinking, social relations, or behavior.	☐
5 Moderate severe - Presence of numerous well-formed delusions that are tenaciously held and occasionally interfere with thinking, social relations, or behavior.	☐
6 Severe - Presence of a stable set of delusions which are crystallized, possibly systematized, tenaciously held, and clearly interfere with thinking, social relations, and behavior.	☐
7 Extreme - Presence of a stable set of delusions which are either highly systematized or very numerous, and which dominate major facets of the patient's life. This frequently results in inappropriate and irresponsible action, which may even jeopardize the safety of the patient or others.	☐

P2. Conceptual disorganization Disorganized process of thinking characterized by disruption of goal-directed sequencing, e.g., circumstantiality, tangentiality, loose associations non sequiturs, gross illogicality, or thought block. Basis for rating: cognitive-verbal processes observed during the course of interview.	
1 Absent - Definition does not apply.	☐
2 Minimal - Questionable pathology; may be at the upper extreme of normal limits.	☐
3 Mild - Thinking is circumstantial, tangential, or paralogical. There is some difficulty in directing thoughts toward a goal and some loosening of associations may be evidenced under pressure.	☐
4 Moderate - Able to focus thoughts when communications are brief and structured, but becomes loose or irrelevant when dealing with more complex communications or when under minimal pressure.	☐
5 Moderate severe - Generally has difficulty in organizing thoughts, as evidenced by frequent irrelevances, disconnectedness. or loosening of associations even when not under pressure.	☐
6 Severe - Thinking is seriously derailed and internally inconsistent, resulting in gross irrelevancies and disruption of thought processes, which occur almost constantly.	☐
7 Extreme - Thoughts are disrupted to the point where the patient is incoherent. There is marked loosening of associations, which results in total failure of communication, e.g., "word salad" or mutism.	☐

P3. Hallucinatory behavior Verbal report or behavior indicating perceptions which are not generated by external stimuli. These may occur in the auditory visual, olfactory, or somatic realms. Basis for rating: Verbal report and physical manifestations during the course of interview, as well as reports of behavior by primary care workers or family.	
1 Absent - Definition does not apply.	☐
2 Minimal - Questionable pathology; may be at the upper extreme of normal limits.	☐
3 Mild - One or two clearly formed but infrequent hallucinations, or else a number of vague abnormal perceptions which do not result in distortions of thinking or behavior.	☐
4 Moderate - Hallucinations occur frequently but not continuously, and the patient's thinking and behavior are affected only to a minor extent.	☐
5 Moderate severe - Hallucinations are frequent, may involve more than one sensory modality, and tend to distort thinking and/or disrupt behavior. Patient may have a delusional interpretation of these experiences and respond to them emotionally and, on occasion, verbally as well.	☐
6 Severe - Hallucinations are present almost continuously, causing major disruption of thinking and behavior. Patient treats these as real perceptions, and functioning is impeded by frequent emotional and verbal responses to them.	☐
7 Extreme - Patient is almost totally preoccupied with hallucinations, which virtually dominate thinking and behavior. Hallucinations are provided a rigid delusional interpretation and provoke verbal and behavioral responses, including obedience to command hallucinations.	☐

P4. Excitement Hyperactivity as reflected in accelerated motor behavior, heightened responsivity to stimuli hypervigilance, or excessive mood lability. Basis for rating: Behavioral manifestations during the course of interview, as well as reports of behavior by primary care workers or family.	
1 Absent - Definition does not apply.	☐
2 Minimal - Questionable pathology; may be at the upper extreme of normal limits.	☐
3 Mild - Tends to be slightly agitated, hypervigilant, or mildly overaroused throughout the interview, but without distinct episodes of excitement or marked mobility. Speech may be slightly pressured.	☐
4 Moderate - Agitation or overarousal is clearly evident throughout the interview, affecting speech and general mobility, or episodic outbursts occur sporadically.	☐
5 Moderate severe - Significant hyperactivity or frequent outbursts of motor activity are observed, making it difficult for the patient to sit still for longer than several minutes at any given time.	☐
6 Severe - Marked excitement dominates the interview, delimits attention, and to some extent affects personal functions such as eating and sleeping.	☐
7 Extreme - Marked excitement seriously interferes in eating and sleeping and makes interpersonal interactions virtually impossible. Acceleration of speech and motor activity may result in incoherence and exhaustion.	☐

P5. Grandiosity Exaggerated self-opinion and unrealistic convictions of superiority, including delusions of extraordinary abilities, wealth, knowledge, fame, power, and moral righteousness. Basis for rating: Thought content expressed in the interview and its influence on behavior.	
1 Absent - Definition does not apply.	☐
2 Minimal - Questionable pathology; may be at the upper extreme of normal limits.	☐
3 Mild - Some expansiveness or boastfulness is evident, but without clear-cut grandiose delusions.	☐
4 Moderate - Feels distinctly and unrealistically superior to others. Some poorly formed delusions about special status or abilities may be present but are not acted upon.	☐
5 Moderate severe - Clear-cut delusions concerning remarkable abilities, status, or power are expressed and influence attitude but not behavior.	☐
6 Severe - Clear-cut delusions of remarkable superiority involving more than one parameter (wealth, knowledge, fame, etc.) are expressed, notably influence interactions, and may be acted upon.	☐
7 Extreme - Thinking, interactions, and behavior are dominated by multiple delusions of amazing ability, wealth knowledge, fame, power, and/or moral stature; which may take on a bizarre quality.	☐

P6. Suspiciousness/persecution Unrealistic or exaggerated ideas of persecution, as reflected in guardedness, a distrustful attitude, suspicious hypervigilance, or frank delusions that others mean one harm. Basis for rating: Thought content expressed in the interview and its influence on behavior.	
1 Absent - Definition does not apply.	☐
2 Minimal - Questionable pathology; may be at the upper extreme of normal limits.	☐
3 Mild - Presents a guarded or even openly distrustful attitude, but thoughts, interactions, and behavior are minimally affected.	☐
4 Moderate - Distrustfulness is clearly evident and intrudes on the interview and/or behavoir, but there is no evidence of persecutorv delusions. Alternatively, there may be indication of loosely formed persecutory delusions, but these do not seem to affect the patient's attitude or interpersonal relations.	☐
5 Moderate severe - Patient shows marked distrustfulness, leading to major disruption of interpersonal relations, or else there are clear-cut persecutory delusions that have limited impact on interpersonal relations and behavior.	☐
6 Severe - Clear-cut pervasive delusions of persecution which may be systematized and significantly interfere in interpersonal relations.	☐
7 Extreme - A network of systematized persecutory delusions dominates the patient's thinking, social relations, and behavior.	☐

P7. Hostility Verbal and nonverbal expressions of anger and resentment, including sarcasm, passive-aggressive behavior, verbal abuse, and assaultiveness. Basis for rating: Interpersonal behavior observed during the interview and reports by primary care workers or family.	
1 Absent - Definition does not apply.	☐
2 Minimal - Questionable pathology; may be at the upper extreme of normal limits.	☐
3 Mild - Indirect or restrained communication of anger such as sarcasm, disrespect, hostile expressions, and occasional irritability.	☐
4 Moderate - Presents an overtly hostile attitude, showing frequent irritability and direct expression of anger or resentment.	☐
5 Moderate severe - Patient is highly irritable and occasionally verbally abusive or threatening.	☐
6 Severe - Uncooperativeness and verbal abuse or threats notably influence the interview and seriously impact upon social relations. Patient may be violent and destructive but is not physically assaultive toward others.	☐
7 Extreme - Marked anger results in extreme uncooperativeness, precluding other interactions, or in eoisede(s) of physical assault toward others.	☐

NEGATIVE SCALE (N)

N1. Blunted affect Diminished emotional responsiveness as characterized by a reduction in facial expression, modulation of feelings, and communicative gestures. Basis for rating: Observation of physical manifestations of affective tone and emotional responsiveness during the course of interview.	
1 Absent - Definition does not apply.	☐
2 Minimal - Questionable pathology; may be at the upper extreme of normal limits.	☐
3 Mild - Changes in facial expression and communicative gestures seem to be stilted, forced, artificial, or lacking in modulation.	☐
4 Moderate - Reduced range of facial expression and few expressive gestures result in a dull appearance.	☐
5 Moderate severe - Affect is generally flat, with only occasional changes in facial expression and a paucity of communicative gestures.	☐
6 Severe - Marked flatness and deficiency of emotions exhibited most of the time. There may be unmodulated extreme affective discharges, such as excitement, rage, or inappropriate uncontrolled laughter.	☐
7 Extreme - Changes in facial expression and evidence of communicative gestures are virtually absent. Patient seems constantly to show a barren or "wooden" expression.	☐

N2. Emotional withdrawal Lack of interest in, involvement with, and affective commitment to life's events. Basis for rating: Reports of functioning from primary care workers or family and observation of interpersonal behavior during the course of interview.	
1 Absent - Definition does not apply.	☐
2 Minimal - Questionable pathology; may be at the upper extreme of normal limits.	☐
3 Mild - Usually lacks initiative and occasionally may show deficient interest in surrounding events.	☐
4 Moderate - Patient is generally distanced emotionally from the milieu and its challenges but, with encouragement, can be engaged.	☐
5 Moderate severe - Patient is clearly detached emotionally from persons and events in the milieu, resisting all efforts at engagement. Patient appears distant, docile, and purposeless, but can be involved in communication at least briefly and tends to personal needs, sometimes with assistance.	☐
6 Severe - Marked deficiency of interest and emotional commitment results in limited conversation with others and frequent neglect of personal functions, for which the patient requires supervision.	☐
7 Extreme - Patient is almost totally withdrawn, uncommunicative, and neglectful of personal needs as a result of profound lack of interest and emotional commitment.	☐

N3. Poor rapport Lack of interpersonal empathy, openess in conversation, and sense of closeness, interest, or involvement with the interviewer. This is evidenced by interpersonal distancing and reduced verbal and nonverbal communication. Basis for rating: Interpersonal behavior during the course of interview.	
1 Absent - Definition does not apply.	☐
2 Minimal - Questionable pathology; may be at the upper extreme of normal limits.	☐
3 Mild - Conversation is characterized by a stilted, strained or artificial tone. It may lack emotional depth or tend to remain on an impersonal, intellectual plane.	☐
4 Moderate - Patient typically is aloof, with interpersonal distance quite evident. Patient may answer questions mechanically, act bored, or express disinterest.	☐
5 Moderate severe - Disinvolvement is obvious and clearly impedes the productivity of the interview. Patient may tend to avoid eye or face contact.	☐
6 Severe - Patient is highly indifferent, with marked interpersonal distance. Answers are perfunctory, and there is little nonverbal evidence of involvement. Eye and face contact are frequently avoided.	☐
7 Extreme - Patient is totally uninvolved with the interviewer. Patient appears to be completely indifferent and consistently avoids verbal and nonverbal interactions during the interview.	☐

N4. Passive/apathetic social withdrawal Diminished interest and initiative in social interactions due to passivity, apathy, anergy, or avolition. This leads to reduced interpersonal involvement and neglect of activities of daily living. Basis for rating: Reports on social behavior from primary care workers or family.	
1 Absent - Definition does not apply.	☐
2 Minimal - Questionable pathology; may be at the upper extreme of normal limits.	☐
3 Mild - Shows occasional interest in social activities but poor initiative. Usally engages with others only when approached first by them.	☐
4 Moderate - Passively goes along with most social activities but in a disinterested or mechanical way. Tends to recede into the background.	☐
5 Moderate severe - Passively participates in only a minority of activities and shows virtually no interest or initiative. Generally spends little time with others.	☐
6 Severe - Tends to be apathetic and isolated, participating very rarely in social activities and occasionally neglecting personal needs. Has very few spontaneous social contacts.	☐
7 Extreme - Profoundly apathetic, socially isolated, and personally neglectful.	☐

N5. Difficulty in abstract thinking Impairment in the use of the abstract-symbolic mode of thinking, as evidenced by difficulty in classification, forming generalizations, and proceeding beyond concrete or egocentric thinking in problem solving tasks. Basis for rating: Responses to questions on similarities and proverb interpretation, and use of concrete vs. abstract mode during the course of the interview.	
1 Absent - Definition does not apply.	☐
2 Minimal - Questionable pathology; may be at the upper extreme of normal limits.	☐
3 Mild - Tends to give literal or personalized interpretations to the more difficult proverbs and may have some problems with concepts that are fairly abstract or remotely related.	☐
4 Moderate - Often utilizes a concrete mode. Has difficulty with most proverbs and some categories. Tends to be distracted by functional aspects and salient features.	☐
5 Moderate severe - Deals primarily in a concrete mode, exhibiting difficulty with most proverbs and many categories.	☐
6 Severe - Unable to grasp the abstract meaning of any proverbs or figurative expressions and can formulate classifications for only the most simple of similarities. Thinking is either vacuous or locked into functional aspects, salient features, and idiosyncratic interpretations.	☐
7 Extreme - Can use only concrete modes of thinking. Shows no comprehension of proverbs, common metaphors or similes, and simple categories. Even salient and functional attributes do not serve as a basis for classification. This rating may apply to those who cannot interact even minimally with the examiner due to marked cognitive impairment.	☐

N6. Lack of spontaneity and flow of conversation Reduction in the normal flow of communication associated with apathy, avolition, defensiveness, or cognitive deficit. This is manifested by diminished fluidity and productivity of the verbal-interactional process. Basis for rating: Cognitive-verbal processes observed during the course of interview.	
1 Absent - Definition does not apply.	☐
2 Minimal - Questionable pathology; may be at the upper extreme of normal limits.	☐
3 Mild - Conversation shows little initiative. Patient's answers tend to be brief and unembellished, requiring direct and leading questions by the interviewer.	☐
4 Moderate - Conversation lacks free flow and appears uneven or halting. Leading questions are frequently needed to elicit adequate responses and proceed with conversation.	☐
5 Moderate severe - Patient shows a marked lack of spontaneity and openness, replying to the interviewer's questions with only one or two brief sentences.	☐
6 Severe - Patient's responses are limited mainly to a few words or short phrases intended to avord or curtail communication (e g., "I don't know," "I'm not at libertv to say."). Conversation is seriously impaired as a result, and the interview is highly unproductive.	☐
7 Extreme - Verbal output is restricted to, at most, an occasional utterance, making conversation not possible.	☐

N7. Stereotyped thinking Decreased fluidity, spontaneity, and flexibility of thinking, as evidenced in rigid, repetitious, or barren thought content. Basis for rating: Cognitive–verbal processes observed during the interview.	
1 Absent - Definition does not apply.	☐
2 Minimal - Questionable pathology; may be at the upper extreme of normal limits.	☐
3 Mild - Some rigidity shown in attitudes or beliefs. Patient may refuse to consider alternative positions or have difficulty in shifting from one idea to another.	☐
4 Moderate - Conversation revolves around a recurrent theme, resulting in difficulty in shifting to a new topic.	☐
5 Moderate severe - Thinking is rigid and repetitious to the point that despite the interviewer's efforts conversation is limited to only two or three dominating topics.	☐
6 Severe - Uncontrolled repetition of demands, statements, ideas, or questions which severely impairs conversation.	☐
7 Extreme - Thinking, behavior, and conversation are dominated by constant repetition of fixed ideas or limited phrases, leading to gross rigidity, inappropriateness, and restrictiveness of patient's communication.	☐

GENERAL PSYCHOPATHOLOGY SCALE (G)

G1. Somatic concern Physical complaints or beliefs about bodily illness or malfunctions. This may range from a vague sense of ill-being to clear-cut delusions of catastrophic physical disease. Basis for rating: Thought content expressed in the interview.	
1 Absent - Definition does not apply.	☐
2 Minimal - Questionable pathology; may be at the upper extreme of normal limits.	☐
3 Mild - Distinctly concerned about health or somatic issues, as evidenced by occasional questions and desire for reassurance.	☐
4 Moderate - Complains about poor health or bodily malfunction, but there is no delusional conviction, and overconcern can be allayed by reassurance.	☐
5 Moderate severe - Patient expresses numerous or frequent complaints about physical illness or bodily malfunction, or else patient reveals one or two clearcut delusions involving these themes but is not preoccupied by them.	☐
6 Severe - Patient is preoccupied by one or a few clearcut delusions about physical disease or organic malfunction, but affect is not fully immersed in these themes, and thoughts can be diverted by the interviewer with some effort.	☐
7 Extreme - Numerous and frequently reported somatic delusions, or only a few somatic delusions of a catastrophic nature, which totally dominate the patient's affect and thinking.	☐

G2. Anxiety Subjective experience of nervousness, worry, apprehension, or restlessness, ranging from excessive concern about the present or future to feelings of panic. Basis for rating: Verbal report during the course of interview and corresponding physical manifestations.	
1 Absent - Definition does not apply.	☐
2 Minimal - Questionable pathology; may be at the upper extreme of normal limits.	☐
3 Mild - Expresses some worry, overconcern, or subjective restlessness, but no somatic and behavioral consequences are reported or evidenced.	☐
4 Moderate - Patient reports distinct symptoms of nervousness, which are reflected in mild physical manifestations such as fine hand tremor and excessive perspiration.	☐
5 Moderate severe - Patient reports serious problems of anxiety which have significant physical and behavioral consequences, such as marked tension, poor concentration, palpitations, or impaired sleep.	☐
6 Severe - Subjective state of almost constant fear associated with phobias, marked restlessness, or numerous somatic manifestations.	☐
7 Extreme - Patient's life is seriously disrupted by anxiety, which is present almost constantly and at times reaches panic proportions or is manifested in actual panic attacks.	☐

G3. Guilt feelings Sense of remorse or self-blame for real or imagined misdeeds in the past. Basis for rating: Verbal report of guilt feelings during the course of interview and the influence on attitudes and thoughts.	
1 Absent - Definition does not apply.	☐
2 Minimal - Questionable pathology; may be at the upper extreme of normal limits.	☐
3 Mild - Questioning elicits a vague sense of guilt or self-blame for a minor incident, but the patient clearly is not overly concerned.	☐
4 Moderate - Patient expresses distinct concern over his responsibility for a real incident in his life but is not preoccupied with it, and attitude and behaviour are essentially unaffected.	☐
5 Moderate severe - Patient expresses a strong sense of guilt associated with self-deprecation or the belief that he deserves punishment. The guilt feelings may have a delusional basis, may be volunteered spontaneously, may be a source of preoccupation and/or depressed mood, and cannot be allayed readily by the interviewer.	☐
6 Severe - Strong ideas of guilt take on a delusional quality and lead to an attitude of hopelessness or worthlessness. The patient believes he should receive harsh sanctions for the misdeeds and may even regard his current life situation as such punishment.	☐
7 Extreme - Patient's life is dominated by unshakable delusions of guilt, for which he feels deserving of drastic punishment, such as life imprisonment, torture, or death. There may be associated suicidal thoughts or attribution of others' problems to one's own past misdeeds.	☐

G4. Tension Overt physical manifestations of fear, anxiety, and agitation, such as stiffness, tremor, profuse sweating, and restlessness. Basis for rating: Verbal report attesting to anxiety and, thereupon, the severity of physical manifestations of tension observed during the interview.	
1 Absent - Definition does not apply.	☐
2 Minimal - Questionable pathology; may be at the upper extreme of normal limits.	☐
3 Mild - Posture and movements indicate slight apprehensiveness, such as minor rigidity, occasional restlessness, shifting of position, or fine rapid hand tremor.	☐
4 Moderate - A clearly nervous appearance emerges from various manifestations, such as fidgety behaviour, obvious hand tremor, excessive perspiration, or nervous mannerisms.	☐
5 Moderate severe - Pronounced tension is evidenced by numerous manifestations, such as nervous shaking, profuse sweating, and restlessness, but conduct in the interview is not significantly affected.	☐
6 Severe - Pronounced tension to the point that interpersonal interactions are disrupted. The patient for example, may be constantly fidgeting, unable to sit still for long, or show hyperventilation.	☐
7 Extreme - Marked tension is manifested by signs of panic or gross motor acceleration, such as rapid restless pacing and inability to remain seated for longer than a minute, which makes sustained conversation not possible.	☐

G5. Mannerisms and posturing Unnatural movements or posture as characterized by an awkward, stilted, disorganized, or bizarre appearance. Basis for rating: Observation of physical manifestations during the course of interview as well as reports from primary care workers or family.	
1 Absent - Definition does not apply.	☐
2 Minimal - Questionable pathology; may be at the upper extreme of normal limits.	☐
3 Mild - Slight awkardness in movements or minor rigidity of posture.	☐
4 Moderate - Movements are notably awkward or disjointed, or an unnatural posture is maintained for brief periods.	☐
5 Moderate severe - Occasional bizarre rituals or contorted posture are observed, or an abnormal position is sustained for extended periods.	☐
6 Severe - Frequent repetition of bizarre rituals, mannerisms, or stereotyped movements, or a contorted posture is sustained for extended periods..	☐
7 Extreme - Functioning is seriously impaired by virtually constant involvement in ritualistic, manneristic, or stereotyped movements or by an unnatural fixed posture which is sustained most of the time.	☐

G6. Depression Feelings of sadness, discouragement, helplessness, and pessimism. Basis for rating: Verbal report of depressed mood during the course of interview and its observed influence on attitude and behavior.	
1 Absent - Definition does not apply.	☐
2 Minimal - Questionable pathology; may be at the upper extreme of normal limits.	☐
3 Mild - Expresses some sadness or discouragement only on questioning. but there is no evidence of depression in general attitude or demeanor.	☐
4 Moderate - Distinct feelings of sadness or hopelessness, which may be spontaneously divulged, but depressed mood has no major impact on behavior or social functioning, and the patient usually can be cheered up.	☐
5 Moderate severe - Distinctly depressed mood is associated with obvious sadness, pessimism, loss of social interest, psychomotor retardation, and some interference in appetite and sleep. The patient cannot be easily cheered up.	☐
6 Severe - Markedly depressed mood is associated with sustained feelings of misery, occasional crying, hopelessness, and worthlessness. In addition, there is major interference in appetite and/or sleep as well as in normal motor and social functions, with possible signs of self-neglect.	☐
7 Extreme - Depressive feelings seriously interfere m most major functions. The manifestations include frequent crying, pronounced somatic symptoms, impaired concentration, psychomotor retardation, social disinterest, self-neglect, possible depressive or nihilistic delusions, and/or possible suicidal thoughts or action.	☐

G7. Motor retardation Reduction in motor activity as reflected in slowing or lessening of movements and speech, diminished responsiveness to stimuli, and reduced body tone. Basis for rating: Manifestations during the course of interview as well as reports by primary care workers or family.	
1 Absent - Definition does not apply.	☐
2 Minimal - Questionable pathology; may be at the upper extreme of normal limits.	☐
3 Mild - Slight but noticeable diminution in rate of movements and speech. Patient may be somewhat underproductive in conversation and gestures.	☐
4 Moderate - Patient is clearly slow in movements, and speech may be characterized by poor productivity, including long response latency, extended pauses, or slow pace.	☐
5 Moderate severe - A marked reduction in motor activity renders communication highly unproductive or delimits functioning in social and occupational situations. Patient can usually be found sitting or lying down.	☐
6 Severe - Movements are extremely slow, resulting in a minimum of activity and speech. Essentially the day is spent sitting idly or lying down.	☐
7 Extreme - Patient is almost completely immobile and virtually unresponsive to external stimuli.	☐

G8. Uncooperativeness Active refusal to comply with the will of significant others, including the interviewer, hospital staff, or family, which may be associated with distrust, defensiveness, stubbornness, negativism, rejection of authority, hostility, or belligerence. Basis for rating: Interpersonal behavior observed during the course of interview as well as reports by primary care workers or family.	
1 Absent - Definition does not apply.	☐
2 Minimal - Questionable pathology; may be at the upper extreme of normal limits.	☐
3 Mild - Complies with an attitude of resentment, impatience, or sarcasm. May inoffensively object to sensitive probing during the interview.	☐
4 Moderate - Occasional outright refusal to comply with normal social demands, such as making own bed, attending scheduled programs, etc. The patient may project a hostile, defensive, or negative attitude but usually can be worked with.	☐
5 Moderate severe - Patient frequently is incompliant with the demands of his milieu and may be characterized by others as an "outcast" or having "a serious attitude problem." Uncooperativeness is reflected in obvious defensiveness or irritability with the interviewer and possible unwillingness to address many questions.	☐
6 Severe - Patient is highly uncooperative, negativistic, and possibly also belligerent. Refuses to comply with most social demands and may be unwilling to initiate or conclude the full interview.	☐
7 Extreme - Active resistance seriously impacts on virtually all major areas of functioning. Patient may refuse to join in any social activities, tend to personal hygiene, converse with family or staff, and participate even briefly in an interview.	☐

G9. Unusual thought content Thinking characterized by strange, fantastic, or bizarre ideas, ranging from those which are remote or atypical to those which are distorted, illogical, and patently absurd. Basis for rating: Thought content expressed during the course of interview.	
1 Absent - Definition does not apply.	☐
2 Minimal - Questionable pathology; may be at the upper extreme of normal limits.	☐
3 Mild - Thought content is somewhat peculiar or idiosyncratic, or familiar ideas are framed in an odd context.	☐
4 Moderate - Ideas are frequently distorted and occasionally seem quite bizarre.	☐
5 Moderate severe - Patient expresses many strange and fantastic thoughts (e.g., being the adopted son of a king, being an escapee from death row) or some which are patently absurd (e.g., having hundreds of children, receiving radio messages from outer space through a tooth filling).	☐
6 Severe - Patient expresses many illogical or absurd ideas or some which have a distinctly bizarre quality (e.g., having three heads, being a visitor from another planet).	☐
7 Extreme - Thinking is replete with absurd, bizarre, and grotesque ideas.	☐

G10. Disorientation Lack of awareness of one's relationship to the milieu, including persons, place, and time, which may be due to confusion or withdrawal. Basis for rating: Responses to interview questions on orientation.	
1 Absent - Definition does not apply.	☐
2 Minimal - Questionable pathology; may be at the upper extreme of normal limits.	☐
3 Mild - General orientation is adequate but there is some difficulty with specifics. For example, patient knows his location but not the street address, knows hospital staff names but not their functions, knows the month but confuses the day of week with an adjacent day, or errs in the date by more than two days. There may be narrowing of interest evidenced by familiarity with the immediate but not extended milieu, such as ability to identify staff but not the Mayor, Governor, or President.	☐
4 Moderate - Only partial success in recognizing persons, places, and time. For example, patient knows he is in a hospital but not its name, knows the name of his city but not the burrough or district, knows the name of his primary therapist but not many other direct care workers, knows the year and season but not sure of the month.	☐
5 Moderate severe - Considerable failure in recognizing persons, place, and time. Patient has only a vague notion of where he is and seems unfamiliar with most people in his milieu. He may identify the year correctly or nearly so, but not know the current month, day of week, or even the season.	☐
6 Severe - Marked failure in recognizing persons, place, and time. For example, patient has no knowledge of his whereabouts, confuses the date by more than one year, can name only one or two individuals in his current life.	☐
7 Extreme - Patient appears completely disoriented with regard to persons, place, and time. There is gross confusion or total ignorance about one's location, the current year, and even the most familiar people, such as parents, spouse, friends, and primary therapist.	☐

G11. Poor attention Failure in focused alertness manifested by poor concentration, distractibility from internal and external stimuli, and difficulty in harnessing, sustaining, or shifting focus to new stimuli. Basis for rating: Manifestations during the course of interview.	
1 Absent - Definition does not apply.	☐
2 Minimal - Questionable pathology; may be at the upper extreme of normal limits.	☐
3 Mild - Limited concentration evidenced by occasional vulnerability, to distraction or faltering attention toward the end of the interview.	☐
4 Moderate - Conversation is affected by the tendency to be easily distracted, difficulty in long sustaining concentration on a given topic, or problems in shifting attention to new topics.	☐
5 Moderate severe - Conversation is seriously hampered by poor concentration, distractibility, and difficulty in shifting focus appropriately.	☐
6 Severe - Patient's attention can be harnessed for only brief moments or with great effort, due to marked distraction by internal or external stimuli.	☐
7 Extreme - Attention is so disrupted that even brief conversation is not possible.	☐

G12. Lack of judgment and insight Impaired awareness or understanding of one's own psychiatric condition and life situation. This is evidenced by failure to recognize past or present psychiatric illness or symptoms, denial of need for psychiatric hospitalization or treatment, decisions characterized by poor anticipation of consequences, and unrealistic short-term and long-range planning. Basis for rating: Thought content expressed during the interview.	
1 Absent - Definition does not apply.	☐
2 Minimal - Questionable pathology; may be at the upper extreme of normal limits.	☐
3 Mild - Recognizes having a psychiatric disorder but clearly underestimates its seriousness, the implications for treatment, or the importance of taking measures to avoid relapse. Future planning may be poorly conceived.	☐
4 Moderate - Patient shows only a vague or shallow recognition of illness. There may be fluctuations in acknowledgement of being ill or little awareness of major symptoms which are present, such as delusions, disorganized thinking, suspiciousness, and social withdrawal. The patient may rationalize the need for treatment in terms of its relieving lesser symptoms, such as anxiety, tension, and sleep difficulty.	☐
5 Moderate severe - Acknowledges past but not present psychiatric disorder. If challenged, the patient may concede the presence of some unrelated or insignificant symptoms, which tend to be explained away by gross misinterpretation or delusional thinking. The need for psychiatric treatment similarly goes unrecognized.	☐
6 Severe - Patient denies ever having had a psychiatric disorder. He disavows the presence of any psychiatric symptoms in the past or present and, though compliant, denies the need for treatment and hospitalization.	☐
7 Extreme - Emphatic denial of past and present psychiatric illness. Current hospitalization and treatment are given a delusional interpretation (e.g.. as punishment for misdeeds, as persecution by tormentors, etc.), and the patient may thus refuse to cooperate with therapists, medication, or other aspects of treatment.	☐

G13. Disturbance of volition Disturbance in the wilful initiation, sustenance, and control of one's thoughts, behavior, movements, and speech. Basis for rating: Thought content and behavior manifested in the course of interview.	
1 Absent - Definition does not apply.	☐
2 Minimal - Questionable pathology; may be at the upper extreme of normal limits.	☐
3 Mild - There is evidence of some indecisiveness in conversation and thinking, which may impede verbal and cognitive processes to a minor extent.	☐
4 Moderate - Patient is often ambivalent and shows clear difficulty in reaching decisions. Conversation may be marred by alternation in thinking, and in consequence verbal and cognitive functioning are clearly impaired.	☐
5 Moderate severe - Disturbance of volition interferes in thinking as well as behavior. Patient shows pronounced indecision that impedes the initiation and continuation of social and motor activities, which also may be evidenced in halting speech.	☐
6 Severe - Disturbance of volition interferes in the execution of simple, automatic motor functions, such as dressing and grooming, and markedly affects speech.	☐
7 Extreme - Almost complete failure of volition is manifested by gross inhibition of movement and speech, resulting in immobility and/or mutism.	☐

G14. Poor impulse control Disordered regulation and control of action on inner urges resulting in sudden, unmodulated, arbitrary, or misdirected discharge of tension and emotions without concern about consequences. Basis for rating: Behavior during the course of interview and reported by primary care workers or family.	
1 Absent - Definition does not apply.	☐
2 Minimal - Questionable pathology; may be at the upper extreme of normal limits.	☐
3 Mild - Patient tends to be easily angered and frustrated when facing stress or denied gratification but rarely acts on impulse.	☐
4 Moderate - Patient gets angered and verbally abusive with minimal provocation. May be occasionally threatening, destructive, or have one or two episodes involving physical confrontation or a minor brawl.	☐
5 Moderate severe - Patient exhibits repeated impulsive episodes involving verbal abuse, destruction of property, or physical threats. There may be one or two episodes involving serious assault, for which the patient requires isolation, physical restraint, or p.r.n. sedation.	☐
6 Severe - Patient frequently is impulsively aggressive, threatening, demanding, and destructive, without any apparent consideration of consequences. Shows assaultive behavior and may also be sexually offensive and possibly respond behaviorally to hallucinatory commands.	☐
7 Extreme - Patient exhibits homicidal attacks, sexual assaults, repeated brutality, or self-destructive behavior. Requires constant direct supervision or external constraints because of inability to control dangerous impulses.	☐

G15. Preoccupation Absorption with internally generated thoughts and feelings and with autistic experiences to the detriment of reality orientation and adaptive behavior. Basis for rating: Interpersonai behavior observed during the course of interview.	
1 Absent - Definition does not apply.	☐
2 Minimal - Questionable pathology; may be at the upper extreme of normal limits.	☐
3 Mild - Excessive involvement with personal needs or problems, such that conversation veers back to egocentric themes and there is diminished concern exhibited toward others.	☐
4 Moderate - Patient occasionally appears self-absorbed, as if daydreaming or involved with internal experiences, which interferes with communication to minor extent.	☐
5 Moderate severe - Patient often appears to be engaged in autistic experiences, as evidenced by behaviors that significantly intrude on social and communicational functions, such as the presence of a vacant stare, muttering or talking to oneself, or involvement with stereotyped motor patterns.	☐
6 Severe - Marked preoccupation with autistic experiences, which seriously delimits concentration, ability to converse, and orientation to the milieu. The patient frequently may be observed smiling, laughing, muttering, talking, or shouting to himself.	☐
7 Extreme - Gross absorption with autistic experiences, which profoundly affects all major realms of behavior. The patient constantly may be responding verbally and behaviorally to hallucinations and show little awareness of other people or the external milieu.	☐

POSITIVE AND NEGATIVE SYNDROME SCALE (PANSS)

G16. Active social avoidance Diminished social involvement associated with unwarranted fear, hostility, or distrust. Basis for rating: Reports of social functioning by primary care workers or family.	
1 Absent - Definition does not apply.	☐
2 Minimal - Questionable pathology; may be at the upper extreme of normal limits.	☐
3 Mild - Patient seems ill at ease in the presence of others and prefers to spend time alone, although he participates in social functions when required.	☐
4 Moderate - Patient begrudgingly attends all or most social activities but may need to be persuaded or may terminate prematurely on account of anxiety, suspiciousness, or hostility.	☐
5 Moderate severe - Patient fearfully or angrily keeps away from many social interactions despite others' efforts to engage him. Tends to spend unstructured time alone.	☐
6 Severe - Patient participates in very few social activities because of fear, hostility, or distrust. When approached, the patient shows a strong tendency to break off interactions, and generally he tends to isolate himself from others.	☐
7 Extreme - Patient cannot be engaged in social activities because of pronounced fears, hostility, or persecutory delusions. To the extent possible, he avoids all interactions and remains isolated from others.	☐

ACKNOWLEDGEMENTS

This work was supported by NIH Award MH077225. We thank Ashley Cain for her assistance in preparing this manuscript.

References

Adams, T. (1997). Mental health care for elderly people. In I. J. Norman, & S. J. Redfern (Eds.), *Dementia* (pp. 183–201). New York, NY: Churchill Livingstone.

APA. (2000). *Diagnositc and statistical manual of mental disorders*. Washington, DC: American Psychiatric Association.

Auslander, L. A., & Jeste, D. V. (2004). Sustained remission of schizophrenia among community-dwelling older outpatients. *Am J Psychiatry*, *161*, 1490–1493.

Brown, G. W., Monck, E. M., Carstairs, G. M., & Wing, J. K. (1962). Influence of family life on the course of schizophrenic illness. *Br J Prev Soc Med*, *16*, 55–68.

Brown, S., Barraclough, B., & Inskip, H. (2000). Causes of the excess mortality of schizophrenia. *Br J Psychiatry*, *177*, 212–217.

Butzloff, R. L., & Hooley, J. M. (1998). Expressed emotion and psychiatric relapse: A meta-analysis. *Arch Gen Psychiatry*, *55*, 547–552.

Cervantes, A. N., Rabins, P. V., & Slavney, P. R. (2006). Onset of schizophrenia at age 100. *Psychosomatics*, *47*, 356–359.

Cohen, C. (2003). *Schizophrenia Into Later Life: Treatment, Research, and Policy*. Washington, DC: American Psychiatric Publishing.

Copeland, J. R. M., Dewey, M. E., Scott, A., Gilmore, C., Larkin, B. A., Cleave, N., et al. (1998). Schizophrenia and delusional disorder in older age: Community prevalence, incidence, comorbidity, and outcome. *Schizophr Bull*, *24*, 153–161.

Craddock, N., & Owen, M. J. (2005). The beginning of the end for the Kraepelinian dichotomy. *Br J Psychiatry*, *186*, 364–366.

Depp, C. A., & Jeste, D. V. (2004). Bipolar disorder in older adults: a critical review. *Bipolar Disorders*, *6*, 343–367.

Diwan, S., Cohen, C. I., Bankole, A. O., Vahia, I., Kehn, M., & Ramirez, P. M. (2007). Depression in older adults with schizophrenia spectrum disorders: prevalence and associated factors. *Am J Geriatr Psychiatry*, *15*, 991–998.

Dolder, C. R., Lacro, J. P., Warren, K. A., Golshan, S., Perkins, D. O., & Jeste, D. V. (2004). Brief evaluation of medication influences and beliefs: development and testing of a brief scale for medication adherence. *J Clinical Psychopharmacology*, *24*, 404–409.

Folsom, D. P., McCahill, M., Bartels, S. J., Lindamer, L. A., Ganiats, T. G., & Jeste, D. V. (2002). Medical comorbidity and receipt of medical care by older homeless people with schizophrenia or depression. *Psychiatr Serv*, *53*, 1456–1460.

Green, M. F., & Nuechterlein, K. H. (2004). The MATRICS initiative: developing a consensus cognitive battery for clinical trials. *Schizophr Research*, *72*, 1.

Harris, M. J., & Jeste, D. V. (1988). Late-onset schizophrenia: An overview. *Schizophr Bull*, *14*, 39–55.

Harvey, P. D., Davidson, M., Mueser, K. T., Parrella, M., White, L., & Powchik, P. (1997). Social-Adaptive Functioning Evaluation (SAFE): A rating scale for geriatric psychiatric patients. *Schizophr Bull*, *23*, 131–145.

Harvey, P. D., Silverman, J. M., Mohs, R. C., Parrella, M., White, L., & Powchik, P. (1999). Cognitive decline in late-life schizophrenia: a longitudinal study of geriatric chronically hospitalized patients. *Biological Psychiatry*, *45*, 32.

Heaton, R. K., Gladsjo, J. A., Palmer, B. W., Kuck, J., Marcotte, T. D., & Jeste, D. V. (2001). Stability and course of neuropsychological deficits in schizophrenia. *Arch Gen Psychiatry*, *58*, 24–32.

Henderson, A. S., Korten, A. E., Levings, C., Jorm, A. F., Christensen, H., Jacomb, P., et al. (1998). Psychotic symptoms in the elderly: a prospective study in a population sample. *International J Geriatr Psychiatry*, *13*, 484–492.

Howard, R., Rabins, P. V., Seeman, M. V., & Jeste, D. V. (2000). Late-onset schizophrenia and very-late-onset schizophrenia-like psychosis: An international consensus. *Am J Psychiatry*, *157*, 172–178.

Jeste, D. V., & Finkel, S. (2000). Psychosis of Alzheimer's disease and related dementias. Diagnostic criteria for a distinct syndrome. *Am J Geriatr Psychiatry*, *8*, 29–34.

Jeste, D. V., Meeks, T. W., Kim, D. S., & Zubenko, G. S. (2006). Research agenda for DSM-V: Diagnostic categories and criteria for neuropsychiatric syndromes in dementia. *J Geriatr Psychiatry Neurol*, *19*, 160–171.

Jeste, D. V., Harris, M. J., Krull, A., Kuck, J., McAdams, L. A., & Heaton, R. (1995). Clinical and neuropsychological characteristics of patients with late-onset schizophrenia. *Am J Psychiatry*, *152*, 722–730.

Jeste, D. V., Twamley, E. W., Zorrilla, L. T. E., Golshan, S., Patterson, T. L., & Palmer, B. W. (2003). Aging and outcome in schizophrenia. *Acta Psychiatrica Scandinavica*, *107*, 336–343.

Jeste, D. V., Alexopoulos, G. S., Bartels, S. J., Cummings, J. L., Gallo, J. J., Gottlieb, G. L., et al. (1999). Consensus statement on the upcoming crisis in geriatric mental health: Research agenda for the next 2 decades. *Arch Gen Psychiatry*, *56*, 848–853.

Jobe, T., & Harrow, M. (2005). Long-term outcomes of patients with schizophrenia: A review. *Canadian J Psychiatry*, *50*, 892–900.

Jones, S. M., Vahia, I. V., Cohen, C. I., Hindi, A., & Nurhussein, M. (2009). A pilot study to assess attitudes, behaviors, and inter-office communication by psychiatrists and primary care providers in the care of older adults with schizophrenia. *International J Geriatr Psychiatry*, *24*, 254–260.

Kang, S. J., Choi, S. H., Lee, B. H., Jeong, Y., Hahm, D. S., Han, I. W., et al. (2004). Caregiver-Administered Neuropsychiatric Inventory (CGA-NPI). *J Geriatr Psychiatry Neurol*, *17*, 32–35.

Kay, S. R., Fiszbein, A., & Opler, L. A. (1987). The Positive and Negative Syndrome Scale (PANSS) for schizophrenia. *Schizophr Bull*, *13*, 261–276.

Keller, J., Flores, B., Gomez, R. G., Solvason, H. B., Kenna, H., & Williams, G. H. (2006). Cortisol circadian rhythm alterations in psychotic major depression. *Biological Psychiatry*, *60*, 275.

Kraeplelin, E. (1919). *Dementia Praecox and Paraphrenia*. New York, NY: Robert E Krieger.

Lacro, J., Dunn, L., Dolder, C., Leckband, S., & Jeste, D. (2002). Prevalence of and risk factors for medication nonadherence in patients with schizophrenia: a comprehensive review of recent literature. *J Clin Psychiatry*, *63*, 892–909.

Lane, R., Glazer, W., Hansen, T., Berman, W., & Kramer, S. (1985). Assessment of tardive dyskinesia using the abnormal involuntary movement scale. *J Nervous Mental Disease*, *173*, 353.

Marder, S. R., Essock, S. M., Miller, A. L., Buchanan, R. W., Casey, D. E., Davis, J. M., et al. (2004). Physical health monitoring of patients with schizophrenia. *Am J Psychiatry*, *161*, 1334–1349.

Mattis, S. (1988). *Dementia Rating Scale. Professional Manual*. Odessa, FL: Psychological Assessment Resources.

Meyers, B. (1995). Late-life delusional depression: Acute and long-term treatment. *International Psychogeriatrics*, *7*, 113–124.

Minsky, S., Vega, W., Miskimen, T., Gara, M., & Escobar, J. (2003). Diagnostic patterns in Latino, African American, and European American psychiatric patients. *Arch Gen Psychiatry*, *60*, 637–644.

Mizrahi, R., Starkstein, S. E., Jorge, R., & Robinson, R. G. (2006). Phenomenology and clinical correlates of delusions in Alzheimer disease. *Am J Geriatric Psychiatry*, *14*, 573–581.

Molinari, V., Chiriboga, D., Branch, L., Cho, S., Turner, K., Guo, J., et al. (2010). Provision of psychopharmalogical services in nursing homes. *J Gerotology: Psychological sciences and Social Sciences, 65* (1). 57–60.

Newcomer, J. (2007). Metabolic considerations in the use of antipsychotic medications: a review of recent evidence. *J CLin Psychiatry*, *68*, 20–27.

Ostling, S., & Skoog, I. (2002). Psychotic symptoms and paranoid ideation in a nondemented population-based sample of the very old. *Arch Gen Psychiatry*, *59*, 53–59.

Ostling, S., Borjesson-Hanson, A., & Skoog, I. (2007). Psychotic symptoms and paranoid ideation in a population-based sample of 95-year-olds. *Am J Geriatric Psych*, *15*, 999–1004, 10.1097/JGP.0b013e31814622b9

Overall, J. (1962). The brief psychiatric rating scale. *Psychological Reports*, *10*, 799–812.

Palmer, B. W., McClure, F., & Jeste, D. V. (2001). Schizophrenia in late life: findings challenge traditional concepts. *Harvard Review of Psychiatry*, *9*, 51–58.

Patterson, T. L., Goldman, S., McKibbin, C. L., Hughs, T., & Jeste, D. V. (2001). UCSD performance-based skills assessment: Development of a new measure of everyday functioning for severely mentally ill adults. *Schizophr Bull*, *27*, 235–245.

Patterson, T. L., Lacro, J., McKibbin, C. L., Moscona, S., Hughs, T., & Jeste, D. V. (2002). Medication management ability assessment: Results from a performance-based measure in older outpatients with schizophrenia. *J Clinical Psychopharmacology*, *22*, 11–19.

Paulson, J. S., Salmon, D. P., Thal, L. J., Romero, R., Weisstien-Jenkins, C., Galasko, D., et al. (2000). Incidence of and risk factors for hallucinations and delusions in patients with probable AD. *Neurology*, *23; 54*(10), 1965–1971.

Randolph, C. C., Tierney, M. M. C., Mohr, E. E., & Chase, T. T. N. (1998). The Repeatable Battery for the Assessment of Neuropsychological Status (RBANS): Preliminary clinical validity. *J Clinical & Experimental Neuropsychology*, *20*, 310.

Reisberg, B., Borestein, J., Salob, S., Ferris, S., Franssen, E., & Georgotas, A. (1987). Behavioral symptoms in Alzheimer's disease: Phenomenology and treatment. *J Clin Psychiatry*, *48*(5 suppl), 9–15.

Richards, C. F., & Gurr, D. E. (2000). Psychosis. *Emergency Medicine Clinics of North America*, *18*, 253.

Robins, L., Helzer, J., Weissman, M., Orvaschel, H., Gruenberg, E., Burke, J., et al. (1984). Lifetime prevalence of specific psychiatric disorders in three sites. *Arch Gen Psychiatry*, *5*, 949–958.

Ropacki, S. A., & Jeste, D. V. (2005). Epidemiology of and risk factors for psychosis of Alzheimer's disease: A review of 55 studies published from 1990 to 2003. *Am J Psychiatry, 162*, 2022–2030.

Schneider, L. S., Tariot, P. N., Dagerman, K. S., Davis, S. M., Hsiao, J. K., Ismail, M. S., et al. (2006). Effectiveness of atypical antipsychotic drugs in patients with Alzheimer's disease. *N Engl J Med, 355*, 1525–1538.

Sheehan, D., Lecrubier, Y., Sheehan, K., Amorim, P., Janavs, J., & Weiller, E. (1998). The Mini-International Neuropsychiatric Interview (M.I.N.I.): the development and validation of a structured diagnostic psychiatric interview for DSM-IV and ICD-10. *J Clin Psychiatry, 59*, 22–33.

Spitzer, R. L., Gibbon, M., & Williams, J. B. (1995). *Structured Clinical Interview for Axis I DSM-IVDisorders (SCID).* Washington, DC: American Psychiatric Association.

Stein, L., & Thienhaus, O. (1993). Hearing impairment and psychosis. *International Psychogeriatrics, 5*, 49–56.

Tariot, P. N., Mack, J. L., Patterson, M. B., Edland, S. D., Weiner, M. F., Fillenbaum, G., et al. (1995). The behavior rating Scale for Dementia of the Consortium to Establish a Registry for Alzheimer's Disease. The Behavioral Pathology Committee of the Consortium to Establish a Registry for Alzheimer's Disease. *Am J Psychiatry, 152*, 1349–1357.

Vahia, I., Bankole, A. O., Reyes, P., Diwan, S., Palekar, N., Sapra, M., et al. (2007). Schizophrenia in later life. *Aging Health, 3*, 383–396.

Vahia, I., Diwan, S., Bankole, A. O., Kehn, M., Nurhussein, M., Ramirez, P., et al. (2008). Adequacy of medical treatment among older persons with schizophrenia. *Psychiatr Serv, 59*, 853–859.

Vega, W., & Lopez, S. (2001). Priority issues in Latino mental health services research. *Mental Health Services Research, 3*, 189–200.

Wallace, C. J., Liberman, R. P., Tauber, R., & Wallace, J. (2000). The independent living skills survey: A comprehensive measure of the community functioning of severely and persistently mentally ill individuals. *Schizophr Bull, 26*, 631–658.

Werner, P. (2003). Psychosis in Parkinson's disease. *Movement Disorders, 18*, 80–87.

Woerner, M. G., Alvir, J. M. J., Saltz, B. L., Lieberman, J. A., & Kane, J. M. (1998). Prospective study of tardive dyskinesia in the elderly: Rates and risk factors. *Am J Psychiatry, 155*, 1521–1528.

CHAPTER

6 Dementia Syndromes in the Older Adult

Carol A. Manning, Jamie K. Ducharme
University of Virginia Health System, Department of Neurology, Charlottesville, VA, USA

The prevalence of age-related dementias will increase dramatically as the number of elderly individuals surges in the coming decades. Currently 5.3 million individuals in the United States are diagnosed with Alzheimer's disease, the most common dementia, and it is predicted that 7.7 million people in the United States will be afflicted with the disease by 2030. The societal and individual burden of caring for these individuals is already a major issue for which we as a nation are unprepared, both financially and in terms of professionals trained in caring for people with dementia.

This chapter will define dementia, describe the most important cognitive domains in neuropsychological assessment, and review and define the most common dementias. Next, assessment measures, current treatments, and, finally, the role of follow-up assessment in geriatric neuropsychology will be discussed. The goal of the chapter is to familiarize psychologists and other mental health professionals with the diagnostic criteria for the most common dementias and with the associated patterns of cognitive and behavioral decline.

DEMENTIA

The term "dementia" describes a constellation of symptoms, not an underlying disease process or etiology. As such, it is an umbrella term that indicates a decline in cognitive functioning relative to previous higher levels of functioning. The most commonly used criteria for dementia come from the DSM-IV-TR, which defines dementia as a decline in memory and a decline in at least one additional area of cognition including aphasia, apraxia, agnosia, or a decline in executive functioning. The term "dementia" is not associated with a particular etiology, prognosis, or treatment, making accurate diagnosis of the type of dementia important, especially in light of our increasing knowledge of specific dementias and as our treatment armamentarium grows.

DESCRIPTION OF COGNITIVE DOMAINS

Neuropsychological assessment is anchored in the assumption that cognition can be both measured and broken down into separate but interconnected parts. These cognitive domains are neuroanatomically connected. As such, deficits in one area of cognitive functioning (e.g., language) implicate an area of brain dysfunction associated with that function (e.g., left temporal lobe). Furthermore, certain patterns of cognitive dysfunction are commonly associated with specific

Handbook of Assessment in Clinical Gerontology. DOI: 10.1016/B978-0-12-374961-1.10006-5

neurological disorders, which helps inform etiology. Initially, descriptors of cognitive functioning were modeled after computer operations including input, storage, processing, and output of information. More current and pragmatic practice uses descriptors of general thinking abilities such as memory, language, attention, praxis, psychomotor processing speed, and executive functioning.

Memory

Many theories have been set forth breaking down the component parts of memory functioning. However, the dual system classification model is perhaps the most aligned with direct observation of behavior, as it defines declarative and procedural memory. Each system is distinct in that it involves independent neural systems. Therefore, dysfunction of one system does not necessarily result in deficit in the other. Declarative memory is highly associated with the hippocampal formation. Dysfunction in this area of the brain is often associated with Alzheimer's disease. Procedural memory involves the dorsolateral prefronto-striatal loop. Therefore, illnesses associated with basal ganglia and prefrontal cortex impairment (e.g., Parkinson's disease) often result in procedural memory deficits.

Declarative or explicit memory involves the conscious awareness and intentional recollection of events, dates, objects, facts, and general engagement in life. This type of memory loss is what patients are most sensitive to and complain of when concerned about dementia. Although there is no shortage of theories available, a three-stage model of declarative memory processing is most distinguishable in the clinical setting. This process involves encoding, storage, and retrieval of material. Disruption to any part of this process results in memory dysfunction; therefore, it is important to clearly identify the true area of weakness. Memory recall is the ability to access stored information when needed. Free recall of information is the unaided recall of information whereas recognition recall involves prompting or cueing of the stored information (e.g., multiple-choice).

Short- and long-term memory recall is also a common descriptor. Recent memory refers to recall of events or information that occurs within minutes up to a few weeks of encoding. Long-term or remote memory refers to events which occurred many years ago, often in childhood or early adulthood. Procedural or implicit memory, the other component of the dual memory system, involves "how to" recall. Conscious awareness is not necessary in procedural recall; examples include walking, dressing, and riding a bicycle. These well-ingrained habits are often retained until the very late stages of dementia.

Language

Expression, reception, and repetition abilities all work to comprise language functioning. Aphasia, meaning "no speech," occurs in response to impairment to certain language areas of the brain. Broca's (expression) and Wernicke's (comprehension) areas are considered to be the main language centers. Damage to either of these structures, or to the connections relaying communication between them, results in language disruption. Neuropsychological evaluation of language functioning assesses verbal capacities such as object naming, word and sentence repetition, verbal comprehension, and speeded word generation to help inform etiology. Additionally, language deficits can serve to mask underlying memory difficulties; therefore, a thorough language evaluation is necessary to tease out deficiencies and their overlap.

Praxis

Praxis involves purposeful expressive functions or coordinated movements. Therefore, apraxia (literally meaning "no work") results in impairment of learned voluntary acts despite capable muscles and sensorimotor coordination pathways. Apraxic disorders usually result from disrupted connections between domain centers in the brain. For example, ideomotor apraxia is commonly associated with lesions disrupting the connection between the speech centers of the brain. This results in an inability to perform skilled tasks on command although the knowledge of the desired action is retained (e.g., pretending to brush hair). Ideational apraxia involves parietal lobe dysfunction resulting in the loss of the understanding of the action itself. Constructional disorders are also sometimes classified as apraxias, but not in the strictest sense of the concept. Constructional disturbances involve compromise of building, drawing, assembling, and space perception abilities.

Motor Speed/Psychomotor Processing

Motor functioning abilities are critical to one's success in everyday capacities. From fine motor skills such as hand-eye coordination and finger dexterity to gross motor requirements such as balance and ambulation, motor functioning is a vital component of daily functioning. The presence of motor disturbance is especially useful in informing etiology and disease stage. Reductions in psychomotor processing speed are often described as mental slowing. One's ability to process information quickly is a salient component of cognitive processing and a common patient complaint relative to a wide range of activities, ranging from driving skills to following a conversation. Psychomotor processing speed is sensitive to age and IQ.

Attention

Attention is variable depending on a number of factors such as novelty, complexity, age, and IQ. Attention is also assumed to have a limited capacity. Thus, only so much processing activity can take place at any given time or speed of intake. Indeed, it is difficult to process information from two sources at once, especially when the information is presented in a rapid fashion. Attention is often described in numerous ways including simple, divided, and sustained attention. Simple immediate attention span is often assessed by asking a person to immediately repeat information (e.g., numbers), and is usually resistant to the effects of aging or illness. Divided attention is more sensitive and involves attending to numerous sensory inputs at once. Sustained attention involves maintaining attention control over a period of time. Attention is especially sensitive to psychiatric, sleep, and pain disturbance.

Executive Functioning

Executive functioning skills are uniquely human capabilities aimed at successful completion of independent, purposive, self-serving behavior (Lezak, Howieson, & Loring, 2004). Executive functioning capacities are somewhat poorly defined and cover a broad range of higher order human behavior. These are often conceptualized into four parts including: (1) volition; (2) planning; (3) purposive action; and (4) effective performance (Lezak et al., 2004). Examples include abilities of abstraction, problem solving, multitasking, planning, conceptualization, sequencing, and responding appropriately to feedback. This includes the ability to effectively respond to social cues and inhibit inappropriate behaviors. Executive functioning skills are closely aligned with self-control, self-direction, and self-care capacities relative to activities of daily living. Reduced executive functioning abilities are associated with frontal lobe dysfunction involving the prefrontal cortex and limbic system. The classic tale of Phineas Gage is an example of the strong association between personality and executive functioning ability.

TYPES OF DEMENTING DISORDERS

Mild Cognitive Impairment

Mrs S is a 73-year-old female with a twelfth grade education who has been an efficient homemaker for 50 years. Within the last year, she has felt that her memory is "slipping." She feels that she is more dependent on her calendar to remember appointments, has a harder time recalling recent events and has difficulty recalling names. She continues to perform all of her usual activities around the house including cooking, cleaning, and paying the bills although she double-checks herself to be sure that she is accurate. She drives without difficulty with the exception of one instance four weeks ago when she became briefly disoriented in a familiar place. She recovered "within minutes" and this has not occurred again since then.

Mild cognitive impairment (MCI) is a relatively new diagnostic term which describes subjective and objective memory decline that is greater than expected given the individual's age and education level, but is insufficient to meet criteria for dementia. The most commonly used criteria for amnestic MCI, defined by Petersen (2000) and Petersen et al., (2001), include complaints of memory decline by the individual which are corroborated by an informant and substantiated by evidence of decline. Relatively intact activities of daily living, mild or no difficulties in non-memory aspects of cognition, and not meeting criteria for dementia are also features of amnestic MCI. Of note: while simple activities of daily living are unchanged, complex or instrumental activities of daily living such as balancing a check book may demonstrate subtle decline (Griffith et al., 2003; Marson et al., 2009). These changes in instrumental activities of daily living may be overlooked given that these individuals are relatively high functioning and the changes are subtle. Non-amnestic MCI refers to relatively intact memory but decline in another area of cognition. Multi-domain MCI indicates decline in more than one area of cognition but of insufficient magnitude to meet criteria for dementia. Pure amnestic MCI may be relatively rare, with multi-domain subtypes occurring more frequently (Lonie, Tierney, & Ebmeier, 2009). Although the definition of MCI does not specifically exclude long-standing cognitive decline due to conditions such as a seizure disorder or brain trauma, MCI representing newly developed cognitive decline has become more commonly accepted (Werner & Korcyzn, 2008).

MCI is of particular interest as a transitional state to dementia. Individuals with dementia are more likely to "convert" to dementia than age-matched healthy controls, with annual conversion rates from MCI to Alzheimer's disease ranging from 2–25% per year (Bowen et al., 1997; Petersen et al., 2001). While MCI has been called early Alzheimer's disease (AD), not all individuals with MCI convert to AD or another dementia. Accurate identification of those who do would present the opportunity to begin early treatment, particularly when disease-modifying treatments become available. Candidate markers for detecting high probability of conversion from MCI to AD include hippocampal volume, hippocampal atrophy, brain amyloid load as assessed via Pittsburgh Compund B (C-PIB), concomitant anxiety and depression, and executive decline (Devanand et al., 2007; Okello et al., 2009). A combination of cognitive tests (Symbol Digit Modalities, Delayed 10 Word List Recall, New York University Paragraph Recall and the Alzheimer's Disease Assessment Cognitive Subscale) have been found to best predict conversion to AD after 36 months (Fleisher et al., 2007).

There is no generally accepted cognitive measure or standard for the diagnosis of MCI. However, a commonly used cut point of decline is 1.5 standard deviations below the mean on a standardized neuropsychological test. A recent meta-analysis of 15 screening measures for detection of MCI determined that none of the screening measures had adequate sensitivity and specificity for accurate diagnosis (Lonie et al., 2009). The authors conclude that, at best, screening measures indicate the need for a referral to specialized services. Treatment options are complicated by the limited ability to predict who will convert to dementia. Although the efficacy of cholinesterase inhibitors which are used in Alzheimer's patients in MCI are equivocal, they appear to be widely used (Weinstein, Barton, Ross, Kramer, & Yaffe, 2009). The potential for identifying early dementia and targeting disease-modifying drugs at early stages make increased interest in MCI likely.

Alzheimer's Disease

Mrs P is a 79-year-old woman who lived with her husband until his death one year ago. Since that time, her children have noticed that she is having difficulty caring for herself, including choosing appropriate clothing. For example, she recently wore winter clothing on a hot summer day. In addition, she wore the same outfit on four consecutive days despite stains. Her children were surprised by this as previously she was fastidious in her appearance. They also noted that her home seems messy and disorganized. Her children have noticed her increasing confusion and difficulty preparing familiar recipes, which is especially disconcerting because she was an accomplished cook. On several occasions she seems to have forgotten conversations with her children regarding upcoming plans and neglected to meet her daughter for lunch despite having discussed it the previous evening. Of note: she denies having difficulty. Initially her children believed that her difficulties were grief but over time they find her difficulties worsening rather than lessening. Upon reflection, her children recall that their father started taking over household responsibilities as long as three years ago. They assumed that it was to share in household responsibilities but they now feel that he was compensating for changes in her.

This vignette demonstrates several typical features of Alzheimer's disease (AD) including memory loss, a decline in the ability to perform over-learned activities such as cooking familiar recipes, and a decline in activities of daily living such as personal care. Alzheimer's disease is associated with an insidious decline and it is not unusual for a family member, such as this woman's husband, to take over responsibilities to compensate. Frequently the decline is not noticed until a critical event occurs, such as her husband's death. It is only in retrospect, often with significant questioning from the health care professional, that the insidious decline is revealed.

Diagnostic criteria for AD include memory loss, which is the hallmark of the disease. In addition to memory loss, cognitive decline in at least one other area of cognition is required for a clinical diagnosis. This can include aphasia, deficits in executive functioning, apraxia, or agnosia (difficulty recognizing objects despite intact sensory abilities). The dementia cannot be due to another illness or condition.

Patients with AD experience rapid forgetfulness, exhibiting an inability to encode and store information. Recognition of previously seen material is poor and typically no better than recall (Welsh et al., 1996). Alzheimer's patients frequently inaccurately identify words as being on a recently seen word list both in recall (intrusions) and on recognition trials (false positives). Individuals with AD might have limited awareness of their memory deficits and might confabulate or respond inaccurately when faced with questions that they cannot answer (Tallberg & Almkvist, 2001). Newer memories appear to be affected first and older memories are affected over time as the disease progresses. Orientation to time and place, which requires recent memory, becomes faulty at early stages of the disease and worsens over time. Eventually recognition of familiar people such as children or spouses becomes impaired in later stages of the disease. Ideomotor apraxias such as problems with bathing, dressing, and using eating utensils emerge as the disease progresses.

Deficits in executive functioning are not prominent features early in the disease. However, when they do occur, they are associated with a marked decline in functional capacity (Boyle et al., 2003; Griffith et al., 2003). Language difficulties in AD often include word finding difficulty, in particular problems retrieving nouns and names of people. It is important to take into account that difficulty recalling names is among the most common complaints of healthy aging and by itself is not a sign of AD. AD patients have more difficulty naming by category, e.g., animals or furniture, than by letter (semantic fluency). It is hypothesized that category fluency is more impaired because it requires access to temporal lobe memory stores which are disrupted by the disease process in AD (Vliet et al., 2003).

Behavioral disturbances accompanying AD can include depression, apathy, and anxiety. The degree of depression varies by disease stage and has been found in up to 50% of AD patients

(Lykestos et al., 1997). Depression in early stages of disease may be associated with awareness of memory loss. As the disease progresses, apathy becomes more prominent.

About two-thirds of individuals with dementia over age 64 have Alzheimer's disease, making it the most commonly occurring dementia (Geldmacher, 2003). Alzheimer's disease occurs more frequently in women than in men, even taking into account the longer lifespan of women. Age remains the biggest risk factor for Alzheimer's disease with prevalance rates as high as 50% among individuals 85 years of age and older. Although several genes for Alzheimer's disease have been identified, they account for only 14% of Alzheimer's disease and they are associated with a younger age of onset. Three new genes (CRU, Picalm, and CR1) were recently identified and they hold promise as significant risk factors for the disease (Harold et al., 2009). Possession of an APOE E4 allele is a significant genetic risk factor, but it is important to note that not all people possessing an E4 allele develop Alzheimer's disease. Other risk factors for AD include a family history of AD, head injury within the last five years, and depression. High educational achievement appears to be a protective factor and is associated with a later age of onset of AD. Other protective factors include physical exercise and a Mediterranean diet. Amyloid plaques and neurofibrillary tangles are the pathological hallmarks of the disease. As such, diagnostic certainty occurs at autopsy or through biopsy, although recent imaging developments assessing amyloid load via C-PIB provide increased certainty *in vivo*.

Vascular Dementia

Mr W is a 69-year-old man with high blood pressure and high cholesterol. Despite his doctor's warnings, he has smoked for 30 years. He has had several "events" in which he has became confused, and on one such occasion he momentarily lost sensation in his right arm. After each "event" he seems to clear from the confusion but his family notices that he never quite goes back to baseline and he continues to have problems with maintaining his concentration and completing tasks. His doctor has diagnosed him with "transient ischemic attacks."

Vascular dementia (VaD) is associated with cerebrovascular disease and is the second most common dementia after AD (O'Brien et al., 2003). The presentation of VaD can vary based on the cause and location of cerebral damage. Significant risk factors for VaD are the same risk factors for stroke and include high blood pressure, high cholesterol, coronary heart disease, peripheral artery disease, diabetes, and smoking. In contrast to AD, the onset of VaD is often sudden and plateaus until another cerebral event occurs, at which time additional cognitive deficits appear. However, not all cognitive decline can be associated with a sudden vascular event. Neurological deficits are more likely to be present than in AD and neuroimaging may reveal areas of infarction or white matter disease.

Relative to AD, memory is more likely to be spared in VaD with better recall and recognition in the latter group (Traykov et al., 2002). Recognition memory is often normal and using recognition cues can significantly aid people with VaD. The most common area of cognitive deficit in VaD is executive functioning. The deficits in executive functioning are related to impaired fronto-subcortical functioning and the result is difficulties with problem solving, focused attention, and speed of processing information. These deficits have been found to negatively impact independent functioning (Cannata, Alberoni, Franceschi, & Mariani, 2002). While semantic aspects of language can be normal, verbal fluency is often impaired (Huff, 1990). Individuals with VaD have been found to have visuospatial deficits, including reading the hands on a clock (Schmidtke & Hull, 2002).

Behavioral changes and psychiatric symptoms are frequently a prominent feature of VaD. Levels of apathy are high and more common in VaD than in AD (Hargrave, Geck, Reed, & Mungas, 2000). The high frequency of apathy is consistent with fronto-subcortical damage found in VaD. Apathy is more highly associated with declines in the ability to perform activities of daily living than the overall level of dementia (Ahron-Peretz, Kliot, & Tomer, 2000; Zawacki et al., 2002). Recently, anxiety was found to be higher in VaD than in AD. Anxiety is associated with decreased quality of life and behavioral difficulties, and occurs with less frequency at later stages of disease (Seignourel, Kunik, Snow, Wilson, & Stanley, 2008). Depression is also a significant problem in VaD and occurs more frequently than in AD (Newman, 1999; Park et al., 2007). Depression in VaD is typically more severe with more vegetative symptoms than in AD (Park et al., 2007).

Fronto-Temporal Dementia

Mr G is a 52-year-old man who worked as a pharmacist until he was let go three months ago due to a series of errors in filling prescriptions. Although his manager states that he was told about each error, Mr G never told his wife that the mistakes occurred. Furthermore he denied any difficulties at work and seemed unconcerned. His wife was shocked because previously he had been a very careful person who took tremendous pride in his work. His wife has noted that he has been less active at home and more likely to sit in his favorite chair for long periods of time. In addition, she described him as "emotionless" seeming to care less about the well-being of her and their children.

The three fronto-temporal dementias subtypes are progressive nonfluent aphasia, semantic dementia, and fronto-temporal dementia (FTD). All three subtypes typically have an earlier age of onset than AD and are associated with fronto-temporal lobar degeneration. In addition, personality or behavioral changes are prominent and are generally noticed prior to cognitive changes. Individuals with FTD are typically distinguishable from AD in terms of a younger age of onset and different cognitive and behavioral difficulties, especially early in the disease (Moretti, Torre, Antonello, & Cazzato, 2001). In the FTD subtype, early behavioral changes are prominent and include loss of social graces especially tactlessness, changes in personal hygiene, emotional blunting, apathy, and disinhibition (Boone, Miller, Swartz, Lu, & Lee, 2003; Snowden et al., 2003). In particular, loss of sympathy and empathy for others and overeating are problematic in FTD (Caycedo, Miller, Kramer, & Rascovsky, 2009). Furthermore, apathy is more frequent in FTD than in AD (Chow et al., 2009). Family members rather than patients are typically more concerned with the changes. Psychiatric disturbance rather than dementia is often suspected initially in FTD in light of the young age of onset and the marked personality changes. Cognitively, deficits in executive functioning are seen early in the disease. Poor attention, concentration and abstract reasoning are early features while memory is relatively intact. Unlike the other FTD variants, language is relatively preserved in the FTD form.

The progressive nonfluent aphasia variant presents with individuals having difficulty with smooth and fluid word production. Stuttering, impaired repetition, and writing difficulties are common. Word production by category is initially better than naming words by letter. Individuals with progressive nonfluent aphasia have increasingly sparer speech, with eventual mutism. Unlike the FTD variant, they have relatively intact social skills at early stages of the disease (Nestor & Hodges, 2000).

In semantic dementia, patients have fluent speech but the speech is often meaningless or devoid of understandable content. In this variant, the patients are unaware of their speech defect and may become frustrated by the other people's inability to understand them. These patients typically have intact comprehension and little awareness of their deficits. Individuals with semantic dementia often have preserved math abilities and a preoccupation with money.

Dementia with Lewy Bodies

Mr L is 72-years-old and six months ago began to be intermittently confused. His wife reports that he seems "perfectly clear" on some days and very confused other days. He also reports that small neighborhood children have come to visit him at night in his room. His wife says that he misperceives his clothes hanging on hooks as the neighborhood children. In the last few months, his walking has become less stable and he has nearly fallen on several occasions.

The criteria for dementia with Lewy bodies (DLB) include fluctuations in cognitive impairment, visual hallucinations, and Parkinsonism. The fluctuations in cognition can occur multiple times within a day or last several days. Caregivers report fluctuations ranging from "normal" cognition to extreme confusion. Although the definition for fluctuating cognition has been difficult to operationalize, it is believed to occur in half to two-thirds of DLB patients. The visual hallucinations are typically non-threatening and are often misperceptions of objects in the room, e.g., a towel hanging on a door knob is seen as a child or small animal. Parkinsonism is seen at disease onset in one-quarter to one-half of DLB patients but cannot occur more than one year prior to cognitive changes. Supportive diagnostic features of DLB include repeated falls, REM behavior sleep disorder, hallucinations in other modalities, and depression. Individuals with DLB do not respond well to antipsychotic medications and are likely to experience extrapyramidal side effects. They do respond well to the cholinesterase inhibitors typically prescribed to AD patients.

Depression is often an early symptom in DLB. Cognitively, individuals with DLB have executive dysfunction early in the disease along with visuospatial and attentional problems. The visuoperceptual disturbances are worse in individuals who have frequent hallucinations (Simard, van Reekum, & Myran, 2003). Cognitive dysfunction becomes more widespread as the disease progresses, and the percentage of time with confusion increases while periods of clarity decrease. Neuropathologically, DLB is associated with widespread cortical Lewy bodies. The cognitive profile of DLB is consistent with fronto-striatal disruption secondary to the depletion of the neurotransmitter dopamine. DLB is the most common dementia associated with a movement disorder. The pathology of DLB and AD can co-occur within individuals. The clinical presentation of mixed DLB-AD appear to be features of both dementias including visual hallucinations, executive dysfunction, and prominent memory deficits.

Parkinson's Dementia

Mr S is a 75-year-old man who has had Parkinson's disease for nine years. Initially he had a tremor on his right side with slowed movements and postural instability. He has had depression for the last several years. More recently, he has had increasing confusion and limited ability to solve simple problems. His thought processes are very slow and he appears to get "stuck" on an idea, with limited ability to come up with alternate solutions.

Parkinson's disease (PD) is traditionally thought of as a movement disorder with few cognitive sequelae. An increasing amount of research indicates that cognitive changes occur in PD, especially in older people. Diagnostic criteria for Parkinson's disease dementia (PDD) include PD with an insidious onset and dementia with a progressive decline. Cognitive impairment must occur in at least two areas and must impair daily functioning. Risk factors for PDD are old age and more severe Parkinsonism (Emre et al., 2007). The onset of dementia is insidious and mild cognitive impairment at diagnosis of PD is considered a risk factor for subsequent dementia. Prevalence rates of PDD vary and the onset of dementia is around 10 years after diagnosis, but this may reflect a diagnostic bias because individuals with dementia occurring around the time of appearance of Parkinsonism are likely to be diagnosed with DLB. Diagnostic criteria stipulate that the diagnosis of DLB is given if the onset of dementia and Parkinsonism occur within a year of each other. DLB and PDD differ by the time-course of the onset of symptoms and the neuropathological distribution of Lewy bodies.

The cognitive changes associated with PD include executive and attentional difficulties. Executive functioning is more impaired in PDD than in AD. In general, attention is impaired in PDD and it appears to fluctuate. Memory is impaired in PDD but less so than in AD. Furthermore, memory retrieval is relatively less affected than is memory recall. Visuospatial construction and perception decline more in PDD than in AD. Language abilities are largely unaffected. Overall, the cognitive deficits found in PDD are similar to those in DLB.

Visual hallucinations are a common problem in PDD and they occur more frequently in PDD and DLB than in AD. Hallucinations in non-demented PD patients are a bad prognostic factor for the onset of dementia. Depression is common in PDD and occurs more frequently than in AD, although dysphoric mood is reported equally by both groups (Emre et al., 2007). Anxiety is frequently comorbid with depression in PDD. Unlike in AD agitation, irritability and anger are not common in PDD. Apathy is a problem in PDD and it appears to increase with dementia severity. Rates of apathy do not differentiate PDD from other dementias. Overall, the behavioral difficulties in PDD are similar to DLB, but behavioral disturbance in DLB is often more severe.

Normal Pressure Hydrocephalus

Mrs L is an 81-year-woman who has had increasing difficulty walking. Her husband complains that she moves more and more slowly and that she loses her balance. In addition, she feels the need to urinate without warning and has had several episodes of incontinence. She is frequently confused, forgets important information, and has trouble concentrating.

Normal pressure hydrocephalus (NPH) presents with a characteristic triad that includes gait disturbance, urinary incontinence, and dementia. The gait disturbance is typically a slow wide-based gait. Step height is frequently diminished. Gait disturbance is typically the first symptom recognized. Urinary incontinence is a frequent urge to urinate that can be aggravated by the slowed gait which prevents the individual from reaching the bathroom rapidly.

Table 6.1 Defining Features of Common Dementias

Type of Dementia	Onset	Primary Cognitive Changes	Behavioral/Psychiatric Changes
MCI	Mild	Do not meet criteria for dementia	Anxiety and depression increase risk of conversion
AD	Insidious, progressive	Memory and at least one other cognitive domain	Depression, apathy, anxiety, agitation in later stages
VaD	Sudden, stepwise	Executive functioning (problem solving, attention, processing speed)	Apathy, depression, anxiety
FTD	Progressive	Executive functioning (attention, abstract reasoning); language depending on subtype	Prominent changes—emotional blunting, loss of social graces, apathy Lack of awareness of deficits
DLB	Progressive cognitive changes within one year of motor changes	Fluctuations in cognition, executive functioning	Visual hallucinations, depression
PDD	Progressive. Motor changes before cognitive	Executive functioning (attention); visuospatial abilities	Depression, anxiety, apathy
NPH	Progressive. Triad of gait disturbance, incontinence, and cognitive changes	Memory, speed of processing	Behavioral features not prominent

Approximately 77% of individuals with NPH experience dementia. The dementia is "subcortical" with prominent memory impairment and slowed speed of processing. Unlike AD, language disturbance and apraxia are rare. Neuroimaging reveals enlarged cerebral ventricles. Evidence for improvement in cognition following shunting is equivocal; however, patients with better verbal memory prior to shunting may be more likely to experience improved cognition following shunting (Thomas et al., 2005).

Other Causes of Dementia

There are multiple causes of dementia that are often overlooked, many of which can be treated. Depression can be the cause of cognitive decline rather than a symptom of a neurodegenerative disease. Even when depression occurs as part of a dementia syndrome, it can cause excess cognitive decline if left untreated. Polypharmacy is a significant problem in the elderly person and can cause confusion and a dementia-like picture. All too frequently prescription medications come from multiple practitioners who are unaware of other medications being taken. Furthermore, over-the-counter drugs and supplements interact with prescribed medications and can contribute to confusion. Hypothyroidism, vitamin deficiencies, and metabolic disturbances can cause cognitive decline. Sleep apnea and other sleep disturbances are associated with cognitive deficits. All of these conditions are more frequent in older people and are more likely to be accompanied by cognitive changes. Ruling out and treating conditions which disturb the more precarious homeostasis in older adults is the first step before diagnosing a neurodegenerative dementia. It is important to treat what is treatable in order to understand the underlying cognitive picture.

STANDARD USES AND GOALS OF ASSESSMENT

Clinical neuropsychology is the study of brain—behavior relationships. This discipline seeks to understand the neural foundations of behavior, often as it relates to a disease process when assessing the older adult. An awareness of both neurological and psychological functioning is required in order to conduct a robust assessment of an individual's cognitive and emotional status and their interplay. Clinical neuropsychology is applied in many fields, often in neurology, psychiatric, or educational settings. The neuropsychological assessment of older adults in outpatient settings has many purposes. The evaluation is often conducted in response to a referral question in pursuit of diagnostic and treatment planning input. Other purposes of neuropsychological evaluation involve research or forensic examination, which will not be covered here (see Horton & Hartlage, 2003; McCaffrey, Williams, Fisher, & Laing, 2004).

A detailed clinical interview, review of medical records, and evaluation of cognitive test performance results in a thorough neuropsychological evaluation aimed at clearly responding to a referral question. Information gleaned from a collateral source is especially critical when assessing possible dementia patients who lack insight into their deficits. Detail regarding the onset, course, and nature of the patient's deficits helps inform diagnosis, treatment, and prognosis. In addition to querying about cognitive capacities (i.e., memory functioning), a detailed report of the patient's independence in activities of daily living is tantamount. Is the patient getting lost while driving on familiar routes? Are they leaving the stove on without awareness when cooking? Are they having problems with financial management, paying bills on time, etc.? A careful review of medical records is also required to help inform differential diagnoses and provide additional data points (e.g., brain imaging). Finally, testing is conducted and the patient's performance is analyzed in comparison to age-related normative data.

Baseline intellectual functioning estimates must also be considered. Given the length and time required to fully assess IQ, abbreviated measures which are resilient to neurocognitive decline are often employed to establish a baseline expected to be consistent with educational level and employment history. This can prove difficult in multicultural contexts given numerous language and cultural barriers. Visual recognition IQ tasks are often utilized so that a verbal component is not required; however, it is possible that the patient has little experience within a test-taking environment, detracting from their cultural understanding of what is required of them. Further, educational and occupational attainment in different cultures may be unequivocal relative to socioeconomic norms. Where available, the use of normative data specific to an individual's racial or cultural identity should be used. For example, standardized normative data have been established for Spanish-speaking individuals through the Spanish normative studies project (NEURONORMA) (see Pena-Casanova et al., 2009).

A comprehensive neuropsychological report should provide a detailed account of the patient's cognitive strengths and weaknesses. Taken together, this should elucidate a clear picture of how the patient responds to cognitive deficits while providing insight into possible compensation strategies and/or rehabilitation. Even when the site and extent of brain lesion is known through imaging, the functional capacities of the patient cannot be fully anticipated without assessment of neuropsychological status. Lastly, but most importantly, detailed feedback of test findings and recommendations should always be provided directly to the patient and caregiver by the neuropsychologist. Results should be described in a non-jargoned, easily digestible fashion that translates test findings into ecologically-valid information for the patient relative to their life experience. Ultimately, the ideal neuropsychological evaluation should clearly contextualize an individual's cognitive and psychological capacities to inform diagnosis, treatment, and recommendations while promoting hope, resilience, and support. Repeat testing over time is also useful to help assess interval change, inform treatment, and provide new recommendations, especially in the setting of a neurodegenerative and progressive disease course.

Dementia Assessment Scales

Cognitive rating scales were created out of the need for at-the-ready bedside exams with an emphasis on pragmatism and simplicity (McDowell, 2006). Brief screening measures have become especially useful in geriatric assessment in which timely evaluations are necessary in the setting of fatigue. Most rating scales have been created with specific populations (e.g., traumatic brain injury, depression) or diagnostic questions (e.g., dementia screening) in mind, resulting in a narrow scope. Numerous criticisms are cited such as the lack of sensitivity to the early or later stages of a disease process and the lack of accountability for cultural factors being given little cross-validation study. Yet, these measures have wide-reaching uses in clinical, research, and forensic settings whether for diagnostic screening, determination of the need for more in-depth assessment, or treatment planning/disposition purposes. More specifically, rating scales are used for purposes of rating disease severity or stage of disease after a diagnosis has been rendered. Rating scales often incorporate collateral source input and behavioral observation to obtain a more robust understanding of the patient's capabilities and level of severity. Cognitive measures, however, focus more upon assessment of the patient's performance on standardized cognitive tasks to help inform diagnosis.

Rating Scales

Clinical Dementia Rating Scale (CDR)

The Washington University Clinical Dementia Rating scale (CDR; Morris, 1993; see Table 6.2) is a structured, clinician-rated interview that collects information on cognitive capacity from both the collateral source and patient for the evaluation of staging severity of dementia. The CDR was developed primarily to assess severity level in persons with dementia but it can be used to stage dementia in other illnesses as well (e.g., Parkinson's disease). Six domains are assessed and then synthesized to assign

Table 6.2 The Clinical Dementia Rating Scale

	None 0	Questionable 0.5	Mild 1	Moderate 2	Severe
Memory	No memory loss or slight; inconsistent forgetfulness	Consistent slight forgetfulness; partial recollection of events; "benign" forgetfulness	Moderate memory loss: more marked for recent events; defect interferes with everyday activity	Severe memory loss, only highly learned material retained: new material rapidly lost	Severe memory loss, only fragments remain
Orientation	Fully oriented	Fully oriented but with slight difficulty with time relationships	Moderate difficulty with time relationships; oriented for place at examination; may have geographic disorientation elsewhere	Severe difficulty with time relationships; usually disoriented to time, often to place	Oriented to person only
Judgment and problem solving	Solves everyday problems and handles business and financial affairs well; judgment good in relation to past performance	Slight impairment in solving problems, similarities and differences	Moderate difficulty in handling problems, similarities and differences; social judgment usually maintained	Severely impaired in handling problems, similarities and differences; social judgment usually impaired	Unable to make judgments or solve problems
Community affairs	Independent function as usual in job, shopping, volunteer, and social groups	Slight impairment in these activities	Unable to function independently at these activities though may still be engaged in some; appears normal to casual inspection	No pretense of independent function outside the home; appears well enough to be taken to functions outside the family home	Appears too ill to be taken to functions outside the family home
Home and hobbies	Life at home, hobbies and intellectual interests well maintained	Life at home, hobbies and intellectual interests slightly impaired	Mild but definite impairment of functions at home; more difficult chores, and complicated hobbies and interests abandoned	Only simple chores preserved; very restricted interests, poorly maintained	No significant function in the home
Personal care	Fully capable of self-care		Needs prompting	Requires assistance in dressing, hygiene and keeping of personal effects	Requires much help with personal care; frequent incontinence

Morris, J.C. (1993). The Clinical Dementia Rating (CDR): current version and scoring rules. Neurology, *43, 2412–2414.*

a Global CDR score. The domains are memory, orientation, judgment and problem solving, community affairs, home and hobbies, and personal care. Impairment is defined only when caused by cognitive loss rather than by physical disability or other non-cognitive factors. Severity ratings range along a 5-point scale (except for the personal care domain):

CDR-0: no cognitive impairment
CDR-0.5: questionable or very mild dementia
CDR-1: mild
CDR-2: moderate
CDR-3: severe

The CDR is frequently utilized in clinical and research settings to describe stage-dependent features of dementia and for use as a clinically-meaningful outcome measure in clinical drug trials. The CDR has been standardized for multicenter use including the Consortium to Establish a Registry for Alzheimer's Disease (CERAD) and the Alzheimer's Disease Cooperative Study. Inter-rater reliability scales have been established at 83% and CDR criterion validity has been found to correlate well with other neuropsychological measures (Morris, 1993). Limitations of the CDR include its length of administration and reliance on collateral source information and clinical judgment. The latter issues have multicultural implications in settings where the primary language and culture of the clinician and informant are dissimilar. The influence of cultural factors must be considered when assessing the informant's estimate of premorbid abilities and certain subjective CDR test items (e.g., home and hobbies, judgment and problem solving). Translations of the CDR have been shown valid and reliable in a number of cultures such as in Asian populations (Lim, Chong, & Sahadevan, 2007).

Cognitive Measures of Dementia

Mini-Mental Status Examination (MMSE)

The Mini-Mental Status Examination (Folstein, Folstein, & McHugh, 1975) is considered the most widely used brief screening measure for dementia. It has been translated into numerous languages and is often used to assess cognitive abilities in epidemiological studies and screen for dementia drug trial participation. Administration takes 5—10 minutes and the following domains are evaluated: concentration or working memory; language and praxis; orientation; memory; and attention span. A total of 30 points is possible and a score below 24 was identified in the original validation MMSE study for identifying cognitive impairment.

A frequently referenced strength of the MMSE is in its psychometric properties. Test—retest reliability is high even with different examiners (Folstein et al., 1975). Yet, the MMSE is often regarded as having good specificity but limited sensitivity. Given its common use as a screening measure, this is problematic. Therefore, the MMSE is limited in its ability to distinguish between mildly demented patients and healthy subjects, but it is effective in identifying moderate to severe dementia. The MMSE total score also does not differentiate among the varying types of dementias, although patterns of performance on certain items are confirmed. For example, Alzheimer's patients perform worse on orientation and word recall compared with Parkinson's patients who perform more poorly on construction.

There are multicultural limitations to consider when using the MMSE. Age and education are shown to impact MMSE scores. Therefore, normative data have been collected to account for age and education stratifications (see Bravo & Hebert, 1997). Furthermore, ethnicity affects MMSE performance. For example, false positive rates are significantly higher in African American and Hispanic American samples compared with European Americans (Espino, Lichtenstein, Palmer, & Hazuda, 2001). Some have recommended lower cutoff levels for certain populations. Bohnstedt, Fox, and

Kohatsu (1994) suggest a cutoff score as low as 19 for identifying cognitive impairment in African Americans. The MMSE is also often criticized for its inadequate assessment of frontal executive functioning capacities. Indeed, skills requiring problem solving, sustained attention, and psychomotor processing speed are not evaluated with the MMSE.

MINI MENTAL STATUS EXAMINATION	NAME: MRN:	DATE: (Or Place Patient Label Here)

EXAMINER:				**SCORE**	
1.	What is the:	Year?		**0**	**1**
		Season?		**0**	**1**
		Month?		**0**	**1**
		Day?		**0**	**1**
		Date?		**0**	**1**
2.	Where are we:	Country?		**0**	**1**
		State		**0**	**1**
		City?		**0**	**1**
		Hospital?		**0**	**1**
		Unit or Floor?		**0**	**1**
3.	I am going to name 3 items. (One second each.) Repeat them please. Give one point for each correct answer. After this repeat the words until the patient can repeat all 3 (stop if unable to learn them after 6 attempts).	**APPLE**		**0**	**1**
		PENNY		**0**	**1**
		TABLE		**0**	**1**
4.	Do serial 7's and the backwards spelling of the 5-letter word "World." The final score is the higher score of the two tests.	**93**	**D**	**0**	**1**
		86	**L**	**0**	**1**
		79	**R**	**0**	**1**
		72	**O**	**0**	**1**
		65	**W**	**0**	**1**
5.	Ask the patient to repeat the words from question 3. Give one point for each correct answer.	**APPLE**		**0**	**1**
		PENNY		**0**	**1**
		TABLE		**0**	**1**
6.	Point at an ink pen and a watch. The patient must name them.	**PEN**		**0**	**1**
		WATCH		**0**	**1**
7.	Repeat after me. "No ifs, ands or buts."			**0**	**1**
8.	Listen carefully because I am going to ask you to do something. The patient must perform a 3-stage task:	"Take this piece of paper with your right hand."		**0**	**1**
		"Fold it in half with both hands."		**0**	**1**
		"Place it on the floor."		**0**	**1**
9.	The patient must read the following sentence and execute the instruction so that you can see that s/he understands it: "CLOSE YOUR EYES."			**0**	**1**
10.	The patient must write a sentence of his/her own. (It must make sense. Spelling mistakes can be ignored.)			**0**	**1**
11.	The patient must copy the diagram below. (Give one point if the corners and sides are drawn correctly and if the sides cross in the shape of a diamond.)			**0**	**1**
TOTAL:				**/ 30**	

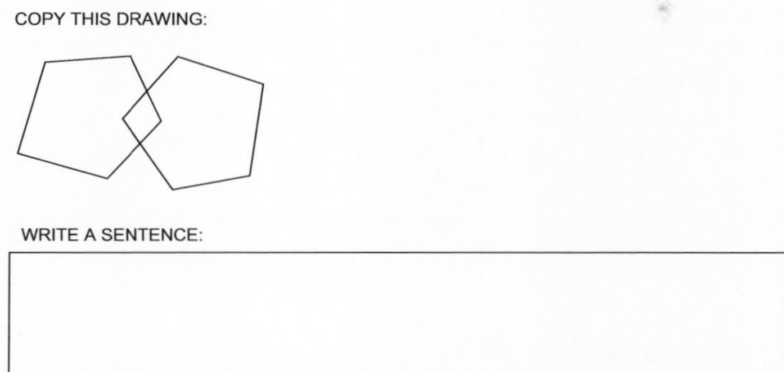

CLOSE YOUR EYES
COPY THIS DRAWING:
WRITE A SENTENCE:

Mattis Dementia Rating Scale (DRS)

The Mattis Dementia Rating Scale (DRS; Mattis, 1976) is a widely used dementia screening measure which examines five areas commonly associated with behavioral change in Alzheimer's disease. These areas include: attention; initiation and perseveration; construction; abstract conceptualization; and memory. A total score is then generated. Administration takes between 20–45 minutes depending upon the level of impairment. Similar to the MMSE, the DRS is negatively correlated with age and education, resulting in the need for comparison to age- and education-stratified normative data. A cutoff score of 123 out of 144 is used to flag possible impairment as it is two standard deviations below the mean of an original sample of 85 healthy adults. This has been further validated in subsequent studies (see Mattis, 1988).

The total DRS score is broadly used to stage severity of dementia while the pattern of subscale performance can inform etiology. Frontal executive functioning is better assessed by the DRS than MMSE. As such, the DRS better identifies frontally-mediated dementias. The construct validity of the attention, conceptualization, and memory subscales has been shown to correlate well with Wechsler scale indices. However, the construction subscale has been found to correlate more strongly with the attention subscale of the DRS than with other measures of visuoconstruction. This is a limiting factor of the DRS and supplementary assessment is advised. The DRS has strong prognostic value, shown to accurately predict rehabilitative outcome and length of survival in Alzheimer's subjects.

Alzheimer's Disease Assessment Scale (ADAS)

The Alzheimer's Disease Assessment Scale (ADAS; Rosen, Mohs, & Davis, 1984) is made up of two parts: cognitive and non-cognitive testing. The ADAS-Cog is more frequently utilized and will be the focus for this discussion. The ADAS-Cog is one of two primary cognitive outcome measures required in all current Food and Drug Administration (FDA) clinical drug trials for Alzheimer's disease in the United States.

The ADAS-Cog consists of items from the following areas chosen for their sensitivity to Alzheimer's disease: language; memory; praxis; and orientation. The test takes 30–35 minutes to administer and the item scores generally range from 1–5. The total ADAS-Cog score ranges from

0–70 with higher scores suggesting greater impairment. In its current form, the ADAS-Cog has been shown successful in not only identifying Alzheimer's patients from healthy elderly controls, but it has also shown to be effective in rating severity between moderate and late stage dementia based on decreasing performance on the orientation items.

Critics charge that the test is less effective in rating severity in MCI and mild dementia cases although it does a better job than the MMSE (Lezak et al., 2004). The addition of word learning with a delayed recall component has been recommended to increase the ADAS-Cog's ability to identify more mild forms of dementia. Inter-rater reliability coefficients are high for the ADAS-Cog (0.82–0.91) following increased standardization of test administration and examiner training. Test–retest reliability is also excellent, reported at 0.91 over a six-week period (Talwalker, Overall, Srirama, & Gracon, 1996). Similar to all cognitive measures reviewed in this chapter, ADAS-Cog outcome scores are shown to negatively correlate with age and education.

Non-Cognitive Measures of Dementia

Neuropsychiatric Inventory (NPI)

The Neuropsychiatric Inventory (NPI; Cummings, et al., 1994) was developed to assess for common behaviors associated with dementia. A structured interview of the caregiver is used to assess 10 behavior domains including delusions, hallucinations, dysphoria, euphoria, anxiety, agitation/aggression, apathy, irritability/lability, disinhibition, and aberrant motor behavior. Sleep and appetite/eating disorder subscales were added in 1997. Screening questions are asked regarding behaviors which have occurred over the past month. If an affirmative response is given, more detailed information is acquired pertaining to the frequency on a 4-point scale and severity on a 3-point scale of the behavior. There is also a useful 6-point caregiver distress scale. Validity scales are high for this measure including inter-rater reliability, internal consistency, and test–retest reliability. Furthermore, all behavior problems have been shown higher in Alzheimer's patients compared with age-matched controls and Parkinson's patients (Mega, Cummings, Fiorello, & Gornbein, 1996). Apathy was found to be the highest indicator of dementia followed by agitation. A self-administered NPI (NPI-Q) has also been created which takes no more than 5 minutes for the caregiver to complete and is highly correlated with the NPI.

Informant ratings

Disability Assessment for Dementia Scale (DAD)

The Disability Assessment for Dementia Scale (DAD; Gelinas, Gauthier, & McIntyre, 1999) was designed to assess functional capacity in a dementia population. The caregiver is asked yes/no questions regarding the patient's independence in the initiation and completion of daily living tasks over the past two weeks. Domains include hygiene, dressing, continence, eating, meal preparation, telephoning, going on an outing, finance/correspondence, medications, and leisure/housework. A total score of all affirmative responses is tallied. The DAD has strong reliability of test–retest, intra-class correlation (0.96), and internal consistency (0.96). Convergent validity has been established well with the Global Deterioration Scale (Gelinas, Gauthier, & McIntyre, 1999). As with other scales involving informant rating, cultural contexts play a role. Aberrant behavior in one culture may not translate to another. Therefore, the main focus is on assessing behavior change from the patient's baseline.

DISABILITY ASSESSMENT FOR DEMENTIA (DAD)

Administration Guidelines

Interview the **caregiver** to measure the actual performance of the patient over the previous 2 weeks. The activities must be performed by the patient without any assistance or reminder. Therefore, to ensure the caregiver answers each question correctly begin with:

"During the past 2 weeks, did the patient, without help or reminder, . . . "

Scoring
- Yes = performed activity in last 2 weeks if only once
- No = did not perform activity or performed with some assistance or reminder
- N/A = individual never previously performed this item or did not have the opportunity to do it in the past 2 weeks. Therefore, it is not relevant.

	Hygiene	**Yes**	**No**	**N/A**
Initiation	Undertake to wash himself/herself or to take a bath or shower			
	Undertake to brush his/her teeth or care for his/her dentures			
	Decide to care for his/her hair (wash and comb)			
Planning and Organization	Prepare the water, towels, and soap for washing, taking a bath or shower			
Effective Performance	Wash and dry completely all parts of his/her body safely			
	Brush his/her teeth or care for his/her dentures appropriately			
	Care for his/her hair (wash and comb)			

	Dressing	**Yes**	**No**	**N/A**
Initiation	Undertake to dress himself/herself			
Planning and Organization	Choose appropriate clothing (with regard to the occasion, neatness, the weather and the color combination)			
	Dress himself/herself in appropriate order (undergarments, trousers/dress, shoes)			
Effective Performance	Dress himself/herself completely			
	Undress himself/herself completely			

	Continence	**Yes**	**No**	**N/A**
Initiation	Decide to use the toilet at appropriate times			
Effective Performance	Use the toilet without "accidents"			

	Eating	**Yes**	**No**	**N/A**
Initiation	Decide that he/she needs to eat			
Planning and Organization	Choose appropriate cutlery and seasonings when eating			
Effective Performance	Eat his/her meals at normal pace and with appropriate manners			

DISABILITY ASSESSMENT FOR DEMENTIA (DAD) (continued)

	Meal Preparation	Yes	No	N/A
Initiation	Undertake to prepare a light meal or snack for himself/herself			
Planning and Organization	Adequately plan a light meal or snack (lingredients, cookware)			
Effective Performance	Prepare or cook a light meal or snack safely			

	Telephoning	Yes	No	N/A
Initiation	Undertake to telephone someone at a suitable time			
Planning and Organization	Find and dial a telephone number correctly			
Effective Performance	Carry out an appropriate telephone conversation			
	Write and convey telephone messages adequately			

	Going on an Outing	Yes	No	N/A
Initiation	Undertake to go out (walk, visit, shop) at an appropriate time			
Planning and Organization	Adequately organize an outing with respect to transportation, keys, destination, weather, necessary money, shopping list			
Effective Performance	Go out and reach a familiar destination without getting lost			
	Safely take the adequate mode of transport (car, bus, taxi)			
	Return from the shops with the appropriate items			

	Finance and Correspondence	Yes	No	N/A
Initiation	Shows an interest in his/her personal affairs such as his/her finances and written correspondence			
Planning and Organization	Organize his/her finance to pay his/her bills (checks, statement, bills)			
	Adequately organize his/her correspondence with respect ro stationery, address, stamps			
Effective Performance	Adequately handle his/her money (make change)			

	Medications	Yes	No	N/A
Initiation	Decide to take his/her medications at the correct time			
Effective Performance	Take his/her medications as prescribed (according to right dosage)			

	Leisure and Housework	Yes	No	N/A
Initiation	Show an interest in liesure activity(ies)			
	Take an interest in the household chores that he/she used to perform in the past			
Planning and Organization	Adequately plan and organize household chores that he/she used to perform in the past			
Effective Performance	Complete household chores adequately as he/she used to perform in the past			
	Stay safely at home himself/herself when needed			

TREATMENT

As addressed earlier, it is important to first rule out and/or treat all possible reversible causes of cognitive disruption such as vitamin deficiency (e.g., B12), thyroid dysfunction, infection (e.g., urinary tract infection, encephalitis), medication effects, dehydration, sleep deprivation, and depression. These factors can fully account for cognitive decline or exacerbate underlying dementia symptoms.

Pharmacological Treatments

Cholinergic medications have been utilized as first line pharmacotherapy for mild to moderate dementia since 1997. Although the efficacy of these medications is well established in research, there is no cure for the progressive loss of function in cognition and daily functioning that is associated with cell death in AD. Current medications on the market serve to treat the symptomatic expression of AD by maximizing neuronal function resulting in a delay in decline. Studies show that treatment with cholinergic medication compared with placebo produces improvements in cognition, activities of daily living, and behavior for three to six months of treatment (Birks, 2006). The desired outcome is the prolonged period at or above the cognitive level at which treatment begins, with anticipated decline from a higher (due to intervention) baseline. Early intervention is critical, ideally initiated at the earliest signs of disease onset (e.g., mild cognitive impairment). A rapid return to pre-treatment baseline has been demonstrated when treatment is stopped. Therefore, long-term use is recommended.

Medications and Efficacy

Cholinesterase inhibitor medications (ChEI) work by blocking acetylcholinesterase, the enzyme responsible for the destruction of acetylcholine. Reduced levels of the neurotransmitter, acetylcholine, are believed to explain extensive cell loss in the basal nuclei of the forebrain found in AD. These medications have also been shown effective in the treatment of VaD and PDD, but less so in the treatment of other forms of dementia, such as FTD. Common cholinergic medications include donepezil (Aricept®), galantamine (Razadyne®; formerly known as Reminyl®), and Rivastigmine (Exelon®).

Memantine HCL (Namenda®) is the only medication approved by the FDA for the treatment of moderate to severe AD. It is not a cholinesterase inhibitor and monotherapy with memantine is not approved in mild to moderate dementia. Memantine functions as a N-methyl-D-aspartate (NMDA)-receptor antagonist. Glutamate-mediated neurotoxicity is thought to be associated with cell death and reduced neuroplasticity in AD. Studies have shown improvement in cognition, daily functioning, and behavioral outcome.

Other Agents

Non-steroidal anti-inflammatory drugs (NSAIDs) are theorized to help treat AD by reducing inflammation of cyclo-oxygenase pathways; however, studies are far from conclusive (Breitner et al., 2009). Another area of investigation has studied the impact of free radicals thought to damage neuronal membranes. There is inconclusive evidence of the efficacy of high-dose vitamin E and selegiline in delaying loss of daily functioning. To date, there is limited research to suggest that other therapies such as estrogen hormone replacement, ginkgo biloba, and nerve growth factor result in positive treatment outcome, nor are any approved by the FDA for use in AD treatment.

Behavioral Strategies

Behavioral symptoms usually occur gradually and in the later stages of AD. However, depression and anxiety are common and can present relatively early. Both pharmacologic and non-pharmacologic treatment has been shown effective in behavioral management. It is important to identify and quantify the problematic behavior in order to help facilitate treatment. Psychotropic agents such as antidepressants, anxiolytics, antipsychotics, and benzodiazapines are commonly used to treat specific symptoms. Behavioral strategies have also been shown to be effective. Sleep disruption and weight loss are commonly associated with dementia. Therefore, improvement of sleep hygiene and nutrition can drastically benefit behavior. Maintenance of a regular routine is also critical. Sundowning is a common feature of AD especially in the moderate to late stages. Sundowning is a syndrome of restlessness often experienced in the late afternoon and evening hours. It is exacerbated by fatigue and dim lighting. Therefore, improvements in sleep quality and brighter lighting can result in decreased behavioral difficulties such as night-time wandering and pacing.

ROLE OF FOLLOW-UP ASSESSMENT

Multidisciplinary Clinic Approach

Ms Jane is an 80-year-old woman presenting with memory complaints. She is accompanied to the appointment by her son who lives out of state and first began noticing his mother's forgetfulness about a year ago. During a recent visit, he noticed that she sometimes repeats herself without awareness and is less oriented to the date. Ms Jane lives alone in her rural home following the recent death of her husband. Her son is concerned about her driving capacities as she recently hit a parked car. She is having more difficulty paying bills on time and there have been episodes of forgetting to turn the stove off when cooking. Ms Jane also appears less interested in her usual activities and time spent with friends since her husband's death.

A holistic approach to dementia treatment is ideal given the complexity of issues associated with cognitive decline. A multidisciplinary approach to care is well suited in meeting patient and caregiver needs throughout the continuum of disease progression. Utilizing the services of a number of specialists from varying backgrounds working together as a team enables effective and efficient care. A multidisciplinary team can be comprised of neurologists, neuropsychologists, geriatric psychiatrists, nurses, social workers, and social service representatives such as from the Alzheimer's Association. As is often the case, the strength of such a team lies in its whole being greater than the sum of its component parts.

Let us return to our vignette about Ms Jane for illustration. Ms Jane is initially evaluated by the team neurologist whose exam is concerned with memory difficulties. The neurologist recommends neuropsychological testing to further assess for cognitive changes outside the realm of normal aging. Brain imaging is ordered to help inform etiology by evaluating for structural change. The neuropsychological evaluation reveals that Ms Jane is a woman of above average intelligence, but her performance on memory testing is significantly below expectation for her age. Other areas of cognition remain generally intact including language skills, executive functioning capacities, attention, processing speed, visual reasoning, and motor functioning. Brain imaging is relatively unremarkable. Test results are consistent with a diagnosis of MCI, and Aricept is prescribed. A referral for follow-up care in the multidisciplinary clinic is recommended.

Ms Jane returns to the clinic with her son. The nursing staff assess her general health and review her medication list for polypharmacy issues. The neurologist is available to discuss brain imaging results, and etiology and treatment. Ms Jane then undergoes brief cognitive testing to evaluate for interval change following treatment initiation of Aricept. Results reveal general stability in cognitive performance compared with the previous evaluation. Serial cognitive assessment is recommended yearly due to the increased risk of conversion to dementia in individuals with MCI.

Neuropsychological test results also indicate the presence of depression, demonstrated in Ms Jane's responses to a mood questionnaire, and evident in behavioral observation. This finding is consistent with the report of decreased social interaction following the recent death of Ms Jane's husband. Therefore, it is recommended that Ms Jane consult with the geriatric psychiatrist regarding psychotropic intervention. Additionally, Ms Jane's son is provided support-oriented psychotherapy services. Finally, community/social work services are required given the report of reductions in activities of daily living and driving skills. The social work representative helps Ms Jane get scheduled for a formal driving evaluation and initiates a discussion of future plans. The Alzheimer's Association representative informs Ms Jane's son of an upcoming seminar on caretaking responsibilities and asset planning which he agrees to attend.

Utility of reassessment in treatment planning

Neuropsychological reassessment is a very effective diagnostic tool for a number of reasons. Primarily it allows for comparison of cognitive performance across time intervals to assess for the presence of cognitive decline, necessary for the diagnosis of a neurodegenerative process. All too often, it is difficult to assess for interval change if baseline testing has not been established for comparison, especially in individuals with high baseline IQs. As in the case of Ms Jane, reassessment is especially warranted to inform diagnosis in cases of MCI given the high rates of conversion to dementia. Reassessment also helps to inform the timing of treatment. As Memantine is the only drug on the market approved for treatment of moderate to severe dementia, neuropsychological re-evaluation is beneficial in assessing the stage of cognitive decline associated with disease progression to inform initiation of treatment. Periodic brief cognitive screening is also useful to assess for acute changes in mental status which would implicate a newly emerged medical problem (e.g., infection). Finally, reassessment can document the stage at which experimental treatment becomes an option.

Drug trials

As mentioned above, current pharmacological treatments are disease slowing, but not preventative or curative. Ongoing clinical trials provide patients with the opportunity to receive medications which have not received FDA approval but may have significant promise. Patients who do not respond well or have achieved maximal benefit from conventional treatment may be appropriate candidates for participation in clinical drug trial research.

CONCLUSION

As our aging population increases, dementia has become an increasing area of focus for mental health professionals serving geriatric populations. Familiarity with the most common dementias is essential. Alzheimer's disease is the most common dementia, followed by VaD and DLB. The type of cognitive decline varies depending on the type of dementia. Behavioral and psychiatric changes are also common. Neuropsychological assessment plays a vital role in accurate diagnosis. Multidisciplinary Memory Disorders clinics provide diagnosis and ongoing care to patients and their families. These clinics can provide a wide array of services including behavioral and pharmacological treatments for the patient, access to clinical research trials, aid in treatment planning, and supportive therapies for patients, families, and other caregivers.

References

Ahron-Peretz, J., Kliot, D., & Tomer, R. (2000). Behavioral differences between white matter lacunar dementia and Alzheimer's disease: A comparison on the Neuropsychiatric Inventory. *Dementia and Geriatric Cognitive Disorders*, *11*(5), 294–298.

Birks, J. (2006). Intervention review: Cholinesterase inhibitors for Alzheimer's disease. *Cochrane Database of Systematic Reviews*, *Issue 1*. Art. No.: CD005593. DOI: 10.1002/14651858.CD005593

Bohnstedt, M., Fox, P. J., & Kohatsu, N. D. (1994). Correlates of Mini-Mental Status Examination scores among elderly demented patients: The influence of race-ethnicity. *Journal of Clinical Epidemiology*, *47*, 1381–1387.

Boone, K. B., Miller, B. L., Swartz, R., Lu, P., & Lee, A. (2003). Relationship between positive and negative symptoms and neuropsychological scores in fronto-temporal dementia and Alzheimer's disease. *Journal of the International Neuropsychological Society*, *9*, 698–709.

Bowen, J., Teri, L., Kukull, W., McCormick, W., McCurry, S., & Larson, E. (1997). Progression to dementia in patients with isolated memory loss. *Lancet*, *349*, 763–765.

Boyle, P. A., Malloy, P. F., Salloway, S., Cahn-Weiner, D. A., Coben, R., & Cummings, J. (2003). Executive dysfunction and apathy predict functional impairment in Alzheimer's disease. *American Journal of Geriatric Psychiatry*, *11*(2), 214–221.

Bravo, G., & Hebert, R. (1997). Age- and education-specific reference values for the mini-mental and modified mini-mental state examinations derived from a non-demented elderly population. *International Journal of Geriatric Psychiatry*, *12*, 1008–1018.

Breitner, J. C., Haneuse, S. J., Walker, R., Dublin, S., Crane, P. K., Gray, S. L., et al. (2009). Risk of dementia and AD with prior exposure to NSAIDs in an elderly community-based cohort. *Neurology*, *72*(22), 1899–1905.

Cannata, A. P., Alberoni, M., Franceschi, M., & Mariani, C. (2002). Frontal impairment in subcortical ischemic vascular dementia in comparison to Alzheimer's disease. *Dementia and Geriatric Cognitive Disorders*, *13*, 101–111.

Caycedo, A. M., Miller, B., Kramer, J., & Rascovsky, K. (2009). Early features in fronto-temporal dementia. *Current Alzheimer Research*, *6*(4), 337–340.

Chow, T. W., Binns, M. A., Cummings, J. L., Lam, I., Black, S. E., Miller, B. L., et al. (2009). Apathy symptom profile and behavioral associations in frontotemporal dementia vs dementia of Alzheimer type. *Arch Neurol*, *66*(7), 888–893.

Cummings, J. L., Mega, M., Gray, K., Rosenberg-Thompson, S., Carusi, D. A., & Gornbein, J. (1994). The Neuropsychiatric Inventory (NPI): Comprehensive assessment of psychopathology in dementia. *Neurology*, *44*(12), 2308–2314.

Devanand, D. P., Pradhaban, G., Liu, X., Khandji, A., De Santi, S., Segal, S., et al. (2007). Hippocampal and entorhinal atrophy in mild cognitive impairment: prediction of Alzheimer disease. *Neurology*, *68*(11), 828–836.

Emre, M., Aarsland, D., Brown, R., Burn, D. J., Duckaerts, C., Mizuno, Y., et al. (2007). Clinical diagnostic criteria for dementia associated with Parkinson's disease. *Movement Disorders*, *22*(12), 1689–1707.

Espino, D. V., Lichtenstein, M. J., Palmer, R. F., & Hazuda, H. P. (2001). Ethnic differences in Mini-Mental State Examination (MMSE) score: Where you live makes a difference. *Journal of the American Geriatrics Society*, *49*, 538–548.

Fleisher, A. S., Sowell, B. B., Taylor, C., Gamst, A. C., Petersen, R. C., & Thal, L. J. (2007). Alzheimer's Disease Cooperative Study: Clinical predictors of progression to Alzheimer's disease in amnestic mild cognitive impairment. *Neurology*, *68*(19), 1588–1595.

Folstein, M. F., Folstein, S. E., & McHugh, P. R. (1975). Mini-mental state: A practical method for grading the cognitive state of patients for the clinician. *J Psychiatr Res*, *12*(3), 189–198.

Geldmacher, D. S. (2003). *Contemporary diagnosis and management of Alzheimer's dementia*. Newtown, PA: Handbooks in Healthcare Co.

Gelinas, I., Gauthier, L., & McIntyre, M. (1999). Development of a functional measure for persons with Alzheimer's disease: the Disability Assessment for Dementia. *American Journal of Occupational Therapy*, *53*, 471–481.

Griffith, H. R., Belue, K., Sicola, A., Krzywanski, S., Zamrini, E., Harrell, L., et al. (2003). Impaired financial abilities in mild cognitive impairment. *Neurology, 60*, 449–457.

Hargrave, R., Geck, L. C., Reed, B., & Mungas, D. (2000). Affective behavioural disturbances in Alzheimer's disease and ischemic vascular disease. *Journal of Neurology, Neurosurgery, and Psychiatry, 68*, 41–46.

Harold, D., Abraham, R., Hollingworth, P., Sims, R., Gerrish, A., Hamshere, M. L., et al. (2009). Genome-wide association study identifies variants at CLU and PICALM associated with Alzheimer's disease. *Nature Genetics, 41*(10), 1088–1093.

Horton, A. M., & Hartlage, L. C. (2003). *Handbook of forensic neuropsychology*. New York, NY: Springer Publishing Company, Inc.

Huff, F. J. (1990). Language in normal aging and age-related neurological diseases. In F. Boller, & J. Grafman (Eds.), *Handbook of Neuropsychology, Vol. 4* (pp. 251–264). Amsterdam: Elsevier.

Lezak, M. D., Howieson, D. B., & Loring, D. W. (2004). *Neuropsychological assessment* (4th edn.). New York, NY: Oxford University Press.

Lim, W. S., Chong, M. S., & Sahadevan, S. (2007). Utility of the Clinical Dementia Rating in Asian populations. *Clinical Medicine and Research, 5*(1), 61–70.

Lonie, J. A., Tierney, K. M., & Ebmeier, K. P. (2009). Screening for mild cognitive impairment: A systematic review. *Int J Geriatr Psychiatry, 24*(9), 902–915.

Lyketsos, C. G., Steele, C., Baker, L., Galik, E., Kopunek, S., Steinberg, M., & Warren, A. (1997). Major and minor depression in Alzheimer's disease: prevalence and impact. *Journal of Neuropsychiatry and Clinical Neuroscience, 9*, 556–561.

Marson, D. C., Martin, R. C., Wadley, V., Griffith, H. R., Snyder, S., Goode, P. S., et al. (2009). Clinical interview assessment of financial capacity in older adults with mild cognitive impairment and Alzheimer's disease. *J Am Geriatr Soc, 57*(5), 806–814.

Mattis, S. (1976). Mental status examination for organic mental syndrome in the elderly patient. In L. Bellack, & T. Karasu (Eds.), *Geriatric Psychiatry* (pp. 77–120). New York, NY: Grune and Stratton.

Mattis, S. (1988). *Dementia Rating Scale: Professional manual*. Odessa, FL: Psychological Assessment Resources.

McCaffrey, R. J., Williams, A. D., Fisher, J. M., & Laing, L. C. (2004). *The practice of forensic neuropsychology: Meeting the challenges in the courtroom*. New York, NY: Plenum Press.

McDowell, I. (2006). *Measuring health: A guide to rating scales and questionnaires* (3rd edn.). New York, NY: Oxford Press.

Mega, M. S., Cummings, J. L., Fiorello, T., & Gornbein, J. (1996). The spectrum of behavioral changes in Alzheimer's disease. *Neurology, 46*(1), 130–135.

Moretti, R., Torre, P., Antonello, R. M., & Cazzato, G. (2001). Fronto-temporal dementia versus Alzheimer's disease. *Archives of Gerentological Geriatrics, supplement, 7*, 273–278.

Morris, J. C. (1993). The Clinical Dementia Rating (CDR): Current version and scoring rules. *Neurology, 43*, 2412–2414.

Nestor, P., & Hodges, J. (2000). Non-Alzheimer's dementias. *Seminars in Neurology, 20*(4), 439–446.

Newman, S. C. (1999). The prevalence of depression in Alzheimer's disease and vascular dementia in a population sample. *Journal of Affective Disorders, 52*(1), 169–176S.

O'Brien, J. T., Erkinjuntti, T., Reisberg, B., Roman, G., Sawada, T., Pantoni, L., et al. (2003). Vascular cognitive impairment. *The Lancet Neurology, 2*, 89–98.

Okello, A., Koivunen, J., Edison, P., Archer, H. A., Turkheimer, F. E., Någren, K., et al. (2009). Conversion of amyloid positive and negative MCI to AD over 3 years: an 11C-PIB PET study. *Neurology, 73*(10), 754–756.

Park, J. H., Lee S. B., Lee T. J., Lee, D. Y., Jhoo, J. H., Youn, J. C., et al. (2007). Depression in vascular dementia is quantitatively and qualitatively different from depression in Alzheimer's disease. *Dement Geriatr Cogn Disord, 23*(2), 67–73.

Pena-Casanova, Blesa, R., Aguilar, M., Gramunt-Fombuena, N., Gomez-Anson, B., Oliva, R., et al. (for the NEURONORMA study team). (2009). Spanish multicenter normative studies (NEURONORMA Project): Methods and sample characteristics. *Archives of Clinical Neuropsychology, 24*(4), 307–319.

Petersen, R. C. (2000). Aging, mild cognitive impairment, and Alzheimer's disease. *Neurologic Clinics, 18*(4), 789–805.

Petersen, R. C., Stevens, J. C., Ganguli, M., Tangalos, E. G., Cummings, J. L., & DeKosky, S. T. (2001). Practice parameter: Early detection of dementia: Mild cognitive impairment (an evidence-based review). *Neurology, 56*, 1133–1142.

Rosen, W. G., Mohs, R. C., & Davis, K. L. (1984). A new rating scale for Alzheimer's Disease. *Am J Psychiatry, 141*(11), 1356–1365.

Schmidtke, K., & Hull, M. (2002). Neuropsychological differentiation of small vessel disease, Alzheimer's disease and mixed dementia. *Journal of Neurological Science, 17*(22), 203–204.

Seignourel, P. J., Kunik, M. E., Snow, L., Wilson, N., & Stanley, M. (2008). Anxiety in dementia: A critical review. *Clin Psychology Rev, 28*(7), 1071–1078.

Simard, M., van Reekum, R., & Myran, D. (2003). Visuospatial impairment in dementia with Lewy bodies and Alzheimer's disease: a process analysis approach. *International Journal of Geriatric Psychiatry, 18*(5), 387–391.

Snowden, J. S., Gibbons, Z. C., Blackshaw, A., Doubleday, E., Thompson, J., Craufurd, D., et al. (2003). Social cognition in fronto-temporal dementia and Huntington's disease. *Neuropsychologia, 41*, 688–701.

Tallberg, I. M., & Almkvist, O. (2001). Confabulation and memory in patients with Alzheimer's disease. *Journal of Clinical and Experimental Neuropsychology, 23*(2), 172–184.

Talwalker, S., Overall, J. E., Srirama, M. K., & Gracon, S. I. (1996). Cardinal features of cognitive dysfunction in Alzheimer's disease: A factor analytic study of Alzheimer's disease Assessment Scale. *Journal of Geriatric Psychiatry and Neurology, 9*, 39–46.

Thomas, G., McGirt, M. J., Woodworth, G., Heidler, J., Rigamonti, D., Hillis, A. E., et al. (2005). Baseline neuropsychological profile and cognitive response to cerebrospinal fluid shunting for idiopathic normal pressure hydrocephalus. *Dement Geriatr Cogn Disord, 20*(2–3), 163–168.

Traykov, L., Baudie, S., Thibaudet, M. C., Rigaud, A. S., Smagghe, A., & Boller, F. (2002). Neuropsychological deficit in early subcortical vascular dementia comparison to Alzheimer's disease. *Dementia and Geriatric Cognitive Disorders, 14*(1), 26–32.

Vliet, E. C., Manly, J., Tang, M. X., Marder, K., Bell, K., & Stern, Y. (2003). The neuropsychological profiles of mild Alzheimer's disease and questionable dementia as compared to age-related cognitive decline. *Journal of the International Neuropsychological Society, 9*(5), 720–732.

Weinstein, A. M., Barton, C., Ross, L., Kramer, J. H., & Yaffe, K. (2009). Treatment practices of mild cognitive impairment in California Alzheimer's Disease Centers. *J Am Geriatr Soc, 57*(4), 686–690.

Welsh, K.A., Mirra, S., Fillenbaum, G., Gearing, M., Beekly, D., & Edland, S. (1996). *Neuropsychological and neuropathological differences of Alzheimer's disease from other dementias: The CERAD experience*. Presented at the 24th annual meeting of the International Neuropsychological Society, Chicago, IL.

Werner, P., & Korczyn, A. D. (2008). Mild Cognitive Impairment: Conceptual, assessment, ethical, and social issues. *Clin Interv Aging, 3*, 413–420.

Zawacki, T. W., Grace, J., Paul, R., Moser, D. J., Ott, B. R., Gordon, N., et al. (2002). Behavioral problems as predictors of functional abilities of vascular dementia patients. *Journal of Neuropsychiatry and Clinical Neuroscience, 14*, 296–302.

CHAPTER

7 Delirium Assessment in Older Adults

Chriscelyn M. Tussey[1], Donna K. Broshek[2], Bernice A. Marcopulos[3]

[1] *Neurocognitive Assessment Laboratory, University School of Medicine, Charlottesville, VA, and Western State Hospital, Staunton, VA, USA,*

[2] *Neurocognitive Assesment Laboratory, University of Virginia School of Medicine, Charlottesville, VA, USA,*

[3] *Psychiatry and Neurobehavioral Sciences, University of Virginia, VA, and Neuropsychology Laboratory, Western State Hospital, Staunton, VA, USA*

Delirium is a severe, and often transient, neuropsychiatric syndrome that is particularly prevalent in elderly, hospitalized patients (Siddiqi, House, & Holmes, 2006). It is a negative prognostic indicator that often results in longer hospitalizations and increased mortality rates (Inouye, 2006; van Zyl & Seitz, 2006). Appropriate identification, evaluation, and treatment of delirium by all health care providers is imperative, especially clinical gerontologists who work predominantly with the aging population. Differential diagnosis can be challenging given the symptom overlap between delirium and other clinical conditions, particularly dementia, and is further complicated by its multiple potential etiologies. Formal cognitive testing is often requested when symptoms emerge, although it should not be initiated until the underlying medical problem causing the delirium has been addressed. When assessment begins, how does a clinician determine if delirium is indeed present? This chapter provides contemporary information regarding the syndrome and its epidemiology, risk factors, diagnostic criteria, and psychosocial interventions. A review of several of the most commonly employed clinical instruments designed to assess delirium and two case studies are included to assist with assessing and understanding this complex syndrome.

HISTORY OF DELIRIUM AS A CLINICAL CONCEPT

Delirium has been recognized as an important medical complication since at least the time of Hippocrates (Lipowski, 1990). The term "delirium" was first used by Celsus in the first century A.D. (Lipowski, 1990), and it was first described in the English literature by Barrough (1583). By the nineteenth century it was viewed as a mental disorder with impairment of consciousness, rather than solely a physical illness (Greiner, 1817). Numerous terms such as "phrenitis," "frenzy," and "febrile insanity" were used to classify the symptoms. Eventually, emphasis was placed on disordered consciousness, rather than only psychiatric states. Bonhoeffer (1912) emphasized that "clouding of consciousness" is a core symptom in delirium resulting from systemic diseases affecting brain functioning. The English neurologist John Hughlings Jackson (Jackson, 1932) espoused a neuropsychological view of delirium as a "dissolution" of the nervous system. From his perspective, the more evolutionarily advanced parts of the brain, such as the neocortex, are affected first, thus releasing the "lower" parts of the brain.

Handbook of Assessment in Clinical Gerontology. DOI: 10.1016/B978-0-12-374961-1.10007-7

Wolff and Curran (1935) conducted the first extensive clinical study of delirious patients. They observed that disturbed consciousness and cognitive impairment were cardinal features. A frequently cited study is Engel and Romano's (1944, 1959) classic work using EEG. They described delirium as a disturbance in level of consciousness manifested by cognitive-attention disturbance. They found that a diffusely slow EEG due to a reduction in brain metabolism was a reliable marker for delirium.

To date, a single pathway leading to delirium is not known. Delirium has been divided into syndromes (i.e., hyperactive, hypoactive, and mixed types) which may illustrate the end product of one or more neurochemical pathways. Dopaminergic excess and cholinergic deficiency along with concomitant disruption of regulatory neurotransmitters, including noradrenaline, GABA, and glutamate, are hypothesized to be the major neurochemical changes that occur in the constellation of a cascade of neurobiological events (Maldonado, 2008). Specific brain lesions most commonly associated with delirium are right parietal and temporal infarcts (Maldonado, 2008). Many complementary theories have been proposed to explain the processes leading to delirium, such as the "oxygen deprivation hypothesis," "neurotransmitter hypothesis," and the "neuronal aging hypothesis" (for a review see Maldonado, 2008).

The etymology of delirium has long impeded communication and education about this syndrome. Semantic confusion continues as numerous terms are used to label delirium symptoms, such as encephalopathy, acute confusional state, and acute organic brain syndrome. The term "subsyndromal delirium" has been added to the vernacular to describe patients who have one or more delirium symptoms but do not meet criteria for full-blown clinical delirium. Ultimately, it appears that the label given to this syndrome varies depending on the specialist applying it (Caine & Lyness, 2000). However, as research on the neuroanatomy of this condition increases, and as the differing pathophysiologies between delirium and conditions with similar symptoms are delineated, the syndrome will continue to be elucidated, with the hopes of improving communication and care for these patients.

EPIDEMIOLOGY

Estimated prevalence and incidence rates vary depending on methodology (e.g., retrospective vs. prospective), instruments used to measure delirium, setting (e.g., intensive care, psychogeriatric, general medical, or surgical units), diagnostic criteria utilized, and whether demented patients were included in the sample. The highest rates of delirium are found in medical inpatient and acute geriatric settings. In fact, delirium represents one of the most common preventable adverse events for older hospitalized patients (Rothschild, Bates, & Leape, 2000). Much lower rates are usually found in outpatient community settings compared with medical settings. For instance, Levkoff, Cleary, Liptzin, and Evans (1991a) reviewed the literature and found a prevalence of 10–30% and an incidence of 4–53.2% in medical outpatients.

More recently, a retrospective cross-sectional study utilizing an administrative database from a large managed care organization examined delirium superimposed on dementia (DSD). Of the total community sample of 76,688 persons aged 65 years or older, 7347 (10%) were diagnosed as having dementia, and an additional 763 (1%) as having delirium alone. Among those with dementia, 976 (13%) had DSD, representing 1.3% of the total sample. Only one episode of delirium was counted per patient, thus the occurrence rates are conservative. On average, the DSD group had 2.9 (± 3.1) claims with a delirium diagnosis, and the delirium-only group had 2.4 (± 3.4) claims with a delirium diagnosis over the three-year study period (Fick, Kolanowski, Waller, & Inouye, 2005)

General Medical Inpatient and Acute Geriatric

In the United States, the care of delirious patients accounts for more than 49% of all hospital days (Department of Health and Human Services, 2000). Prospective studies of medical inpatients show a prevalence of delirium (cases present at the time of hospital admission) of 12–31%, with measures of incidence (new cases arising during hospital admission) from 3–25% (Adamis, Treloar, MacDonald, & Martin, 2005; Cole, Dendukuri, McCusker, & Ling, 2003). According to Marcantonio, Flacker, Michaels, and Resnick (2000) delirium is the most common post-operative complication occurring in between 15–25% of older patients following elective surgery and 25–65% of older patients following emergency admission and surgery.

The reported incidence of delirium in the intensive care unit (ICU) also ranges vastly, from 16–89% (Devlin, Fong, Fraser, & Riker, 2007). A prospective, observational cohort study conducted by Balas et al. (2007) examined 114 English-speaking participants and their surrogates, aged 65 and older, admitted to a surgical intensive care unit (SICU). Chart reviews and surrogate interviews were conducted within 24 hours of SICU admission and participants were screened for delirium daily throughout their hospitalization with either the Confusion Assessment Method-Intensive Care Unit (CAM-ICU) while in the SICU, or the standard Confusion Assessment Method (CAM) while on medical/surgical units. The authors found 18.4% of participants had evidence of dementia on admission to the SICU. Few older adults (2.6%) were admitted to the hospital with evidence of pre-existing delirium, but 28.3% developed delirium in the SICU and 22.7% during the post-SICU period. A total of 52 of 114 (45.6%) participants were delirious 24 hours before hospital admission (as measured by the CAM-Short Version, which was administered to surrogates) or some-time during their hospital stay. These findings support the notion that older adults are at high risk for developing delirium during hospitalization.

Prospective studies have documented delirium prevalence rates of 28–42% upon admission to a palliative care unit. Longitudinal studies indicate that delirium may occur in as high as 90% of all patients with a terminal illness (Lawlor et al., 2000; Harris, 2008).

Psychiatric

Ritchie, Steiner, and Abrahamowicz (1996) studied the incidence and risk factors for delirium among hospitalized psychiatric patients. They conducted a chart review of 199 psychiatric patients admitted to Montreal General Hospital, excluding patients with dementia and alcohol delirium. The overall incidence was 14.6% and the occurrence of delirium was associated with advanced age, a diagnosis of bipolar disorder, and treatment with anticholinergic, antiparkinsonian medications. The incidence rate obtained by Ritchie and colleagues was very high and discordant compared with the findings of subsequent studies (Huang, Tsai, Chan, Hwang, & Sim, 1998; Patten, Williams, Haynes, McCruden, & Arboleda-Florez, 1997).

Koponen and Riekkinen (1993) also conducted a prospective study of delirium in elderly psychiatric patients, but they included patients with dementia. They found that 13.4 % of all admitted patients to the psychogeriatric ward had delirium, using DSM-III criteria. The majority (81%) of their delirious patients had CNS pathology, usually Parkinson's disease, dementia of the Alzheimer's type, or vascular dementia. A Taiwanese study of 2512 psychiatric admissions found that 1.4% of the inpatients were delirious. Results indicated higher rates in patients over age 65 (9.6%), and medications were identified as the likely cause of delirium in many cases. However, an epidemiological evaluation of associations between delirium and specific medication exposures was not attempted (Huang et al., 1998).

Patten et al. (1997) conducted a prospective study evaluating the epidemiology of delirium in general hospital psychiatric inpatients. They examined 401 patients, who were not delirious at the time of admission, during 420 admissions. There were nine cases in which delirium onset occurred during their hospital stay, leading to an estimated incidence proportion of 2.14%. Unfortunately, due to the insuffient number of delirium cases, a pharmacoepidemiological risk factor analysis could not be performed.

Patten, Williams, Petcu, and Oldfield (2001) sought to identify the clinical and pharmacological determinants of delirium in psychiatric inpatients. They found, as previously mentioned, that exposure to lithium, anticholinergic medications, and antipsychotics was significantly associated with the occurence of delirium, although exposure to antidepressants and anticonvulsant mood stabilizers was not. They declared that the effects were multiplicative, and there was no evidence of interaction between the exposures to each medication. However, they acknowledged that they may have had inadequate power to detect such interactions.

ETIOLOGY/RISK FACTORS

The etiology of delirium typically stems from a combination of both predisposing and precipitating risk factors (Inouye & Charpentier, 1996). There is an ample body of literature that suggests that age, dementia, psychoactive drug use, and medical comorbidity may increase the likelihood of delirium (Bohner et al., 2003; Galanakis, Bickel, Gradinger, Von Gumppenberg, & Forstl, 2001)

Like epidemiological research, risk factors differ across studies depending upon the age of the patients and the setting. It is important to consider whether delirium was present at the time of admission, developed during admission, or emerged after discharge. Risk factors can be categorized as: (1) a pre-existing condition of the patient; (2) an acute condition of the patient; or, (3) an iatrogenic or environmental factor. Potential pre-existing conditions include age >70, transfer from a nursing home, visual or hearing impairment, history of depression, dementia, stroke, epilepsy, or use of psychoactive drugs. Acute conditions may include drug overdoses or illicit drug use, metabolic issues, sepsis, or serum urea nitrogen. Iatrogenic/environmental factors may include medications (particularly anticholinergics, sedatives, and analgesics), tube feeding, or catheter use (Devlin et al., 2007).

The severity of delirium is another important risk factor that warrants attention. Voyer, McCusker, Cole, St-Jacques, and Khomenko (2007) investigated whether the factors associated with delirium varied according to the severity of the delirium experienced among new long-term care admissions. Upon admission, patients were screened for delirium with the CAM, and the severity of delirium symptoms was determined by the Delirium Index. Of the 71 delirious older patients, 32 (45.1%) had moderate–severe delirium while 39 (54.9%) presented with mild delirium. A significant positive relationship was observed between premorbid cognitive impairment and delirium severity. Additional factors were significantly associated with delirium, including low Mini-Mental State Examination (MMSE) scores and the presence of severe illness at the time of admission, as well as low functional autonomy. Interestingly, older patients suffering from mild delirium used significantly more drugs, notably narcotics, than those with moderate–severe delirium. However, stepwise regression revealed that the MMSE score at admission and narcotic medication use were the factors most strongly associated with the severity of delirium symptoms.

Given the cross-sectional design of this study, it is difficult to ascertain whether the drug precipitated the delirium or if the physician prescribed a drug in response to behavioral symptoms of delirium. This might, in part, account for the lower number of drugs used by patients displaying moderate–severe symptoms of delirium. The authors concluded that factors associated with moderate–severe delirium were different from those associated with mild delirium and that, as would be expected, moderate–severe delirium is associated with poorer outcomes (Voyer, et al., 2007).

In addition to the aforementioned risk factors, it is important to consider the impact of psychological health on delirium. McAvay et al. (2007) conducted a prospective cohort study of patients 70 and older who were at intermediate or high risk for delirium and were not taking antidepressants at hospital admission. They found that patients who developed delirium reported a higher rate of depressive symptoms than those without. After controlling for measures of physical and mental health, depressive symptoms, including dysphoric mood and hopelessness, were predictive of incident delirium. In contrast, symptoms of withdrawal, apathy, and vigor were not associated with delirium.

CLINICAL FEATURES

The core diagnostic features of delirium include fluctuating alteration in consciousness and a change in cognition or a perceptual disturbance (APA, 2000). However, the manifestation of delirium can be rather idiosyncratic. The heterogenous presentation increases the complexity of symptom recognition.

Lipowski (1989) described several types of delirium based on psychomotor behavior and level of arousal: hypoactive; hyperactive; and mixed. The typical elderly patient with delirium is the hypoactive type, presenting as quietly confused, disoriented, lethargic, mildly anxious, and perplexed (Inouye, 1994). In the palliative care setting, hypoactive delirium is most common and it is frequently misdiagnosed as depression or severe fatigue (Spiller & Keen, 2006). For example, in a hospice setting, 29 out of 100 acute admissions were found to have delirium; 86% of these had the hypoactive subtype. The hyperactive type who is overtly agitated and floridly hallucinating is less common, though often more easily recognized by clinicians. For instance, Francis, Martin, and Kapoor (1990) found that disruptive behaviors and hallucinations occurred in less than half of their elderly patients with delirium. Incontinence was the most common behavioral marker for this group of patients. Individuals with a mixed presentation vacillate between hypo- and hyper-psychomotor symptom expression.

There is evidence suggesting that the subtypes of delirium may be related to different etiologies and may have different treatment responses. For instance, hypoactive delirium has most commonly been associated with hypoxia, metabolic disturbances, and hepatic encephalopathies, and a higher mortality risk than the hyperactive subtype (Meagher, O'Hanlon, O'Mahony, Casey, & Trzepacz, 2000). Hyperactive delirium is often associated with alcohol and drug withdrawal or drug intoxication.

The onset of delirium is typically rapid and may include a variety of neuropsychiatric symptoms, which typically increase at night. A patient may have fluctuating levels of awareness and orientation, impaired memory, and poor attention. There are typically disturbances in the sleep—wake cycle and activity level (Brown & Boyle, 2002). The patient may report symptoms of uneasiness, headache, irritability, fatigue, restlessness, anxiety, or depression (Beresin, 1988). Also, perceptual distortions and visual hallucinations are a common feature of delirium. Visual hallucinations are more common than auditory hallucinations (Trzepacz, 1996). Neurologic abnormalities may include tremors, asterixis, myoclonus, frontal release signs, and changes in muscle tone. Emotional reactions typically involve fear and depression.

Outcome Studies

Patients who develop delirium during their hospital stay have a poorer prognosis. An association has been found between delirium and functional decline, increased hospital stay, and higher mortality rates (Dasgupta & Dumbrell, 2006; Inouye, 2006; van Zyl & Seitz, 2006;). According to Siddiqi et al. (2006), death rates have ranged from 14.5—37%. McCusker, Cole, Abrahamowicz, Primeau, and Belzile (2002) found that compared with older patients with mild delirium, those with severe delirium, as defined by the Delirium Index, had a greater likelihood of dying within 12 months.

As previously indicated, a patient's subtype of delirium may be related to outcome. In a prospective study of patients aged 65 and older who were hospitalized for acute hip fracture surgery, Marcantonio,

Ta, Duthie, and Resnick (2002) found that patients with subsyndromal delirium had outcomes similar to those with mild delirium, suggesting that the presence of delirium symptoms may be more important than the DSM-IV-TR diagnosis of delirium, per se. Pure hypoactive delirium accounted for over 70% of all cases, although delirium with hyperactive features tended to be more severe, was more likely to be treated with sedating medications, and in general had poorer outcomes. Even after adjusting for the severity of delirium, hyperactivity was an independent correlate of nursing home placement or death one month after surgery.

With regard to the course of delirium, McAvay et al. (2006) found that of 433 study patients, 24 (5.5%) had delirium at discharge, 31 (7.2%) had delirium that resolved during hospitalization, and 378 (87.3%) were never delirious. The average length of hospital stay was 15.4 days for patients discharged delirious, followed by 14.3 days for those with delirium that resolved, and 7.3 days for those who were never delirious. After one year of follow-up, 20 of 24 patients (83.3%) discharged with delirium, the delirium in 21 of 31 patients (67.7%) was resolved, and 157 of 378 patients (41.5%) who were never delirious had been placed in a nursing home or had died. The authors concluded that delirium at discharge is associated with a high rate of nursing home placement and mortality over a one-year follow-up period. This finding is consistent with previous research (e.g., Adamis, Treloar, Martin, & MacDonald, 2006).

Neuropsychological Test Findings

The psychopathology of delirium remains "remarkably under-studied" (Bhat & Rockwood 2007, p. 1167). Although cognitive impairment is known to occur, characterization of its neuropsychological profile is lacking (Brown et al., 2009). Patients with delirium often demonstrate gross impairments of attentional functioning and a high frequency of psychiatric perceptual disturbances (Meagher et al., 2007).

Often the Mini-Mental State Examination (MMSE) is used as a cognitive screener in studies of delirious patients. Most studies find that the total score of a delirious patient is similar to scores received by dementia patients. However, the MMSE score typically fluctuates significantly during the hospital course, which does not occur in those patients with dementia only (Francis et al., 1990). Lower MMSE scores and lowered performance on tasks of executive functioning, attention, and processing speed suggest a link between delirium and long-term cognitive impairment (Fann, Roth-Roemer, Katon, & Syrjala, 2007; McCusker, Cole, & Dendukuri, 2001). However, it is important to emphasize that the MMSE is a cognitive screener, and is not specifically designed for the detection of delirium, a concern that will be addressed below in the review of frequently employed instruments used to measure delirium.

Brown et al. (2009) explored the perceptual differences found in individuals with delirium. They hypothesize that patients with delirium may have deficits in the cognitive systems that underlie visual perception. The researchers administered five neuropsychological tests of visual perception to 17 older patients with delirium and two control groups comprising 14 patients with Alzheimer's dementia and 18 cognitively normal patients. Also, the MMSE and the Consortium to Establish a Registry for Alzheimer's Disease (CERAD) verbal memory test assessed the specificity of any perceptual impairments. Results revealed that patients with delirium scored significantly lower than cognitively normal patients on all perceptual tasks and significantly lower than patients with dementia on three of these tasks. Mini-Mental State Examination scores did not differ between the delirium and dementia groups, and patients with delirium showed significantly better verbal recognition performance than those with dementia. Overall, the results suggested that individuals with delirium have specific visual perceptual deficits that cannot be fully explained by general cognitive impairment.

In addition to attention, memory, and visual deficits, language disturbance is a prominent neuropsychological finding in delirium. Deficits may include paraphasias, dysarthria, dysnomia, reduced fluency, and tangential, circumstantial, and disorganized speech (Baranowski & Patten, 2000). Wallesch and Hundsalz (1994) examined naming and word comprehension performance in both delirious patients and patients with Alzheimer's disease (AD). They found that although both groups had similar levels of impairment, they had differences in types of errors. In particular, the delirious patients produced more unrelated misnaming errors, which the authors interpreted as misperceptions. Visual hallucinations were more common in delirium than Alzheimer's disease. Also, unlike the AD patients in which word frequency was related to misnaming, there was a lack of correlation between word frequency and misnaming in delirious patients. Intrusions were also more prominent in delirious patients.

Rudolph et al. (2008) conducted research to determine if post-operative delirium was associated with early and long-term Post-operative Cognitive Dysfunction (POCD). It was hypothesized that patients with post-operative delirium would be more likely to meet criteria for diagnosis of POCD and that subjects with long-lasting delirium (3 days) would be more likely to have early and long-term POCD. International recruitment of 1218 participants aged 60 who were undergoing non-cardiac surgery was conducted. Participants were excluded if they had a score of 23 on the MMSE, a central nervous system disease including dementia or Parkinson's disease, previous neuropsychological testing, illiteracy, inability to understand the language of the test administration, administration of tranquilizers or antidepressants prior to admission, cardiac or neurosurgery, severe hearing or vision disorders, life expectancy less than three months, or refusal to comply with the protocol. POCD is often accessed via neuropsychological tests that measure a variety of cognitive domains, including attention, memory, executive function, visuospatial abilities, psychomotor, and language function (Silverstein, Steinmetz, Reichenberg, Harvey, & Rasmussen, 2007). As such, the Visual Verbal Learning Test, the Concept Shifting Test, the Stroop Color-Word Test, and the Letter—Digit Substitution were completed upon entry into the study, post-operatively at seven days or hospital discharge (whichever came first), and at three months.

Results indicated that patients with postoperative delirium had a higher incidence of early POCD, although conclusions about long-term POCD were impossible to render due to limited power and missing data. Early POCD was more common in participants who developed long-duration (3 days) delirium. Given that inattention is a predominant cognitive symptom of delirium, and that attention is important for optimal performance on all neuropsychological tests (Stuss & Levine, 2002), it is important to note that delirium and POCD are not necessarily independent conditions. Nevertheless, the data highlight the importance of neuropsychological testing for assessing delirium and related conditions.

THE IMPORTANCE OF ASSESSING DELIRIUM

Delirium is often undiagnosed, despite its high frequency in elderly medical patients (Francis, Strong, Martin, & Kapoor, 1988; Inouye, Foreman, Mion, Katz, & Cooney, 2001; Lewis, Miller, Morley, Nork, & Lasater, 1995). One of the reasons that delirium is not identified is because older patients frequently present with hypoactivity and lethargy, rather than with agitation and hallucinations (Inouye, 1994). Also, cognitive function is rarely formally assessed in medical evaluations. Perhaps as a result of both of these factors, recent research found that emergency physicians (EP) missed delirium in 76% of the cases (Han et al., 2009). Also, the researchers found that of admitted patients whose delirium the EP missed, over 90% of these cases were also missed by the hospital physician at the time of admission. This is particularly concerning given that if delirium is missed in the ED, there is a potential delay in diagnosing delirium in the hospital setting. Kakuma et al.

(2003) found that older patients whose delirium was unrecognized by the EP had the highest death rate, compared with ED patients whose delirium was recognized and patients without delirium. Han et al. (2009) offer additional support for the importance of diagnosing delirium. For example, ED patients with underlying life-threatening illnesses may receive inappropriate diagnostic evaluations and be discharged home. Once home, they may be unable to comprehend their discharge instructions, thus leading to non-adherence and medical errors.

Although cognitive function is rarely formally assessed in medical evaluations, similarly medical factors are at times unfortunately not taken into consideration during a cognitive evaluation. Although the literature on cognitive assessment in dementia often includes an overview of delirium, rarely is the frequency of delirium addressed or how to adequately screen for it before attempting an extensive battery of cognitive tests. Inouye (1994) suggests that any deterioration in mental status in a hospitalized elderly patient should be considered to be delirium unless determined otherwise. Given that Treloar and MacDonald (1997a; 1997b) found that the symptoms most associated with reversible cognitive dysfunction were "quiet" symptoms, such as slowness of thought, speech incoherence, fluctuating attention, and plucking at bedclothes, formal assessment appears to be critical to the identification of delirium.

It is crucial to distinguish dementia from delirium. Delirium is usually associated with a potentially life-threatening medical condition that needs to be addressed immediately by appropriate medical personnel. Delirium is prevalent in persons with dementia (Voyer, Cole, McCusker, & Belzile, 2006). Subjective memory complaints, newly diagnosed dementia, and need for long-term care have been associated with delirium in elderly patients after hospitalization (Rahkonen, Luukkainen-Markkula, Paanila, Sivenius, & Sulkaya, 2000) or hip surgery (Bickel, Gradinger, Kochs, & Forstl, 2008). This highlights the notion that delirium does not merely have short-term sequalae; rather, it may predict a future cognitive decline that is associated with an increased risk of dementia.

Delirium superimposed on dementia (DSD) ranges from 22–89% in hospitalized and community-dwelling older adults aged 65 and older with dementia (Fick, Agostini, & Inouye, 2002). Previous studies have found DSD may lead to increased rates of re-hospitalization within 30 days (Fick & Foreman, 2000). In addition to DSD, factors which are typically associated with missed or misdiagnosed delirium include: inconsistencies in the terminology used to describe delirium; failure to conduct an objective test of cognition screening; presence of the hypoactive or hypoalert subtype, which is frequently misdiagnosed as depression; and fluctuation in the intensity of symptoms with periods of apparent lucidity (McAvay et al., 2007).

One of the most important and clear distinctions between dementia and delirium is that dementia occurs in the presence of a normal level of consciousness (Rabins & Folstein, 1982). The presence of hallucinations and delusions does not reliably distinguish between the two groups (Rabins & Folstein, 1982), although other authors (Beresin, 1988; Roth, 1991) have asserted that hallucinations are usually less florid in dementia. Delirium typically has an acute onset and a shorter duration than dementia, which usually has an insidious onset. Orientation and memory are typically impaired in both conditions and cannot be used to reliably distinguish the two. An abnormal EEG (grade II or III) was found in 59.1% of psychogeriatric inpatients diagnosed with delirium in contrast to abnormal EEGs found in 40.1% of patients with dementia, or other organic disorders, and 12% of psychiatric patients without delirium or dementia (Rosen et al., 1994).

DIAGNOSTIC CRITERIA

Diagnostic criteria for delirium first appeared in DSM-III (Trzepacz, 1996). In the DSM-III, delirium was listed as an organic brain syndrome with the essential feature of a "clouded state of consciousness (reduced clarity or awareness of the environment), with reduced capacity to shift, focus, and sustain attention to environmental stimuli" (APA, 1980). Additional criteria included perceptual disturbances, incoherent speech, disturbed sleep–wake cycle, alterations in psychomotor activity, memory impairment and disorientation, a fluctuating course, and evidence of a presumably etiologically-related specific organic factor.

The diagnostic criteria for delirium in DSM-III-R emphasized difficulty maintaining and appropriately shifting attention and disorganized thinking, rather than the vague "clouded state of consciousness" used in the DSM-III (APA, 1987). Also included were a reduced level of consciousness, perceptual disturbances, disturbed sleep–wake cycle, alterations in psychomotor activity, disorientation, impaired memory, and a fluctuating course. The DSM-III-R diagnosis also required evidence of a specific organic factor or a presumed organic factor that was considered to be etiologically related.

Similar to the DSM-III criteria, the DSM-IV required a "disturbance of consciousness (i.e., reduced clarity of awareness of the environment) with reduced ability to focus, sustain, and shift attention" (APA, 1994). The diagnosis also required a change in cognitive ability or a new perceptual disturbance that could not be explained by a dementia and an acute onset with a fluctuating course. Specific etiologies were to be identified in the diagnosis, including "delirium due to a general medical condition" (which had to be specified), "substance intoxication delirium," "substance withdrawal delirium," "substance-induced delirium" (associated with medication or exposure to toxins), and "delirium due to multiple etiologies." When the etiology was suspected, but had not been established, the diagnosis was "delirium not otherwise specified." The latter category was also appropriate when the etiology did not fall into one of the other categories, such as "delirium secondary to sensory deprivation."

Additional features of delirium presented in the DSM-IV indicated that disorientation to time may be the first symptom to appear in mild delirium and that sensory misperceptions are primarily visual, although they could occur in other sensory modalities. Associated features included a disturbed sleep–wake cycle, increased or decreased psychomotor behavior, and emotional disturbances, which tended to occur most often at night when fewer environmental cues were present. It was also noted that EEGs were often abnormal with evidence of generalized slowing or fast activity. The DSM-IV criteria have been criticized for not accurately portraying delirium as a diffuse disorder of the brain with multiple cognitive and behavioral deficits, with a resultant higher risk of misdiagnosis (Trzepacz, 1996).

In its most recent edition, the DSM-IV-TR contains much of the same diagnostic criteria but several changes have been made. Specifically, in the "Associated Features" section, modifications were made to emphasize the presence of two varieties of delirium: hyperactive and hypoactive. Text was also added to the "Specific Age Features" section to reflect the finding that advanced age has been found to be a risk factor for delirium in a variety of study populations, even after controlling for other risk factors (such as concomitant illness). Prevalence data on delirium in a variety of medically ill populations are now available (e.g., up to 60% of nursing home residents aged 75 or older may develop delirium). Also, in the current DSM-IV-TR, the importance of early recognition and treatment of delirium is added to the Course section of the text. Furthermore, under the criteria for "delirium due to a general medical condition," the list of associated general medical conditions was reorganized and updated. Under "substance-induced delirium," text was added to clarify that the onset and offset may be affected by various factors such as brain damage, older age, and substance half-life (APA, 2000).

Despite these changes, the DSM-IV-TR continues to be criticized. For example, the current criteria for delirium do not address the prodromal or affective symptoms (e.g., depressed mood) of delirium, which might be more prominent in patients with delirium in palliative care settings and also associated with worse outcomes (Alici & Breitbart, 2009). Further, subsyndromal delirium is not recognized in

DSM-IV-TR, nor are guidelines offered for when post-delirium cognitive impairment is better attributed to dementia. It is hoped that the DSM-V will rectify some of these deficits. Meagher and Trzepacz (2007) proposed that the neuropsychiatry of dementia and delirium should be highlighted in the upcoming DSM-V and suggest the following: (1) dementia research should carefully research any delirium component and utilize instruments that capture differentiating characteristics; (2) categorization of the differing courses of delirium symptoms (e.g., acute transient versus recurring); (3) inclusion of phenomenological detail regarding syndromal and subsyndromal delirium; (4) inclusion of phenomenological detail and relative frequency of symptoms for major types of dementias; and (5) emphasis on the differential diagnosis of delirium and subsyndromal delirium in the dementia sections as possible reasons for the clinical presentation during the course of illness in those who are treatment refractory.

REVIEW OF DELIRIUM ASSESSMENT MEASURES

Abbreviated Mental Test

The Abbreviated Mental Test (AMT; Hodkinson, 1972; Jitapunkuel, Pillay, & Ebrahim, 1991) consists of 10 items that assess orientation, memory, and mental control, and is a frequently used measure of mental status in the United Kingdom. A validity study revealed no significant difference in AMT scores between elderly patients pre-surgically, while those who subsequently developed delirium had a significantly greater decline in AMT score post-operatively (Chonchubhair, Valacio, Kelly, & O'Keefe, 1995). A decline of two points on the 10-point scale yielded a 93% sensitivity and an 84% specificity for diagnosis of postoperative delirium, with an AMT score of less than 8 proposed as an indicator of delirium. No data were provided on the ethnicity of the sample used to validate the measure. The authors also did not provide information on the effects of age and education on the scale.

The validity of the AMT was examined in Spain among individuals chosen randomly from census data and outpatients diagnosed with dementia (Sarasqueta et al., 2001). In the community sample, 11 were diagnosed with dementia and 85 without. In the total sample, a score of 7 maximized the efficacy of the test. The sensitivity for this cutoff point was 91.5% (78.7–97.2%) and the specificity was 82.4% (72.2–89.5%). Although a score of 9 offered 100% sensitivity, it increased the proportion of false positives to 66%. Similar research conducted in Germany (Linstedt, Berkau, Meyer, Kropp, & Zenz, 2002) found congruent results.

In follow-up studies, Swain, O'Brien, & Nightingale, (1999) and Swain, O'Brien, and Nightingale (2000) examined the relationship between the AMT and the MMSE, and the AMT, the AMT4, a 4-item version of the AMT (AMT4), and the MMSE, respectively. The prospective studies examined 276 patients admitted to an elderly medicine unit at an inner city teaching hospital. In the first study (Swain, O'Brien, & Nightingale, 1999), the positive predictive value of the AMT was 92.7%. In the second project, the AMT4 had a predictive efficiency of 83.3% for the AMT and 73.2% for the MMSE. The results support the notion that the AMT4 may be useful in the initial assessment of cognition in elderly patients, with minimal loss of accuracy in detecting marked cognitive impairment when compared with the AMT.

Cognitive Test for Delirium

The cognitive test for delirium (CTD) was designed to assess cognitive functioning for the purpose of identifying delirium in an intensive care unit (Hart et al., 1996). The two alternate forms of the CTD consist of five subtests that assess orientation, attention span, memory for words and pictures of objects, comprehension, and vigilance. Items are included from the Wechsler Memory Scale-Revised and the Boston Diagnostic Aphasia Examination and conversion formulas for scoring the subtests are provided. The scores for each subtest range from 0–6 and are summed to produce a maximum score of 30. The CTD requires approximately 10–15 minutes administration time and was designed to accommodate medically ill patients who may have significant functional limitations, such as intubation, motor restrictions, or illiteracy. Items are presented to enhance the patient's attention, visual stimuli are enlarged, memory testing uses both verbal codes and pictures to facilitate encoding, and only nonverbal responses are required by patients.

Internal consistency was demonstrated by a coefficient alpha of 0.87 and the first factor in a principal components analysis accounted for 73% of the variability (Hart et al., 1996). An intraclass correlation coefficient of 0.90 revealed high agreement between the two alternate forms. Performance on the CTD was compared for patients with delirium (n = 22; mean age = 62.5, SD = 14.4), dementia (n = 26; mean age = 64.9, SD = 12.3), schizophrenia (n = 25; mean age = 34.4, SD = 14.6), and depressive illness (n = 30; mean age = 38.8, SD = 14.6). A MANCOVA, which covaried gender, age, and education, found a significant difference between the groups on the CTD and MMSE with post hoc tests revealing poorer performance for the patients with delirium. A receiver operator characteristic (ROC) curve analysis identified an optimal cutoff score of <18, yielding sensitivity of 100% and specificity of 95.1%. The four patients incorrectly classified by the CTD had severe dementia. A shortened and simplified version of the Delirium Rating Scale (Trzepacz, Baker, & Greenhouse, 1988) completed by ICU nurses correlated −0.02 with the CTD in patients with delirium. A follow-up study revealed that the CTD could be administered to patients who were not able to complete the MMSE due to functional limitations. The effect of education on CTD scores was not assessed. Approximately half of the patient sample was African American.

In a more recent study, the reversibility of delirium and mortality was assessed in terminally ill patients (Leonard, Agar, Mason, & Lawlor, 2008). The researchers found clinical utility in the CTD, noting that irreversible delirium was associated with greater disturbance of CTD attention, and survival time was predicted by CTD score ($P < 0.001$), age ($P = 0.01$), and organ failure ($P = 0.01$).

Although the CTD does not assess diagnostic features such as acuteness of onset or fluctuating course, its use as a measure of the cognitive features of delirium is promising. The design of the CTD, which enables administration to patients who are intubated, not verbally responsive, or motorically restricted, is a strength, as is the emphasis on maximizing the patient's ability to attend and encode test stimuli. Additional research is needed to assess the effect of education on CTD performance and its utility in quantifying delirium severity.

Confusion Assessment Method

The confusion assessment method (CAM) consists of nine operationalized criteria from DSM-III-R and was created to allow non-psychiatric clinicians to perform rapid detection of delirium in high risk geriatric patients (Inouye et al., 1990). The criteria include acute onset, inattention, disorganized thinking, altered level of consciousness, disorientation, memory impairment, perceptual disturbances, psychomotor agitation, psychomotor retardation, and disturbed sleep–wake cycle. Diagnosis is based on an algorithm which requires the presence of an acute onset, fluctuating course and inattention, and either disorganized thinking or an altered level of consciousness as indicated by positive answers to select items. The CAM is based on directly observable behaviors and requires approximately five minutes to complete.

The original validation study of the CAM was performed on outpatients at a geriatric assessment center and elderly patients admitted to general medical wards at two urban teaching hospitals with a total sample of 56 patients (Inouye et al., 1990). The racial composition of the two samples was different: 21% caucasian at site 1 and 4% caucasian at site 2. No data were provided regarding whether age and education affected CAM scores for the two samples. Patients with dementia, psychiatric disorders, and variable severity levels of dementia were assessed to determine sensitivity and specificity of the CAM. An expert panel of four geriatricians, two psychiatrists, and two neurologists determined that the CAM possessed high face validity, but was concerned about the diagnostic algorithm's ability to differentiate between delirium and dementia. Inter-rater reliability calculated between independent blind evaluations by the researchers yielded 100% agreement (kappa = 1.0) for the presence or absence of delirium, 88% agreement (kappa = 0.67) for the nine clinical features, and 93% agreement (kappa = 0.81) for the four diagnostic features in the algorithm. Assessment of convergent validity revealed that the CAM was significantly correlated ($p < 0.001$) with the MMSE (kappa = 0.64), Story Recall (kappa = 0.59), Digit Span (kappa = 0.66), and Visual Analog Scale for Confusion (kappa = 0.82). The latter appears to be the same analog rating used in adjunct with the MMSE and also known as the Global Accessibility Rating (Anthony, LeResche, Von Korff, Niaz, & Folstein, 1985; Folstein, Folstein, & McHugh, 1975).

CAM ratings were also validated by comparing the results with independent, blind clinical assessments made by a psychiatrist yielding sensitivity of 100% and 94% and specificity of 95% and 90%, depending upon the site (Inouye et al., 1990). Positive predictive values were 91% and 94%, and negative predictive accuracy values were 100% and 90%, again depending upon the site. Discrepancies were noted to occur in the evaluation of patients with severe underlying dementia. Scores on a modified CAM were found to correlate with patient mortality and were superior to emergency room physicians in detecting delirium in geriatric patients presenting to an emergency room (Lewis et al., 1995).

Overall, the CAM has become the most widely used instrument for detection of delirium worldwide, and its use in the palliative care population is growing (Hjermstad, Loge, & Kaasa, 2004). The measure has been deemed valid when administered by different medical specialists, with an agreement between different interviewers for the presence of delirium equal to 100% (Inouye, 2001). However, the importance of training and education cannot be underestimated, given that some research has revealed that nurses using the CAM, for example, have under-recognized delirium (Inouye et al., 2001).

Confusion Assessment Method for the Intensive Care Unit

The CAM has been adapted to facilitate rapid (approximately two minutes), objective assessment for use with nonverbal, mechanically ventilated patients in an intensive care unit (Ely et al., 2001). In this version (the CAM-ICU) the MMSE component was replaced with an Attention Screening Examination (ASE). If patients cannot participate in the picture-recognition ASE (e.g., due to visual impairment), a verbal random letter test is administered. In two studies of 38 ICU patients (33 of whom developed delirium based on an independent physician DSM-IV diagnosis) and 96 ICU patients (80 of whom developed delirium based on an independent physician DSM-IV diagnosis), the nurse-rated CAM-ICU showed a high sensitivity (93–100%) and specificity (93–100%), and excellent inter-rater reliability (K-R 20 = 84-0.96). The CAM-ICU requires minimal training and is easy to use (Schuurmans, Deschamps, Markham, Shortridge-Baggett, & Duursma, 2003b). Of note, in verbal, non-intubated ICU patients, the standard CAM may be better at detecting subtle cases of delirium (McNicoll, Pisani, Ely, Gifford, & Inouye, 2005).

Delirium Index

The Delirium Index (DI) was adapted from the CAM and is intended as a measure of the severity of delirium for use in delirium research that a research assistant (non-clinician) could score according to patient observation, without additional information from family members, nursing staff, or the patient's medical chart. The DI includes seven of the ten symptom domains of the CAM (disorders of attention, thought, consciousness, orientation, memory, perception, and psychomotor activity), each scored on a scale from 0 (absent) to 3 (present and severe) using operational criteria for each score. The total DI score may vary from 0–21, with a higher score indicating greater severity. The remaining three domains of the CAM (acute onset, sleep–wake disturbance, fluctuation) were excluded because they do not assess severity (acute onset) and cannot be assessed using patient observation only (fluctuation, sleep–wake disturbance).

In a prospective cohort study, the reliability and validity of the DI was evaluated with repeated patient assessments at multiple points in the hospital, at eight weeks after discharge, and at 6 and 12 months after admission. The sample included medical admissions of patients aged 65 and older: 165 with delirium and dementia; 57 with delirium only; 55 with dementia only; and 41 with neither. Study patients had a mean age of 83.5, 64% were female, 52% had not completed high school, and 71% lived in their own home. The severity of delirium symptoms was measured using the DI. Delirium was diagnosed using the CAM. Other measures included the Mini-Mental State Examination, Informant Questionnaire on Cognitive Decline in the Elderly, Barthel Index (BI), premorbid instrumental activities of daily living, Charlson Comorbidity Index, Clinical Severity of Illness scale (CSI), and the Acute Physiology Score (APS). The first five items of the MMSE were used as the basis of observation for the DI. Additional questions were asked as needed (McCusker, Cole, Dendukuri, & Belzile, 2004).

With respect to reliability, the Cronbach alpha for the DI was 0.74 overall, suggesting good internal consistency. The alpha coefficient increased to 0.82 after exclusion of perceptual disturbances, a symptom whose severity was essentially unrelated to the severity of any of the other symptoms. The values of the alpha coefficient in the subgroups of patients, including and excluding perceptual disturbances, were delirium and dementia F = 0.69 and 0.79; delirium only F = 0.67 and 0.78; dementia only F = 0.55 and 0.59; and neither delirium nor dementia, F = 0.44 and 0.52, respectively. The inter-rater reliability of the DI was assessed for a sample of 26 patients, some of whom were evaluated multiple times, resulting in a total of 39 pairs of ratings. The intra-class correlation coefficient was 0.98 (SD 50.06). Regarding validity of the DI, both measures of fluctuation were significantly higher in those with delirium than in those without delirium, regardless of the presence of dementia. The means of the SDs (and 95% CIs) were 2.35 (2.11–2.61) and 1.36 (1.18–1.52) for patients with and without delirium, respectively. Similar results were found for the MMSE (McCusker et al., 2004). "Internal responsiveness" was defined as "the ability of a measure to change over a prespecified time" and "external responsiveness" was defined as "the extent to which change in a measure reflects change in a reference measure of health status (McCusker et al., 2004, p. 1745)." Internal responsiveness at eight weeks in delirious patients with and without dementia was measured by effect sizes (−0.60 and −0.74 respectively). Also, low to good levels of external responsiveness were found.

The results of this prospective study supported the use of the DI as a reliable and valid measure of the severity of delirium, with or without dementia. The DI is unique compared with other measures of delirium severity because it can be completed via patient observation alone. Furthermore, although the MMSE performed similarly to the DI, the DI appeared slightly more responsive to patients with delirium, whereas the MMSE was more responsive for non-delirious patients, supporting the more specific usefulness of the DI for monitoring the severity of symptoms in delirious patients, whereas the MMSE is a more generic measure of cognitive function suitable for use with different types of patients (McCusker et al., 2004).

Delirium Observation Screening Scale

The Delirium Observation Screening Scale (DOS) was designed to facilitate early recognition of delirium (Schuurmans, Shortridge-Bagget, & Duursma, 2003a). It was developed according to the

DSM-IV criteria for delirium and tested for content validity by a group of experts in the field of delirium. At the development stage, the DOS Scale was designed with 25 behavioral items that were rated on a 5-point Likert scale (Schuurmans et al., 2003b). After reviewing studies of geriatric and hip fracture patients, the scale was reduced to 13 items that can be rated as present or absent in less than 5 minutes (Schuurmans, Donders, Shortridge-Bagget, & Duursma 2002). A score of 0 is defined as "normal behavior," suggesting the absence of behavioral alterations. Three items (3, 8, and 9) are reverse-scored. The highest total score is 13, and three or more points indicate probable delirium.

In two prospective studies with high risk groups of patients, the DOS Scale showed high internal consistency (0.93–0.96) (Schuurmans et al., 2003a; Schuurmans et al., 2002). Predictive validity was good in both studies. Correlations of the DOS Scale with the MMSE were −0.66 and −0.79. Concurrent validity, as tested by comparison of the research nurse's ratings of the DOS Scale and the CAM was 0.63. Construct validity of the DOS has been tested against the Informant Questionnaire of Cognitive Decline in Elderly (IQCODE; 0.33 and 0.74) and the Barthel Index (−0.26 and −0.55). An algorithm of 13 items rated over three consecutive shifts has been developed. The sensitivity of this algorithm is 0.94 and specificity is 0.77 (Schuurmans et al., 2002).

van Gemert and Schuurmans (2007) conducted a study to determine which of the two delirium observation screening scales, the NEECHAM Confusion Scale or the DOS scale, had the best discriminative capacity for diagnosing delirium and which was more practical for daily use by nurses. The research was conducted at a university hospital and included 87 patients who were observed and rated on both scales for symptoms of delirium during three shifts. A DSM-IV diagnosis of delirium was made or rejected by a geriatrician, and nurses were asked to rate the practical value of both scales using a structured questionnaire. The sensitivity (0.89–1.00) and specificity (0.86–0.88) of the DOS and the NEECHAM were high for both scales. Nurses rated the practical use of the DOS scale as significantly easier and more relevant to their practice than the NEECHAM.

The Delirium Rating Scale-Revised-98

The predecessor of the Delirium Rating Scale-Revised-98 (DRS-R-98) is the Delirium Rating Scale (DRS), which deserves a brief discussion. The DRS is a 10-item clinician-rated scale based upon a 24-hour period of time that utilizes all available information, including patient interview, nursing reports, medical history and tests, and family report (Trzepacz et al., 1988). The presence and severity of symptoms are rated and scores range from 0 (no impairment) to 32 (severe impairment). Items assessed include temporal onset of symptoms, perceptual disturbances, hallucinations, delusions, psychomotor behavior, cognitive testing, physical disorder, disturbed sleep–wake cycle, mood lability, and fluctuations in symptoms. The cognitive testing item requires the administration of a mental status examination to be used in conjunction with the DRS and the item on hallucinations distinguishes between auditory and visual hallucinations with the latter purported to be more typical of delirium. Overall, the DRS was considered sensitive to delirium, but specificity depended upon the setting. It had limited use for diagnosis in psychogeriatric settings and reduced validity for patients with dementia (Rosen et al., 1994). The DRS has been criticized for its lack of emphasis on assessing attention and its reliance on clinical judgment, and was not recommended for use by lay interviewers (Levkoff, Liptzin, Cleary, Reilly, & Evans, 1991b; Rockwood, Goodman, Flynn, & Stolee, 1996; Smith, Breitbart, & Platt, 1995). Also, the requirement of the DRS to include administration of an adjunctive measure of cognitive functioning made it more time-consuming (Smith et al., 1995; Trzepacz, 1994).

Although the original DRS (Trzepacz et al., 1988) continues to be widely used to measure symptom severity in delirium, as indicated above, it has several limitations, including grouping cognitive disturbances into a single item, not distinguishing motoric disturbances, and not assessing thought process or language disorder (Meagher et al., 2007). It was revised in order to address some of these issues. The DRS-R-98 is a 16-item scale. Each item is rated 0 (absent/normal) to 3 (severe impairment), with descriptions anchoring each severity level. The maximum total score is 46 points, and severity scale scores range from 0—39, with higher scores indicating more severe delirium (Trzepacz et al., 2001). Delirium typically involves scores above 15 points (severity scale) or 18 points (total scale). DRS-R-98 assessment can be repeated after a 24-hour period. The measure was originally validated among elderly patients with pre-existing dementia, schizophrenia, depression, and other psychiatric illnesses as both a total scale (16 items) and a severity scale (13 items) for repeated assessment.

de Rooij et al. (2006) recently conducted a validation study of the Dutch version of the DRS-R-98. The authors found that the Dutch DRS-R-98 effectively differentiated between patients with delirium, patients with dementia, and non-psychiatric patients. Furthermore, the DRS-R-98 was deemed a valid and reliable measure of severity as demonstrated by high intra-class correlation (0.97) and high internal consistency (Cronbach's alpha = 0.94). This measure offers something unique over its predecessor—the ability to detect non-hypoactive delirium. Specifically, positive scores on the affect liability and motor agitation items predicted the presence of non-hypoactive delirium with 89% specificity and 57% sensitivity.

Delirium Symptom Interview

The Delirium Symptom Interview (DSI) is a structured interview originally based on the seven symptom domains (disorientation, disturbance of consciousness, sleep disruption, perceptual disturbance, speech incoherence, alteration in psychomotor activity, and fluctuating behavior) specified in the DSM-III criteria for delirium, a literature review, and the clinical experience of the investigators (Albert et al., 1992). The interview consists of 17 items which require a response from the patient and 16 items based on behavioral observations, which are scored immediately following the interview. The final item requires an indication of whether the patient meets the criteria for delirium. According to the authors, administration time is approximately 10—15 minutes, although this time may be lengthened when patients are inattentive or tangential. The interview is designed to be administered by a trained lay interviewer.

In the original study, 50 medical or surgical inpatients, aged 65 or older, in an acute care hospital were assessed by a lay interviewer using the DSI (Albert et al., 1992). Patients were seen on the same day by a psychiatrist and neurologist who conducted independent clinical assessments which focused on three critical symptoms—disorientation, disturbance of consciousness, and perceptual disturbance—and then discussed their findings to reach a consensus. In order to evaluate inter-rater reliability, 21 patients were evaluated by two lay interviewers simultaneously with one interview administering the DSI and the other independently coding the responses and behavioral observations.

The inter-rater reliability between two lay interviewers produced a kappa coefficient of 0.90 (Albert et al., 1992). The kappa coefficient for agreement between the DSI and the consensus of the physicians on one of the three critical symptoms was 0.93. Internal consistency within each symptom domain was assessed by Cronbach's coefficient alpha with the following results: disturbance of consciousness, 0.80; disorientation, 0.75; incoherent speech, 0.61; psychomotor activity, 0.56; perceptual disturbance, 0.53; fluctuating behavior, 0.50; and sleep disturbance, 0.45.

Patients with dementia were included in the sample and, according to the authors, were identified as "cases" of delirium by both the DSI and the physicians, which might account for the high percentage (60%) of cases identified in this sample (Albert et al., 1992). Also, no mention is made of whether patients were screened for pre-existing psychiatric illness. As a result, it is not clear whether the DSI assesses unique symptoms of delirium or global cognitive impairment secondary to other pre-existing factors. The sensitivity of the DSI was reported to be 0.90 and the specificity to be 0.80. The authors did not indicate whether the DSI was affected by race, age, or education.

A strength of the DSI is that the interview format allows administration by a trained lay interviewer and may be particularly useful in epidemiologic studies or for longitudinal assessments (Levkoff et al., 1991b; Trzepacz, 1994). Although it can be used to make reliable diagnoses and may be of benefit in clinical research, it has been criticized for being cumbersome for many research purposes (Smith et al., 1995). A drawback is that the DSI does not assess the temporal onset of symptoms because this information must typically be obtained from secondary sources, such as relatives or caretakers. According to the authors, in their practice the DSI is used in conjunction with a chart review form "to identify true cases of delirium, as opposed to patients with symptoms of delirium that could be due to dementia or pre-existing psychoses" (Albert et al., 1992, p. 17). This suggests that the original DSI was not sufficient to provide a diagnosis of delirium and may not discriminate between individuals with delirium or dementia (Trzepacz, 1994).

Consistent with the current DSM-IV-TR (2000) definition of delirium, modifications were made in the original DSI instrument to separate the symptom of "disturbance of attention" from that of "disturbance of consciousness." Items addressing informal observations of inattention were redirected as triggers to the presence of inattention, a new eighth symptom. Additionally, an item was added to incorporate and rate performance on formal tasks of attention (Kiely et al., 2003).

High Sensitivity Cognitive Screen

The High Sensitivity Cognitive Screen (HSCS) was designed to address the limitations of most cognitive screening measures in the identification and measurement of mild delirium and "prodromal disorders" (Fogel, 1991). The HSCS may be administered to patients whose first language is English, have a minimum of eight years of education, and do not demonstrate gross cognitive impairment or aphasia. Patients with suspected delirium or moderate to severe dementia should be prescreened with the MMSE. The HSCS is not administered to those scoring 20 or less. The HSCS consists of six subtests that assess memory, language, visuomotor and visuospatial functions, attention and concentration, self-regulation, and planning. The items were derived from standard mental status procedures, the Bender-Gestalt (Bender, 1946), and the Woodcock-Johnson Psycho-Educational Battery (Woodcock & Johnson, 1975). It can be administered and scored by a research assistant with two days of training and supervision, and administration time ranges from 20–30 minutes. A numerical score is produced for each item, but interpretations are not made on a total summary score. Instead, an "interpretive algorithm" is used to classify scores as normal, borderline, or abnormal with the latter classified as mild, moderate, or severe.

Reliability assessment revealed an inter-rater reliability of 0.98 and test–retest reliability of 0.95 (Fogel, 1991). Compared with a comprehensive neuropsychological assessment, the HSCS yielded an accuracy rate of 93% using a normal versus borderline or abnormal dichotomy and a Pearson product moment correlation of 0.71 on a 4-point severity rating scale. A determination of cognitive functioning using the normal versus borderline or abnormal dichotomy in a sample of neurological patients resulted in a sensitivity of 87%, specificity of 75%, a false positive rate of 7%, and a false negative rate of 40%. Item correlations with age and education were not significant with the exception of a significant correlation between age and sentence completion, and education and writing to dictation. The average education of the validation sample subjects was 12.8 years (SD = 2.7, range = 4–17). Fogel (1991) reported a significant decline in scores with age in subjects 60–85 years. Race and education were examined in a younger group of HIV patients. No association was found between race and a brief version of the HSCS. Patients with less than high school education had a significantly greater rate of failing the brief HSCS, but no difference was found between high school graduates with varying levels of post high school education. A study of construct validity revealed a strong association between moderate to severe impairment on the HSCS and EEG abnormalities (Fogel, 1991).

Fogel (1991) cautions that the HSCS was not designed to diagnose cognitive impairment, but that it may be helpful in identifying relatively mild cognitive deficits, including mild delirium, prodromal states, and cognitive impairment, which might persist after resolution of delirium. Although it is not as brief as most screening instruments and its length may preclude its use with select populations, the HSCS has demonstrated good reliability and validity in assessing milder cognitive impairment (Smith et al., 1995). The HSCS was not designed to diagnose dementia (Fogel, 1991), but has been described as "very probably the instrument of choice for studies on cognitive phenomenology in delirium" (Smith et al., 1995, p. 51).

The Intensive Care Delirium Screening Checklist (ICDSC)

The ICDSC is an 8-item list based on DSM-IV criteria and other features of delirium, and includes assessment of consciousness, attentiveness, orientation, the presence of hallucinations or delusions, psychomotor agitation or retardation, inappropriate speech or mood, sleep—wake cycle disturbances, and overall symptom fluctuation (Bergeron, Dubois, Dumont, Dial, & Skrobik, 2001). The ICDSC was developed as an easy, bedside screening tool that circumvents the communication limitations of ICU patients, incorporates data that are gathered during routine patient care, and can be completed quickly by the patient's nurse or physician. The ICDSC was constructed using observations from a three-month pilot study that evaluated the use of a number of previously validated delirium assessment tools (e.g., CAM, DRS, and CTD) in the ICU.

During the evaluation process 1 point is given towards each domain that is present, with a score of 4 or higher out of 8 signaling the presence of delirium. A total of 93 consecutive patients admitted over a three-month period to a mixed medical—surgical ICU, without delirium at admission, were evaluated with the ICDSC every eight hours by the primary care nurse as well as independently, but consecutively, each morning (for a maximum of five days) by a research nurse, an intensivist, and a "gold standard" psychiatrist. Delirium was observed in 16% of the study cohort with an ICDSC score or 4 or higher accounting for 93% of these patients. Fifteen false positives occurred, but in 14 out of 15 patients other concomitant conditions were able to explain the ICDSC result [i.e., another psychiatric diagnosis ($n = 4$), dementia ($n = 3$), a structural neurological abnormality ($n = 6$), or cirrhosis ($n = 1$)]. A ROC curve was 0.9017 and the calculated sensitivity was 99% and specificity was 64%. When item reliability for the checklist was evaluated over the five days, alpha homogeneity coefficients ranged from 0.71—0.79 (Bergeron et al., 2001).

The first item of the ICDSC—level of consciousness—was found to be the factor that most weakened homogeneity with the alpha homogeneity coefficient improving to 0.78—0.85 when level of consciousness was removed. Inter-observer reliability between nurses, and between nurses and physicians was high, thus demonstrating that nurses can screen ICU patients as well as physicians using this measure, though training is recommended for all (Bergeron et al., 2001).

High agreement rates were found between the ICDSC and the CAM-ICU (Plaschke et al., 2008). Furthermore, each of the eight ICDSC items has been found to be highly discriminating for the diagnosis of delirium, highlighting the promise of this instrument and suggesting that perhaps any screening or diagnostic scale should incorporate these individual features of delirium (Marquis, Ouimet, Riker, Cossette, & Skrobik, 2007).

Memorial Delirium Assessment Scale

The Memorial Delirium Assessment Scale (MDAS) was uniquely created to quantify the severity of delirium symptoms in medical patients with particular utility for clinical intervention trials

(Breitbart et al., 1997). The MDAS is a 10-item scale with each item rated from 0 (no impairment) to 3 (severe impairment) and is designed for use by clinicians. The items assess awareness, disorientation, short-term memory, digit span, ability to shift and maintain attention, disorganized thinking, perceptual disturbance, delusions, alterations in psychomotor behavior, and disturbed sleep–wake cycles. The items are scored based on observations, information provided by nursing staff and/or family members, and the medical chart, as well as by brief cognitive assessment. For example, the disorientation scale requires that the patient respond to 10 orientation items (e.g., date, season, city) and the short-term memory scale requires the recall of three items after five minutes.

Assessment of inter-rater reliability yielded an intra-class correlation coefficient of 0.92 with the intra-class correlation coefficients of individual items varying from 0.64–0.99 (Breitbart et al., 1997). Analysis of internal consistency produced a Cronbach's alpha coefficient of 0.91. Only two items—perceptual disturbance and delusions—yielded item-total correlations below 0.60 (correlations of 0.44 and 0.31, respectively). The authors suggested that the lower correlations on the latter two items might be partially due to the fact that some patients had already begun treatment of their delirium prior to the administration of the MDAS.

According to Breitbart et al. (1997), medical patients with delirium had significantly higher MDAS scores than patients with non-delirium cognitive disorders or non-cognitive psychiatric disorders. Scores on the MDAS were significantly correlated with the MMSE ($r = -0.91$, $p < 0.0001$), DRS ($r = 0.88$, $p < 0.0001$), and the clinicians' global rating of dementia severity ($r = 0.89$, $p < 0.0001$). Analysis of covariance indicated that the MDAS scores significantly predicted the clinicians' global rating and that adding DRS or MMSE scores did not add incremental predictive value. Even after controlling for the DRS and MMSE scores, the MDAS scores continued to significantly predict the clinicians' global rating scores. Using a cutoff score of 13, with scores of 13 or higher reflective of delirium, the sensitivity was 70.6, specificity was 93.8, positive predictive accuracy was 93.3, and negative predictive accuracy was 75.0. More recent research in advanced cancer patients suggest a score of 7 will yield a sensitivity of 98% and specificity of 76% (Lawlor et al., 2000).

Studies indicate that the MDAS is a reliable and valid instrument for the detection of delirium severity in medical patients based on small samples (Breitbart et al., 1997; Smith et al., 1995) in a variety of countries, including Japan (Matsuoka et al., 2001) and Italy (Grassi et al., 2001). Also, it may be useful in palliative care settings as long as administrators of the measure follow adequate training and guidelines (Fadul, Kaur, Zhang, Palmer, & Bruera, 2007).

Research on the MDAS has been lacking with regard to the effects of race, age, or education effects on the instrument. And, although the MDAS was designed for repeated administration, it has not yet been validated for that purpose, although it shows promise for rapid serial assessments (Trzepacz, 1994). Unlike the DRS, it incorporates brief assessment of cognitive functioning within the measure and, thus, does not require the use of other clinical measures such as the MMSE. It has been suggested, however, that the MDAS would benefit from concurrent administration of brief cognitive measures, such as the Trail Making Test (Trzepacz, 1994). Breitbart et al. (1997) suggested that the MDAS also demonstrated some usefulness in the diagnosis of dementia, but caution that additional validity studies are needed in this area and to establish the most appropriate cutoff score.

NEECHAM Confusion Scale

The NEECHAM Confusion Scale was developed for quick use by nurses using information that is routinely available as a standard part of nursing assessments (Champagne, Neelon, McConnell, & Funk,

1987; Neelon, Champagne, McConnell, Carlson, & Funk, 1992). The scale consists of three levels—responsiveness, behavior, and physiologic control—with each level having three components. Of note, the third level (physiological control) assesses vital functions stability, urinary continence, and oxygen saturation measured via a pulse oximeter. The physiological measures are a distinguishing aspect of this scale and patients with low levels of oxygen may benefit from oxygen supplementation (Williams, 1991). Total scores range from 0–30 with the latter denoting the lack of impairment and scores of 24 or less indicative of confusion.

The NEECHAM has been noted to have high internal consistency with a Cronbach's alpha of 0.85, test–retest reliability of 0.96, and inter-rater reliability of 0.96 (Neelon et al., 1992). It is not clear if the latter was corrected for chance agreement. Inter-rater correlation in another study was 0.97 without correction for chance agreement (Siemsen, Miller, Newman, & Lucas, 1992).

The NEECHAM has been found to correlate significantly with the MMSE, a positive score on six out of eight DSM-II items, and history of mental status deficits obtained from admission records in elderly hospitalized patients (Neelon et al., 1992). Scores on the NEECHAM were not associated with a psychiatric diagnosis. Using history of mental status problems, the MMSE, and DSM-III as a comparison, the NEECHAM had a sensitivity of 95%, a specificity of 78%, a false positive rate of 17%, and a false negative rate of 3%. Very different results were obtained with a small sample, which found a sensitivity of 30% and specificity of 0.92 when compared with the MMSE (Siemsen et al., 1992).

Immers, Schuurmans, & van de Bijl (2005) conducted a prospective study that examined the reliability and validity of the NEECHAM in ICU settings. Results revealed high sensitivity (97%) and good specificity (83%). Concurrent validity with DSM-IV criteria indicated a strong link (chi square 67.52, $p < 0.001$) and there was high inter-rater reliability (Cohen's Kappa 0.60) and internal consistency (Cronbach's alpha 0.88). These findings suggested that the NEECHAM may be equally as effective for use with ICU patients, even those who are intubated, as it is in the general hospital population. Rompaey et al. (2008) compared the CAM-ICU and the NEECHAM in non-intubated patients. The observational study included a consecutive sample of 172 non-intubated patients who had been in a mixed ICU at least 24 hours. All adult patients with a Glasgow Coma Scale score of greater than 9 were included. A nurse researcher simultaneously utilized both scales once daily in the morning. A total of 599 paired observations were conducted. The CAM-ICU revealed a 19.8% incidence of delirium. The NEECHAM scale detected incidence rates of 20.3% for delirious, 24.4% for confused, 29.7% for at risk, and 25.6% for normal patients. The majority of the positive CAM-ICU patients were detected by the NEECHAM scale. The sensitivity of the NEECHAM scale was 87% and the specificity was 95%. The positive predictive value and the negative predictive value were 79% and 97%, respectively. Interestingly, the diagnostic capability in cardiac surgery patients proved to be lower than in other patients.

Hattori et al. (2009) serially examined post-operative psychiatric symptoms/behavioral abnormalities using the NEECHAM. The incidence of post-operative delirium was approximately 80% in patients showing a pre-operative MMSE score of 25 points or lower or a NEECHAM score of 27 points or lower, supporting utility of the NEECHAM Confusion Scale for evaluating the risk of post-operative delirium, the post-operative state, and treatment response.

A major strength of the NEECHAM is that is can be easily utilized by nursing staff to monitor changes in patient cognitive status. The use of oxygen saturation as an item may aid in the early assessment of delirium, although factor analyses have revealed that the physiological subtest does not load on the general factor which includes the other items (see Smith et al., 1995). Further more the scale has been criticized because the physiology subscale, particularly oxygen saturation, limits its use in different clinical settings and with varying delirium etiologies, and it has been described as "too complicated" for busy clinical nurses (Trzepacz, 1994).

Conclusions regarding delirium measures

Delirium is inherently a difficult condition to diagnose, given its high overlap with other conditions such as dementia. Although delirium research has proliferated in the past decade, congruent with the conclusions drawn in the first edition of this book, the current methods used to assess delirium need more research. Many of the aforementioned measures are different with regard to content, goal, type of ratings, the expertise of the rater, and rating time. While these differences are expected given the many possible combinations of these factors, a challenge is that many of these instruments have calculated the reliability and validity in different ways, and the quality of the testing procedures varies as well.

The current state of delirium assessment is particularly plagued by its many methodological limitations. Several of the measures described above have questionable psychometric properties and unfortunately only some of the instruments have been recently empirically investigated. Also, many instruments do not assess the effects of age, education, and ethnicity, all variables that are important when interpreting results (Strauss, Sherman, & Spreen, 2006). Furthermore, most studies are conducted using a hospitalized sample, despite the reality that delirium also develops at home and in nursing home patients.

Another significant problem with many of the aforementioned numerical rating scales is their inability to distinguish between severe dementia and delirium on the basis of cutoff scores. Clinical assessment should include a determination of acuteness of onset, or additional rapid decline in patients with underlying dementia, regardless of whether this is assessed by the rating scale. It is particularly difficult to identify delirium in patients with severe dementia on measures of cognitive functioning (Hart et al., 1996). It is necessary that screening measures are recognized as only one part of a clinical assessment and must be considered in conjunction with history, examination, and interview or observed behavior (Strain et al., 1988).

Ultimately, the delirium assessment measure that one chooses is contingent on the reason for which it is needed (e.g., diagnosis or screening, research, severity rating, etc.). For example, although the NEECHAM Confusion Scale and the Delirium Observation Screening Scale were judged as fairly equal with regard to sensitivity and specificity, nurses perceived the DOS scales as easier to use and more relevant to their practice (van Gemert & Schuurmans, 2007). Also, the DRS-R-98 is considered ideal for longitudinal research and has advantages over the original DRS with regard to flexibility and breadth of symptom coverage. Some measures may be better suited for rapid ICU assessment than others. Regardless of the measure chosen, or its purpose, it is imperative that the clinician utilizing the tool is appropriately trained to use the instrument. Given the many potentially detrimental sequelae of failing to diagnose, or inaccurately diagnosing delirium, diagnostic error should be minimized to the greatest extent possible.

CASE STUDIES

Case Study 1—Ms M

Ms M is a 71-year-old retired accountant who was admitted to a local hospital for knee surgery. The surgery and post-operative recovery were unremarkable, although she had not slept well since the night prior to surgery. Eventually, Ms M pulled out her IV and became agitated and confrontational when nurses arrived to replace it. She began accusing the nurses of trying to kill her, and ultimately called the police out of fear for her life. At one point in the night, staff became concerned that she may need to be transferred to the psychiatric unit and a neuropsychologist was consulted. A thorough clinical interview was conducted, along with review of Ms M's presentation upon admission. A previous mental health history, substance abuse issues, and medication interactions were ruled out. The possibility of a urinary tract infection was raised; however, medical testing ruled this out as well as other potential medical concerns.

Collateral information was obtained from Ms M's daughter, who explained that her mother experienced a similar episode during another knee surgery two years prior. In that instance, Ms M eventually returned to baseline. Neuropsychological testing revealed deficits in memory, attention, and orientation. The CAM revealed the presence of many delirium features. Given her current symptoms, in addition to her older age, major surgery, and what appeared to be a previous episode of delirium, Ms M was diagnosed with delirium. It is possible that the etiology of this diagnosis was multi-factorial, and potentially the result of sleep deprivation in combination with opiate analgesia and low sodium and albumin levels. Haloperidol was administered orally and the opiate analgesia was titrated as soon as clinically possible. After these changes, along with several nights of sleep, Ms M returned to baseline.

Case 2—Mr B

Mr B was a 69-year-old retired military veteran. He presented to a Veteran's Affairs Hospital emergency room and was diagnosed with pneumonia. He was an anxious man, and his worrying intensified after his admission, despite efforts by his medical team to comfort him. His anxiety negatively affected his sleeping, which had been poor since admission. After three days, Mr B began talking to an empty chair, demanding, "You get out of here—I do not know your wife." He pulled out his nasal oxygen and argued with nurses when they tried to replace the canula, insisting that they were not to listen to the "man in the chair." A neuropsychologist was consulted. A clinical interview was conducted; however, little information could be obtained due to Mr B's acute confusion. The DRS-R-98 revealed severe symptoms consistent with delirium.

Mr B's son reported that his father's memory had been increasingly poor for the past two years, including losing track of conversations, forgetting to take his medications, and occasionally forgetting medical appointments. His son was most concerned because Mr B recently had difficulty finding the VA Hospital, a route which he had taken many times in his later life. In fact, Mr B was driving so erratically that he was pulled over by the police and ultimately escorted to the VA hospital. Mr B's son added that his mother, Mr B's wife, passed away one year ago, and that his memory difficulties became significantly more obvious after her death. Also, Mr B was quite depressed after her death. His son denied that Mr B had any difficulties with alcohol or drug abuse or any similar behavior. Regarding potential medication interactions, he was taking antibiotics for pneumonia.

Blood tests revealed a raised white cell count and a physical evaluation indicated that Mr B was hypoxic. Pseudodementia was ruled out, even though Mr B appeared to have residual sadness related to the loss of his wife. He was eventually diagnosed with delirium superimposed on dementia. Potential causes for the delirium might have been the hypoxia caused by the pneumonia in the context of dementia and unfamiliar circumstances, which contributed to his disorientation. Mr B continued treatment for pneumonia and initially his delirium was addressed non-pharmacologically. Unfortunately, his symptoms became increasingly worse, particularly at night. Psychosocial intervention included psychoeducation and support for the family, as well as comfort care for the patient. Mr B's delirium eventually remitted after the pneumonia was treated, and he returned home. However, due to his deteriorating ability to care for himself, he was eventually transferred to a nursing home.

PSYCHOSOCIAL INTERVENTIONS

In addition to assisting in the identification of delirium, clinical gerontologists are well equipped to help the patient, family, and staff manage the symptoms of delirium. As has been described, delirium is intrinsically a multi-factorial syndrome with a complex and dynamic interrelationship between a patient's predisposing and precipitating factors. As a result, in order to ensure efficacy of an intervention, the multi-factorial origins of delirium must be addressed via multi-component interventions. Thus, in addition to pharmacological treatments such as haloperidol to treat psychotic symptoms associated with delirium, psychosocial (non-pharmacological) interventions should be employed for the patient and their family.

Attard, Ranjith, and Taylor (2008) suggested that delirium may be addressed psychosocially by providing the patient with support and orientation, an unambiguous environment, and maintaining competence, to the greatest extent possible. Support and orientation can be provided by communicating clearly and concisely, placing clear signposts in the patient's living area, such as a clock, calendar, daily activities schedule, etc., having familiar objects from the patient's home in the room (e.g., favorite picture, pillow), ensuring consistency in staff, and involving family and caregivers to elicit feelings of security and orientation. Attard and colleagues noted that physical restraints should be avoided, if possible. An unambiguous environment can be facilitated by simplifying care areas. Removal of unnecessary objects and extreme sensory stimulation, avoiding frequent changes in the location of the patient's bed or other furniture, avoiding the use of medical jargon in front of the patient, and ensuring that lighting is adequate will likely be helpful. The patient's competence may be maintained by identifying and correcting any sensory impairments (e.g., ensure that eyeglass prescription is correct, hearing aids are functional, etc.). If language barriers exist, an interpreter may be used. Consistent efforts to encourage self-care and participation in treatment will help make the patient feel self-efficacious.

In a systematic study that explored the experiences of the family members of cancer patients with terminal delirium, Namba et al. (2007) found that each intervention must be tailored to the individual needs of the patient and family. However, families consistently discussed several strategies that they perceived as helpful. These included:

- respecting the patients' subjective world;
- treating patients the same as before;
- exploring unmet physiological needs underlying delirium symptoms;
- considering ambivalent emotions when using psychotropics;
- coordinating care to achieve meaningful communication according to fluctuating levels of consciousness throughout the day;
- facilitating preparations for the patient's death;
- alleviating the patient's feelings of being a burden on others;
- relieving the family's physical and psychological burden; and
- providing information support.

Specific strategies to help the family may include:

- providing education about delirium;
- reassuring them that they can leave the patient's care to the staff;
- making the hospital environment comfortable;
- coordinating support from other members of the family;
- reassuring them that they did their best and made the right decisions; and
- allowing them to share their experiences with other families who are experiencing similar circumstances and who are open to the information.

CONCLUSION

Clinical gerontologists consulting in hospitals and, to a lesser extent, outpatient settings, are likely to encounter delirious elderly patients. Delirium is a complex neuropsychiatric syndrome that is difficult to diagnose. This challenge is particularly concerning given prevalence rates ranging from 12–89% (depending on the setting), and the many potential consequences of undiagnosed and untreated delirium (e.g., institutionalization, mortality). Although research regarding delirium has increased, measures used to screen for delirium continue to have limitations, including questionable reliability, validity, and clinical utility.

Given the challenges with delirium measures, it appears that identification of delirium is a task best addressed from a multidisciplinary approach, perhaps involving physicians, nurses, and psychologists, as well as other medical staff. Assessment should include a thorough review of a patient's medical history and current medical status, and the patient's behavior should be observed over time. The combination of a brief cognitive screening measure and a longitudinally administered behavioral observation checklist is warranted. The clinical gerontologist should give careful consideration to the possibility of delirium before undertaking an extensive cognitive evaluation of an elderly hospital patient. In many cases, it might be best to briefly assess the patient with a carefully chosen delirium instrument, and then recommend that the patient have an extensive cognitive evaluation after stabilization and discharge from the hospital to avoid confounding the effects of dementia and delirium.

The assessment instrument that is used is contingent on many factors, such as setting and the expertise of the rater. Current research suggests that the CAM and DRS are among the most frequently used by non-clinical staff to diagnose delirium, likely because of ease of use and sound validation. The CAM may be the most useful scale for diagnosing delirium, and the DRS may be best for rating symptom severity and tracking the course of delirium. The NEECHAM and the DOS are recommended as screeners for patients at high risk for delirium. The CAM-ICU is strongly recommended over the CAM for ICU patients. Regardless of which instrument is utilized, successful delirium assessment is imperative. Improved detection of this syndrome can enhance intervention and the chance of patient survival.

APPENDIX A: MEMORIAL DELIRIUM ASSESSMENT SCALE (MDAS)

(Breitbart et al., 1997)

Instructions: Rate the severity of the following symptoms of delirium based on current interaction with subject or assessment of his/her behavior or experience over past several hours (as indicated in each time.)

ITEM 1—REDUCED LEVEL OF CONSCIOUSNESS (AWARENESS): Rate the patient's current awareness of an interaction with the environment (interviewer, other people/objects in the room; for example, ask patients to describe their surroundings).

0: none	Patient spontaneously fully aware of environment and interacts appropriately
1: mild	Patient is unaware of some elements in the environment, or not spontaneously interacting appropriately with the interviewer; becomes fully aware and appropriately interactive when prodded strongly; interview is prolonged but not seriously disrupted
2: moderate	Patient is unaware of some or all elements in the environment, or not spontaneously interacting with the interviewer; becomes incompletely aware and inappropriately interactive when prodded strongly; interview is prolonged but not seriously disrupted
3: severe	Patient is unaware of all elements in the environment with no spontaneous interaction or awareness of the interviewer, so that the interview is difficult-to-impossible, even with maximal prodding

ITEM 2—DISORIENTATION: Rate current state by asking the following 10 orientation items: date, month, day, year, season, floor, name of hospital, city, state, and country.

0: none	Patient knows 9–10 items
1: mild	Patient knows 7–8 items
2: moderate	Patient knows 5–6 items
3: severe	Patient knows no more than 4 items

ITEM 3—SHORT-TERM MEMORY IMPAIRMENT: Rate current state by using repetition and delayed recall of 3 words (patient must immediately repeat and recall words 5 min. later after an intervening task). Use alternate sets of 3 words for successive evaluation (for example, apple, table, tomorrow; sky, cigar, justice).

0: none	All 3 words repeated and recalled
1: mild	All 3 repeated, patient fails to recall 1
2: moderate	All 3 repeated, patient fails to recall 2
3: severe	Patient fails to repeat 1 or more words

ITEM 4—IMPAIRED DIGIT SPAN: Rate current performance by asking subjects to repeat first 3, 4, then 5 digits forward and then 3, then 4 backwards; continue to the next step only if patient succeeds at the previous one.

0: none	Patient can do at least 5 numbers forward and 4 backward
1: mild	Patient can do at least 5 numbers forward, 3 backward
2: moderate	Patient can do 4–5 numbers forward, cannot do 3 backward
3: severe	Patient can do no more than 3 numbers forward

ITEM 5—REDUCED ABILITY TO MAINTAIN AND SHIFT ATTENTION: As indicated during the interview by questions needing to be rephrased and/or repeated because patient's attention wanders, patient loses track, patient is distracted by outside stimuli or over-absorbed in a task.

0: none	None of the above; patient maintains and shifts attention normally
1: mild	Above attentional problems occur once or twice without prolonging the interview
2: moderate	Above attentional problems occur often, prolonging the interview without seriously disrupting it
3: severe	Above attentional problems occur constantly, disrupting and making the interview difficult-to-impossible

ITEM 6—DISORGANIZED THINKING: As indicated during the interview by rambling, irrelevant or incoherent speech, or by tangential, circumstantial, or faulty reasoning. Ask patient a somewhat complex question (for example, "Describe your current medical condition.").

0: none	Patient's speech is coherent and goal-directed
1: mild	Patients speech is slightly difficult to follow; responses to questions are slightly off target but not so much as to prolong the interview
2: moderate	Disorganized thoughts or speech are clearly present, such that interview is prolonged but not disrupted
3: severe	Examination is very difficult or impossible due to disorganized thinking or speech

ITEM 7—PERCEPTUAL DISTURBANCE: Misperceptions, illusions, hallucinations inferred from inappropriate behavior during the interview or admitted by subject, as well as those elicited from nurse/family/chart accounts of the past several hours or of the time since last examination.

0: none	No misperceptions, illusions, or hallucinations
1: mild	Misperceptions or illusions related to sleep, fleeting hallucinations on 1–2 occasions without inappropriate behavior
2: moderate	Hallucinations or frequent illusions on several occasions with minimal inappropriate behavior that does not disrupt the interview
3: severe	Frequent or intense illusions or hallucinations with persistent inappropriate behavior that disrupts the interview of interferes with medical care

ITEM 8—DELUSIONS: Rate delusions inferred from inappropriate behavior during the interview or admitted by the patient, as well as delusions elicited from nurse/family/chart accounts of the past several hours or of the time since the previous examination.

0: none	No evidence of misinterpretations or delusions
1: mild	Misinterpretations or suspiciousness without clear delusional ideas or inappropriate behavior
2: moderate	Delusions admitted by the patient or evidenced by his/her behavior that do not or only marginally disrupt the interview or interfere with medical care
3: severe	Persistent and/or intense delusions resulting in inappropriate behavior, disrupting the interview or seriously interfering with medical care

ITEM 9—DECREASED OR INCREASED PSYCHOMOTOR ACTIVITY: Rate activity over past several hours, as well as activity during interview, by circling (a) hypoactive, (b) hyperactive, or (c) elements of both present.

0: none	Normal psychomotor activity
a b c 1: mild	Hypoactivity is barely noticeable, expressed as slight slowing of movement. Hyperactivity is barely noticeable or appears as simple restlessness.
a b c 2: moderate	Hypoactivity is undeniable, with marked reduction in the number of movements or marked slowness of movement; subject rarely spontaneously moves or speaks. Hyperactivity is undeniable, subject moves almost constantly; in both cases, exam is prolonged as a consequence.
a b c 3: severe	Hypoactivity is severe; patient does not move or speak without prodding or is catatonic. Hyperactivity is severe; patient is constantly moving, overreacts to stimuli, requires surveillance and/or restraint; getting through the exam is difficult or impossible.

ITEM 10—SLEEP–WAKE CYCLE DISTURBANCE (DISORDER OF AROUSAL): Rate patient's ability to either sleep or stay awake at the appropriate times. Utilize direct observation during the interview, as well as reports from nurses, family, patient, or charts describing sleep–wake cycle disturbance over the past several hours or since last examination. Use observations of the previous night for morning evaluations only.

0: none	At night, sleeps well; during the day, has no trouble staying awake
1: mild	Mild deviation from appropriate sleepfulness and wakefulness states: at night, difficulty falling asleep or transient night awakenings, needs medication to sleep well; during the day, reports periods of drowsiness or, during the interview, is drowsy but can easily fully awaken him/herself
2: moderate	Moderate deviations from appropriate sleepfulness and wakefulness states: at night, repeated and prolonged night awakening; during the day, reports of frequent and prolonged napping or, during the interview, can only be roused to complete wakefulness by strong stimuli
3: severe	Severe deviations from appropriate sleepfulness and wakefulness states: at night, sleeplessness; during the day, patient spends most of the time sleeping or, during the interview, cannot be roused to full wakefulness by any stimuli

REFERENCES

Adamis, D., Treloar, A., MacDonald, A., & Martin, F. (2005). Concurrent validity of two instruments (The Confusion Assessment Method and Delirium Rating Scale) in the detection of delirium among older medical inpatients. *Age and Ageing*, *34*, 72–75.

Adamis, D., Treloar, A., Martin, F., & MacDonald, A. (2006). Recovery and outcome of delirium in elderly medical inpatients. *Archives of Gerontology and Geriatrics*, *43*(2), 289–298.

Albert, M. S., Levkoff, S. E., Reilly, C., Liptzin, B., Pilgrim, D., Clearly, P. D., et al. (1992). The Delirium Symptom Interview: An interview for the detection of delirium symptoms in hospitalized patients. *Journal of Geriatric Psychiatry and Neurology*, *5*, 14–21.

Alici, Y., & Breitbart, W. (2009). Delirium in Palliative Care. *Clinical Focus—Primary Psychiatry, 16*(5), 42—48.

Anthony, J. C., LeResche, L. A., Von Korff, M. R., Niaz, U., & Folstein, M. F. (1985). Screening for delirium on a general medical ward: The tachistoscope and a global accessibility rating. *General Hospital Psychiatry, 7*, 36—42.

APA. (1980). *Diagnostic and statistical manual of mental disorders* (3rd ed.). Washington, DC: APA.

APA. (1987). *Diagnostic and statistical manual of mental disorders* (3rd edn, revised). Washington, DC: American Psychiatric Association.

APA. (1994). *Diagnostic and statistical manual of mental disorders* (4th ed.). Washington, DC: American Psychiatric Association.

APA. (2000). *Diagnostic and statistical manual of mental disorders* (4th edn, text-revision). Washington, DC: American Psychiatric Association.

Attard, A., Ranjith, G., & Taylor, D. (2008). Delirium and its treatment. *CNS Drugs, 22*(8), 631—644.

Balas, M., Deutschman, C., Sullivan-Marx, E., Strumpf, N., Alston, R., & Richmond, T. (2007). Delirium in older patients in surgical intensive care units. *Journal of Nursing Scholarship, 39*(2), 147—154.

Baranowski, S., & Patten, S. (2000). The predictive value of dysgraphia and constructional apraxis for delirium in psychiatric inpatients. *Canadian Journal of Psychiatry, 45*, 75—79.

Barrough, P. (1583). *The method of physick*. London, England: Field.

Bender, L. (1946). *Bender-Gestalt test*. New York, NY: American Orthopsychiatric Association.

Beresin, E. V. (1988). Delirium in the elderly. *Journal of Geriatric Psychiatry and Neurology, 1*, 127—143.

Bergeron, N., Dubois, M., Dumont, M., Dial, S., & Skrobik, Y. (2001). Intensive Care Delirium Screening Checklist: Evaluation of a new screening tool. *Intensive Care Medicine, 27*, 859—864.

Bhat, R., & Rockwood, K. (2007). Delirium as a disorder of consciousness. *Journal of Neurology, Neurosurgery, and Psychiatry, 78*, 1167—1170.

Bickel, H., Gradinger, R., Kochs, E., & Forstl, H. (2008). High risk of cognitive and functional decline after post-operative delirium: A three-year prospective study. *Dementia: Geriatric and Cognitive Disorders, 26*, 26—31.

Böhner, H., Hummel, T., Habel, U., Miller, C., Reinbott, S., Yang, Q., et al. (2003). Predicting delirium after vascular surgery: A model based on pre- and intra-operative data. *Annals of Surgery, 238*(1), 149—156.

Bonhoeffer, K. (1912). Die psychosen in Gefolge von akuten Infektionen, Allgemeinerkrankungen und inneren Erkrankungen. In G. L. Aschaffenburg (Ed.), *Handbuch der psychiatrie*. Leipzig: Deuticke.

Breitbart, W., Rosenfeld, B., Roth, A., Smith, M. J., Cohen, K., & Passik, S. (1997). The Memorial Delirium Assessment Scale. *Journal of Pain and Symptom Management, 13*(3), 128—137.

Brown, T. M., & Boyle, M. F. (2002). Delirium. *BMJ, 325*, 644—647.

Brown, L., McGrory, S., McLaren, L., Starr, J., Deary, I., & MacLullich, A. (2009). Cognitive visual perceptual deficits in delirium. *Journal of Neurology, Neurosurgery, and Psychiatry, 80*, 594—599.

Caine, E., & Lyness, J. (2000). Delirium, dementia, and amnestic and other cognitive disorders. In M. B. Sadock, & M. V. Sadock (Eds.), *Comprehensive textbook of psychiatry* (pp. 854—923). New York, NY: Lippincott Williams & Wilkins.

Champagne, M. T., Neelon, V. J., McConnell, E. S., & Funk, S. G. (1987). The NEECHAM Confusion Scale: Assessing acute confusion in the hospitalized and nursing home elderly. *The Gerontologist, 27*, 3A.

Chonchubhair, A. N., Valacio, R., Kelly, J., & O'Keefe, S. (1995). Use of the Abbreviated Mental Test to detect postoperative delirium in elderly people. *British Journal of Anaesthesia, 75*, 481—482.

Cole, M., Dendukuri, N., McCusker, J., & Ling, H. (2003). An empirical study of different diagnostic criteria for delirium among elderly medical inpatients. *Journal of Neuropsychiatry and Clinical Neuroscience, 15*, 200—207.

Dasgupta, M., & Dumbrell, A. (2006). Preoperative risk assessment for delirium after non-cardiac surgery: A systemic review. *Journal of the American Geriatric Society, 54*, 1578—1589.

Department of Health and Human Services. (2000). *Administration on aging: A profile of older Americans*. Washington, DC: Department of Health and Human Services.

de Rooij, S., van Munster, B., Korevaar, J., Casteelen, G., Schuurmans, M., van der Mast, R., et al. (2006). Delirium subtype identification and the validation of the Delirium Rating Scale-Revised-98 (Dutch Version) in hospitalized elderly patients. *International Journal of Geriatric Psychiatry, 21*, 876—882.

Devlin, J., Fong, J., Fraser, G., & Riker, R. (2007). Delirium assessment in the critically ill. *Intensive Care Medicine*, *33*, 929–940.

Ely, E., Margolin, R., Francis, J., May, L., Truman, B., Dittus, R., et al. (2001). Evaluation of delirium in critically ill patients: Validation of the Confusion Assessment Method for the Intensive Care Unit (CAM-ICU). *Critical Care Medicine*, *29*, 1370–1379.

Engel, G., & Romano, J. (1944). Studies of delirium II: Reversibility of the encephalogram with experimental procedure. *Archives of Neurology and Psychiatry*, *51*, 378–392.

Engel, G., & Romano, J. (1959). Delirium—A syndrome of cerebral insufficiency. *Journal of Chronic Disease*, *9*, 260–277.

Fadul, N., Kaur, G., Zhang, T., Palmer, J. L., & Bruera, E. (2007). Evaluation of the Memorial Delirium Assessment Scale (MDAS) for the screening of delirium by means of simulated cases by palliative care health professionals. *Supportive Care in Cancer*, *15*, 1271–1276.

Fann, J., Roth-Roemer, S., Katon, W., & Syrjala, K. (2007). Impact of delirium on cognition, distress, and health-related quality of life after hematopiet stem-cell transplantation. *Journal of Clinical Oncology*, *25*, 1223–1231.

Fick, D. M., & Foreman, F. D. (2000). Consequences of not recognizing delirium superimposed on dementia in hospitalized elderly individuals. *Journal of Gerontological Nursing*, *26*, 30–40.

Fick, D. M., Agostini, J. V., & Inouye, S. K. (2002). Delirium superimposed on dementia: A systematic review. *Journal of the American Geriatrics Society*, *50*, 1723–1732.

Fick, D. M., Kolanowski, A., Waller, J., & Inouye, S. K. (2005). Delirium superimposed on dementia in a community-dwelling managed care population: A 3-year retrospective study of occurence, cost, and utilization. *Journal of Gerontology*, *60*, 748–753.

Fogel, B. S. (1991). The High Sensitivity Cognitive Screen. *International Psychogeriatrics*, *3*(2), 273–288.

Folstein, M. F., Folstein, S. E., & McHugh, P. R. (1975). "Mini-mental State." A practical method for grading the cognitive state of patients for the clinician. *Journal of Psychiatric Research*, *12*, 189–198.

Francis, J., Martin, D., & Kapoor, W. N. (1990). A prospective study of delirium in hospitalized elderly. *Journal of the American Medical Association*, *263*, 1097–1101.

Francis, J., Strong, S., Martin, D., & Kapoor, W. (1988). Delirium in elderly general medical patients: Common but often unrecognized. *Clinical Research*, *36*, 711A.

Galanakis, P., Bickel, H., Gradinger, R., Von Gumppenberg, S., & Forstl, H. (2001). Acute confusional state in the elderly following hip surgery: Incidence, risk factors, and complications. *International Journal of Geriatric Psychiatry*, *16*, 349–355.

Grassi, L., Caraceni, A., Beltrami, E., Borreani, C., Zamorani, M., Maltoni, M., et al. (2001). Assessing delirium in cancer patients. The Italian versions of the Delirium Rating Scale and the Memorial Delirium Assessment Scale. *Journal of Pain and Symptom Management*, *21*, 59–68.

Greiner, F. C. (1817). *Der traum und das fieberhafte irreseyn*. Altenburg: Brockhaus.

Han, J., Zimmerman, E., Cutler, N., Schnelle, J., Morandi, A., Dittus, R., et al. (2009). Delirium in older emergency department patients: Recognition, risk factors, and psychomotor subtypes. *Society for Academic Emergency Medicine*, *16*, 193–200.

Harris, D. (2008). Delirium in advanced disease. *Postgraduate Medical Journal*, *83*, 525–528.

Hart, R. P., Levenson, J. L., Sessler, C. N., Best, A. M., Schwartz, S. M., & Rutherford, L. E. (1996). Validation of a cognitive test for delirium in medical ICU patients. *Psychosomatics*, *37*(6), 533–546.

Hattori, H., Kamiya, J., Shimada, H., Akiyama, H., Yasui, A., Kuroiwa, K., et al. (2009). Assessment of the risk of postoperative delirium in elderly patients using E-PASS and the NEECHAM Confusion Scale. *International Journal of Geriatric Psychiatry*, *24*, 1304–1310.

Hjermstad, M., Loge, J., & Kaasa, S. (2004). Methods for assessment of cognitive failure and delirium in palliative care patients: Implications for practice and research. *Palliative Medicine*, *18*, 494–506.

Hodkinson, H. M. (1972). Evaluation of a mental test score for assessment of mental impairment in the elderly. *Age and Ageing*, *1*, 233–238.

Huang, S., Tsai, S., Chan, C., Hwang, J., & Sim, C. (1998). Characteristics and outcome of delirium in psychiatric inpatients. *Journal of Psychiatry and Clinical Neuroscience*, *52*(1), 47–50.

Immers, H., Schuurmans, M., & van de Bijl, J. (2005). Recognition of delirium in ICU patients: A diagnostic study of the NEECHAM Confusion Scale in ICU patients. *BMC Nursing*, *4*(7), 1–6.

Inouye, S. K. (1994). The dilemma of delirium: Clinical and research controversies regarding diagnosis and evaluation of delirium in hospitalized elderly medical patients. *American Journal of Medicine*, *97*, 278–288.

Inouye, S. K. (2001). Nurses' recognition of delirium and its symptoms: Comparison of nurse and researcher ratings. *Archives of Internal Medicine*, *161*, 2467–2473.

Inouye, S. (2006). Delirium in older persons. *New England Journal of Medicine*, *354*, 1157–1165.

Inouye, S. K., & Charpentier, P. A. (1996). Precipitating factors for delirium in hospitalized elderly persons. *Journal of the American Medical Association*, *275*, 852–857.

Inouye, S., Foreman, M., Mion, L., Katz, K., & Cooney, L. (2001). Nurses' recognition of delirium and its symptoms: Comparison of nurse and researcher ratings. *Archives of Internal Medicine*, *161*, 2467–2473.

Inouye, S. K., van Dyck, C. H., Alessi, C. A., Balkin, S., Siegal, A. P., & Horwitz, R. I. (1990). Clarifying confusion: The Confusion Assessment Method. A new method for detection of delirium. *Annals of Internal Medicine*, *113*, 941–948.

Jackson, J. H. (1932). Selected writings. In J. Taylor (Ed.), London, England: Hodder & Stoughton.

Jitapunkuel, S., Pillay, I., & Ebrahim, S. (1991). The Abbreviated Mental Test: Its use and validity. *Age and Ageing*, *20*, 332–336.

Kakuma, R., du Fort, G., Arsenault, L., Perrault, A., Platt, R., Monette, J., et al. (2003). Delirium in older emergency department patients discharged home: Effect on survival. *Journal of American Geriatric Society*, *51*, 443–450.

Kiely, D. K., Bergman, M. A., Murphy, K. M., Jones, R. N., Oray, J. E., & Marcantonio, E. R. (2003). Delirium among newly admitted postacute facility patients: prevalence, symptoms, and severity. *Journal of Gerontology*, *58*(5), 441–445.

Koponen, H. J., & Riekkinen, P. J. (1993). A prospective study of delirium in elderly patients admitted to a psychiatric hospital. *Psychological Medicine*, *23*, 103–109.

Lawlor, P. G., Gagnon, B., Mancini, I. L., Pereira, J. L., Hanson, P. J., Bruera, E. D., & Suarez-Almazor, M. E. (2000). Occurrence, causes, and outcome of delirium in patients with advanced cancer. A prospective study. *Archives of Internal Medicine*, *160*, 786–794.

Leonard, M., Agar, M., Mason, C., & Lawlor, P. (2008). Delirium issues in palliative care settings. *Journal of Psychosomatic Research*, *65*, 289–298.

Levkoff, S., Cleary, P., Liptzin, B., & Evans, D. A. (1991a). Epidemiology of delirium: An overview of research issues and findings. *International Psychogeriatrics*, *3*, 149–167.

Levkoff, S., Liptzin, B., Cleary, P., Reilly, C. H., & Evans, D. (1991b). Review of research instruments and techniques used to detect delirium. *International Psychogeriatrics*, *3*(2), 253–271.

Lewis, L. M., Miller, D. K., Morley, J. E., Nork, M. J., & Lasater, L. C. (1995). Unrecognized delirium in ED geriatric patients. *American Journal of Emergency Medicine*, *13*(2), 142–145.

Linstedt, U., Berkau, A., Meyer, O., Kropp, P., & Zenz, M. (2002). The Abbreviated Mental Test in a German version for detection of postoperative delirium. *Anasthesiol Intensivmed Notfallmed Schmerzther*, *37*, 205–208.

Lipowski, Z. J. (1989). Delirium in the elderly patients. *New England Journal of Medicine*, *320*, 578–582.

Lipowski, Z. J. (1990). *Delirium; Acute confusional states*. New York, NY: Oxford University Press.

Maldonado, J. R. (2008). Pathoetiological model of delirium: A comprehensive understanding of the neurobiology of delirium and an evidence-based approach to prevention and treatment. *Critical Care Clini*, *24*, 789–856.

Marcantonio, E. R., Flacker, J. M., Michaels, M., & Resnick, N. M. (2000). Delirium is independently associated with poor functional recovery after hip fracture. *Journal of American Geriatrics Society*, *48*, 618–624.

Marcantonio, E. R., Ta, T., Duthie, E., & Resnick, N. (2002). Delirium severity and psychomotor types: Their relationship with outcomes and hip fracture repairs. *Journal of the American Geriatrics Society*, *50*, 850–857.

Marquis, F., Ouimet, S., Riker, R., Cossette, M., & Skrobik, Y. (2007). Individual delirium symptoms: Do they matter? *Critical Care Medicine*, *35*, 2533–2537.

Matsuoka, Y., Miyakeb, Y., Arakakia, H., Tanakas, K., Saekic, K., & Yamawakic, S. (2001). Clinical utility and validation of the Japanese version of Memorial Delirium Assessment Scale in a psychogeriatric inpatient setting. *General Hospital Psychiatry*, *23*, 36–40.

McAvay, G., Van Ness, P., Bogardus, J. S., Zhang, Y., Leslie, D. L., Leo-Summers, L., et al. (2006). Older adults discharged from the hospital with delirium: 1-year outcomes. *Journal of American Geriatric Society*, *54*, 1245–1250.

McAvay, G., Van Ness, P., Bogardus, S., Zhang, Y., Leslie, D., Leo-Summers, L., et al. (2007). Depressive symptoms and the risk of incident delirium in older hospitalized adults. *Journal of the American Geriatric Society*, 684–691.

McCusker, J., Cole, M., & Dendukuri, N. B. (2001). Delirium in older medical inpatients and subsequent cognitive and functional status: A prospective study. *Canadian Medical Association Journal*, *165*, 575–583.

McCusker, J., Cole, M., Dendukuri, N. B., & Belzile, E. (2004). The Delirium Index, a measure of the severity of delirium: New findings on reliability, validity, and responsiveness. *Journal of the American Geriatrics Society*, *52*, 1744–1749.

McCusker, J., Cole, M., Abrahamowicz, M., Primeau, F., & Belzile, E. (2002). Delirium predicts 12-month mortality. *Archives in Internal Medicine*, *162*, 457–463.

McNicoll, L., Pisani, M., Ely, E., Gifford, D., & Inouye, S. (2005). Detection of delirium in the Intensive Care Unit: Comparison of Confusion Assessment Method for the Intensive Care Unit with Confusion Assessment Method ratings. *Journal of the American Geriatrics Society*, *53*(3), 495–500.

Meagher, D., & Trzepacz, P. (2007). Phenomenological distinctions needed in DSM-V: Delirium, subsyndromal delirium, and dementias. *Journal of Neuropsychiatry and Clinical Neuroscience*, *19*, 468–470.

Meagher, D., O'Hanlon, D., O'Mahony, E., Casey, P., & Trzepacz, P. (2000). Relationship between symptoms and motoric subtype of delirium. *Journal of Neuropsychiatry and Clinical Neuroscience*, *12*, 51–56.

Meagher, D., Moran, M., Raju, B., Gibbons, D., Donnely, S., Saunders, J., et al. (2007). Phenomenology of delirium: Assessment of 100 adult cases using standardised measures. *British Journal of Psychiatry*, *190*, 135–141.

Namba, M., Morita, T., Imura, C., Kiyohara, E., Ishikawa, S., & Hirai, K. (2007). Terminal delirium: Families' experience. *Palliative Medicine*, *21*, 587–594.

Neelon, V. J., Champagne, M. T., McConnell, E., Carlson, J., & Funk, S. G. (1992). Use of the NEECHAM Confusion Scale to assess acute confusional states of hospitalized older patients. In S. G. Funk, E. M. Tornquist, M. T. Champagne, & R. A. Wiese (Eds.), *Key aspects of elder care: Managing falls, incontinence, and cognitive impairment*. New York, NY: Springer Publishing.

Patten, S. B., Williams, J. V., Petcu, R., & Oldfield, R. (2001). Delirium in psychiatric inpatients: A case-control study. *Canadian Journal of Psychiatry*, *46*, 162–166.

Patten, S., Williams, J., Haynes, L., McCruden, J., & Arboleda-Florez, J. (1997). The incidence of delirium in psychiatric inpatient units. *Canadian Journal of Psychiatry*, *42*, 858–863.

Plaschke, K., von Haken, R., Scholz, M., Engelhardt, R., Brobeil, A., Martin, E., et al. (2008). Comparison of the Confusion Assessment Method for the Intensive Care Unit (CAM-ICU) with the Intensive Care Delirium Screening Checklist (ICDSC) for delirium in critical care patients gives high agreement rate(s). *Intensive Care Medicine*, *34*, 431–436.

Rabins, P. V., & Folstein, M. F. (1982). Delirium and dementia: Diagnostic criteria and fatality rates. *British Journal of Psychiatry*, *140*, 149–153.

Rahkonen, T., Luukkainen-Markkula, R., Paanila, S., Sivenius, J., & Sulkaya, R. (2000). Delirium episode as a sign of undetected dementia among community dwelling elderly subjects: A 2-year follow-up study. *Journal of Neurology, Neurosurgery and Psychiatry*, *69*, 519–521.

Rothschild, J., Bates, D., & Leape, L. (2000). Preventable medical injuries in older patients. *Archives of Internal Medicine*, *160*, 2717–2728.

Rockwood, K., Goodman, J., Flynn, M., & Stolee, P. (1996). Cross-validation of the Delirium Rating Scale in older patients. *Journal of the American Geriatrics Society*, *44*, 839–842.

Rompaey, B. V., Schuurmans, M. J., Shortridge-Baggett, L. M., Truijen, S., Elseviers., M., & Bossaert, L. (2008). A comparison of the CAM-ICU and the NEECHAM Confusion Scale in intensive care delirium assessment: An observational study in non-intubated patients. *Critical Care*, *12*(1), 1–8.

Rosen, J., Sweet, R. A., Mulsant, B. H., Rifai, A. H., Pasternak, R., & Zubenko, G. S. (1994). The Delirium Rating Scale in a psychogeriatric inpatient setting. *The Journal of Neuropsychiatry and Clinical Neurosciences*, *6*, 30–35.

Roth, M. (1991). Clinical perspectives. *International Psychogeriatrics*, *3*, 309–317.

Ritchie, J., Steiner, W., & Abrahamowicz, M. (1996). Incidence of and risk factors for delirium among psychiatric inpatients. *Psychiatric Services*, *47*, 727–730.

Rudolph, J., Marcantonio, E., Culley, D., Silverstein, J., Rasmussen, L., Crosby, G., et al. (2008). Delirium is associated with early postoperative cognitive dysfunction. *Anaesthesia*, *63*(9), 941–947.

Sarasqueta, C., Bergareche, A., Arce, A., Lopez de Munain, A., Poza, J., De La Puente, E., et al. (2001). The validity of Hodkinson's Abbreviated Mental Test for dementia screening in Guipuzcoa, Spain. *European Journal of Neurology*, *8*, 435–440.

Schuurmans, M. J., Shortridge-Bagget, L. M., & Duursma, S. A. (2003a). The Delirium Observation Screening Scale: A screening instrument for delirium. *Research & Theory for Nursing Practices*, *17*, 31–50.

Schuurmans, M. J., Donders, Shortridge-Bagget, & Duursma. (2002). Delirium case findings: Pilot testing of a new screening scale for nurses. *Journal of the American Geriatric Society*, *50*(Suppl. A8), S3.

Schuurmans, M. J., Deschamps, P., Markham, S., Shortridge-Baggett, L., & Duursma, S. (2003b). The measurement of delirium: Review of Scales. *Research and Theory for Nursing Practice: An International Journal*, *17*(3), 207–225.

Siddiqi, N., House, A., & Holmes, J. (2006). Occurence and outcome of delirium in medical in-patients: A systematic literature review. *Age Ageing*, *35*, 350–364.

Siemsen, G. C., Miller, J., Newman, A. H., & Lucas, C. M. (1992). The predictive value of the NEECHAM scale. In S. G. Funk, E. M. Tornquist, M. T. Champagne, & R. A. Wiese (Eds.), *Key aspects of elder care: Managing falls, incontinence, and cognitive impairment*. New York, NY: Springer Publishing.

Silverstein, J., Steinmetz, J., Reichenberg, A., Harvey, P., & Rasmussen, L. (2007). Postoperative cognitive dysfunction in patients with preoperative cognitive impairment: Which domains are most vulnerable? *Anesthesiology*, *106*, 431–435.

Smith, M. J., Breitbart, W. S., & Platt, M. M. (1995). A critique of instruments and methods to detect, diagnose, and rate delirium. *Journal of Pain and Symptom Management*, *10*(1), 35–77.

Spiller, J., & Keen, J. (2006). Hypoactive delirium: Assessing the extent of the problem for inpatient specialist palliative care. *Palliative Medicine*, *20*, 17–23.

Strain, J. J., Fulop, G., Lebovits, A., Ginsberg, B., Robinson, M., Stern, A., et al. (1988). Screening devices for diminished cognitive capacity. *General Hospital Psychiatry*, *10*, 16–23.

Strauss, E., Sherman, E. M., & Spreen, O. (2006). *Compendium of neuropsychological tests: Administration, norms, and commentary* (3rd ed.). New York, NY: Oxford University Press.

Stuss, D., & Levine, B. (2002). Adult clinical neuropsychology: Lessons from studies of the frontal lobes. *Annual Review of Psychology*, *53*, 401–433.

Swain, D. G., O'Brien, A. G., & Nightingale, P. G. (1999). Cognitive assessment in elderly patients admitted to hospital: The relationship between the Abbreviated Mental Test and the Mini-Mental State Examination. *Clinical Rehabilitation*, *13*, 503–508.

Swain, D. G., O'Brien, A. G., & Nightingale, P. G. (2000). Cognitive assessment in elderly patients admitted to hospital: The relationship between the shortened version of the Abbreviated Mental Test and the Abbreviated Mental Test and Mini-Mental State Examination. *Clinical Rehabilitation*, *14*, 608–610.

Treloar, A. J., & MacDonald, A. J. D. (1997a). Outcome of delirium: Part 1. Outcome of delirium diagnosed by DSM-III-R, ICD-10, and CAMDEX and derivation of the Reversible Cognitive Dysfunction Scale among acute geriatric inpatients. *International Journal of Geriatric Psychiatry*, *12*, 609–613.

Treloar, A. J., & MacDonald, A. J. D. (1997b). Outcome of delirium: Part 2. Clinical features of reversible cognitive dysfunction—Are they the same as accepted definitions of delirium? *International Journal of Geriatric Psychiatry*, *12*, 614–618.

Trzepacz, P. T. (1994). A review of delirium assessment instruments. *General Hospital Psychiatry*, *16*, 397–405.

Trzepacz, P. T. (1996). Delirium: Advances in diagnosis, pathophysiology, and treatment. *The Psychiatric Clinics of North America*, *19*(3), 429–448.

Trzepacz, P. T., Baker, R. W., & Greenhouse, J. (1988). A symptom rating scale for delirium. *Psychiatry Research*, *23*, 89–97.

Trzepacz, P. T., Mittal, D., Torres, R., Kanary, K., Norton, J., & Jimerson, N. (2001). Validation of the Delirium Rating Scale-Revised-98: Comparison with the Delirium Rating Scale and the Cognitive Test for Delirium. *Journal of Neuropsychiatry and Clinical Neuroscience*, *13*, 229–242.

van Gemert, L., & Schuurmans, M. (2007). The Neecham Confusion Scale and the Delirium Observation Screening Scale: Capacity to discriminate and ease of use in clinical practice. *BMC Nursing*, *6*, 1–6.

van Zyl, L., & Seitz, D. (2006). Delirium concisely: Condition is associated with increased morbidity, mortality, and length of hospitalization. *Geriatrics*, *61*(3), 18–21.

Voyer, P., Cole, M., McCusker, J., & Belzile, E. (2006). Prevalence and symptoms of delirium superimposed on dementia. *Clinical Nursing Research*, *15*, 46–66.

Voyer, P., McCusker, J., Cole, M., St-Jacques, S., & Khomenko, L. (2007). Factors associated with delirium severity among older patients. *Journal of Clinical Nursing*, *16*, 819–831.

Wallesch, C. W., & Hundsalz, A. (1994). Language function in delirium: A comparison of single word processing in acute confusional states and probable Alzheimer's disease. *Brain and Language*, *46*, 592–606.

Williams, M. A. (1991). Delirium/acute confusional states: Evaluation devices in nursing. *International Psychogeriatrics*, *3*(2), 301–307.

Woodcock, R. W., & Johnson, M. B. (1975). *Woodcock-Johnson Psycho-Educational Battery.* Hingham, MA: Teaching Resources.

Wolff, H. G., & Curran, D. (1935). Nature of delirium and allied states: The dysergastic reaction. *Archives of Neurology and Psychiatry*, *51*, 378–392.

CHAPTER

Assessment of Cognitive Training

8

George W. Rebok, Jeanine M. Parisi, Alden L. Gross, Adam P. Spira
Department of Mental Health, Johns Hopkins Bloomberg School of Public Health, Baltimore, MD, USA

INTRODUCTION

Memory loss is a common concern among older adults, but it is not an inevitable part of cognitive aging. Research findings suggest that behavioral interventions may help individuals maintain or improve memory and cognitive performance in later life. The challenge for the geriatric clinician is to comprehensively assess an individual in order to determine the nature and severity of impairment and best determine the most appropriate course of treatment, including which type of cognitive training program(s) may be most beneficial.This chapter is structured to guide a clinician through: (1) the assessment of cognitive impairment; (2) selection of the most appropriate cognitive training program; and (3) evaluation of the effects of cognitive training, both in cognitively normal older adults and in those with mild cognitive impairment (MCI) and dementia. Although several types of cognitive training programs are available, the focus of this chapter is on ways to assess changes resulting from memory training programs.

The aging process is accompanied by numerous neuropsychological and cognitive changes. Many cognitive abilities, such as processing speed, working memory, inductive reasoning, spatial orientation, and word fluency are subject to age-related decline (Salthouse, 1996; Schaie, 2005). However, other abilities (e.g., language, semantic knowledge, memory for emotional events, implicit or procedural memory) do not decline appreciably in normal aging (Baltes, 1997; Schaie, 2005; Zacks & Hasher, 2006).

Many older adults are concerned about memory loss and declining cognitive health (Connell, Roberts, & McLaughlin, 2007). This may be because cognitive function is strongly related to the ability to perform tasks of daily living (Allaire & Marsiske, 2002; Owsley, Sloane, McGwin, & Ball, 2002) and, in turn, to live independently. However, normative age-related changes in cognitive abilities are qualitatively different than memory impairments typically associated with Alzheimer's disease and related dementias (Whalley, Deary, Appleton, & Starr, 2004). Whereas occasionally forgetting a name or where one put the car keys typically is not cause for concern, memory loss that affects day-to-day function (e.g., difficulty performing familiar tasks, disorientation of time and place, poor or decreased judgment, changes in mood and behavior) is much more problematic.

In the past, cognitive decline was commonly considered an inevitable consequence of aging. Several research findings, however, have demonstrated the plasticity of the aging brain. We now know that older adults are able to learn new skills or develop compensatory mechanisms for the skills they already possess, even among individuals with pre-existing memory impairments (e.g., Belleville, 2008; Belleville et al., 2006; Camp, Foss, Stevens, & O'Hanlon, 1996; Cavallini, Pagnin, & Vecchi,

Handbook of Assessment in Clinical Gerontology. DOI: 10.1016/B978-0-12-374961-1.10008-9

2003; De Vreese, Neri, Fioravanti, Belloi, & Zanetti, 2001; Grandmaison & Simard, 2003; Rapp, Brenes, & Marsh, 2002; Rasmusson, Rebok, Bylsma, & Brandt, 1999; Rebok, 2008; Verhaeghen, Marcoen, & Goossens, 1992; Woolverton, Scogin, Shackelford, Black, & Duke, 2001). This research has uncovered several effective behavioral interventions to help maintain or improve cognitive performance. The challenge for the geriatric clinician is to comprehensively assess an individual, to determine the nature and severity of impairment, and to identify the training program(s) that are most likely to be beneficial.

TOOLS AND TECHNIQUES FOR INITIAL ASSESSMENT OF MEMORY AND COGNITION IN LATE ADULTHOOD

Before selecting or implementing a cognitive training program, the clinician should assess the client's neuropsychological, physical, and psychological status, as well as other contextual and life-event information. A full history is needed because the nature and severity of the cognitive impairment can render particular treatment options inappropriate. A patient's lifestyle or personal preferences might also determine the course of treatment.

Memory Assessments

There are many neuropsychological tools and techniques available not only for evaluating effects of memory training on clients, but also for determining the need for specific kinds of training. Table 8.1 lists the major types of memory and a few of the most common measures used to assess each type, but it is by no means comprehensive. For a more complete treatment of neuropsychological assessment, please refer to Lezak (2004) or Craik and Tulving (2000). Neuropsychologists typically test several different memory domains in order to best understand the nature and severity of memory impairment because different memory abilities may show differential age decline and responsiveness to training. For instance, a patient with early signs of dementia will show deficits on delayed recall components of verbal memory tests, but their prospective memory might be relatively unaffected (Albert, 2008).

The term "working memory" refers to the short-term storage and manipulation of information (Baddeley, 1990). Neuropsychological tests that assess working memory include serial digit learning (Benton et al., 1994) and digit span backwards (Wechsler, 1987) tests. In contrast, memory for information that is retrieved after a longer time frame (e.g., over several days or years) is often referred to as long-term memory. Long-term memory can be further divided into declarative (explicit) and procedural (implicit) memory.

Episodic memory falls under the category of declarative long-term memory, and is most easily assessed with a long-delay recall trial from any word-list learning test such as the Hopkins Verbal Learning Test–Revised (Brandt & Benedict, 2001). This type of memory best discriminates persons with Alzheimer's disease from cognitively normal older adults because a defining feature of the disease is rapid information loss after only brief delays. Once a person has dementia, however, severity cannot be measured with this type of assessment because episodic memory is impaired early in the disease course (Albert, 2008).

Semantic memory is also a form of declarative memory and refers to memory for meanings using general knowledge about the world. Semantic memory can be assessed through recognition tests such as the Portland Digit Recognition test (Binder, 1993) or the Word Memory Test (Green, Allen, & Astner, 1996). Because semantic memory, unlike episodic memory, does not decline with age (Craik, 1977; Zacks & Hasher, 2006), strategies that take advantage of such existing abilities may be easier for older adults to learn with training.

Table 8.1 Memory Domains and Measures

Memory Type	Description	Measures
Working memory	Brain's workbench where environmental stimuli are encoded	Brown-Peterson Technique (Peterson & Peterson, 1959) Telephone Test (Crook, Ferris, McCarthy, & Rae, 1980) Serial Digit Learning (Benton et al., 1994) Digit Span Test (Wechsler, 1987)
Episodic memory	Memory for new learning	California Verbal Learning Task (Delis, Kramer, Kaplan, & Ober, 1987) Hopkins Verbal Learning Task-Revised (Brandt & Benedict, 2001 Rey Auditory Verbal Learning Test (Rey, 1941) Logical Memory Test (Wechsler, 1987) Rivermead Behavioural Memory Test (Wilson, Cockburn, & Baddeley, 1985)
Semantic memory	Memory for meanings	Word Memory Test (Green, Allen, & Astner, 1996) Portland Digit Recognition Test (Binder, 1993)
Procedural memory	Memory for processes	Lexical Decision Task (Meyer & Schvaneveldt, 1971) Implicit Association Test (Greenwald, McGhee, & Schwarz, 1998) Word Stem Completion (Light, 1991)
Prospective memory	Memory for future events	Cambridge Prospective Memory Test (Wilson et al., 2005)

Procedural (implicit) memory is a type of long-term memory for skills such as riding a bicycle or typing on a keyboard that one may not consciously think about. Tests of procedural memory include the Implicit Association Task (Greenwald, McGhee, & Schwarz, 1998) and Lexical Decision Task (Meyer & Schvaneveldt, 1971).

Prospective memory is memory for future events, such as performing a task at a certain time (e.g., attending a doctor's appointment on Tuesday, after lunch). Although prospective memory may be assessed fairly easily (such as by asking a patient to call your office in four days), validated assessments, such as the Cambridge Prospective Memory Test (Wilson et al., 2005), are also available.

Consideration of Table 8.1 is only the beginning of a clinician's decision-making process about memory assessment. As some tasks are more burdensome and time-consuming than others, a clinician should consider how much time they have to allocate for assessments. For example, verbal memory tests such as the Auditory Verbal Learning Test (AVLT; Rey, 1941) or the California Verbal Learning Test (CVLT; Delis, Kramer, Kaplan, & Ober, 2000) have good psychometric properties (reliability, validity), and are well-established tests. However, they take longer to administer compared with the Hopkins Verbal Learning Test-Revised (HVLT-R; Brandt & Benedict, 2001). The HVLT-R also has well-established reliability and validity, and is well tolerated, even by significantly impaired individuals. Finally, it provides environmental support for memory through semantic categories that can serve as cues for memory recall.

Other Cognitive Assessments

In addition to assessing memory function, it is equally important to assess related cognitive constructs (e.g., attention, perception, language, executive functioning) as these abilities are often related to memory performance. Further, certain cognitive impairments can limit the options for memory training. For instance, many memory-training programs, such as the ACTIVE memory training intervention, focus on attention and concentration skills (Jobe et al., 2001). Therefore, an individual demonstrating pre-existing impairment in these cognitive domains may not have the skills and abilities to adhere to, or potentially benefit from, a memory training intervention (Cahn-Weiner, Malloy, Rebok, & Ott, 2003; Unverzagt et al., 2007).

Table 8.2 presents some common assessments for cognitive domains other than memory, as well as general cognitive status. *General* or *global cognitive status* is measured by tests such as the Mini-Mental State Exam (MMSE; Folstein, Folstein, & McHugh, 1975) that assess multiple cognitive domains, using domain-specific cognitive items. For instance, the MMSE includes items that separately assess verbal memory, visuospatial ability, and orientation. Measures of general cognition can be a quick and efficient way to assess a patient's cognitive state, but are not as sensitive as domain-specific measures of cognition in identifying particular cognitive deficits (Leroi, Sheppard, & Lyketsos, 2002;

Table 8.2 Cognitive Domains and Measures

Cognitive Domain	Description	Measures
Global cognition	General cognitive status	Mini-Mental Status Exam (Folstein, Folstein, & McHugh., 1975)
		Telephone Interview for Cognitive Status (Brandt et al., 1988)
		Cognitive Abilities Screening Instrument (Teng et al., 1994)
		WAIS-III (Wechsler, 1987)
Attention	Selective concentration	Brief Test of Attention (Schretlen, 1989)
		Digit Symbol Substitution Test (Wechsler, 1987)
		Paced Auditory Serial Attention Test (Crawford, Obonsawin, & Allan, 1998)
		Digit Span Forward Test (Wechsler, 1987)
Visuospatial or perceptual ability	Capacity to transform visual and spatial stimuli	Rey-Osterrieth Complex Figure Draw (Osterrieth, 1944; Woodrome & Fastenau, 2005)
		Brief Visuospatial Memory Test-revised (Benedict, 1997)
		Benton Line Orientation (Warrington & Rabin, 1970)
		Clock Drawing Task (Shulman, 2000)
		Pattern Comparison (Salthouse & Babcock, 1991)
Language	Verbal fluency and expression of speech	Boston Naming Test (Kaplan, Goodglass, & Weintraub, 1983)
		Verbal Fluency Test (Harrison et al., 2000)
Executive function	Shifting	Trail-Making Test (Armitage, 1946)
		Wisconsin Card Sort Test (Berg, 1948)
	Inhibition	Stroop Test (Kindt, Biermanm, & Brosschot, 1996)
		Wisconsin Card Sort Test (Berg, 1948)
	Planning/problem solving	Candle Problem (Duncker, 1945)

Lyketsos, Chen, & Anthony, 1999). Additionally, global measures are subject to ceiling effects among cognitively intact older adults (Leroi et al., 2002).

Tests of *attention* are typically tasks that measure an individual's ability to concentrate and sustain focus over time and ignore irrelevant stimuli. Examples include the Brief Test of Attention (Schretlen, 1989) and the Digit Symbol Substitution task (Wechsler, 1987). Low performance on such tasks implies problems with sustained attention. Such an impairment could obviously affect performance on other cognitive tasks, such as those involving memory. Patients with mild dementia show little impairment when given simple attention tasks like the Digit Span Forward test (Wechsler, 1987), but impairment is more apparent as tasks become increasingly more complex.

Tests of *visuospatial* or *perceptual ability* include the Pattern Comparison and Rey–Osterrieth Complex Figure Draw tasks (Osterrieth, 1944; Salthouse & Babcock, 1991). They test the mental capacity to remember or mentally manipulate visual and spatial stimuli, and deficits may suggest neurological injury, presence of dementia, or an agnosia of some sort (Colcombe & Kramer, 2003).

Tests of *language ability*, such as the Verbal Fluency Test (Harrison et al., 2000) or the Boston Naming Test (Kaplan, Goodglass, & Weintraub, 1983), assess the verbal production and expression of speech. Semantic and phonemic fluency are two types of fluency measured by the Verbal Fluency Test (Harrison et al., 2000). Semantic or category fluency is tested by giving the patient a semantic category upon which to draw, such as animals. Phonemic fluency taps into memory functions but also requires executive information processing functions to initiate and maintain systematic memory search strategies for information given an ambiguous cue. Both types of fluency are predictive of dementia (Chan, Butters, Salmon, & Maloney, 1993; Henry, Crawford, & Phillips, 2004).

Finally, *executive abilities* are a broad category of cognitive functions that encompasses cognitive control and coordination of multiple cognitive capacities (Duncan, Emslie, Williams, Johnson, & Freer, 1996). Examples include set-shifting and multi-tasking (Kramer & Madden, 2008; Salthouse, Hambrick, Lukas, & Dell, 1996), problem solving, inhibition (Metcalfe & Mischel, 1999; Salthouse & Meinz, 1995), and goal-directed behaviors like meal preparation and shopping (Kramer, Hahn, & Gopher, 1999; Kray, Eber, & Lindenberger, 2004).

DIAGNOSTIC ISSUES

When administering clinical assessments to both cognitively healthy and impaired (e.g., mild cognitive impairment, Alzheimer's disease) older adults, the clinician should remain flexible and adjust which tests are used as needed. This may be especially true when working with individuals with moderate to severe cognitive impairments. Factors such as age, educational level, and cultural influences can affect how well patients perform on assessments and should be taken into account when administering tests and interpreting results. Such characteristics are important in order to establish a reliable measure of the patient's baseline ability, because not all older adults will perform in line with published norms of neuropsychological tests.

Another issue that frequently arises in the diagnosis of memory impairments is the presence of comorbid conditions. An individual may complain of memory deficits, which are secondary to other issues, such as depression or anxiety (Verhaeghen, Geraerts, & Marcoen, 2000). Therefore, the patient should be screened for these and other comorbid mental conditions that may co-occur with memory impairment. Clinicians should also take into account self-reports as well as surrogate reports of a client's memory problems, as these complaints may be an early marker of deteriorating cognition. These reports may also help determine the types of tasks with which older adults have difficulty and identify their self-perceived strengths and weaknesses.

In summary, cognitive assessments should be used in combination with other assessment tools and techniques (e.g., physical, neurological, and psychological assessments), and findings should be considered in the context of the individual's life history. Further, the clinician may use this information to recommend a training approach and individually tailor the training program to best meet the needs and preferences of the client.

COGNITIVE TRAINING PROGRAMS AND INTERVENTIONS

Cognitive training interventions have provided much of the evidence supporting the notion of developmental plasticity later in life. These interventions typically involve guided practice on standard tasks designed to engage particular cognitive functions, such as memory, attention, processing speed, or executive functions (Clare & Woods, 2004). The largest training study to date, ACTIVE (Advanced Cognitive Training for Independent and Vital Elderly), is an ongoing randomized clinical trial designed to examine the effectiveness and durability of cognitive interventions on basic measures of cognition, as well as immediate and long-term transfer effects to everyday activities (Ball et al., 2002; Willis et al., 2006). Participants were randomized into one of four treatment groups (memory, reasoning, speed of processing training, or a no-contact control group). Each type of training involved strategy instruction and practice exercises, and was provided in ten 60–75 minute group sessions distributed over the course of five to six weeks. Results indicated that each intervention immediately improved the targeted cognitive ability compared with baseline, and the improvements were durable at least until a five-year follow-up.

Moreover, these training gains transferred to more distal outcomes related to everyday cognitive functioning, including better instrumental activities of daily living, increased mobility, improved locus of control, and improved health-related quality of life (Bherer et al., 2006; Edwards et al., 2002; Edwards et al., 2005; Jennings, Webster, Kleykamp, & Dagenbach, 2005; Roenker, Cissell, Ball, Wadley, & Edwards, 2003; Willis et al., 2006; Wolinsky et al., 2009). Therefore, these results provide evidence for the long-term benefits of cognitive interventions, potentially delaying cognitive and functional decline later in life.

Other types of training programs involve multi-factorial approaches. In addition to strategy training, these programs also focus on emotional states (Neely & Bäckman, 1993; Yesavage, Sheikh, Tanke, & Hill, 1988), cognitive beliefs (Lachman, Weaver, Bandura, Elliott, & Lewkowicz, 1992; Valentijn et al., 2005; West, Bagwell, & Dark-Freudeman, 2008), attentional skills (Stigsdotter & Bäckman, 1989; West et al., 2003; Yesavage & Rose, 1983), or educating individuals about their cognitive health (West et al., 2008). For instance, meta-memory training teaches self-monitoring routines and self-regulation of behavior, facilitates improved understanding of memory impairments, and provides external feedback (Dunlosky, Cavallini, Roth, McGuire, Vecchi, & Hertzog, 2007). In this educational approach, clients are taught to recognize cognitive/memory problems and may benefit from improved understanding of the nature and effects of their problems. Training through such comprehensive approaches in addition to traditional memory training may be more advantageous than memory training alone (Neely & Bäckman, 1993; Stigsdotter & Bäckman, 1989; Woolverton et al., 2001), perhaps increasing the transfer and generalization of skills (Shute & Gawlick, 1995).

The majority of training interventions have been conducted in a group format led by trained facilitators, who provide instruction, practice, and feedback (Rebok, Carlson, & Langbaum, 2007). These sessions typically last from 60–90 minutes and are distributed over the course of a few weeks (Rebok, 2008; Verhaghen et al., 1992). Implementing these interventions is costly and relies on coordinating schedules of group members and facilitators, as well as the availability of a suitable location, limiting their practical utility. As such, there has been recent interest in exploring alternative ways to implement and disseminate cognitive training interventions. Training platforms, such as audiotape and videotape training (Rebok, Rassmusson, Bylsma, & Brandt, 1997; West & Crook, 1992), and computerized and online training (Hermann & Plude, 1998; Mahncke, Bronstone, & Merzenich, 2006; Morrell et al., 2006; Saczynski, Rebok, Whitfield, & Plude, 2004), have yielded promising results (Bottiroli & Cavallini, 2009). There are advantages and disadvantages of different training approaches (e.g., web-based vs. in-person training, one-on-one vs. small-group training). However, results suggest that improvements on memory tasks frequently occur as a result of memory training, regardless of the type of training program provided (Cavallini et al., 2003; Rasmusson et al., 1999; Verhaeghen et al., 1992).

With so many types of interventions available, how does a clinician decide on the most effective type of memory program for a given individual? Several considerations should factor into the clinician's selection, such as the client's cognitive and functional ability, ease of strategy use, and personal preferences, including how much time the individual is willing to devote to learning and practicing the training techniques. Furthermore, the type of intervention that may be most appropriate and yield the most benefit for any given individual may depend on age, education, the nature and severity of the cognitive impairment, as well as other physical or mental health conditions (Bagwell & West, 2008; Bissig & Lustig, 2007; Verhaeghen et al., 1992; Yesavage, Sheikh, Friedman, & Tanke, 1990). For instance, among cognitively healthy older adults, interventions typically focus on training cognitive skills to enhance current function, with the goal of postponing or preventing future decline (Acevedo & Loewenstein, 2007). On the other hand, when individuals demonstrate pre-existing cognitive impairment, the goal is to make the most of remaining cognitive and functional skills (Acevedo & Loewenstein, 2007; Camp et al., 1996; Camp & Stevens, 1990; Clare, Wilson, Carter, & Hodges, 2003) or to adjust environmental demands so that cognitive load is reduced (e.g., by providing external memory aids) (Bourgeois, 1990; Clare & Woods, 2004) in hopes that everyday functioning will benefit.

As mentioned earlier, there are many different types of cognitive training programs available, but the focus of this chapter is on programs involving memory training. We now turn the discussion to specific memory techniques and strategies that may be effective in the maintenance or optimization of memory performance.

MEMORY TRAINING TECHNIQUES

Several studies have suggested that both healthy and cognitively impaired older adults are capable of learning and applying new memory techniques that improve their memory performance (Cavallini et al., 2003; Rasmusson et al., 1999; Sitzer, Twamley, & Jeste, 2006; Woolverton et al., 2001). Multiple memory training strategies exist, including mnemonic strategy training, prospective memory training, spaced-retrieval, procedural memory training, and training in the use of external memory aids. Below we describe several options for both cognitively healthy and impaired older adults who wish to improve their cognitive health and well-being (Floyd & Scogin, 1997; Rebok et al., 2007; Verhaeghen et al., 1992).

Mnemonic Strategy Training

Many cognitive training intervention studies have sought to improve memory skills through the training of mnemonic techniques. The idea behind using mnemonics is to encode difficult-to-remember information in a way that is meaningful and easier to remember. These strategies include rehearsal, the use of imagery, the association or categorization of items, and the method of loci (visualizing items to be remembered in a sequence of specific, well-learned locations).

Rehearsal emphasizes the importance of repetition and practice to facilitate learning and improve recall (Gordon & Berger, 2003; Heun, Burkart, & Benkert, 1997). *Visual imagery* entails mentally picturing items to be remembered in logical or illogical contexts (Rankin, Karol, & Tuten, 1984; Rasmusson et al., 1999; Sharps & Price-Sharps, 1996). *Organization/categorization* involves grouping (also referred to as chunking or clustering) items into meaningful categories. *Association* entails making connections between items or pieces of information, and might be made with respect to time (e.g., remembering to take morning medications with breakfast), environment (e.g., mentally retracing steps through the house to locate lost keys), or specific characteristics of a person (e.g., "Kyle with the nice smile"). The more personally meaningful the association is to the individual, the greater the likelihood that the association will be remembered.

These simple strategies are often combined to form more complex mnemonic strategies, such as face—name recognition, name-learning name-recall, number and story mnemonics, and the method of loci. *Face—name recognition, name-learning, and name-recall* involve learning to couple faces with names by integrating mnemonic devices, phonemic aids, and visual imagery. *Number mnemonics* are used to remember strings of numbers like dates, phone numbers, and addresses (Derwinger, Neely, MacDonald, & Bäckman, 2005; Hill, Campbell, Foxley, & Lindsay, 1997), whereas *story* or *sentence mnemonics* involve creating a story or sentence using to-be-remembered items to enable later recall (e. g., Hill, Allen, & McWhorter, 1991). The *method of loci* is a mnemonic link system based on places, such as locations on the body or sites along one's route to work. Each location is paired with a to-be-remembered item, and this structured sequence of images provides memory cues to enable recall (e.g., Cavallini et al., 2003; Hill et al., 1991; Kliegl, Smith, & Baltes, 1989; Rebok & Balcerak, 1989; Yesavage & Rose, 1984).

Prospective Memory Training/Spaced-Retrieval Training

During early stages of dementia, interventions may target well-preserved skills to prevent further decline (Bäckman, 1992; Heindel, Salmon, Shults, Walicke, & Butters, 1989). In fact, Alzheimer's disease patients show normal implicit memory abilities in several situations and are able to learn certain skills such as motor, perceptual, and cognitive skills (Deweer et al., 1994). Using *prospective memory training* or *spaced-retrieval training* the clinician asks the client to remember information or to carry out a target task in a specified number of minutes. The goal is to increase the intervening delay systematically according to a learner's performance (e.g., Camp, 1989; Camp & Stevens, 1990; Camp et al., 1996), thereby building the skills that the person needs to complete daily activities.

Procedural Memory Training

Through repeated practice, *procedural* (*implicit*) *memory training* enables individuals to learn or improve performance of a motor task (e.g., hand washing, brushing teeth, using the telephone, opening and closing a door, dressing) (Saint-Cyr, Taylor, & Lang, 1988; Ullman, 2001; Zanetti et al., 1997; Zanetti et al., 2001). This type of training is usually individually tailored to the needs of the client and centered on specific activities of daily life, such as getting to appointments on time, medication adherence, or remembering names (Acevedo & Loewenstein, 2007; Clare & Woods, 2004; Woods, Thorgrimsen, Spector, Royan, & Orrell., 2006). When the individual has severe memory impairments, family members or primary caregivers are essential resources in the implementation of at-home practice of these memory training programs (Davis, Massman, & Doody, 2001; De Vreese et al., 2001).

External Memory Aids

Both healthy and impaired older adults may compensate for normal memory losses and acquired difficulties through the use of external aids like calendars, reminder notes, and recorded messages. The Internet and other computer resources also serve as external aids that can assist one's memory and ability to function independently in one's community. The beneficial effects of training with external aids can be enhanced if the individual plays an active role in the identification of the problem to be treated and is motivated to use the external aids. Research has suggested that the use of external aids in combination with internal memory strategies may be particularly effective for impaired individuals (Bourgeois & Mason, 1996; Fleming, Shum, Strong, & Lightbody, 2005; West, 1985).

Although we present several options for memory training, we cannot provide an exact prescription for the type of training that should be administered in any particular case. Instead, a clinician needs to assess each individual's personal preferences and determine what strategies can be learned, maintained, and generalized outside of the training context to improve everyday functioning. With this said, it is often those who need training the most who seem to benefit the least. For instance, training gains tend to be reduced for older individuals (over 75 years of age) and those with lower initial cognitive ability (Verhaeghen et al., 1992).

MEMORY AND COGNITIVE ASSESSMENT AND INTERVENTIONS IN DIVERSE POPULATIONS

As culture shapes one's values, perceptions, and beliefs, it may also affect the identification of memory impairment and response to treatment. Therefore, an additional challenge for the clinician is to provide effective and culturally appropriate assessments and interventions for racial/ethnic minorities (Falicov, 1998; Tharp, 1991).

Identifying Cognitive Impairment: Screening Assessments

Several considerations need to be addressed when identifying appropriate clinical outcome measures to be used with ethnically diverse clients (Faison et al., 2007). Standard neuropsychological measures are often influenced by variables related to cultural background and ethnicity, and rely on literacy skills, knowledge, invalidity or education (Manly et al., 1998). This may lead to elderly members of minority groups being misdiagnosed as a result of inaccurate or culturally inappropriate testing methods (Dilworth-Anderson, Hendrie, Manly, Khachaturian, & Fazio, 2008; Loewenstein, Acevedo, Czaja, & Dura, 2004). Therefore, researchers need to develop more sensitive screenings that take into account variations in both culture and language to produce meaningful results (Manly, 2005). For instance, the Cognitive Abilities Screening Instrument was developed as a general cognitive ability measure sensitive to dementia in Asian American populations (Teng et al., 1994). There is some evidence, however, that screening assessments, such as the Mini-Mental State Examination, the Alzheimer's Disease Assessment Scale, and the Clinical Dementia Rating Scale, may be equally sensitive among different ethnic groups (Sano et al., 1997; Bell, Sano, Jin, Thomas, & Thal, 1999); however, there is still much work to be done in this area.

Treatment of Cognitive Impairment: Interventions

A second concern is how to most appropriately take cultural factors into consideration in the development of the treatment plan. The clinician should ask the individual which group they self-identify with and attempt to understand the beliefs and practices of that culture. The clinician should also try to understand how cultural elements could affect adherence to the treatment. Increasing the cultural relevance of interventions may increase the likelihood of adherence (Hepworth, Rooney, Rooney, Strom-Gottfried, & Larsen, 2006). Some research suggests that the value placed on meaningful activities and rewarding relationships varies by racial and ethnic group membership (e.g., Gaines, 1989). Therefore, the support of friends and family may play a substantive role in treatment progress and maintenance of activities. Furthermore, different racial or ethnic groups may be more likely to adhere to the interventions if held in familiar and comfortable surroundings, such as local churches or community centers (McCabe, Varricchio, & Padberg, 1994).

It is also important to explore options for improving communication within diverse communities. When English is not the primary language, it is essential to include bilingual members on an intervention team, as well as provide bilingual materials (McCabe et al., 1994; Olin, Dagerman, Fox, Bowers, & Schneider, 2002). Additionally, when illiteracy is an issue, information can be provided through the use of videotape or other graphic tools (Millon-Underwood, Sanders, & Davis, 1993).

Although it is important to be aware of cultural differences, clinicians should make certain that they do not stereotype their clients based on racial or ethnic group membership. The clinician also should take into account other attributes (e.g., gender, religion) that may contribute to the successful implementation of memory training programs (Falicov, 1998; Paradis, Friedman, Hatch, & Ackerman, 1996).

USE OF REASSESSMENT IN CLINICAL WORK

For all clients, the clinician should follow up at intervals congruent with the expected rate of change in the training's target abilities. The standard neuropsychological approach to assessing memory problems is to test someone once and to compare their scores with how most people of a similar age and background would perform (Lezak, 2004). However, this ignores the client's pre-morbid level of cognitive function (Manly, 2005). Individual changes in cognitive and memory function can only be detected by periodically evaluating memory performance, as one's own previous abilities may be more important than how an individual currently measures up to peers (Nesselroade & Baltes, 1979).

During treatment, an ongoing assessment of memory performance and attitudes to the training program would allow the clinician to determine if the selected course of treatment was appropriate and identify modifications that need to be made. A clinician would also be able to determine the level of adherence or compliance with the treatment program. For instance, patients with MCI may initially respond to mnemonic strategies but, as problems progress to Alzheimer's disease, other techniques such as spaced-retrieval may have to be implemented. Additionally, periodically assessing memory over the course of treatment would allow a clinician to identify memory changes that may be related to changes in other medical or psychological conditions, which may alter course of treatment or treatment outcomes.

If a client does not appear to benefit from training there are several options. The clinician may want to begin with an open and sincere conversation with the client or primary caregiver to gain a better understanding of recent medical or cognitive changes that may affect results of training, as well as to determine if the type if training is not well-matched to the client's background and skills. Also, treatment decisions should be part of a larger collaborative effort and, if possible, consultation with the individual's primary care physician may help determine if a memory training program would be appropriate for use with a client. There are several reasons why training may not benefit a client, including medical conditions, limited cognitive ability, and low motivation or adherence to treatment regimen. Once the reasons are determined, the clinician may need to modify the current training program or switch to a different training program. In some cases, this may simply involve additional practice or incorporating new memory techniques; other cases may require redesigning the training program. If neither of these options present viable solutions, the clinician may choose to end training sessions altogether. If there are noted instances of worsening cognitive impairment, the clinician should end training immediately and refer the individual to follow-up with their primary care physician.

Once a training program is complete, ongoing cognitive assessment enables the clinician to monitor the maintenance of training gains and determine whether "booster session" are needed (Hertzog, Kramer, Wilson, & Lindenberger, 2008; Rebok, 2008). In addition to tracking and documenting a patient's memory change, reassessment might indicate a need for continued practice with training materials to sustain any gains reaped from training. Retraining or reminding clients periodically about what they learned in training has been shown to help maintain training benefits (Willis et al., 2006). How often a client should be reassessed depends on how long it takes to show reliable change in the aspect of memory that was tested and the target of intervention (Hoffman & Stawski, 2009). It is important to identify these relevant time intervals in order to detect meaningful change over time rather than transient, within-person fluctuations (Nesselroade, 1991).

CLINICAL CASE STUDY

We present a case study below to summarize the previously discussed information. We will describe an older adult with memory complaints and depressed mood but cognitively normal for his age. The scenario will portray how the clinician could conduct an initial assessment, make a diagnosis, determine a treatment/intervention approach, and monitor and evaluate changes in memory and cognitive performance.

Case Study 1

Mr A is an 81-year-old white male with 18 years of education, whose wife died several years ago after a 10-year course of Alzheimer's disease. At a recent check-up appointment with his primary care physician, Mr A reported experiencing depressed mood and memory problems over the prior two months. Mr A's physician contacted Dr B, a clinical psychologist with extensive experience working with older adults. The primary care physician informed Dr B that Mr A was in very good health; his only medical problems were mild arthritis and well-controlled hypertension. Mr A agreed to meet with Dr B and in their initial session Mr A explained that he had experienced these same mood and cognitive symptoms after his wife passed away, but that they had resolved in the year following her death. Dr B administered a depression screening measure and referred Mr A to a neuropsychologist colleague for a cognitive evaluation. Consistent with his complaints, results indicated that Mr A had moderate depressive symptoms and noteworthy deficits in verbal memory that were probably due to depression. Dr B explained to Mr A that his deficits might be explained by his mood disturbance, and they completed 12 weeks of cognitive behavioral therapy aimed at improving his depressive symptoms.

Mr A's depressive symptoms decreased substantially with treatment, and eventually went into full remission, yet he still complained of forgetfulness. Further neuropsychological testing indicated that Mr A's memory was within the normal range for an individual of his age and level of education. Based on Mr A's complaints and his desire to do something to improve his memory, Dr B suggested that they begin a memory training program. Mr A was enthusiastic about this suggestion and after Dr B explained more about the program, and Mr A consented, they completed a comprehensive baseline memory assessment. This included standardized tests of visual, verbal, spatial, and procedural memory (see Table 8.1), as well as an assessment of Mr A's beliefs about how good his memory was, relative to most of his peers. Mr A also completed a memory diary, in which he recorded instances of memory successes and memory lapses over one week. Although Mr A often failed to record memory successes, to his surprise, completing this diary exercise revealed that he had relatively few memory lapses, and that these tended to occur in particular contexts. Specifically, Mr A had difficulty recalling the names of new acquaintances, and he found this awkward and embarrassing when he subsequently encountered them.

Based on Mr A's neuropsychological test results (indicating normal cognition), the pattern of his self-reported memory lapses, and the existing evidence base, Dr B decided that a multi-component intervention, involving both face–name and name-learning interventions, would be the most appropriate and he obtained Mr A's informed consent to begin this treatment. Prior to implementing the intervention, Dr B conducted a pre-treatment assessment by presenting Mr A with 10 pictures of individuals he had cut out of magazines, telling Mr A their (made-up) names, and instructing him to remember them. Twenty minutes later, Dr B showed Mr A the same photos and asked him to recall these individuals' names. He recorded the number that Mr A named correctly, to serve as a measure of baseline performance.

Dr B explained that learning to remember names was similar to many other skills, i.e., it required consistent practice. In addition to encouraging Mr A to practice face–name and name-learning methods in his everyday life, Dr B provided him with in-home practice materials, which he prepared by cutting 50 different faces out of magazines, pasting them to the back of index cards, and writing names for each individual on the back of the cards. They agreed that Mr A would learn the names of 10 individuals each week on his own, and that Dr B would quiz him during their weekly session. Mr A consistently completed these in-home exercises, and he and Dr B plotted his progress on a chart at each of their weekly sessions. Over the next six weeks, Mr A showed steady improvement on his quiz scores.

After 10 sessions, to assess changes in subjective memory, Dr B asked Mr A to complete the memory diary once again over the course of one week. Consistent with his objective improvement on the objective name-learning exercises, Mr A recorded fewer name-related memory failures and more successes. He noted that these gains enhanced his confidence and his desire to socialize. Given the resolution of his depressive symptoms and his memory improvement, Dr B suggested that they stop meeting weekly but that they check in once every six months, to evaluate Mr A's mood and to complete a booster session to review name-learning and face–name strategies as needed.

CONCLUSION

As the population of individuals aged 65 years and older is expected to double by 2030 (He, Sengupta, Velkoff & DeBarros 2005), we will inevitably observe an increase in the prevalence of cognitive impairment and dementia. Although the majority of older adults will not demonstrate significant cognitive impairments, many older adults will seek the guidance of clinicians about current memory concerns, as well as about how to avoid future decline. It is crucial that clinicians are equipped with the tools and knowledge to assess normative age-related changes as well as cognitive impairments, and make informed treatment decisions in clinical settings.

To summarize, assessment should be concerned with a variety of test scores and observed behaviors, contextualized within a person's life history. Further consideration of the patient's needs, abilities, preferences, and cultural background will allow for the most appropriate design and implementation of a cognitive training program. Ongoing assessment helps ensure that training is appropriate and well tolerated, and that other medical and cognitive issues which may have arisen during treatment have been taken into account when interpreting training results. The clinician may use this information to recommend a training approach and individually tailor the training program to best meet the needs and preferences of the client. After training, periodic assessment is also important for the long-term maintenance and transfer of training gains to everyday function.

References

Acevedo, A., & Loewenstein, D. A. (2007). Nonpharmacological cognitive interventions in aging and dementia. *Journal of Geriatric Psychiatry and Neurology*, *20*, 239–249.

Albert, M. (2008). The neuropsychology of the development of Alzheimer's disease. In F. I. M. Craik, & T. A. Salthouse (Eds.), *The Handbook of Aging and Cognition* (4th ed., pp. 97–132). London, UK: Academic Press.

Allaire, J. C., & Marsiske, M. (2002). Well- and ill-defined measures of everyday cognition: Relationship to older adults' intellectual ability and functional status. *Psychology and Aging*, *17*, 101–115.

Armitage, S. G. (1946). An analysis of certain psychological tests used for the evaluation of brain injury. *Psychological Monographs*, *60*, 277.

Bäckman, L. (1992). Memory training and memory improvement in Alzheimer's disease: Rules and exceptions. *Acta Neurologia Scandinavica*, *139*, 84–89.

Baddeley, A. D. (1990). *Human memory: Theory and practice*. Hove, UK: Lawrence Erlbaum Associates.

Bagwell, D. K., & West, R. L. (2008). Assessing compliance: Active versus inactive trainees in a memory intervention. *Clinical Interventions in Aging*, *3*, 371–382.

Ball, K., Berch, D. B., Helmers, K. F., Jobe, J. B., Leveck, M. D., Marsiske, M., et al. (2002). Effects of cognitive training interventions with older adults: A randomized controlled trial. *Journal of the American Medical Association*, *288*, 2271–2281.

Baltes, P. B. (1997). On the incomplete architecture of human ontogeny: Selection, optimization, and compensation as foundation of developmental theory. *American Psychologist*, *52*, 366–380.

Bell, K. L., Sano, M. C., Jin, S., Thomas, R. G., & Thal, L. J. (1999). Ethnic differences in clinical measures among participants in Alzheimer's disease clinical trials. *Neurology*, *52*, 396.

Belleville, S. (2008). Cognitive training for persons with mild cognitive impairment. *International Psychogeriatrics/IPA*, *20*, 57–66.

Belleville, S., Gilbert, B., Fontaine, F., Gagnon, L., Menard, E., & Gauthier, S. (2006). Improvement of episodic memory in persons with mild cognitive impairment and healthy older adults: Evidence from a cognitive intervention program. *Dementia and Geriatric Cognitive Disorders*, *22*, 486–499.

Benedict, R. (1997). *Brief Visuospatial Memory Test-Revised*. Odessa, FL: Psychological Assessment Resources.

Benton, A. L., Sivan, A. B., Hamsher, K. de S. et al. (1994). *Contributions to neuropsychological assessment. A clinical manual* (2nd ed.). New York, NY: Oxford University Press.

Berg, E. A. (1948). A simple objective treatment for measuring flexibility in thinking. *Journal of General Psychology*, *39*, 15–22.

Bherer, L., Kramer, A. F., Peterson, M. S., Colcombe, S., Erickson, K., & Becic, E. (2006). Testing the limits of cognitive plasticity in older adults: Application to attentional control. *Acta Psychologica*, *123*, 261–278.

Binder, L. M. (1993). *Portland Digit Recognition Test manual* (2nd ed.). Portland, OR: Private publication

Bissig, D., & Lustig, C. (2007). Who benefits from memory training? *Psychological Science*, *18*, 720–726.

Bottiroli, S., & Cavallini, E. (2009). Can computer familiarity regulate the benefits of computer-based memory training in normal aging? A study with an Italian sample of older adults. *Aging, Neurospychology, Cognition*, *16*, 401–418.

Bourgeois, M. S. (1990). Enhancing conversation skills in patients with Alzheimer's disease using a prosthetic memory aid. *Journal of Applied Behavioral Analysis*, *23*, 29–42.

Bourgeois, M. S., & Mason, L. A. (1996). Memory wallet intervention in an adult day care setting. *Behavioral Interventions*, *11*, 3–18.

Brandt, J., & Benedict, R. H. B. (2001). *Hopkins Verbal Learning Test-Revised: Professional manual*. Odessa, FL: Psychological Assessment Resources.

Cahn-Weiner, D. A., Malloy, P. F., Rebok, G. W., & Ott, B. R. (2003). Results of a randomized placebo-controlled study of memory training for mildly impaired Alzheimer's disease patients. *Applied Neuropsychology*, *10*, 215–223.

Camp, C. J. (1989). Facilitation of new learning in Alzheimer's disease. In G. Gilmore, P. Whitehouse, & M. Wykle (Eds.), *Memory and aging: Theory, research, and practice* (pp. 212–225). New York, NY: Springer.

Camp, C. J., & Stevens, A. B. (1990). Spaced-retrieval: A memory intervention for dementia of the Alzheimer's type (DAT). *Clinical Gerontologist*, *10*, 58–60.

Camp, C. J., Foss, J. W., Stevens, A. B., & O'Hanlon, A. M. (1996). Improving prospective memory task performance in Alzheimer's disease. In M. Brandimonte, G. Einstein, & M. McDaniel (Eds.), *Prospective memory: Theory and applications*. Mahwah, NJ: Lawrence Erlbaum Associates.

Cavallini, E., Pagnin, A., & Vecchi, T. (2003). Age and everyday memory: The beneficial effect of memory training. *Archives of Gerontological Geriatrics*, *37*, 241–257.

Chan, A. S., Butters, N., Salmon, D. P., & Maloney, L. T. (1993). An assessment of the semantic network in patients with schizophrenia. *Journal of Cognitive Neuroscience*, *5*, 254–261.

Clare, L., & Woods, R. T. (2004). Cognitive training and cognitive rehabilitation for people with early-stage Alzheimer disease: A review. *Neuropsychological Rehabilitation*, *14*, 385–401.

Clare, L., Wilson, B. A., Carter, G., & Hodges, J. R. (2003). Cognitive rehabilitation as a component of early intervention in dementia: A single case study. *Aging and Mental Health*, *7*, 15–21.

Colcombe, S., & Kramer, A. F. (2003). Fitness effects on the cognitive function of older adults: A meta-analytic study. *Psychological Science*, *14*, 125–130.

Connell, C. M., Roberts, J. S., & McLaughlin, S. J. (2007). Public opinion about Alzheimer disease among Blacks, Hispanics, and Whites: Results from a national survey. *Alzheimer Disease & Associated Disorders*, *21*, 232–240.

Craik, F. I. M. (1977). Age differences in human memory. In J. E. Birren, & K. W. Schaie (Eds.), *Handbook of the psychology of aging* (pp. 384–420). New York, NY: Van Nostrand.

Craik, F. I. M., & Tulving, E. (2000). *The Oxford handbook of memory.* London, UK: Oxford University Press.

Crawford, J. R., Obonsawin, M. C., & Allan, K. M. (1998). PASAT and components of WAIS-R performance: Convergent and discriminant validity. *Neuropsychological Rehabilitation*, *8*, 255–272.

Crook, T., Ferris, S., McCarthy, M., & Rae, D. (1980). Utility of digit recall tasks for assessing memory in the aged. *Journal of Consulting and Clinical Psychology*, *48*, 228–233.

Davis, R. N., Massman, P. J., & Doody, R. S. (2001). Cognitive intervention in Alzheimer's disease. *Alzheimer Disease and Associated Disorders*, *15*, 1–9.

Delis, D. C., Kramer, J. H., Kaplan, E., & Ober, B. A. (2000). *California Verbal Learning Test* (2nd ed.). San Antonio, TX: The Psychological Corporation.

Derwinger, A., Neely, A. S., MacDonald, S., & Bäckman, L. (2005). Forgetting numbers in old age: Strategy and learning speed matter. *Gerontology*, *51*, 277–284.

De Vreese, L., Neri, M., Fioravanti, M., Belloi, L., & Zanetti, O. (2001). Memory rehabilitation in Alzheimer's disease: A review of progress. *International Journal of Geriatric Psychiatry*, *16*, 794–809.

Deweer, B., Ergis, A., Fossati, P., Pillon, B., Boller, F., Agid, Y., et al. (1994). Explicit memory, procedural learning, and lexical priming in Alzheimer's disease. *Cortex*, *30*, 113–126.

Dilworth-Anderson, P., Hendrie, H. C., Manly, J. J., Khachaturian, A. S., & Fazio, S. (2008). Diagnosis and assessment of Alzheimer's disease in diverse populations. *Alzheimer's & Dementia*, *4*, 305–309.

Duncan, J., Emslie, H., Williams, P., Johnson, R., & Freer, C. (1996). Intelligence and the frontal lobe: The organization of goal-directed behavior. *Cognitive Psychology*, *30*, 257–303.

Duncker, K. (1945). On problem-solving. *Psychological Monographs*, *58*, 270.

Dunlosky, J., Cavallini, E., Roth, H., McGuire, C. L., Vecchi, T., & Hertzog, C. (2007). Do self-monitoring interventions improve older adult learning? *The Journal of Gerontology: Psychological Sciences and Social Sciences*, *62*, 70–76.

Edwards, J. D., Wadley, V. G., Myers, R. S., Roenker, D. L., Cissell, G. M., & Ball, K. K. (2002). Transfer of a speed of processing intervention to near and far cognitive outcomes. *Gerontology*, *48*, 329–340.

Edwards, J. D., Wadley, V. G., Vance, D. E., Wood, K., Roenker, D. L., & Ball, K. K. (2005). The impact of speed of processing training on cognitive and everyday performance. *Aging and Mental Health*, *9*, 262–271.

Faison, W. E., Schultz, S. K., Aerssens, J., Alvidrez, J., Anand, R., & Farrer, L. A. (2007). Potential ethnic modifiers in the assessment and treatment of Alzheimer's disease: Challenges for the future. *International Psychogeriatrics*, *19*, 539–558.

Falicov, C. J. (1998). *Latino families in therapy.* New York, NY: Guilford.

Fleming, J. M., Shum, D., Strong, J., & Lightbody, S. (2005). Prospective memory rehabilitation for adults with traumatic brain injury: A compensatory training programme. *Brain Injury*, *19*, 1–10.

Floyd, M., & Scogin, F. (1997). Effects of memory training on the subjective memory functioning and mental health of older adults: A meta-analysis. *Psychology and Aging*, *12*, 150–161.

Folstein, M. F., Folstein, S. E., & McHugh, P. R. (1975). Mini-mental state: A practical guide for grading the cognitive state of patients for the clinician. *Journal of Psychiatric Research*, *12*, 189–198.

Gaines, A. D. (1989). Alzheimer's disease in the context of Black (southern) culture. *Health Matrix*, *6*, 4.

Gordon, B., & Berger, L. (2003). *Intelligent Memory.* New York, NY: Viking Press.

Grandmaison, E., & Simard, M. (2003). A critical review of memory stimulation programs in Alzheimer's disease. *The Journal of Neuropsychiatry and Clinical Neurosciences*, *15*, 130–144.

Green, P., Allen, L., & Astner, K. (1996). *Manual for Computerised Word Memory Test.* Durham: CogniSyst.

Greenwald, A. G., McGhee, D. E., & Schwarz, J. L. K. (1998). Measuring individual differences in implicit cognition: The Implicit Association Test. *Journal of Personality and Social Psychology*, *74*, 1464–1480.

Harrison, J. E., Buxton, P., Husain, M., & Wise, R. (2000). Short test of semantic and phonological fluency: Normal performance, validity and test–retest reliability. *British Journal of Clinical Psychology, 39*, 181–191.

He, W., Sengupta, M., Velkoff, V. A., & DeBarros, K. A. (2005). U.S. Census Bureau, Current Population Reports, 65+ in the United States, 2005. (pp. 23–209). Washington, DC: U.S. Government Printing Office.

Heindel, W. C., Salmon, D. P., Shults, C. W., Walicke, P. A., & Butters, N. (1989). Neuropsychological evidence for multiple implicit systems: A comparison of Alzheimer's, Huntington's, and Parkinson's disease patients. *Journal of Neuroscience, 9*, 582–587.

Henry, J. D., Crawford, J. R., & Phillips, L. H. (2004). Verbal fluency performance in dementia of the Alzheimer's type: a meta-analysis. *Neuropsychologia, 42*, 1212–1222.

Hepworth, D. H., Rooney, R. H., Rooney, G. D., Strom-Gottfried, K., & Larsen, J. A. (2006). *Direct social work practice: Theory and skills* (7th ed.). Belmont, CA: Thomson Brooks.

Herrmann, D. J., & Plude, D. (1998). *The effectiveness of face–name mnemonic training as a function of training technologies and learning ability, Technical Report 1*. Terre Haute, IN: Practical Memory Institute.

Hertzog, C., Kramer, A. F., Wilson, R. S., & Lindenberger, U. (2008). Enrichment effects on adult cognitive development: Can the functional capacity of older adults be preserved and enhanced? *Psychological Science in the Public Interest, 9*, 1–65.

Heun, R., Burkart, M., & Benkert, O. (1997). Improvement of picture recall by repetition in patients with dementia of Alzheimer type. *International Journal of Geriatric Psychiatry, 12*, 85–92.

Hill, R. D., Allen, C., & McWhorter, P. (1991). Stories as a mnemonic aid for older learners. *Psychology and Aging, 6*, 484–486.

Hill, R. D., Campbell, B. W., Foxley, D., & Lindsay, S. (1997). Effectiveness of the number-consonant mnemonic for retention of numeric material in community-dwelling older adults. *Experimental Aging Research, 23*, 275–286.

Hoffman, J., & Stawski, R. S. (2009). Persons as contexts: Evaluating between-person and within-person effects in longitudinal analysis. *Research in Human Development, 6*, 97–120.

Jennings, J. M., Webster, L. M., Kleykamp, B. A., & Dagenbach, D. (2005). Recollection training and transfer effects in older adults: Successful use of a repetition-lag procedure. *Aging, Neuropsychology, & Cognition, 12*, 278–298.

Jobe, J. B., Smith, D. M., Ball, K., Tennstedt, S. L., Marsiske, M., Willis, S. L., et al. (2001). ACTIVE: A cognitive intervention trial to promote independence in older adults. *Controlled Clinical Trials, 22*, 453–479.

Kaplan, E. P., Goodglass, H., & Weintraub, S. (1983). *The Boston Naming Test* (2nd ed.). Philadelphia, PA: Lea & Febiger.

Kindt, M., Biermanm, D., & Brosschot, J. F. (1996). Stroop versus Stroop: Comparison of a card format and a single-trial format of the standard color-word Stroop task and the emotional Stroop task. *Personality and Individual Differences, 21*, 653–661.

Kliegl, R., Smith, J., & Baltes, P. B. (1989). Testing the limits and the study of adult age differences in cognitive plasticity of a mnemonic skill. *Developmental Psychology, 25*, 247–256.

Kramer, A. F., & Madden, D. (2008). Attention. In F. I. M. Craik, & T. A. Salthouse (Eds.), *The handbook of aging and cognition* (3rd ed., pp. 189–250). Mahwah, NJ: Erlbaum.

Kramer, A. F., Hahn, S., & Gopher, D. (1999). Task coordination and aging: Explorations of executive control processes in the task switching paradigm. *Acta Psychologia, 101*, 339–378.

Kray, J., Eber, J., & Lindenberger, U. (2004). Age differences in executive functioning across the lifespan: The role of verbalization in task preparation. *Acta Psychologica, 115*, 143–165.

Lachman, M. E., Weaver, S. L., Bandura, M., Elliott, E., & Lewkowicz, C. J. (1992). Improving memory and control beliefs. *Journal of Gerontology, 47*, 293–299.

Leroi, I., Sheppard, J. M., & Lyketsos, C. G. (2002). Cognitive function after 11.5 years of alcohol use: Relation to alcohol use. *American Journal of Epidemiology, 156*, 747–752.

Lezak, M. (2004). *Neuropsychological assessment* (4th ed.). New York, NY: Oxford University Press.

Light, L. L. (1991). Memory and aging: Four hypothesis in search of data. *Annual Review of Psychology, 42*, 333–376.

Loewenstein, D. A., Acevedo, A., Czaja, S. J., & Duara, R. (2004). Cognitive rehabilitation of mildly impaired Alzheimer disease patients on cholinesterase inhibitors. *American Journal of Geriatric Psychiatry, 12*, 395–402.

Lyketsos, C. G., Chen, L. S., & Anthony, J. C. (1999). Cognitive decline in adulthood: An 11.5-year follow-up of the Baltimore Epidemiologic Catchment Area study. *American Journal of Psychiatry, 156*, 58–65.

Mahncke, H. W., Bronstone, A., & Merzenich, M. M. (2006). Memory enhancement in healthy older adults using a brain plasticity-based training program: A randomized, controlled study. *Proceedings of the National Academy of Sciences, 103*, 12523–12528.

Manly, J. J. (2005). Advantages and disadvantages of separate norms for African Americans. *The Clinical Neuropsychologist, 19*, 270–275.

Manly, J. J., Jacobs, D. M., Sano, M., Bell, K., Merchant, C. A., Small, S. A., et al. (1998). Cognitive test performance among nondemented elderly African Americans and Whites. *Neurology, 50*, 1238–1245.

McCabe, M. S., Varricchio, C. G., & Padberg, R. M. (1994). State of the art care: Efforts to recruit the economically disadvantaged to national clinical trials. *Seminars in Oncology Nursing, 10*, 123–129.

Metcalfe, J., & Mischel, W. (1999). A hot/cool-system analysis of delay of gratification: Dynamics of willpower. *Psychological Review, 106*, 3–19.

Meyer, D. E., & Schvaneveldt, R. W. (1971). Facilitation in recognizing pairs of words: Evidence of a dependence between retrieval operations. *Journal of Experimental Psychology, 90*, 227–234.

Millon-Underwood, S., Sanders, E., & Davis, M. (1993). Determinants of participation in state-of-the-art cancer prevention, early detection/screening, and treatment trials among African-Americans. *Cancer Nursing, 16*, 25–33.

Morrell, R. W., Rager, R., Harley, J. P., Herrmann, D. J., Rebok, G. W., & Parenté, R. (2006). Developing an online intervention for memory improvement: The Sharper Memory Project. *Cognitive Technology, 11*, 34–46.

Neely, A. S., & Bäckman, L. (1993). Long-term maintenance of gains from memory training in older adults: Two 3½ year follow-up studies. *Journal of Gerontology, 48*, 233–237.

Nesselroade, J. R. (1991). The warp and the woof of the developmental fabric. In R. M. Downs, L. S. Liben, & D. S. Palermo (Eds.), *Visions of aesthetics, the environment and development: The legacy of Joachim Wohlwill* (pp. 213–240). Hillsdale, NJ: Erlbaum.

Nesselroade, J. R., & Baltes, P. B. (1979). *Longitudinal research in the study of behavior and development*. New York, NY: Academic Press.

Olin, J. T., Dagerman, K. S., Fox, L. S., Bowers, B., & Schneider, L. S. (2002). Increasing ethnic minority participation in Alzheimer disease research. *Alzheimer Disease and Associated Disorders, 16*, 82–99.

Osterrieth, P. A. (1944). Filetest de copie d'une figure complex: Contribution a l'etude de la perception et de la memoire [The test of copying a complex figure: A contribution to the study of perception and memory]. *Archives de Psychologie, 30*, 286–356.

Owsley, C., Sloane, M., McGwin, G., & Ball, K. (2002). Timed instrumental activities of daily living tasks: Relationship to cognitive function and everyday performance assessments in older adults. *Gerontology, 48*, 254–265.

Paradis, C., Friedman, S., Hatch, M., & Ackerman, R. (1996). Cognitive behavioral treatment of anxiety disorders in Orthodox Jews. *Cognitive and Behavioral Practice, 3*, 271–288.

Peterson, L. R., & Peterson, M. J. (1959). Short-term retention of individual verbal items. *Journal of Experimental Psychology, 58*, 193–198.

Rankin, J. L., Karol, R., & Tuten, C. (1984). Strategy use, recall, and recall organization in young, middle-aged, and elderly adults. *Experimental Aging Research, 10*, 193–196.

Rapp, S., Brenes, G., & Marsh, A. P. (2002). Memory enhancement training for older adults with mild cognitive impairment: A preliminary study. *Aging & Mental Health, 6*, 5–11.

Rasmusson, D. X., Rebok, G. W., Bylsma, F. W., & Brandt, J. (1999). Effects of three types of memory training in normal elderly. *Aging, Neuropsychology, and Cognition, 6*, 56–66.

Rebok, G. W. (2008). Cognitive training: Influence on neuropsychological and brain function in later life. *State-of-Science Review.* SR: E22. UK Government Foresight Mental Capital and Mental Wellbeing Project. Government Office for Science.

Rebok, G. W., & Balcerak, L. J. (1989). Memory self-efficacy and performance differences in young and old adults: Effect of mnemonic training. *Developmental Psychology*, *25*, 714–721.

Rebok, G. W., Carlson, M. C., & Langbaum, J. B. S. (2007). Training and maintaining memory abilities in healthy older adults: Traditional and novel approaches. *Journal of Gerontology: Psychological Sciences*. Spec No.1, 53–61.

Rebok, G. W., Rasmusson, D. X., Bylsma, F. W., & Brandt, J. (1997). Memory improvement tapes: How effective for elderly adults? *Aging, Neuropsychology, and Cognition*, *4*, 304–311.

Rey, A. (1941). L'examen psychologique dans les cas d'encephalopathie tramatique. *Archives de Psychologie*, *28*, 286–340.

Roenker, D. L., Cissell, G. M., Ball, K. K., Wadley, V. G., & Edwards, J. D. (2003). Speed-of-processing and driving simulator training result in improved driving performance. *Human Factors*, *45*, 218–233.

Saczynski, J. S., Rebok, G. W., Whitfield, K. E., & Plude, D. J. (2004). Effectiveness of CD-ROM memory training as a function of within-session autonomy. *Cognitive Technology*, *9*, 24–32.

Saint-Cyr, J. A., Taylor, A. E., & Lang, A. E. (1988). Procedural learning and neostriatal dysfunction in man. *Brain*, *111*, 941–960.

Salthouse, T. A. (1996). The processing-speed theory of adult age differences in cognition. *Psychological Review*, *103*, 403–428.

Salthouse, T. A., & Babcock, R. L. (1991). Decomposing adult age differences in working memory. *Developmental Psychology*, *27*, 763–776.

Salthouse, T. A., & Meinz, E. J. (1995). Aging, inhibition, working memory, and speed. *Journal of Gerontology: Psychological Sciences*, *50*, 297–306.

Salthouse, T. A., Hambrick, D. Z., Lukas, K. E., & Dell, T. C. (1996). Determinants of adult age differences on synthetic work performance. *Journal of Experimental Psychology: Applied*, *2*, 305–329.

Sano, M., Mackell, J. A., Ponton, M., Ferreira, P., Wilson, J., Pawluczyk, S., et al. (1997). The Spanish Instrument Protocol: Design and implementation of a study to evaluate treatment efficacy. Instruments for Spanish-speaking patients with Alzheimer's disease. The Alzheimer's disease Cooperative Study. *Alzheimer Disease and Associated Disorders*, *11*, 57–64.

Schaie, K. W. (2005). *Developmental influences on adult intelligence: The Seattle Longitudinal Study*. New York, NY: Oxford University Press.

Schretlen, D. (1989). *Brief Test of Attention*. Odessa, FL: Psychological Assessment Resources.

Sharps, M. J., & Price-Sharps, J. L. (1996). Visual memory support: an effective mnemonic device for older adults. *The Gerontologist*, *36*, 706–708.

Shulman, K. I. (2000). Clock-drawing: Is it the ideal cognitive screening test? *International Journal of Geriatric Psychiatry*, *15*, 548–561.

Shute, V. J., & Gawlick, L. A. (1995). Practice effects on skill acquisition, learning outcome, and retention. *Human Factors*, *37*, 781–803.

Sitzer, D. I., Twamley, E. W., & Jeste, D. V. (2006). Cognitive training in Alzheimer's disease: A meta-analysis of the literature. *Acta Psychiatrica Scandinavia*, *114*, 75–90.

Stigsdotter, A., & Bäckman, L. (1989). Multifactorial memory training with older adults: How to foster maintenance of improved performance. *Gerontology*, *35*, 260–267.

Teng, E. L., Hasegawa, K., Homma, A., Imai, Y., Larson, E., Graves, A., et al. (1994). The cognitive abilities screening instrument (CASI): A practical test for cross-cultural epidemiological studies of dementia. *International Psychogeriatrics*, *6*, 45–58.

Tharp, R. G. (1991). Cultural diversity and treatment of children. *Journal of Consulting and Clinical Psychology*, *59*, 799–812.

Ullman, M. T. (2001). The declarative/procedural model of lexicon and grammar. *Journal of Psycholinguistic Research*, *30*, 37–69.

Unverzagt, F., Kasten, L., Johnson, K. E., Rebok, G. W., Marsiske, M., Koepke, K. M., et al. (2007). Effect of memory impairment on training outcomes in ACTIVE. *Journal of the International Neuropsychological Society*, *13*, 953–960.

Valentijn, S. A. M., van Hooren, S. A. H., Bosma, H., Touh, D. M., Jolles, J., van Boxtel, M. P. J., et al. (2005). The effect of two types of memory training on subjective and objective memory performance in healthy individuals aged 55 years and older: A randomized controlled trial. *Patient Education and Counseling*, *57*, 106–114.

Verhaeghen, P., Geraerts, N., & Marcoen, A. (2000). Memory complaints, coping, and well-being in old age: A systematic approach. *The Gerontologist*, *40*, 540–548.

Verhaeghen, P., Marcoen, A., & Goossens, L. (1992). Improving memory performance in the aged through mnemonic training: A meta-analytic study. *Psychology and Aging*, *7*, 242–251.

Warrington, E., & Rabin, P. (1970). Perceptual matching in patients with cerebral lesions. *Neuropsychologia*, *8*, 475–487.

Wechsler, D. (1987). *Wechsler memory scale revised manual.* San Antonio, TX: Psychological Corporation.

West, R. (1985). *Memory fitness over 40.* Gainesville, FL: Triad Publishing.

West, R. L., & Crook, T. H. (1992). Video training and imagery for mature adults. *Applied Cognitive Psychology*, *6*, 307–320.

West, R. L., Bagwell, D. K., & Dark-Freudeman, A. (2008). Self-efficacy and memory aging: The impact of a memory intervention based on self-efficacy. *Aging, Neuropsychology, and Cognition*, *15*, 302–329.

West, R. L., Thorn, R. M., & Bagwell, D. K. (2003). Memory performance and beliefs as a function of goal setting and aging. *Psychology and Aging*, *18*, 111–125.

Whalley, L. J., Deary, I. J., Appleton, C. L., & Starr, J. M. (2004). Cognitive reserve and the neurobiology of cognitive aging. *Ageing Research Reviews*, *3*, 369–382.

Willis, S. L., Tennstedt, S. L., Marsiske, M., Ball, K., Elias, J., Koepke, K. M., et al. (2006). Long-term effects of cognitive training on everyday functional outcomes in older adults. *Journal of the American Medical Association*, *296*, 2805–2814.

Wilson, B. A., Cockburn, J., & Baddeley, A. (1985). *The Rivermead Behavioral Memory Test.* Gaylord, MI: National Rehabilitation Services.

Wilson, B. A., Emslie, H., Foley, J., Shiel, A., Watson, P., Hawkins, K., et al. (2005). *The Cambridge Prospective Memory Test.* London, UK: Harcourt.

Wolinsky, F. D., Vander Weg, M. W., Martin, R., Unverzagt, F. W., Willis, S. L., Marsiske, M., et al. (2009). Does cognitive training improve locus of control among older adults? *Journal of Gerontology: Social Sciences.* DOI: 10.1093/geronb/gbp117

Woodrome, S. E., & Fastenau, P. S. (2005). Test–retest reliability of the Extended Complex Figure Test-Motor independent administration (ECFT-MI). *Archives of Clinical Neuropsychology*, *20*, 291–299.

Woods, B., Thorgrimsen, L., Spector, A., Royan, L., & Orrell, M. (2006). Improved quality of life and cognitive stimulation therapy in dementia. *Aging and Mental Health*, *10*, 219–226.

Woolverton, M., Scogin, F., Shackelford, J., Black, S., & Duke, L. (2001). Problem-targeted memory training for older adults. *Aging, Neuropsychology, and Cognition*, *8*, 241–255.

Yesavage, J. A., & Rose, T. L. (1984). The effects of a face–name mnemonic in young, middle-aged, and elderly adults. *Experimental Aging Research*, *10*, 55–57.

Yesavage, J. A., & Rose, T. L. (1983). Concentration and mnemonic training in elderly with memory complaints: A study of combined therapy and order effects. *Psychiatry Research*, *9*, 156–167.

Yesavage, J. A., Sheikh, J. I., Friedman, L., & Tanke, E. (1990). Learning mnemonics: Roles of aging and subtle cognitive impairment. *Psychology and Aging*, *5*, 133–137.

Yesavage, J., Shiekh, J. I., Tanke, E. D., & Hill, R. (1988). Response to memory training and individual differences in verbal intelligence and state anxiety. *American Journal of Psychiatry*, *145*, 636–639.

Zacks, R. T., & Hasher, L. (2006). Aging and long-term memory: Deficits are not inevitable. In E. Bialystok, & F. I. M. Craik (Eds.), *Lifespan cognition: Mechanisms of change* (pp. 162–177). New York, NY: Oxford University Press.

Zanetti, O., Binetti, G., Magni, E., Rozzini, L., Bianchetti, A., & Trabucchi, M. (1997). Procedural memory stimulation in Alzheimer's disease: Impact of a training programme. *Acta Neurologica Scandinavia*, *95*, 152–157.

Zanetti, O., Zanieri, G., DiGiovanni, G., De Vreese, L. P., Pezzini, A., Metitieri, T., et al. (2001). Effectiveness of procedural memory stimulation in mild Alzheimer's disease patients: A controlled study. *Neuropsychological Rehabilitation*, *11*, 263–272.

CHAPTER

9

The Assessment of Elder Abuse

Elizabeth J. Santos, Deborah A. King

University of Rochester Medical Center, Rochester, NY, USA

INTRODUCTION AND HISTORY

Elder abuse is a significant public health problem estimated to affect up to 10% of Americans aged 65 years or older. Elder abuse causes enormous emotional costs to the individual and family and, as society ages, the problem will be compounded. By the year 2030, the number of adults over the age of 65 years is expected to double. The U.S. Senate Special Committee on Aging estimates that elder abuse already affects 5 million elders yearly. Worldwide, the World Health Organization (WHO) estimates that the number of older adults affected by abuse is 4–6% and this is widely believed to be an underestimation. In this chapter, we will address the topic of elder abuse assessment by first considering the history of the problem, fundamental research challenges in studying elder abuse, definitions and terms, epidemiology of the problem, and notable clinical sequelae and risk indicators of elder abuse. We will also incorporate exemplary case studies and provide descriptions of several important screening tools.

Family violence, such as spouse and child abuse, surfaced to the nation's consciousness in the early to middle twentieth century. Laws to establish adult and child protective services emerged in the 1960s, but the focus was on younger, impaired adults. It was not until the 1970s that elder abuse started to gain recognition as a societal problem. British scientific journals first described "granny battering" in 1975. In 1978, the U.S. House Select Committee on Aging held the first congressional hearings on elder abuse. The term "elder abuse" was purposefully chosen to capture and galvanize public opinion. However, little action was taken on political, legislative or research fronts to advance the understanding of elder abuse or formulate a public response until the early 1990s.

The Social Security Act of 1974 established the requirement for each state to protect vulnerable adults, focusing especially on developmentally disabled adults. Adult Protective Services (APS) around the United States are mandated to serve adults aged 18 and over who are vulnerable to mistreatment, unable to protect themselves, and have no designated caregiver. The scope of APS depends on the legal mandates of each specific state. A few APS organizations limit their services to those 18–59 years old; others restrict service to those 60 years of age and above. In 2004, a national survey of APS data was conducted and a report generated that focused specifically on clients aged 60 years and older (Teaster & Otto, 2006). Twenty-four states reported 88,455 substantiated cases of abuse; 19 states reported 36.7% of their cases involved self-neglect. Unfortunately, only eight states provided reasons for case closure, including 6.3% entering long-term care facilities and 2.4% dying.

In 1992, the Older Americans Act was re-authorized and amended to address elder abuse under Titles III and VII. The Vulnerable Elder Rights Protection Program was established and the National Center on Elder Abuse (NCEA) was created and funded by the U.S. Administration on Aging (AoA). In parallel fashion in 1992, the National Center for Injury Prevention and Control (NCIPC), widely

Handbook of Assessment in Clinical Gerontology. DOI: 10.1016/B978-0-12-374961-1.10009-0

recognized as the "lead federal agency for injury prevention" that studies issues of violence and abuse of women, children and older adults, was created as part of the Centers for Disease Control (CDC). Although the CDC and the AoA both were organized under the Department of Health and Human Services (HHS), this parallel structure increased the complexity of the funding process for elder abuse initiatives. Moreover, the magnitude of funding was been small relative to the estimated magnitude of the problem.

In 2002, the NCEA was funded with only $3.5 million dollars. In the same year, it was estimated that only $153 million dollars were spent by the federal government to address elder abuse, neglect, and financial exploitation, mostly distributed through block grants to support adult protective services programs (Baker, 2003). This represented only 0.08% of the amount spent on abuse prevention for women and children. Similarly, for the fiscal year 2004, NCIPC received $153.6 million dollars of the CDC's $7.1 billion dollar budget.

DEFINITIONS AND SCOPE OF THE PROBLEM

The definition of elder abuse has been a subject of debate for decades, making it difficult to conduct and evaluate research in a systematic fashion. For the purposes of this chapter, we will utilize the framework and definitions of the NCEA as follows (http://www.ncea.aoa.gov/ncearoot/Main_Site/index.aspx - fact sheet):

- **Physical Abuse**—Inflicting, or threatening to inflict, physical pain or injury on a vulnerable elder, or depriving them of a basic need.
- **Emotional Abuse**—Inflicting mental pain, anguish, or distress on an elder person through verbal or nonverbal acts.
- **Sexual Abuse**—Non-consensual sexual contact of any kind.
- **Exploitation**—Illegal taking, misuse, or concealment of funds, property, or assets of a vulnerable elder.
- **Neglect**—Refusal or failure by those responsible to provide food, shelter, health care, or protection for a vulnerable elder.
- **Abandonment**—The desertion of a vulnerable elder by anyone who has assumed the responsibility for care or custody of that person.

Unfortunately, the legal definitions of these terms vary from state to state, causing clinical researchers to adopt different definitions and terms to conform to their state's regulations. Noting this barrier to scientific rigor in the field, the U.S. National Academy of Sciences proposed the following definition of "elder mistreatment" in 2003:

- Intentional actions that cause harm or create a serious risk of harm (whether or not harm is intended) to a vulnerable elder by a caregiver or other person who stands in a trust relationship to the elder; or
- Failure by a caregiver to satisfy the elder's basic needs or to protect the elder from harm; or
- "Mistreatment" conveys two ideas: that some injury, deprivation, or dangerous condition has occurred to the elder person and that someone else bears responsibility for causing the condition or failing to prevent it.

Importantly, this definition eliminates "self-neglect" as a form of elder mistreatment and emphasizes the responsibility of the caregiver. Additionally, victimization by strangers is eliminated from the definition of "elder mistreatment" in order to highlight the "trusting relationships" that they believe should be the focus of studies of elder abuse. This new research definition should be integrated into future studies to facilitate dialog and comparability of research methods and results.

EPIDEMIOLOGY OF THE PROBLEM—WHAT WE KNOW AND WHAT WE DON'T KNOW

In addition to confusion about the definition of elder abuse, there are other reasons why the true incidence and prevalence of the problem is as yet unknown. Epidemiological studies of diagnosable conditions often begin by using the International Classification of Diseases (ICD) codes. In ICD-9, the current coding schema used by hospitals and billing services, there is a code (995.8) for "adult maltreatment" with additional specifiers for the types of abuse. However, a White Paper commissioned by the NCEA and released in May 2006 underscored problems with using this method (Wood, 2006). First of all, most health care professionals use codes to bill for a specific injury or illness, such as fracture or pneumonia. Yet there is little-to-no reimbursement for abuse codes and therefore less incentive for their use. Moreover, practitioners may not be prepared to recognize or identify family violence as there are few specialty training programs to prepare them for this problem, and even fewer focused on elder abuse. Additionally, practitioners are trained to diagnose and treat problems.

Elder mistreatment is a complex systemic problem which takes an extraordinary amount of time to assess with no easy remedy for resolution. Sometimes victims and health care professionals are reluctant to address this uncomfortable and complicated issue as they feel powerless to address it. Therefore, surveys which rely on ICD-9 data are of limited use because the codes are rarely used. Other data sources are scarce, as many important national surveys, such as the CDC's National Ambulatory Medical Care Survey (NAMCS) and the National Health Interview Survey (NHIS), do not even contain any questions related to abuse.

The World Health Organization (WHO), along with the International Network for the Prevention of Elder Abuse (INPEA) and other partners, used focus groups and meetings with professionals in five developing and three developed countries to better understand the problem of elder abuse. Argentina, Brazil, India, Kenya, Lebanon, Canada, Austria, and Sweden participated in this investigation. Similar to previous reports, this study noted many problems with existing methods of identifying victims. The importance of cultural context was underlined, as it was found that definitions of abuse were not consistent worldwide. Making matters worse, participants often used ambiguous terms such as "emotional problems," "lack of emotional support," "loss of dignity," and "disrespect by the family" to describe potential abuse.

The report also acknowledged that larger social and political contexts of older adults' lives must be understood to adequately address the problem of abuse. For example, issues such as retirement, social roles of elders and their caretakers, and public policy towards taking care of older adults must be understood in each culture. The report identified categories of "societal abuse" pertaining to finances (i.e., "inadequate pensions") and housing problems (i.e., poor "accommodation"). Finally, culture-specific "patterns of abandonment" were identified in Kenya and Brazil when, during family holidays, older adults were routinely left at hospitals.

CLINICAL SEQUELAE OF ELDER ABUSE AND NEGLECT

The sequelae of elder abuse are especially noteworthy for those working with older adults. Most tragically, abused older adults have heightened mortality risk. One study (Lachs, Williams, O'Brien, Pillemer, & Charlson, 1998) reported that abused older adults were three times more likely to die within three years than their non-abused counterparts. A recent study by Dong and colleagues (Dong et al., 2009) also found increased mortality for abused elders with a hazard ratio of 2.06 for confirmed cases of abuse.

Another study by Lachs and colleagues (Lachs, Williams, O'Brien, & Pillemer, 2002) analyzed the relationship between adult protective service (APS) use and nursing home placement. They found that elder mistreatment and self-neglect, with referral to APS, were the strongest predictors of placement, far exceeding other medical, social, and functional impairments. Unfortunately, case reports and studies of institutionalized abuse victims often end in nursing home placements, without characterizing what happens to the victims after placement. Research to date has stopped short of tracking victims clinically through the course of institutionalization in order to better understand components of nursing home care that could be most effectively modified to successfully respond to their specialized needs.

As the older adult population continues to expand, the number of mistreated elders in the community who are subsequently admitted to nursing homes will also rise. It is now clear that providers of geriatric care must offer services that enhance residents' quality of life, but this can be a difficult task. Nursing home residents are a heterogeneous group whose needs must be evaluated with consideration given to financial and ethical concerns, and evidence-based practice. Clinical experience, case reports, and studies suggest that nursing homes have many residents who have a history of mistreatment. Title VII of the Older Americans Act (OAA) established Ombudsman programs in every state to advocate for residents of long-term care facilities. Long-term care (LTC) ombudsmen are responsible for investigating complaints, providing information about LTC, representing resident interests, and educating the public about resident welfare. Nursing home residents who have been mistreated represent a noteworthy group that may differ from other residents in terms of their mental and physical needs. Further research is needed to better understand this group and adapt practices to better serve them in a more efficacious and compassionate manner.

Efforts to better understand how mistreated older adults differ from other older adults have largely consisted of clinical case studies and anecdotal reports. Therefore, risk indicators have been inferred without the use of control groups or longitudinal follow-up. Nevertheless, these reports have suggested a few risk factors common to victims, including a shared living situation, social isolation, and dementia (Fulmer et al., 2003; Lachs, Williams, O'Brien, Hurst, & Horwitz, 1997; National Research Council 2003). Risk factors that may be common to abusers include mental illness, hostility and alcohol/drug abuse. There is even less evidence for other hypothesized risk factors such as female gender, history of spousal abuse, physical impairment, victim dependence, and caregiver stress (Fulmer et al., 2005). Characteristics of self-neglecting older adults may include depression, dementia, substance abuse, low socioeconomic status, and social isolation (Brandl, & Dyer, 2007).

In the current economic climate, many people have to work outside the home to provide for their families, leaving no one to care for their aging parents. Changes in social roles and lack of external social resources contribute to caregiver stress. Unfortunately, this reality is often used as an excuse for abuse, even by the victims who blame themselves for being burdens. When discussing an incident of financial exploitation by adult children during one of the WHO focus groups in Canada (WHO/INPEA, 2002), one participant did label the act abuse, but justified it by saying, "He must have needed the money." A paper by the Neglect Assessment Team (NAT) at Mount Sinai Medical Center in New York City emphasizes that health status of the caregiver and the caregiver's ability to provide care must also be assessed (Kahan, 2003). Victims are often reluctant to admit abuse and may even blame themselves because of shame and a desire to protect the abuser. Many victims believe they have no alternative but to return to the abusive situation. Abusers who may not want outside intervention may be reluctant to bring the victim to care, causing both parties to miss out on potentially valuable resources and services.

Another clinically useful perspective is presented by Ramsey-Klawsnik (2000), who identified five types of perpetrators. The "overwhelmed" perpetrator is a caregiver who means to provide good care for their loved one, but becomes frustrated and lashes out at the older adult in their care. When elder abuse research was in its infancy, this was a common perception and preventive interventions were aimed at reducing caregiver stress. However, subsequent research has shown that caregiver stress is much less important as a potential cause of mistreatment and that other factors must be considered. "Impaired" perpetrators are those who are similarly well meaning, but due to their own deficits cannot adequately care for the older adult in their care. Examples include caregivers who have physical or mental illness and are unaware of their limitations. In the institutional setting, inadequate training or skills can impair employees' ability to manage the needs of the residents.

Three additional proposed categories of abuser share the characteristic of personal gain (Ramsey-Klawsnik, 2000). "Narcissistic" perpetrators put their personal needs above those of the victim. Their only goal in caregiving is anticipated secondary gain, typically financial in nature. "Domineering or bullying" perpetrators believe that their maltreatment of older adults is justified. Control of the older adult is rationalized, and often ageism and the belief that the older adult is weak and undeserving of respect contribute to the justification and continued victimization. The most brutal type of perpetrator, the "sadistic" offender, is described as lacking remorse and deriving pleasure from making others experience pain. The older adult is intimidated, tormented, and terrorized to please the perpetrator.

Case Study 1—Financial Exploitation

Ms Gordon is a 75-year-old female who has never married and lives alone. Her niece, Ms Norris, has been getting a few dollars for helping her with household chores and shopping for many years. Recently, Ms Norris began asking for more and more money to help with these chores, citing the rising price of gas and food. Ms Gordon noticed checks missing from her checkbook and asked Ms Norris if she knew anything about them. Ms Norris became infuriated, blamed Ms Gordon's "failing memory" and stormed out of the house. Ms Norris did not come back for several weeks, leaving Ms Gordon without much food and no transportation. When Ms Norris did come back, Ms Gordon was so happy for the company and the help that she did not ask about the checks again.

Several months later, a bank teller who had known Ms Gordon for over 20 years became suspicious when she noted several large withdrawals in Ms Gordon's name coming through the drive-thru window. The bank teller knew Ms Gordon did not drive and was usually quite careful with her money. The teller told her manager of her suspicions and the manager contacted the bank's legal department for advice. They were advised to call APS to investigate. When APS came to her home, Ms Gordon was not aware of the withdrawals in her name and became quite upset. At this point, the police and the assistant district attorney for elder affairs became involved and were able to prosecute Ms Norris for stealing money from Ms Gordon. APS helped Ms Gordon link with the local aging services agency who arranged help with shopping, transportation, and social activities.

Case Study 2—Elder Neglect

Mr Zemans is an 88-year-old male whose wife died over 10 years ago. His daughters have never been close to him or each other, but agree to split up the responsibilities of taking care of him. When his youngest daughter, Mrs Thomas comes over to bring him groceries and meals, Mr Zemans is insulting and verbally abusive. Eventually, Mrs Thomas stops visiting Mr Zemans altogether. Mrs Franklin, Mr Zemans oldest daughter, usually brings him to his doctor appointments, but when she has a heart attack, she cannot drive and no one comes to take Mr Zemans to appointments or to refill his medications. APS is eventually called by Mr Zemans neighbors who haven't seen him in several weeks. They find him emaciated with no food in the pantry, swollen legs, and difficulty breathing. APS brings him to a hospital where he is later discharged to a nursing home.

Case Study 3—Physical Abuse

Mrs Stamford is an 82-year-old Caucasian widow whose husband died last year. She was diagnosed with Alzheimer's dementia three years ago and her husband was her primary caregiver. Her daughter agreed to take care of Mrs Stamford and after several months Mrs Stamford moved in with her daughter, Mrs Kaminsky, and son-in-law who had just lost his job and would be able to look after her during the day. Mrs Stamford's physician, Dr Mann, noticed bruising on her arms and legs, but Mrs Stamford would only say that she was clumsy and fell. Dr Mann was suspicious and called APS to check on Mrs Stamford. When the APS social worker came to the door, Mr Kaminsky would not let them in until the police arrived. The APS social worker observed Mr Kaminsky throwing away many beer cans before the police arrived. When they were finally able to question Mrs Stamford, she remained mute and refused to answer any of their questions for fear she would be placed in a nursing home. Mrs Stamford continued to live with her daughter and son-in-law.

During Mrs Stamford's next visit, Dr Mann was able to speak with her daughter alone. Dr Mann focused his questions on Mrs Kaminsky's well-being. Mrs Kaminsky broke down in tears and admitted that her husband was an alcoholic who abused her as well. Dr Mann helped Mrs Kaminsky call the local abused women's shelter from the office and helped connect her with services. Mrs Kaminsky was isolated from friends and family by her husband, but finally realizing the danger that she and her mother were in, Mrs Kaminsky confided in them that her husband was abusive. With help from the local women's shelter, friends, and family, Mrs Kaminsky and her mother moved into their own apartment and Mrs Stamford went to an adult day care center during the day when her daughter was at work.

Case Study 4—Psychological Abuse

Mr Kline is a 67-year-old male who has never been married. He has multiple medical problems including several heart attacks, strokes, and diabetes, which have left him with right-sided paralysis. He now needs 24-hour care and hemodialysis three times a week. In order to stay in his own home, he has arranged for a combination of visiting nurse services paid by insurance, and private pay aide services to help with household chores and personal hygiene. His evening aide, Mr Joseph bathes him and puts him to bed. But, when Mr Kline's medication is changed and he begins soiling the bed at night, Mr Joseph becomes annoyed and yells at Mr Kline. As this night-time soiling becomes more consistent, Mr Joseph begins to ignore Mr Kline's calls for help for over an hour and then shames him by letting him lie in his feces, and insults him. Eventually, Mr Kline regresses, ceases calling for help at night and develops a decubitus ulcer. His visiting nurse transfers him to a hospital where his decubitus ulcer develops into systemic sepsis and he dies.

Case Study 5—Sexual Abuse

Mrs Lee is a 70-year-old female who has been widowed and has lived alone for over 20 years. As her memory begins to fail, her children try to find a solution to keep her in her home. Mrs Lee's grandson, J.T., agrees to move in with her. J.T. stays out very late and comes in at all hours. As Mrs Lee becomes more confined to her room, J.T. takes over the house and invites friends over who begin a methamphetamine lab in Mrs Lee's kitchen. People are coming in and out of Mrs Lee's house all the time. J.T. has become addicted to methamphetamine and Mrs Lee has also been exposed by the production in her kitchen. When J.T. is intoxicated, he becomes aggressive and bursts into his grandmother's room where he sexually assaults her. Mrs Lee cannot defend herself and this pattern of intoxication and sexual abuse occurs several times a month. Several months later, her children visit during the holidays and discover what has been happening. Mrs Lee is brought to the hospital and then transferred to a nursing home. At the nursing home, she is quite agitated and screams out whenever a male aide or resident approaches her. A therapist is hired to work with Mrs Lee on her symptoms of post-traumatic stress disorder. The therapist is also able to help the staff by educating them about post-traumatic stress disorder and together they create a behavior plan suited to decrease Mrs Lee's distress and modify their approach to decrease her hypervigilance.

SCREENING FOR ELDER ABUSE

Screening does not equal assessment. The goal of an elder abuse screening tool is to identify older adults who *may* be suffering from abuse and neglect. The goal of elder abuse assessment is to *confirm* or verify victimization. A screening tool is ideally a quickly administered questionnaire. As previously described, elder abuse is a complicated, frequently multi-level phenomenon, which is not often easy to recognize. Assessment of elder abuse requires many man hours and investigation by specialists.

As the WHO points out, we must also be cognizant of cultural contexts when investigating possible cases of elder abuse. There are reportedly violent practices and customs within social structures which are not considered abusive and must be taken into account when examining abuse. Examples include societies where older widows are abandoned and their property taken as a matter of course, or where the daughters-in-law take over the household and marginalize the parents. These acts are considered abusive in Western culture, but may not be noted as abuse in other societies as described above.

Training in elder abuse assessment is quite disparate among the various professions who take care of older adults. Most clinicians are not trained to identify elder mistreatment. Eight percent of primary care physicians in Ohio reported that they were not trained to diagnose elder mistreatment and only 13% recalled any training about elder mistreatment (Kennedy, 2005). In a survey of all U.S. medical schools, 77% of medical schools deans reported elder abuse was included as part of the curriculum, but only 38% of the medical students agreed (Alpert, Tonkin, Seeherman, & Holtz, 1998). This discrepancy highlights the disconnection between the purveyors of medical education and the practicing physicians that they will become. The National Elder Abuse Incidence Survey (National Center on Elder Abuse, 1998), using APS data from 1996, reported that 8.4% of APS referrals came from a combination of physicians, nurses, and clinics. In 2004, a national survey of APS data produced a report specifically about those clients 60 years and older. Physicians generated only 1.4% of the referrals, and they did not generate any data about reporting by psychologists. To our knowledge, there is no information about psychologists' reporting statistics.

Review of Existing Screening Tools and Assessment Methods

Although the American Medical Association (AMA) recommends screening all geriatric patients for abuse, screening instruments are not yet standardized, easily accessible, or easy to use. Due to the lack of sufficient evidence proving that screening for abuse and intimate partner violence in older adults actually prevents harm or decreases disability or death rates, the U.S. Preventive Services Task Force (USPSTF) could neither recommend nor discourage screening for elder abuse (USPSTF, 2004). Nevertheless, we will discuss here the tools that are the most well known and available to clinicians at this point in time, including both screening and assessment approaches. It should be recognized that useful application of these tools must be tied to a coordinated response that includes access to medical, mental health and social services.

The Brief Abuse Screen for the Elderly (BASE) is only five questions long, making it appealing to clinicians working in fast-paced clinical settings (Reis, Nahmiash, & Shrier 1993). It has also demonstrated an 86–90% inter-rater reliability. However, this tool requires specialized training in order to be applied appropriately, and there are no clear guidelines as to the nature of that training. The Caregiver Abuse Screen (CASE) was developed by the same group to be a brief, 8-item questionnaire completed by caregivers themselves (Reis & Nahmiash, 1995). Internal consistency among six of the eight abuse items was fair (Chronbach's alpha = 0.71). However, the authors of the tool have noted that use of the CASE alone was insufficient and recommend that it be augmented with other measures.

Another recognized screening measure is the Indicators of Abuse Screen (Reis & Nahmiash, 1998), which has been studied in home settings and found to have adequate internal consistency (Chronbach's alpha = 0.92). Although 78–84% of cases are reported to be successfully identified as victims using this tool, experience and specialized training are required for valid use. Moreover, it takes two to three hours to complete the measure, making it impractical to use in most settings.

The Conflict Tactics Scale (CTS) has been used since 1978 to identify victims of intimate partner violence, but it is heavily weighted toward identification of physical violence. Moreover, it is not specific to the older adult and does not include neglect. Recently, a modified version of the CTS (MCTS) was studied among caregivers of dementia patients in the United Kingdom (Cooper, Manela, Katona, & Livingston, 2008; Cooper, Maxmin, Selwood, Blanchard, & Livingston, 2009). Using weighted physical abuse scores, the modified measure was compared with the findings of an expert panel. The weighted MCTS with a cutoff point of four out of five demonstrated 100% sensitivity, 98% specificity, 79% positive predictive value, and 100% negative predictive value. Internal consistency using Chronbach's alpha was 0.83. However, there are many modified versions of the CTS and, according to the published reports, it is unclear which has the greatest validity.

The Hwalek-Sengstock Elder Abuse Screening Test (H-S/EAST) was originally designed in 1986 as a 15-item self-report tool which could be used quickly to identify older adults who were victims of abuse (Neale, Hwalek, Scott, Sengstock, & Stahl 1991). The 15-item scale had a false positive rate of 9.3%, and a false negative rate of 35.7% in the original validation. Another study showed a correct classification in 67–74% of cases (Nelson, Nygren, McInerney, & Klein 2004). A study using the H-S/EAST in the Australian Longitudinal Study on Women's Health led to further refinement of the instrument to six items focused on the factors of vulnerability and coercion. Unfortunately, the refined version lacked comparison to a gold standard assessment, and sensitivity and specificity could not be evaluated (Schofield, Reynolds, Mishra, Powers & Dobson, 2002).

The BASE, CASE, IOA, CTS and H-S/EAST are just a few examples of the many instruments being developed and used in studies. No one instrument has been proven to have adequate psychometric properties and utility in everyday practice. Without such an instrument, it remains a challenge to efficiently and successfully identify victims in need of help and participants for much-needed research. The current clinical and research standard is still reliant on clinical observation and identification of cases based on practitioners' varied experiences.

In 2004, the Ohio Elder Abuse Task Force produced a manual to guide development of Interdisciplinary Teams (I-Team) to address the problems of elder mistreatment (Elder Abuse Task Force, 2004). This major undertaking required the coordination and efforts of many organizations around the country. The I-Team model capitalizes on the need for unique approaches and coordinated interdisciplinary interventions. The ideal team meets at least eight times annually per county and includes representatives with expertise in social work, legal issues, medicine, law enforcement, domestic violence, finances, clergy, animal control, and housing. In addition, there is a representative from the state ombudsman's office for institutional abuse. It is also recommended that there be representation of community minority groups within the I-Team. At each meeting, presentation of each case lasts 20–30 minutes. Although comprehensive in addressing the complex, systemic nature of elder abuse, this coordinated effort is time-consuming and requires considerable effort to coordinate the multiple professional areas represented by such a diverse team. Nevertheless, this is a promising area for future study within settings where resources exist to launch a multi-faceted, multidisciplinary approach.

SPECIAL ISSUES

Given the estimated high prevalence of elder abuse and the concomitant stresses for individuals, families, and providers, it is important to address several special issues that are frequently challenging to clinical providers.

Many clinicians may be hesitant to report suspected cases of abuse because of the risk of disrupting the patient–therapist rapport. There is no easy solution to this predicament either. It is the responsibility of clinicians to ensure the safety of their patients, and in the case of children, the lines are more clearly drawn; we all must call Child Protective Services (CPS) when a child is in danger. But, most older adults have the ability to make choices related to their own care, and free will is a prized right that clinicians must respect. There are cases where an older adult patient does not realize the danger they face when the clinician must intervene, but each case must be considered on an individual basis.

The clinician must take into account the type and immediacy of risk toward the patient, the patient's understanding of this risk, and the patient's ability to modify the situation on their own. Clearly, thinking about cases in this way will make the continuum of abuse and responses to abuse apparent. Discussion and supervision with colleagues can really help the clinician deal with this challenge. Development of relationships with providers of services for older adults, such as care managers, visiting nurses, APS, and contacts with a local area agency on aging can help provide the clinician with resources to rely upon when a suspected case of abuse is encountered.

Unfortunately, there seems to be a profound misunderstanding of the role APS can actually play in most instances of suspected elder abuse. Most professionals are more familiar with the Child Protective Services (CPS) than APS, in part due to mandatory reporting laws and required training. For example, physicians in New York State must complete child abuse training before their licenses are issued. CPS has a mandate to remove children from abusive environments immediately, but because adults have rights to self-determination, APS often cannot remove abused elders.

In many states, APS takes only cases for clients that meet three specific criteria: (1) must be above the age of 18; (2) must be unable to care for him/herself due to a physical or mental disability; and (3) must not have an available caregiver. These strict criteria eliminate many of the patients that physicians see in a hospital setting since in the hospital an older adult has active caregivers and is in a safe place. If the client is in the community, they often have a designated caregiver and are not eligible for APS. If it is determined that the client does not meet the three criteria, the case is closed. This limitation of services, in addition to the perceived delay of response, has turned many professionals away from utilizing APS.

Another dilemma clinicians may face when a case of abuse is suspected is who has legal jurisdiction over the case. A number of areas have developed police and district attorneys' offices with specialized expertise on cases involving older adults, and interest in this area continues to grow. Clinicians can now call and ask for specialized legal professionals to investigate suspected cases of abuse. Also, many areas have developed coalitions of groups concerned with the welfare of older adults, which one can contact for help and information. In the United States, one can contact the National Committee for the Prevention of Elder Abuse (NCPEA) at www.preventelderabuse.org for lists of member organizations. Internationally, the International Network for the Prevention of Elder Abuse (INPEA) at www.inpea.net has additional contact information for groups throughout Africa, Japan, and Europe.

CONCLUSION AND FUTURE DIRECTIONS

Although elder abuse is becoming more recognized in our society, there is still uncertainty about the actual prevalence of the problem and a paucity of well-validated, efficient, and effective measures for the identification of potential cases. Researchers continue to develop new tools and to refine existing approaches. Success in this effort depends in great part on the use of common terminology and definitions, such as that proposed by the National Center on Elder Abuse (1998). In addition, screening and assessment approaches must be standardized and adapted in a manner consistent with the social and cultural context in which the elder lives. As the USPSTF has already declared, research needs to be done to determine whether the tools that we use are helpful or harmful for victims.

One means of increasing the likely effectiveness of screening approaches is to assure that they are applied within a coordinated system of care prepared to respond to the complex, systemic challenges presented by abused elders and their families or caregivers. Aging services provide one such context. Community-dwelling older adults often encounter care managers for help with a variety of services, from help with coordinating in-home services and grocery shopping to help with paying heating bills. Care managers often meet the older adult in his or her home, giving the care manager the opportunity to see the older adult in an environment that a therapist or physician cannot imagine from their offices. This access allows the aging services care manager to ask private, sensitive questions about all parts of the older adult's life, including questions about elder abuse.

Through a grant from the National Institute on Aging, in partnership with the largest aging services provider in our area, we are developing a screening tool for aging services care managers to use as part of their routine screening interviews. This screening tool development includes a number of qualitative interviews to assess the acceptability and understandability of the questions to older adults and to the care managers as well.

Only when safe screening becomes standardized as part of routine care of older adults will we be equipped to intervene early on and prevent the most egregious forms of abuse and neglect of our elders.

APPENDIX A

Brief Abuse Screen for the Elderly (BASE)

Please respond to every question (as well as you can estimate) concerning all clients ____ years or over who are caregivers (give regular help of any kind) or care receivers:

1. Is the client an older person or caregiver? ☐ Yes ☐ No
2. Is the client a caregiver of an older person? ☐ Yes ☐ No
3. Do you suspect abuse? ☐ Yes ☐ No

i) By caregiver (comments) ____________________

1	2	3	4	5
No, not at all	Only slightly, doubtful	Possibly, probably, somewhat	Yes, quite likely	Definitely

ii) By care receiver or other (comments) ____________________

1	2	3	4	5
No, not at all	Only slightly, doubtful	Possibly, probably, somewhat	Yes, quite likely	Definitely

4. If any answer for #3 except "no, not at all," indicate what kind(s) of abuse(s) is (are) suspected.

i) physical ____ ii) psychosocial _____ iii) financial _____ iv) neglect _______ (include passive and active)

5. If abuse is suspected, about how soon do you estimate that intervention is needed?

1	2	3	4	5
Immediately	Within 24 hours	24-72 hours	1 week	2 or more weeks

Scoring information was not provided.

APPENDIX B

CAREGIVER ABUSE SCREEN (CASE)

Purpose: To screen for abuse through multiple sources, for instance, through caregivers, care-receivers, and/or abuse interveners, rather than only through professional reporting. It is designed specifically for community use.

Instructions: The CASE has eight items to ask informal caregivers of which "yes" or "no" are the answers. A caregiver may complete the questionnaire. A score of four or more on the CASE may be conservatively considered as suggestive of a higher risk for abuse. However, even a score of one can be indicative of abuse.

Please answer the following questions as a helper or caregiver:

	YES	NO
1. Do you sometimes have trouble making (___________ [name of person]) control his/her temper or aggression?	____	____
2. Do you often feel you are being forced to act out of character or do things you feel bad about?	____	____
3. Do you find it difficult to manage (______'s) behavior?	____	____
4. Do you sometimes feel that you are forced to be rough with (____)?	____	____
5. Do you sometimes feel you can't do what is really necessary or what should be done for (______)?	____	____
6. Do you often feel you have to reject or ignore (_____)?	____	____
7. Do you often feel so tired and exhausted that you cannot meet (_____'s) needs?	____	____
8. Do you often feel you have to yell at (____)?	____	____

APPENDIX C

INDICATORS OF ABUSE (IOA)

Indicators of abuse are listed below, numbered in order of importance.* After a two- to three-hour home assessment (or other intensive assessment) please rate each of the following items on a scale of 0 to 4. Do not omit any items. Rate according to your current opinion.

Scale: Estimated extent of problem:
0 = nonexistent
1 = slight
2 = moderate
3 = probably/moderately severe
4 = yes/severe
00 = non applicable
000 = don't know

Caregiver Age _____ years
Caregiver and Care Receiver Kinship ____ spouse
____ nonspouse

Caregiver

____ 1. Has behavior problems
____ 2. Is financially dependent
____ 3. Has mental/emotional difficulties
____ 6. Has an alcohol/substance abuse problem
____ 7. Has unrealistic expectations
____ 9. Lacks understanding of medical condition
____ 10. Caregiving reluctancy
____ 12. Has marital/family conflict
____ 13. Has poor current relationship
____ 14. Caregiving inexperience
____ 17. Is a blamer
____ 24. Had poor past relationship

Care Receiver

____ 4. Has been abused in the past
____ 5. Has marital/family conflict
____ 8. Lacks understanding of medical condition
____ 11. Is socially isolated
____ 15. Lacks social support
____ 16. Has behavior problems
____ 18. Is financially dependent
____ 19. Has unrealistic expectations
____ 20. Has alcohol/medication problem
____ 21. Has poor current relationship
____ 22. Has suspicious falls/injuries
____ 23. Has mental/emotional difficulties
____ 25. Is a blamer
____ 26. Is emotionally dependent
____ 27. No regular doctor

APPENDIX D

(From Hwalek & Sengstock, 1986)

ELDER ABUSE SCREENING TEST

1. ** Do you have anyone who spends time with you, taking you shopping or to the doctor?[1]
2. *** Are you helping to support someone?
3. ** Are you sad or lonely?
4. * Who makes decisions about your life—like how you should live or where you should live?
5. *** Do you feel uncomfortable with anyone in your family?
6. ** Can you take your own medication and get around by yourself?
7. *** Do you feel that nobody wants you around?
8. *** Does anyone in your family drink a lot?
9. * Does someone in your family make you stay in bed or tell you you're sick when you're not?
10. * Has anyone forced you to do things you didn't want to do?
11. * Has anyone taken things that belonged to you without your OK?
12. *** Do you trust most of the people in your family?

13. *** Does anyone tell you that you give them too much trouble?
14. *** Do you have enough privacy at home?
15. * Has anyone close to you tried to hurt you or harm you recently?

References

Alpert, E. J., Tonkin, A. E., Seeherman, A. M., & Holtz, H. A. (1998). Family Violence Curricula in U.S. Medical Schools. *American Journal of Preventive Medicine*, *14*, 273–282.

Baker, J. U. (2003). *Elder abuse: Problem in search of a policy.* Loyola University Chicago.

Brandl, B., & Dyer, C. B. (2007). *Elder Abuse Detection and Intervention*. New York, NY: Springer.

Cooper, C., Manela, M., Katona, C., & Livingston, G. (2008). Screening for elder abuse in dementia in the LASER-AD study: prevalence, correlates and validation of instruments. *International Journal of Geriatric Psychiatry*, *23*, 283–288.

Cooper, C., Maxmin, K., Selwood, A., Blanchard, M., & Livingstone, G. (2009). The sensitivity and specificity of the Modified Conflict Tactics Scale for detecting clinically significant elder abuse. *International Psychogeriatrics*, *21*(4), 774–778.

Dong, X. Q., Simon, M., Mendes de Leon, C., Fulmer, T., Beck, T., Hebert, L., et al. (2009). Elder self-neglect and abuse and mortality risk in a community-dwelling populations. *JAMA*, *302*(5), 517–526.

Elder Abuse Task Force. (2004). Ohio Elder Abuse Interdisciplinary Team (I-Team) Manual.

Fulmer, T., Firpo, A., Guadagno, L., Easter, T. M., Kahan, F., & Paris, B. (2003). Themes from a grounded theory analysis of elder neglect assessment by experts. *Gerontologist*, *43*(5), 745–752.

Fulmer, T., Paveza, G., van de Weerd, C., Fairchild, S., Guadagno, L., Bolton-Blatt, M., et al. (2005). Dyadic vulnerability and risk profiling for elder neglect. *Gerontologist*, *45*(4), 525–534.

Hwalek, M. A., & Sengstock, M. C. (1986). Assessing the probability of abuse of the elderly: Toward development of a clinical screening instrument. *Journal of Applied Gerontology*, *5*(2), 153–173.

Kahan, F. S., & Paris, B. E. C. (2003). Why elder abuse continues to elude the health care system. *Mount Sinai Journal of Medicine*, *70*(1), 62–68.

Kennedy, R. D. (2005). Elder abuse and neglect: The experience, knowledge, and attitudes of primary care physicians. *Family Medicine*, *37*(7), 481–485.

Lachs, M. S., Williams, C. S., O'Brien, S., & Pillemer, K. A. (2002). Adult protective service use and nursing home placement. *Gerontologist*, *42*(6), 734–739.

Lachs, M. S., Williams, C., O'Brien, S., Hurst, L., & Horwitz, R. (1997). Risk factors for reported elder abuse and neglect: A nine-year observational cohort study. *Gerontologist*, *37*(4), 469–474.

Lachs, M. S., Williams, C. S., O'Brien, S., Pillemer, K. A., & Charlson, M. E. (1998). The mortality of elder mistreatment. *JAMA*, *280*(5), 428–432.

National Center on Elder Abuse. (1998). *The National Elder Abuse Incidence Study, Final Report*. Prepared for the Administration on Aging in collaboration with Westat, Inc.

National Research Council. (2003). Elder Mistreatment: Abuse, Neglect, and Exploitation in an Aging America. Panel to Review Risk and Prevalence of Elder Abuse and Neglect. In R. J. Bonnie, & R. B. Wallace (Eds.), *Committee on National Statistics and Committee on Law and Justice, Division of Behavioral and Social Sciences and Education*. Washington, DC: The National Academies Press.

Neale, A. V., Hwalek, M. A., Scott, R. O., Sengstock, M., & Stahl, C. (1991). Validation of the Hwalek-Sengstock Elder Abuse Screening Test. *Journal of Applied Gerontology*, *10*, 406–418.

Nelson, H. D., Nygren, P., McInerney, Y., & Klein, J. (2004). Screening women and elderly adults for family and intimate partner violence: A review of the evidence for the U.S. Preventive Services Task Force. *Annals of Internal Medicine*, *140*, 387–396.

[1] A response of "no" to items 1, 6, 12, and 14; a response of "someone else" to item 4; and a response of "yes" to all others was scored in the "abused" direction.

Identified factors: *violation of personal rights or direct abuse, **characteristics of vulnerability, and ***potentially abusive situation.

Ramsey-Klawsnik, H. (2000). Elder-abuse offenders: A typology. *Generations*, *24*(2), 17–22.

Reis, M., & Nahmiash, D. (1998). Validation of the Indicators of Abuse (IOA) screen. *Gerontologist*, *38*, 471–480.

Reis, M., Nahmiash, D., & Shrier, R. (1993). *A Brief Abuse Screen for the Elderly (BASE): Its validity and use*. Paper presented at the 22nd Annual Scientific and Educational Meeting of the Canadian Association on Gerontology. Montreal, Quebec, Canada.

Reis, M., & Nahmiash, D. (1995). When seniors are abused: An intervention model. *Gerontologist*, *35*, 666–671.

Schofield, M. J., Reynolds, M., Mishra, G. D., Powers, J. R., & Dobson, A. J. (2002). Screening for vulnerability to abuse among older women: Women's Health Australia Study. *Journal of Applied Gerontology*, *21*, 24–39.

Teaster, P. B., & Otto, J. (2006). Abuse of Adults Age 60+: The 2004 Survey of Adult Protective Services – Abuse of Adults 60 Years of Age and Older (report, online resource). http://www.apsnetwork.org/Resources/docs/AbuseAdults60.pdf

U.S. Preventive Services Task Force. (2004). Screening for Family and Intimate Partner Violence: Recommendation Statement. *Annals of Family Medicine*, *2*, 156–160.

WHO/INPEA. (2002). *Missing voices: views of older persons on elder abuse*. Geneva: World Health Organization.

Wood, E. F. (2006). The Availability and Utility of Interdisciplinary Data on Elder Abuse: A White Paper for the National Center on Elder Abuse. Washington, DC: National Center on Elder Abuse.

CHAPTER

Assessment of Dementia Family Caregivers

10

Carey Wexler Sherman[1], **Louis D. Burgio**[2], **Jennifer D. Kowalkowski**[3]

[1] *Institute for Social Research, University of Michigan, Ann Arbor, MI, USA*

[2] *School of Social Work, Institute of Gerontology, University of Michigan, Ann Arbor, MI, USA*

[3] *Psychology Department, Eastern Michigan University, Ypsilanti, MI, USA*

The integral role of the family caregiver (CG) is well established in the research and treatment literature (Aneshensel, Pearlin, Mullan, Zarit, & Whitlatch, 1995; Feinberg, 2002; Schulz & Beach, 1999; Vitaliano, Zhang, & Scanlan, 2003). Such family care has been shown to be protective for care recipients with dementia who, as a result, remain longer in the community and delay institutionalization (Pruchno, Michaels, & Potashnik, 1990; Whitlatch, Feinberg, & Stevens, 1999). Extensive research demonstrates, however, that prolonged and challenging family caregiving can induce a litany of adverse physical and mental health effects (see reviews by Gaugler, Davey, Pearlin, & Zarit, 2000; Pinquart & Sorensen, 2003, 2005; Vitaliano, Zhang, & Scanlon, 2003). Public policy in the United States relies heavily on the provision of home-based intensive and long-term family care for relatives with chronic health concerns (Stone, 2000; Thompson, 2004). Family caregivers currently provide over $250 billion dollars in unpaid labor (Arno, Levine, & Memmott, 1999), and the numbers of families impacted by lengthy periods of caregiving will only increase as the population ages and dementia prevalence increases (Herbert, Scherr, Bienias, Bennett, & Evans, 2003).

Negative physical health outcomes that have been associated with caregiving include weaker immune response (Kiecolt-Glaser, Glaser, Gravenstein, Malakey & Sheridan, 1996), chronic sleep disturbance (Rausch, Baker, & Boonmee, 2007), cognitive decline (Caswell et al., 2003), and greater risk for morbidity and mortality (Schulz & Beach, 1999). Such adverse effects can also threaten the quality of care provided to the patient. Family caregiving has also been associated with deleterious mental health effects, including higher rates of depression and anxiety (Pearlin & Aneshensel, 1994), caregiver burden and stress (Zarit, Davey, Edwards, Femia, & Jarrott, 1998; Vitaliano,Young & Russo, 1991), and increased isolation and loneliness (Beeson, Horton-Deutsch, Farran, & Neundorfer 2000; Bergman-Evans, 1994). Research in recent years has also highlighted the positive outcomes of caregiving. Many caregivers report feelings of satisfaction, fulfillment and growth from their contributions to assuring the well-being of their care recipient (Buffum & Brod, 1998; Farran, Keane-Hagerty, Salloway, Kupferer, & Wilken, 1991; Roff, et al., 2004).

Recent caregiving meta-analyses and reviews increasingly recognize and reflect the complex, transactional, and multifaceted nature of the caregiving experience for patients and their family members (Pinquart & Sorenson, 2005). At the same time, a recent report by the National Center on Caregiving at the Family Caregiver Alliance (Family Caregiving Alliance, 2006) reiterated

Handbook of Assessment in Clinical Gerontology. DOI: 10.1016/B978-0-12-374961-1.10010-7

concerns that systematic assessment of the circumstances or well-being of family caregivers in community settings is still under-utilized and under-examined (Baxter, 2000; Feinberg, Whitlatch, & Tucke, 2000). Zarit, Femia, Kim and Whitlatch (2010) highlight the growing recognition that "caregivers possess unique combinations of risk factors and outcomes that suggest the need for individualized or tailored interventions" (p. 2). Similarly, researchers have noted that the array of personal and situational stressors, and the presence or lack of resources, combine in distinctive and influential ways to either mediate or moderate outcomes (Lazarus & Folkman, 1984; Pearlin, Mullan, Semple, & Skaff, 1990).

Therefore, a primary reason for conducting a systematic assessment of CGs is as a prerequisite for greater specificity and sophistication in intervention and practice efforts. Indeed, evidence-based intervention studies have helped identify which skills, supports, and strategies best serve the needs of particular groups of caregivers. Such research has demonstrated that caregivers do better—or, at least less badly—when they have a solid working knowledge of their family member's disease, are taught various skills to manage the stress and burden of caregiving (Belle et al., 2006; Hepburn, Lewis, Sherman, & Tornatore, 2003) and/or when interventions address personal psychological needs such as depression or anxiety (Mittleman, Roth, Coon, & Haley, 2004).

BACKGROUND ON ASSESSMENT

Practitioners have a vast variety of caregiver assessments to choose from. The key to successful integration and implementation of caregiver assessment relies on selecting those measures that reflect the goals of a service program or a treatment plan, as well as the types of CGs who are being served. It is also critical to determine how the assessment information will be used. The focus of this chapter is on the assessments used for clinical purposes and care planning.

The Family Caregiver Alliance's review of CG assessment utilization (FCA, 2006) states that any assessment should serve to: improve CGs' understanding of their role; provide practitioners with relevant information to establish a care or treatment plan with achievable outcomes; and assist practitioners in providing referrals for appropriate services. This involves assessment of CGs' characteristics and problems, but also their perceptions of stress and burden related to the care recipients' (CR) behavior and limitations.

The important domains of information provided by CG assessment include general background on the CG and their situation, the CG's physical and emotional health, the perceptions of burden and stress associated with CRs' functional and behavioral status, and the CG's salient cultural or personal caregiving values, preferences, and style. In addition, a primary focus of many caregiver assessments is to determine the CG's knowledge of relevant caregiving skills or strategies relevant to their CG role, as well as personal, family, and community resources available to the caregiver (FCA, 2006). An often neglected but critical variable is the CG's report of overall quality of life (Frisch, 1988; Frisch et al., 2005). Finally, it is also valuable to inquire about the caregiver's evaluation of the quality of the care relationship as part of a client-specific assessment.

A primary goal of this chapter, then, is to suggest and review psychometrically sound assessments that the authors have found helpful in guiding the clinicians to effective interventions. We have attempted to select measures that are accessible, widely used and, with a few exceptions, in the public domain. We include in the chapter a few "exemplar" measures in their entirety, for illustration. While these measures represent the current "gold standard," the scope of this chapter does not allow a truly exhaustive review. More detailed information on caregiver assessments can be found at: http://www.dementiacoalition.org/pdfs/ca_grid.pdf and at http://caregiver.org/caregiver/jsp

ASSESSMENT STRATEGY AND PROPOSED MEASURES

Assessment measures are designed to provide a systematic method of collecting information to describe a client's circumstances with respect to specific issues, concerns, problems, strengths, and resources. Given the dynamic and complex nature of family caregiving for relatives with chronic or progressive disease, such as dementia, these assessments will provide timely information on all aspects of CG well-being, which may impact their current ability to provide high quality care to their family member. In this chapter, we propose two categories of assessment: core assessments with global information on such factors as emotional level, physical health, and quality of life; as well as characteristics on the care dyad. The ideal is to provide the core assessment to all CGs who are seeking help. The client-specific assessments, triggered by the core assessments and clinical interviews, are intended to provide more targeted information. The information from the core and client-specific assessments is used to: (1) tailor the intervention to each CG's needs; and (2) when conducted pre- and post-interventions, to provide information on client progress and intervention effectiveness.

First Steps: The Core Assessment Battery

Gathering a general assessment of a caregiver's general circumstances is the optimal place to begin any clinical or service relationship. Therefore, it is important to utilize a measure or instrument that has been constructed to provide a "wide angle" yet detailed view of the caregiving dyad's circumstances with respect to their social, emotional, physical, and financial status, as well as their current service use.

The stressors associated with caregiving have broad impacts across all domains of life. While negative effects are not universal, nor uniform across caregivers, practitioners will want to determine areas of concern in order to develop and provide the most appropriate assistance plan. It is, therefore, crucial in the initial stages of the development of an intervention plan to consider the general personal health and well-being of the caregiver. Extensive research has documented that caregivers often de-emphasize the effects of caregiving upon their own health (Hepburn et al., 2003; Mittleman et al., 2004: Schulz et al., 2003). When caregivers do not attend to their own health issues, or ignore the deleterious effects of caregiving, they can risk their own long-term health and can even put their care recipients at risk of premature and permanent institutionalization. Older caregivers often present with existing health issues, but it is equally important to conduct initial and follow-up assessment of physical and mental health status with middle-aged caregivers, such as adult children. Adult child caregivers often have to manage multiple, and competing, roles and responsibilities. Using information from a global core assessment can identify those areas of the caregiver's life that are in most need, and that are most amenable, to support services.

We recommend that all CGs presenting with significant stress and burden be administered the Core Assessment Battery (see Table 10.1). One such core assessment is the Uniform Assessment Tool (UAT) (California Caregiver Resource Center, 2003 [revised]). The UAT provides an abundance of information that assists the clinician in developing an intervention plan. However, like all assessments provided in this chapter, it is an excellent outcome measure that should, ideally, be administered pre- and post-intervention. Other core assessments include the Quality of Life Inventory (Frisch, 1988; Frisch et al., 2005), a multi-faceted assessment of quality of life, and the SF-36 Health Survey (Ware, Kosinski, & Keller, 1994; Ware, Kosinski, & Dewey, 2000), which provides information on physical and emotional health.

The California Caregiver Resource Center's Uniform Assessment Tool is a highly regarded example of a caregiver-specific omnibus assessment questionnaire. This tool was assembled by

Table 10. 1 Assessment measures

Core Assessment Battery	Reference	# of Items	Scales/Factors
California Caregiver Resource Center— Uniform Assessment Tool			
Survey of demographics			
Caregiving situation		6	
Functional level of care recipient		17	
The revised memory and behavior problems	Teri et al., 1992	24	
CR health		4	
CG health and well-being		15	
Adapted Zarit Burden Interview	Bedard et al., 2001	12	
Caregiver relationship issues		1	
Desire to institutionalize	Morycz, 1985		
CH information and service needs			
Plan of action (completed by staff)			
Caregiver questionnaire (CES-D)	Radloff, 1977	20	
Quality of Life Inventory (QOLI)	Frisch, 1988; Frisch, 1994	32	16 dimensions (scales) including: health, self-esteem, goals and values, money, work, play, learning, creativity, helping, love, friends, children, relatives, home, neighborhood, community, overall score
SF-36 Health Survey	Ware et al., 2000	36	Eight scales including: physical functioning, role-physical, bodily pain, general health, vitality, social functioning, role-emotional, mental health
Client-Specific Assessments: Negative Sequelae of Caregiving			
Caregiver Stressor Scale—Revised	Zarit, Stephens, Townsend, & Green, 1998		
Role captivity	Zarit et al., 1998	3	
Worry and strain	Zarit et al., 1998	8	
Overload	Pearlin et al., 1990	7	
Anger	Derogatis & Spencer, 1982;	3	
	Pearlin et al., 1990	1	
CES-D	Radloff, 1977	20	
Positive and Negative Affect Schedule (PANAS-SF)	Watson, Clark, & Tellegen, 1988	10	
Patient Health Questionnaire Brief Depression Scale (PHQ-9)	Spitzer, Kroenke, & Williams, 1999	9	

Table 10. 1 Assessment measures *(continued)*

Core Assessment Battery	Reference	# of Items	Scales/Factors
REACH-Adapted Functional Independence Scale (FIM, now CAFU)	Gitlin et al., 2005	17	Two factor structure: ADL's and IADL's (Gitlin et al., 2005)
Zarit Burden Interview	Zarit, Reever, & Bach-Peterson, 1980	22	Three subscales: embarrassment/anger, reaction to patient's dependency, and self-criticism (Knight, Fox, & Chou, 2000)
Client-Specific Assessments: Positive Aspects of Caregiving			
Positive Aspects of Caregiving	Tarlow et al., 2004	9	Two factors: self-affirmation and outlook on life (Tarlow et al., 2004)
CG Self-Efficacy Scale	Steffan, McKibbin, Zeiss, Galaagher-Thompson, & Bandura, 2002		
Resilience Scale	Wagnild & Young, 1993	25	Two factors: personal competence and acceptance of self and life
The Duke University Religion Index (DUREL)	Koenig, Parkerson, & Meador, 1997	5	

a state-funded caregiver support program that serves 11 California Resource Centers. The UAT is designed to examine the needs and situations of family caregivers to aid in care planning and service support, and includes both survey-style and open-ended questions. It includes two "gold standard" measures of caregiving-specific burden and stress, the adapted Zarit Burden Scale (Bedard et al., 2001) and the Memory and Behavioral Problems (Teri et al., 1992). These well-established scales are described in greater detail below.

The UAT asks the CG for general demographics, but also to report on the overall care situation, including information on the care dyad's living situation, duration and intensity of care, financial status, medical insurance coverage, and the willingness to institutionalize. Questions also ask about the CR's health and disease status, and the CG's self-reported physical and mental health, and availability of social support. Examples of open-ended questions include, "Are other family members or friends involved in the care of (CR)?" "If family or friends are involved, how are they working together to provide care for (CR)?" and "What functional problems cause you the most concern in caring for (CR)?" Finally, the UAT includes a Care Plan and Service Recommendation Form, which allows the practitioner to directly link a caregiver's scores on the UAT to available programs and/or support services.

The UAT represents an easily accessible and comprehensive tool for clinicians to use in both initial and follow-up assessment of a caregiver's overall status. The instrument is designed to be administered by a practitioner and could be readily integrated into a more in-depth clinical or support service interview. Given its more extensive and open-ended format, it is difficult to estimate exact administration time, but allowing sufficient time for a caregiver to respond to the questions would be an important consideration in interview planning.

The Quality of Life Inventory (QOLI) provides both an overall and domain-specific assessment of the client's satisfaction with life. Feelings of satisfaction are based on the extent to which a person feels that their needs, goals, and wishes are being met in the important areas of life (Frisch et al., 2005). The QOLI measures strengths, assets, and "real life" challenges in a non-pathological manner. Given that CGs who report high strain also report more problems with emotional distress, worse physical functioning, and fewer social contacts than non-caregivers (Roth, Perkins, Wadley, Temple, & Haley, 2009), eliciting information on quality of life issues through instruments like the QOLI can serve as the basis of an intervention plan, as well as an effective way to measure treatment progress.

The QOLI's 32 items reflect a client's generalized assessment of life satisfaction through 16 scales focusing on the individual's health, self-esteem, goals and values, finances, work and leisure, learning, creativity, support, affection, family and friends, home, neighborhood, and community. A score is obtained for each scale, which combine for an overall score. The QOLI can be administered either through a paper—pencil or computer format, takes only 15 minutes to complete, and is accessible to individuals with only a sixth grade reading level. It is worth noting that the QOLI is currently not in the public domain and must be purchased, and that there is a service for scoring and preparing comprehensive patient profiles. (For further information on the QOLI, refer to http://pearsonassess.com.)

As stated earlier, it is always important to determine the CG's health status. While caregivers should be directed to consult with their primary care physicians, many caregivers may postpone preventive health visits or procedures due to time or financial constraints that result from their caregiving role. Inquiring about current physical health problems can be a valuable opportunity to promote family members' essential self-care and reinforce how their well-being guarantees the highest quality care for their loved one. In addition, recent research has also demonstrated the importance of assessing caregiver cognition. As CGs are expected to manage all aspects of their loved one's medical care, decision-making, and logistics of daily life, it is crucial that the caregiver's own cognitive abilities are intact and not overly stressed by the demands (Caswell et al., 2003).

To this end, the SF-36 Health Inventory is a multi-purpose, short-form health survey that can also be used meaningfully with caregivers. As with the QOLI, the SF-36 has been used and examined extensively in medical and intervention studies across a diverse range of patient and non-clinical populations. The SF-36 has been used in studies of over 200 diseases and conditions to determine disease burden and disease-specific benchmarks. In fact, a recent meta-analysis of generic "quality of life" measures recently judged the SF-36 to be the most widely evaluated generic patient-assessed health outcome measure (Garratt, Schmidt, Mackintosh, & Fitzpatrick, 2002).

The SF-36 is noted for being brief yet comprehensive, and for its well-documented psychometric properties (for full history of development and psychometric evaluations see Ware, Snow, Kosinski, & Gandek, 1993 and Ware et al., 2000). The items included in the current questionnaire represent multiple operational indicators of health, including behavioral function and dysfunction, distress and well-being, objective reports and subjective ratings, and both favorable and unfavorable self-evaluations of general health status (Ware et al., 1993). Now available in over 100 languages, the SF-36's questions provide an 8-scale profile of functional health and well-being scores for physical functioning, role of physical status, bodily pain, general health, vitality, social functioning, role of emotional status, and mental health. Questions include, "Does your health now limit you in the (following) activities? If so, how much?" Response options in these questions range from "Yes, limited a lot" to "No, not limited at all." Other examples of questions include, "During the past four weeks, to what extent have your physical or emotional problems interfered with your normal social activities with family, friends, neighbors or groups?" Questions such as this include a multi-level response option, ranging from "Not at all" to "Extremely." Such questions are highly relevant to caregiving adults, yet non-pathologizing in their tone and style.

The SF-36 can be administered either through an interview format, by the client, or via computerized administration. It generally takes only 10–15 minutes to administer and has been used effectively and reliably with patients over the age of 14 years. It has been used successfully in young and old populations, and in many countries. Computer administered and telephone voice recognition interactive systems are currently being evaluated, according to the SF-36 websites (http://www.sf-36.org and http://qualitymetric.com).

Next Steps: Targeted Assessments

It is expected that results from core assessments, such as those described above, will identify central areas of concern and areas where assistance is needed, and guide the practitioner toward their next steps of intervention. At the same time, a CGs scores may indicate the need for additional, more focused assessment. For example, if a caregiver's SF-36 scores suggest that their emotional well-being is limiting their ability to sustain the needed level of care or self-care, the clinician will want to obtain a more focused assessment of caregiver depression, anxiety, and/or burden.

The potential for negative effects resulting from caregiving has been extensively documented in research and intervention studies. Caregivers are at risk of elevated depression, anxiety, isolation, caregiver strain and grief (Meuser & Marwit, 2001; Vitaliano et al., 1991), and family conflict (Semple, 1992). In addition, dementia caregiving is considered to be among the most intensive and challenging form of care (Vitaliano et al., 1991; Zarit, Orr & Zarit, 1985). For these reasons, targeted mental health assessment is often an important aspect of caregiver clinical and support services.

Caregiver Depression

Caregivers have been shown to have significantly higher rates of depression and anxiety relative to the non-caregiving population. Informal caregivers are at nearly three times higher risk for depression compared with the general populations of similar age (Schulz & Beach, 1999). As many as 60% of caregivers report depressive symptomology (National Family Caregivers Association, 2001). Depression in caregivers is costly. Depression contributes to early institutionalization, neglect, and elder abuse of the care recipient. Dementia caregivers in particular appear to be at risk for mental health concerns, even compared with other caregivers.

There are many depression measures available. Most research and practice relies on a few widely used measures for determining the presence or degree of depressive symptomotology, including the Center for Epidemiologic Studies Depression Scale (CES-D); (Radloff, 1977) and the Geriatric Depression Scale (Yesavage et al., 1983). A newer measure of depression, the Physical Health Questionnaire (PHQ-9) has been well validated in medical and practice research, and offers a very reliable and brief screen adept at distinguishing the presence and severity of depression (Kroenke, Spitzer & Williams, 2001; Kroenke & Spitzer, 2002). The PHQ-9 was recently highlighted by the MacArther Initiative on Depression and Primary Care (http://depression-primary care.org).

This 9-item depression scale has been shown to be a powerful predictive tool for primary care clinicians in diagnosing depression. It is also suggested as a valuable tool for selecting and monitoring treatment progress. Based on the hallmark diagnostic criteria for major depressive disorder as delineated in the Diagnostic and Statistical Manual, Fourth Edition (DSM-IV), it assesses symptoms and functional impairment, and derives a severity score to help direct care plans. The respondent is asked, "Over the last two weeks, how often have you been bothered by the following problems?" Problems include, "little interest or pleasure in doing things," "poor appetite or overeating," or "feeling bad about yourself, that you are a failure or have let your family down." Questions have a 4-point response option, ranging from "not at all" to "nearly every day." In addition, there is a separate question that asks "how difficult have any of these problems made it for the respondent to do his/her work, take care of things at home, or get along with other people?" The scale is brief and easy to administer and can be completed by the patient directly, with the score tabulated by a clinical staff member. Higher scores indicate more severe depressive symptoms. The PHQ-9 is being used extensively in medical and dementia research and intervention, and is readily available (see http://www.pfizer.com for terms of use).

Caregiver Burden

Caregiver burden is defined as the all-encompassing challenges felt by caregivers with respect to their physical and emotional well-being, family relations, and work and financial status (Pearlin et al., 1990; Zarit et al., 1985). Zarit and colleagues have designed a series of exemplary measures to assess burden that have guided measurement and research in the caregiving field. The Zarit Burden Interview (ZBI; Zarit, Reever, & Bach-Paterson, 1980) and an abridged 12-item version with similar psychometric properties to the longer version (Bedard et al., 2001; see Appendix A) is the most widely referenced scale in studies of caregiver burden, and often serves as the primary outcome measure for negative affect. Questions on the ZBI-12 include, "Do you feel stressed between caring for your relative and trying to meet other responsibilities for your family or work?" with response options ranging from "never" to "nearly always". Other questions include, "Do you feel that you have lost control of your life since your relative's illness?" and "Do you feel you should be doing more for your relative?" A second measure, the Caregiver Stressors Scale-Revised (Zarit, Davey, Edwards, Femia, & Jarrott, 1998) is a 25-item measure of caregiving competency, strain, role overload, role captivity, and emotional control. Higher scores on this measure indicate greater caregiver stress.

Behavioral Challenges for Caregivers

While subjective caregiver burden has not been shown to correlate necessarily with the duration of caregiving or the stage of disease, nor functional impairment of the care recipient (CR), it is closely associated with the degree of problem behaviors among dementia care recipients. It may be essential, therefore, to gather current information on the functional level of the care recipient to best understand the nature and demands on the caregiver.

At the same time, documenting the caregiver's activities of daily living (ADLs) or instrumental activities of daily living (IADLs) (Katz, 1983) is a first step, as was demonstrated in the CCRC-UAT. ADL and IADL measures are critical because they are highly associated with use of medical and hospital services, admission to nursing homes (Branch & Jette, 1981), living arrangements (Bishop, 1986), and even mortality (Manton, 1988). As the basic tasks of everyday life, ADLs and the more specific IADLs, give a quick but essential measure of the person's functionality. Among older caregivers, certainly, a good measure of function is critical.

A measure that examines this aspect of caregiving is the REACH-adapted Functional Independence Measure (Gitlin et al., 2005; see Appendix B), now referred to as the Caregiver Assessmant of Function and Upset (CAFU). The REACH CAFU is a 17-item measure in which caregivers rate the ADLS and IADLs of the CR over the past week. Questions about functioning are scored "Yes/No," and each question has a follow-up of whether the caregiver has helped the CR with that area of function (again, "Yes/No"). There is also an additional question about the overall change or improvement in ADLs or IADLs. The CAFU also assesses burden associated with providing care for ADLs and IADLs. Dependence has been associated with the number of years of caregiving and the CR's general level of cognitive function. Psychometric analysis has determined this measure to have good internal consistency.

Care planning may, in certain circumstances, also benefit from more in-depth information about the CR behaviors, as well as the caregiver's response to the behaviors, or level of "bother." The Revised Memory and Behavioral Problems Checklist (RMBPC) (Teri et al., 1992) assessment is considered a valuable tool for measuring the care recipient's particular behavioral and cognitive deficits and the degree to which those behaviors adversely affect or bother the caregiver. Generally, memory-related problems cluster on distinct factors that are separate from emotional difficulties or other emotional problems. This tool asks the caregiver to account for the presence or absence of a set of 24 care recipient behaviors in the past week. Behaviors include, "asking the same question over and over again" and "forgetting what day it is," or "threats to hurt self/others." For each behavior, caregivers rate the degree of frequency, ranging from "Never occurred" to "Daily or more often." The caregiver is then asked for each behavior to gauge how bothered they find that behavior to be, on a scale ranging from "Not at all" to "Extremely." Higher scores indicate a greater level of behavioral disturbance and caregiver bother. This measure has been found to be highly predictive of caregiver depression and burden, and is used in most caregiver intervention studies.

Finally, another newer measure that practitioners may find very helpful in assessing care planning decisions is the Desire to Institutionalize Scale (DTI; Morycz, 1985). This has been used to assess the DTI among caregivers of persons with dementia in the United States (Belle et al., 2006) and internationally (Hébert, Dubois, Wolfson, Chambers & Cohen, 2001). This measure has demonstrated good internal consistency and reliability across White, African American and Hispanic caregivers. This study represents an important and much needed step in caregiving assessment research, but also reveals that the DTI can be a very useful tool for clinician care planning and support of caregivers by revealing caregivers' desire to institutionalize their CR.

Positive Rewards of Caregiving

In addition to assessing adverse psychological impacts of caregiving, it has become increasingly clear that practitioners should identify and document caregiver's appraisals of rewards and positive aspects of the caregiving experience. Positive rewards have been shown to mediate, or buffer, the adverse effects of CG burden. For example, caregiver depression, daily burden, and subjective health problems have been shown to be significantly lower in CGs reporting greater positive rewards of caregiving (Hilgeman, Allen, DeCoster, Burgio, 2007). Positive dimensions of caregiving include the sense of gratification, fulfillment, and feeling needed, and being able to attend to and "repay" loved ones for their support (Farran, 1997; Hepburn, et al., 2003; Picot, Youngblut, & Zeller, 1997; Switzer et al., 2000; Tarlow et al., 2004). The assessment of positive aspects of caregiving, therefore, is recommended as an integral aspect of CG intervention to support a more strengths-based and positive reward orientation to any clinical practice with caregivers.

One assessment that demonstrates this focus is the REACH Positive Aspects of Caregiving (PAC) (Tarlow et al., 2004; see Appendix C) measure. This brief measure includes nine items and uses language that is readily accessible and allows for greater response variability. The measure is designed to assess subjectively perceived gains from, desirable aspects of, or positive affective returns from providing care for their care recipient. Tested among a diverse large sample, caregivers generally perceived that caregiving provides a variety of positive and satisfying experiences, such as enhanced attitudes and greater appreciation toward life and strengthened relationships with others. This tool asks caregivers to rate how much they agree with statements about caregiving, such as caregiving "made me feel useful; needed," "enabled me to develop a more positive attitude toward life," and "strengthened my relationships with others." Response options are on a 5-point scale ranging from "disagree a lot" to "agree a lot." Gathering a client's level of endorsement of such statements gives a practitioner a useful means of capturing and responding to a caregiver's identification of any positive aspects to the caregiving experience.

Other constructs that tap into positive or strengths-based responses to caregiving include caregiver self-efficacy, resilience, and personal religiosity. These constructs, which represent personal "traits" and cultural preferences or styles, differ from the other health or outcome measures in that they are less likely to change as a result of clinical or training interventions. Nonetheless, we suggest measuring these aspects of CG coping styles may be very useful to planning the most effective, person-focused, and culturally sensitive plan of intervention or support.

Self-efficacy is defined as a person's beliefs about their capacity to respond and perform in ways that influence events that affect their life (Bandura, 1994). People with confidence in their capabilities are better able to approach difficulties as challenges to be mastered, and are more likely to recover from setbacks or failures. Research has found greater self-efficacy is associated with better coping responses, greater levels of accomplishment, and lower stress and depression (Aneshensel et al., 1995). There is growing evidence that self-efficacy is domain or role-specific (ie., parent, cognitive functioning, caregiver) and that it is responsive to reappraisal or refinement as a result of intervention (Bandura, 1997; Steffan et al., 2002).

The Caregiver Self-Efficacy Scale (Steffan et al., 2002) was developed with dementia caregivers to assess perceived self-efficacy for caregiving tasks. It measures three facets of caregiving efficacy: ability to obtain respite; response to disruptive patient behaviors; and controlling upsetting thoughts. Construct validity of the measure was supported by relationships between these three facets of perceived caregiving efficacy and depression, anxiety, anger, perceived social support, and criticism. The scale contains 15 items, with questions such as "How confidently do you feel you can … ask a friend/family member to do errands for you." Respondents are asked to rate their confidence on a scale from 0 (cannot do at all) to 100 (certain can do). While the measure was originally intended to be administered by a clinician, it is feasible for CGs to fill out this measure independently for later review by the clinician. Obtaining the CG's self-report on their ability to manage various aspects of the care role helps clinicians to identify areas of potential strength and concern, and provides valuable insight into the caregiver's perceived ability to cope and respond.

The construct of resilience has been examined by developmental and social psychologists in individuals across the life course. Resilient individuals are thought to exhibit emotional stamina through adaptability and courage, and demonstrate the ability to prosper in the face of extraordinary and chronic challenges (Bonanno, 2004; Masten, 2001; Ramsey & Blieszner, 1999). Another hallmark of resilience is to be able to seek out and obtain support from interpersonal and institutional support systems in order to effectively cope with those challenges.

The Resilience Scale (Wagnild & Young, 1993), which is designed for use by older adults, includes 25 items. Respondents are asked to indicate their level of agreement with such statements as, "I usually manage one way or another." Factor analysis of this scale yielded two factors: personal competence and acceptance of self and life. The scale has high concurrent validity with measures of life satisfaction and morale. While it is not assumed that resilience scores will change dramatically, or at all, in response to intervention, it is extremely valuable for the practitioner to assess their client's level of resilience as a potential gauge of how emotionally sturdy or able to adapt a caregiver may be in the face of a chronic and demanding care trajectory. A person-centered clinical relationship will benefit from tailoring an intervention approach to the person's resilience style. Practitioners can leverage a caregiver's innate sense of resilience, work to address areas of strength that may nurture more resilient responses, or consider whether a client is at greater emotional risk due to lower levels of resilience.

Finally, research has documented that religiosity can play a significant role in personal and cultural coping, particularly in certain racial and ethnic communities (Dilworth-Anderson, Williams, & Gibson, 2002). For example, African American caregivers have been shown to cope with difficulties of caregiving with prayer, faith in God, and religion (Picot et al., 1997; Wood & Parham, 1990). In fact, African American caregivers, compared to White caregivers, often consider God as a part of their informal support network to the same extent as family, friends, and neighbors. Coping through religious belief and/or ritual is likely in other ethnic or cultural group members, depending on their level of affiliation. Therefore, assessing a caregiver's level of religiosity may provide the practitioner with salient information regarding a caregiver's preferred resources and/or style of coping. Of course, it is equally essential to inquire about a client's perceived level of affiliation to their racial or ethnic tradition. Being a particular race or religion (as shown on a demographic form) does not mean that the person necessarily values religion as a primary resource. The culturally sensitive and person-focused practitioner will make no such assumptions, but will open up communication, via an assessment or in the course of clinical dialog, to establish if in fact religion is a meaningful resource for the individual.

A particularly well-regarded measure is the Duke University Religion Index (DUREL) (Koenig et al., 1997). This index was created to measure those aspects of religiousness that are frequently related to health outcomes, while avoiding topics (i.e., well-being) that could contaminate the scale. This brief measure contains only five items, and so is very quick to administer, and has demonstrated relatively high internal consistency reliability. The respondent's frequency rates are obtained for organizational religiosity (e.g., church or temple attendance), non-organizational religiosity (e.g., reading religious texts), and intrinsic aspects of religiosity (e.g., incorporation into daily life). Frequency response options range from 1 (low) to 6 (high). It has been suggested that scores be interpreted into three levels: minimal (1, 2); moderate (3, 4); and high (5, 6).

ASSESSING CONTEXTUAL VARIABLES: THE FAMILY UNIT AND SOCIAL SUPPORT

Although items on the Uniform Assessment Tool ask for contextual variables, time allowing, the clinician may want additional information. We consider the assessment of these factors supplemental—not because they are of secondary importance—but because, due to their complexity, they are factors that are likely beyond the clinician's ability to change substantially.

The Family Unit

Family members can provide critical support to the primary caregiver, thus reducing the amount of stress and burden experienced by the CG. Perceived social support is understood as a protective resource in health and well-being (Antonucci, Fuhrer, & Dartigues, 1997; Oxman, Berkman, Kasl, Freeman, & Barrett, 1992), and most people, especially older adults, report preferring to get assistance from close family members compared with friends or formal agencies. Conversely, conflict within the family can be a major source of stress and burden (Semple, 1992), ambivalence (Luescher & Pillemer, 1998), and guilt (Murphy, Hanrahan, & Luchins, 1997) for CGs.

As marital and family histories continue to become increasingly complex across the life course (Bornat, Dimmock, Jones, & Peace, 1999; De Jong Gierveld & Peeters, 2003; Sherman & Boss, 2007), practitioners are advised to recognize that family membership or proximity may not guarantee assistance. Similarly, close social ties often include non-family members, especially in different groups. African American, immigrant and gay/lesbian families are often comprised of both biological and fictive kin. Identifying and incorporating a broad and responsive approach to clients' support networks is essential to successful intervention with CGs in diverse ethnic, racial, religious or affinity communities.

In addition, social isolation is a genuine risk factor for many CGs. In many cases, however, CGs may not be able or willing to acknowledge the degree to which they are isolated from or in conflict with their close social ties. For that reason, measurements which assess this dimension of the caregiving experience can offer targeted, yet non-pathologizing information for intervention planning.

When it is relevant to assess social networks and support for a CG, there are a variety of measures to consider. The Family Environment Scale (FES; Moos & Moos, 1994) measures social and environmental characteristics of families and has been used extensively in clinical settings to diagnose and intervene in family issues. The FES measures people's perceptions of their actual family environments. For CGs presenting family focused concerns or conflicts, the FES could provide valuable assessment of a CG's perceived family situation. The FES includes 10 subscales measuring three underlying dimensions of the family environment: relationship; personal growth; system maintenance; and change. The scale has been shown to have respectable internal and test—retest reliability.

The quality of the pre-existing and current CG—CR relationship can also provide critical information to the clinician. Caregivers reporting higher satisfaction in their premorbid relationships with the CR report significantly less burden and less reactivity to CR memory and behavioral problems, and have higher problem solving and more effective communication with the CR (Steadman, Tremont, & Davis, 2007).

Similarly, CGs who frame their role primarily in terms of their ongoing relationship to the CR appear to fare better over the duration of caregiving (Lewis, Hepburn, Narayan, & Kirk, 2005). Therefore, tapping into client-specific and defining aspects of a particular care relationship is essential to the provision of support services that address CG's unique and specific needs and care experience. For example, the Burns Relationship Satisfaction Scale (BRSS; Burns & Sayers, 1988) is a brief 7-item self-report inventory that assesses the degree of overall and specific relationship satisfaction, including communication, openness, conflict resolution style, degree of affection, intimacy, closeness and caring, and role satisfaction. Responses range from 0 (very dissatisfied) to 6 (very satisfied) to give an overall summed score (0—42). This measure has high internal consistency and is highly correlated with other measures of relationship satisfaction.

Two other brief social support instruments include the Multidimensional Scale of Perceived Social Support (MSPSS; Zimet, Dahlem, Zimet, & Farley, 1988) and the Lubben Social Network Scale (LSNS-6). The MSPSS asks respondents to indicate level of agreement with 12 statements reflecting perceived social support from family, friends and close social ties. The revised Lubben Social Network Scale (LSNS-6) is a brief 6-item tool that assesses perceived social support received from family and friends in order to gauge degree or risk of social isolation (Lubben et al., 2006; Lubben & Gironda, 2004). Recent evaluations of the LSNS-6 found it to have high internal consistency, stable factor structures, and good predictive power. This tool offers a valuable addition to a clinician's targeted assessment of a CG's perceived and experienced social isolation in the caregiving role.

THE PRACTICE OF ASSESSMENT

It is common for clinicians to conduct assessment at or near the beginning of their therapeutic contact with clients. The purpose of these assessments is to provide critical information that will help the clinician to better understand the issues and problems facing the caregiver. By administering the core assessment, which is usually followed by selected client-specific assessments, information is gleaned that informs the overall care plan and helps identify interventions that target the most pressing problems.

We believe that a single administration of an assessment package is necessary, but no longer sufficient when providing clinical support in either a private practice or in a community agency setting. Given that change is a fundamental characteristic of any caregiving experience, some method of periodic reassessment provides critical and systematic means by which to monitor changes in caregiver status, well-being or care demands. It is incumbent on all clinicians, therefore, to provide at least pre- and post-intervention assessments to ascertain whether they have helped the CG reach their therapeutic and/or caregiving strategy goals; reduce overall CG burden, depression, and bother related to CR behavioral disturbances, the provision of ADL care, or relational issues. Most preferable, although perhaps less feasible, is for clinicians to also conduct reassessments mid-treatment to assess whether the intervention is in fact having the desired effects on the identified areas of greatest concern.

While reassessments often involve using more focused or abridged measures to monitor progress on a care plan, practitioners should recognize that if reassessments are too narrow, they may miss the identification of new or emerging concerns or issues. Changes in the CG or CR's status may precipitate new caregiving challenges that, if undetected, could adversely affect CG well-being and/or affect the quality of care for the CR.

By reassessing the CG, one can discover whether the therapeutic contacts are, in essence, cost- and time-effective. Cost-effectiveness can be measured in terms of investment in staff time (community settings) and the clients' time. In situations where monetary reimbursements are involved, cost is measured in terms of the amount of money invested to obtain a certain level of improvement in the presenting symptoms. Community agencies are often under intense pressure from funding sources to "increase accountability," i.e., show that they have been effective in changing client outcomes in a positive direction. In an economic climate where more effective services will be expected with fewer dollars, it may not be long before even clinicians in private practice will be required to "prove their worth" and efficacy via assessment measures in order to obtain reimbursement.

The setting in which assessments take place should also be carefully considered to address travel and access constraints faced by CGs. When possible, a home visit as part of an assessment interview, or on its own, offers the practitioner the opportunity to directly observe the care context. Assessments are often administered in an agency or clinician's office, but can also be conducted by telephone, if needed, to minimize additional travel and disruption for the CG. As a rule, assessments are best conducted without the immediate presence of the CR to assure that CGs may speak openly about their caregiving situation or concerns. To this end, some form of coverage for the CR, either in the home or at an agency, may be necessary to assure the collection of the highest quality assessment information.

Cultural/Racial Issues in Assessment

There are three cultural issues that require consideration when administering assessments to CGs from various cultural backgrounds. One crucial rule is to never assume or assign an individual's race or gender. The CG should be allowed to self-select both race and gender, with the use of a brief demographic form that is completed by the CG. If assessment procedures are altered based on race or gender, the CG's self-selection should guide the assessment. In addition, race and gender, at least for the purpose of assessment and intervention, are determined by the individual's identification with the cultural values associated with that race and gender. Although we are not suggesting that practitioners must employ cultural identification or affiliation scales, such scales do exist (e.g., the Cultural Justification for Caregiving Scale; Dilworth-Anderson et al., 2004), and may be relevant depending on the CG's presenting issues or situation.

Second, we recommend strongly that individuals who administer assessments receive cultural sensitivity training and subsequently demonstrate cultural competence. Excellent on-line resources on multicultural training and ethnogeriatric practice and training can be found at http://apa.org/pi/multiculturalguidelines.html and http://www.standford.edu/group/etnoger. To demonstrate cultural competence, we recommend using the Multicultural Awareness Knowledge Skills Survey (MAKSS; D'Andrea, Daniels, & Heck, 1991).

Finally, relatively few CG assessments have been normed on a multicultural sample. Consequently, one cannot be certain that results of an assessment of a non-majority culture CG are comparable with that of White/Caucasian CGs. However, over the last few years, an increasing amount of research has been done comparing the psychometrics and factor structures of CG measures completed by White, African

American and Latino caregivers. Two measures included in this chapter, for example, have been shown to have similar psychometrics and factor structures among these three ethnic/racial groups: the RMBPC (Roth et al., 2003) and the Modified FIM, now refered to as the CAFU (Gitlin et al., 2005). Such research represents an important consideration of cultural influences on assessment and on the CG experience itself.

CONCLUSION

Medical, health, and social science experts have recognized the need to promote the need for a national commitment to integrating family-centered and systematic caregiver assessment into the broader care delivery system. We know that even well-intentioned intervention will not ameliorate depressive symptomotology among caregiver participants if those caregivers are, in fact, not clinically depressed to start with (Zarit & Femia, 2008). Increasingly, clinicians and practitioners need to take caregivers' broader contextual factors into greater account if they are to provide the most targeted and effective intervention. Caregiver's levels of acculturation, cultural values, personal and relational characteristics are important to assess in order to provide services that are genuinely sensitive and relevant to the particular needs of our society's growing number of caregivers.

Pearlin and Aneshensel (1994) wisely cautioned that caregiver outcomes are "best thought of not as end-states but as patterns of continuity and change that parallel continuities and changes in the conditions of caregiving" (p. 18). The use of well-established and appropriate caregiver assessments will play a growing and critical role in identifying, optimizing, and matching individual caregiver's needs and capacities with available resources and support.

CASE STUDIES

Below are three case studies to illustrate how caregiver assessment can be integrated appropriately and meaningfully into clinical practice.

Case Study 1—Spouse caregiver

Edna Stephens, a 75-year-old Caucasian woman, is the primary caregiver for her 82-year-old husband, Dale. Edna and Dale have been married for 56 years and have two adult children. Always having led a very active lifestyle, Edna became concerned when Dale began withdrawing from their regular social events. She had also noticed that he began missing regular meetings at the senior center and forgetting his doctor's appointments. After consultation with their primary care physician, Dale was referred for further testing with a geriatric team. During the period of Dale's assessment appointments, Edna's psychological well-being began to decline significantly. She began to lose weight because she had little appetite and found herself rarely sleeping through the night. She worried constantly about the results of Dale's evaluation and their future together. Their children lived several states away and were very busy with their own lives. She did not want to bother them with the details of the problems until she knew for sure what was happening. Edna tried to keep her worries to herself, as she was afraid to worry Dale and create more stress in their lives.

A few months later, doctor's finally confirmed Dale's diagnosis of Mild Cognitive Impairment (MCI). MCI is often thought of as a transition stage between the normal cognitive decline associated with the aging process and more serious disease processes, such as Alzheimer's disease. Edna called her children and gave them the news about Dale's diagnosis. Edna's daughter, Rebecca, had asked her mother how she was handling everything. Although Edna replied that she was managing just fine, Rebecca was still concerned. Edna had suffered from some minor depressive episodes in her lifetime, particularly around times of stress and transition; the last time occurring when her younger sister passed away seven years ago from breast cancer. Rebecca continued to call Edna on a daily basis and grew more concerned when her mother began to show more signs of depression. Rebecca spoke to her father and they agreed that Edna needed to consult with someone regarding her own emotional state.

Despite some resistance, Dale and Rebecca eventually convinced Edna to speak with their family physician. The physician told Edna that he would be glad to run some blood work and rule out any underlying illness. The nurse in his practice also administered The California Caregiver Resource Center Uniform Assessment Tool as a core assessment to ascertain Edna's general status and the caregiving situation. Edna's scores on the CES-D portion of the UAT were high, suggesting the need for further intervention. Both she and the doctor noticed Edna's flat affective state. Based on the overall UAT results, the physician encouraged Edna to seek counseling at a nearby mental health practice.

During Edna's first appointment, the psychologist, Ms Altrez, conducted a semi-structured interview and administered several assessment measures, including the PHQ-9, the depression severity screen. Ms Altrez recognized a number of important risk factors for depression in Edna's profile; most notably, her history of previous depressive episodes and current life stressors. Based on Edna's scores and history, Ms Altrez recommended Edna continue to work with her for short-term counseling for her depression and for coping with her transition to caregiving. After 12 sessions of cognitive-behavioral treatment for depression, Ms Altrez repeated the PHQ-9 to gauge change, if any, in Edna's depression. Edna's score indicated sufficient decrease in depressive symptom severity for Ms Altrez to recommend reducing clinical visits. At the same time, she encouraged Edna to join the local MCI support group to learn more about how to manage her husband's MCI and to make social contacts with other caregivers and with local support care counselors who assist spouse caregivers.

Case Study 2—Adult Child Caregiver: Issues of Placement

Enrique Garcia is a divorced 39-year-old Latino male with no children. Enrique lives alone as he completes his internal medicine residency in the hospital. His mother, Carmen Garcia, is 62-years-old and lives about 45 minutes from Enrique's house. Carmen has a history of heart disease and hypertension, and has recently been diagnosed with vascular dementia. Enrique's one sister lives on the west coast with her family. Carmen's husband died over 15 years ago.

Although Enrique understood the dementia disease process, he found it very difficult to deal with his mother's personality changes. He began visiting her several times per week because of her frantic requests to perform household chores or to intervene with Carmen's neighbor, who she was convinced was stealing from her. His workplace was accommodating the occasional requests to leave early, but he realized that he needed to make some more sustainable decisions. When Enrique took his mother to her recent doctor appointment, the geriatrician advised Enrique that he would eventually need to make some decisions regarding her long-term care. He feared that she would soon become unable to safely care for herself and would need 24-hour supervision, either in an assisted living facility or a family member's home.

In accordance with traditional Latinos' cultural values, Enrique felt a great sense of responsibility for his mother's care. He strongly resisted the idea of institutionalization out of respect for his mother and avoided discussing the topic with his sister. His own work demands, and his mother's increasing needs, however, made him realize that he needed to make some tough decisions. Enrique's situation is not unique. Many Latino Americans struggle to balance contemporary demands of work and family with the cultural preference in the Latino community for family to provide care for loved ones in the home. Growing up, Enrique witnessed his own mother care for his grandparents in their old age. He felt great shame at his inability to provide the same level of care to his own mother, but realized that he could not provide the level of care she was going to require.

Enrique discussed his predicament with Carmen's neurologist at her next appointment, who encouraged him to speak with the geriatric social worker in the practice. At his first appointment, the social worker interviewed Enrique about his mother's current functioning levels and his own feelings about the situation. As part of the intake interview, the social worker had Enrique fill out the CCRC-UAT. Based on Enrique's responses regarding his family history and his presenting concerns, she also asked him to complete several targeted assessment measures, including the Desire to Institutionalize measure and the Duke University Religion Index (DUREL).

Given Enrique's responses on these instruments and the clinical interview, the social worker focused their subsequent sessions on exploring potential care options that could fulfill Enrique's value and cultural system. Over the course of their sessions, she supported Enrique's successful selection of an assisted living facility that was accustomed to working with Latino elders. This facility had Spanish-speaking staff and activities that reflected residents' religious and cultural preferences. In addition, the social worker connected Enrique with an outreach group that served members of the Latino community. She also connected him with an adult–child caregiver training class that highlighted strategies to balance caregiving and personal roles in a culturally sensitive context.

After three months, Enrique returned to the social worker for a follow-up session. During this meeting, she asked him to complete several measures, including the DTI, to reassess his caregiving situation and how he felt regarding his decisions. With the changes he had made regarding his mother's living situation, Enrique endorsed her institutionalization and also reported less subjective burden and increased positive aspects of caregiving. He was able to express relief that his mother enjoyed the facility's activities and the other residents, and that he could feel confident that, with his ongoing involvement, his mother was being well taken care of at her new facility.

Case Study 3—Spouse Caregiver

Edward Smith is an 82-year-old who has been married to his wife Margaret, 80, for 60 years. Edward and Margaret live together in a rural community. Four years ago, Margaret was diagnosed with Alzheimer's disease. Their three grown children acknowledged Margaret's failing memory, but because they didn't live nearby, they didn't really comprehend the changes in her behavior and the demands of caregiving that their father was facing.

In the early stages of the disease, Edward and Margaret tried very hard to maintain their regular social engagements and lifestyle as much as possible. As Margaret's condition worsened, however, Edward needed to take more control of managing their everyday life, for example coordinating the doctor's appointments and medications, taking care of household chores, and keeping up with shopping and finances. Except for holidays with family, Margaret and Edward had always led an independent lifestyle. They knew how busy their children were with their own families and careers, and didn't want to be a burden on their adult children.

As Margaret's mental status declined, it became more difficult for Edward physically to manage household tasks and monitor Margaret's behavior at the same time. Edward had his own health concerns, with hypertension and cardiovascular disease. He also had arthritis which made doing household tasks challenging. Margaret was also exhibiting behaviors that were worrisome and bothered Edward a great deal: she was very restless at nights; had forgotten to turn off the stove several times; and she repeatedly asked the same questions during each day.

Edward was increasingly feeling that he was not able to handle the demands of care on his own and was worried for her safety. On the advice of a close friend from church, Edward contacted the caregiver support group that met at the church. At the first meeting, Edward received useful information about day-to-day coping, but also learned about nursing home placement, an option he had never really considered. He was glad to talk with other caregivers, but was sorry that he was the only husband in the group. When Edward stayed after the meeting to talk about his special concerns, the group facilitator suggested he would benefit from talking with a care counselor at the local dementia support association.

During his first appointment, Edward described the challenge of caregiving and his growing concern that he would not be able to manage their house and keep Margaret safe. He expressed feeling lonely since their social contacts had dwindled. He felt he was not able to keep up his natural wish to have "everything under control" and to "not depend on anyone else."

In the early stages, the clinician administered several brief assessments to Edward. The core assessment included the Quality of Life Inventory and the SF-36, given Edward's own health, age, and history. Based on the results, the clinician recognized Edward's need for more time and flexibility to attend to his own social and medical needs. She discussed the importance of caregiver self-care, and they discussed steps Edward could take to get some in-home care assistance to help with housework and other caregiving chores. With this extra assistance, Edward would be able to have some time to socialize, lessen the physical burdens of care, and make time for his own doctor appointments. The care counselor advised that Edward might enjoy attending a special husband caregiver group that was held in a nearby town. In addition, the clinician took some session time to discuss with Edward about how he might speak with his children about potential institutional placement when the demands of care became too physically challenging. She discussed with Edward about setting up a family meeting with his children to discuss Margaret's disease trajectory and future care options, including institutionalization options in the region.

After five months of periodic sessions with Edward, the counselor re-administered the QOLI and the SF-36. Edward's scores indicated that despite Margaret's disease progression, he reported higher overall quality of life. Edward had found genuine friendship and support in the husband support group, and reported feeling that with the help of the in-home health aide, he was able to better manage his own health needs and stay connected with old friends and the church community. Edward still expressed feeling concerned and apprehensive about any future nursing home placement for Margaret, but reported relief in knowing that his family now understood and supported his need for greater assistance, and that they were informed about care options when Margaret's condition would require that level of care.

APPENDIX A: ZARIT BURDEN INTERVIEW-12

(Zarit, Reever, & Bach-Paterson, 1980)

ZARIT BURDEN INTERVIEW

INSTRUCTIONS: The following is a list of statements, which reflect how people sometimes feel when taking care of another person. After each statement, indicate how often you feel that way; never, rarely, sometimes, quite frequently, or nearly always. There are no right or wrong answers.

	Never	Rarely	Sometimes	Quite Frequently	Nearly Always
1) Do you feel that because of the time you spend with your relative that you don't have enough time for yourself?	0	1	2	3	4
2) Do you feel stressed between caring for your relative and trying to meet other responsibilities for your family or work?	0	1	2	3	4
3) Do you feel angry when you are around the relative?	0	1	2	3	4
4) Do you feel that your relative currently affects your relationships with other family members or friends in a negative way?	0	1	2	3	4
5) Do you feel strained when you are around your relative?	0	1	2	3	4
6) Do you feel that your health has suffered because of your involvement with your relative?	0	1	2	3	4
7) Do you feel that you don't have as much privacy as you would like because of your relative?	0	1	2	3	4
8) Do you feel that your social life has suffered because you are caring for your relative?	0	1	2	3	4
9) Do you feel that you have lost control of your life since your relative's illness?	0	1	2	3	4
10) Do you feel uncertain about what to do about your relative?	0	1	2	3	4
11) Do you feel you should be doing more for your relative?	0	1	2	3	4
12) Do you feel you could do a better job in caring for your relative?	0	1	2	3	4

WN22018
ZARIT BURDEN INTERVIEW

Page 1 of 1

ZBI-12 - United States/English
ZBI-12_AU1.0_eng-USori.doc

For more information contact Mapi Research Trust, Lyon, France. Email: trust@mapi.fr or mapi-trust.org

APPENDIX B: CAREGIVER ASSESSMENT OF FUNCTION AND UPSET (CAFU)

(Selected items; Gitlin et al., 2005)

Subject ID _ _ _ _ _ _ _ _

CAREGIVER ASSESSMENT OF FUNCTION AND UPSET (CAFU)

Now I am going to ask you some questions about the specific kinds of difficulties your (CR) might have been having this past week. For each area I will ask whether he/she has needed any kind of help. "Help" means supervision, direction, or personal assistance provided by you or someone else. (Show card #8)

IADLS

1. During the past week has your (CR) needed any kind of help using the telephone? (This includes answering the telephone, dialing, holding the phone, and hanging up.)

0 ( ) No →

> Does your (CR) need an assistive device (*for example large numbers on the face or hearing augmentation)* for __________, does he/she take more than reasonable time for __________, or is there a concern for safety?
>
> 7 ( ) No
> 6 ( ) Yes

1 ( ) Yes →

> IF HELP REQUIRED: What type of help is provided?
>
> 5 ( ) Only supervision, directing, setting-up items (oversight), or reminding (cueing)
> 4 ( ) a little physical help
> 3 ( ) a moderate amount of physical help
> 2 ( ) a lot of physical help
> 1 ( ) complete help (or activity no longer attempted)

Subject ID __ __ __ __ __ __ __ __

2. During the past week has your (CR) needed any kind of help with shopping (such as going to the store for a bag of groceries)?

0 ( ) No →

> Does your (CR) need an assistive device (*for example a cart to transport personal items)* for __________, does he/she take more than reasonable time for __________, or is there a concern for safety?
>
> 7 ( ) No
> 6 ( ) Yes

1 ( ) Yes →

> IF HELP REQUIRED: What type of help is provided?
>
> 5 ( ) Only supervision, directing, setting-up items (oversight), or reminding (cueing)
> 4 ( ) a little physical help
> 3 ( ) a moderate amount of physical help
> 2 ( ) a lot of physical help
> 1 ( ) complete help (or activity no longer attempted)

3. During the past week has your (CR) needed any kind of help with food preparation (making lunch or a light meal)?

0 ( ) No →

> Does your (CR) need an assistive device (*for example adapted utensils, dycem, reacher)* for __________, does he/she take more than reasonable time for __________, or is there a concern for safety?
>
> 7 ( ) No
> 6 ( ) Yes

1 ( ) Yes →

> IF HELP REQUIRED: What type of help is provided?
>
> 5 ( ) Only supervision, directing, setting-up items (oversight), or reminding (cueing)
> 4 ( ) a little physical help
> 3 ( ) a moderate amount of physical help
> 2 ( ) a lot of physical help
> 1 ( ) complete help (or activity no longer attempted)

Subject ID _ _ _ _ _ _ _ _

6. During the past week has your (CR) needed any kind of help traveling by car, bus, etc.? (This includes getting into and out of a care as well as planning a trip.)

0 ( ) No →

> Does your (CR) need an assistive device (*for example seating adaptation)* for __________, does he/she take more than reasonable time for __________, or is there a concern for safety?
> 7 ( ) No
> 6 ( ) Yes

1 ( ) Yes

> IF HELP REQUIRED: What type of help is provided?
>
> 5 ( ) Only supervision, directing, setting-up items (oversight), or reminding (cueing)
> 4 ( ) a little physical help
> 3 ( ) a moderate amount of physical help
> 2 ( ) a lot of physical help
> 1 ( ) complete help (or activity no longer attempted)

7. During the past week has your (CR) needed any kind of help taking his/her medications? (This includes setup, correct time, and dosage.)

0 ( ) No →

> Does your (CR) need an assistive device (*for example pill dispenser or crusher)* for __________, does he/she take more than reasonable time for __________, or is there a concern for safety?
> 7 ( ) No
> 6 ( ) Yes

1 ( ) Yes

> IF HELP REQUIRED: What type of help is provided?
>
> 5 ( ) Only supervision, directing, setting-up items (oversight), or reminding (cueing)
> 4 ( ) a little physical help
> 3 ( ) a moderate amount of physical help
> 2 ( ) a lot of physical help
> 1 ( ) complete help (or activity no longer attempted)

Subject ID __ __ __ __ __ __ __ __

ADLS

Now here are some additional questions about the activities your (CR) may need help with.

10. During the past week has your (CR) needed any kind of help getting into or out of a bed, chair or wheelchair?

0 ( ) No →

> Does your (CR) need an assistive device (*for example a hospital bed, lift chair, transfer board)* for __________, does he/she take more than reasonable time for __________, or is there a concern for safety?
> 7 ( ) No
> 6 ( ) Yes

1 ( ) Yes

> IF HELP REQUIRED: What type of help is provided?
>
> 5 ( ) Only supervision, directing, setting-up items (oversight), or reminding (cueing)
> 4 ( ) a little physical help
> 3 ( ) a moderate amount of physical help
> 2 ( ) a lot of physical help
> 1 ( ) complete help (or activity no longer attempted)

11. During the past week has your (CR) needed any kind of help eating meals? (This includes getting food from plate to mouth.)

0 ( ) No →

> Does your (CR) need an assistive device (*for example rocker knife, dycem, or adapted utensils)* for __________, does he/she take more than reasonable time for __________, or is there a concern for safety?
> 7 ( ) No
> 6 ( ) Yes

1 ( ) Yes

> IF HELP REQUIRED: What type of help is provided?
>
> 5 ( ) Only supervision, directing, setting-up items (oversight), or reminding (cueing)
> 4 ( ) a little physical help
> 3 ( ) a moderate amount of physical help
> 2 ( ) a lot of physical help
> 1 ( ) complete help (or activity no longer attempted)

Subject ID __ __ __ __ __ __ __ __

12. During the past week has your (CR) needed any kind of help bathing, (such as rinsing or drying the body) either in the tub, shower, or a sponge bath,?

0 ( ) No →

Does your (CR) need an assistive device (*for example a tub bench, handheld shower, or grab bars)* for ___________, does he/she take more than reasonable time for ___________, or is there a concern for safety?

7 ( ) No
6 ( ) Yes

1 ( ) Yes

IF HELP REQUIRED: What type of help is provided?

5 ( ) <u>Only</u> supervision, directing, setting-up items (oversight), or reminding (cueing)
4 ( ) a little physical help
3 ( ) a moderate amount of physical help
2 ( ) a lot of physical help
1 ( ) complete help (or activity no longer attempted)

13. During the past week has your (CR) needed any kind of help dressing above the waist? (This includes dressing and undressing the upper body and obtaining clothes from drawers/closets.)

0 ( ) No →

Does your (CR) need an assistive device (*for example a reacher, button hooks, Velcro clothing)* for ___________, does he/she take more than reasonable time for ___________, or is there a concern for safety?

7 ( ) No
6 ( ) Yes

1 ( ) Yes

IF HELP REQUIRED: What type of help is provided?

5 ( ) <u>Only</u> supervision, directing, setting-up items (oversight), or reminding (cueing)
4 ( ) a little physical help
3 ( ) a moderate amount of physical help
2 ( ) a lot of physical help
1 ( ) complete help (or activity no longer attempted)

Subject ID __________

14. During the past week has your (CR) needed any kind of help dressing from the waist down? (This includes dress and undressing the lower body, including shoes and socks, and obtaining clothes from drawer/closets.)

0 ( ) No →

> Does your (CR) need an assistive device (*for example a reacher, stocking donner)* for __________, does he/she take more than reasonable time for __________, or is there a concern for safety?
>
> 7 ( ) No
> 6 ( ) Yes

1 ( ) Yes

> IF HELP REQUIRED: What type of help is provided?
>
> 5 ( ) Only supervision, directing, setting-up items (oversight), or reminding (cueing)
> 4 ( ) a little physical help
> 3 ( ) a moderate amount of physical help
> 2 ( ) a lot of physical help
> 1 ( ) complete help (or activity no longer attempted)

15. During the past week has your (CR) needed any kind of help toileting, such as adjusting clothing before and after toilet use or cleansing?

0 ( ) No →

> Does your (CR) need an assistive device (*for example grab bars, commode, raised toilet seat)* for __________, does he/she take more than reasonable time for __________, or is there a concern for safety?
>
> 7 ( ) No
> 6 ( ) Yes

1 ( ) Yes

> IF HELP REQUIRED: What type of help is provided?
>
> 5 ( ) Only supervision, directing, setting-up items (oversight), or reminding (cueing)
> 4 ( ) a little physical help
> 3 ( ) a moderate amount of physical help
> 2 ( ) a lot of physical help
> 1 ( ) complete help (or activity no longer attempted)

APPENDIX C: POSITIVE ASPECTS OF CAREGIVING

(Tarlow et al., 2004)

Positive Aspects of Caregiving Subject ID _ _ _ _ _ _ _

POSITIVE ASPECTS OF CAREGIVING

Some caregivers say that, in spite of all the difficulties involved in giving care to a family member with memory or health problems, good things have come out of their caregiving experience too. I'm going to go over a few of the good things reported by some caregivers. I would like you to tell me how much you agree or disagree with these statements. Please refer to the responses listed on this card. **[Give card to respondent.]**

	Providing help to (CR) has.....	***Disagree a lot***	***Disagree a little***	***Neither agree nor disagree***	***Agree a little***	***Agree a lot***	Unknown	Refused
1. (RC27)	***made me feel more useful.***	0 ( )	1 ( )	2 ( )	3 ( )	4 ( )	-3 ( )	-4 ( )
2. (RC27)	***made me feel good about myself.***	0 ( )	1 ( )	2 ( )	3 ( )	4 ( )	-3 ( )	-4 ( )
3. (RC27)	***made me feel needed.***	0 ( )	1 ( )	2 ( )	3 ( )	4 ( )	-3 ( )	-4 ( )
4. (RC27)	***made me feel appreciated.***	0 ( )	1 ( )	2 ( )	3 ( )	4 ( )	-3 ( )	-4 ( )
5. (RC27)	***made me feel important.***	0 ( )	1 ( )	2 ( )	3 ( )	4 ( )	-3 ( )	-4 ( )
6. (RC27)	***made me feel strong and confident.***	0 ( )	1 ( )	2 ( )	3 ( )	4 ( )	-3 ( )	-4 ( )
7. (RC27)	***given more meaning to my life.***	0 ( )	1 ( )	2 ( )	3 ( )	4 ( )	-3 ( )	-4 ( )
8. (RC27)	***enabled me to learn new skills.***	0 ( )	1 ( )	2 ( )	3 ( )	4 ( )	-3 ( )	-4 ( )
9. (RC27)	***enabled me to appreciate life more.***	0 ( )	1 ( )	2 ( )	3 ( )	4 ( )	-3 ( )	-4 ( )
10. (RC27)	***enabled me to develop a more positive attitude toward life.***	0 ( )	1 ( )	2 ( )	3 ( )	4 ( )	-3 ( )	-4 ( )
11. (RC27)	***strengthened my relationships with others.***	0 ( )	1 ( )	2 ( )	3 ( )	4 ( )	-3 ( )	-4 ( )

References

Aneshensel, C. A., Pearlin, L. I., Mullan, J. T., Zarit, S. H., & Whitlatch, C. (1995). *Profiles in Caregiving: The Unexpected Career.* New York, NY: Academic Press.

Antonucci, T. C., Fuhrer, R., & Dartigues, J. F. (1997). Social relations and depressive symptomatology in a sample of community-dwelling French older adults. *Psychology & Aging*, *12*, 189–195.

Arno, P. S., Levine, C., & Memmott, M. M. (1999). The economic value of informal caregiving. *DataWatch: Health Affairs*, *18*, 182–188.

Bandura, A. (1994). Self-efficacy. In V. S. Ramachaudran (Ed.), *Encyclopedia of human behavior*, *Vol. 4.* (pp. 71–81). New York, NY: Academic Press. (Reprinted in H Friedman (Ed.), *Encyclopedia of mental health.* San Diego, CA: Academic Press, (1998)).

Bandura, A. (1997). *Self-efficacy: The Exercise of Control.* New York, NY: WH Freeman & Co.

Baxter, E. C. (2000). Caregiver assessment: learn about the caregiver, distinct from the person with dementia. *Alzheimer's Care Quarterly*, *1*, 62–70.

Bedard, M., Molloy, D. W., Squire, L., Dubois, S., Lever, J. A., & O'Donnell, M. (2001). The Zarit Burden Interview: A new short version and screening version. *The Gerontologist*, *41*, 652–657.

Beeson, R., Horton-Deutsch, S., Farran, C., & Neundorfer, M. (2000). Loneliness and depression in caregivers of persons with Alzheimer's disease or related disorders. *Issues in Mental Health Nursing*, *21*(8), 799–806.

Belle, S. H., Burgio, L., Burns, R., Coons, D., Czaja, S. J., Gallagher-Thompson, D., et al. (2006). Enhancing the quality of life of dementia caregivers from different ethnic or racial groups: A randomized, controlled trial. *Annals of Internal Medicine*, *145*, 727–746.

Bergman-Evans, B. (1994). A health profile of spousal Alzheimer's caregivers: Depression and physical health characteristics. *Journal of Psychosocial Nursing & Mental Health Services*, *32*, 25–30.

Bishop, C. (1986). Living arrangement choices of elderly singles. *Health Care Financing Review*, *7*, 65–73.

Bonanno, G. A. (2004). Loss, trauma, and human resilience. *American Psychologist*, *59*, 20–28.

Bornat, J., Dimmock, B., Jones, D., & Peace, S. (1999). Stepfamilies and older people: Evaluating the implications of family change for an ageing population. *Ageing and Society*, *19*, 239–261.

Branch, L. G., & Jette, A. M. (1981). A prospective study of long-term care institutionalization among the aged. *American Journal of Public Health*, *72*, 1373–1379.

Buffum, M. D., & Brod, M. (1998). Humor and well-being in spouse caregivers of patients with Alzheimer's disease. *Applied Nursing Research*, *11*, 12–18.

Burns, D. D., & Sayers, S. L. (1988). *Cognitive and affective components of marital satisfaction: Development and validation of a brief relationship satisfaction scale.* Unpublished manuscript.

California Caregiver Resource Center. (2003). *The Uniform Assessment Tool.* <www.caregiver.org/caregiver/jsp/. .../tk_california_assessment_tool.pdf> Accessed 1.5.09.

Caswell, L. W., Vitaliano, P., Croyle, K., Scanlan, J. M., Zhang, J., & Daruwala, A. (2003). Negative associations of chronic stress and cognitive performance in older adult spouse caregivers. *Experimental Aging Research*, *29*, 303–318.

D'Andrea, J., Daniels, R., & Heck, R. (1991). Evaluating the impact of multicultural counseling training. *Journal of Counseling and Development*, *70*(1), 143–150.

De Jong Gierveld, J., & Peeters, A. (2003). The interweaving of repartnered older adults' lives with their children and siblings. *Ageing & Society*, *23*, 187–205.

Derogatis, L. R., & Spencer, P. M. (1982). *The Brief Symptom Inventory (BSI): Administration, and Procedures Manual-I.* Baltimore, MD: Clinical Psychometric Research.

Dilworth-Anderson, P., Goodwin, P., & Williams, S. (2004). Can culture help explain the physical health effects of caregiving over time among African American caregivers? *Journal of Gerontology: Social Sciences*, *59B*, S138–S145.

Dilworth-Anderson, P., Williams, I. C., & Gibson, B. (2002). Issues of race, ethnicity and culture in caregiving research: A 20 year review. *The Gerontologist*, *42*, 237–272.

Family Caregiving Alliance. (2006). *Caregiver Health: A population at risk.* <http://www.caregiver.org> Accessed 12.10.09.

Farran, C. J., Keane-Hagerty, E., Salloway, S., Kupferer, S., & Wilken, C. S. (1991). Finding meaning: An alternative paradigm for Alzheimer's disease family caregivers. *The Gerontologist*, *31*, 483–489.

FCA (see Family Caregiving Alliance).

Feinberg, L. F. (2002). *The state of the art: Caregiver assessment in practice settings*. San Francisco, CA: Family Caregiver Alliance. Available at http://www.caregiver.org

Feinberg, L. F., Whitlatch, C. J., & Tucke, S. (2000). *Making hard choices: Respecting both voices. Final report to the Robert Wood Johnson Foundation*. San Francisco, CA: Family Caregiver Alliance. Available at. http://www.caregiver.org.

Frisch, M. B. (1988). Quality of life therapy and assessment in health care. *Clinical Psychology: Science and Practice*, *5*, 19–40.

Frisch, M. B. (1994). *Quality of life inventory manual and treatment guide*. Minneapolis, MN: CS Pearson, Inc.

Frisch, M. B., Clark, M. P., Rouse, S. V., Rudd, M. D., Paweleck, J., & Greenstone, A. (2005). Predictive and treatment validity of life satisfaction and the quality of life inventory. *Assessment*, *12*, 66–78.

Garratt, A., Schmidt, L., Mackintosh, A., & Fitzpatrick, R. (2002). Quality of life measurement: Bibliographic study of patient assessed health outcome measures. *British Medical Journal*, *324*, 1417–1421.

Gaugler, J. E., Davey, A., Pearlin, L., & Zarit, S. H. (2000). Modeling caregiver adaptation over time: The longitudinal impact of behavior problems. *Psychology and Aging*, *15*, 437–450.

Gitlin, L. N., Roth, D. L., Burgio, L. D., Loewenstein, D. A., Winter, L., Nichols, L., et al. (2005). Caregiver appraisals of functional dependence in individuals with dementia and associated caregiver upset: Psychometric properties of a new scale and response patterns by caregiver and care recipient characteristics. *Journal of Aging and Health*, *17*, 148–171.

Hébert, R., Dubois, M.-F., Wolfson, C., Chambers, L., & Cohen, C. (2001). Factors associated with long-term institutionalization of older people with dementia: data from the Canadian Study of Health and Aging. *Journal of Gerontology: Medical Sciences*, *56A*, M693–M699.

Herbert, L. E., Scherr, P. A., Bienias, J. L., Bennett, D. A., & Evans, D. A. (2004). State-specific projections through 2025 of Alzheimer disease prevalence. *Neurology*, *62*, 1645.

Hepburn, K., Lewis, M., Sherman, C. W., & Tornatore, J. (2003). The Savvy caregiver program: Developing and testing a transportable dementia family caregiver training program. *The Gerontologist*, *43*(6), 908–915.

Hilgeman, M. M., Allen, R. S., DeCoster, J., & Burgio, L. D. (2007). Positive aspects of caregiving as a moderator of treatment outcome over 12 months. *Psychology and Aging*, *22*, 361–371.

Katz, S. (1983). Assessing self-maintenance: Activities of daily living, mobility, and instrumental activities of daily living. *Journal of the American Geriatrics Association*, *31*, 721–727.

Kiecolt-Glaser, J., Glaser, R., Gravenstein, S., Malarkey, W., & Sheridan, J. (1996). Chronic stress alters the immune response to influenza virus vaccine in older adults. *Proceedings of the National Academy of Science (Medical)*, *93*, 3043–3047.

Knight, B. G., Fox, L. S., & Chou, C. (2000). Factor structure of the Burden Interview. *Journal of Clinical Geropsychology*, *6*(4), 249–258.

Koenig, H., Parkerson, G. R., & Meador, K. G. (1997). Religion index for psychiatric research. *American Journal of Psychiatry*, *154*, 885–886.

Kroenke, R., & Spitzer, R. L. (2002). The PHQ-9: A new depression and diagnostic severity measure. *Psychiatric Annals*, *32*, 509–521.

Kroenke, R., Spitzer, R. L., & Williams, J. B. (2001). The PHQ-9: Validity of a brief depression severity measure. *Journal of General Internal Medicine*, *16*, 606–613.

Lazarus, R. S., & Folkman, S. (1984). *Stress appraisal and coping*. New York, NY: Springer.

Lewis, M. L., Hepburn, K. W., Narayan, S., & Kirk, L. (2005). Relationship matters in dementia caregiving. *American Journal of Alzheimer's Disease and Other Dementias*, *20*(6), 341–347.

Lubben, J., & Gironda, M. (2004). Measuring social networks and assessing their benefits. In C. Phillipson, G. Allen, & D. Morgan (Eds.), *Social Networks and Social Exclusion: Sociological and Policy Perspectives*. Aldershot, UK: Ashgate.

Lubben, J., Blozik, E., Gillman, G., Iliffe, S., Renteln Kruse, W., Beck, J., et al. (2006). Performance of an abbreviated version of the Lubben social network scale among three European community-dwelling other adult populations. *The Gerontologist*, *46*, 503–513.

Luescher, K., & Pillemer, K. (1998). Intergenerational ambivalence: A new approach to the study of parent—child relations in later-life. *Journal of Marriage and Family, 60*, 412—425.

Manton, K. G. (1988). A longitudinal study of functional change and mortality in the United States. *Journal of Gerontology: Social Science, 43*, S153—S161.

Masten, A. (2001). Ordinary magic: Resilience processes in development. *American Psychologist, 56*, 227—238.

Meuser, T. M., & Marwit, S. J. (2001). A comprehensive, stage-sensitive model of grief in dementia caregiving. *The Gerontological Society of America, 41*, 658—670.

Mittleman, M. S., Roth, D. L., Coon, D. W., & Haley, W. E. (2004). Sustained benefit of supportive intervention for depressive symptoms in caregivers of patients with Alzheimer's disease. *American Journal of Psychiatry, 161*(5), 850—856.

Moos, R.H., & Moos, B.S. (1994). *Family Environment Scale Manual—Development Application, Research—Third Edition*. Palo Alto, CA: Consulting Psychologist Press.

Morycz, R. K. (1985). Caregiving strain and desire to institutionalize family members with Alzheimer's disease: Possible predictors and model development. *Research on Aging, 7*, 329—361.

Murphy, K., Hanrahan, P., & Luchins, D. (1997). A survey of grief and bereavement in nursing homes: The importance of hospice grief and bereavement for the end-stage Alzheimer's disease patient and family. *Journal of the American Geriatrics Society, 45*, 1104—1107.

National Family Caregivers Association. (2001). *Survey of self-identified caregivers*. http://caregiver.org

Oxman, T. E., Berkman, L. F., Kasl, S., Freeman, D. H., & Barrett, J. E. (1992). Social support and depressive symptoms in the elderly. *American Journal of Epidemiology, 135*, 356—368.

Pearlin, L. I., & Aneshensel, C. S. (1994). Caregiving: The unexpected career. *Social Justice Research, 7*, 373—390.

Pearlin, L. I., Mullan, J. T., Semple, S. J., & Skaff, M. M. (1990). Caregiving and the stress process: An overview of concepts and their measures. *The Gerontologist, 30*, 583—594.

Picot, S. J. F., Youngblut, J., & Zeller, R. (1997). Development and testing of a measure of perceived rewards in adults. *Journal of Nursing Measurement, 5*, 33—52.

Pinquart, P., & Sorensen, S. (2003). Associations of stressors and uplifts with caregiver burden and depressive mood: A meta-analysis. *Journals of Gerontology: Psychological Sciences, 58B*, P112—P128.

Pinquart, P., & Sorenson, S. (2005). Ethnic differences in stressors, resources, and psychological outcomes of family caregiving: A meta-analysis. *The Gerontologist, 45*, 90—106.

Pruchno, R. A., Michaels, J. E., & Potashnik, S. L. (1990). Predictors of institutionalization among Alzheimer disease victims with caregiving spouses. *Journal of Gerontology, 45*, S259—266.

Radloff, L. S. (1977). The CES-D Scale: A self-report depression scale for research in the general population. *Applied Psychological Measures, 1*, 385—401.

Ramsey, J. L., & Blieszner, R. (1999). *Spiritual Resiliency in Older Women: Models of Strength for Challenges through the Life Span*. Thousand Oaks, CA: Sage.

Rausch, S. M., Baker, K., & Boonmee, J. (2007). Sleep disturbances in caregivers of patients with end-stage congestive heart failure: Part II—Assess and intervene. *Progress in Cardiovascular Nursing, 22*, 93—96.

Roff, L. L., Burgio, L. D., Gitlin, L., Nichols, L., Chaplin, W., & Hardin, J. M. (2004). Positive aspects of Alzheimer's caregiving: The role of race. *Journals of Gerontology, Series B: Psychological Sciences and Social Sciences, 59*, 185—190.

Roth, D. L., Burgio, L. D., Gitlin, L. N., Gallagher-Thompson, D., Coon, D. W., Belle, S. H., et al. (2003). Psychometric analysis of the Revised Memory and Behavior Problems Checklist: Factor structure of occurrence and reaction ratings. *Psychology and Aging, 18*, 906—915.

Roth, D. L., Perkins, M., Wadley, V. G., Temple, E. M., & Haley, W. E. (2009). Family caregiving and emotional strain: associations with quality of life in a large national sample of middle-aged and older adults. *Quality of Life Research, 18*(6), 679—688.

Schulz, R., & Beach, S. R. (1999). Caregiving as a risk factor for mortality. *Journal of the American Medical Association, 282*, 2215—2219.

Schulz, R., Burgio, L., Burns, R., Eisdorfer, C., Gallagher-Thompson, D., Gitlin, L. N., et al. (2003). Resources for Enhancing Alzheimer's Caregiver Health (REACH): Overview, site-specific outcomes, and future directions. *The Gerontologist, 43*, 514—520.

Semple, S. J. (1992). Conflict in Alzheimer's caregiving families: Its dimensions and consequences. *The Gerontologist, 32*(5), 648–655.

Spitzer, R. L., Kroenke, K., & Williams, J. B. W. (1999). Validation and utility of a self-report version of PRIME-MD. *Journal of the American Medical Assocation (JAMA), 282*, 1737–1744.

Sherman, C. W., & Boss, P. (2007). Spousal dementia caregiving in the context of late-life remarriage. *Dementia, 6*, 245–270.

Steadman, P. L., Tremont, G., & Davis, J. D. (2007). Premorbid relationship satisfaction and caregiver burden in dementia caregivers. *Journal of Geriatric Psychiatry and Neurology, 20*, 115–119.

Steffan, A. M., McKibbin, C., Zeiss, A. M., Galaagher-Thompson, D., & Bandura, A. (2002). The revised scale for caregiving self-efficacy: Reliability and validity studies. *Journal of Gerontology, Psychological Sciences, 57B*, P74–86.

Stone, R. I. (2000). *Long-term care for the elderly with disabilities: Current policy, emerging trends, and implications for the 21st century.* New York, NY: Milbank Memorial Fund.

Switzer, G. E., Wishniewski, S. R., Belle, S. H., Burns, R., Winter, L., Thompson, L., et al. (2000). Measurement issues in intervention research. In R. Schulz (Ed.), *Handbook on Dementia Caregiving*. New York, NY: Springer.

Tarlow, B. J., Wishniewski, S. R., Belle, S. H., Rubert, M., Ory, M. G., & Gallacher-Thompson, D. (2004). Positive aspects of caregiving: Contributions of the REACH Project to the development of new measures for Alzheimer's caregiving. *Research on Aging, 26*, 429–453.

Teri, L., Truex, P., Logsdon, R., Uomoto, J., Zarit, S., & Vitaliano, P. P. (1992). Assessment of behavioral problems in dementia: The revised memory and behavior problems checklist. *Psychology and Aging, 7*, 622–631.

Thompson, L. (2004). *Long-term care: Support for family caregivers: Issue brief.* Washington, DC: Georgetown University Long-term Care Financing Project.

Vitaliano, P. P., Young, H. M., & Russo, J. (1991). Burden: A review of measures used among caregivers of individuals with dementia. *The Gerontologist, 31*, 67–75.

Vitaliano, P., Zhang, J., & Scanlan, J. M. (2003). Is caregiving hazardous to one's physical health? A meta-analysis. *Psychological Bulletin, 129*, 946–972.

Wagnild, G. M., & Young, H. M. (1993). Development and psychometric evaluation of the resilience scale. *Journal of Nursing Measurement, 1*, 165–178.

Ware, J., Kosinski, M., & Dewey, J. (2000). *How to Score Version Two of the SF-36 Health Survey.* Lincoln, RI: QualityMetric Inc.

Ware, J. E., Jr., Kosinski, M., & Keller, S. D. (1994). *SF36: Physical and Mental Summary Scales: A User's Manual*. Boston, MA: The Health Institute, New England Medical Center.

Ware, J. E., Jr., Snow, K. K., Kosinski, M., & Gandek, B. (1993). *SF-36 health survey. Manual and interpretation guide*. Boston, MA: The Health institute, New England Medical Center.

Watson, D., Clark, L. A., & Tellegen, A. (1988). Development and validation of brief measures of positive and negative affect: The PANAS scales. *Journal of Personality and Social Psychology, 54*, 1063–1070.

Whitlatch, C. J., Feinberg, L. F., & Stevens, E. J. (1999). Predictors of institutionalization for persons with Alzheimer's disease and the impact on family caregivers. *Journal of Mental Health and Aging, 5*, 275–288.

Wood, J. B., & Parham, I. A. (1990). Coping with perceived burden: Ethnic and cultural issues in Alzheimer's family caregiving. *Journal of Applied Gerontology, 9*, 325–339.

Yesavage, J. A., Brink, T. L., Rose, T. L., Lum, O., Huang, V., Adey, M., & Leirer, V. O. (1983). Development and validation of a geriatric screening scale; a preliminary report. *Journal of Psychiatric Research, 17*, 37–49.

Zarit, S. H., & Femia, E. E. (2008). A future for family care and dementia intervention research? Challenges and strategies. *Aging and Mental Health, 12*, 5–13.

Zarit, S. H., Orr, N. K., & Zarit, J. M. (1985). *The hidden victims of Alzheimer's disease: Families under stress.* New York, NY: New York University Press.

Zarit, S. H., Reever, K. E., & Bach-Peterson, J. (1980). Relatives of the impaired elderly, correlates of feelings of burden. *The Gerontologist, 20*, 649–655.

Zarit, S. H., Femia, E. E., Kim, K., & Whitlatch, C. J. (2010). The structure of risk factors and outcomes for family caregivers: Implications for assessment and treatment. *Aging and Mental Health, 14*(2), 220–231.

Zarit, S. H., Stephens, M. A., Townsend. A., & Greene, R. (1998). Stress reductions for family caregivers: Effects of adult day care use. *Journal of Gerontology Series B: Psychological and Social Science*, *53*, S267–277.

Zarit, S. H., Davey, A., Edwards, A. B., Femia, E. E., & Jarrott, S. E. (1998). Family caregiving: Research findings and clinical implications. In B. Edelstein (Ed.), *Clinical Geropsychology* (pp. 499–523). Oxford, UK: Elsevier.

Zimet, G. D., Dahlem, N. W., Zimet, S. G., & Farley, G. K. (1988). The multidimensional scale of perceived social support. *Journal of Personality Assessment*, *52*, 30–41.

CHAPTER

Assessment with Late-Life Families: Issues and Instruments

11

Brian D. Carpenter, Elizabeth A. Mulligan

Department of Psychology, Washington University, St. Louis, Mo, USA

INTRODUCTION

Of all the groups we join throughout the lifespan, one of the most important and enduring is our family. We all start in one, most of us all live within one, and many of us extend the tradition and create our own. Yes, the shape, size, and significance of our families may differ, but we share the experience of being part of this very intimate group. Family bonds are important at every phase of life yet seem particularly meaningful at both the beginning and end of life, when dependency on family is more common. They, in turn, can exert a powerful influence—positive or negative—on the quality of our lives. In later life, families can be a key source of support as older adults face the challenges of aging. And they can be an impediment to successful aging, in ways both direct and indirect, intentional and unintentional. Families can be both helpful and hurtful; indeed, even the same family can be both. This chapter is designed to help clinicians and researchers assess what features of the family are likely to influence how they manage events later in the lifespan.

We have two main goals in the chapter. The first is to help clinicians and researchers think about the range of issues that can influence the format, structure, content, interpretation, and implementation of an assessment with late-life families. Our second goal is to review a number of assessment models and tools that may be useful. Frankly, there are few assessment instruments that have been designed specifically for late-life families or adapted for them with sufficient validation. Still, we believe there are some instruments that have the potential to be useful with late-life families, with certain caveats in mind. We provide a summary of those instruments, after first discussing general issues in late-life family assessment.

RATIONALE FOR A CHAPTER ON FAMILY ASSESSMENT

Four realities of contemporary life make family assessment important in clinical gerontology. Perhaps the most obvious is the now familiar aging of the population. As the number of older adults grows, so too will the number of families supporting them. One estimate suggested that 34 million adults—a full 16% of the population—are providing care to people over age 50 (National Alliance for Caregiving & AARP, 2004), and that number will continue to rise. If care for older adults was a “normative experience” for families in the past (Brody, 1985), it is likely to become near universal in the coming decades. In a related change, the growth in the number of very old people (aged 85 and older) will be the most rapid of all, doubling to 9.6 million by 2030, and doubling again to 20.9 million by 2050 (He, Sengupta, Velkoff, & DeBarros, 2005). This group may have unique and potentially intensive care needs that demand even more assistance from family members. At the same time, with three-, four-, and even

Handbook of Assessment in Clinical Gerontology. DOI: 10.1016/B978-0-12-374961-1.10011-9

five-generation families becoming more common, older adults are likely to find *themselves* caring for even older parents.

It is also worth noting that while the number of older adults will increase in the coming decades, the number of younger family members available to take care of them will not increase at the same pace (Mack, Lee, & Friedland, 2001), meaning further burden on the family members who are available. These are not singular developments. Further out on the horizon is the New Boomer generation (born 1983–2001), which includes almost as many people as the original Baby Boom (Carlson, 2009). When they reach old age, beginning around the year 2048, we are likely to experience a repeat of current challenges. Therefore, now is a good time to start developing and using assessments with late-life families.

A second reality is that the majority of support to older adults is provided not by formal caregivers, agencies, or institutions, but by spouses, adult children, siblings, and a variety of other family members (National Alliance for Caregiving & AARP, 2004; National Family Caregiving Alliance, 2000). Families are the ones doing the work. Therefore, any attempt to understand how best to support older adults must include the people who provide the majority of that support.

A third issue is that assistance to older adults is typically provided not by one person working in isolation, but rather by multiple family members collaborating. Families are a team in their work, and the impact of elder care is felt throughout the family system (Connidis, 2001; Qualls, 2000), taking place in an intricate "life event web" (Pruchno, Blow, & Smyer, 1984). Changes in one person's life ripple within and across generations. Consequently, an approach that takes into account the perspective and circumstance of each person in the family is essential.

A final reality is that providing support to older adults brings with it many challenges that are likely to test the family and its resources. Families are called upon to provide a wide range of assistance—financial, housing, transportation, personal care, emotional, and decision support. And they do so while navigating complicated and discontinuous medical, social service, and entitlement benefit systems; while balancing elder care with competing work, family, and personal responsibilities; while figuring out how to provide support in the context of an often long and complex family history; and while negotiating with everyone in the family on how caregiving will change roles, responsibilities, and relationships. In an outrageous understatement, elder care is demanding work, both physically and psychologically, for the entire family. Assessment is an important way to understand the stresses and resources within the family, and the help they need to be successful. For professionals from many disciplines who collaborate with families in later life, assessment is the first step in learning what the family wants, what the family needs, how the family functions, and how others can interact effectively with the family. To be more specific, assessment with late-life families can:

- Identify families who may be vulnerable or at risk for suboptimal functioning in their relationships and supportive activities;
- Highlight individual and family strengths that can enhance family relationships and facilitate elder support;
- Clarify individual and family expectations and preferences for what and how support should be provided;
- Assist clinicians and formal service providers in knowing how to tailor interventions and programs best to support families;
- Track changes and growth in families over time as interventions and services are implemented, and as the circumstances of the family evolve;
- Guide researchers in identifying important causal processes and outcomes in the family system.

The value of assessment will differ for each family, depending on the family's circumstances and needs. Indeed, by virtue of their idiosyncratic histories and developmental trajectories, families in later life are probably more diverse than at any other time in the lifespan. Attention to differences is essential, and we turn to this issue of diversity next.

DIVERSITY IN LATE-LIFE FAMILIES

Differences in family structure, sexual orientation, gender, socioeconomic status, race and ethnicity, culture, and values are becoming more apparent both within and between late-life families. For assessment, this means there is a need for instruments whose content is sensitive to differences and whose norms reflect the various populations with which the instruments are used. There is a parallel demand for clinicians and researchers who are knowledgeable about diversity later in life and who are skilled in the application and interpretation of appropriate assessment tools (American Psychological Association, 2003). Below we discuss some key facets of diversity, with an emphasis on their implications for late-life family assessment.

One obvious change in families that has been unfolding for decades is increased diversity in family structure. Longer life expectancies combined with lower fertility rates have resulted in families composed of more living generations, with fewer people in each generation, resulting in a "beanpole" family structure, in contrast to the previously dominant "pyramidal" structure (Bengtson, Rosenthal, & Burton, 1990). Multigenerational relationships have become more important in light of this population trend. In some cases these relationships are a welcome resource (e.g., a niece providing instrumental support to a childless older adult), but in other cases they create additional stress in the life of an older adult (e.g., a grandparent taking care of a grandchild because of substance abuse in the middle generation). This has obvious implications for the number of people who are likely to be part of a family system that is the target of assessment, and it broadens the range of issues a late-life family may face.

Another byproduct of longer life expectancies is that family relationships are likely to evolve over many decades. Developmental models that explain the evolution of prolonged family relationships have not yet emerged. Assessment tools also have lagged, and measures that were developed and validated with younger, more condensed families, may not have adequate content coverage and may not come equipped with adequate norms.

Inadequate norms are also an issue in light of the changing composition of late-life families. Higher rates of divorce and remarriage have made blended families more common, and, within them, family norms, expectations, and roles may be less clear. For example, adult children may not feel as obligated to care for a stepfather in comparison with a biological parent (Ganong & Coleman, 2006). Patterns of communication and decision-making also may differ. Not only are there more people to communicate with, but psychological residue from a divorce or remarriage may strain communication and collaborative decision-making.

Remaining unmarried and choosing not to have children also have become more common. About 4% of the current population of older adults have never been married, and about 20% are childless (Connidis, 2001; He et al., 2005). These older adults typically receive emotional and instrumental support from siblings and fictive kin, that is, neighbors and friends who are invited to fulfill the role of family (Barresi & Hunt, 1990; Gironda, Lubben, & Atchison, 1999). In some cases, formal care providers, such as home health aides and private duty nurses, also may develop close relationships with older adults and take on family-like roles (Piercy, 2000).

Fictive kin are also a source of support for other groups of older adults, including lesbian, gay, bisexual, and transgender individuals (Savin-Williams & Esterberg, 2000). Because the current cohort of older adults lived through a historical period when homosexuality was not accepted, they may have faced criticism and estrangement from their family. As a result, friends may be their primary (and preferred) source of support. An additional consideration with this group of older adults is that same-sex couples face unique legal challenges, including restrictions regarding taxation and inheritance, and surrogate decision-making. These challenges may place a strain on the entire family system.

Another epidemiologic trend that affects family structure is the greater life expectancy for women relative to men. Older women of all ages are less likely to be married: by age 75, only 29% of women are married, compared with 67% of men (He et al., 2005). In addition, because the current cohort of older women spent less time in the workforce, they are more likely to struggle financially during late life (He et al., 2005). Consequently, older women may be more likely to turn to their children for emotional and instrumental help, and the characters who are the focus of the assessment and the stressors that arise are likely to reflect this.

In addition to more varied family structures, late-life families also are becoming more diverse in terms of racial, ethnic, and cultural background. By 2050, ethnic minorities over age 55 will make up a greater proportion of the population, increasing from 8% to 12% for African Americans, 6% to 18% for Hispanics, and 3% to 8% for Asian Americans (He et al., 2005). These trends are important because people from different racial and ethnic backgrounds may have distinct issues in late life, may have unique patterns of relating and communicating, and may respond differently to assessment measures, making clear the need to validate tools and develop norms for specific populations. For example, in Asian American and Latino families, adult children often feel a strong obligation to provide care for their parents, although these beliefs may vary depending on the family's level of acculturation (Knight et al., 2002; Pinquart & Sorensen, 2005). Consequently, for measures of filial responsibility, separate norms would be needed.

As a final point, we want to emphasize that diversity *within* families also has important implications for assessment. For example, in a recent study, older adults were more likely to have traditional family structures than even their own offspring (Blieszner, 2009). Members within the same family may be diverse in terms of their experiences, viewpoints, stages in life, and even their race and ethnicity, in the case of interracial and multiracial children. Likewise, differences in values and differences in resources (psychological, financial) within the family may make collaboration across generations more difficult (Fingerman, 2001).

We highlight these facets of family life in order to heighten sensitivity to differences as people prepare, administer, and interpret assessments. To paraphrase a well-worn axiom, "If you've seen one family, you've seen one family." Despite the intention of most assessment instruments to aggregate and summarize, assessment means also being prepared for idiosyncrasy and difference.

OTHER RELEVANT DEMOGRAPHIC AND SOCIAL TRENDS

We next highlight other demographic, social, and contextual trends that can influence the dynamics, resources, and vulnerabilities of late-life families. Clinicians and researchers who are aware of these trends may be better equipped to choose appropriate assessment instruments, interpret their results accurately, and offer relevant, effective recommendations.

Although there is some debate about whether geographic dispersion of family members is increasing (Wolf & Longino, 2005), the reality is that distance matters in families. The majority of family members live within 20 minutes of older care recipients (Wagner, 1997), but it is not uncommon to have family members living in different parts of the country or world. Distance makes it more challenging for families to identify when older adults need assistance, judge what level of assistance they need, locate and manage trustworthy and dependable support resources in the local community, negotiate the division of responsibility and the logistics of caregiving among multiple family members, and maintain communication with everyone involved. In terms of assessment, geographic distance can hinder obtaining information from the full family system, even though long-distance family members may be very involved in care decisions. Distance also makes it difficult to observe interpersonal dynamics that may be important to understanding the family's strengths and weaknesses.

One feature of modern society that might counteract the effects of dispersion is the rapid development and dissemination of technology, which has changed the way assessment data can be obtained. Web-based home and personal monitoring systems, for instance, enable clinicians and researchers (and families, for that matter) to observe older adults from a distance via live video stream from the home; track behavior such as refrigerator, cupboard, and pill bottle activity; and monitor physiological indicators of health such as heart rate and blood sugar. Of course these technologies raise important issues about confidentiality, but they do provide an additional resource for assessment and intervention.

Monitoring technologies are complemented by an expanding array of communication tools, such as cell phones, text messaging, e-mail, and videoconferencing, along with social networking products such as Facebook, MySpace, and Twitter. Some of these tools can enhance the assessment process, by facilitating access to people's opinions (e.g., e-mailing questionnaires) and their behavior (e.g., conducting behavioral observations via videoconferencing). And some of these tools might be the topic of assessment themselves. For example, when appraising the social support resources of a family, electronic communication and on-line acquaintances need to be considered. Many of these tools have become ubiquitous among younger generations, with more gradual adoption by older adults (Jones & Fox, 2009). Consequently, it may be useful to assess, when relevant, the availability, receptivity, and familiarity with different communication technologies. A family may be willing to invest in cable Internet access for an older adult's home computer, a reasonable intervention to encourage social connection, but if the older adult is resistant, and if sufficient training and technical support are not provided, the effort may be doomed.

Another trend with a more uncertain trajectory is related to current health and illness in the population. Because of improved public health, in recent years some evidence has emerged to suggest that people in the United States are not only living longer, but also healthier, with fewer, better managed chronic diseases and greater functional independence (He et al., 2005). At the same time, there are other trends that could undermine these gains. Increasing rates of diabetes and obesity, for example, could cancel out improvements in other areas. In this case, people may need family assistance earlier and for longer periods of time, and younger family members, now with their own health problems, may find it difficult to care for aging relatives. These trends highlight the importance of incorporating broad medical factors across all generations in family assessment.

A final note of emphasis about these demographic and social changes is that they are not universal. Whether because of location, finances, knowledge or other reasons, access to the Internet, an ability to travel by plane, adequate health insurance coverage, and financial resources are dispersed unevenly in our society. Conscientious assessment keeps this additional facet of diversity in mind.

KEY ASSESSMENT ISSUES

When planning and executing an assessment, some issues are common across age groups, and some are unique to late-life families. Keeping this in mind the following questions can help guide the pragmatics of administration, and the interpretation and application of results.

What is the Purpose of the Assessment?

The scope and content of an assessment are naturally influenced by its purpose. A clinical assessment may use different instruments and procedures than an assessment designed to address a research hypothesis.

As for clinical assessments, a key first step is to grasp the referral question. What is the main issue or problem that needs clarification or the primary question that needs to be answered? Is it a "family" issue that involves the entire system (e.g., How prepared is the family as a group to coordinate transportation for an older father's physical therapy appointments?) or a "family-related" issue (e.g., How is an adult survivor of child abuse reacting to her father's diagnosis of prostate cancer?) (Feetham, 1991)? The level of analysis is likely to affect which instruments are chosen and who takes part in the assessment.

Who is the Target of the Assessment?

The purpose of the assessment will, to some degree, influence who is assessed. But the theoretical orientation of the clinician and goal of the researcher also may guide who takes part. A family systems approach would attempt to include all key family members in the assessment, but that does not mean it is necessary to talk with every family member in every situation.

Consider the case of an older woman who is dealing with end-stage renal disease. Disease management tasks likely include frequent dialysis, symptom monitoring, and lifestyle modifications, all of which have an impact on the life of both the person with the disease and her partner. In this case a dyadic assessment may be sufficient to answer a question about how best to support this couple. In other circumstances a more expansive assessment may be appropriate. An older adult with severe and worsening chronic obstructive pulmonary disease may be considering home hospice, and an assessment of the broader family system—adult children, grandchildren, other relatives, friends—may be important to determine the extent to which the family will be able to manage the older adult's care needs at home, above and beyond the support provided by the hospice agency.

What Should be Told to the Participants?

An early step in the assessment process includes describing to the family what they are about to undertake. Family assessment raises a number of ethical considerations in this arena that deserve mention (American Psychological Association, 2002). First, principles of informed consent demand that family members are told what information will be gathered and what will be done with it. That means telling people what kinds of questions they will be asked, what kinds of tasks they may be asked to do, which family members will be involved, and how and with whom results will be shared. Informed consent may be challenging when working with older adults who have some degree of cognitive impairment. Using clear, simple language, with adequate repetition and clarification, may help maximize understanding. In some cases, proxy consent, along with assent from the older adult, may be required. In all cases, informed consent should be considered a *process* rather than an *event*, meaning that consent should be evaluated throughout the assessment.

Consent and feedback also raise the issue of confidentiality, when people are asked about others in the family. If a sibling is going to be asked about changes in his brother's functional abilities, his brother should know. If an adult child is going to be asked to offer an opinion about a parent's decision-making style, their parent should know. Indeed, in the case of research, many Institutional Review Boards require special consent procedures when family members are asked to provide information about someone else in the family, whether or not that third party is also involved in the research (National Institute of Health, 2001). A related issue has to do with mandatory reporting when an assessment raises suspicions about elder abuse or neglect. Clinicians and researchers must be clear in their own minds, and clear with the people they are assessing, about their obligations to disclose to appropriate authorities when there are concerns about the safety and welfare of a family member.

Another ethical issue is the responsible use of assessment materials. A clinician or researcher should use only instruments that are within their scope of expertise. In addition, the user should be aware of the boundaries of the instruments based on their reliability, validity, and applicability to individual families (e.g., availability of relevant norms). Information about the limitations of assessment also should be shared with families when providing feedback.

How Will Information About the Family be Obtained?

Assessment information can be obtained via three primary methods: self-report questionnaires; behavioral observations; and clinician-rated scales. Each offers its own unique perspective on the family, and each comes with its own strengths and weaknesses. Self-report questionnaires are relatively brief and efficient, and directly tap a family member's opinion or subjective experience. At the same time, they rely on a person's ability to be aware of and reflect upon complex phenomena (e.g., family norms, emotions, communication patterns), are vulnerable to social desirability bias (positive or negative), and often result in a relatively restricted range of responses (most families think they function relatively well).

Observational assessments provide relatively objective information but are more time consuming, potentially intrusive, and complex to conduct, often requiring trained raters to code interactions among family members. Finally, clinician-rated scales enable an "expert" to weigh in on how the family is functioning, but are often based on extensive individual and family interviews, which are themselves vulnerable to bias. Ideally, family assessments are conducted with multiple people, in multiple ways, although in reality, resource constraints are likely to dictate what kind of information can be obtained.

When an Instrument Developed Specifically for Late-Life Families does not Exist, What are the Issues in Using Something that has been Developed for Other Groups?

As we mentioned earlier, there are few instruments designed specifically for late-life families, particularly instruments developed for clinical purposes, so it is often necessary to modify and adapt existing instruments. This may not be entirely wasted effort, because many models of family functioning (and the assessment tools that emerge from those models) are intended to represent general features or processes that are presumably applicable to all families. Good communication is good communication, regardless of whether you are evaluating a Caucasian or African American family, a straight or gay family, a young or old family.

Having said that, there are limits to the generalizability of adapted tools: constructs relevant to late-life families may be missing (e.g., caregiving norms), and some individual items within existing subscales may not be relevant (e.g., "The grown-ups in this family understand and agree on family decisions"). Consequently, whether existing scales adequately capture the experience of late-life families and whether their scores are reliable and valid remain unclear. In general, instruments that have not been validated with late-life families should be used with caution until adequate empirical evidence is gathered to show that the instruments (or their adapted versions) are appropriate for late-life families.

How will Assessment Information from Multiple People be Combined and Integrated?

Assessments with multiple family members can yield a great deal of information that needs to be combined into a cohesive summary (Sawin, Harrigan, & Woog, 1995). If you administer the Family Assessment Measure (Skinner, Steinhauer, & Santa-Barbara, 1995) to two older parents and their three adult children, for each person you end up with scores on seven family dimensions, meaning you would have 35 subscale scores to digest.

In a research study, multilevel modeling (Raudenbush & Bryk, 2002) would be one technique for examining variability at different levels (e.g., within generations, families, or family subsystems). In a clinical context, one approach would be to create aggregate scores (a sum or average) to reflect the overall functioning of the family. For instance, when preparing for family therapy, it may be sufficient to know the overall family's perception of their style of affective expression. However, one feature of aggregate scores is that they obscure potentially meaningful differences among people within the family. As an alternative, when differences within the family are of interest, discrepancy scores can be calculated (subtracting one person's score from another's). As an example, when families are considering housing alternatives for a frail parent, it may be useful to know whether family members have different ideas about co-residence. The challenge of discrepancy scores, though, is to determine what discrepancies—and what size discrepancies—are most meaningful.

When choosing an assessment instrument, it is also important to notice whether the instrument asks respondents to do their own mental aggregating. For instance, on the Family Assessment Device (Epstein, Baldwin, & Bishop, 1983) people rate items according to "how well it describes your own family." The instruction forces people to aggregate across different relationships, resulting in a loss of important within-family variability and frustrating respondents who have different relationships with different members of their family. If the goal is to capture those unique relationships, the question would need to be asked for each one. Manuals and instructions for most instruments do not provide explicit guidance on how to combine information from multiple family members, so users must think carefully about what information they want.

At What Point in History Does the Assessment Take Place?

With this question we refer to the timing of the assessment relative to: (1) the developmental stage of the family; (2) the developmental stage of individuals within the family; and (3) the point in history when the assessment occurs, with its concomitant social, financial, and political context. This idea of age, cohort, and period effects is portrayed in Figure 11.1 (adapted from Glenn, 2004).

Consider this example. Imagine that an older parent is diagnosed with an aggressive form of cancer, and she is told her life expectancy is 6–9 months. This woman and her family will face a number of challenges in the months ahead that span issues of medical care, housing, financial planning, and psychological and spiritual adaptation. An assessment of her family's resources and ability to manage this hallmark event will differ depending on when the family hears about the cancer diagnosis. Family A in Figure 11.1 receives the news when the older parent is 60 years old. Her adult children are in their 40s, attending to their own work and family responsibilities, with their own young children.

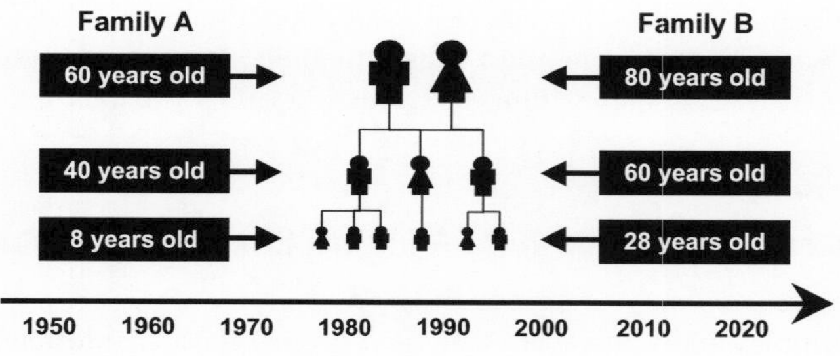

FIGURE 11.1

Assessment in the Context of Lifespan and Sociocultural Contexts.

In contrast, in Family B, the parent is diagnosed when she is 80. Her children are in their 60s, retired with more free time and financial resources, with children who are out of college and living independently. Each family is in a unique developmental phase, as is each member of the family. Because of those developmental differences, each family is likely to approach this new cancer diagnosis with different expectations, experiences, resources, and competing demands.

Family support in late-life will intersect with a variety of events and circumstances: marriage or divorce (or remarriage); the birth of subsequent generations; education and work responsibilities; relocation to another part of the country or world in the case of a job transfer or military deployment; and illness and death in any generation. Any of these events can complicate the resources that families can contribute to elder care, just as they can complicate the psychological and practical picture for people throughout the family.

Another layer to consider is the particular time in history when family events occur. An assessment happening today (August, 2009) as we write this chapter would need to account for family functioning in the context of a global economic downturn, tense political situations in Iraq and Afghanistan, health care reform efforts in the new Obama presidential administration, and concern about an H1N1 flu pandemic. Historical events can influence the issues and stressors that are urgent for the family, can guide the questions we therefore ask during an assessment, and can shape the focus of interventions we subsequently recommend. Although it may not be possible or necessary to conduct a systematic assessment of all these factors, keeping them in mind can enrich the understanding of how a family might face a new challenge.

ASPECTS OF FAMILY FUNCTIONING

What is important to know about a late-life family? What features of the family predict its ability to meet late-life challenges? And what features might be a useful focus for treatment and intervention? In this section we describe several aspects of functioning that recur across family theories and assessment instruments. Not every assessment will need to address all of them; we describe them here simply to identify common features that influence family functioning.

Family Structure

Family structure includes the people who are considered part of the family—present members, as well as important figures from the past—and the quality of the relationships among them. This information can help identify who should be included in an assessment, who might be sources of support for older adults, and what relationships are flashpoints for potential conflict. One way to document family structure is by constructing a genogram. A genogram is a visual representation of a family's composition, structure, and relationships, constructed with a set of standard symbols to depict the family (McGoldrick, Gerson, & Petry, 2008 is an excellent instructional resource). Although there is no ideal or suboptimal family structure, a genogram can provide preliminary but valuable information about the important personalities in the family and their relationships.

Family History

In addition to structure, the process of constructing a genogram also can evoke information about key events in a family's history, such as births, divorces, and deaths. These past events provide a context for understanding the current functioning of the family. In addition, more subtle, subjective, longstanding interpersonal dynamics often persist within the family of origin, even as people grow older

(Fingerman & Bermann, 2000; Rossi & Rossi, 1990; Whitbeck, Hoyt, & Huck, 1994). With their long emotional half-life, disappointments and slights, unresolved conflicts or outright abuse can flare up many decades later, complicating a family's ability to make decisions or engage in care at all (Qualls & Segal, 2003). On the other hand, reviewing important events in the family's history also can identify strengths in how families have coped with challenges in the past.

Family Roles

Family roles reflect how responsibilities and tasks have been divided within the family. These roles become apparent with direct questions about who is responsible for specific tasks, such as who manages family finances, who provides assistance with indoor housekeeping and outside home/yard maintenance, who arranges appointments, and even who typically hosts family functions (Epstein et al., 1983). Sometimes these roles are divided based on occupational expertise within the family: everyone defers legal matters to the adult daughter who is a lawyer; medical questions are directed toward the sister who worked as a nurse; financial issues are seen as the purview of the son in investment banking. Other roles are based on temperament or aptitude: one daughter is the "kin keeper" who always arranges holiday gatherings and hosts them at her home; a nephew with a flexible work schedule is the dependable one who can be counted on to stop by and check in on someone; the remote adult child overseas writes a check to help pay for in-home care.

The most efficient way to get this information is through careful questioning and observation, not with the standardized assessment instruments that currently exist. Indeed, family roles emerge even during a simple clinical interview. One person does most of the talking, taking on a leadership role. Another makes jokes or changes the subject or acts as the peacemaker whenever conflicts are mentioned. Identifying family roles can help clarify who might do what in support of an older adult, and how the negotiations might unfold.

Flexibility

Flexibility refers to a family's ability to adapt in response to stressors. In older families, changes in how the family interacts may be necessary as individual needs change (Qualls, 1999). An older parent may need to become more comfortable asking for and receiving help from her children; an adult child may need to make peace with an older in-law to facilitate caregiving; a grandchild may need to assume more responsibility around the house so their parents can tend to an aging parent. If family members resist changing in the face of a new stressor, or if they continue to use coping skills that worked at one time but are no longer effective, important support and supervision may be missing, care responsibilities may be unevenly divided, and family members may place themselves at greater risk for anger, depression, and burnout (Fingerman & Bermann, 2000; Mitrani et al., 2006). Family theories also suggest, however, that too much flexibility can be harmful. A family with no clear rules or roles will find it difficult to make decisions or develop a coherent, organized plan of care (Beavers & Hampson, 1990; Olson, 2000).

Family Contact and Support

Contact and shared activities are one set of indicators of family closeness (Bengtson & Roberts, 1991). Types of support include instrumental (e.g., financial assistance, childcare, transportation), emotional (e.g., empathy, affection), and informational (e.g., advice, information) (Cohen & Wills, 1985; House, Umberson, & Landis, 1988). Questions about the type, amount, and direction of support exchange are useful, as are subjective ratings of the quality of interactions, because even if a family is in frequent contact, their interactions could be tense and destructive.

Family Closeness

Family closeness is a broad construct that encompasses emotional bonds, affection, trust, and respect. Healthy families are characterized by a balance between being invested in each other's lives and maintaining some degree of differentiation and independence (Beavers & Hampson, 1990; Bowen, 1978; Olson, 2000). For example, a family who is not close might remain disconnected even in a time of crisis, such as a new dementia diagnosis in a parent. At the other end of the spectrum, a family who is too emotionally close may have trouble inviting in outside resources or supports. Balanced closeness involves an adaptive level of emotional support and involvement that maximizes functioning for all members of the family.

Decision-Making Skill

Effective decision-making skills are essential to the functioning of late-life families, who are likely to face an increasing pace and magnitude of decisions over time. These skills involve the ability to recognize that a decision is needed, gather information to weigh options, consider the benefits and risks of those options, and make and implement a decision. This is another area where current standardized assessment instruments provide little information; the most innovative approaches have used observations of couples or families (e.g., Henry, Berg, Smith, & Florsheim, 2007), but these methods are often impractical in clinical situations.

Communication

Communication in late-life families involves both verbal and nonverbal behavior toward one another and takes place over an increasingly diverse set of platforms (e.g., in-person interactions, telephone conversations, e-mail exchanges, text messages, etc.). Healthy families speak to one another in a way that is clear and direct (Epstein et al., 1983; Olson, 2000). It is obvious to whom messages are intended, and it is obvious what is being said or asked. Healthy communication also means being open and respectful of the opinions of others; family members feel comfortable expressing an opinion, even if it contradicts someone else. Disagreements can occur without fear that they will cause irreparable damage. Healthy families are also able to stay on topic when important issues are discussed. In contrast, in a less functional family, members may make assumptions about each other's feelings and preferences, speak in vague terms, and be unreceptive to differences in opinion (Epstein et al., 1983; Olson, 2000). Many of the standard instruments reviewed later include subscales focused on communication.

Knowledge of Preferences

When older adults are no longer able to make decisions on their own, family members are often called upon to be a surrogate and state preferences for them and act upon them. Healthy families are knowledgeable about each other's preferences, or are at least willing to investigate and consider those preferences. Knowledge is to some degree based on good communication skills, but also genuine curiosity and respect for the wishes of others in the family.

Norms and Expectations

Norms reflect the responsibilities that family members feel toward one another. When norms are congruent, family members are likely able to collaborate more efficiently and effectively because of a shared vision and sense of purpose; when norms are incongruent, conflict is more likely, as goals diverge (Bengtson & Roberts, 1991). That is not to suggest that family members must all think alike. Indeed, some amount of ambivalence in family relationships is common, often arising from conflicting normative expectations (Connidis & McMullin, 2002; Luescher & Pillemer, 1998). For example, an adult daughter-in-law may feel torn between her desire support her ill mother-in-law and her desire to dedicate her time to her husband and children.

ASSESSMENT INSTRUMENTS

In this next section we provide a brief synopsis of instruments. With one exception discussed later, we have chosen not to discuss instruments based on clinician ratings, e.g., Structural Global Assessment of Relational Functioning (American Psychiatric Association, 2000) or observational coding systems, e.g., Structural Analysis of Social Behavior—Composite Observational Coding Scheme (Florsheim & Benjamin, 2001) and Structural Family Systems Ratings—Dementia Caregiver (Mitrani, Feaster, McCabe, Czaja, & Szapocznik, 2005). The aforementioned either have not been used widely with late-life families or present pragmatic limitations, despite their potential utility in some circumstances. Instead, we concentrate on self-report instruments because of their relative ease of administration and scoring.

We have divided the instruments into two categories. The first includes instruments that have a strong theoretical foundation, extensive previous use in both clinical and research contexts, and adequate or better psychometric properties, although previous work with these instruments has concentrated on younger families. The second category includes instruments that also have a sound theoretical foundation and have been designed for and used with late-life families, although they lack the depth of previous use and documented psychometric strengths of the other instruments. For all these scales we provide a brief description of the instrument and evaluation of its utility, and refer the reader to Table 11.1 for technical details.

Section I: Instruments with Extensive Support for Use with Younger Families

Family Assessment Device

The Family Assessment Device (FAD; Epstein et al., 1983; Ryan, Epstein, Keitner, Miller, & Bishop, 2005; see Appendix A) is a self-report instrument based on the McMaster Model of Family Functioning, which highlights basic functions important to family health. Given its emphasis on functionality, "healthy" refers to a family's ability to provide basic resources for its members (e.g., food, security) and accomplish common, critical developmental tasks (e.g., accommodate role transitions, cope with unexpected crises).

The McMaster Model (and thus the FAD) focuses on six dimensions of family functioning: problem solving; communication; roles; affective responsiveness; affective involvement; and behavior control. In addition, the FAD also includes a General Functioning scale which can be used as a brief, overall assessment of the family. The scale's developers acknowledge that the McMaster Model is not an exhaustive list of important facets of the family, but does include clinically useful features. The FAD, therefore, has a definite clinical focus, is designed to differentiate healthy from unhealthy families, and can provide practitioners with information to guide family treatment.

There has been some debate about the factor structure of the FAD, with some authors suggesting that factor analysis supports only the use of the General Functioning and Behavior Control subscales (Ridenour, Daley, & Reich, 1999). But the developers of the scale point to the clinical utility and validity of all seven subscales, and argue each provides important information (Miller, Ryan, Keitner, Bishop, & Epstein, 2000a, 2000c). The scale has been translated into 24 languages, and there is evidence that it is useful in different cultures (Miller, Ryan, Keitner, Bishop, & Epstein, 2000b; Ryan et al., 2005), although this information is sparse and extensive norms do not exist for diverse populations based on ethnicity, socioeconomic status, or age. In addition, it is not clear how reports from multiple family members should be integrated. Nonetheless, on its face, the FAD addresses constructs that are relevant to late-life families who face developmental challenges that demand communication, shared problem solving, role adjustment, and affective expression, among other skills. Moreover, the extensive history of the development of the McMaster Model and the FAD suggest they have some utility in family assessment and treatment.

Another notable strength of the McMaster Model and the instruments associated with it is the integration between assessment and treatment. Indices from the FAD and the McMaster Clinical Rating Scale can be used to guide treatment planning using Problem Centered Systems Therapy of the Family. There is good evidence for the efficacy of this manualized, short-term, systems-oriented treatment, although not with late-life families.

Family Assessment Measure

The Family Assessment Measure (FAM-III) (Skinner, Steinhauer, & Santa-Barbara, 1983; Skinner et al., 1995) is a self-report instrument designed to assess perceptions of family strengths and weaknesses. The FAM-III is based on the Process Model of Family Functioning (Steinhauer, Santa-Barbara, & Skinner, 1984), a transtheoretical framework that describes seven broad domains of family functioning: task accomplishment; role performance; communication; affective expression; involvement; control; and values and norms. According to the developers, these domains represent basic, interdependent, and dynamic features of the family. Because these domains are thought to be universally important to family functioning, the FAM-III is presumed to be useful across clinical theoretical orientations and research goals.

There are three forms of the FAM-III. The General Scale examines overall family health, the Dyadic Relationship Scale examines how one family member views their relationship with another family member, and the Self-Rating Scale enables one person to evaluate their own functioning within the family. The General Scale also includes indices of social desirability and defensiveness. An abridged version of the instrument, the Brief FAM, exists for each form and was designed for screening or tracking change with repeated, brief assessments. The three forms can be used separately, or together for a more comprehensive portrait of the family (with an obvious increase in time needed for administration).

The psychometrics of this instrument are adequate, although reliability is less strong for some subscales. Validity coefficients are generally acceptable, although as with many family instruments, predictive validity is less well established. The original validation of the FAM included norms for relatively young families (mean age of the adults=38.6), and though subsequent research has provided expanded norms for specific clinical groups, no studies have focused on late-life families. In addition, use of the instrument with families of varying structures and racial/cultural backgrounds has been limited. Still, the transtheoretical framework helps make this instrument applicable to families of many types, at any stage of development.

With its many forms, the FAM-III can provide a great deal of data about a family, which brings the benefit of comprehensiveness and the burden of integrating so much information. In addition to the profile provided by the FAM-III, which depicts areas of relative strength and weakness, the instrument also enables comparisons of perceptions within the family when family members complete the same form. For instance, an adult child may have a different perception of communication within the family compared with her older father, which can provide a point for discussion or intervention. Some approximation of this is possible with the other instruments reviewed in this section, although the FAM-III is already constructed for this purpose.

Table 11.1 Assessment Instrument Properties

Instrument	Focus	Source	Scales	Format	Source of Information
Instruments with strong clinical and research support, but limited use to date with late-life families					
Family Assessment Device (FAD)	Structural and organizational properties of families.	Epstein, N.B., Baldwin, L.M., & Bishop, D.S. (1983). The McMaster Family Assessment Device. *Journal of Marital and Family Therapy, 9,* 171–180.	General Functioning Problem Solving Communication Roles Affective Responsiveness Affective Involvement Behavior Control	60 statements rated on a 4-point scale	Self-report
Family Assessment Mesasure - III (FAM)	Family systems processes critical to accomplishing basic, developmental, and crisis-related tasks.	Skinner, H.A., Steinhauer, P.D., & Santa-Barbara, J. (1995) *Family Assessment Measure-III Manual*. Toronto, Canada: Multi Health Systems.	Task Accomplishment Role Performance Communication Affective Expression Involvement Control Values and Norms Social Desirability Defensiveness	General Scale (50 items); Dyadic Relationship Scale (42 items); Self-Rating Scale (42 items); Brief FAM (14 items; brief form exists for each of the 3 scales), Each item rated on a 4-point scale.	Self-report
Family Adaptability and Cohesion Scales (FACES IV)	Cohesion and flexibility dynamics within the family.	Olson, D.H., Gorall, D.M., & Tiesel, J. (2007). FACES IV and the Circumplex Model: Validation study. Retrieved July 6, 2009 from Life Innovations, Inc. Web site: http://www.faceive.com/home.html	Balanced Cohesion Balanced Flexibility Disengaged Enmeshed Rigid Chaotic Dimensional and ratio scores calculated that take into account relative amounts of balanced and unbalanced traits endorsed.	42 items rated on a 5-point scale.	Self-report
Self-Report Family Inventory (SFI)	Competence of the family system to carry out tasks and manage itself, and functional and behavioral styles of relating and interacting.	Beavers, W.R. & Hampson, R.B. (1990) *Successful Families: Assessment and Intervention*. New York: W. W. Norton	Health/Competence Conflict Cohesion Leadership Emotional Expressiveness	34 items rated a 5-point scale to indicate how much each statement fits a family; 2 items rated on a 5-point scale to indicate overall family fuctioning and level of independence in the family.	Self-report
Family Environment Scale (FES)	Social environment of the family, within an Interactionist framework.	Moos, R. & Moos, B. (1994). *Family Environment Scale Manual: Development, applications, research* (3rd ed.). Palo Alto, CA: Consulting Psychologist Press.	Relationship: Cohesion Expressiveness Conflict Personal Growth: Independence Achievement Orientation Intellectual-Cultural Orientation Active-Recreational Orientation Moral-Religious Emphasis System Maintenance: Organization Control	Long Form: 90 true/false items (10 per subscale) which can be reworded to inquire about the real, Ideal, or expected family. Short Form: 40 items from across each subscale. Family Relationship Index (FRI): 30 items from the Cohesion, Expressiveness, and Conflict subscales.	Self-report
Family APGAR	Perception of the value of the family as a psychosocial support.	Smilkstein, G. (1978). The Family APGAR: A proposal for a family function test and its use by physicians. *Journal of Family Practice, 6,* 1231–1239.	Adaptation Partnership Growth Affection Resolve	5 questions rated on a 3-point scale.	Self-report

Typical Administration Duration	Reading/ Age Level	Sample Items	Reliability†	Validity†	Availability
15–20 minutes	Age 12+	Individuals are accepted for what they are. We don't say what we mean. We discuss who is responsible for household jobs. We are able to make decisions about how to solve problems. We express tenderness.	***	***	Available online at http://chipts. ucla. edu/ assessment/ IB/Lis
Full FAM = 20–45 minutes, Brief FAM = 5–10 minutes per scale	Age 10+	We argue about who said what in our family. We tell each other about things that bother us. We can rely on family members to do their part. We agree about who should do what in our family. When our family gets upset, we take too long to get over it.	***	***	Psychological Assessment Resources, Inc.
10 minutes	Age 9+	Our family tries new ways of dealing with problems. There is no leadership in this family. We resent family members doing things outside the family. Family members are supportive of each other during difficult times.	***	***	Life Innovations, Inc.
10 minutes	Age 11+	There is a closeness in my family but each person is allowed to be special and different. Our family members would rather do things with other people than together. Our family is good at solving problems together. We all have a say in family plans. We argue a lot.	**	**	In primary citation
20–40 minutes	Age 12+	Family members really help and support one another. Family members often keep their feelings to themselves. If there's a disagreement in our family, we try hard to smooth things over and keep the peace. Family members have strict ideas about what is right and wrong. We feel it is important to be the best at whatever you do.	**	**	Consulting Psychologists Press, Inc.
Less than 5 minutes	Age 10+	I am satisfied that my family accepts my wishes to take on new activities or make changes in my lifestyle. I am satisfied with the way my family expresses affection and responds to my feelings, such as anger, sorrow, and love.	**	**	In primary citation

†Key for reliability and validity information:
*** = *substantial evidence, good psychometrics*
** = *some evidence, variable psychometrics across studies or subscales*
* = *little evidence, poor or unavaliable psychometrics*

Table 11.1 *(continued)*

Instrument	Focus	Source	Scales	Format	Source of Information
		Instruments with limited clinical and research support but designed for late-life families			
Checklist of Family Relational Abilities (CFRA)	Family's relational skills in domains relevant to the care of ill patients.	Wilkins, V. M., Quill, T. E., & King, D. A. (2009). Assessing families in palliative care: A pilot study of the Checklist of Family Relational Abilities. *Journal of Palliative Medicine, 12*, 517–519.	Attachment Bonds Openness of Communication Regarding the Current Illness Collaborative Decision Making Regarding the Current Illness Overall Level of Family Relational Abilities	3 domain reted on 3- or 4-point descriptive anchors; 4-point overall rating of relational abilities.	Clinician rated
Paternalism and Respect for Autonomy	Attitudes regarding filial obligation and the relative importance of parental autonomy.	Cicirelli, V.G. (1992). *Family caregiving: Autonomous and paternalistic decision making*. Newbury Park, CA: Sage Publications, Inc.	Paternalism Independent autonomy Shared autonomy	30 items/scale rated on a 4-point scale.	Self-report
Hamon Filial Responsibility Scale	Filial responsibility expectations for emotional, instrumental, contact, and communication support to older parents.	Hamon, R.R., & Blieszner, R. (1990). Filial responsibility expectations among adult child-older parent pairs. *Journals of Gerontology: Psychological Sciences, 45*, P110–112.	Overall breadth of felt responsibility	16 items rated on a 4-point scale.	Self-report
Intergenerational Ambivalence	Conflicting attitudes or emotions towards family members or family relationships.	Luescher, K. & Pillemer, K. (1998). Intergeneration ambivalence. A new approach to the study of parent-child relations in later life. *Journal of Marriage and the Family, 60*, 413–425. Willson, A.E., Shuey, K. M., & Elder, G.H. (2003). Ambivalence in the relationship of adult children to aging parents and in-laws. *Journal of Marriage and the Family, 65*, 1055–1072.	Positive feelings or relationship characteristics Negative feelings or relationship characteristics	6 items rated on 4-point scale.	Self-report
Prereferences for Everyday Living Inventory (PELI)	Psychosocial preferences of older adults.	Carpenter, B. D., Van Haitsma, K., Ruckdeschel, K., & Lawton, M. P. (2000). The psychosocial preferences or older adults: A pilot examination of content and structure. *The Gerontologist, 40*, 335–348.	Social Contact Growth Activities Diversionary Activities Self Dominion Enlisting Others in Care	48 general preference items rated on a 5-point scale; 358 specific preference items answered yes/no, with the exception of some that are open-ended.	Selp-report

Typical Administration Duration	Reading/ Age Level	Sample Items	Reliability†	Validity†	Availability
1–2 minutes, but based on previous interactions with the family	n/a	Openness of Communication Regarding the Current Illness: ___ Communication between all or nearly all family members is open and includes expression of emotional reactions to the illness. ___ Most family members discuss the illness openly but some individuals are excluded and/or family members avoid expression of emotional reactions. ___ Some family members discuss the facts of the illness but few family members are involved in the discussions and/or emotional reactions are not shared. ___ There is little if any discussion of the illness between family members.	*	*	In primary citation
60 minutes	Unspecified	No matter how much an elderly parent objects, the adult child should do whatever he or she thinks is best in the long run for the parent's health. When an elderly parent becomes forgetful about financial matters, the adult child should take over and run things as he or she thinks best. If an elderly parent of sound mind decides not to see the doctor about a chronic condition, the adult child should support the parent's decision. If an elderly parent who is emotionally unstable wants to donate money to charity, the adult child should help the parent decide how much to give.	**	**	In primary citation
5 minutes	Unspecified	Rate the degree to which you agree that adult children should help their older parents in the following areas: Give emotional support. Give financial help. Live close to parent.	*	*	In primary citation
Less than 5 minutes	Unspecified	How much does he or she make you feel appreciated, loved, or cared for How often does he or she make too many demands for help and support?	*	**	In primary citation
20–25 minutes for general items, 60–90 minutes for general and specific items	8th grade+	General, followed by specific, items: A. Do you like to take a bath or shower at a specific time? 1. Which do you prefer, a bath or a shower? 2. How often do you like to take a bath or shower? B. Do you like animals? 1. What kind of animals do you like? 2. What kind of contact would you like to have with animals? C. Do you want to have family or friends involved in major decisions about your life, such as decisions about medical care, where you live, and decisions about your finances? 1. Which specific family members do you want to have involved in these kinds of decisions? 2. Which specific family members do you NOT want to have involved in these kinds of decisions?	**	**	Authors of primary citation

Family Adaptability and Cohesion Scales

The Family Adaptability and Cohesion Scales-IV (FACES-IV; Olson, Gorall, & Tiesel, 2007) is a self-report measure based on the Circumplex Model (Olson, 2000), which focuses on three domains of family functioning: communication; cohesion; and flexibility (previously known as "adaptability"). Only cohesion and flexibility are assessed with the FACES-IV. According to the model, healthy families balance both connectedness with independence, and stability with flexibility, and this balance is achieved with effective communication. The FACES-IV includes two scales to measure healthy family functioning (balanced cohesion, balanced flexibility), and four scales to measure unhealthy family functioning (disengaged, enmeshed, rigid, and chaotic).

Olson and colleagues (2007) recommend using the FACES-IV as part of a larger assessment packet that includes both the Family Communication Scale (adapted from Barnes & Olson, 1989) and the Family Satisfaction Scale (Olson & Wilson, 1989). They also recommend using the self-report measures in combination with the corresponding observational measure, the Clinical Rating Scale (Thomas & Olson, 1993). One caution we might mention is that the self-report and observational measures frequently provide discrepant results (Olson, 2000), and it is not clear how best to combine results from these two tools. Additionally, how to combine scores across family members is not clear.

Although the Circumplex Model has been applied to a diverse group of families, including single parent households, stepfamilies, and gay and lesbian couples (Olson et al., 2007), the newly developed FACES-IV has not. Moreover, the validation sample for the FACES-IV was homogeneous: approximately two-thirds of the sample was female, 90% was Caucasian, and the average age was 28 (Olson et al., 2007). Finally, some items may not be applicable for use with older families (e.g., "Children have a say in their discipline"). Therefore, in spite of the strong research support for the Circumplex Model with younger families, the utility of the FACES-IV with late-life and diverse families has yet to be determined.

Self-Report Family Inventory

The Self-Report Family Inventory (SFI; Beavers & Hampson, 1990) is a measure of family functioning based on the Beavers Systems Model. This model includes two orthogonal dimensions: family health/competence and family style. According to the model, healthy families are structured but also willing to alter their structure in response to developmental changes or specific stressors. In addition, family members are able to derive satisfaction both from within and from outside of their families, take responsibility for their actions, respect each other's perspectives and choices, and resolve conflicts easily.

In general, the SFI has good psychometric properties, although some subscales have low test—retest reliability. The SFI also has been used with a diverse group of families, both in terms of culture and structure (Beavers & Hampson, 2003). As of 2003, the SFI had been translated into nine languages and used in 15, primarily European, countries. In spite of these strengths, the SFI has not been used with late-life families, and some items may need to be removed or adapted for use with this population (e.g., "In our home, we feel loved"). Another potential limitation is that some items are used for more than one subscale, leading to intercorrelations among subscales. Finally, Beavers and Hampson recognize that family members often disagree about their perceptions of their family and thus end up with different scale scores; examining the pattern of scores within families is presumably of some clinical utility. Yet research on the best way to combine various ratings within a family is limited.

Family Environment Scale

The Family Environment Scale (FES; Moos & Moos, 1994) was developed from an interactionist framework with the purpose of describing the social environment of the family. As such, although the constructs tapped by the FES overlap with some of those in other instruments, the underlying focus of the FES is on how family members relate to and behave with one another, all within the larger social context. Families are assessed on three dimensions, within which there are a number of subscales: relationship (cohesion, expressiveness, and conflict subscales); personal growth (independence, achievement orientation, intellectual-cultural orientation, active-recreational orientation, and moral-religious emphasis); system maintenance (organization and control). In addition to the long form of the FES, other forms enable assessment of perceptions of the current (real form), wished for (ideal form), and expected (expectations form) family. A short form also exists as a subset of items from each subscale. An even briefer form, the Family Relationships Index (FRI), includes just three subscales (cohesiveness, expressiveness, and conflict).

The FES provides a comprehensive family assessment that is quite different in terms of some aspects of its content than the other instruments in this section. For instance, its attention to interest in political and cultural engagement places the family squarely in a larger social context, which may be valuable information when working with late-life families. Still, use of the instrument with late-life families and diverse families has been limited. Another disadvantage is the instrument's relative length, although users could isolate specific subscales of interest. Moreover, in recent years there has been some debate about the reliability of some subscales, perhaps highlighting the measurement error inherent in true/false items. This has been particularly true in research with families from diverse ethnic and cultural backgrounds, e.g., Puerto Ricans, Vietnamese (Munet-Vilaro & Egan, 1990). In addition, although factor analytic studies have consistently found 2—3 solutions, these factors have not usually mapped onto the three dimensions proposed by the scale's authors. Therefore, for researchers using the FES it is important to calculate and report reliability indices for each sample and to consider how unstable validity might affect associations with other dependent and independent variables. Likewise, clinicians may need to keep in mind how low reliability and validity might cloud interpretation and prediction.

Family APGAR

Based on the brief assessment used to judge the health of newborns, the Family APGAR (Smilkstein, 1978) is intended to provide an efficient way to characterize the "health" of the family. The scale consists of five questions posed to family members about their satisfaction with family relationships. Questions address perceptions of the family in five domains: adaptation (use of resources for problem solving when the family is under stress); partnership (sharing of decision-making and responsibilities); growth (mutual support and guidance to encourage maturation); affection (expressions of love and caring); and resolve (commitment of time, space, and wealth). It is important to keep in mind that items are rated in terms of a person's *satisfaction* with family functioning. Therefore, the Family APGAR score indicates subjective contentment with family functioning, not family functioning per se. For instance, a family may not communicate much about problems, and a respondent may be satisfied with that, even if it may not be helpful to the family from an outsider's perspective.

Scale content covers many of the same constructs addressed in lengthier instruments, and its brevity makes it easy to use for repeated assessments. In addition, the psychometrics of the instrument are generally sound (Smilkstein, Ashworth, & Montano, 1982), although there have been some questions about validity (Gardner et al., 2001), and the scale has not been used extensively outside of health care contexts or with diverse samples (including families beyond those with young children). The scale's developer has recommended that a 5-point response scale provides greater discriminatory power and should be used for research purposes, while the original 3-point scale is sufficient for clinical use (Smilkstein, 1993). A number of authors have pointed out the potential utility of this scale when working with older adults (e.g., Burke & Laramie, 2004; Ebersole, Hess, Touhy, & Jett, 2005) and, because of its efficiency, this scale may be useful with further validation.

Section II: Instruments with Support for Use with Late-Life Families

Checklist of Family Relational Abilities

The Checklist of Family Relational Abilities (CFRA; Wilkins, Quill, & King, 2009, see Appendix B) is one of the more recently developed instruments available to assess the family system. A clinician-rated index, the CFRA enables clinicians to gauge a family's readiness to manage key tasks in a health care situation. Although it was developed to assess families in a particular clinical context (i.e., palliative care), it is based on some of the same theoretical foundations as other scales and taps overlapping constructs. The instrument is based on an epigenetic model of family relational functioning (Wynne, 1984), which takes a developmental perspective and cites the formation of attachment bonds as an initial foundation upon which more complex relational abilities (e.g., open communication, collaborative decision-making) are based. These skills come to bear when families are faced with serious illness in a family member, specifically when they need to talk about and decide upon a plan of care.

Attachment, communication, and problem solving are rated on descriptively anchored scales. The checklist also includes a 4-point ranking of overall functioning, with an indication for family intervention. With that information, clinicians may be able to tailor information and decisions for a family, and be better prepared for how to interact with them when presenting treatment options and decisions.

This instrument's strengths are its brevity and attempt to provide a concise, objective assessment that could assist any provider on an interdisciplinary care team. The mean age of participants in the pilot validation sample was 58 ($SD = 12$ years, range = 39–81) and included many different family relations (spouses, adult children, siblings, and in-laws), suggesting relevance to late-life families. Still, the scale was developed based on just 13 family members, mostly Caucasian, suggesting additional validation is clearly needed. Nevertheless, the instrument was developed by a group of clinicians and researchers with extensive experience working with late-life families in a health care context, and the tool holds promise.

Paternalism and Respect for Autonomy

As part of research focused on family functioning in late life, Cicirelli (1992) developed two scales to assess beliefs about paternalism and respect for autonomy in family caregiving. These scales, developed specifically for use with adult children and older parents, are useful to measure the extent to which older parents and their adult children agree about who should make decisions about parent care. Elements of incongruence may indicate the potential for discord in the family when care coordination is needed, as beliefs about autonomy and paternalism are likely antecedents to how family members actually behave when older adults need assistance. Similarly, incongruence could indicate points for intervention to help the family be better prepared for upcoming decisions.

The Paternalism scale consists of brief scenarios that inquire about the extent to which people believe adult children know what is best for an older parent and should be able to force a parent to accept decisions made for them. Attitudes reflect a continuum from direct paternalism (i.e., it is acceptable for adult children to intervene in parents' decisions without the parents' request or consent) to paternalism by default (i.e., it is acceptable for adult children to intervene when parents are indifferent about making their own decisions). Scenarios in the Respect for Autonomy scale address both negative autonomy (i.e., refraining from interfering with a parent's decisions) and positive autonomy (i.e., actively promoting a parent's decision-making). Two factor-derived subscales include Independent Autonomy (parent making decisions independently) and Shared Autonomy (parent making decisions with adult children).

These scales may be of interest to researchers who are exploring attitudinal congruence across generations as either independent variables (e.g., Is congruence related to choices that parents and children make or how they interact when making decisions?) or dependent variables (e.g., Is gender or geographical proximity or communication style predictive of attitudinal congruence?). Likewise, these scales may be useful to clinicians for pinpointing potential areas of conflict and tailoring family education or treatment. To offer a caveat, however, the scales were developed with a relatively homogeneous, Caucasian sample and have not been widely used since their original publication.

Hamon Filial Responsibility Scale

The Hamon Filial Responsibility Scale (HFRS; Hamon & Blieszner, 1990) is a brief, self-report instrument designed to assess expectations regarding care that adult children should provide to their aging parents. The scale is designed to provide a comprehensive assessment of filial obligations and addresses emotional, instrumental, contact, and communication responsibilities. A common way of using the HFRS is to compare perceived obligations across generations in order to highlight points of agreement and disagreement. Incongruencies may indicate areas of potential conflict that could be addressed in family education or therapy. Limited psychometric properties of the HFRS have been reported, though those that have are good. As with many instruments, validation samples have been restricted in their diversity. The scale is narrow in its purpose but is comprehensive in its content, and may be useful for examining this specific facet of family life.

Intergenerational Ambivalence

Because of its importance in family functioning, we discuss intergenerational ambivalence, even though no one standard way to assess this construct has yet emerged. Intergenerational ambivalence is defined as the presence of contradictions in parent–child relationships that arise from conflicting normative expectations and/or conflicting emotions and attitudes about each other (Connidis & McMullin, 2002; Luescher & Pillemer, 1998). For example, an adult daughter may feel torn between a desire to provide support to her chronically ill mother and a desire to focus on her relationships with her husband and her children. Ambivalence is common in late-life relationships (Pillemer & Suitor, 2002; Willson, Shuey, & Elder, 2003) and is associated with diminished well-being and increased physiological response to stressors (Fingerman, Pitzer, Lefkowitz, Birditt, & Mroczek, 2008; Uchino, Holt-Lunstad, Uno, & Flinders, 2001). The presence of ambivalence may alert clinicians to a potentially difficult caregiving situation.

Despite the clinical relevance, scales to measure intergenerational ambivalence have been used exclusively in research contexts. Direct measures of ambivalence include asking people if they have mixed feelings toward family members, or if they feel conflicted about their family relationships (Pillemer & Suitor, 2002; Pillemer et al., 2007). Indirect measures include asking questions about both positive and negative perceptions of intergenerational relationships and then calculating an ambivalence score that is a combination of responses to these questions (Fingerman, Chen, Hay, Cichy, & Lefkowitz, 2006; Fingerman et al., 2008; Thompson, Zanna, & Griffin, 1995; Willson et al., 2003; Willson, Shuey, Elder, & Wickrama, 2006). Psychometric information about these methods is limited. However, both direct and indirect measures have been used in ethnically, culturally, and nationally diverse samples (Fingerman et al., 2008; Lowenstein, 2007).

Preferences for Everyday Living Inventory

The Preferences for Everyday Living Inventory (PELI; Carpenter, Van Haitsma, Ruckdeschel, & Lawton, 2000) is a tool that enables older adults to describe their priorities and preferences related to daily activities and care. We review this tool because it can be helpful to clinicians and family members as they plan for and implement care for an older adult. The instrument grew out of research and practice in long-term and home-based care settings, where the culture change movement has emphasized individualized care that reflects the values and wishes of care recipients.

With its self-report format, the PELI enables older adults to describe a broad range of both general preferences (e.g., "Do you like to exercise?") and specific likes and dislikes (e.g., "Do you have an interest in walking for exercise?"). The general questions fall into five empirically derived content domains: social contact; growth activities (personal growth and development); diversionary activities (leisure pursuits); self-dominion (personal expression in living environment and routine); and enlisting others in care. The PELI can be administered in its entirety, or in subsections, and the questions can be answered in a semi-structured interview or by self-report.

Comprehensive information about an older adult's psychosocial preferences may be used to tailor recreational and educational activities, to personalize a living environment, to individualize personal care routines, and to guide the extent of involvement by others in care. In our work with families, we have used the PELI to compare preferences articulated by older adults with presumed preferences estimated by their adult children (Carpenter, Lee, Ruckdeschel, Van Haitsma, & Feldman, 2006). Discrepancies between actual and presumed preferences then serve as a foundation for family education (Carpenter & Mulligan, 2009). Incongruencies about preferences (as with incongruencies on attitudes measured by other instruments in this review) provide information about family knowledge and can guide family intervention.

The PELI is a relatively new instrument, and although its preliminary psychometric properties appear promising, it has been used to date with relatively homogenous samples of older adults receiving residential and home health care. The breadth of the instrument is both a strength and liability: the content coverage is extensive, but administration of the full instrument takes, on average, an hour. Older adults have responded favorably to the instrument, appreciating the respect the questions pay to their preferences, and family members and formal caregivers have reported enhanced knowledge upon reviewing PELI results. The scale is obviously focused in its purpose but does provide comprehensive information that can inform supportive services.

CASE STUDY

Background Information

Silvia Ramirez is a 73-year-old woman who was admitted to a rehabilitation center after a hip replacement following a fall outside her home. Silvia's attending physician has concerns about her ability to return home, given two other recent falls and comorbidities including hypertension, diabetes, and severe arthritis in both knees. In addition, Silvia recently stopped driving due to worsening vision associated with macular degeneration. Discharge planning will include input from many disciplines at the rehabilitation center, and the staff psychologist, Dr Clarke, has been consulted to help clarify Silvia's wishes and the ability of her family to offer Silvia support.

Before talking with Silvia, Dr Clarke spoke with the physician to clarify the purpose of the consult, and with the social worker to gather preliminary information about the family and the discharge options that were being considered. Next, Dr Clarke visited with Silvia in her room, introduced himself, described the purpose of his visit, and obtained consent from Silvia to gather additional information from her and her adult children.

Silvia was friendly and cooperative with the clinical interview and provided the following information as Dr Clarke drew a genogram with Silvia's input. According to Silvia, she has been living in California since she emigrated from Mexico 20 years ago. Her husband passed away two years ago after living with Alzheimer's disease for seven years, during which time Silvia was his primary caregiver. Since her husband's death, Silvia has been living in the small house they shared. She said she manages all household responsibilities on her own, but acknowledged increasing difficulty getting up and down the stairs of her basement and finding things she puts down around the house because of her poor vision.

Silvia has been a homemaker her whole life, and her current income comes solely from her husband's small pension and Social Security benefits. Medicare covers most of her medical costs and prescriptions. Silvia spent the majority of their savings on care for her husband, so her resources are limited. She has considered selling her house, which she owns outright, and moving to an apartment, but she is afraid that money from the sale of her home would be inadequate over time.

There are three adult children in the Ramirez family: Alicia, 51, lives in New York City; Carlos, 48, lives about 15 minutes away from Silvia; and Ana, 42, lives about an hour away with her two children. In terms of her own family of origin, Silvia is the youngest of five siblings, but only two of her siblings are still living. Her older brother, Luis, lives in Mexico, and her younger sister, Maria, lives about 10 minutes away from Silvia. Silvia describes her relationship with her sister as very close. They are both recently widowed. In addition to her family, Silvia has close friends in her neighborhood and church, where she volunteers regularly.

With Silvia's permission, Dr Clarke tried to contact all three of her children by telephone to gather additional information. He was unable to reach Alicia despite leaving several messages; he talked with Carlos one afternoon when he was visiting his mother; and he spoke with Ana briefly on the telephone. According to Carlos, both he and Ana understand the concerns of the physician and have considered asking Silvia to move in with them. Carlos said his mother would be reluctant to live with him because he is gay and lives with his partner of 12 years. For her part, Ana does not think she has the time or energy to care for her mother. She is a single mother of two school-aged children, and she is currently working two jobs. Moreover, Ana has sought treatment for depression in the past, and she is concerned about becoming depressed again if she takes on the added responsibility of providing a home to her mother. According to Carlos, relations are strained between everyone and Alicia, who "left us to move east." Silvia said she does not want to live with any of her children and prefers to stay in her own home, although she would consider living with Ana if necessary.

With this background, Dr Clarke decided it would be useful to obtain standardized assessments of some family features to round out his understanding of the family and to offer more targeted recommendations to the family and the treatment team about how best to support the Ramirez family.

Assessment Targets and Instruments

Dr Clarke is interested in getting more detailed information from each member of the Ramirez family regarding current patterns of support within the family and expectations regarding filial responsibilities. He has each family member complete the Family Assessment Device (FAD) to gather information about family functioning, and has a separate interview with each family member. In preparing his consultation report, he also rates the family on the Checklist of Family Relational Abilities (CFRA) based on his clinical interviews and observations of family interactions.

Case Analysis and Summary

The Ramirez family has many features that characterize modern, late-life families. Silvia has outlived her husband and now survives on a fixed income, limiting her ability to pay for in-home supportive services. However, she has a wide network of family and friends who are, to varying degrees, willing and able to help her. Within her family, Silvia's close relationship with her sister is a powerful source of emotional support, although her sister is not able to provide much practical assistance because of her own physical limitations. Her children, meanwhile, have their own busy lives, and while they are mostly eager to help Silvia in whatever way they can, they wonder how they will balance care with their other responsibilities. Equally important, everyone in the family is feeling stressed about decisions regarding Silvia's placement, decisions that need to be made soon. All this is taking place in a family that has deep ties to its Hispanic culture. Silvia feels the most connection to her cultural heritage and in fact visits her *curandero*, or folk healer, for medical care. Carlos and Ana feel strong filial obligations toward their mother and identify with some features of Mexican culture, though not as strongly as their mother.

Interpretation of the FAD suggested mostly agreement within the family about its relatively good functioning, with some notable discrepancies in opinion. Most obviously, Alicia did not return the FAD. Her siblings said they were not surprised, as Alicia had been distant from the family for years, in terms of both geography and contact. In fact, both siblings noted that they had made ratings on the FAD without considering Alicia; as Ana said, "If I included her, my ratings would have been a lot worse. She just doesn't contribute and makes things hard for the rest of us with her criticism." In contrast, Silvia seemed to protect Alicia, excusing her behavior by noting "how busy she is with her important job." When pressed, however, Silvia acknowledged that Alicia has not been involved much in the family, even missing last summer's family reunion.

The remaining family members agreed that their family is comfortable expressing a range of emotions, that those emotions tend to be reasonable and appropriate for the circumstances, and that the family is able to handle both routine and emergent situations that require family collaboration. Silvia and Ana said they felt family members took an active interest in each other's lives and respected their activities and choices, although Carlos's view of the family in this area was less positive. He explained that his sexual orientation continued to cause uneasiness in the family, obvious from his mother's vocal prayers for him and his sister's concerns about the influence Carlos and his partner might have on her children.

Still, all family members felt communication in the family was open regarding everyday matters, if not more emotional topics. In addition, they felt people in the family were clear and direct in their communication and said what they needed to say to the right person, rather than talking behind their back. Finally, there was general agreement that the family's biggest challenge was in the area of problem solving. Silvia, Carlos, and Ana all felt that the family was often disorganized and stuck when action was needed. They said they had trouble formulating a list of alternatives, with pros and cons. Dr Clarke also noted the responses from Carlos and Ana regarding unclear roles and responsibilities in the family. Although Silvia believes everyone pitches in and fulfills his or her own jobs in the family, Carlos and Ana see more confusion and disorder in how things get done. The family has not had explicit conversations about who should be doing what tasks, and, when something is left unattended to, family members tend to ignore it or stew, without addressing it openly.

In reviewing the results from the FAD, along with his multiple family interviews, Dr Clarke felt the Ramirez family was functioning relatively well but possessed some vulnerabilities that could make Silvia's upcoming discharge more complicated. On the CFRA he rated the family as having strong, positive attachment bonds, capable of having open communication about Silvia's current medical situation, able to reach mutually satisfying decisions, but still temporarily overwhelmed by what to do regarding discharge.

Silvia, Carlos, and Ana appeared to have mostly positive feelings toward one another and were capable of sharing their thoughts, opinions, and feelings. They were likely to be interested and involved in discharge planning meetings with the staff, and seemed capable of participating in these conversations with openness and emotional maturity. At the same time, Dr Clarke thought they might benefit from more assistance laying out a clear plan for Silvia's discharge and putting that plan into action. He believed that, for this family, staff might need to be more active and forceful in helping the family generate options and weigh those options. Responsibilities for gathering information could be assigned to specific people in the family, with clear expectations about what information is needed and when. An explicit conversation about Silvia's specific post-discharge needs and who could fulfill them would be important. According to everyone in the family, Alicia was not likely to offer much help, though she might be willing to provide financial support to Silvia. Carlos and Ana, meanwhile, would need to divide day-to-day caregiving roles, perhaps with complementary help from Silvia's friends, church, and local service organizations. Keeping Silvia connected with her sister and folk healer was also a priority.

Based on information from the assessment and interviews, in his consultation report to the staff and the Ramirez family Dr Clarke recommended several sessions of problem solving-focused family therapy. Goals of the brief therapy included:

1. Discuss results of the FAD and the CFRA, noting family strengths but also potential vulnerabilities in diffuse roles and discrepancies in perceptions of family involvement.
2. Review Silvia's preferences and values regarding housing and autonomy. Likewise, discuss each individual's beliefs about filial obligations for parent care.
3. With input from the interdisciplinary care team, outline caregiving support that Silvia is likely to need and the discharge options that are available.
4. Weigh the discharge options and reach consensus on a plan.
5. Develop a post-discharge plan that outlines responsibilities for each person in the family and a timeline for specific tasks.
6. Reinforce the family's already effective communication and problem solving skills.

Dr Clarke conducted four sessions of family therapy, addressing each goal. In addition, he gathered information from the physician, occupational therapist, and physical therapist regarding Silvia's progress and likely care needs at discharge. He also spoke with the social worker to clarify the range of discharge options available to Silvia, given her financial resources and available services in her local community. Finally, he facilitated a family meeting at which all disciplines met with the Ramirez family to finalize a discharge plan.

Upon discharge, Silvia went to live for four weeks with Ana. After some emotional conversations, Ana agreed to let her children stay with Carlos and his partner on the weekends, to provide her with a break from childcare. In addition, Silvia spoke with members of her congregation, and the Women's Group brought by occasional meals to Ana's house for the family. Carlos was able to take time off work to transport Silvia to her outpatient appointments, including a visit to her folk healer. When Silvia returned to her own home, Carlos organized housekeeping services for her three times per week, and, after a frank discussion by telephone, Alicia agreed to pay for the service. Dr Clarke continued to check in with Silvia and Carlos during Silvia's outpatient rehabilitative therapy appointments.

CONCLUSION

With current instruments, assessment with late-life families is like cooking in someone else's kitchen: they have all the basic implements and ingredients a kitchen should have but perhaps not exactly what you need. Many of the instruments described in this chapter have not been used with late-life families, and most have not been validated with ethnic/racial minority groups or diverse family structures. Still, it is striking that again and again, across different models of family functioning and different assessment instruments, similar constructs appear useful for differentiating healthy from unhealthy families. Some consensus appears to be emerging about what makes for optimal family functioning, despite the diversity of families, and despite the different methods that are currently available for measuring it. Much work needs to be done, particularly with late-life families; we hope this chapter encourages clinicians to think carefully about how to create and adapt tools, and prompts researchers to begin the arduous but critical process of validating instruments specifically for this group.

APPENDIX A: FAMILY ASSESSMENT DEVICE

(RYAN et al., 2005)

INSTRUCTIONS:

This assessment contains a number of statements about families. Read each statement carefully, and decide how well it describes your family. You should answer according to how you see your family.

For each statement there are four (4) possible responses:

Strongly Agree (SA)	Check SA if you feel that the statement describes your family very accurately.
Agree (A)	Check A if you feel that the statement describes your family for the most part.
Disagree (D)	Check D if you feel that the statement does not describe your family for the most part.
Strongly Disagree (SD)	Check SD if you feel that the statement does not describe your family at all.

These four responses will appear below each statement like this:

41. We are not satisfied with anything short of perfection.

______SA	______A	______D	______SD	______

The answer spaces for statement 41 would look like this. For each statement, there is an answer space below. Do not pay attention to the blanks at the far right-hand side of each space. They are for office use only.

Try not to spend too much time thinking about each statement, but respond as quickly and as honestly as you can. If you have difficulty, answer with your first reaction. Please be sure to answer every statement and mark all your answers in the space provided below each statement.

1. Planning family activities is difficult because we misunderstand each other.
   ____SA ____A ____D ____SD ____
2. We resolve most everyday problems around the house.
   ____SA ____A ____D ____SD ____

3. When someone is upset the others know why.
____SA ____A ____D ____SD ____
4. When you ask someone to do something, you have to check that they did it.
____SA ____A ____D ____SD ____
5. If someone is in trouble, the others become too involved.
____SA ____A ____D ____SD ____
6. In times of crisis we can turn to each other for support.
____SA ____A ____D ____SD ____
7. We don't know what to do when an emergency comes up.
____SA ____A ____D ____SD ____
8. We sometimes run out of things that we need.
____SA ____A ____D ____SD ____
9. We are reluctant to show our affection for each other.
____SA ____A ____D ____SD ____
10. We make sure members meet their family responsibilities.
____SA ____A ____D ____SD ____
11. We cannot talk to each other about the sadness we feel.
____SA ____A ____D ____SD ____
12. We usually act on our decisions regarding problems.
____SA ____A ____D ____SD ____
13. You only get the interest of others when something is important to them.
____SA ____A ____D ____SD ____
14. You can't tell how a person is feeling from what they are saying.
____SA ____A ____D ____SD ____
15. Family tasks don't get spread around enough.
____SA ____A ____D ____SD ____
16. Individuals are accepted for what they are.
____SA ____A ____D ____SD ____
17. You can easily get away with breaking the rules.
____SA ____A ____D ____SD ____
18. People come right out and say things instead of hinting at them.
____SA ____A ____D ____SD ____
19. Some of us just don't respond emotionally.
____SA ____A ____D ____SD ____
20. We know what to do in an emergency.
____SA ____A ____D ____SD ____
21. We avoid discussing our fears and concerns.
____SA ____A ____D ____SD ____
22. It is difficult to talk to each other about tender feelings.
____SA ____A ____D ____SD ____
23. We have trouble meeting our bills.
____SA ____A ____D ____SD ____
24. After our family tries to solve a problem, we usually discuss whether it worked or not.
____SA ____A ____D ____SD ____
25. We are too self-centered.
____SA ____A ____D ____SD ____
26. We can express feelings to each other.
____SA ____A ____D ____SD ____
27. We have no clear expectations about toilet habits.
____SA ____A ____D ____SD ____
28. We do not show our love for each other.
____SA ____A ____D ____SD ____

29. We talk to people directly rather than through go-betweens.
____SA ____A ____D ____SD ____
30. Each of us has particular duties and responsibilities.
____SA ____A ____D ____SD ____
31. There are lots of bad feelings in the family.
____SA ____A ____D ____SD ____
32. We have rules about hitting people.
____SA ____A ____D ____SD ____
33. We get involved with each other only when something interest us.
____SA ____A ____D ____SD ____
34. There's little time to explore personal interests.
____SA ____A ____D ____SD ____
35. We often don't say what we mean.
____SA ____A ____D ____SD ____
36. We feel accepted for what we are.
____SA ____A ____D ____SD ____
37. We show interest in each other when we can get something out of it personally.
____SA ____A ____D ____SD ____
38. We resolve most emotional upsets that come up.
____SA ____A ____D ____SD ____
39. Tenderness takes second place to other things in our family.
____SA ____A ____D ____SD ____
40. We discuss who is to do household jobs.
____SA ____A ____D ____SD ____
41. Making decisions is a problem for our family.
____SA ____A ____D ____SD ____
42. Our family shows interest in each other only when they can get something out of it.
____SA ____A ____D ____SD ____
43. We are frank with each other.
____SA ____A ____D ____SD ____
44. We don't hold to any rules or standards.
____SA ____A ____D ____SD ____
45. If people are asked to do something, they need reminding.
____SA ____A ____D ____SD ____
46. We are able to make decisions about how to solve problems.
____SA ____A ____D ____SD ____
47. If the rules are broken, we don't know what to expect.
____SA ____A ____D ____SD ____
48. Anything goes in our family.
____SA ____A ____D ____SD ____
49. We express tenderness.
____SA ____A ____D ____SD ____
50. We confront problems involving feelings.
____SA ____A ____D ____SD ____
51. We don't get along well together.
____SA ____A ____D ____SD ____
52. We don't talk to each other when we are angry.
____SA ____A ____D ____SD ____
53. We are generally dissatisfied with the family duties assigned to us.
____SA ____A ____D ____SD ____
54. Even though we mean well, we intrude too much into each others' lives.
____SA ____A ____D ____SD ____

55. There are rules about dangerous situations.
____SA ____A ____D ____SD ____
56. We confide in each other.
____SA ____A ____D ____SD ____
57. We cry openly.
____SA ____A ____D ____SD ____
58. We don't have reasonable transport.
____SA ____A ____D ____SD ____
59. When we don't like what someone has done, we tell them.
____SA ____A ____D ____SD ____
60. We try to think of different ways to solve problems.
____SA ____A ____D ____SD ____

Note. See Ryan et al. (2005) for scoring instructions, a case study using the instrument, and norms from a variety of patient groups and cultures.

APPENDIX B: CHECKLIST OF FAMILY RELATIONAL ABILITIES

(WILKINS et al., 2009)

For each category below, mark the best description of the family you are working with. The term "family members" is used to include the patient as well as any other involved individual who has biological, legal or emotional ties to the patient.

Attachment Bonds

________ Strong, positive bonds of affection are apparent between all or nearly all family members.
________ Attachment bonds appear to be weak, ambivalent or "mixed" (i.e., both positive bonds and conflictual relationships in the family).
________ Intense conflict or "wounded" relationships are apparent between most or all family members.

Openness of Communication Regarding the Current Illness

________ Communication between all or nearly all family members is open and includes expression of emotional reactions to the illness.
________ Most family members discuss the illness openly but some individuals are excluded AND/OR family members avoid expression of emotional reactions.
________ Some family members discuss the facts of the illness but few family members are involved in the discussions AND/OR emotional reactions are not shared.
________ There is little if any discussion of the illness between family members.

Collaborative Decision-Making Regarding the Current Illness

________ Most or all family members participate in decision-making and most seem satisfied with decisions that are made.
________ Decisions are made by a minority of family members (e.g., the patient alone or one or two family members) but others accept or have grown to accept the decisions.
________ Decisions are made by a minority of family members, causing others to feel left out and unsatisfied with the decisions on an ongoing basis.
________ The family has great difficulty making decisions AND/OR there is serious, ongoing conflict about decisions that are made.

Overall Level of Family Relational Abilities
Circle the number below which best describes the overall capabilities and needs of the family:

4	**"Naturally Resilient"**: Predominately strong, positive bonds of attachment; clear and open communication; effective, collaborative decision-making (LITTLE IF ANY FAMILY INTERVENTION NEEDED).
3	**"Overwhelmed"**: Predominately strong relational abilities but temporarily stymied by intensity and/or complexity of the patient's situation (BRIEF FAMILY SUPPORT MAY HELP ENGAGE NATURAL ABILITIES).
2	**"Closed" or "Fixed"**: Significant difficulties with communication and/or decision-making (TARGETED INTERVENTION OR FAMILY CONSULTATION MAY HELP OPEN COMMUNICATION AND/OR FACILITATE DECISION-MAKING).
1	**"Wounded"**: Damaged bonds of attachment, intensely negative or conflictual communication and/or decision-making (FAMILY THERAPY INDICATED TO ADDRESS LONGSTANDING GRIEVANCES BETWEEN FAMILY MEMBERS).

REFERENCES

American Psychiatric Association. (2000). *Diagnostic and statistical manual of mental disorders-IV-TR*. Washington DC: Author.

American Psychological Association. (2002). Ethical principles of psychologists and code of conduct. *American Psychologist*, *57*, 1060–1073.

American Psychological Association. (2003). Guidelines for psychological practice with older adults. *American Psychologist*, *59*, 236–260.

Barnes, H., & Olson, D. H. (1989). Parent–adolescent communication scale. In D. H. Olson, H. I. McCubbin, H. Barnes, A. Larsen, M. Muxen, & M. Wilson (Eds.), *Family Inventories* (pp. 438–447). St. Paul, MN: Family Social Science, University of Minnesota.

Barresi, C. M., & Hunt, K. (1990). The unmarried elderly: Age, sex, and ethnicity. In T. H. Brubaker (Ed.), *Family relationships in later life* (2nd ed., pp. 169–192). Thousand Oaks, CA: Sage Publications Inc.

Beavers, W. R., & Hampson, R. B. (1990). *Successful families: Assessment and intervention*. New York, NY: W.W. Norton & Co.

Beavers, W. R., & Hampson, R. B. (2003). Measuring family competence: The Beavers Systems Model. In F. Walsh (Ed.), *Normal family processes* (3rd ed., pp. 549–580). New York, NY: The Guilford Press.

Bengtson, V. L., & Roberts, R. E. L. (1991). Intergenerational solidarity in aging families: An example of formal theory construction. *Journal of Marriage & the Family*, *53*, 856–870.

Bengtson, V. L., Rosenthal, C., & Burton, L. (1990). Families and aging: Diversity and heterogeneity. In R. H. Binstock, & L. K. George (Eds.), *Handbook of aging and the social sciences* (3rd ed., pp. 263–287). New York, NY: Academic Press.

Blieszner, R. (2009). Who are the aging families? In S. H. Qualls, & S. H. Zarit (Eds.), *Aging families and caregiving* (pp. 1–18). Hoboken, NJ: John Wiley & Sons Inc.

Bowen, M. (1978). *Family therapy in clinical practice*. New York, NY: Jason Aronson.

Brody, E. M. (1985). Parent care as a normative family stress. *The Gerontologist*, *25*, 19–29.

Burke, M. M., & Laramie, J. A. (2004). *Primary care of the older adult: a multidisciplinary approach* (2nd ed.). St. Louis, MO: Elsevier Mosby.

Carlson, E. (2009). 20th-Century U.S. generations. In *Population Bulletin 64, No. 1*. Washington DC: Population Reference Bureau.

Carpenter, B. D., & Mulligan, E. (2009). Family, know thyself: A workbook-based intergenerational intervention to improve parent care coordination. *Clinical Gerontologist*, *32*, 147–163.

Carpenter, B. D., Van Haitsma, K., Ruckdeschel, K., & Lawton, M. P. (2000). The psychosocial preferences of older adults: A pilot examination of content and structure. *The Gerontologist*, *40*, 335–348.

Carpenter, B. D., Lee, M., Ruckdeschel, K., Van Haitsma, K. S., & Feldman, P. H. (2006). Adult children as informants about parent's psychosocial preferences. *Family Relations*, *55*, 552–563.

Cicirelli, V. G. (1992). *Family caregiving: Autonomous and paternalistic decision-making*. Newbury Park, CA: Sage Publications, Inc.

Cohen, S., & Wills, T. A. (1985). Stress, social support, and the buffering hypothesis. *Psychological Bulletin*, *98*, 310–357.

Connidis, I. A. (2001). *Family ties and aging*. Thousand Oaks, CA: Sage Publications, Inc.

Connidis, I. A., & McMullin, J. A. (2002). Ambivalence, family ties, and doing sociology. *Journal of Marriage and Family*, *64*, 594–601.

Ebersole, P., Hess, P., Touhy, T., & Jett, K. (2005). *Gerontological nursing and healthy aging*. St. Louis, MO: Elsevier Mosby.

Epstein, N. B., Baldwin, L. M., & Bishop, D. S. (1983). The McMaster Family Assessment Device. *Journal of Marital & Family Therapy*, *9*, 171–180.

Feetham, S. (1991). Conceptual and methodological issues in research of families. In A. Whall, & J. Fawcett (Eds.), *Family theory development in nursing: State of the science and art* (pp. 55–68). Philadelphia, PA: F.A. Davis.

Fingerman, K. L. (2001). *Aging mothers and their adult daughters: A study in mixed emotions*. New York, NY: Springer Publishing Co.

Fingerman, K. L., & Bermann, E. (2000). Applications of family systems theory to the study of adulthood. *International Journal of Aging & Human Development*, *51*, 5–29.

Fingerman, K. L., Chen, P.-C., Hay, E., Cichy, K. E., & Lefkowitz, E. S. (2006). Ambivalent reactions in the parent and offspring relationship. *Journals of Gerontology: Series B: Psychological Sciences and Social Sciences*, *61B*, P152–P160.

Fingerman, K. L., Pitzer, L., Lefkowitz, E. S., Birditt, K. S., & Mroczek, D. (2008). Ambivalent relationship qualities between adults and their parents: Implications for the well-being of both parties. *Journals of Gerontology: Series B: Psychological Sciences and Social Sciences*, *63B*, P362–P371.

Florsheim, P., & Benjamin, L. S. (2001). The Structural Analysis of Social Behavior Observational Coding Scheme. In P. K. Kerig, & K. M. Lindahl (Eds.), *Family observational coding systems: Resources for systemic research* (pp. 127–150). Mahwah, NJ: Lawrence Erlbaum Associates Publishers.

Ganong, L., & Coleman, M. (2006). Obligations to stepparents acquired in later life: Relationship quality and acuity of needs. *Journals of Gerontology: Series B: Psychological Sciences and Social Sciences*, *61B*, S80–S88.

Gardner, W., Nutting, P. A., Kelleher, K. J., Werner, J. J., Farley, T., Stewart, L., et al. (2001). Does the Family APGAR effectively measure family functioning? *Journal of Family Practice*, *1*, 19–25.

Gironda, M., Lubben, J. E., & Atchison, K. A. (1999). Social networks of elders without children: Erratum. *Journal of Gerontological Social Work*, *31*, 197.

Glenn, N. D. (2004). Distinguishing age, period, and cohort effects. In J. T. Mortimer, & M. J. Shanahan (Eds.), *Handbook of the life course* (pp. 465–476). New York, NY: Springer.

Hamon, R. R., & Blieszner, R. (1990). Filial responsibility expectations among adult child–older parent pairs. *Journals of Gerontology*, *45*, P110–P112.

He, W., Sengupta, M., Velkoff, V. A., & DeBarros, K. A. (2005). 65+ in the United States: 2005. In *Current population reports* (*U.S. Census Bureau*) (pp. 23–209). Washington, DC: U.S. Government Printing Office.

Henry, N. J. M., Berg, C. A., Smith, T. W., & Florsheim, P. (2007). Positive and negative characteristics of marital interaction and their association with marital satisfaction in middle-aged and older couples. *Psychology and Aging*, *22*, 428–441.

House, J. S., Umberson, D., & Landis, K. R. (1988). Structures and processes of social support. *Annual Review of Sociology*, *14*, 293–318.

Jones, S., & Fox, S. (2009). *Generations online in 2009*. <http://www.pewinternet.org/Reports/2009/Generations-Online-in-2009.aspx> Accessed 05.22.09.

Knight, B., Robinson, G., Longmire, C., Chun, M., Nakao, K., & Kim, J. (2002). Cross cultural issues in caregiving for persons with dementia: Do familism values reduce burden and distress? *Ageing International*, *27*, 70–94.

Lowenstein, A. (2007). Solidarity-conflict and ambivalence: Testing two conceptual frameworks and their impact on quality of life for older family members. *Journals of Gerontology: Series B: Psychological Sciences and Social Sciences*, *62B*, S100–S107.

Luescher, K., & Pillemer, K. (1998). Intergenerational ambivalence: A new approach to the study of parent–child relations in later life. *Journal of Marriage & the Family*, *60*, 413–425.

Mack, K., Lee, T., & Friedland, R. (2001). *Family caregivers of older persons: Adult children*. Washington, DC: The Center on an Aging Society, Georgetown University.

McGoldrick, M., Gerson, R., & Petry, S. (2008). *Genograms: Assessment and intervention*. New York, NY: W.W. Norton & Company.

Miller, I. W., Ryan, C. E., Keitner, G. I., Bishop, D. S., & Epstein, N. B. (2000a). 'Factor analyses of the family assessment device,' by Ridenour, Daley, & Reich. *Family Process*, *39*, 141–144.

Miller, I. W., Ryan, C. E., Keitner, G. I., Bishop, D. S., & Epstein, N. B. (2000b). The McMaster Approach to Families: Theory, assessment, treatment and research. *Journal of Family Therapy*, *22*, 168–189.

Miller, I. W., Ryan, C. E., Keitner, G. I., Bishop, D. S., & Epstein, N. B. (2000c). Why fix what isn't broken? A rejoinder to Ridenour, Daley, & Reich. *Family Process*, *39*, 381–384.

Mitrani, V. B., Feaster, D. J., McCabe, B. E., Czaja, S. J., & Szapocznik, J. (2005). Adapting the Structural Family Systems Rating to assess the patterns of interaction in families of dementia caregivers. *The Gerontologist*, *45*, 445–455.

Mitrani, V. B., Lewis, J. E., Feaster, D. J., Czaja, S. J., Eisdorfer, C., Schulz, R., et al. (2006). The role of family functioning in the stress process of dementia caregivers: a structural family framework. *The Gerontologist*, *46*, 97–105.

Moos, R., & Moos, B. (1994). *Family Environment Scale Manual: Development, applications, research* (3rd ed.). Palo Alto, CA: Consulting Psychologist Press.

Munet-Vilaro, F., & Egan, M. (1990). Reliability issues of the Family Environment Scale for cross-cultural research. *Nursing Research*, *39*, 244–247.

National Alliance for Caregiving & AARP. (2004). *Caregiving in the U.S.* Author.

National Family Caregiving Alliance. (2000). *Caregiver survey – 2000*. Kensington, MD: Author.

National Institute of Health. (2001). *Protection of third party information in research: Recommendations of the National Institutes of Health to the Office for Human Research Protections*. <http://bioethics.od.nih.gov/nih_third_party_rec.html> Accessed 05.15.09.

Olson, D. H. (2000). Circumplex Model of marital and family systems. *Journal of Family Therapy*, *22*, 144–167.

Olson, D. H., & Wilson, M. (1986). Family satisfaction. In D. H. Olson, H. I. McCubbin, H. Barnes, A. Larsen, M. Muxen, & M. Wilson (Eds.), *Family Inventories* (pp. 25–31). St. Paul, MN: Family Social Science, University of Minnesota.

Olson, D. H., Gorall, D. M., & Tiesel, J. W. (2007). *FACES IV and the Circumplex Model: Validation study*. Minneapolis, MN: Life Innovations, Inc.

Piercy, K. W. (2000). When is it more than a job: Close relationships between home health aides and older clients. *Journal of Aging and Health*, *12*, 362–387.

Pillemer, K., & Suitor, J. J. (2002). Explaining mothers' ambivalence toward their adult children. *Journal of Marriage and Family*, *64*, 602–613.

Pillemer, K., Suitor, J. J., Mock, S. E., Sabir, M., Pardo, T. B., & Sechrist, J. (2007). Capturing the complexity of intergenerational relations: Exploring ambivalence within later-life families. *Journal of Social Issues*, *63*, 775–791.

Pinquart, M., & Sorensen, S. (2005). Ethnic differences in stressors, resources, and psychological outcomes of family caregiving: A meta-analysis. *The Gerontologist*, *45*, 90–106.

Pruchno, R. A., Blow, F. C., & Smyer, M. A. (1984). Life events and interdependent lives: Implications for research and intervention. *Human Development*, *27*, 31–41.

Qualls, S. H. (1999). Family therapy with older adult clients. *Journal of Clinical Psychology*, *55*, 977–990.

Qualls, S. H. (2000). Therapy with aging families: Rationale, opportunities and challenges. *Aging & Mental Health*, *4*, 191–199.

Qualls, S. H., & Segal, D. L. (2003). Assessment of older adults and their families. In K. Jordan (Ed.), *Handbook of couple and family assessment* (pp. 111–127). Hauppauge, NY: Nova Science Publishers.

Raudenbush, S. W., & Bryk, A. S. (2002). *Hierarchical linear models: Applications and data analysis methods*. Thousand Oaks, CA: Multi-Health Systems.

Ridenour, T. A., Daley, J. G., & Reich, W. (1999). Factor analyses of the Family Assessment Device. *Family Process*, *38*, 497–510.

Rossi, A. S., & Rossi, P. H. (1990). *Of human bonding: Parent–child relations across the life course*. Hawthorne, NY: Aldine de Gruyter.

Ryan, C. E., Epstein, N. B., Keitner, G. I., Miller, I. W., & Bishop, D. S. (2005). *Evaluating and treating families: The McMaster approach*. New York, NY: Routledge.

Savin-Williams, R. C., & Esterberg, K. G. (2000). Lesbian, gay, and bisexual families. In D. H. Demo, K. R. Allen, & M. A. Fine (Eds.), *Handbook of family diversity* (pp. 197–215). New York, NY: Oxford University Press.

Sawin, K. J., Harrigan, M. P., & Woog, P. (1995). *Measures of family functioning for research and practice*. New York, NY: Springer Publishing Co.

Skinner, H. A., Steinhauer, P. D., & Santa-Barbara, J. (1983). The Family Assessment Measure. *Canadian Journal of Community Mental Health*, *2*, 91–105.

Skinner, H. A., Steinhauer, P. D., & Santa-Barbara, J. (1995). *Family Assessment Measure, Version III (FAM-III)*. Toronto, ON: Multi-Health Systems.

Smilkstein, G. (1978). The Family APGAR: A proposal for a family function test and its use by physicians. *The Journal of Family Practice*, *6*, 1231–1239.

Smilkstein, G. (1993). Family APGAR analyzed. *Family Medicine,* 293–294.

Smilkstein, G., Ashworth, C., & Montano, D. (1982). Validity and reliability of the Family APGAR as a test of family function. *The Journal of Family Practice*, *15*, 303–311.

Steinhauer, P. D., Santa-Barbara, J., & Skinner, H. (1984). The process model of family functioning. *The Canadian Journal of Psychiatry/La Revue canadienne de psychiatrie*, *29*, 77–88.

Thomas, V., & Olson, D. H. (1993). Problem families and the Circumplex Model: Observational assessment using the Clinical Rating Scale (CRS). *Journal of Marital & Family Therapy*, *19*, 159–175.

Thompson, M. M., Zanna, M. P., & Griffin, D. W. (1995). Let's not be indifferent about (attitudinal) ambivalence. In R. E. Petty, & J. A. Krosnick (Eds.), *Attitude strength: Antecedents and consequences* (pp. 361–386). Hillsdale, NJ: Lawrence Erlbaum Associates Inc.

Uchino, B. N., Holt-Lunstad, J., Uno, D., & Flinders, J. B. (2001). Heterogeneity in the social networks of young and older adults: Prediction of mental health and cardiovascular reactivity during acute stress. *Journal of Behavioral Medicine*, *24*, 361–382.

Wagner, D. L. (1997). *Long-distance caregiving for older adults*. Washington, DC: National Council on the Aging.

Whitbeck, L. B., Hoyt, D. R., & Huck, S. M. (1994). Early family relationships, intergenerational solidarity, and support provided to parents by their adult children. *Journals of Gerontology*, *49*, S85–S94.

Wilkins, V. M., Quill, T. E., & King, D. A. (2009). Assessing families in palliative care: A pilot study of the checklist of family relational abilities. *Journal of Palliative Medicine*, *12*, 517–519.

Willson, A. E., Shuey, K. M., & Elder, G. H., Jr. (2003). Ambivalence in the relationship of adult children to aging parents and in-laws. *Journal of Marriage and Family*, *65*, 1055–1072.

Willson, A. E., Shuey, K. M., Elder, G. H., Jr., & Wickrama, K. A. S. (2006). Ambivalence in mother–adult child relations: a dyadic analysis. *Social Psychology Quarterly*, *69*, 235–252.

Wolf, D. A., & Longino, C. F., Jr. (2005). Our "Increasingly Mobile Society?" The curious persistence of a false belief. *The Gerontologist*, *45*, 5–11.

Wynne, L. C. (1984). The epigenesis of relational systems: A model for understanding family development. *Family Process*, *23*, 297–318.

PART

2

Behavioral Disorders

CHAPTER

Screening, Assessing and Intervening for Alcohol and Medication Misuse in Older Adults

12

Kristen Lawton Barry, Frederic C. Blow

University of Michigan Department of Psychiatry, and Department of Veterans Affairs National Serious Mental Illness Treatment Research and Evaluation Center (SMITREC), Ann Arbor, MI, USA

INTRODUCTION

The misuse and abuse of alcohol, medications, and illicit drugs in older adults present unique challenges in terms of recognition, interventions, and determining the most appropriate treatment options. Substance use problems in this age group are often not recognized and, if recognized at all, are generally undertreated. Additionally, there are concerns in the field that the standard diagnostic criteria for abuse/dependence are difficult to apply to older adults, leading to underidentification. Substance misuse/abuse, in particular among elders, is an increasing problem. Older adults with these problems are a special and vulnerable population.

From the standpoint of recognition, older adults are more likely than younger adults to seek services from their primary and specialty care providers, which opens the door to greater recognition and treatment for those who drink/use drugs at hazardous levels. Health care providers who work with geriatric patients have a unique opportunity to observe and treat the repercussions of alcohol, drug, and medication misuse problems.

Therefore, the purpose of this chapter is to describe the state-of-the-art in terms of: (1) definitions of substance use risk (alcohol, drugs, medications); (2) pertinent screening instruments and techniques; (3) elements of assessments for older adults; (4) screening and assessment for physical, mental, and functional health; and (5) use of brief interventions, brief treatments, and formal specialized treatments.

PREVALENCE OF ALCOHOL AND DRUG USE/MISUSE/ABUSE

Alcohol

Over a number of years, community surveys have estimated the prevalence of problem drinking among older adults to range from 1 to 16% (Adams, Barry, & Fleming, 1996; Barry, 1997; Fleming, Manwell, Barry, Adams, & Stauffacher, 1999; Menninger, 2002; Moore et al., 1999; Office of Applied Studies, 2004, 2007). These rates vary widely depending on the definitions of older adults, at-risk and problem drinking, alcohol abuse/dependence, and the methodology used in obtaining samples. The National Survey on Drug Use and Health (2002–2003) found that, for individuals age 50+, 12.2% were heavy drinkers, 3.2% were binge drinkers, and 1.8% used illicit drugs (Huang et al., 2006; Office of Applied Studies, 2007). The 2005–2006 National Survey on Drug Use and Health showed a significant level of

Handbook of Assessment in Clinical Gerontology. DOI: 10.1016/B978-0-12-374961-1.10012-0

binge drinking among those age 50 to 64 (Blazer & Wu, 2009). They also found that 19% of the men and 13% of the women had two or more drinks a day, considered heavy or "at-risk" drinking. The survey also found binge drinking in those over 65, with 14% of men and 3% of women engaging in binge drinking.

Estimates of alcohol problems are much higher among health care-seeking populations, because problem drinkers are more likely to seek medical care (Oslin, 2004). Early studies in primary care settings found 10–15% of older patients met criteria for at-risk or problem drinking (Barry, CSAT, 1999; Callahan & Tierney, 1995). In a large primary care study of 5065 patients over 60, Adams, Barry, and Fleming (1996) found that 15% of the men and 12% of the women sampled regularly drank in excess of National Institute of Alcoholism and Alcohol Abuse limits, >7 drinks/week for women and >14 drinks/week for men; the guidelines recommend no more than one drink a day for both men and women over 65 [National Institute of Alcholism and Alcohol Abuse (NIAAA), 1995a,b].

These guidelines are consistent with some empirical evidence for risk-free drinking among older adults (Chermack, Blow, Hill, & Mudd, 1996). Clinicians who are finding fewer cases of problem drinkers and alcohol or drug disorders in their own practices may want to begin screening programs. Because patients with a previous history of problems with alcohol or other drugs are at risk for relapse, establishing a history of use can provide important clues for future problems. The health costs of untreated alcohol problems have been well described but may be even greater among the elderly, who are already at increased risk for many health problems.

In terms of meeting criteria for abuse/dependence, two studies in nursing homes reported that 29–49% of residents had a lifetime diagnosis of alcohol abuse or dependence, with 10–18% reporting active dependence symptoms in the past year (Joseph, Atkinson, & Ganzini, 1995; Oslin, Streim, Parmelee, Boyce, & Katz, 1997). In 2002, over 616,000 adults age 55 and older reported alcohol dependence in the past year (DSM-IV definition): 1.8% of those age 55–59; 1.5% of those age 60–64; and 0.5% of those age 65 or older (Office of Applied Studies, 2002). Although alcohol and drug/medication dependence are less common in older adults when compared to younger adults, the mental and physical health consequences are serious.

Medication Misuse

Misuse of medications by older adults is perhaps a more challenging issue to identify. Despite high rates of medication use among older adults, few studies have specifically examined the prevalence and nature of medication misuse and abuse in this population. The existing literature on this topic, while scant, indicates that medication misuse affects a small but significant minority of the elderly population. Older adults are at higher risk for inappropriate use of medications than younger groups. Adults aged 65 years and older comprise about 13% of the population, but account for 36% of all prescription medication in the United States (Cook, 1999). Older adults use more prescriptions and over-the-counter medications than other age groups and studies show that about a quarter of older adults use psychotherapeutic drugs, with 27% of all tranquilizer prescriptions and 38% of sedative hypnotics written for older adults. A relatively recent study found that 25% of older adults use prescription psychoactive medications that have abuse potential (Simoni-Wastila & Yang, 2006). There over 2 million serious adverse drug reactions yearly with 100,000 deaths per year. Adverse drug reactions are especially prominent among nursing home patients with 350,000 events each year (Gurwitz et al., 2000; Lazarou, Pomeranz, & Corey, 1998). A survey of social services agencies indicated that medication misuse affects 18–41% of the older clients served, depending on the agency (Schonfeld et al., 2009; Schonfeld, Rohrer, Zima, & Spiegel, 1994).

In addition, prescription drug abuse has been the second most common type of substance abuse among older adults for a number of years (after alcohol abuse) (Finlayson & Davis, 1994; Holroyd & Duryee, 1997). Three percent of VA geropsychiatric inpatients were diagnosed with dependence or abuse disorders involving prescription drugs (Edgell, Kunik, Molinari, Hale, & Orengo, 2000); 5% of a community-based, high-risk elderly population were referred for prescription drug abuse (Jinks & Raschko, 1990); and 11% of patients at an outpatient geriatric psychiatry clinic were diagnosed with benzodiazepine dependence (Holroyd & Duryee, 1997). By 2020, the non-medical use of psychotherapeutic drugs among older adults is projected to increase from 1.2% (911,000) to 2.4% (2.7 million) (Colliver, Compton, Gfroerer, & Condon, 2006).

Several aspects of prescription misuse and abuse among the elderly differ both quantitatively and qualitatively from those found in younger populations. Misuse and abuse of prescription drugs by older adults is not typically done to "get high" (Blow, Bartels, Brockmann, & van Citters, 2006). Problematic use by older adults is usually unintentional (Simoni-Wastila & Yang, 2006), and most abused medications are obtained legally (Blow et al., 2006).

Correlates of Prescription Drug Abuse in Older Adults

There are a number of correlates that have been linked to prescription drug misuse/abuse. Female gender (Finlayson & Davis, 1994; Jinks & Raschko, 1990; Simoni-Wastila & Yang, 2006), social isolation (Jinks & Raschko, 1990; Simoni-Wastila & Yang, 2006), and a history of substance abuse or another mental health disorder (Jinks & Raschko, 1990; Simoni-Wastila & Strickler, 2004; Simoni-Wastila & Yang, 2006; Solomon, Manepalli, Ireland, & Mahon, 1993) are all associated with increased risk of problems related to medications. One study indicates that older adults with prescription drug dependence are even more likely than their younger counterparts to have a dual diagnosis (Solomon et al., 1993).

Prolonged use of psychotropic medications, especially benzodiazepines, has been associated with depression and cognitive decline (Dealberto, McAvay, Seeman, & Berkman, 1997; Hanlon et al., 1998; Hogan, Maxwell, Fung, & Ebly, 2003). Benzodiazepine use is also positively correlated with confusion, falls, and hip fractures in the elderly (Leipzig, Cumming, & Tinetti, 1999). Further, the use of opiate analgesics can lead to increased sedation and impairment in vision, attention, and coordination among older patients (Ray, Thapa, & Shorr, 1993; Solomon et al., 1993).

In addition to the concerns regarding the misuse of medications alone, combined alcohol and medication misuse has been estimated to affect up to 19% of older Americans (National Institute on Alcohol Abuse and Alcoholism, 1998). Substance abuse problems among elderly individuals often occur from misuse of over-the-counter and prescription drugs. Drug misuse can result from the overuse, underuse or irregular uses of either prescription or over-the-counter drugs. Misuse can relatively easily become abuse (Patterson & Jeste, 1999; Schonfeld et al., 2009).

Illicit Drugs

The use of illicit drugs is relatively rare in the current cohort of older adults. The National Survey on Drug Use and Health (2002–2003) found that, for individuals age 50+, 1.8% used illicit drugs (Huang et al., 2006; Office of Applied Studies, 2007). However, research suggests that the number of illicit drug users (and those with problems related to alcohol) in older adulthood is likely to increase due to the aging of the "baby boom" generation. Blow, Barry, Fuller, & Booth (2002) analyzed the National Health and Nutrition Examination Survey (NHANES) data which suggested that the Baby Boom cohort, as it continues to age, could maintain a higher level of alcohol consumption than in previous older adult cohorts. Consequently, a larger percentage of future older adults may have alcohol use patterns that place their health at risk.

MENTAL AND PHYSICAL HEALTH RISKS ASSOCIATED WITH USE/MISUSE/ABUSE

Drinking at hazardous levels increases the risk of hypertension (Chermack et al., 1996; National Institute of Alcholism and Alcohol Abuse, 1995) and may increase the risk of breast cancer (Baker, 1985; Rosin & Glatt, 1971) and diabetes (Vestal et al., 1977), among other medical conditions in this population. Hazardous drinking can significantly affect a number of other conditions in this age group (Fleming & Barry, 1992) including mood disorders and sleep, as well as general health functioning (Blow et al., 2000). Depression has been linked to relapse in drinking and increased alcohol intake. Blow et al. (2000) found a main effect of drinking status on general health, physical functioning, physical role functioning, pain, vitality, mental health, emotional role and social functioning, controlling for race and gender, with low-risk drinkers scoring better than abstainers and better than hazardous drinkers.

Symptoms of harmful drinking are often less visible among older adults because they may be masked by social, medical, or psychological conditions. Tolerance of ethanol can be reduced by the physiological aging processes (Rosin & Glatt, 1971) and by health conditions common to old age (Baker, 1985). Comparable amounts of alcohol produce higher blood alcohol levels in older adults than in younger persons, and may exacerbate other health problems (Vestal et al., 1977). Drinking produces higher blood alcohol levels in older adults than in younger persons when comparable amounts of alcohol are drunk, and many problems common among older people, such as chronic illness, poor nutrition, and polypharmacy, may be exacerbated by even small amounts of alcohol (Rosin & Glatt, 1971; Vestal et al., 1977).

What might be considered light or moderate drinking for individuals in their thirties may have multiple negative health effects in an older person. Therefore, clinicians who treat older patients need to assess alcohol use levels and be aware of health implications of their patients' alcohol use.

Practitioners from a variety of disciplines, including those who provide home health care and extended care, as well as those who manage community-based social programs for the elderly, can play a crucial role in detecting and treating alcohol problems in this age group. One of the challenges to all clinicians who work with older adults is meeting these goals within the context of a managed care environment, where providers are expected to deliver quality medical and mental health care across a wide variety of problems with greater time constraints. As more physical and mental health care is delivered within managed health care, the costs of treatment and the effectiveness of interventions for alcohol problems will benefit from new innovative technologies and techniques which require less provider intervention time and are more targeted to each patient's particular set of symptoms and health patterns. Fleming et al. (1999) conducted a brief intervention trial to reduce hazardous drinking with older adults using brief advice in primary care settings. This study showed that older adults can be engaged in brief intervention protocols, the protocols are acceptable in this population, and there is a substantial reduction in drinking among the at-risk drinkers receiving the interventions. One procedure found to identify large numbers of heavy drinkers who are likely to be motivated to change is routine health and lifestyle screening in medical settings (Adams et al., 1996; Skinner, Holt, & Israel, 1981).

DEFINITIONS OF SUBSTANCE USE RISK IN OLDER ADULTHOOD

The terms presented in this chapter are derived from both the clinical and research expertise of professionals in the field of addictions. The term *alcohol use disorders* includes the clinical problems of alcohol abuse and dependence. However, many older adults have alcohol problems without meeting any standardized criteria for abuse and/or dependence. In order to address the range of alcohol problems in older adults screening and assessment procedures need to focus on a range of drinking levels. Decisions regarding interventions and treatment may need to be made partly based on level of alcohol/medication use and misuse, and partly based on problems manifested regardless of amount used.

To diagnose alcohol use disorders clinicians look for behavioral factors such as the inability to cut down or stop, social and emotional consequences such as family problems, and physiological symptoms such as insomnia, gastrointestinal pain, liver toxicity, tolerance (over time it takes more of the substance to feel an effect), and withdrawal. A limitation for the alcohol field, particularly in medical settings, is the lack of laboratory tests to make a definitive diagnosis of alcohol abuse or dependence. Liver function and other laboratory tests detect end organ damage but do not detect the primary disorder. Only about 20% of people with alcohol abuse or dependence have elevated serum gamma-glutamyl transferase (GGT; Babor, De La Fuente, Saunders, & Grant, 1989). Research has indicated a positive relationship between level of drinking (consumption) and severity of alcohol-related problems. This relationship is often true for younger adults but is not as applicable for all older adults with alcohol-related problems. In older adults, problems with alcohol can occur with relatively low levels of use. Screening and intervention efforts should include both an evaluation of medical and psychosocial problems that can be related to alcohol and a determination of consumption levels.

Because of the potential for interactions between alcohol and medications in this age group, the definitions of low-risk, at-risk, problem use, and abuse/dependence should always include an evaluation of medication use (prescription and over-the-counter) along with the use of alcohol. Additionally, it is important to understand the broad range of problematic use of prescription medications that can be found in this population. Culberson and Ziska (2008) provided a breakdown of the various types of medication misuse and abuse that can occur among older adults. Discussion of those definitions are included in the risk categories below.

Low-Risk Use

Alcohol use that does not lead to problems is called *low-risk use* (see Case Study 1). Persons in this category can set reasonable limits on alcohol consumption and do not drink when driving a car or boat, operating machinery, or using contraindicated medications. They also do not engage in binge drinking (National Institute of Alcholism and Alcohol Abuse, 1995). In this age group, low-risk use of medications could include using an anti-anxiety medication for an acute anxiety state following the physician's prescription with no use of alcohol, or drinking one drink three times/week without the use of any contraindicated medications.

Case Study 1

Marie Howell is a 67-year-old retired teacher who drinks one glass of wine when out to dinner with friends once or twice a week. She has a relatively large social network, walks in the mall with a friend three times/week for exercise, and is active in volunteer work in a literacy program. She has no family history of alcoholism and does not take contraindicated medications. She receives routine health care from a primary care physician and attends a senior center where she has contact with other health care personnel including a social worker and a nurse. Ms Howell would benefit from prevention messages regarding her alcohol use in the context of her overall health and well being. "*I know that one of your goals is to prevent health problems. Your exercise program looks good. You continue to be active with friends and in the community. You have no family history of alcohol problems, are taking no medication to interfere with alcohol, and don't exceed a glass of wine once or twice a week. These are all good things that you have been doing to stay as healthy as you can.*"

At-Risk Use

At-risk use is use that increases the chances that a person will develop problems and complications related to the use of alcohol. These individuals consume more than 7 drinks/week, or drink in risky situations (see Case Study 2). They do not currently have health problems caused by alcohol but if this drinking pattern continues, problems may result.

There are two types of medication misuse that may fit into at-risk use or problem use (below) depending on severity. The types are "misuse by the patient" and "misuse by the practitioner." Misuse by the patient includes: taking more or less medication than prescribed; hoarding or skipping doses of a medication; use of medication for purposes other than those prescribed; and use of the medication in conjunction with alcohol or other contraindicated medications. Misuse by the practitioner includes: prescribing medication for an inappropriate indication; prescribing a dosage that is unnecessarily high; or failure to monitor or fully explain the appropriate use of a medication (Culberson & Ziska, 2008).

Case Study 2

Jack Hendrick is a 64-year-old executive with a large marketing firm. He is a hard-driving person who works long hours and has few hobbies and interests outside of work. Although the company has a policy that employees retire at 65, he has not planned what he will do. He is slightly overweight, does not exercise except for occasionally playing golf, and drinks two drinks/day during the week and three to four drinks/day on the weekends. He has no diagnosed health problems related to alcohol use but his wife worries about his drinking and would like him to spend more time in activities with her that do not involve alcohol. He has gone to a psychologist at his wife's urging. The message from his psychologist would include a statement regarding his use of alcohol and concern about potential problems. "*You indicated that, on average, you drink alcohol every day and drink two drinks at a time during the week and drink more than that on the weekends. You and I have talked about your stresses at work, your wife's concerns about your use of alcohol and your own worries about retirement. National guidelines recommend that men your age drink no more than (seven drinks/week: no more than one/day). I am concerned that your pattern of alcohol use fits into the at-risk drinking category.*"

Problem Use

Problem use refers to a level of use that has already resulted in adverse medical, psychological, or social consequences as in Case Study 3. Although most problem drinkers consume more than the low-risk limits, some older adults who drink smaller amounts may experience alcohol-related problems. As mentioned above, medication misuse can also fit into the problem use category. Assessment to determine severity is needed.

Case Study 3

Catherine Jones is a 70-year-old widow living alone in a small apartment in a large city. She has developed few interests and outside activities since her husband died four years ago. In a routine visit to her primary care clinic, the nurse practitioner asked some questions about her general health and Mrs Jones reported that she was tired all the time and, because she did not sleep well, she was using over-the-counter sleeping pills. When asked, she said that she generally drinks one glass of wine a day before dinner just as she and her husband did when they were younger. She had been taking prescription medicine for stomach pain for six months but the pain has not improved. The effect of alcohol is exacerbated by age, by the use of some medications for stomach pain like Zantac, and by over-the-counter sleeping pills. Her nurse practitioner discussed with her the potential problems of mixing some medications with alcohol, provided information about the senior center in her neighborhood and the name of a contact person at the center, and suggested she try the center for some activities and that she stop the use of alcohol since it could be starting to cause problems that would get worse with time."*I am concerned about your use of alcohol with the medications for your stomach and the sleeping pills. The stomach medicine you take and the sleeping pills can increase the effect of the alcohol. I'm also concerned that you may not have a lot of options to see other people and that can be pretty lonely. I'm giving you the number for the senior center in your neighborhood and the name of the person to call at the center. In the next month, I'd like you to stop the use of alcohol and the sleeping pills to see how you feel, and I'd like you to try out the senior center. I'll see you in one month so we can determine together how things are going.*" Mrs Jones felt that she would be able to follow these recommendations. The nurse practitioner made an appointment with her in one month to check on progress.

Alcohol and Other Drug Dependence

Those who use at the level of *alcohol dependence* have a medical disorder characterized by loss of control, are preoccupied with alcohol, continue to use despite adverse consequences, and suffer physiological symptoms such as tolerance and withdrawal as in Case Study 4 (American Psychiatric Association, 1994). A wide range of legal and illegal substances can be addictive.

Medication abuse involves medication use that results in diminished physical or social functioning; medication use in risky situations; and continued medication use despite adverse social or personal consequences (Culberson & Ziska, 2008). Dependence includes medication use that results in tolerance or withdrawal symptoms; unsuccessful attempts to stop or control medication use; and preoccupation with attaining or using a medication.

Case Study 4

Joe Thompson is a 68-year-old retired electrician. He has had chronic abdominal pain and unresolved hypertension for the past ten years. He has a history of alcohol problems and had one admission to alcohol treatment 15 years ago. Four years ago, after experiencing withdrawal symptoms during a hospital admission for a work-related injury, he again entered an alcohol treatment program. After two years of abstinence, Mr. Jackson began drinking again. He now drinks approximately five beers a day plus some additional liquor once a week. His physician and social worker in the primary care clinic are aware that this is a chronic relapsing disorder and continue to work with Mr Jackson to help him stabilize his medical conditions and find longer-term help for his primary alcohol dependence. "*Mr Jackson, your high blood pressure and your stomach pains have not improved. The amount you are drinking can certainly interfere with them getting better and can make other physical and family problems worse. I know you've tried hard to deal with your alcohol problems and you kept those problems in check for a long time, but now they are getting in the way of your health and well-being again. I know it takes a lot to stay sober and that relapses can occur when stresses increase. I'm worried about your health and would like you to talk to someone from the alcohol program. Would you be willing to talk with them if we call and make the appointment together?*"

SCREENING: ASKING THE FIRST QUESTIONS

To be able to practice prevention and early intervention with older adults, clinicians need to screen for alcohol and alcohol/medication interaction problems. Screening can be done as part of a routine mental and physical health care and updated annually, before the older adult begins taking any new medications, or in response to problems that may be alcohol or medication related.

Alcohol

The common signs and symptoms of alcohol problems in older adults are listed in Table 12.1. However, because of the relationship between alcohol consumption and health problems, questions about consumption (quantity and frequency of use) provide a method to categorize patients into

Table 12.1 Signs and Symptoms of Alcohol and Medication Problems in Older Adults

Alcohol	
anxiety	increased tolerance to alcohol
blackouts, dizziness	legal difficulties
depression	memory loss
disorientation	new difficulties in decision making
excessive mood swings	poor hygiene
falls, bruises, burns	poor nutrition
family problems	seizures, idiopathic
financial problems	sleep problems
headaches	social isolation
incontinence	unusual response to medications

Medications
excessive worry about whether psychoactive medications are working
extensive knowledge of and preference for a specific psychoactive medication
excessive anxiety about the supply and timing of a medication
continued use of a medication or refill requests after the indicated medical condition has been resolved
complaints about physicians who refuse to prescribe a preferred medication or do not take symptoms seriously
excessive sleeping
changes in personal grooming or hygiene
withdrawal from family, friends, and social activities

(Adapted from Fleming & Barry, 1992)
(Adapted from Blow & Barry 2001)

levels of risk for alcohol use. The traditional assumption that all patients who drink have a tendency to underreport their alcohol use is not supported by research (Babor et al., 1989). People who are not alcohol dependent often give accurate answers.

Clinicians can get more accurate histories by asking questions about the recent past; embedding the alcohol use questions in the context of other health behaviors (i.e., exercise, weight, smoking, alcohol use); and paying attention to non-verbal cues that suggest the patient is minimizing use (i.e., blushing, turning away, fidgeting, looking at the floor, change in breathing pattern).

Screening questions can be asked by verbal interview, by paper-and-pencil questionnaire, or by computerized questionnaire. All three methods have equivalent reliability and validity (Barry & Fleming, 1990; Greist et al., 1987). Any positive responses can lead to further questions about consequences. *To successfully incorporate alcohol (and other drug) screening into clinical practice, it should be simple and consistent with other screening procedures already in place.*

Before asking any screening questions the following conditions are needed: (1) the interviewer needs to be friendly and non-threatening; (2) the purpose of the questions should be clearly related to their health status; (3) the patient should be alcohol free at the time of the screening; (4) the information should be confidential; and (5) the questions should be easy to understand. Screening questions can be used with the older adult who may have alcohol-related problems as well as to guide an interview with a concerned friend, spouse, or family member. In some settings (such as waiting rooms), screening instruments are given as self-report questionnaires, with instructions for the patient to discuss the meaning of the results with their health care provider.

In addition to these general considerations, the following interviewing techniques can be used. Try to interview patients under the best possible circumstances. For patients requiring emergency treatment or who are severely impaired, it is best to wait until their condition has stabilized and they have become accustomed to the health setting where the interview is to take place. Look for signs of alcohol or drug intoxication. Patients who have alcohol on their breath or who appear intoxicated give unreliable responses. Consider conducting the interview at a later time. If this is not possible, make note of these findings on the patient's record.

If the alcohol questions are embedded in a longer health interview, a transitional statement is needed to move into the alcohol-related questions. The best way to introduce alcohol questions is to give the patient a general idea of the content of the questions, their purpose, and the need for accurate answers. The following is an illustrative introduction: *"Now I am going to ask you some questions about your use of alcoholic beverages during the past year. Because alcohol use can affect many areas of health (and may interfere with certain medications), it is important to know how much you usually drink and whether you have experienced any problems with your drinking. Please try to be as accurate as you can be"* (Center for Substance Abuse Treatment, 1998). This statement should be followed by a description of the types of alcoholic beverages typically consumed (e.g., *"By alcoholic beverages we mean your use of wine, beer, vodka, sherry, and so on"*). If necessary, include a description of beverages that may not be considered alcoholic (e.g., cider, low alcohol beer). Determinations of consumption are based on "standard drinks." A standard drink is a 12 ounce bottle of beer, a 4 ounce glass of wine, or $1\frac{1}{2}$ ounces (a shot) of liquor (e.g., vodka, gin, whiskey).

When using standardized alcohol screening questionnaires in an interview format, it is important to read the questions as written and in the order indicated. By following the exact wording, better comparability will be obtained between your results and those obtained by other interviewers. This section of the chapter will focus on four widely used screening instruments: the Michigan Alcoholism Screening Test-Geriatric version (MAST-G); its shortened version the SMAST-G; the CAGE; and the Alcohol Use Disorders Identification Test (AUDIT).

The *Michigan Alcoholism Screening Instrument-Geriatric Version (MAST-G)* (see Figure 12.1) was developed at the University of Michigan (Blow et al., 1992a) as an elderly alcoholism screening instrument for use in a variety of settings. Psychometric properties of this instrument are superior to other screening tests for the identification of elderly persons with alcohol abuse/dependence. The MAST-G was the first major elderly-specific alcoholism screening measure to be developed with items unique to older problem drinkers. The MAST-G was developed in two phases: the pilot testing/development phase and the validation phase. From various resources, a total of 94 items were developed and refined for the MAST-G. The initial items were pilot tested for wording and understandability using 125 adults over age 55 who were recruited from various community and clinical care locations. In addition to the MAST-G items, demographic data, several health questions, the CAGE, and the MAST were administered to all study participants so that comparisons could be made to these instruments.

After pilot testing the original items, they were then administered to 840 individuals over age 55 (average age was 65.9 years; SD = 7.5; range = 55–91). Item reduction was accomplished by item analyses and by a factor analysis of items. Similar items tapping underlying dimensions from the factor analyses, and those items with very low or very high positive response rates, were removed. These procedures resulted in 32 items being retained for final validation.

During the validation phase of the study, the reduced 32-item instrument was refined using a stratified sample of 290 aged subjects (the mean age was 66.1 years; SD = 7.3) that included five groups: (1) those currently meeting criteria for alcohol dependence, but not in treatment; (2) those currently in treatment for alcoholism; (3) those with a previous history of alcoholism and currently in recovery; (4) social drinkers; and (5) abstainers. The sample was stratified by these groups to ensure

	Yes	No
1. After drinking have you ever noticed an increase in your heart rate or beating in your chest?	____	____
2. When talking with others, do you ever underestimate how much you actually drink?	____	____
3. Does alcohol make you sleepy so that you often fall asleep in your chair?	____	____
4. After a few drinks, have you sometimes not eaten or been able to skip a meal because you didn't feel hungry?	____	____
5. Does having a few drinks help decrease your shakiness or tremors?	____	____
6. Does alcohol sometimes make it hard for you to remember parts of the day or night?	____	____
7. Do you have rules for yourself that you won't drink before a certain time of the day?	____	____
8. Have you lost interest in hobbies or activities you used to enjoy?	____	____
9. When you wake up in the morning, do you ever have trouble remembering part of the night before?	____	____
10. Does having a drink help you sleep?	____	____
11. Do you hide your alcohol bottles from family members?	____	____
12. After a social gathering, have you ever felt embarrassed because you drank too much?	____	____
13. Have you ever been concerned that drinking might be harmful to your health?	____	____
14. Do you like to end an evening with a nightcap?	____	____
15. Did you find your drinking increased after someone close to you died?	____	____
16. In general, would you prefer to have a few drinks at home rather than go out to social events?	____	____
17. Are you drinking more now than in the past?	____	____
18. Do you usually take a drink to relax or calm your nerves?	____	____
19. Do you drink to take your mind off your problems?	____	____
20. Have you ever increased your drinking after experiencing a loss in your life?	____	____
21. Do you sometimes drive when you have had too much to drink?	____	____
22. Has a doctor or nurse ever said they were worried or concerned about your drinking?	____	____
23. Have you ever made rules to manage your drinking?	____	____
24. When you feel lonely does having a drink help?	____	____

FIGURE 12.1

Michigan Alcoholism Screening Test-Geriatric Version (MAST-G).

that there was adequate representation of the variety of older drinking behavior for maximum generalizability of the MAST-G. In addition to the MAST-G, the CAGE Questions and the MAST, all subjects in the validation phase were interviewed using the Substance Abuse Module of the Diagnostic Interview Schedule (DIS) to allow us to make alcohol dependence diagnoses. The diagnosis of alcohol dependence (DSM-III-R) was used as the validation standard. This process yielded a final MAST-G version of 24 items.

The MAST-G has a sensitivity of 94.9%, specificity of 77.8%, positive predictive value of 89.4%, and negative predictive value of 88.6%. Similar values were found after excluding those subjects who did not currently drink. Therefore, when considering only those who had an opportunity to meet criteria for a current diagnosis, the psychometric properties were stable.

High internal consistency as measured by Cronbach's coefficient alpha (0.92) for the total MAST-G was shown. Item-total correlations ranged from 0.30 to 0.69. Only four items had item-total correlations below 0.40. In addition, factor analysis identified five underlying symptom domains: Loss and Loneliness; Relaxation; Dependence; Loss of Control with Drinking; and Rule-Making. These five factors have reliability coefficients of 0.89, 0.83, 0.81, 0.64, and 0.77, respectively. Most of the inconsistency within the fourth factor is due to the men (0.60).

The *Short Michigan Alcoholism Screening Test-Geriatric version* (*SMAST-G*) (see Figure 12.2) is the short form of the MAST-G and was developed for use in busy clinical settings and in research settings where brevity is an issue (Blow, Gillespie, Barry, Mudd, & Hill, 1998). Major barriers to using the longer scale in busy clinical settings are length and administration time. To address these issues, a short version of the MAST-G was developed. The 10 items on the short version of the MAST-G (SMAST-G) were selected by factor analysis. The initial sensitivity and specificity of the SMAST-G were tested in a sample of 50 older adult subjects (age range 55–81). The testing criteria were DSM-III-R diagnoses of alcohol abuse and/or dependence as measured by the Diagnostic Interview Schedule-Revised. Twenty-six percent of the sample were diagnosed with alcohol abuse and/or dependence. Based on an ROC analysis, an SMAST-G cutpoint between 3 and 4 yielded a sensitivity of 0.85 and specificity of 0.97. The SMAST-G fared as well as the AUDIT, and may be more acceptable to elderly individuals. In this sample, SMAST-G is also an acceptable alternative to the MAST-G for elderly-specific brief alcohol screening and is superior to other screening instruments developed in younger populations. A score of two or more (e.g., two "yes" responses) indicates probable alcohol problems. The SMAST-G questions ask about participants' experiences within the last year.

	YES (1)	NO (0)
1. When talking with others, do you ever underestimate how much you actually drink?	____	____
2. After a few drinks, have you sometimes not eaten or been able to skip a meal because you didn't feel hungry?	____	____
3. Does having a few drinks help decrease your shakiness or tremors?	____	____
4. Does alcohol sometimes make it hard for you to remember parts of the day or night?	____	____
5. Do you usually take a drink to relax or calm your nerves?	____	____
6. Do you drink to take your mind off your problems?	____	____
7. Have you ever increased your drinking after experiencing a loss in your life?	____	____
8. Has a doctor or nurse ever said they were worried or concerned about your drinking?	____	____
9. Have you ever made rules to manage your drinking?	____	____
10. When you feel lonely, does having a drink help?	____	____

TOTAL S-MAST-G SCORE (0–10) ____

FIGURE 12.2

Short Michigan Alcoholism Screening Test–Geriatric Version.

The *CAGE* (Mayfield, McLeod, & Hall, 1974) is the most widely used alcohol problem screening test in clinical practice. It contains four items regarding alcohol use: wanting to *C*ut down; feeling *A*nnoyed that people criticized one's drinking; feeling *G*uilty about others criticizing drinking; and having a drink upon waking in the morning to get rid of a hangover—an *E*ye-opener. Two positive responses are considered a positive screen and indicate that further assessment is warranted. The sensitivity and specificity of the CAGE varies from 60 to 90% and from 40 to 90%, respectively (Ewing, 1984; Mayfield et al., 1974). CAGE alcohol items can be asked alone, but are sometimes embedded along with CAGE-like items about exercise, smoking, and weight (Fleming & Barry, 1991). For example, participants were asked consecutively if in the last year they felt guilty about their: smoking, lack of exercise, weight, or alcohol use. The instrument most widely promoted as the standard screening test for clinical practice is the CAGE (Bush, Shaw, Cleary, Delbanco, & Aronson, 1987; Ewing, 1984; King, 1986). Like most of the screening instruments reviewed, the sensitivity and specificity of the CAGE varies from 60 to 95% and 40 to 95%, respectively (Beresford, Blow, Singer, Hill, & Lucey, 1990; Bush et al., 1987). The variability of these reports may be related to: (1) different criterion; (2) assessment of lifetime use as compared to current use; (3) varying the cutoff score from 1 to 4 positive responses; and (4) differences in population samples. Major deficiencies of this test include its inability to assess current problems, levels of consumption, or binge drinking. It has also not been well validated with at-risk drinkers, women, older adults and non-Caucasian ethnic groups. Older adults may not screen positive on the CAGE while still having problems with alcohol use. Others may not have annoyed them about their drinking because family may not know and they may not have close contact with friends. In addition, very few older adults need a drink upon rising in the morning, an "eye-opener." They may consume alcohol at a level they used when younger and not believe they need to cut down. On the other hand, older women have been more likely to say they feel guilty while using very little alcohol. Follow-up questions are always needed for positive screens on these questions to determine what prompted each positive response.

The *Alcohol Use Disorders Identification Test (AUDIT)* (see Figure 12.3) is well validated in adults under 65 (Babor et al., 1989; Blow et al., 1998; Fleming & Barry, 1991; Fleming, Barry, & MacDonald, 1991; Schmidt, Barry, & Fleming, 1995) and has had initial validation in a study of older adults (Blow et al., 1998). The AUDIT is comprised of two sections: a 10-item scale (see Appendix) with alcohol-related information for the *previous year only*; and a "Clinical Screening Procedure" which includes a trauma history and a clinical examination. The questionnaire is introduced by a section explaining to the respondent that questions about alcohol use in the *previous year only* are included.

The recommended cut-off score for the AUDIT has been 8, but Blow et al. (1998) found a Cronbach's alpha reliability of 0.95, sensitivity of 0.83, and specificity of 0.91 in a sample of older adults with a cut-off score of 7. Most of the questions in AUDIT are phrased in terms of "how often" symptoms occur. If the clinician is using the AUDIT as part of an interview, it is useful to offer several examples of the response categories (for example, "Never," "Several times a month," "Daily") to suggest how he might answer. When the patient has responded, it is useful to probe during the initial questions to be sure that the most accurate response has been selected (for example, "*You say you drink several times a week. Is this just on weekends or do you drink more or less every day?*"). If responses are ambiguous or evasive, continue asking for clarification and ask the patient to choose the response closest to their experience. If the patient does not drink on a regular basis, recording the drinking pattern can be difficult. For example, if the patient was drinking heavily in the one month before an accident, but has not had any alcohol since, it will be difficult to characterize the "typical" drinking pattern. Using the amount of drinking and related symptoms for the heaviest drinking period of the past year will provide the most useful information. However, clinicians need to make a note of the special circumstances and time period assessed for that particular patient.

Medications

The "brown bag approach" is often recommended to determine medication use. The practitioner can ask older adults to bring every medication they take in a brown paper bag, including over-the-counter and prescription medications, vitamins, and herbs. Home health care providers can check medications and other remedies used by an older adult in the course of a regular home visit. Unfortunately, no screening measures have been developed and validated for assessment of prescription drug misuse and abuse in the elderly. There are some signs and symptoms, however, to consider (see Table 12.1; Blow, CSAT, 1998).

The following questions are about **the past year**.	**(Score)**
1. How often do you have a drink containing alcohol?	
❑ Never	(0)
❑ Monthly or less	(1)
❑ 2 to 4 times a month	(2)
❑ 2 to 3 times a week	(3)
❑ 4 or more times a week	(4)
2. How many drinks containing alcohol do you have on a typical day when you are drinking?	
❑ None	(0)
❑ 1 or 2	(1)
❑ 3 or 4	(2)
❑ 5 or 6	(3)
❑ 7 or 9	(4)
10 or more	(5)
3. How often do you have six or more drinks on one occasion?	
❑ Never	(0)
❑ Less than monthly	(1)
❑ Monthly	(2)
❑ Weekly	(3)
❑ Daily or almost daily	(4)
4. How often during the last year have you found that you were unable to stop drinking once you had started?	
❑ Never	(0)
❑ Less than monthly	(1)
❑ Monthly	(2)
❑ Weekly	(3)
❑ Daily or almost daily	(4)
5. How often during the last year have you failed to do what was normally expected from you because of drinking?	
❑ Never	(0)
❑ Less than monthly	(1)
❑ Monthly	(2)
❑ Weekly	(3)
❑ Daily or almost daily	(4)
6. How often during the last year have you needed a first drink in the morning to get yourself going after a heavy drinking session?	
❑ Never	(0)
❑ Less than monthly	(1)
❑ Monthly	(2)
❑ Weekly	(3)
❑ Daily or almost daily	(4)
7. How often during the last year have you had a feeling of guilt or remorse after drinking?	
❑ Never	(0)
❑ Less than monthly	(1)
❑ Monthly	(2)
❑ Weekly	(3)
❑ Daily or almost daily	(4)

FIGURE 12.3

Alcohol Use Disorders Identification Test (Audit).

8. How often during the last year have you been unable to remember what happened the night before because you had been drinking?

- ❑ Never (0)
- ❑ Less than monthly (1)
- ❑ Monthly (2)
- ❑ Weekly (3)
- ❑ Daily or almost daily (4)

9. Have you or someone else been injured as the result of your drinking?

- ❑ Never (0)
- ❑ Less than monthly (1)
- ❑ Monthly (2)
- ❑ Weekly (3)
- ❑ Daily or almost daily (4)

10. Has a relative, friend, or a doctor or other health worker been concerned about your drinking or suggested you cut down?

- ❑ Never (0)
- ❑ Less than monthly (1)
- ❑ Monthly (2)
- ❑ Weekly (3)
- ❑ Daily or almost daily (4)

FIGURE 12.3—*Continued*

Additionally, there are special considerations when evaluating medication use in the elderly. Aging may affect the body's ability to develop tolerance (Patterson & Jeste, 1999). Accordingly, older adults could experience more severe drug-related problems without changing their patterns of substance use or exceeding recommended therapeutic dosages (Adams & Cox, 1995; Fingerhood, 2000). Specifically, benzodiazepine dependence may arise even in the absence of apparent abuse (Finfgeld-Connett, 2004).

Coupled with potential increased tolerance, older adults may naturally become less active, rendering it difficult for clinicians to detect substance abuse-related declines in functioning or social involvement (Fingerhood, 2000). Substance abuse in the elderly may coincide with other mental disorders, including other substance-related disorders, which increases the likelihood of experiencing an adverse drug interaction. Solomon and colleagues (1993) found that 75% of substance-dependent older adults were also diagnosed with another mental disorder, compared to 36% of young adults (Solomon et al., 1993). Data from the National Epidemiologic Survey on Alcohol and Related Conditions (NESARC) indicated that non-medical prescription drug use disorders were highly comorbid with anxiety, mood, and personality disorders, as well as other substance use disorders (Huang et al., 2006). Patients, caregivers, and clinicians could mistakenly characterize adverse effects of a medication, such as confusion or discoordination, as symptoms of a new illness or age-related decline (Dowling, Weiss, & Condon, 2008).

Careful screening for alcohol, medications, and other drugs is a key to providing needed interventions and treatments to the vulnerable and growing population of older adults who are experiencing problems related to substances.

BROAD-BASED ASSESSMENT OF ALCOHOL PROBLEMS IN OLDER ADULTS

Assessment helps the clinician to determine the severity of the alcohol problem—whether or not the patient is an at-risk drinker, a problem drinker, or alcohol dependent. The following are some general guidelines for clinicians to adapt to each particular patient and situation. Clinicians can follow up the brief questions about consumption and consequences such as those in the AUDIT and the CAGE with a few more in-depth questions about consequences, health risks, and social/family issues.

To assess dependence, ask questions about alcohol-related problems, a history of failed attempts to stop or cut back, or withdrawal symptoms such as tremors. Clinicians should refer any patient thought to be alcohol dependent for a diagnostic evaluation and possible specialized alcohol treatment with an emphasis on treatment targeted at older adults. Medication assessments include questions about prescriptions, particularly antidepressants, benzodiazepines, codeine, over-the-counter medications, and herbal remedies. If there is evidence of prescription drug problems, the patient should also be referred to a specialist for a diagnostic assessment and possible specialized treatment.

For older adults with positive alcohol screens, assessments are needed to confirm the problem, to characterize the dimensions of the problem, and to develop individualized treatment plans. For purposes of insurance or other funding resources, the assessment should follow criteria in the Diagnostic and Statistical Manual of Mental Disorders, Fourth Edition (DSM-IV) (American Psychiatric Association, 1994) or other relevant criteria, keeping in mind that these criteria may not apply directly to planning older adults' treatment. The unqualified application of such criteria is problematic in older adult populations because the symptoms of other medical diseases and psychiatric disorders overlap to a considerable extent with substance-related disorders.

Problems with DSM-IV Criteria for Older Adults

Most clinicians use the model defined in the American Psychiatric Association's Diagnostic and Statistical Manual of Mental Disorders, Fourth Edition (DSM-IV; American Psychiatric Association, 1994) for classifying the signs and symptoms of alcohol-related problems. The DSM-IV uses specific criteria to distinguish between those drinkers who abuse alcohol and those who are dependent on alcohol.

Although widely used, the DSM-IV criteria may not apply to many older adults who experience neither the legal, social nor psychological consequences specified. For example, "a failure to fulfill major role obligations at work, school, or home" is less applicable to a retired person with minimal familial responsibilities. Nor does the criterion "continued use of the substance(s) despite persistent or recurrent problems" always apply. Many older alcoholics do not realize that their persistent or recurrent problems are in fact related to their drinking, a view likely to be reinforced by health care clinicians who may attribute these problems, in whole or in part, to the aging process or age-related comorbidities.

Even though tolerance is one of the DSM-IV criteria for a diagnosis of substance dependence, the thresholds of consumption often considered by clinicians as indicative of tolerance may be set too high for older adults because of their altered sensitivity to and body distribution of alcohol (Atkinson, 1990). The lack of tolerance to alcohol does not necessarily mean that an older adult does not have a drinking problem or is not experiencing serious negative effects as a result of their drinking. Furthermore, many late onset alcoholics have not developed physiological dependence, and they do not exhibit signs of withdrawal. Table 12.2 presents the DSM-IV criteria for substance dependence as they apply to older adults with alcohol problems (Center for Substance Abuse Treatment, 1998).

The drinking practices of many older adults who do *not* meet the diagnostic criteria for abuse or dependence still place them at risk of complicating an existing medical or psychiatric disorder. Consuming one or two drinks per day, for example, may lead to increased cognitive impairment in patients who already have Alzheimer's disease, may lead to worsening of sleep problems in patients with sleep apnea, or may interact with medications rendering them less effective or causing adverse side effects. A barrier to good clinical management in these cases may be the lack of understanding of the risks of so-called "moderate drinking." Limiting access to treatment because symptoms do not meet the rigorous diagnostic criteria of the DSM-IV may preclude an older patient from making significant improvements in their life.

Table 12.2 Applying DSM-IV Criteria to Older Adults

Criteria	Special Considerations for Older Adults
1. Tolerance	May have problems with even low intake due to increased sensitivity to alcohol and higher blood alcohol levels
2. Withdrawal	Many late onset alcoholics do not develop physiological dependence
3. Taking larger amounts or over a longer period than was intended	Increased cognitive impairment can interfere with self-monitoring; drinking can exacerbate cognitive impairment and monitoring
4. Unsuccessful efforts to cut down or control use	Same issues across lifespan
5. Spending much time to obtain and use alcohol and to recover from effects	Negative effects can occur with relatively low use
6. Giving up activities due to use	May have fewer activities, making detection of problems more difficult
7. Continuing use despite physical or psychological problem caused by use	May not know or understand that problems are related to use, even after medical advice

(From Blow, CSAT Treatment Improvement Protocol, 1998)

The changing social roles and circumstances of older adults may further reduce the applicability of the criteria. Problems with occupational activities or work obligations may no longer be relevant in terms of functioning; however, an emphasis on maintaining a dwelling, managing finances, or participating in social or recreational activities is still salient. "Recurrent substance use in situations in which it is physically hazardous," a substance abuse criteria in the DSM-IV (American Psychiatric Association, 1994), does not always mean driving while intoxicated, but can include other activities that may be dangerous for an older frail adult (e.g., climbing a ladder, crossing a street, or taking a bath while impaired by alcohol). Assessment can take place in one visit, if time permits, or in stages if the patient is not in immediate danger from their behavior.

Case Study 5

John Anderson is a 68-year-old man with a regularly scheduled appointment at the primary care clinic to monitor his blood pressure. He completed the screening questionnaire while seated in the waiting room. He had four glasses of wine the previous evening and had a history of binge drinking (generally four to five drinks per occasion) two to three times/week. An assessment of his drinking would follow DSM-IV criteria. After assessing DSM-IV domains the physician assistant said, "*Mr Anderson, in the screening questionnaire you said you were drinking four drinks/day three times a week. You also reported experiencing some issues related to your drinking such as other people criticizing your drinking. As you age you become more sensitive to the effects of alcohol. The organs that clear alcohol through the body do not work as efficiently. You can have some negative consequences of drinking with lower levels of use than when you were younger. You mentioned that you had experienced such things as problems with your health including high blood pressure. You have also been unable to follow through on some of your obligations at the senior center. These problems can occur with even lower levels of alcohol use than you could manage when you were younger. Sometimes people also drink to help cope with changes in life. For now, I recommend that you should drink no more than one drink per day, no more than three times a week. Also, drinking more than three drinks on any occasion is considered binge drinking for men over 60. Binge drinking can cause negative consequences such as medication interactions, and can lead to problems controlling high blood pressure. Maintaining independence and staying as healthy as possible are important goals for a good quality of life and we want you to stay as healthy as possible. Are you willing to try cutting back on your drinking to the level I am recommending? Let's see how this goes for a month and we can re-evaluate your alcohol use again at your next appointment.*"

Substance Abuse Assessment Instruments

The use of validated substance abuse assessment instruments can be of great help to clinicians by providing a structured approach to the assessment process, as well as a checklist of items that should be evaluated with each patient receiving an alcohol assessment. Specialized assessments are generally conducted by treatment program personnel or trained mental and physical health care providers. Structured assessment interviews "possess (at least potentially) the desired qualities of quantifiability, reliability, validity, standardization, and recordability" (Institute of Medicine, 1990).

Two structured assessment instruments are recommended for use with older adults (Center for Substance Abuse Treatment, 1998): the *Structured Clinical Interview for DSM-III-R* (*SCID*; Spitzer & Williams, 1985), and the *Diagnostic Interview Schedule* (*DIS*) for DSM-IV. This instrument was originally developed by Robins, Helzer, Croughan, & Ratcliff, (1981), with DSM-III criteria and has been updated as DSM criteria have evolved. The SCID is a multimodule assessment that covers disorders of: substance use; psychotic; mood; anxiety; somatoform; eating; adjustment; and personality. It takes a trained clinician approximately 30 minutes to administer the 35 SCID questions that probe for alcohol abuse or dependence.

The DIS is a highly structured interview that does not require clinical judgment and can be used by non-clinicians. The DIS assesses both current and past symptoms and is available in a computerized version. It has been translated into a number of languages including Spanish and Chinese.

SCREENING AND ASSESSMENT FOR PHYSICAL, MENTAL, AND FUNCTIONAL HEALTH

Many older adults require a full assessment of their physical, mental, and functional health to be able to adequately understand the impact of their alcohol use. Older adults with medical and psychiatric disorders are more likely to have impairments in functional abilities. Ninety percent of adults over the age of 65 require the use of glasses and 50% of adults over 65 have some degree of hearing loss (Hull, 1989; Plomp, 1978). Sensory impairments affect older adults in subtle ways that are not always immediately obvious but should be incorporated into any treatment planning. Older adults need to be able to read prescriptions or hear what is said in a group therapy session. When clinicians do not help their older patients compensate for sensory impairments, they can interfere with interventions and treatments. As an example, an evening program should not be recommended to older adults who cannot drive at night and do not have someone else to drive them.

Assessing Functional Health

Functional health refers to a person's capacity to perform two types of everyday tasks: activities of daily living (ADLs), which include ambulating, bathing, dressing, feeding, and using the toilet; and instrumental activities of daily living (IADLs), which include managing finances, preparing meals, shopping, taking medications, and using the phone. Limitations in these domains can result in an inadequate diet, mismanagement of medications or finances, or other serious problems.

Activities of daily living (ADLs) and instrumental activities of daily living (IADLs) can be impaired due to alcohol use. Although alcohol-related functional impairments are potentially reversible, they should be considered when planning treatments. There are known complications of and differences between alcohol use in men and women related to compromised functional abilities and ADLs. In a recent study of older adults with a former history of alcohol abuse, impairment in ADLs was twice as common in women as in men (Ensrud et al., 1994). In addition, alcohol use was more strongly correlated with functional impairment than were smoking, age, use of anxiolytics, stroke, or diminished grip strength.

The *Medical Outcomes Study 36-Item Short Form Health Survey (SF-36)* is a recommended self-report questionnaire that measures health-related quality of life, including both ADLs and IADLs (McHorney, War, Lu, & Sherbourne, 1994). Although this instrument is more comprehensive, it is also more difficult to use because of complex scoring of the various subscales. The SF-36 does provide, however, a comprehensive assessment of health and not just functional abilities. This instrument can be used by health care providers in a range of settings. There is now a shorter validated version of this instrument available, the SF-12 (see Appendix).

Assessing Comorbid Disorders

There is a complex relationship between alcohol use and coexisting physical or mental disorders. Medical and psychiatric problems can coexist with alcohol use with no specific relationship to drinking. On the other hand, those problems may be precursors or maintaining factors for drinking. The use of alcohol to anesthetize pain is an example of a factor that maintains a problem. In this instance, alcohol can be a problem by itself and can also interact with medications used for pain. The assessment of comorbid medical and/or psychiatric disorders can require the cooperation of a treatment team consisting of providers who treat primarily physical health problems and those who work with mental health problems. Treatment teams may be part of routine care in some clinical settings, but they may also need to be brought together on an ad hoc basis for particular cases.

Studies have shown that the most common health problem among alcohol-dependent older adults is alcoholic liver disease. Chronic obstructive pulmonary disease, peptic ulcer disease, and psoriasis also are found much more frequently in older alcoholics than in older adults with no alcohol problems. Alcohol also appears to be a risk factor for myopathy, cerebrovascular disease, gastritis, diarrhea, pancreatitis, cardiomyopathy, sleep disorders, HIV/AIDS-related diseases, and both intentional and unintentional injuries (Tobias, Lippmann, & Pary, 1989).

Of importance for clinicians who work with older adults is the finding that acute alcohol withdrawal syndrome is more protracted and severe in older adults than in younger adults (Brower, Mudd, Blow, Young, & Hill, 1994; Liskow, Rinck, Campbell, & DeSouza, 1989). Because there is no research on the recent practice of outpatient detoxification for older adults, very careful assessment is warranted before detoxification from any drug; outpatient detoxification may not be appropriate for older adults who are frail or who have a comorbidity.

Assessing Psychiatric Comorbidity

Data from the Epidemiologic Catchment Area (ECA) study have strengthened support for a possible link between alcohol use and abuse and the development of other psychiatric illnesses (Regier et al., 1990). Adults with a lifetime diagnosis of alcohol abuse or dependence had nearly three times the risk of being diagnosed with another mental disorder. Comorbid disorders associated with alcohol use include anxiety disorders, affective illness, cognitive impairment, schizophrenia, and antisocial personality disorder (Blazer & Williams, 1980; Blow, Cook, Booth, Falcon, & Friedman, 1992b; Finlayson, Hurt, Davis, & Morse, 1988; National Institute of Alcholism and Alcohol Abuse, 1995a,b; Saunders et al., 1991; Wagman, Allen, & Upright, 1977). According to one study, older alcohol abusers are more likely to have triple diagnoses (alcohol, depression, and personality disorders) whereas younger substance abusers are more likely to have diagnoses of schizophrenia (Speer & Bates, 1992). Psychiatric comorbidities should be assessed by trained mental health providers and/or using instruments such as the SCID or the DIS (see section on alcohol assessment instruments).

Assessing Depression

Affective disorders, particularly depression and anxiety, are quite common in older patients and will influence intervention and treatment options. For instance, patients who take psychotropic medications need to be treated by staff familiar with these medications. Suicidal patients require intensive inpatient programs and an immediate intervention. Major depressive symptoms are common after detoxification and are often worse in older adults. These patients may need prescribed medicines to alleviate the depression before the abuse or addiction therapy is resumed.

Instruments used to screen and assess depression can be extremely useful as methods of detecting significant affective illness and for monitoring changes in affective states. The *Geriatric Depression Scale* (*GDS*) *Short Form* (Sheikh & Yesavage, 1986) and the *Center for Epidemiological Studies Depression Scale* (*CES-D*; Radloff, 1977) have been validated in older age groups although not specifically in older adults with addiction problems. The CES-D may be most useful in general outpatient settings as a screen for depression among older patients. DSM-IV criteria is used as part of the assessment of depression.

Assessing Cognitive Impairments

The presence of cognitive impairment or dementia significantly alters treatment decisions. It is particularly important to distinguish between dementia and delirium, which are often mistaken for each other by clinicians diagnosing older patients. Dementia is a chronic, progressive, and generally irreversible cognitive impairment sufficient to interfere with an individual's daily living. Dementia will also limit an individual's ability to interact in traditional group settings. Common causes of dementia include Alzheimer's disease, vascular disorders (e.g., multi-infarct dementia), and alcohol-related dementia. Dementia also makes it more difficult to monitor outcomes of drinking (patients may forget they drank), to get into treatment, and to benefit from the treatment. Delirium is a potentially life-threatening illness that requires acute intervention—usually hospitalization. The cognitive losses experienced with delirium, unlike the effects of dementia, can often be reversed with proper medical treatment. Patients who appear to have memory loss, impaired abstract thinking, confusion, difficulty communicating, extreme emotional reactions and outbursts, and disorientation to time, place, and person need to be evaluated for signs of cognitive impairment, since these symptoms are not part of the normal aging process.

Two instruments are recommended to assess cognitive impairment, the *Orientation/Memory/ Concentration Test* (Katzman et al., 1983), which is simple and can be completed in the office, and the *Folstein Mini-Mental Status Exam* (*MMSE*; Folstein, Folstein, & McHugh, 1975), which is an acceptable alternative. The MMSE can be insensitive to subtle cognitive impairments in the assessment of older problem drinkers who have been sober for 30–60 days in an outpatient setting. Because the MMSE is weaker on visual-spatial testing and does not include screening tests of abstract thinking and visual memory, using the "*draw-a-clock task*" (Watson, Arfken, & Birge, 1993) and the *Neurobehavioral Cognitive Status Examination* (*NCSE*; Kiernan, Mueller, Langston, & Van, 1987) as supplements is recommended by the CSAT Treatment Improvement Protocol (1998) for drinking in older adulthood.

Treatment Options

After determining that an older adult may benefit from a reduction in or complete abstention from alcohol use, the clinician should assess the patient's understanding of the situation. Many older adults may not know that their alcohol use is affecting their health. Because patient understanding and cooperation are essential both in eliciting accurate information and following through on the treatment plan prescribed, clinicians should use the assessment process as an opportunity to educate the older adult and to motivate him or her to accept treatment.

CULTURAL ISSUES IN SCREENING AND ASSESSMENT

Any screening, assessment, and intervention strategies for older adults with alcohol-related problems need to be sensitive to age, gender, and cultural issues. Studies on the use of screening questions for health promotion in primary care settings have found that, although providers agree with recommendations for screening, they are less likely to perform the screening, especially with elderly patients (Black, Sefcik, & Kapoor, 1990; Radecki & Cowell, 1990). Additionally, in cultures where the traditional role of the older individual is as an authority figure, health care providers from that culture have more favorable attitudes toward elderly patients. In an alcohol treatment population, Booth, Blow, Cook, Bunn, and Fortney (1992) found that members of some minorities and elderly, particularly Hispanic and African Americans, were more likely to seek inpatient care for diagnoses other than alcoholism and that, as a result, such individuals need targeted interventions to encourage them to seek alcohol-specific care. All treatment strategies need to be culturally competent and, to the extent possible, incorporate appropriate ethnic considerations (e.g., rituals). Health care providers may need the help of experienced non-medical personnel to adequately assess cultural issues in determining the best methods to screen older individuals for alcohol problems, and the best intervention and treatment options for those who screen positive. An awareness of specific cultural issues related to working with older adults about alcohol or medication problems will ensure continuity of care and provide the best opportunity to achieve positive outcomes.

SUMMARY

Recent research indicates that at-risk drinking and alcohol-related problems are common in older adults. Clinicians can expect that approximately 15% of the men and 12% of the women in this age group will drink above recommended guidelines. Since most alcohol-related problems occur in non-dependent drinkers (Institute of Medicine, 1990), mental and physical health care providers can have a substantial impact on a potentially serious problem through identification and treatment of these patients. Alcohol screening and assessment can be done quickly and efficiently in most health care settings. The key is the development of a system in each unique setting to insure that all older adults receive baseline screening and that patients who present with physical or mental health problems which could be alcohol-related receive differential assessments to determine if alcohol or alcohol/medication interactions play a part in the presenting problem. With changes in the health care system to managed models of care, the time is right to move forward into systematic, cost-effective approaches to identifying treating one of the most vulnerable and fastest growing segments of the U.S. population.

REFERENCES

Adams, W. L., Barry, K., & Fleming, M. (1996). Screening for problem drinking in older primary care patients. *JAMA*, *276*(24), 1964.

Adams, W. L., & Cox, N. S. (1995). Epidemiology of problem drinking among elderly people. *International Journal of the Addictions*, *30*(13–14), 1693–1716.

American Psychiatric Association. (1994). *Diagnostic and Statistical Manual of Mental Disorders* (4th ed.). Washington, DC: APA.

Atkinson, R. M. (1990). Aging and alcohol use disorders: diagnostic issues in the elderly. *International Psychogeriatrics*, *2*(1), 55–72.

Babor, T., De La Fuente, J., Saunders, J., & Grant, M. (1989). *AUDIT: the alcohol use disorders identification test: guidelines for use in primary health care*. Geneva, Switzerland: World Health Organization.

Baker, S. L. (1985). Substance abuse disorders in aging veterans. In E. Gottheil, R. A. Druley, T. E. Skiloday, & H. Waxman (Eds.), *Alcohol, Drug Addiction and Aging* (pp. 303–311). Springfield, IL: Charles C. Thomas.

Barry, K. L. (1997). Alcohol and drug abuse. In *Fundamentals of Clinical Practice: A Textbook on the Patient, Doctor, and Society*. New York, NY: Plenum Medical Book Company.

Barry, K. L. (Chair) (1999). *Treatment Improvement Protocol: Brief Alcohol Interventions and Therapies in Substance Abuse Treatment (TIP 34)*. Rockville, MD: Center for Substance Abuse Treatment, Substance Abuse and Mental Health Services Administration.

Barry, K. L., & Fleming, M. F. (1990). Computerized administration of alcoholism screening tests in a primary care setting. *Journal of the American Board of Family Practice*, *3*(2), 93–98.

Beresford, T., Blow, F., Singer, K., Hill, E., & Lucey, M. (1990). Comparison of CAGE questionnaire and computer-assisted laboratory profiles in screening for covert alcoholism. *The Lancet*, *336*(8713), 482–485.

Black, J., Sefcik, T., & Kapoor, W. (1990). Health promotion and disease prevention in the elderly: comparison of house staff and attending physician attitudes and practices. *Archives of Internal Medicine*, *150*(2), 389.

Blazer, D. G., & Williams, C. (1980). Epidemiology of dysphoria and depression in an elderly population. *American Journal of Psychiatry*, *137*(4), 439.

Blazer, D. G., & Wu, L. T. (2009). The epidemiology of at-risk and binge drinking among middle-aged and elderly community adults: National Survey on Drug Use and Health. *American Journal of Psychiatry*, *166* (10), 1162.

Blow, F. C., & Barry, K. L. (2001). Alcoholism. In G. Maddox (Ed.), *The Encyclopedia of Aging,* Vol. 1, (3rd ed.) (pp. 56–58). New York, NY: Springer Publishing.

Blow, F. C., Barry, K. L., Fuller, B., & Booth, B. (2002). Analysis of the National Health and Nutrition Examination Survey (NHANES): Longitudinal analysis of drinking over the lifespan. In S. P. Korper, & C. L. Council (Eds.), *Substance use by Older Adults: Estimates of Future Impact on the Treatment System* (pp. 125–141). Rockville, MD: Substance Abuse and Mental Health Services Administration, Office of Applied Studies.

Blow, F. C., Bartels, S. J., Brockmann, L. M., & van Citters, A. D. (2006). *Evidence-based practices for preventing substance abuse and mental health problems in older adults*. Washington, DC: Older Americans Substance Abuse and Mental Health Technical Assistance Center, SAMHSA.

Blow, F. C., Brower, K., Schulenberg, J., Demo-Dananberg, L., Young, J., & Beresford, T. (1992a). The Michigan alcoholism screening test–geriatric version (MAST–G): a new elderly-specific screening instrument. *Alcoholism, Clinical and Experimental Research*, *16*(2), 372.

Blow, F. C., Cook, C., Booth, B., Falcon, S., & Friedman, M. (1992b). Age-related psychiatric comorbidities and level of functioning in alcoholic veterans seeking outpatient treatment. *Hospital and Community Psychiatry*, *43*(10), 990–995.

Blow, F. C., Gillespie, B. W., Barry, K. L., Mudd, S. A., & Hill, E.M. (1998). *Brief screening for alcohol problems in elderly populations using the Short Michigan Alcoholism Screening Test–Geriatric Version (SMAST–G)*. Poster presented at the Research Society on Alcoholism Annual Scientific Meeting, Hilton Head Island, SC.

Blow, F. C., Walton, M., Chermack, S., Barry, K. L., Coyne, J., Gomberg., E., & Mudd, S. (2000). The relationship between alcohol problems and health functioning of older adults in primary care settings. *Journal of the American Geriatrics Society*, *48*(7), 769–774.

Blow, F. C. (Chair), & Center for Substance Abuse Treatment. (1998). *Treatment improvement protocol #26: substance abuse among older adults*. [DHHS Publication No. (SMA) 98-3179]. Rockville, MD: Department of Health and Human Services.

Booth, B., Blow, F., Cook, C., Bunn, J., & Fortney, J. (1992). Age and ethnicity among hospitalized alcoholics: a nationwide study. *Alcoholism, Clinical and Experimental Research*, *16*(6), 1029–1034.

Brower, K., Mudd, S., Blow, F., Young, J., & Hill, E. (1994). Severity and treatment of alcohol withdrawal in elderly versus younger patients. *Alcoholism, Clinical and Experimental Research, 18*(1), 196–201.

Bush, B., Shaw, S., Cleary, P., Delbanco, T., & Aronson, M. (1987). Screening for alcohol abuse using the CAGE questionnaire. *American Journal of Medicine*, *82*(2), 231–235.

Callahan, C. M., & Tierney, W. M. (1995). Health services use and mortality among older primary care patients with alcoholism. *Journal of the American Geriatrics Society, 43*(12), 1378–1383.

Chermack, S., Blow, F., Hill, E., & Mudd, S. (1996). The relationship between alcohol symptoms and consumption among older drinkers. *Alcoholism, Clinical and Experimental Research, 20*(7), 1153–1158.

Colliver, J., Compton, W., Gfroerer, J., & Condon, T. (2006). Projecting drug use among aging baby boomers in 2020. *Annals of Epidemiology, 16*(4), 257–265.

Cook, A. E. (1999). Strategies for containing drug costs: implications for a Medicare benefit. *Health Care Financing Review, 20*(3), 29–37.

Culberson, J., & Ziska, M. (2008). Prescription drug misuse/abuse in the elderly. *Geriatrics, 63*(9), 22–31.

Dealberto, M. J., McAvay, G. J., Seeman, T., & Berkman, L. (1997). Psychotropic drug use and cognitive decline among older men and women. *International Journal of Geriatric Psychiatry, 12*(5), 567–574.

Dowling, G., Weiss, S. R. B., & Condon, T. (2008). Drugs of abuse and the aging brain. *Neuropsychopharmacology, 33*(2), 209–218.

Edgell, R. C., Kunik, M. E., Molinari, V. A., Hale, D., & Orengo, C. A. (2000). Nonalcohol-related use disorders in geropsychiatric patients. *Journal of Geriatric Psychiatry and Neurology, 13*(1), 33–37.

Ensrud, K., Nevitt, M., Yunis, C., Cauley, J., Seeley, D., Fox, K., et al. (1994). Correlates of impaired function in older women. *Journal of the American Geriatrics Society, 42*(5), 481–489.

Ewing, J. (1984). Detecting alcoholism. The CAGE questionnaire. *JAMA, 252*(14), 1905–1907.

Finfgeld-Connett, D. (2004). Treatment of substance misuse in older women: using a brief intervention model. *Journal of Gerontological Nursing, 30*(8), 30–37.

Fingerhood, M. (2000). Substance abuse in older people. *Journal of the American Geriatrics Society, 48*(8), 985–995.

Finlayson, R. E., & Davis, L. J. (1994). Prescription drug dependence in the elderly population: demographic and clinical features of 100 inpatients. *Mayo Clinic Proceedings, 69*(12), 1137–1145.

Finlayson, R. E., Hurt, R., Davis, L., Jr., & Morse, R. (1988). Alcoholism in elderly persons: a study of the psychiatric and psychosocial features of 216 inpatients. *Mayo Clinic Proceedings*, *63*, 761–768.

Fleming, M. F., & Barry, K. (1991). The effectiveness of alcoholism screening in an ambulatory care setting. *Journal of Studies on Alcohol, 52*(1), 33–36.

Fleming, M. F., Barry, K., & MacDonald, R. (1991). The Alcohol Use Disorders Identification Test (AUDIT) in a college sample. *Substance Use and Misuse*, *26*(11), 1173–1185.

Fleming, M. F., & Barry, K. L. (Eds.). (1992). *Addictive Disorders*. St. Louis, MO: Mosby Yearbook Medical Publishers.

Fleming, M. F., Manwell, L. B., Barry, K. L., Adams, W., & Stauffacher, E. A. (1999). Brief physician advice for alcohol problems in older adults: a randomized community-based trial. *The Journal of Family Practice*, *48* (5), 378–384.

Folstein, M., Folstein, S., & McHugh, P. (1975). Mini-Mental State: a practical method for grading the cognitive state of patients for the clinician. *Journal of Psychiatric Research, 12*(3), 189–198.

Greist, J., Klein, M., Erdman, H., Bires, J., Bass, S., Machtinger, P., et al. (1987). Comparison of computer- and interviewer-administered versions of the Diagnostic Interview Schedule. *Psychiatric Services*, *38*(12), 1304.

Gurwitz, J. H., Field, T. S., Avorn, J., McCormick, D., Jain, S., Eckler, M., et al. (2000). Incidence and preventability of adverse drug events in nursing homes. *The American Journal of Medicine*, *109*(2), 87–94.

Hanlon, J. T., Horner, R. D., Schmader, K. E., Fillenbaum, G. G., Lewis, I. K., Wall, W. E., et al. (1998). Benzodiazepine use and cognitive function among community-dwelling elderly. *Clinical Pharmacology and Therapeutics*, *64*(6), 684–692.

Hogan, D., Maxwell, C., Fung, T., & Ebly, E. (2003). Prevalence and potential consequences of benzodiazepine use in senior citizens: results from the Canadian Study of Health and Aging. *The Canadian Journal of Clinical Pharmacology, 10*(2), 72–77.

Holroyd, S., & Duryee, J. J. (1997). Substance use disorders in a geriatric psychiatry outpatient clinic: prevalence and epidemiologic characteristics. *Journal of Nervous and Mental Disease*, *185*(10), 627–632.

Huang, B., Dawson, D., Stinson, F., Hasin, D., Ruan, W. J., Saha, T., et al. (2006). Prevalence, correlates, and comorbidity of nonmedical prescription drug use and drug use disorders in the United States: results of the National Epidemiologic Survey on Alcohol and Related Conditions. *Journal of Clinical Psychiatry*, *67*(7), 1062–1073.

Hull, R. (1989). Incidence of selected language, speech and hearing disorders among the elderly. In R. Hull, & K. M. Griffin (Eds.), *Communication Disorders in Aging*. Newbury Park, CA: Sage.

Institute of Medicine. (1990). *Broadening the base of treatment for alcohol problems*. Washington, DC: National Academy Press.

Jinks, M. J., & Raschko, R. R. (1990). A profile of alcohol and prescription drug abuse in a high-risk community-based elderly population. *DICP*, *24*(10), 971–975.

Joseph, C., Atkinson, R., & Ganzini, L. (1995). Problem drinking among residents of a VA nursing home. *International Journal of Geriatric Psychiatry*, *10*(3), 243–248.

Katzman, R., Brown, T., Fuld, P., Peck, A., Schechter, R., & Schimmel, H. (1983). Validation of a short orientation–memory–concentration test of cognitive impairment. *American Journal of Psychiatry*, *140*(6), 734.

Kiernan, R. J., Mueller, J., Langston, J. W., & Van, D. (1987). The Neurobehavioral Cognitive Status Examination: a brief but differentiated approach to cognitive assessment. *Annals of Internal Medicine*, *107*(4), 481.

King, M. (1986). At risk drinking among general practice attenders: validation of the CAGE questionnaire. *Psychological Medicine*, *16*(1), 213–217.

Lazarou, J., Pomeranz, B. H., & Corey, P. N. (1998). Incidence of adverse drug reactions in hospitalized patients: a meta-analysis of prospective studies. *JAMA*, *279*(15), 1200–1205.

Leipzig, R. M., Cumming, R. G., & Tinetti, M. E. (1999). Drugs and falls in older people: a systematic review and meta-analysis: I. Psychotropic drugs. *Journal of the American Geriatrics Society*, *47*(1), 30–39.

Liskow, B., Rinck, C., Campbell, J., & DeSouza, C. (1989). Alcohol withdrawal in the elderly. *Journal of Studies on Alcohol*, *50*(5), 414–421.

Mayfield, D., McLeod, G., & Hall, P. (1974). The CAGE questionnaire: validation of a new alcoholism screening instrument. *American Journal of Psychiatry*, *131*(10), 1121.

McHorney, C., War, J. Jr., Lu, J., & Sherbourne, C. (1994). The MOS 36-item Short-Form Health Survey (SF-36): III. Tests of data quality, scaling assumptions, and reliability across diverse patient groups. *Medical Care*, *32*(1), 40–66.

Menninger, J. A. (2002). Assessment and treatment of alcoholism and substance-related disorders in the elderly. *Bulletin of the Menninger Clinic*, *66*(2), 166–183.

Moore, A. A., Morton, S. C., Beck, J. C., Hays, R. D., Oishi, S. M., Partridge, J. M., et al. (1999). A new paradigm for alcohol use in older persons. *Medical Care*, *37*(2), 165–179.

National Institute of Alcholism and Alcohol Abuse (1995a). *The Physician's Guide to Helping Patients with Alcohol Problems* (NIH Publ. No. 95–3769).

National Institute of Alcholism and Alcohol Abuse (NIAAA) (1995b). *The Physician's Guide to Helping Patients with Alcohol Problems* (NIH Publ. No. 95–3769).

National Institute on Alcohol Abuse and Alcoholism (1998). Drinking in the United States: main findings from the 1992 National Longitudinal Alcohol Epidemiologic Survey (NLAES).

Office of Applied Studies. (2002). *Summary of findings from the 2002 National Survey on Drug Use and Health*. Rockville, MD: Substance Abuse and Mental Health Services Administration, Department of Health and Human Services.

Office of Applied Studies. (2004). *Results from the 2003 National Survey on Drug Use and Health: National Findings* NSDUH Series H-25. Rockville, MD: Substance Abuse and Mental Health Services Administration.

Office of Applied Studies. (2007). The DASIS Report. Older adults in substance abuse treatment: update. Retrieved October 30, 2007, from http://oas.samhsa.gov/2k5/olderAdultsTX/olderAdults.TX.

Oslin, D. W. (2004). Late-life alcoholism: issues relevant to the geriatric psychiatrist. *The American Journal of Geriatric Psychiatry*, *12*(6), 571–583.

Oslin, D. W., Streim, J., Parmelee, P., Boyce, A., & Katz, I. (1997). Alcohol abuse: a source of reversible functional disability among residents of a VA nursing home. *International Journal of Geriatric Psychiatry, 12*(8), 825–832.

Patterson, T. L., & Jeste, D. V. (1999). The potential impact of the baby-boom generation on substance abuse among elderly persons. *Psychiatric Services, 50*(9), 1184–1188.

Plomp, R. (1978). Auditory handicap of hearing impairment and the limited benefit of hearing aids. *The Journal of the Acoustical Society of America, 63*, 533.

Radecki, S. E., & Cowell, W. G. (1990). Health promotion for elderly patients. *Family Medicine, 22*(4), 299–302.

Radloff, L. (1977). The CES-D scale: a self-report depression scale for research in the general population. *Applied Psychological Measurement, 1*(3), 385.

Ray, W. A., Thapa, P. B., & Shorr, R. I. (1993). Medications and the older driver. *Clinics in Geriatric Medicine, 9* (2), 413–438.

Regier, D., Farmer, M., Rae, D., Locke, B., Keith, S., Judd, L., et al. (1990). Comorbidity of mental disorders with alcohol and other drug abuse. Results from the Epidemiologic Catchment Area (ECA) Study. *Journal of the American Medical Association, 264*(19), 2511.

Robins, L., Helzer, J., Croughan, J., & Ratcliff, K. (1981). National Institute of Mental Health diagnostic interview schedule: its history, characteristics, and validity. *Archives of General Psychiatry, 38*(4), 381–389.

Rosin, A., & Glatt, M. (1971). Alcohol excess in the elderly. *Quarterly Journal of Studies on Alcohol, 32*(1), 53.

Saunders, P., Copeland, J., Dewey, M., Davidson, I., McWilliam, C., Sharma, V., et al. (1991). Heavy drinking as a risk factor for depression and dementia in elderly men. Findings from the Liverpool longitudinal community study. *The British Journal of Psychiatry, 159*(2), 213.

Schmidt, A., Barry, K., & Fleming, M. (1995). Detection of problem drinkers: the alcohol use disorders identification test (AUDIT). *Southern Medical Journal, 88*(1), 52.

Schonfeld, L., King-Kallimanis, B., Duchene, D., Etheridge, R., Herrera, J., Barry, K., et al. (2009). Screening and brief intervention for substance misuse among older adults: The Florida BRITE Project. *American Journal of Public Health, 99*(7), 1–7.

Schonfeld, L., Rohrer, G., Zima, M., & Spiegel, T. (1994). Alcohol abuse and medication misuse in older adults as estimated by service providers. *Journal of Gerontological Social Work, 21*(1), 113–126.

Sheikh, J., & Yesavage, J. (1986). Geriatric Depression Scale (GDS): recent findings and development of a shorter version. *Clinical Gerontologist, 5*(2), 165–173.

Simoni-Wastila, L., & Strickler, G. (2004). Risk factors associated with problem use of prescription drugs. *American Journal of Public Health, 94*(2), 266–268.

Simoni-Wastila, L., & Yang, H. (2006). Psychoactive drug abuse in older adults. *American Journal of Geriatric Pharmacotherapy, 4*(4), 380–394.

Skinner, H., Holt, S., & Israel, Y. (1981). Early identification of alcohol abuse: 1. Critical issues and psychosocial indicators for a composite index. *Canadian Medical Association Journal, 124*(9), 1141.

Solomon, K., Manepalli, J., Ireland, G. A., & Mahon, G. M. (1993). Alcoholism and prescription drug abuse in the elderly: St. Louis University grand rounds. *Journal of the American Geriatrics Society, 41*(1), 57–69.

Speer, D., & Bates, K. (1992). Comorbid mental and substance disorders among older psychiatric patients. *Journal of the American Geriatrics Society, 40*(9), 886.

Spitzer, R. L., & Williams, J. B. (1985). *Structured Clinical Interview for DSM-III (SCID)*. New York, NY: Biometrics Research Division, New York State Psychiatric Institute.

Tobias, C., Lippmann, S., & Pary, R. (1989). Dementia in the elderly. *Postgraduate Medicine, 86*(6), 97.

Vestal, R., McGuire, E., Tobin, J., Andres, R., Norris, A., & Mezey, E. (1977). Aging and ethanol metabolism. *Clinical Pharmacology and Therapeutics, 21*(3), 343.

Wagman, A., Allen, R., & Upright, D. (1977). Effects of alcohol consumption upon parameters of ultradian sleep rhythms in alcoholics. *Advances in Experimental Medicine and Biology, 85*, 601.

Watson, Y., Arfken, C., & Birge, S. (1993). Clock completion: an objective screening test for dementia. *Journal of the American Geriatrics Society, 41*(11), 1235.

CHAPTER

13 Assessment and Conceptualization of Sexuality Among Older Adults

Linda R. Mona[1], Gali Goldwaser[2], Maggie L. Syme[3], Rebecca P. Cameron[4], Colleen Clemency[5], Aletha R. Miller[6], Larry Lemos[7], Michelle S. Ballan[8]

[1] *Long Beach Healthcare System, Long Beach, CA, USA,*

[2] *PTSD and Stress-related Disorders, Research Service (151), VA San Diego Healthcare System, San Diego, CA, USA,*

[3] *VA Boston Healthcare System, Psychology Service, Boston, MA, USA,*

[4] *Psychology, California State University, Sacramento, CA, USA,*

[5] *Edith Nourse Rogers Memorial Veterans Hospital, Bedford, MA,*

[6] *Deer Oaks Mental Health Associates-Behavioral Health Organization, Fort Worth, TX, USA,*

[7] *Community Living Center, VA Long Beach Healthcare System, Long Beach, CA, USA,*

[8] *Columbia University School of Social Work, New York, NY, USA*

INTRODUCTION

Mental health practitioners and researchers have recently begun to focus on the sexual experiences and physically intimate relationships of older adults as important topics for assessment, psychotherapy, and investigation. This recent change has been brought about by two main factors. Clinicians have been called to examine personal beliefs about diversity and multiculturalism and to more seriously consider age as an important aspect of diversity throughout an individual's lifespan (Hays, 2001). There has also been an increase in ease around discussing sexuality over the past 10 years that has been brought forth by broadened public perceptions about an individual's right to sexual pleasure, more flexible thinking about gender roles and identities, and increased attention to the intimate lives of sexual minorities (i.e., people with disabilities, transgendered individuals, and intersexed people) (Garnets & Peplau, 2006; Mona et al., 2009; Wierzalis, Barret, Pope, & Rankins, 2006). The reality is that many older adults enjoy satisfying and vibrant sexual lives. However, the unique psychological and physiological factors that affect intimate relationships and physical sexual expression change as individuals age. Furthermore, these changes can significantly influence level of sexual satisfaction and the meaning of sexual experiences.

The literature suggests that a majority of older adults are engaged in intimate relationships and regard sexuality as an important part of life. Lindau and colleagues (2007) found that frequency of sexual activity reported by older adult respondents who were sexually active was similar to that reported among adults 18 to 59 years of age in the 1992 National Health and Social Life Survey (NHSLS) (Laumann, Gagnon, Michael & Michaels, 1994). Interestingly, frequency of sexual activity among older adults decreased only minimally with increasing age through age 74, despite a high rate of sexual problems (>50%) (Lindau et al., 2007). Thus, getting older and experiencing age-related physiological

Handbook of Assessment in Clinical Gerontology. DOI: 10.1016/B978-0-12-374961-1.10013-2

and biological changes does not equate with a decrease in sexual activity. Instead, it appears that older adults are simply facing shifts in their experiences with sexual expression and their subjective evaluation of intimate relationships.

This chapter will address the sexual lives of older adults from various psychological, physiological, and diversity perspectives. We begin this exploration by highlighting significant social, political, and medical advances that have shaped the pursuit of sexual satisfaction for older adults. Next we consider age as a diverse factor and further examine the ways in which other multicultural experiences affect the sexual experiences of older adults. A significant portion of the chapter is devoted to a review of the varying contexts in which sexual assessments might be completed with older adults, including suggestions for assessment measures and strategies that clinicians could utilize with this unique population. The intent of this section is to aid the reader in the development of broader case conceptualizations for sexual functioning and to provide guidance in choosing measures for use with older adults. We close the chapter with a case study highlighting a comprehensive approach to psychosexual assessment. Older adults are living fulfilling sexual lives and experiencing sexual expression differently due to age-related changes. Mental health professionals are therefore called to pay attention to this important life experience and to prioritize and conduct clinical sexual assessment in a comprehensive and ethically responsive manner.

OLDER ADULT SEXUALITY AND CURRENT TIMES

Older adults of the early 21st century have experienced many extraordinary events and participated in the shaping and evolution of society throughout their lifespan. There have been key social and political events, major advances and changes in health care, and economic fluctuations and adversities that have required adaptation and resilience from this generation. This sociopolitical environment has in turn shaped older adults as a cohort, including their sexual beliefs and behaviors, as well as how society views older adult sexuality.

The sexual lives of older adults have undoubtedly been affected by changes in the health care arena. Significant health care advances have led to improved physical health and increased longevity. According to recent statistics, average life expectancy in the United States is 78.1 years (U.S. Census Bureau, 2009). The growth of the long-term care industry has coincided with these changes, as older adults are living longer and many need some form of assistance in their older age. A congressional report given by the U.S. Health and Human Services and U.S. Department of Labor (2003) reported that an estimated 15 million Americans received long-term care services in 2000, both in community and institutional settings. Further, it was reported that a projected 27 million Americans will need long-term care services by 2050. As increased numbers of older adults require care, challenges for families arise such as the shifting of roles when younger cohorts become involved in health care decision-making and caregiving. The way sexuality is expressed will likely need to be negotiated in situations where the older adult is not completely independent and may be bound by rules, beliefs, and attitudes of an institution or residence in which they receive care (Hajjar & Kamel, 2004). Furthermore, it is essential for providers to recognize and understand the degree to which gender-specific factors may influence sexual health and sexual expression of older adults.

WOMEN, AGING, AND FACTORS AFFECTING SEXUAL FUNCTIONING

A recent global study of women aged 40–80 found that 43% had at least one problem with sexual functioning (Laumann et al., 2005). Several concerns are commonly reported, such as lack of interest in sexual activities, difficulty achieving orgasm, dyspareunia and other sexual pain disorders, partner's health and sexual functioning (Addis et al., 2006; Kaiser, 2003; Laumann, Glasser, Neves, & Moreira, 2009), lack of partner (DeLamater & Sill, 2005; Meston, 1997), and psychological issues such as body image and sexual self-esteem (DeLamater & Sill, 2005; Nusbaum, Helton, & Ray, 2004). Several factors are involved in the manifestation of these issues for older adult women, including physiological, psychological, and social contributions.

Physiological Factors

A primary influence on sexual functioning is the change in hormones that women experience after menopause. Post-menopausal effects on the endocrine system include an almost complete cessation of principal estrogen, which affects blood flow, atrophy of the vaginal wall, vaginal narrowing, and decreases in lubrication. The resultant impact on sexual activities may include fewer and weaker muscle contractions, decreasing the intensity or presence of orgasm, as well as increased vaginal dryness, which can cause painful intercourse. Also, lowered levels of testosterone have been implicated in decreased libido for older adult women (DeLamater & Sill, 2005; Kaiser, 2003; Walsh & Berman, 2004). Estrogen and testosterone medications, including oral and topical agents, as well as lubricating products, have been used as treatment options. Research has also found that women who maintained regular sexual activity prior to and up to menopause had less marked changes (Kaiser, 2003).

Good health is associated with increased sexual activity, improved sexual functioning, and more liberal sexual attitudes in older adults (Johnson, 1996; Lindau et al., 2007). For older adult women, the physical health and sexual functioning of their partners also affects their own level of sexual activity and functioning (Nusbaum, Singh, & Pyles, 2004). The presence of chronic and other medical conditions such as degenerative and rheumatoid arthritis (DeLamater & Sill, 2005; Kaiser, 2003), diabetes, hyper/hypotension, myocardial infarction, stroke, kidney disease, cancer, and spinal cord injury (Cohen & Alfonso, 1997; DeLamater & Sill, 2005; Kaiser, 2003; Walsh & Berman, 2004) is often associated with decreased sexual activity and impaired sexual functioning. Additionally, many medications have sexual side effects, which have been reported more often in older adults than in the general population (Wade & Bowling, 1986 as cited in DeLamater & Sill, 2005), including antihypertensives, antiandrogens, steroids, antidepressants, and mood stabilizers. In addition to medication side effects, specific medical conditions are either specific to or differentially affect women, including hysterectomies and gynecological and breast cancers. Surgical and other medical treatments to either remove or treat part of the sexual anatomy have both a physical (e.g., post-surgical pain, lower estrogen levels inducing vaginal dryness and atrophy) as well as a psychological impact (body image, sexual self-esteem, depression) (Kagan, Holland, & Chalian, 2008; Kaiser, 2003; Meston, 1997).

Psychological Factors

For a significant number of older adult women, medical treatment does not suffice due to psychosocial factors, implicating a need to look beyond the medical model of assessment and treatment (DeLamater & Sill, 2005; Walsh & Berman, 2004). For example, body image is inexorably linked to sexual interest, participation, and satisfaction in women. The natural changes in the body as a result of aging (e.g., graying of hair, facial and body wrinkles) may be viewed as unattractive and affect a woman's desire and interest in sexual activity, depending in part on her beliefs about sex and aging and/or her previous level of self-esteem (Kingsberg, 2000). Conditions such as incontinence, or the loss of or alterations in sexual anatomy (e.g., mastectomy) can add to body image concerns and should be addressed when appropriate (Tannenbaum, Corcos, & Assailan, 2006).

Attitudes and beliefs about sex are also imperative to address with older adult women. Many of today's older adults were socialized to view sex as a reproductive act and masturbation and/or sex outside marriage as unacceptable. The research is beginning to document a shift in this perspective as older and younger women tend towards equally liberal sexual attitudes (Nussbaum et al., 2004). Currently, older adult women tend to report significantly less interest, participation, and satisfaction in activities, such as masturbation, oral sex, erotic reading and movies, and sexual daydreams, when compared to their male counterparts (Johnson, 1996). Understanding a client's attitudes is critically important to treatment planning because interventions may involve prescribing behaviors that are outside her comfort zone.

Social Factors

Another phenomenon affecting older adult women is the lack of intimate partners (DeLamater & Sill, 2005; Lindau et al., 2007; Meston, 1997). Across age groups of older adults, women are less likely to be partnered, and the gender disparity widens with increased age. A recent national study reported that only 38.4% of women over the age of 75 were partnered, compared to 72% of their male contemporaries (Lindau et al., 2007). Presence of a partner may be connected to sexual activity in that only 4% of older adult women who were unpartnered were sexually active, while 22% of their unpartnered male counterparts reported engaging in sexual activities (Lindau et al., 2007). When considering low rates of sexual engagement of unpartnered females, potential explanatory factors may include attitudes about sex without an identified marital partner, limited range of intimate activities in older adult women, sexual self-esteem and body image, grief and other mood disturbances due to loss of partner, and/or loss of physical functioning.

MEN, AGING, AND FACTORS AFFECTING SEXUAL FUNCTIONING

Since the introduction of Viagra® in 1998, widespread attention has been placed on the "epidemic" of male sexual dysfunction. As a result, changes in the male sexual experience that had previously been viewed as normative have been increasingly pathologized (Pesce, Seidman, & Roose, 2002). In the past decade, the Viagra® boom has led to the identification of a worried-well population, as men aged 18–45 are the fastest growing consumers of pharmaceutical interventions for erectile dysfunction (ED; Marshall, 2006). Despite the increasing numbers of clients with concerns about sexual dysfunction and/or decreased sexual desire, a recent study by Kontula and Haavio-Mannila (2009) indicated that almost two-thirds of men reported no frequent problems with erection, even at the age of 70. As a result, for the older male client presenting with concerns of sexual functioning, close attention in an assessment should be placed on physiological, psychological, and social factors related to their identified problem.

Physiological Factors

As men age, a variety of changes occur that affect the male sexual response. Older men may experience reduced libido, frequency in morning erections, penile sensitivity, arousal, and ejaculation volume or force, as well as prolonged plateau phases and refractory periods (Pesce et al., 2002). Increased attention in the past decade has been placed on the role of testosterone in the older male sexual experience. In adulthood, testosterone is associated with the maintenance of sexual functioning, mood, libido, and anabolic effects on bone and muscle (Gooren, 2006). Andropause, or late onset hypogonadism (LOH), is the decline of testosterone with increasing age (Gooren, 2006; Morley et al., 2000). Medical research has noted considerable variability in the amount of testosterone lost over the course of one's life and how this impacts functioning (Gooren, 2006; Morley et al., 2000). Healthy men experience a gradual decline of 30% in plasma testosterone levels between the ages of 25 and 75, and considerably larger declines in these levels have been observed in men with chronic illness (Gooren, 2006). As a result, it is imperative that men presenting with concerns of sexual dysfunction be assessed both medically and psychologically.

In addition to normative or pathological declines in testosterone, health concerns in the older adult male are frequently a reason for sexual inactivity. In fact, one-third of older men report that illness has disturbed their sex life (Kontula & Haavio-Mannila, 2009). Chronic illnesses such as diabetes, hypertension, arthritis, and prostate disease, and the treatments associated with these illnesses have been shown to contribute to reduced sexual desire and/or ED (Kontula & Haavio-Mannila, 2009). In a study by DeLamater and Sill (2005), hypertension and enlarged prostate were negatively correlated with sexual desire. Anticoagulants and hypertensive medications were additionally related to low sexual desire, but medications for cardiovascular disease and elevated cholesterol were not significantly correlated with desire.

Psychological Factors

Attitudes towards sexual activity and general mental health have frequently been found to be predictors of sexual desire and activity (DeLamater & Sill, 2005; Kontula & Haavio-Mannila, 2009; Pesce et al., 2002). In addition to age, Kontula and Haavio-Mannila (2009) found that the strongest predictors of sexual activity were high sexual self-esteem, good health, active (and positive) sexual history, frequent alcohol use, and finding sex important in a relationship. Men who believe that sexual activity is important to their overall quality of life are significantly more likely to disagree with the concept that sex is only for young people (DeLamater & Sill, 2005).

The complex interaction of mental disorders, treatments for mental disorders, and ED has additionally been noted (Pesce et al., 2002). It does appear that depression and anti-depressant medications may lead to sexual dysfunction (reduced libido, ED, delayed orgasm, anorgasmia), and erectile problems may have serious emotional and psychological effects (Marshall, 2006; Pesce et al., 2002). It is estimated that approximately one-third of men experiencing ED meet criteria for a psychiatric diagnosis, most commonly affective disorders (Pesce et al., 2002). Additionally, men with sexual concerns frequently have subsyndromal depression and anxiety (Pesce et al., 2002). Likewise, up to 75% of depressed clients report decreased libido as a symptom of their mental health concerns. It is clear that both medical and psychiatric factors that may be contributing to ED must be appropriately assessed in order to best ensure the appropriate treatment is delivered.

Social Factors

Similarly to their female counterparts, the presence of a regular sexual partner is the greatest predictor of frequency of sexual activity in older male adults (Kontula & Haavio-Mannila, 2009). Because men are more likely to have a partner than women, they often report more frequent sexual activity in adulthood, with one-fourth of men reporting weekly sexual activity at the age of 70 (Kontula & Haavio-Mannila, 2009). Interestingly, DeLamater and Sill (2005) found that in contrast to women, the presence of a partner is not associated with greater desire in older men. According to this study, men preserve their level of sexual desire as they age regardless of partner status.

Kontula and Haavio-Mannila (2009) also examined the impact of length of relationship on sexual activity frequency and desire. In relationships lasting longer than 40 years, one-third of men report weekly sexual encounters whereas 14% reported that they had not had sex in the past year (Kontula & Haavio-Mannila, 2009). Thirty-five percent of men (compared to 20% of women) in relationships lasting over 40 years indicated a desire for more frequent sexual intercourse in their relationship. Additionally, in contrast to the popular view that longer relationships would be related to lower levels of desire as men get "bored" with their partners, only one-fourth of men in relationships lasting more than 40 years reported lower desire. These relationships were additionally regularly faced with difficulties in sexual functioning and increasing illness as partners aged (Kontula & Haavio-Mannila, 2009).

RECENT ADVANCES IN PHARMACOTHERAPY FOR SEXUAL DISORDERS

Since the first edition of this book (Zeiss, Zeiss, & Davies, 1999), significant advances in our understanding of pharmacological treatment options for sexual dysfunction in older adults have been made. With the discovery and subsequent release of phosphodiesterase type 5 (PDE5) inhibitors, effective treatment options for some sexual disorders, mainly male ED, have become increasingly available in the United States and Europe. Since the initial release of sildenafil citrate (Viagra®) in 1998, two more effective PDE5 inhibitors (i.e., Levitra® and Cialis®) have been released and are all considered to be well tolerated and effective (i.e., decreasing symptoms of erectile dysfunction) treatments for ED. This class of medications has recently been considered for treatment of other sexual disorders, including women's sexual disorders such as female sexual arousal disorder (FSAD), which is characterized by difficulty in obtaining sufficient vaginal lubrication and/or genital swelling, or maintenance of these sexual responses for completion of sexual activity, leading to significant psychosocial distress.

A recent randomized crossover study comparing the efficacy of the three PDE5 inhibitors demonstrated overall equivalence among the three agents (Viagra®, Levitra®, and Cialis®) (Jannini et al., 2009). Although only a small number of studies (e.g., Sipski, Rosen, Alexander, & Hamer, 2000) have been completed examining the effectiveness of PDE5 inhibitors for use with women, some support for the inclusion of these medications into treatment plans for women with sexual disorders has been demonstrated. Moderate levels of effectiveness, such as for treatment of FSAD (Schoen & Bachmann, 2009), have so far been found, including increases in subjective arousal (Sipski et al., 2000), frequency of arousal, fantasies, penile-vaginal intercourse and enjoyment, and overall improvement in sexual health (Caruso, Intelisano, Lupo, & Agnello, 2001). More recent follow-up studies have shown differing, less promising results (e.g., Caruso, Intelisano, Farina, Di Mari, & Angello, 2003). However, some studies also point to the role that PDE5 inhibitors have for women experiencing decreased libido because of the side effects associated with treatment for depression with SSRIs (Nurnberg et al., 2008). The evidence supporting unlicensed use of PDE5 inhibitors in women with sexual disorders remains inconclusive due to contradictory findings across studies (Foster, Mears, & Goldmeier, 2009). As a result, there is the need for further research on the use of PDE5 inhibitors to treat women with sexual dysfunction, particularly for postmenopausal women.

Significant work in the area of hormone replacement therapy (HRT) has been completed during the past ten years, including some large randomized controlled trials (RCTs; Palacios, 2008). The risk/benefit ratio for the use of HRT in men (Stanworth & Jones, 2008) and women (Palacios, 2008), continues to be examined, but most studies point to the sexual health benefits that are obtained from HRT for both men and women. Men's testosterone levels peak somewhere in early adulthood and continue to decline throughout the lifespan, eventually leading to andropause in many men. Such biological changes (e.g., hypogonadism) are associated with decreased sexual desire and ED (Haren, Kim, Tariq, Wittert & Morley, 2006; Swerdloff & Wang, 2004). Older men may benefit from improved sexual health by seeking testosterone therapy alone, or in combination with a PDE5 inhibitor (Greco, Spera, & Aversa, 2006). Menopause and the hormonal changes associated with normal aging also impact women's sexual health, as evidenced by vasomotor and vaginal sexual health-related symptoms including: vaginal dryness; narrowing of the vaginal wall; and delayed response to stimuli. Women can obtain sexual health benefits from treatment with HRT, although much more work needs to be done to elucidate which hormones and combinations of hormones best fit particular individuals to maximize the risk/benefit ratio.

Although the research on the use of PDE5 inhibitors for women lags behind that for men, slowly more research is being conducted testing the efficacy and value of this class of medications for women. We will likely see continued success with these and newer medications in the near future. Additional studies will be needed to demonstrate the safety, tolerance, and efficacy of newer medications with an older adult population. Lastly, with the increasing availability of pharmacotherapy treatment options for sexual dysfunction in older adult men and women, providers working with this population will need to remain up-to-date so as to communicate the most current information possible to their clients.

The complexities of the sexual lives of older adults have been detailed above and serve to illustrate the unique individual, social, and physiological similarities and differences that affect women and men as they age. What is of equal interest is the degree to which other diverse variables play a role in the intimate lives of older adults. That is, how do non-majority identities influence aging and, furthermore, how do multiple diverse factors interact to affect the erotic and romantic lives of older adults? The individual, family, and non-majority social experiences of older adults are reviewed below with particular attention paid to the ways in which clinicians may assess for multiple identities as they begin the process of case conceptualization.

DIVERSITY AND MULTICULTURAL CONSIDERATIONS IN OLDER ADULTS

Given advances in health care interventions and increasing emphasis on disease prevention, the older adult population is rapidly growing and the proportion of ethnic minority older adults is growing at an even faster rate than that of European Americans (Dilworth-Anderson & Cohen, 2009). Although multicultural competence has received increased attention within mental health training programs and service delivery settings in recent years (Hays, 2008), not all forms of diversity are routinely acknowledged. Specifically, recognition of the cultural identities of sexual minorities and people with disabilities often lags behind awareness of ethnic or racial diversity, and our understanding of the interaction among multiple identities (e.g., older adult, bisexual, Asian American) is frequently rudimentary (Hays, 2008). Thus, health care providers must continue to develop their multicultural awareness and competence in order to effectively meet the needs of diverse older adults. Providing multiculturally sensitive *sexual* health care may prove particularly challenging due to providers' potential for bias in light of deep-seated culturally based beliefs and attitudes about sexuality, particularly as it relates to diversity (Mulholland, 2007).

Cultural factors significantly affect sexual health and well-being (Wincze, Bach, & Barlow, 2008). Clinicians must systematically consider the full range of cultural identities and contexts that may affect their clients, including race, ethnicity, immigration status, socioeconomic status, religion, gender and gender identity, sexual orientation, disability status, and age, as well as the interactions among multiple identity statuses, as each of these may affect the client's experience of sexuality, sexual dysfunction, and options for ameliorating sexual problems. Cultural factors were not integrated into psychiatric diagnoses in general (Smart & Smart, 1997) nor assessment of sexual dysfunction in particular (see, for example, Sbrocco, Weisbery, & Barlow, 1995) until recently. In an effort to respond to criticism that the DSM-III and III-R (APA, 1980, 1987) failed to adequately address cultural factors in psychiatric diagnosis, the DSM-IV (APA, 1994) included more attention to cultural factors throughout several areas of the manual (e.g., discussion of cultural features of several disorders, modifications to Axis IV, etc.), and provided a list of culture-bound syndromes and an outline for cultural formulation.

The cultural formulation outline, found in Appendix I of the DSM-IV-TR (APA, 2000), is organized around four broad domains, as well as an overall assessment summarizing the impact of culture on diagnosis and care.

The first domain is cultural identity, which refers to the client's ethnic and cultural reference groups and subgroups; extent of participation in the culture of origin and the larger culture; language proficiency and preference; and the role of culture in development (APA, 2000; Lewis-Fernández & Díaz, 2002). Mona, Romesser-Scehnet, Cameron, and Cardenas (2006) discuss the case of Frank, a Salvadoran American man with cerebral palsy who struggled with various sexual issues. During his marriage, his wife, a Peruvian American, initially rejected penile-vaginal intercourse with him due to her concerns that cerebral palsy was heritable. Once she communicated her reason for avoiding sex, he was able to arrange for a physician to allay her concerns. They went on to develop a sexual relationship, but he never resolved his concerns about the impact of his disability on their sexual interactions, particularly given his perception that he did not live up to Latino cultural ideals of masculine sexuality. Frank's marriage ended and he then received therapy that helped him to begin to integrate and positively reframe his identity as a person with a disability.

Clients with disabilities who have been able to develop a positive disability identity and to connect with facets of disability culture ideals (e.g., acceptance of human differences, willingness to accept help and to assume interdependence, tolerance for uncertainty and imperfect outcomes, an appreciation of humor and the absurd, skills for managing systems) (Gill, 1995) bring significant strengths to the sexual problems that may develop in, or persist into, older age. Mona et al., (2009) presented the case of Annie, a Latina who experienced anxiety about sexual activity following a spinal cord injury. Over time, she developed an appreciation for the flexibility and intimacy possible in her new relationship because the focus of sexual activity was broader and more mutual than it had been in her previous relationships.

Religious traditions provide one important context in which individuals experience their sexuality. Although some religious traditions emphasize the impurity of sex and/or the primary relationship of sexual behavior to procreation, it should not be assumed that a client who is deeply religious shares those views. For example, Bhui and colleagues (1994) discuss the cultural framework that accompanies Islamic and Hindu religious traditions, which they see as generally sex-positive in relation to sex within heterosexual marriage. Sexual pleasure within marriage is highly valued, although prohibitions against masturbation and extramarital sex are also present. Attention to the religious dimensions of cultural views about sexuality is critically important, accompanied as always by an idiographic perspective due to the heterogeneity of beliefs and teachings within broad religious traditions.

The second domain has to do with cultural explanations of illness. This includes the way the client and their social group conceptualize the client's symptoms, the ways in which symptoms and distress are communicated, and the relationship of the symptoms to cultural group norms, including an understanding of what the symptoms mean, how severe they are, and whether they fit a culture-specific syndrome pattern. In addition, culturally based etiological explanations need to be explored, as do the history of and orientation to various forms of treatment (professional and traditional).

Bhui, Herriot, Dein, and Watson (1994) studied ethnically Asian clients along with a matched sample of ethnically English clients at a sex and marital therapy clinic in Britain. Both groups of clients were predominantly male, and most of the Asian clients in their sample were Indian, Pakistani, or Bangladeshi. Bhui and colleagues (1994) did not find demographic differences in education and occupational status or diagnostic differences between the ethnically Asian and British clients. However, Asian clients were more likely to describe their presenting complaint in somatic terms. One case highlighted by Bhui and colleagues (1994) illustrates a basic diagnostic challenge: even a culturally informed diagnosis can be inaccurate when assessment is not thorough! This client was referred by a urology clinic based on a psychological interpretation of his symptoms, which were consistent with a diagnosis of a culture-bound syndrome, dhat (which includes fatigue and anxiety about semen loss). However, it was discovered that his difficulties were associated with a fibrosis of the penis that caused a bend in its shaft when erect, leading to his re-referral to urology.

Within the third domain, the client's social support networks and their role in or relationship to the client's distress and potential for recovery should be evaluated. Roles, expectations, and responsibilities among kin, religious, and other network members need to be understood in light of the client's culture. Examining the culture of sexuality among lesbians, Garnets and Peplau (2006) review research that suggests lesbians masturbate more frequently, engage in erotic communication more readily, and experience orgasm more frequently than heterosexual women. However, they also discuss the controversy about findings that lesbian relationships may involve less frequent sexual behavior over time, and the difficulty in determining whether that is problematic or simply culturally normative. Research reviewed by Garnets and Peplau (2006) suggests that serial monogamy is characteristic of lesbian relationship patterns, and, interestingly, single lesbians appear to be more fully integrated into communities and friendship networks with other lesbians than partnered lesbians. Clinicians need to assess sexual behavior and social embeddedness in light of these and other possible cultural variations that accompany lesbian identity.

The sociocultural context of sexuality for aging gay men as portrayed by Wierzalis et al. (2006) may typically include a desire to continue being sexual, with concomitant concerns about isolation due to the loss of youth, attractiveness, and virility, as well as possible unresolved grief over the loss of friends and lovers to the AIDS epidemic. However, these authors describe a positive developmental trajectory for many gay men who invest in and value the intimacy and connection available in relationships. They note the availability of gay subcultural contexts in which older men are valued, as either objects of sexual desire to younger men or as carriers of cultural wisdom. Important considerations when assessing gay men include attention to cohort effects, particularly the political context of their youth in relation to the gay civil rights movement, and for gay men, lesbians, and bisexuals, an awareness of the clients' developmental history with respect to coming out (Wierzalis et al., 2006).

Lastly, the fourth domain, cultural elements of the relationship between the individual and the clinician, should be considered. This may include relatively straightforward attention to ensuring the availability of interpreters, or the more difficult tasks of understanding the client's experience of the health care interaction, the clinician's awareness of her own culturally based attitudes and expectations, and the avoidance of a stereotype-based formulation of the client. Mulholland (2007) analyzed interview data from 25 White sex therapists who were members of the British Association of Sexual and Relationship Therapy. His findings suggest that White sexual health care providers run the risk of stereotyped thinking about non-White clients that may limit their understanding of the client. He noted a tendency to minimize ethnic differences in favor of viewing gender differences as universal. Additionally, he noted clinicians' attitudes toward non-Western men and women. Specifically, providers expressed ambivalence between viewing women in other cultures as passive and oppressed, but also potentially sexually demanding and powerful. There was a tendency to view men from non-Western cultures as oppressive toward women, which was seen as accompanied by either tremendous responsibility to reproduce and to provide (among Asian men) or by promiscuity in the case of African and Caribbean men. Further, Mulholland (2007) found that therapists attributed generally good sexual satisfaction and health to heterosexuals of African descent, were more nonspecific in their characterization of sexual problems among White British individuals, and saw ethnically Asian men as more likely to suffer from premature ejaculation and masturbation anxieties, whereas ethnically Asian women were seen to experience low libido. Such generalizations may impede clinicians' efforts to consider all possible diagnostic issues; in contrast, an awareness of the natural tendency to generalize and a willingness to go beyond one's expectations can be invaluable. Clinicians need to monitor their own values and belief systems (Davies, Zeiss, Shea, & Tinklenberg, 1998) as well as their potential stereotypes as they undertake sexual assessment of clients of all cultures, but especially when the client/clinician encounter is cross-cultural (including age, ethnicity, etc.).

Ensuring a culturally sensitive therapeutic relationship is challenging, as Lewis-Fernández and Díaz (2002) discuss, emphasizing ethnic matching of client and provider can lead to the assumption that cultural differences are being acknowledged, when in fact the provider's cultural framework may be very different from the client's, despite language or ethnic similarities. Particularly challenging areas include judgment calls about the degree of pathology evidenced by particular symptoms, including, for example, non-traditional sexual practices; creating a therapeutic relationship that is consistent with the client's cultural expectations; and choosing treatment modalities that fit the client's understanding of what will be helpful (Lewis-Fernández & Díaz, 2002).

Finally, the cultural formulation advocates summarizing the overall cultural assessment as it relates to the client's identity, symptoms or syndrome, social context, interaction with the system of treatment and care, and prognosis (APA, 2000). Attention to the cultural formulation as it relates to multiple facets of a client's identity will assist clinicians in providing a thorough and thoughtful analysis of issues that might otherwise be overlooked. Practitioners faced with complex intersections of identity (e.g., configurations of generational, religious, and socioeconomic status) will need to educate themselves about the impact of these statuses on sexuality and sexual health care, while remaining vigilant about their own potential to substitute generalizations for an individualized understanding of the client's experience.

INITIAL STAGES OF ASSESSMENT

Before discussing specific assessment strategies for the older adult population, we would like to highlight treatment setting issues that often create a crucial context for services delivery. Considering the myriad of access points to this population and the diversity of roles and settings for providers including integrated primary care, enhanced-referral systems, and multi- and interdisciplinary team settings, it would be impossible to give universal advice regarding assessment of sexual functioning in older adults. Frequently mental health providers serve as consultants, referral sources, and/or members of a larger team, which may place them in the role of advocate and educator to other professionals and teams. Thus, when advocating for or implementing assessment services, it is important to keep in mind that the type of assessment and the role of the mental health provider will change as a function of the setting.

Primary care is one of the most frequent points of access to health care for older adults. Assessing for healthy sexual functioning in this setting is often overlooked and frequently avoided in this population. Older adults rarely introduce the topic of sexual expression because of beliefs that their problems are a normal process of aging, lack of knowledge about available services/treatment, embarrassment, concerns about providers being disgusted and/or disinterested in their sexual functioning, and a perception that general practitioners hold negative attitudes toward older adult sexuality (Gott & Hinchcliff, 2003; Laumann et al., 2009). Further, physicians often report additional barriers including time constraints, fear of opening the "floodgate" or offending the older adult, lack of training in sexual functioning assessment, and embarrassment (Bartlik, Rosenfeld, & Beaton, 2005; Bonds et al., 2007; Gott, Hinchcliff, & Galena, 2004; Verhoeven et al., 2003). These and other factors contribute to low rates of identification of sexual problems in older adults presenting in primary care settings.

Clinicians can play a significant role in advocating for screening questions and tools to use in an enhanced-referral primary care setting, as well as provide education on how to utilize a permission-giving and trusting style, specifically to clinics, physicians, and/or teams that have a high volume of older adult referrals. In an enhanced-referral setting the physicians, pharmacists, mental health providers, and other team members are not located in the same physical space, but may be part of the same care team and may meet on a semi-regular basis. Changes can be as simple as adding one question aimed at identifying potential sexual functioning problems with a few follow-up questions to rule-in or rule-out medical treatment. Examples include: (1) "What questions or concerns might you have with your sexual functioning?"; (2) "Many of my clients have noticed changes in erections/painful intercourse/sexual functioning. Are you noticing any changes in those areas?"; and (3) "Sexual health is an important part of overall health, and I ask all clients about their sexual functioning. May I ask you some questions about your sexual functioning?" (Hatzichristou, et al. 2004; Sadovsky, 2000).

Mental health providers may also work as part of an interdisciplinary team. For example, they may deliver assessment services in a community setting such as a hospice, nursing home, or other assisted living facilities. Administrators and staff of such settings may have negative attitudes, beliefs, and policies regarding sexual relationships for residents, which create barriers to sexual expression (Drench & Losee, 1996; Hajjar & Kamel, 2004). Families' embarrassment and problematic beliefs about older adult sexuality might also inadvertently hinder sexual expression (Rheaume & Mitty, 2008; Zeiss & Kasl-Godley, 2001). Mental health providers may need to assume the role of advocate for older adult clients, promoting the right to participate in sexual activities, or educating staff and family about older adult sexuality (Rheaume & Mitty, 2008; Zeiss & Kasl-Godley, 2001). Assessment of intimate relationships and sexuality can be easily incorporated into the facility's intake interview under the psychosocial or social support sections. If the clinician is an active participant on the interdisciplinary team and routinely sees all clients, this can be integrated into their assessment process, as described above for primary care settings. As with an enhanced-referral primary care setting, mental health providers should educate staff as necessary about questions to ask, referral services available, and permission-giving and trusting styles of communication. Sexuality assessment in a long-term care facility has specific considerations and should include areas such as privacy of information and proposed activities, types of assistance needed for desired activities, and capacity evaluations focused on sexuality.

Assessment of Sexual Consent Capacity in Older Adults

Rationale and Definitions

Assessment in the older adult population often includes the evaluation of capacity, given the prevalence of dementing disorders (e.g., mild cognitive impairment, Alzheimer's disease), neurocognitive threats such as stroke, and other neurodegenerative diseases in this population. According to a *Global Burden of Disease* report released by the World Health Organization in 2000, the occurrence of dementia in adults 65 years and older in the US is 6–10%, with Alzheimer's disease accounting for 50–70% of these cases. Also, an integrative global analysis revealed that rates of dementia begin at approximately 1% for 60- to 69-year-olds and this rate doubles for every five-year increase in age (WHO, 2000).

Capacity is a clinical term referring to a clinician's assessment of an individual's ability to make decisions and perform certain functions within a specific domain (e.g., driving, giving consent to participate in research, testifying). It is essential to understand that the clinician's conclusion about capacity is not a legal finding, but often serves as evidence in a legal proceeding (American Bar Association/American Psychology Association, 2008).

Sexual consent capacity is the ability to voluntarily make a reasoned decision whether or not to engage in sexual activity. There is limited research on this issue among older adults, and a related lack of uniform clinical and legal standards for use in this population. Many existing legal standards have emerged from criminal proceedings involving the developmentally disabled population; consequently, many sexual consent capacity assessment tools have been developed and normed on the developmentally disabled population. The literature on developmentally disabled individuals cannot be generalized to older adults; however, the two areas of research may be able to converge as more studies applying existing assessment standards to older adults emerge (Bogacki, Armstrong, & Stuempfle, 2004; Kennedy, 1999).

The decision whether or not to engage in sexual activities differs from other domains of decisional capacity. One central difference is temporal, in that an older adult choosing whether or not to have a medical procedure or execute a financial decision may have time to weigh the risks and benefits and may consult with others, whereas in a sexual consent scenario the opportunity to consult others and take time to make decisions is often absent. Also, in sexual consent there is no conservator or guardian appointed that can serve as a deputy decision-maker for the individual with diminished capacity (American Bar Association/American Psychology Association, 2008; Kennedy, 1999, 2003; Kennedy & Niederbuhl, 2001). In the case that an individual has been appointed a guardian for other decision-making domains, the concept of limited guardianship serves to protect the individual's autonomy. In fact, many state laws specifically address limiting the guardian in making social and sexual decisions unless the adult is found incapable. Thus, older adults may be considered to have capacity for sexual decision-making even if they have been determined to lack capacity for another area, such as financial decision-making.

Legal and Ethical Standards

Awareness of the legal and ethical standards governing sexual consent capacity is critical when conducting assessments in this area. Constitutional, civil, and criminal law each has an effect on legal rulings in this area, and legal standards vary from state to state (Lyden, 2007; Stavis, 1991). Although there are no universally accepted criteria in the U.S., the majority of state laws regarding sexual consent capacity generally involve three widely accepted elements of capacity (Lyden, 2007). The first is *knowledge* of relevant facts needed to make the decision. Second is the *rationality or mental capacity* to realize and reason through the risks and benefits of engaging or not engaging in sexual activity. The third element is *voluntariness*, which indicates that the older adult can take self-protective measures against coercion when making the decision (American Bar Association/American Psychology Association, 2008; Lichtenberg & Strzepek, 1990; Lyden, 2007; Stavis, 1991). Even states that have not adopted these three elements often use a variation on them, such as requiring only rationality and voluntariness, or adding another requirement such as understanding the moral implications of sexual expression (e.g., Alabama, Colorado, Hawaii, Idaho, and New York).

It is suggested that practitioners consult state guardianship laws regarding capacity, and specifically sexual consent capacity, in order to structure the assessment process in such as way as to satisfy legal standards. Consulting with a legal professional who is familiar with or works with guardianship, conservatorship, and competency cases may be helpful. Once the legal standards have been investigated, it is recommended that clinicians document the relationship of their assessment protocols to the legal elements of capacity set forth by the state.

Clinicians must consider the ethical implications of their approach to sexual capacity assessment. Specifically, when making a clinical decision in sexual consent capacity the clinician is often balancing the ethical principles of: (1) autonomy—Principle E: Respect for People's Rights and Dignity; and (2) protecting the client from harm—Principle A: Beneficence and Nonmaleficence (APA, 2002; Lichtenberg & Strzepek, 1990). Consultation with other professionals, including through state associations and organizations serving older adults, may serve to ensure that ethical requirements related to the assessment process are fulfilled.

Across settings, older adults are affected by the decisions of caregivers, guardians, staff, family, and friends, and may often lack the opportunity and/or ability to advocate for themselves. It is important to understand the organizational context in which the assessment is being undertaken in order to ensure a systemic approach to balancing the client's needs and rights with those of the organization. Clinicians have an important opportunity to protect their older adult clients, as well as to give them a voice when it comes to sexual expression.

Assessment Standards and Considerations

Currently, there is one known assessment tool specifically intended for measuring sexual consent capacity in older adults. Lichtenberg and Strzepek (1990) developed a structured interview aimed at establishing sexual consent capacity with dementia clients in a long-term care facility (Table 13.1). The authors designed the questions to assess: (1) basic cognitive functions (memory, recognition); (2) reasoning and planning skills; (3) affective stability; and (4) social judgment skills. Also, the assessment was structured as a two-part process: (1) asking the client the assessment questions and (2) relaying the client's answers to the interdisciplinary team to gather any feedback and/or behavioral evidence that may be supportive or contradictory. Other attempts to standardize sexual consent capacity have been undertaken by researchers working with individuals with development disabilities (e.g., Kennedy, 1999). As mentioned, these populations are distinct in many ways and the generalizability of these assessment tools for older adults has not been established.

Considerations for sexual consent capacity assessment include whether or not to involve staff, family, and/or interdisciplinary team resources in the assessment process (e.g., adult children, administrative staff, and/or nursing at a long-term care facility). These sources can provide important collateral information, as well as a comforting and familiar presence for the older adult. An emerging concept in the literature is the importance of assessing whether decisions the client makes are consistent with formerly articulated values; collateral information can be particularly helpful in determining the client's longstanding value system. However, collateral sources may serve as a hindrance to the clinician's evaluation and advocacy to the extent they hold negative attitudes toward older adult sexuality and experience discomfort about the possibility of sexual expression in long-term care facilities (Gott & Hinchcliff, 2003; Lyden, 2007; Roach, 2004; Walker & Harrington, 2002).

Other assessment considerations include the use of tools (e.g., manikins, diagrams, videos) and adaptive techniques with older adults who may have difficulties reading, hearing, and/or who may not have full physical functioning. As with other capacity domains, the clinician should view the declaration of capacity or incapacity as a temporary decision and keep in mind the possibility of gaining capacity with further education and/or rehabilitation (American Bar Association/American Psychology Association, 2008; Kennedy, 1999).

Table 13.1 Assessment Guidelines (Lichtenberg & Strzepek, 1990)

1. Patient's Awareness of the Relationship
   a. Is the patient aware of who is initiating sexual contact?
   b. Does the patient believe that the other person is a spouse and thus acquiesce out of a delusional belief, or are they cognizant of the other's identity and intent?
   c. Can the patient state what level of sexual intimacy they would be comfortable with?
2. Patient's Ability to Avoid Exploitation
   a. Is the behavior consistent with formerly held values/beliefs?
   b. Does the patient have the capacity to say no to any uninvited sexual contact?
3. Patients Awareness of Potential Risks
   a. Does the patient realize that this relationship may be time limited (placement on unit temporary, one-time interest, etc.)?
   b. Can the patient describe how they will react when the relationship ends?

Providers may additionally need to be sensitive to the importance of assessing sexual capacity when working with clients without dementia diagnoses. As outlined below, intimacy and sexuality are lifelong needs. For clients at end-of-life with limited physical functioning, providers may need to be sensitive to ethical and legal implications of promoting partner intimacy.

DEATH, DYING, AND SEXUALITY IN OLDER ADULTS

The importance of addressing sexuality at end-of-life is not a new concept, but rather an often overlooked one (Wasow, 1977). It is a widespread assumption that individuals with chronic and/or terminal illnesses have reduced sexual needs, and/or that it would be "abnormal" to have sexual urges when dealing with a life-threatening illness (Mercer, 2008). Even more frequently ignored is sexuality in older adults at the end-of-life, as the limited research on this topic has predominately focused on sexuality and sexual functioning among middle-aged cancer patients. Qualitative studies conducted in the last ten years in hospice settings have included sexuality issues among older adults. In fact, in one study, an 81-year-old male with metastatic lung cancer discussed the importance of his sexual identity and ongoing sexual experiences only four days before his death (Lemieux, Kaiser, Pereira, & Meadows 2004). While the importance of discussing sexuality at end-of-life has begun to receive attention, there is still a paucity of research examining how intimacy is encouraged, facilitated, or assessed during this unique phase of life (Stausmire, 2004).

The assessment of sexuality among individuals at end-of-life can be a difficult topic, and participants in qualitative studies encouraged providers to be sensitive to the timing of their assessment (Lemieux et al., 2004; Stausmire, 2004). In particular, for clients with a newly diagnosed terminal illness, they encouraged providers to wait until after the first round of treatments are over to begin exploring sexual functioning and desire (Lemieux et al., 2004). This sensitivity to timing allows for the client and/or their partners to deal with the immediate needs of treatment and identify potential side effects before re-evaluating and re-establishing intimacy. Illness and aggressive treatment regimens may lead to progressive loss of body function, which may affect energy level, body image, and self-esteem, and may result in the need for a caregiver to assist with activities of daily living (Stausmire, 2004). It is important to recognize that while the *form* of intimacy may change with an individual's progressing weakness at end-of-life, the *importance* of oneself as a sexual being remains stable.

If a partner is available, conducting a sexual assessment conjointly with the client and their partner can be especially helpful. For couples who have experienced a dramatic decrease in their sexual intimacy, it is important to explore the reasons behind this rather than assume it is related to decreased physical functioning. For example, a healthy partner may assume that the dying partner is too ill to engage in intimate sexual acts, or may be concerned about causing pain (Stausmire, 2004). In contrast, the dying partner may view the healthy partner's unwillingness to initiate sexual contact to mean loss of attraction. Such breakdowns in communication may further distance the couple and lead to less frequent intimate contact. Allowing the assessment process to be a place where client and partner can explore the importance of their sexual relationship, how illness/injury has impacted the relationship and the ability to function sexually can promote positive communication and, subsequently, sexual connectivity (Stausmire, 2004).

ASSESSMENT TOOLS AND GUIDELINES

Of primary importance in the assessment of sexual functioning and intimate relationships in older adults is the ability to build rapport and establish a comfortable, non-threatening environment to discuss this often very personal topic. Due to generational factors and individual beliefs about sexuality, older adults may be reluctant to initiate this conversation within a therapy session, and instead look to their providers to lead the discussion. Throughout this section we will identify and describe semi-structured interviews that promote the disclosure of comprehensive sexually related information, in addition to describing various psychometrically supported measures that may serve as a means of supplementing the clinical interview. O'Connor and colleagues (2008) discuss the relative merits of structured interviews versus self-report questionnaires for the assessment of sexual dysfunction in older adults. A comprehensive sexual assessment incorporates both of these methods of assessment thereby enhancing the client/clinician relationship and reducing misinformation acquired during the assessment. Interview data combined with detailed information about sexual behavior and relationship patterns allow respondents to take the needed time to independently formulate and/or expand upon answers to sensitive questions. To date, few measures have been validated on older adults. As a result, some of the measures discussed below are measures of sexual functioning, interest, and attitudes that may have useful application to the older adult community with appropriate modifications.

Various practitioners and researchers have emphasized the importance of assessing both the clients and, if applicable, their partners in order to best ascertain the nature of the presenting concerns (Sbrocco, Weisberg, & Barlow, 1995; Zeiss, Zeiss, & Davies, 1999). According to Sbrocco and colleagues (1995), a large part of the clinical interview should consist of educating clients. In particular, they emphasize the importance of teaching positive communication skills around sexuality, as well as providing education about a realistic understanding of "normal" sexual functioning. For example, many older adults may feel uncomfortable disclosing their masturbation and self-stimulation practices, out of concern that these are abnormal or immoral. The interviewer may put the client at ease by normalizing these practices (after all, almost 99% of the population engages in masturbation practices (Sbrocco et al., 1995)) while eliciting information about the client's history and/or beliefs around masturbation (Sbrocco et al., 1995). These authors encourage interviewers to frame questions in a manner that normalizes sexual activity while providing information and alleviating the client's discomfort about discussing this topic. Sbrocco and colleagues (1995) additionally remind practitioners that it is not uncommon for these interviews to be conducted by providers who are 30—40 years younger than the client. Particularly in training settings, they suggest interviewers remain sensitive to this age discrepancy and normalize client discomfort as applicable (Sbrocco et al., 1995).

A Semi-Structured Interview for Thorough Assessment of Sexual Dysfunction

Zeiss, Zeiss, and Davies (1999) outlined a model for the assessment of sexual functioning among older adults (see Table 13.2). This model provides a solid framework for an initial assessment by examining psychological, medical, social, and cognitive factors in sexual function and dysfunction through open-ended questions. Recent developments, including the increased focus on medical interventions for treatment of sexual dysfunction and an improved understanding among providers of sexuality as a significant component of quality of life, have made it timely to expand on the interview outlined above.

Whereas Zeiss, Zeiss, and Davies (1999) specifically emphasize the importance of avoiding the assumption of heterosexuality and encouraging neutrality towards sexual activity that is often considered socially taboo (e.g., use of sex workers/prostitutes), increased focus should be placed on sensitivity to various diversity issues. For example, when assessing a person with a disability, inquiring specifically about if/how sexual positions are limited and whether the client incorporates assistive devices (e.g., sex toys and other adaptive products) into their sexual encounters may be warranted. Additionally, assessment must include the client's past experiences with pharmacological interventions and openness to explore other options. For example, for an older adult male client who has had limited

Table 13.2 A Semi-structured Interview for Thorough Assessment of Sexual Dysfunction (Zeiss, Zeiss, & Davies, 1999)

1. General Background
   a. Explanation of clinic procedures
   b. Request for explicit, specific information, while providing permission for patient to be uncomfortable
   c. Life situation
      i. Age
      ii. Relationship—status, length, prior relationships, sexual orientation
      iii. Family—kids, living situation
      iv. Work—status, history
   d. Drug and alcohol status
      i. Current use of alcohol, cigarettes, other drugs
      ii. Prior use
   e. Medical situation—very quick review
      i. Major medical problems
      ii. Menopausal status, if female patient, or menopausal status of female partner, if relevant
2. Nature of Sexual Difficulty
   a. Description of problem(s) and current functioning
      i. Desire problems
         1. Sexual thoughts, fantasies, feelings, urges
         2. What percentage of the time is this a problem?
      ii. Excitement phase problems
         1. Erection problems
            a. What percentage of the time is this a problem?
            b. Percent erection obtained typically and maximally
            c. Frequency of attempts
            d. When do problems occur—during which sexual activities? During foreplay? During intromission? Prior to ejaculation? With which partner(s)?
            e. Pain with erection, intromission, or ejaculation
            f. Nocturnal or A.M. erections? Nocturnal emissions?
            g. Erectile experience during masturbation
         2. Lubrication/vasocongestion problems
            a. What percentage of the time is this a problem?
            b. Percent lubrication, labia engorgement obtained typically and maximally
            c. Frequency of attempts
            d. When do problems occur—during which sexual activities? During foreplay? During intromission? Prior to ejaculation? With which partner(s)?
            e. Pain with intercourse
            f. Experience during masturbation
      iii. Orgasm phase problems
            a. Rapid ejaculation
               i. Frequency of sexual activity; any changes in frequency?
               ii. Duration of erection until ejaculation
               iii. Duration of intercourse/sexual activity
               iv. Behavior after ejaculation (patient's and partner's)
               v. Masturbation frequency and style
               vi. What influences latency until ejaculation
            b. Lack of orgasm
               i. Aroused during foreplay? Intercourse? Other sexual activity?
               ii. Percent of time orgasmic with partner and typical timing when orgasmic
               iii. Percent of time orgasmic in masturbation; typical timing when orgasmic
               iv. If uncertain regarding orgasm, ask if experience is pleasant: How would you describe your sensations during arousal? When are you having an orgasm?
               v. How relationship with partner affects the problem

Table 13.2 A Semi-structured Interview for Thorough Assessment of Sexual Dysfunction (Zeiss, Zeiss, & Davies, 1999) *Continued*

Note: Questions about any other sexual problems, such as vaginismus, dyspareunia, or sexual aversion, should follow the same pattern: describe current functioning in detail and examine what currently influences the occurrence of the problem

- a. History of the problem
  - i. Baseline sexual functioning
    1. When was the last period of sexual function with no major problems?
    2. What was the pattern of activity at that time—frequency, partner(s), type of sexual activities, etc.?
  - ii. Pattern of onset
    1. Gradual vs. abrupt
    2. What aspects of the problem changed first (e.g., if erection, was percent of typical erection or percentage of time able to get erection first affected?)
    3. Circumstances on first occasion(s)
    4. If there are multiple problems, what was the sequence of onset, e.g., if erection or orgasm problems, did they precede or follow desire problems in onset?
    5. If erection or orgasm problems could be resolved, what is patient's expectation of likely desire level?
  - iii. How does the couple handle the problem?
  - iv. What have they tried to resolve the problem?
  - v. Any upsetting experiences caused by the problem (intra-psychic or between the couple; e.g., is the identified patient distressed/depressed as a consequence of the sexual problem?
- b. Causal beliefs and goals (this section is vital; do not omit)
  - i. Patient's and partner's beliefs about causes of the problem
    1. Primary hypotheses
    2. Other possible contributing factors
    3. Openness to a multifactorial explanation
  - ii. Goals
    1. Do not assume the goal is the opposite of the problem—ask what the patient's goals are. How much change in quality of life does the patient expect if sexual problems are resolved?
    2. How do the patient's goals match the goals of his/her partner (if there is one)?
  - iii. Current attitudes and beliefs
    1. The purpose of this section is to find out
       - a. Current sexual values and behaviors
       - b. The degree of integration of segregation of sex from other aspects of the patient's life
       - c. What areas might be particularly difficult for him/her/them to change
    2. Current attitudes toward sex
       - a. General attitudes, concern re: "normalcy"
       - b. Positive/negative/neutral feelings about: genital area, menstruation, vaginal/penile secretions, masturbation, oral-genital contact, foreplay, intercourse, manual stimulation to orgasm, sexual fantasy
       - c. Beliefs about partner's attitudes re: a and b above
       - d. Beliefs about sex and aging
       - e. Should men and women have different roles in sexual activities? Nonsexual activities? Patients' views on sex-specific roles compared to his/her current situation
       - f. Conflicts between attitudes about sex and those of peer groups, religion, partner(s)
       - g. Place of sex in patient's relationship: how important?
  - iv. Current behavior (some of this is redundant. Pursue according to nature of problem and clarity of information already derived from other questions. Some repetition is useful to check reliability and to allow patients to share some information they may not have recalled earlier)
    1. Relationship with primary partner, if relevant
       - a. Feelings about the relationship: positives and negatives
       - b. Physical and non-physical expression of affection in relationship

(*Continued*)

Table 13.2 A Semi-structured Interview for Thorough Assessment of Sexual Dysfunction (Zeiss, Zeiss, & Davies, 1999) *Continued*

c. Partner's health status
d. Is divorce or separation a possibility?
e. Impact of sexual problems on relationship
f. Communication: Generally; about difficult or conflictual topics; specifically about sex
g. Patterns of sexual initiation
h. Other problem areas
i. Use of contraception, if relevant
j. If partner not present, will he/she come in? Discuss in details, emphasizing the importance of couples' interview as next step

2. Sexual activity with partners other than a primary partner
   a. Group rules in the primary relationship, if relevant
   b. Occurrences of intimacy and sexual activity
   c. Experience of the presenting problem in relationships other than a primary relationship
   d. Gender of other partners
   e. Safe sex practices
3. Activity with partner of gender opposite from primary orientation, whether patient has a primary partner or not (e.g., same-sex sexual activity if patient presents as heterosexual; heterosexual activity if he/she presents as homosexual)
   a. Sexual experiences with non-primary gender: fantasies and behaviors
   b. Feelings about these experiences
   c. Safe sex practices

success with Viagra® and other medical interventions, examining the client's willingness to try a penile pump or a penile ring may provide the client with more options for achieving an erection. Finally, assessment of cultural factors is needed to facilitate a comprehensive understanding of how diverse factors may or may not be significant to the meaning of sexual functioning and experiences.

The Derogatis Interview for Sexual Functioning (DISF/DISF-SR)

The Derogatis Interview for Sexual Functioning (DISF; Derogatis, 1997) is a 25-item semi-structured interview designed to assess multidimensional sexual functioning in both men and women. As described by Meston and Derogatis (2002), this measure is comprised of five domains: sexual cognition/fantasy; sexual arousal; sexual behavior/experience; orgasm; and sexual drive/relationship. The DISF has an additional self-report version of the interview, the DISF-SR, which is similarly constructed. These measures were initially normed on community samples aged 19–64. As a result, the appropriateness of using this measure with older adults experiencing sexual dysfunction has not yet been determined. The structured interview does provide a useful and comprehensive framework for gaining insight into the nature of a client's complaints in order to inform treatment planning and intervention, and developing norms for older adults is essential for its clinical utility in this population.

Sexual Beliefs and Information Questionnaire (SBIQ-R)

The Sexual Beliefs and Information Questionnaire (SBIQ-R; Adams et al., 1996) was developed to determine whether lack of information regarding sexuality and sexual functioning might impair performance and satisfaction among aging males and their female partners. Normed on 271 older male veterans and 116 female partners referred for treatment of sexual dysfunction to a psychology department in a rural area, the SBIQ-R was demonstrated to be internally consistent ($\alpha = 0.82$). Male participants who were administered this survey were an average of 56.6 years old (*SD* = 14.13), and their female counterparts were an average of 52.9 years old (*SD* = 17.16). The SBIQ-R consists of five domains including: time/patience; stress/pressure; aging; sexual satisfaction; and miscellaneous/basic knowledge. Initial examination of the scale revealed that most participants had adequate knowledge of sexual functioning as a whole; however, a large percentage held erroneous views about the ability to have a sexually satisfying relationship without intercourse. Participants additionally had incorrect or incomplete knowledge of the role of hormones in impotence. Studies examining the effectiveness of psychoeducation regarding sexual function and communication among partners demonstrated that individual results on the SBIQ-R are sensitive to change over time (Adams et al., 1996). The complete SBIQ-R is provided in Table 13.3.

Table 13.3 Sexual Beliefs and Information Questionnaire (SBIQ-R; Adams et al., 1996)

For each of these items, circle "T" if you think the statement is true, circle "F" if you think it is false, and circle "?" if you are not sure. Some of the questions do not have one right or wrong answer. The answers you choose will help us understand how you feel or what you think is right.

1.	T	F	?	The penis must be totally erect before a man can have an orgasm (climax) and ejaculate
2.	T	F	?	A couple can have a good sexual relationship even if they never have their orgasm (climax) at the same time
3.	T	F	?	A condom (rubber) protects against pregnancy and many diseases
4.	T	F	?	Lubrication (getting wet) in the female shows sexual excitement like the erection does in the male
5.	T	F	?	Anal sex without a condom increases the possibility of getting a sexual disease
6.	T	F	?	Masturbation by either a man or a woman is a sign that something is wrong with his or her sex life
7.	T	F	?	Sex problems often occur because men and women are too embarrassed to tell their partner what stimulation they need to get aroused
8.	T	F	?	Most women are able to be sexually satisfied even if their partner cannot maintain an erection
9.	T	F	?	Deep in the vagina is the most sensitive area of the woman's sexual organs
10.	T	F	?	The larger the penis the more physically satisfying it is to the woman during intercourse
11.	T	F	?	If a couple cannot have intercourse, there is no way for them to have a satisfying sexual relationship
12.	T	F	?	Erections in healthy older men are often not as hard as in healthy younger men
13.	T	F	?	As a man gets older, his orgasm (climax) and ejaculation may become less powerful or he may not ejaculate at all on some occasions
14.	T	F	?	After middle age, some women may need a longer time to get aroused and may need to use lubricant to have sex without discomfort
15.	T	F	?	As a man gets older, his penis usually requires much more touching and a longer time to get erect
16.	T	F	?	Stress and fear of failure can cause a man to lose his ability to get or maintain an erection
17.	T	F	?	Drinking and smoking have no effect on a man's sexual abilities
18.	T	F	?	Most men begin to experience some erection problems by the time they reach their 40s or 50s

(Continued)

Table 13.3 Sexual Beliefs and Information Questionnaire (SBIQ-R; Adams et al., 1996) *Continued*

19.	T	F	?	A couple's sex life can often be improved by taking more time to please the other both in and out of bed
20.	T	F	?	Most of the time impotence is the result of the man not having enough male hormones
21.	T	F	?	Sexual pleasure without intercourse is against my religion
22.	T	F	?	Sex for most people is not like in the movies—it takes time and effort
23.	T	F	?	Some medications can cause men to have problems with erections
24.	T	F	?	A man or woman should always be ready to have intercourse if the partner wants it
25.	T	F	?	If a man or woman is not able to have intercourse, it is best for the couple to avoid all physical affection.

The Aging Sexual Knowledge and Attitudes Scale (ASKAS)

The Aging Sexual Knowledge and Attitudes Scale (ASKAS; White, 1982) was designed to assess sexual attitudes and informational knowledge among older adults, people who work with older adults, and families of older adults (White, 1982). The scale consists of 61 items including 35 true/false questions that measure knowledge of sexuality among older adults and 26 seven-point Likert-type items that assess the respondent's attitudes (described as permissiveness) towards sexuality in older persons. Initially normed on older adults in nursing homes and the community, nursing home staff, and families of older adults, split—half, alpha and test—retest reliabilities for older adults were all in the acceptable range (0.90, 0.91, and 0.97, respectively, on knowledge items and 0.83, 0.76, and 0.96, respectively, on attitude items). White (1982) suggests the use of the ASKAS among clinicians who are interested in exploring how information known to and attitudes held by older adults may serve to exacerbate their experience of sexual dysfunction.

Overall, the assessment of sexual functioning in older adults requires a delicate approach in order to promote the development of rapport, provide practical education, make an accurate diagnosis, and offer the most fitting treatment options. It is our view that a comprehensive assessment necessitates a thorough clinical interview and supplemental measures that are interpreted in light of available empirical support. The clinical interview provides clients an opportunity to explore topics and concerns that may not have been previously discussed with other providers, and can provide practitioners with clinical information not readily available in psychometric scales. Likewise, inclusion of appropriate quantitative measures may provide more detailed information about client functioning, attitudes, and knowledge not otherwise addressed in an interview. In the last ten years, there has been an increased focus on the development of validated assessment measures for sexual functioning. Continued work is needed to develop and validate appropriate measures with older adults. Older adults presenting with concerns related to sexual functioning are complex, diverse individuals, and their needs and problems are unique. As a result, it is imperative that interviewers take time to understand the client in the context of their individuality, personal and relationship history, and presenting concerns.

Case Study

Teresa and Joe present for an initial psychotherapy assessment session indicating, "We just don't do it anymore! Sex used to be a regular and good part of our marriage and now it never seems to happen and when it does happen, we don't enjoy it the way we have in the past." The couple, Teresa, age 72, and Joe, age 78, report that they have been married for 50 years and had originally met through friends at a Catholic Church event. Teresa stated that they dated for one year before getting married and then approximately two years after being married they had their first child. The couple has four children. Joe and Teresa identify as having "different backgrounds" from each other, explaining that Teresa was born in El Salvador, to a family with few monetary resources, while Joe was born in the United States to middle class African American parents. Even though both members of the couple identified as having different ethnic, cultural, and socioeconomic backgrounds, both strongly reported that the Catholic faith was important in their lives growing up and at present. Teresa's health has been fairly good throughout most of her life with the exception of late-onset diabetes about two years ago. She has been able to manage this condition with the proper medication. Joe has had difficulties with high blood pressure for over 20 years and also manages this condition with medication. Joe indicates that, "Sex has always been an exciting part of our relationship, but it doesn't seem like my wife is interested anymore. And, when she is, my body doesn't always cooperate the way that I would like." Teresa agrees with Joe's account of their difficulty with this aspect of their relationship. Both members of the couple would like to "go back to having more sex and enjoying it the way that it used to be." Both Teresa and Joe are retired; Teresa worked as high school teacher for many years while Joe worked as an engineer for an aerospace company for over 40 years.

Teresa and Joe posed a unique challenge for the clinician as they presented a complex and diverse picture. A thorough clinical interview was an essential tool and helped the clinician, along with the couple, to elucidate key issues that contributed to the diagnostic and conceptual process. The semi-structured interview outlined by Zeiss, Zeiss, and Davies (1999) was selected for this case as it covers several important domains: psychological; medical; social; and cognitive factors in sexual function and dysfunction. The clinician also considered the four domains of cultural formulation outlined in the DSM-IV-TR when conducting the assessment (APA, 2000). Specifically, the cultural formulation guided the clinician to consider the following four areas. First, the clinician approached the interview with sensitivity to domains of diversity such as each individual's racial/ethnic background, religion, and socioeconomic status. Cultural explanations of sexual functioning and sexual problems were also explored with the couple, which addressed the second domain of cultural formulation. The potential impact of the couple's social network and the expectations that go with the roles they play within those systems were also examined in order to attend to the third domain. Finally, the clinician concentrated on becoming aware of his or her own beliefs and attitudes about sexual expression in older adults, as well as background factors that may have affected interactions with the couple. The four domains were woven into the assessment process and aided the clinician in developing a more culturally informed conceptualization and treatment.

As mentioned, a fundamental task for the clinician was to establish a safe and comfortable environment in order to facilitate rapport building. Sexuality, for some, can be a sensitive subject, and although Teresa and Joe appear to be at ease talking about their sexual lives, there are multiple factors that surfaced and influenced rapport. To increase the likelihood of developing a comfortable rapport, the clinician utilized concepts consistent with contextually focused therapies (e.g., Feminist Therapy) that included establishing a non-hierarchical relationship with the couple by directly addressing issues of power in the therapeutic relationship, elucidating the assessment process, and directly collaborating with them to form the goals of the assessment. Also, a key component of developing a therapeutic relationship with Teresa and Joe was normalizing their experiences and providing them with education about sexual functioning across the lifespan and particular issues relevant to their situation.

To more directly address the presenting issues, the clinician utilized an open and encouraging style allowing for candid discussion of the problems Teresa and Joe have been experiencing. Questions were presented in an open-ended manner, helping to elicit a richer narrative including the various sexual difficulties experienced by the couple. When examining the nature and history of the couple's sexual issues, the Derogatis Interview for Sexual Functioning (DISF; Derogatis, 1997) was a useful semi-structured inventory, particularly because its design targeted toward both partners in a relationship facilitated assessment of the current level of sexual functioning in both Teresa and Joe. The DISF provided additional information regarding sexual cognition/fantasy, sexual arousal, sexual behavior/experience, orgasm, and sexual drive/relationship. The clinician also had the option to more specifically tailor the assessment by administering the self-report version (DISF-SR) to both Teresa and Joe.

Both Teresa and Joe reported medical issues that are known to affect sexual functioning. A follow-up was conducted in order to gather more detailed information such as onset, symptom severity, any functional impairment in daily activities, and specific medications they were each taking. For Teresa, the clinician focused on information about diabetes and talked with the couple about its impact on vascular and hormonal health, which can affect blood flow, muscle contraction, estrogen production, and other key functions for female sexual health. For Joe, the clinician asked further questions about the degree to which his hypertension has been addressed clinically, knowing that this and other vascular conditions are highly correlated with erectile function and desire, and may be particularly relevant to his current issues.

Given the couple's age and various health conditions and medications that may affect cognition, it was essential to incorporate basic memory and thought processing questions within the context of the intake. Cognitive functioning of both Teresa and Joe was explored first with brief questions such as, "Have you had any difficulties with remembering things like names and places?" or "Have you noticed that you have been forgetting things that you would usually remember?" Neither Teresa nor Joe endorsed issues with cognitive function; however, if they had, it would be imperative to pursue this further with screenings and potentially further testing to address issues related to capacity to consent to sexual activities.

An integral area to assess is the psychological impact of aging on sexual functioning. Teresa and Joe had questions and concerns for the clinician about body image and loss of physical functioning. Other issues that might arise in the future for this couple include caregiving and potentially loss of a partner. The clinician also asked questions that concern the couple's beliefs and attitudes about sex, as this often plays an important role in the sex lives of older adults. This was also a time to inquire about past sexual scripts, sexual behaviors that are "off limits" for the couple, and approach more sensitive issues such as monogamy, relationship rules, and safer sex practices. The clinician also focused on what Teresa and Joe want for the future of their relationship, including physical and emotional aspects of intimacy.

After the comprehensive assessment was completed, a treatment plan was developed in collaboration with the couple. This included a referral to a sex therapist who is experienced with older adults, as the couple decided to pursue therapy. It was also recommended that Teresa and Joe discuss changes in physical functioning and sexual activity with their physicians, given that they have comorbid medical issues. The clinician thoroughly discussed any referrals and recommendations with the couple so that they have the opportunity to ask questions, voice any concerns, and understand their role in the next steps of treatment.

References

Adams, S. G., Jr., Dubbert, P. M., Chupurdia, K. M., Jones, A., Jr., Lofland, K. R., & Leermakers, E. (1996). Assessment of sexual beliefs and information in aging. Couples with sexual dysfunction. *Archives of Sexual Behavior, 25*(3), 249–260.

Addis, I. B., Van Den Eeden, S. K., Wassel-Fyr, C. L., Vittinghoff, E., Brown, J. S., & Thom, D. H. Reproductive Risk Factors for Incontinence Study at Kaiser (RRISK) Study Group. (2006). Sexual activity and function in middle-aged and older women. *Obstetrics and Gynecology, 107*(4), 755–764.

American Bar Association/American Psychological Association. (2008). *Assessment of Older Adults with Diminished Capacity: A Handbook for Psychologists*. Washington, DC: Author.

American Psychiatric Association. (1980). *Diagnostic and Statistical Manual of Mental Disorders* (3rd ed.). Washington, DC: Author.

American Psychiatric Association. (1987). *Diagnostic and Statistical Manual of Mental Disorders* (3rd ed., rev.). Washington, DC: Author.

American Psychiatric Association. (1994). *Diagnostic and Statistical Manual of Mental Disorders* (4th ed.). Washington, DC: Author.

American Psychiatric Association. (2000). *Diagnostic and Statistical Manual of Mental Disorders* (4th ed., text rev.). Washington, DC: Author.

American Psychological Association. (2002). *Ethical Principles of Psychologists and Code of Conduct*. Washington. DC: Author.

Bartlik, B. D., Rosenfeld, S., & Beaton, C. (2005). Assessment of sexual functioning: sexual history taking for health care practitioners. *Epilepsy and Behavior, 7*, 15–21.

Bhui, K., Herriot, P., Dein, S., & Watson, J. P. (1994). Asians presenting to a sex and marital therapy clinic. *International Journal of Social Psychiatry, 40*(3), 194–204.

Bogacki, D. F., Armstrong, D. J., & Stuempfle, P. (2004). The Social Sexual Awareness Scale (SSAS): development and validation of an instrument to measure capacity to consent to high risk sexual behavior. *American Journal of Forensic Psychology, 22*(2), 5–38.

Bonds, D. E., Ellis, S. D., Weeks, E., Lichstein, P., Burke, K., & Posey, C. (2007). Patient attitudes toward screening. *North Carolina Medical Journal, 68*(1), 23–29.

Caruso, S., Intelisano, G., Farina, M., Di Mari, L., & Angello, C. (2003). The function of sildenafil on female sexual pathways: a double-blind, cross-over, placebo-controlled study. *European Journal of Obstetrics and Gynecology and Reproductive Biology*, *110*, 201–206.

Caruso, S., Intelisano, G., Lupo, L., & Agnello, C. (2001). Premenopausal women affected by sexual arousal disorder treated with sildenafil: a double-blind, cross-over, placebo-controlled study. *BJOG*, *108*, 623–628.

Cohen, M. A., & Alfonso, C. A. (1997). A comprehensive approach to sexual history-taking using the biopsychosocial model. *International Journal of Mental Health*, *26*(1), 3–14.

Davies, H. D., Zeiss, A. M., Shea, E. A., & Tinklenberg, J. R. (1998). Sexuality and intimacy in Alzheimer's patients and their partners. *Sexuality and Disability*, *16*(3), 193–203.

DeLamater, J. D., & Sill, M. (2005). Sexual desire in later life. *Journal of Sex Research*, *42*(2), 138–149.

Derogatis, L. R. (1997). The Derogatis Interview for Sexual Functioning (DISF/DISF-SR): an introductory report. *Journal of Sex and Marital Therapy*, *23*, 291–304.

Dilworth-Anderson, P., & Cohen, M. D. (2009). Theorizing across cultures. In V. L. Bengston, D. Gans, N. M. Pulney, & M. Silverstein (Eds.), *Handbook of Theories of Aging* (2nd ed., pp. 487–498). New York, NY: Springer.

Drench, M. E., & Losee, R. H. (1996). Sexuality and sexual capacities of elderly people. *Rehabilitation Nursing*, *21*(3), 118–123.

Foster, R., Mears, A., & Goldmeier, D. (2009). A literature review and case reports series on the use of phosphodiesterase inhibitors in the treatment of female sexual dysfunction. *International Journal of STD and Aids*, *20*, 152–157.

Garnets, L., & Peplau, L. A. (2006). Sexuality in the lives of aging lesbian and bisexual women. In D. Kimmel, T. Rose, & S. David (Eds.), *Lesbian, Gay, Bisexual, and Transgender Aging* (pp. 70–90). New York, NY: Columbia.

Gill, C.J. (Fall, 1995). A psychological view of disability culture. *Disability Studies Quarterly*. Retrieved Feb. 24, 2004 from http://www.independentliving.org/docs3/gill1995.html

Gooren, L. (2006). The characteristics of late-onset hypogonadism, its prevalence, symptoms and diagnosis. *Journal of Men's Health and Gender*, *3*(2), 187–191.

Gott, M., & Hinchliff, S. (2003). Barriers to seeking treatment for sexual problems in primary care: a qualitative study with older people. *Family Practice*, *20*(6), 690–695.

Gott, M., Hinchliff, S., & Galena, E. (2004). General practitioner attitudes to discussing sexual health issues with older people. *Social Science and Medicine*, *58*, 2093–2103.

Greco, E. A., Spera, G., & Aversa, A. (2006). Combining testosterone and PDE5 inhibitors in erectile dysfunction: basic rationale and clinical evidence. *European Urology*, *50*, 940–947.

Hajjar, R. R., & Kamel, H. K. (2004). Sexuality in the nursing home, part 1: Attitudes and barriers to sexual expression. *Journal of the American Medical Directors Association*, *5*(2), 42–47.

Haren, M. T., Kim, M. J., Tariq, S. H., Wittert, G. A., & Morley, J. E. (2006). Andropause: a quality-of-life issue in older males. *Medical Clinics of North America*, *90*, 1005–1023.

Hatzichristou, D., Rosen, R., Broderick, G., Clayton, A., Cuzin, B., & Derogatis, L., et al. (2004). Clinical evaluation and management strategy for sexual dysfunction in men and women. *Journal of Sexual Medicine*, *1*(1), 49–57.

Hays, P. (2001). *Addressing cultural complexities in practice: a framework for clinicians and counselors*. Washington, DC: American Psychological Association.

Hays, P. (2008). *Addressing cultural complexities in practice: assessment, diagnosis, and therapy* (2nd ed.). Washington, DC: American Psychological Association.

Jannini, E. A., Isidori, A. M., Gravina, G. L., Aversa, A., Balercia, G., & Bocchio, M., et al. (2009). The ENDOTRIAL study: a spontaneous, open-label, randomized, multicenter, cross-over study on the efficacy of sildenafil, tadalafil, and vardenafil in the treatment of erectile dysfunction. *Journal of Sexual Medicine*, *6*(9), 2547–2560.

Johnson, B. K. (1996). Older adults and sexuality: a multidimensional perspective. *Journal of Gerontological Nursing*, *22*(2), 6–15.

Kagan, S. H., Holland, N., & Chalian, A. A. (2008). Sexual issues in special populations: geriatric oncology—sexuality and older adults. *Seminars in Oncology Nursing*, *24*(2), 120–126.

Kaiser, F. E. (2003). Sexual function and the older woman. *Clinics in Geriatric Medicine*, *19*, 463–472.

Kennedy, C. H. (1999). Assessing competency to consent to sexual activity in the cognitively impaired population. *Journal of Forensic Psychology*, *1*(3), 17–33.

Kennedy, C. H. (2003). Legal and psychological implications in the assessment of sexual consent and the cognitively impaired population. *Assessment*, *10*(4), 352–358.

Kennedy, C. H., & Niederbuhl, J. (2001). Establishing criteria for sexual consent capacity. *American Journal on Mental Retardation*, *106*(6), 503–510.

Kingsberg, S. A. (2000). The psychological impact of aging on sexuality and relationships. *Journal of Women's Health and Gender-Based Medicine*, *9*(1), 33–38.

Kontula, O., & Haavio-Mannila, E. (2009). The impact of aging on human sexual activity and sexual desire. *Journal of Sex Research*, *46*(1), 46–56.

Laumann, E. O., Gagnon, J. H., Michael, R. T., & Michaels, S. (1994). *The Social Organization of Sexuality: Sexual Practices in the United States* (P. 88). Chicago, IL: University of Chicago Press.

Laumann, E. O., Glasser, D. B., Neves, R. C. S., Moreira, E. D., Jr., & Global Study of Sexual Attitudes and Behaviors (GSSAB) Investigators' Group. (2009). A population-based survey of sexual activity, sexual problems and associated help-seeking behavior patterns in mature adults in the United States of America. *International Journal of Impotence Research*, *21*, 171–178.

Laumann, E. O., Nicolosi, A., Glasser, D. B., Paik, A., Gingell, C., Moreira, E., Wang, T., & Global Study of Sexual Attitudes and Behaviors (GSSAB) Investigators' Group. (2005). Sexual problems among women and men aged 40–80: prevalence and correlates identified in the Global Study of Sexual Attitudes and Behaviors. *International Journal of Impotence Research*, *17*(1), 39–57.

Lemieux, L., Kaiser, S., Pereira, J., & Meadows, L. M. (2004). Sexuality in palliative care: patient perspectives. *Palliative Medicine*, *18*, 630–637.

Lewis-Fernández, R., & Díaz, N. (2002). The cultural formulation: a method for assessing cultural factors affecting the clinical encounter. *Psychiatric Quarterly*, *73*(4), 271–295.

Lichtenberg, P. A., & Strzepek, D. M. (1990). Assessments of institutionalized dementia patients' competencies to participate in intimate relationships. *Gerontologist*, *30*(1), 117–120.

Lindau, S. T., Schumm, P., Laumann, E. O., Levinson, W., O'Muircheartaigh, C. A., & Waite, L. J. (2007). A study of sexuality and health among older adults in the United States. *New England Journal of Medicine*, *357* (8), 762–774.

Lyden, M. (2007). Assessment of consent capacity. *Sexuality and Disability*, *25*, 3–20.

Marshall, B. L. (2006). The new virility: Viagra, male aging, and sexual function. *Sexualities*, *9*(3), 345–362.

Mercer, B. (2008). Interviewing people with chronic illness about sexuality: and adaptation of the PLISSIT model. *Journal of Clinical Nursing*, *17*(11c), 341–351.

Meston, C. M. (1997). Aging and sexuality. *Western Journal of Medicine*, *167*, 285–290.

Meston, C. M., & Derogatis, L. R. (2002). Validated instrument for assessing female sexual function. *Journal of Sex and Marital Therapy*, *28*, 155–164.

Mona, L. R., Romesser-Scehnet, J. M., Cameron, R. P., & Cardenas, V. (2006). Cognitive-behavioral therapy and people with disabilities. In P. Hays, & G. Y. Iwamasa (Eds.), *Culturally Responsive Cognitive-Behavioral Therapy: Assessment, Practice, and Supervision* (pp. 199–222). Washington, DC: American Psychological Association.

Mona, L. R., Cameron, R. P., Goldwaser, G., Miller, A. R., Syme, M. L., & Fraley, S. S. (2009). Prescription for pleasure: exploring sex positive approaches in women with spinal cord injury. *Topics in Spinal Cord Injury Rehabilitation*, *15*, 15–29.

Morley, J. E., Charlton, E., Patrick, P., Kaiser, F. E., Cadeau, P., McCready, D., & Perry, H. M. (2000). Validation of a screening questionnaire for androgen deficiency in aging males. *Metabolism*, *49*(9), 1239–1242.

Mulholland, J. (2007). The racialisation and ethnicisation of sexuality and sexual problems in sex therapeutic discourse. *Sex and Relationship Therapy*, *22*(1), 27–44.

Nurnberg, H. G., Hensley, P. L., Heiman, J. R., Croft, H. A., Debattista, C., & Paine, S. (2008). Sildenafil treatment of women with antidepressant-associated sexual dysfunction. *JAMA*, *300*(4), 395–404.

Nusbaum, M. R. H., Helton, M. R., & Ray, N. (2004). The changing nature of women's sexual health concerns through the midlife years. *Maturitas*, *49*, 283–291.

Nusbaum, M. R. H., Singh, A. R., & Pyles, A. A. (2004). Sexual healthcare needs of women aged 65 and older. *Journal of the American Geriatrics Society, 52*, 117–122.

O'Connor, D. B., Corona, G., Forti, G., Tajar, A., Lee, D. M., & Finn, J. D., et al. (2008). Assessment of sexual health in aging men in Europe: Development and validation of the European Male Ageing Study Sexual Function Questionnaire. *Journal of Sexual Medicine, 5*, 1374–1385.

Palacios, S. (2008). Advances in hormone replacement therapy: making the menopause manageable. *BMC Women's Health, 8*, 22.

Pesce, V., Seidman, S. N., & Roose, S. P. (2002). Depression, antidepressants and sexual functioning in men. *Sexual and Relationship Therapy, 17*(3), 281–287.

Rheaume, C., & Mitty, E. (2008). Sexuality and intimacy in older adults. *Geriatric Nursing, 29*(5), 342–349.

Roach, S. (2004). Sexual behaviour of nursing home residents: staff perceptions and responses. *Journal of Advanced Nursing, 48*(4), 371–379.

Sadovksy, R. (2000). Integrating erectile dysfunction treatment into primary care practice. *American Journal of Medicine, 109*(9A), 22–28.

Sbrocco, T., Weisberg, R. B., & Barlow, D. H. (1995). Sexual dysfunction in the older adult: assessment of psychological factors. *Sexuality and Disability, 13*(3), 201–218.

Schoen, C., & Bachmann, G. (2009). Sildenafil citrate for female sexual arousal disorder: a future possibility? *Nature Reviews Urology, 6*, 216–222.

Sipski, M. L., Rosen, R. C., Alexander, C. J., & Hamer, R. M. (2000). Sildenafil effects on sexual and cardiovascular responses in women with spinal cord injury. *Urology, 55*, 812–815.

Smart, D. W., & Smart, J. F. (1997). DSM-IV and culturally sensitive diagnosis: some observations for counselors. *Journal of Counseling and Development, 75*, 392–398.

Stanworth, R. D., & Jones, T. H. (2008). Testosterone for the aging male; current evidence and recommended practice. *Clinical Interventions in Aging, 3*(1), 25–44.

Stausmire, J. M. (2004). Sexuality at the end of life. *American Journal of Hospice and Palliative Care, 21*(1), 33–39.

Stavis, P. F. (1991). Sexual activity and the law of consent. Retrieved March 5th, 2009, from http://www.cqcapd.state.ny.us/counsels_corner/cc50.htm

Swerdloff, R. S., & Wang, C. (2004). Androgens and the ageing male. *Best Practice and Research Clinical Endocrinology and Metabolism, 18*(3), 349–362.

Tannenbaum, C., Corcos, J., & Assalian, P. (2006). The relationship between sexual activity and urinary incontinence in older women. *Journal of the American Geriatrics Society, 54*, 1220–1224.

U.S. Census Bureau, International Population Reports. (2009). An aging world: 2008 (Publication No. P95/09-1). Retrieved from http://www.census.gov/prod/2009pubs/p95-09-1.pdf

U.S. Department of Health and Human Services & US Department of Labor. (2003). The future supply of long-term care workers in relation to the aging baby boom generation: report to congress. Retrieved from http://aspe.hhs.gov/daltcp/reports/ltcwork.htm

Verhoeven, V., Bovijn, K., Helder, A., Peremans, L., Hermann, I., & Van Royen, P., et al. (2003). Discussing STI's: doctors are from Mars, patients from Venus. *Family Practice, 20*(1), 11–15.

Walker, B. L., & Harrington, D. (2002). Effects of staff training on staff knowledge and attitudes about sexuality. *Educational Gerontology, 28*, 639–654.

Walsh, K. E., & Berman, J. R. (2004). Sexual dysfunction in the older woman: an overview of the current understanding and management. *Drugs and Aging, 21*(10), 655–675.

Wasow, M. (1977). Human sexuality and terminal illness. *Health and Social Work, 2*(2), 104–121.

White, C. B. (1982). A scale for the assessment of attitudes and knowledge regarding sexuality in the aged. *Archives of Sexual Behavior, 11*(6), 491–502.

Wierzalis, E. A., Barret, B., Pope, M., & Rankins, M. (2006). Gay men and aging: sex and intimacy. In D. Kimmel, T. Rose, & S. David (Eds.), *Lesbian, Gay, Bisexual, and Transgender Aging* (pp. 70–90). New York, NY: Columbia.

Wincze, J. P., Bach, A. K., & Barlow, D. H. (2008). Sexual dysfunction. In D. H. Barlow (Ed.), *Clinical Handbook of Psychological Disorders: A Step-by-Step Treatment Manual* (4th ed., pp. 615–661). New York, NY: Guilford.

World Health Organization. (2000). Global burden of dementia in the year 2000: summary of methods and data sources. Retrieved from http://www.who.int/healthinfo/statistics/bod_dementia.pdf

Zeiss, A. M., & Kasl-Godley, J. (2001). Sexuality in older adults' relationships. *Generations*, *25*(2), 18–25.

Zeiss, A. M., Zeiss, R. A., & Davies, H. (1999). Assessment of sexual function and dysfunction in older adults. In P. Lichtenberg (Ed.), *Handbook of Assessment in Clinical Gerontology* (pp. 270–296). New York, NY: John Wiley & Sons, Inc.

CHAPTER 14

Nutrition in the Elderly

Kathryn E. Brogan[1], K-L. Catherine Jen[2]

[1] *Department of Nutrition and Food Science and Department of Pediatrics, Wayne State University, Detroit, MI, USA,*

[2] *Department of Nutrition and Food Science Wayne State University Detroit, MI, USA*

INTRODUCTION

Nutrition status is fundamental to the quality of life in the aging person as it is closely associated with an older person's functionality and ability to remain independent. By self report, the top nine chronic health conditions in older persons include hypertension (53.3%), arthritis (49.5%), heart disease (30.9%), any types of cancer (21.2%), diabetes (18.0%), asthma (10.6%), emphysema or chronic bronchitis (10.0%), and stroke (9.3%). Each of these health conditions has nutritional implications (http://www.agingstats.gov/agingstatsdotnet/Main_Site/Data/2008_Documents/tables/Tables.aspx). Early identification of nutritional deficiencies can improve length and quality of years. Additionally, maintenance of a healthy body weight in the face of aging, with the prevention of both underweight and obesity, can reduce the symptoms of chronic health conditions and have a protective effect against mortality (Yan et al., 2004). This chapter will discuss the current nutrition recommendations for the well elderly person, the impact of aging on appetite, the nutrition risks faced by the elderly related to specific chronic diseases, in addition to the influence of medications on food intake and tools for the assessment of nutrition status.

PHYSIOLOGICAL CHANGES ASSOCIATED WITH AGING

As humans age, a series of physiological changes inevitably occur. These changes may lead to reduced appetite and food intake, body weight loss, malnutrition, and a compromised immune system. Table 14.1 summarizes the effects of aging on organ systems.

In the gastrointestinal (GI) tract specifically, the overall aging effects alter the sensory response and GI motility, and decrease muscle strength and digestive enzyme secretions. Ultimately, decreased absorption of both macronutrients (energy) and micronutrients (vitamins and minerals) is seen. The eating process is negatively affected with sensory losses even before the internalization of foods. Sensory losses tend to progress more rapidly after 70 years of age, but can become noticeable around 60 years (Schiffman & Graham, 2000). Decreases in the acuity of eyesight, smell, and taste often lead to deficits in energy consumption with direct associations for impaired protein and micronutrient status. These possible deficiencies impact function and immunity. While chemosensory losses occur naturally with age, certain disease states (such as cancer), medications, surgical interventions, malnutrition and environmental exposure also complicate the situation.

Along with taste impairments, dentition can greatly influence consumption. Loss of teeth and gum diseases are common in the elderly. These conditions make chewing more difficult and limit the food

Handbook of Assessment in Clinical Gerontology. DOI: 10.1016/B978-0-12-374961-1.10014-4

Table 14.1 Physiological Changes Associated with Normal Aging

Organ System	Aging Effect
Skin	Dryness, wrinkling, mottled pigmentation, loss of elasticity, dilation of capillaries
Head and neck	Macular degeneration, hearing loss
Cardiovascular	Thickening heart wall and valves, increased collagen, increased collagen rigidity, alteration in heart size, decreased elasticity of blood vessels with calcification
Pulmonary	Stiffening of tissue, decreased vital capacity, decrease maximum oxygen consumption, decreased breathing capacity, decreased propulsive effectiveness of cough reflex
Renal	Decreased size, decreased glomerular filtration rate (GFR), decreased renal blood flow, decreased active tubular secretion and reabsorption, decreased renal concentrating ability
Endocrine	Altered circulating hormone levels and actions
Nervous	Decreased sensory perception, decreased muscle response to stimuli, decreased cognition and memory, loss of brain cells
Musculoskeletal	Progressive loss of skeletal muscle, degeneration of joints, decalcification of bone

Adapted from McGee & Jensen (2000), with permission.

choices. Plant-based foods, like fresh fruits and vegetables, are often eliminated from the daily menu. Soft and easy to chew replacement foods are usually low in dietary fibers, making this population more prone to constipation, as well as vitamin and mineral deficiencies. Without the mechanical manipulation of meats available, a large protein and energy source may be missed. In order to prevent teeth loss at a later stage of life, a lifetime of dental hygiene must be practiced. Assessments of nutritional status include routine checks on oral health and, as appropriate, denture evaluation for proper fit.

The swallowing difficulties in the elderly may be a result of the natural aging process and are also highly prevalent in those with neuromuscular diseases or structural abnormalities of the esophagus. Any disordered swallowing, or dysphagia, is defined as difficulty moving food from the mouth to the stomach accompanied by varying levels of aspiration (Easterling & Robbins, 2008). This occurs in 16–22% of persons older than 50 years, 60% of persons in nursing facilities (Firth & Prather, 2002), and in an estimated 45% of institutionalized dementia patients (Easterling & Robbins, 2008). Dysphagia is also associated with increased risk of choking, pneumonia, decreased intake of macro- and micronutrients, dehydration and death. A multidisciplinary team, which includes physician specialists, speech pathologists, nurses, and dietitians, is involved in the evaluation of the individual's ability to ingest different textures and types of foods. The American Dietetic Association published the National Dysphagia Diet (NDD) in order to establish standard terminology and practice applications of dietary texture modification in dysphagia management (National Dysphagia Diet Task Force, 2002). The labeled levels for liquid viscosity in the NDD (Thin, Nectar-like, Honey-like, and Spoon-thick) are acknowledged to be "a commonsense approach" and "a catalyst for more research" (McCullough, Pelletier, & Steele, 2003). Guidelines regarding the four levels of semisolid/solid foods are as follows:

National Dysphagia Diet Semisolid/Solid Food Levels

- NDD Level 1: Dysphagia—Pureed (homogeneous, very cohesive, pudding-like, requiring very little chewing ability)
- NDD Level 2: Dysphagia—Mechanical Altered (cohesive, moist, semisolid foods, requiring some chewing)
- NDD Level 3: Dysphagia—Advanced (soft foods that require more chewing ability)
- Regular: (all foods allowed)

As food moves through the body and begins the process of digestion and absorption, one of the significant changes in the GI system in the elderly is a decrease in the relaxation of the stomach. This results in declining regulation of the satiation system, which is linked to a decrease in nitric oxide and subsequent decrease in the gastric emptying of large meals; leading to an earlier and greater development of fullness (Morley & Thomas, 1999). In addition, circulating concentrations of cholecystokinin (CCK), a GI hormone that signals satiety during digestion, appear to be increased with aging (MacIntosh et al., 2001). The accessory organs (pancreas, gallbladder, liver) and the organs of the GI tract itself (stomach, intestines) produce smaller amounts of enzymes needed for digestion. This results in impaired nutrient absorption leading to energy deficiency in addition to the already reduced intake. Certain specific nutrients are affected more than others by changes in GI function. More than 20% of the population older than 60 years of age may suffer from atrophic gastritis (Park & Johnson, 2006). Inflamed stomach, increased bacteria growth, reduced secretion of hydrochloric acid and intrinsic factors are the characteristics of atrophic gastritis, which will result in reduced appetite and nutrient absorption, such as calcium, iron, zinc, folate, and especially vitamin B12. Vitamin B12 deficiency, also related specifically to a decreased secretion of the *intrinsic factor*, is a common cause of anemia (macrophagic anemia) in the elderly. Deficiencies from poor intakes of iron (from meats) and folate (from green leafy vegetables) will further worsen the anemic status. Calcium deficiency will make the bone fragile and prone to fractures. Reduced gastric motility due to loss of intestinal wall elasticity with aging is also very commonly seen in this population. Resulting constipation not only affects the quality of life, but also decreases appetite.

As humans age, there is a change in body composition. It is common to see older adults losing lean body mass (muscle and skeletal, referred to as sarcopenia) and gaining body fat, even if a person maintains a constant body weight during adult life. Other notable changes include a decrease in intracellular fluid and a change in the distribution of fat stores. All of these changes negatively correlate with altered physiological responses such as reduced cellular capacity to store water, a decline in strength, balance and muscle mass, and increased abdominal obesity. Clinically, older people are predisposed to dehydration, reduced basal metabolism, falls and injury, and central (metabolic syndrome enhancing) weight gain (Brownie, 2006). Due to the changes in body composition, a high waist circumference may be a better predictor for all-cause mortality than a high body mass index and a high waist/hip ratio (Seidell & Visscher, 2000).

Two thirds of the U.S. adult population is either overweight [body mass index (BMI) $>25.0\ \text{kg/m}^2$] or obese (BMI $>30.0\ \text{kg/m}^2$) (Ogden et al., 2006), and the BMI generally increases with age until age 55 years for men and 65 years for women (Cornoni-Huntley et al., 1991). Even though BMI levels over $25\ \text{kg/m}^2$ are a health hazard for adults, particularly those with chronic health conditions, a slightly elevated BMI in the elderly may have some protective effects (Bouillanne et al., 2009). Increased body weight is associated with increased bone mineral density and decreased osteoporosis and hip fracture in older men and women (Felson, Zhang, Hannan, & Anderson, 1993). Weight loss therapy that minimizes muscle and bone loss is recommended for older persons who are obese and who have functional impairments or metabolic complications that can benefit from weight loss (Villareal, Apovian, Kushner, & Klein, 2005).

Unintentional weight loss in the elderly is linked to increased morbidity and mortality (Huffman, 2002). Low food consumption combined with poor appetite and chewing problems are associated with the development of malnutrition (Feldblum et al., 2007). Malnourishment, or undernutrition, is a broad term indicating that the intake of dietary nutrients is less than adequate to sustain health (Furman, 2006). The prevalence of undernutrition in older adults ranges from 5% (Sullivan, 2000) to 85% (Kayser-Jones, 2000) depending on the study's setting, with rates being higher in nursing home residents. Anorexia of aging increases the risk for older persons to develop severe anorexia and weight loss when disease occurs (Morley & Thomas, 1999). In patients with Alzheimer's disease, for example, weight loss correlates with disease progression and a weight loss of at least 5% is a significant predictor of death (White, Pieper, & Schmader, 1998). Diet therapy is often directed at the treatment of protein-energy malnutrition, which may improve the functional capacity in elderly adults with multiple disorders (Akner & Cederholm, 2001).

Social and cultural factors also influence the development of malnutrition in the elderly. Poverty, loneliness, and social isolation are the predominant social factors that contribute to decreased food intake in the elderly (Donini, Savina, & Cannella, 2003). Depression is one of the most common reversible causes of weight loss in elderly persons, accounting for up to 30% of undernutrition in medical outpatients (Wilson, Vaswani, Liu, Morley, & Miller, 1998). Memory-related illnesses like dementia or Alzheimer's can exacerbate malnutrition.

NUTRITION RECOMMENDATIONS FOR OLDER AMERICANS

The 2005 Dietary Guidelines for Americans emphasize a diet rich in both fruits and vegetables; fluids; whole grains; low-fat milk; and foods high in potassium. Further recommendations include decreasing sodium intake, and increasing vitamins B12 and D from fortified foods, supplements or both (www.health.gov/dietaryguidelines). In 2005 the United States Department of Agriculture (USDA) also released an updated Food Guide Pyramid and website MyPyramid.gov as an aid for the general population to interpret and follow these guidelines. In order to meet the increased nutritional needs of the elderly an adaptation known as the Modified MyPyramid for Older Adults (MFGP) was developed by Tufts University and the USDA (Lichtenstein, Rasmussen, Yu, Epstein, & Russell, 2008) (Figure 14.1). The modified MFGP is set up to be used in conjunction with the MyPyramid.gov website. The MFGP attends to the increased nutrient needs in this population that are not addressed by MyPyramid.gov (because recommendations are based on calorie levels and not life stage). Specifically, higher Daily Reference Intakes (DRIs) exist for those 70+ years for vitamins B12, D, and B6, and the mineral calcium. It also addresses the fact that elderly individuals are less likely to utilize the internet.

Current data suggest that the older adult population is at risk for not meeting the nutrients visually emphasized by the MFGP. The recommendations include:

1. Low-fat and non-fat dairy as well as low-lactose and lactose-free forms, which are depicted to increase calcium intakes.
2. Food icons for deeply colored vegetables and fruits and a wide range of food packaging (i.e., frozen, resealable bags) encourage intakes of vitamins E, K, and potassium. Positive health outcomes including bone health, lower blood pressure, and decreased incidence of cardiovascular disease associated with higher fruit and vegetable intakes are emphasized.
3. High-fiber plant-based foods in both fresh and stewed/canned forms provide micronutrient and laxative benefits even if dentition difficulties exist (fiber supplements are not recommended related to risk of decreased gut mineral absorption).
4. A dietary supplement/fortification flag at the top of the MFGP indicates that supplements or fortified foods containing calcium and vitamin D or vitamin B12 may be needed.

Further visual adjustments that address other needs in the elderly include a row of glasses at the base of the pyramid to represent the importance of meeting fluid needs and a second row depicting a variety of age-appropriate physical activities to remind and encourage active lifestyles during the older years.

Another guide emphasizing adequate nutrient consumption is called the Dietary Reference Intakes (DRIs). DRIs for macronutrients for elderly have been established. Table 14.2 lists the DRIs for individuals aged 51 or older and can be used as a guideline for diet planning.

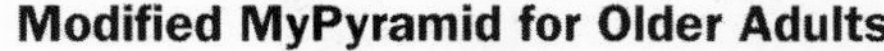

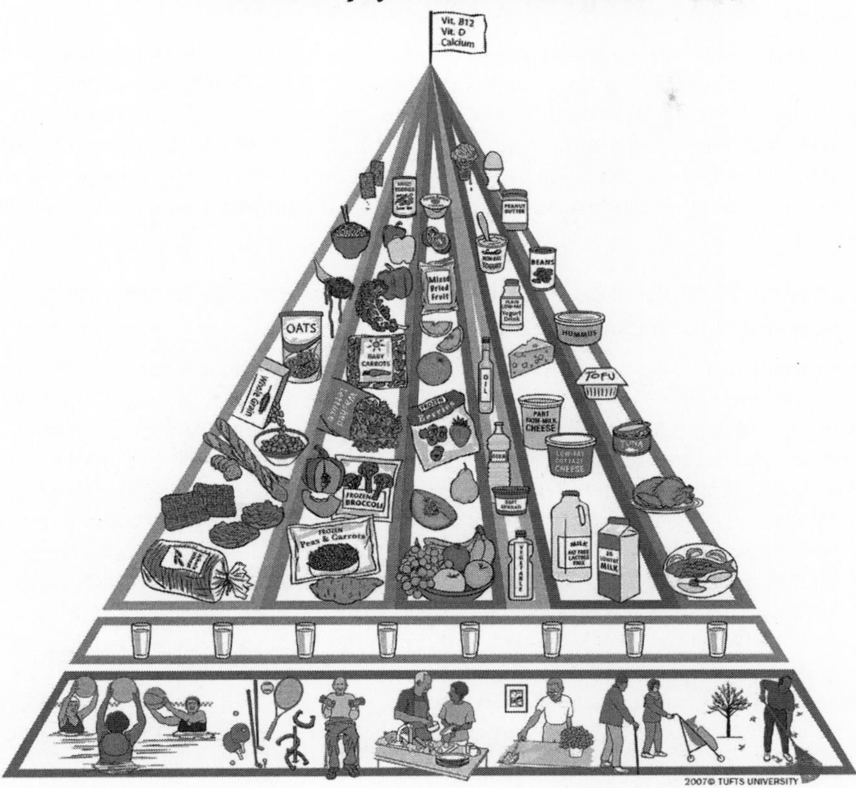

FIGURE 14.1

Modified MyPyramid for Older Adults.

http://nutrition.tufts.edu/docs/pdf/releases/ModifiedMyPyramid.pdf

Table 14.2 Dietary Reference Intakes (DRI) for Macronutrients for Adults Aged 51 Years or Older

				Fat[a] (g)	
Gender and Age (yr)	**Protein (g)**	**CHO (g)**	**Fiber (g)**	**Linoleic Acid**	**α-Linolenic Acid**
Men 51–70	56	130	30	14	1.6
>70	56	130	30	14	1.6
Women 51–70	46	130	21	11	1.1
>70	46	130	21	11	1.1

There is no DRI for total fat intake due to lack of sufficient data. Adequate intake, determined by averaging the observed and experimentally determined approximations, is used for total fat and essential fatty acids.

NUTRITIONAL ASSESSMENT FOR THE ELDERLY

Since poor nutrition and unintentional weight loss are associated with increased morbidity and mortality (Ensrud et al., 2003; Fischer & Johnson, 1990; Huffman, 2002; Newman et al., 2001), it is important to detect the undernourished and/or malnourished elderly before a significant amount of weight has been lost. The American Dietetic Association, the American Academy of Family Physicians and the National Council on Aging have promoted nutritional screening and early nutritional intervention for the elderly in the last two decades. The commonly used nutritional assessment tools include the following.

The Anthropometric Measures, Biochemical Data, Clinical Assessment, Dietary Data and Economic Assessment (the ABCDEs)

1. **Anthropometric data.** Body weight, height, skinfold thickness, and waist circumference provide a general nutritional status of the individual. These data are easy to obtain and can be collected from large populations without much financial burden by trained health care personnel. These data can then be compared to age- and gender-specific standards or previous measures from the same individual (longitudinal measures). The longitudinal measures will reveal the trend of a person's overall health status. Even though obesity is a major health hazard in the general population and in the elderly, weight loss is also common in this population and is associated with reduced functionality and increased mortality (Gazewood & Mehr, 1998; Huffman, 2002). The most frequently reported anthropometric data is BMI, which is based on body weight and height [body weight (kg)/height $(m)^2$]. BMI has been widely used to indicate the disease risks. BMI is classified into the categories as shown in Table 14.3.
2. **Biochemical data.** These measurements are usually obtained from an individual's blood, urine or feces samples. The concentrations of nutrients, metabolic byproducts of these nutrients, as well as hormone and some enzymes, can be measured from these samples. Some commonly used biochemical data include blood or urine glucose (as an indicator for diabetes), blood lipid levels (as indicators for cardiovascular diseases), red blood cell count, hemoglobin level or hematocrit percent (as indicators for anemia), blood urea nitrogen (for kidney function), and stool blood (for colorectal cancer), etc. Medical equipment and trained personnel are required to operate the necessary equipment and interpret the results.
3. **Clinical assessment.** This assessment, performed by health care professionals, examines physical signs of nutrient-related diseases. Every part of the body, such as eyes, hair, neck, fingernails, skin,

Table 14.3 Classification of Overweight and Obesity

			Disease Risk Relative to Normal Weight and Waist Circumference	
	BMI >102 cm	Obesity Class Men <102 cm		
			Women < 88 cm	>88 cm
Underweight	<18.5		–	–
Normal	18.5–24.9		–	–
Overweight	25.0–29.9		Increased	High
Obesity	30.0–34.9	I	High	Very high
	35.0–39.9	II	Very high	Very high
Extreme obesity	≥40.0	III	Extremely high	Extremely high

etc., can provide a clue for nutrient deficiencies or toxicity. Poor wound healing indicates a potential vitamin C deficiency. Prolonged bleeding signals vitamin K deficiency. Trained personnel with knowledge in nutrients and their functions are required to make these observational data accurate.

4. **Dietary data collection to confirm the dietary issues.** All the anthropometric, biochemical, and clinical data only provide a clue for the potential diet-related problems. In order to accurately identify the sources of the health problems, a dietary history is required. There are several assessment methods to obtain dietary records. The most commonly used includes: a 24-hour dietary recall; three-day dietary recalls (two weekdays and one weekend day); and the food frequency questionnaires. The 24-hour recall only provides food items consumed in a 24-hour period, hence deviation to the individual's typical food intake is high. Due to variations in daily intake, a three-day 24-hour recall is more representative of an individual's typical intake pattern. One example of a 24-hour dietary record is shown in Table 14.4.

   The dietary recall is only necessary when the elderly still have the ability to consume ordinary foods by mouth. The recall procedure may pose some difficulties for the elderly. They must be able to see, read, and write in order to record the food items. With the memory loss common in the elderly, the records may not be accurate. Hence, sometimes it is the caregiver's responsibility to record the food intake in order to make the records meaningful. This complication can also decrease the accuracy if the caregiver is overburdened or not present for all eating episodes.

   Food frequency questionnaires ask individuals how many servings of the following foods they consume in a typical day/week/month: breads, cereals or grain products; vegetables; fruits; meat, poultry, fish or alternative protein products; dairy products; fats; oils; and sweets. The Block Food Frequency Questionnaire is the most validated and frequently used questionnaire. The full questionnaire contains 110 questions and takes about 30—40 minutes to complete. The brief version contains 70 questions and takes about 15—20 minutes to complete, although it may underestimate

Table 14.4 Example of a 24-hour Dietary Recall

	Food	Method of Preparation	Method of Cooking or Brand	Amount Consumed
Breakfast	Bread	Whole wheat	Toasted	2 slices
	Butter	Unsalted		1 tablespoon
	Eggs	w/1 T butter	Scrambled	2
Mid-morning snack	Apple		Fresh	1 medium
Lunch	Pepperoni pizza	Thin crust	Tony's	2 slices of a medium pizza
	Soft drink	Regular cola	Faygo	12 oz
Afternoon snack	Chocolate chip cookies	3.5″ diameter	Pepperidge Farm	1 piece
Dinner	Chicken breast	Skin and fat removed	Roasted	½ of a breast
	Broccoli flowerets		Steamed with 1 T butter	1 cup
	Dinner roll	3″ diameter	Baked	1
	Ice cream, vanilla		Eddy's	0.5 cup
Before bed snack	Milk	Skim	Borden's	8 oz

the nutrient intake levels (http://www.nutritionquest.com/products/questionnaires_screeners.htm). The food frequency questionnaire in combination with dietary recall provides a more accurate description of each individual's nutrient intake patterns. The USDA maintains a database for the analysis of food composition (http://www.ars.usda.gov/Services/docs.htm?docid=5720). There are other software programs to be used for diet analysis, such as Food Processor SQL (ESHA Research, Salem, OR).

5. **Economic assessment.** The latest survey in 2007 indicates that 3.6 million elderly (9.7%) are living below the poverty level (http://www.census.gov/prod/2008pubs/p60-235.pdf) and another 2.4 million living at "near-poor" level. Financial condition affects an individual's ability to purchase and prepare foods (Klesges et al., 2001). This is especially important when examining the nutritional status of the elderly because most of the elderly are living on a fixed income and may not be able to afford purchasing fresh fruits or vegetables as well as other high-quality foods.

The Mini Nutritional Assessment (MNA®)

The MNA® (Table 14.5, Guigoz, 2006; Rubenstein, Harker, Salva, Guigoz, & Vellas, 2001; Vellas et al., 2006, reproduced with permission from Nestlé Nutrition Institute, Société des Produits Nestlé SA, Vevey, Switzerland, Trademark Owners) was established in the early 1990s by an international panel of experts for the purpose of establishing an accurate and simple evaluation of the nutritional status in the elderly older than 65 years of age (Guigoz, 2006; Guigoz, Vellas, & Garry, 1994). In the last decade, MNA® has been extensively validated with elderly living in different environments (hospitals, nursing homes, geriatric clinics, community-based nursing program, and physician's office), with a variety of mental capacities, and with different nutritional status (Guigoz, 2006; Guigoz et al., 1994). The MNA® has been translated into different languages and used in countries with Western-style health care settings (Chumlea, 2006). There are two steps in administrating the MNA®. The first step is the short form of MNA® (MNA-SF) which contains six questions and can be completed within 6 minutes. This MNA-SF (questions A to F, below) can be used as a screen tool.

Case Study

Mr Wolfson just recently lost his wife of 52 years. As an 80-year-old widower, he lives alone in an apartment and far from his two adult children and grandchildren. His height is 5 ft and 10 inches and his current weight is 175 lbs, down from 185 lbs three months ago. His calculated BMI is 25.11 kg/m^2. He feels lonely and depressed. Although Mr Wolfson does cook simple dishes, without his wife cooking and eating meals with him, he has lost his appetite. Mr Wolfson also has a history of hypertension and type 2 diabetes. In the last couple of weeks, he has felt lethargic too. His children are concerned about his health status and decided to take him to the doctors for a check-up. Upon entering the office, he was evaluated using the MNA.

The first part of the MNA is for screening purpose. There are six questions:

(A) Question A asks whether the food intake decline over the last three months is due to loss of appetite or physical difficulties. A score of 0 is given when the answer is severe loss of appetite, while a score of 2 is given when there is no change in appetite. Since Mr Wolfson has been eating, but not as much as several months before, he received a score of "1."

(B) Question B deals with weight status, with weight loss of more than 3 kg receiving a 0 and no weight loss receiving a score of 3. Mr Wolfson lost about 10 lbs (4.5 kg), therefore he scored a "0."

(C) Question C concerns mobility with scores from 0 (bed or chair bound) to 2 (goes out). Since Mr Wolfson still goes out once in a while and is mobile, he receives a "2."

(D) Question D deals with psychological stress in the past three months with a yes or no answer. Mr Wolfson has suffered psychological stress due to the loss of his wife; therefore he received "0" for yes.

Table 14.5 The Mini Nutritional Assessment (with permission from Nestlé Nutrition Institute, Vevey, Switzerland)

Nestlé Nutrition INSTITUTE

Mini Nutritional Assessment MNA®

Last name: First name: Sex: Date:

Age: Weight, kg: Height, cm: I.D. Number:

Complete the screen by filling in the boxes with the appropriate numbers.
Add the numbers for the screen. If score is 11 or less, continue with the assessment to gain a Malnutrition Indicator Score.

Screening

A Has food intake declined over the past 3 months due to loss of appetite, digestive problems, chewing or swallowing difficulties?
0 = severe loss of appetite
1 = moderate loss of appetite
2 = no loss of appetite ☐

B Weight loss during the last 3 months
0 = weight loss greater than 3 kg (6.6 lbs)
1 = does not know
2 = weight loss between 1 and 3 kg (2.2 and 6.6 lbs)
3 = no weight loss ☐

C Mobility
0 = bed or chair bound
1 = able to get out of bed/chair but does not go out
2 = goes out ☐

D Has suffered psychological stress or acute disease in the past 3 months
0 = yes 2 = no ☐

E Neuropsychological problems
0 = severe dementia or depression
1 = mild dementia
2 = no psychological problems ☐

F Body Mass Index (BMI) (weight in kg) / (height in m²)
0 = BMI less than 19
1 = BMI 19 to less than 21
2 = BMI 21 to less than 23
3 = BMI 23 or greater ☐

Screening score (subtotal max. 14 points) ☐ ☐
12 points or greater Normal – not at risk – no need to complete assessment
11 points or below Possible malnutrition – continue assessment

Assessment

G Lives independently (not in a nursing home or hospital)
0 = no 1 = yes ☐

H Takes more than 3 prescription drugs per day
0 = yes 1 = no ☐

I Pressure sores or skin ulcers
0 = yes 1 = no ☐

Ref. Vellas B, Villars H, Abellan G, et al. Overview of the MNA® - Its History and Challenges. J Nut Health Aging 2006;10:456-465.
Rubenstein LZ, Harker JO, Salva A, Guigoz Y, Vellas B. Screening for Undernutrition in Geriatric Practice: Developing the Short-Fom Mini Nutritional Assessment (MNA-SF). J. Geront 2001;56A: M366-377.
Guigoz Y. The Mini-Nutritional Assessment (MNA®) Review of the Literature - What does it tell us? J Nutr Health Aging 2006; 10:466-487.

For more information : www.mna-elderly.com

J How many full meals does the patient eat daily?
0 = 1 meal
1 = 2 meals
2 = 3 meals ☐

K Selected consumption markers for protein intake
• At least one serving of dairy products (milk, cheese, yogurt) per day yes ☐ no ☐
• Two or more servings of legumes or eggs per week yes ☐ no ☐
• Meat, fish or poultry every day yes ☐ no ☐
0.0 = if 0 or 1 yes
0.5 = if 2 yes
1.0 = if 3 yes ☐.☐

L Consumes two or more servings of fruits or vegetables per day?
0 = no 1 = yes ☐

M How much fluid (water, juice, coffee, tea, milk…) is consumed per day?
0.0 = less than 3 cups
0.5 = 3 to 5 cups
1.0 = more than 5 cups ☐.☐

N Mode of feeding
0 = unable to eat without assistance
1 = self-fed with some difficulty
2 = self-fed without any problem ☐

O Self view of nutritional status
0 = views self as being malnourished
1 = is uncertain of nutritional state
2 = views self as having no nutritional problem ☐

P In comparison with other people of the same age, how does the patient consider his/her health status?
0.0 = not as good
0.5 = does not know
1.0 = as good
2.0 = better ☐.☐

Q Mid-arm circumference (MAC) in cm
0.0 = MAC less than 21
0.5 = MAC 21 to 22
1.0 = MAC 22 or greater ☐.☐

R Calf circumference (CC) in cm
0 = CC less than 31 1 = CC 31 or greater ☐

Assessment (max. 16 points) ☐ ☐.☐

Screening score ☐ ☐

Total Assessment (max. 30 points) ☐ ☐.☐

Malnutrition Indicator Score
17 to 23.5 points at risk of malnutrition ☐
Less than 17 points malnourished ☐

(E) Question E is related to neuropsychological problems, with a score of 0 meaning severe dementia or depression and a score of 2 meaning no psychological problem. Mr Wolfson received a "0" for severe depression.

(F) Question F is related to body mass index. When BMI is less than 19, a 0 is assigned and BMIs equal to or greater than 23 are scored a 3. Mr Wolfson's BMI is 25.11; therefore he received a "3" for Question F.

For these six screening questions (short form), the maximal score is 14 points. When an individual scores 12 points or more in the screen, there is no concern about the nutritional risk and there is no need to go to step 2 to complete the full length MNA. If the total score is less than 11 points, then a continued assessment in step 2 is indicated, for this individual may be at risk of malnutrition. Mr Wolfson had a total score of 6; therefore he runs the risk of malnutrition and needs to be assessed in step 2 with the full length MNA.

In step 2 (full length, assessment):

(G) Question G asks if the individual lives independently or not. Mr Wolfson received a "1" for living independently.

(H) Question H asks if the individual takes more than three prescription drugs per day. The answer for Mr Wolfson was yes, a "0" was entered into the MNA form.

(I) Question I is related to pressure sores or skin ulcers. Mr Wolfson has none of these; therefore for an answer of "no" he received a "1."

(J) Question J assesses the number of full meals the individual eats daily. Mr Wolfson usually does not eat breakfast with the exception of a glass of juice in the morning. He does eat lunch and dinner each day, even though the serving size is smaller compared to before his wife passed away several months ago. Therefore he scored a "1" for two meals.

(K) Question K asks selected consumption markers for protein intake. Three sub-questions include a yes or no answer:

At least one serving of dairy products (milk, cheese, yogurt) per day?
Two or more servings of legumes or eggs per week?
Meat, fish or poultry every day?

If 0–1 sub-questions are answered "yes" then a score of "0.0" is assigned. If two questions are answered yes, then a score of "0.5" is assigned. If all three sub-questions received a "yes" response then a score of "1.0" is assigned. Mr Wolfson received 0.5 for Question K since he does not consume any dairy products.

(L) Question L addresses whether the individual consumes two or more servings of fruits or vegetables per day. Mr Wolfson consumes more than two servings of vegetables or fruits; therefore he received a "1."

(M) Question M asks how much fluid (water, juice, coffee, tea, milk, etc.) is consumed per day. Mr Wolfson loves to have soup for lunch and drinks a glass of juice each morning. In addition, he drinks a couple cups of tea throughout the day; his score for this question was 0.5 for 3–5 cups (0 = 1–2 cups, 0.5 = 3–5 cups, 1.0 = greater than 5 cups).

(N) Question N deals with mode of feeding, with "0" for unable to eat without assistance, "1" for self-fed with some difficulty, and "2" for self-fed without any problem. Mr Wolfson received a "2" for being able to self-feed without any problem.

(O) Question O explores the self-view of nutritional status. A "0" is entered if the individual views self as being malnourished, "1" for uncertain of nutritional state, and "2" is for viewing self as have no nutritional problem. Since Mr Wolfson is not sure about his nutritional status, he received a "1" for this question.

(P) Question P asks the individual to compare the health status of himself/herself with other people of the same age. A "0" score indicates not as good, "0.5" for does not know, "1.0" for as good, and "2.0" as better than others. Mr Wolfson believes that his health status is as good as others of the same age, so he received a "1.0."

(Q) Question Q measures the mid-arm circumference (MAC) in cm, with "0" for less than 21 cm, "0.5" for between 21 and 22 cm, and "1.0" for 22 cm or greater. Mr Wolfson's MAC was 23 cm, hence he scored a "1.0" for this question.

(R) Question R measures calf circumference (CC). Mr Wolfson received a score of "1" for a CC measurement of 32 cm, greater than the cutoff point of 31 cm.

For the assessment part, Mr Wolfson receives a score of "11.0" out of a potential maximal score of 16. For the total assessment (maximal score of 30 points), his score is 17.

The scoring system is as follows:

- Normal, no risk of malnutrition: equal or greater than 23.5 points
- At risk of malnutrition: 17 to 23.5 points
- Malnourished: less than 17 points

Mr Wolfson's total assessment score was 17. He is at risk of malnutrition. Early nutritional intervention is recommended before protein-energy malnutrition sets in. A dietary history should be obtained by a registered dietitian (RD). Each medication Mr Wolfson is taking should be carefully examined to identify its effects on appetite, smell, and taste, as well as on cognitive function.

Older adults receiving scores less than 17 points require immediate nutritional intervention. The primary care provider and the RD should be consulted in order to calculate the energy needs and to plan a balanced menu which provides adequate energy and nutrients. With this scoring system, MNA detects the malnutrition risks before other physiological alterations are apparent. It can be administered repeatedly to screen the nutritional status and body weight changes in an individual longitudinally. However, it cannot be used as a monitoring tool even though it can be used to re-screen the individuals after a nutritional intervention. It has been recommended to re-screen nursing home residents at risk of malnutrition every three months.

Council on Nutrition Appetite Questionnaire (CNAQ) and Simplified CNAQ (SNAQ)

Unintentional weight loss of 5–10% in the previous 12 months predicts a poor health status and prognosis in elderly patients (Huffman, 2002). Loss of appetite has been shown to be a natural aging phenomenon, especially in men (Morley, 2001), and is one of the causes of unintentional weight loss (Rolland et al., 2006). Therefore, assessing the appetite has become one of the important screen tools. CNAQ is an eight-item questionnaire that has been validated for older adults living in community settings and in long-term care facilities. It was also validated against another validated questionnaire, Appetite Hunger and Sensory Perception Questionnaire (AHSP; Wilson et al., 2005). Due to its length (29 items, with 10 minutes completion time) and complexity, the AHSP has little clinical use (Mathey, 2001). CNAQ, on the other hand, can be completed in about 3 minutes. The answer to each question is scored from 1 (worse) to 5 (best) in a Likert-type scale. The total score for the CNAQ is from 8 to 40. A score of <28 indicates a potential for weight loss of a significant amount. After further validation of the CNAQ, four questions were eliminated due to low reliability, resulting in the Simplified CNAQ (SNAQ, Table 14.6). This four-item questionnaire can be easily administered in the clinician's office. A score of less than 14 identifies early signs of reduced appetite and risk of weight loss in the near future (Wilson et al., 2005). The SNAQ should be a major component of the screening. It should be repeated periodically in order to detect any changes in appetite before significant weight loss occurs.

Geriatric Nutritional Risk Index (GNRI)

Nutrition Risk Index (NRI) is a tool used to identify patients at risk for malnutrition (Buzby, Knox et al., 1988a; Buzby et al., 1988b). The calculation is based on weight, height, and blood albumin levels. Its applicability to the elderly has been limited due to the difficulty in accurately measuring weight and height in this population. Bouillanne et al. (2005) proposed to use ideal body weight in place of the actual body weight. As for the height (H), it is estimated according to the following equations formulated by Chumlea and Guo (1992) using knee height (KH) versus stature, due to the fact that some elderly cannot stand straight, are handicapped, or have very limited mobility.

Table 14.6 Simplified Nutritional Appetite Questionnaire (SNAQ)

Name: ______________________ Sex (circle): Male Female

Age: ____________ Weight: ____________ Height: ____________

Date: ________

Administration Instructions: Ask the subject to complete the questionnaire by circling the correct answers and then tally the results based upon the following numerical scale: a = 1, b = 2, c = 3, d = 4, e = 5. The sum of the scores for the individual items constitutes the SNAQ score. *SNAQ score ≤ 14 indicate significant risk of at least 5% weight loss within six months*

1. My appetite is
   a. very poor
   b. poor
   c. average
   d. good
   e. very good
2. When I eat
   a. I feel full after eating only a few mouthfuls
   b. I feel full after eating about a third of a meal
   c. I feel full after eating over half of a meal
   d. I feel full after eating most of a meal
   e. I hardly ever feel full
3. Food tastes
   a. very bad
   b. bad
   c. average
   d. good
   e. very good
4. Normally I eat
   a. less than one meal a day
   b. one meal a day
   c. two meals a day
   d. three meals a day
   e. more than three meals a day

$$\text{For men: H (cm)} = [2.02 \times \text{KH(cm)}] - [0.04 \times \text{age(y)}] + 64.19$$

$$\text{For women: H (cm)} = [1.83 \times \text{KH(cm)}] - [0.24 \times \text{age(y)}] + 84.88$$

The ideal body weight is calculated using the Lorentz equation (WLo) (Bouillanne et al., 2005):

$$\text{For men: WLo} = \text{H} - 100 - [(\text{H} - 150)/4]$$

$$\text{For women: WLo} = \text{H} - 100 - [(\text{H} - 150)/2.5]$$

The GNRI is then calculated as follows:

$$\text{GNRI} = [1.489 \times \text{albumin(g/L)}] + [41.7 \times (\text{measured weight/WLo})]$$

The resulting GNRI scores are classified into four categories:

- <82, major risk
- 82–92, moderate risk

- 92–98, low risk
- >98, no risk

It should be pointed out that this GNRI requires albumin levels before it can be calculated. Therefore it is an accurate tool to assess the nutritional status and the risk of morbidity and mortality in hospitalized patients. However, for routine clinical evaluation or in a community setting, it may have limited application due to lack of serum albumin data.

Case Study

Mrs Harrington, a 77-year-old woman, broke her hip and is hospitalized for hip replacement surgery. In addition she has been complaining that she has no appetite for food recently and has been losing weight. Currently her weight is at 68 kg and serum albumin level is 35 g/L. Since she has a difficult time standing straight, knee height (50.8 cm) is used to calculate her height.

$$
\begin{aligned}
\text{Height} &= [1.83 \times \text{KH}] - [0.24 \times \text{age}] + 84.88 \\
&= [1.83 \times 50.8] - [0.24 \times 77] + 84.88 \\
&= 92.96 - 18.48 + 84.88 \\
&= 159\ \text{cm}
\end{aligned}
$$

The Lorentz weight (WLo) is calculated:

$$
\begin{aligned}
\text{WLo} &= \text{height} - 100 - ((\text{H} - 150)/2.5) \\
&= 159 - 100 - ((159 - 150)/2.5) \\
&= 159 - 100 - 3.6 \\
&= 55.4\ \text{kg}
\end{aligned}
$$

$$
\begin{aligned}
\text{GNRI} &= (\text{albumin} \times 1.489) + (41.7 \times \text{measured weight/WLo}) \\
&= (35 \times 1.489) + (41.7 \times 68/55.4) \\
&= 52.12 + 61.12 \\
&= 113.24
\end{aligned}
$$

Thus, although Mrs Harrington was losing weight, there was no immediate risk for malnutrition. It is recommended that the same measures be conducted after three months.

AGING AND CHRONIC DISEASE STATES

There is high probability that an elderly adult will, in addition to aging, be suffering the effects of chronic health issues. In the United States, approximately 80% of all persons 65 years of age and older have at least one chronic condition, and 50% have at least two chronic conditions (Goulding, Rogers, & Smith, 2003). Persons aged over 65 years represented just over 12% of the total population in 2006, yet they accounted for more than 30% of the country's health care costs, utilizing more hospital services and consuming more than 40% of all prescription drugs (http://www.agingstats.gov/agingstatsdotnet/Main_Site/Data/Data_2008.aspx). The successful management of a chronic condition can both increase quality of life and decrease medical costs.

Often a nutrition prescription accompanies the medication and treatment plan for an individual with a chronic disease as recommended by the medical care team. These recommendations are frequently restrictive in nature and some can be complex concepts for individuals to learn and follow, regardless of age. Clinical judgment must be used individually in all cases of older adults to determine how aggressively nutrition restrictions should be used to prevent malnutrition and preserve the social enjoyment of eating. A 2005 position paper published by the American Dietetic Association (ADA) states that nutrition in the aging has two primary goals: maintenance of health and promotion of quality of life. The ADA recognizes that liberalization of the diet or nutrition prescription may improve both of these in older adults and advocates the use of qualified dietetics professionals to assess and evaluate the need for medical nutrition therapy in each individual (American Dietetic Association, 2005). The Institute of Medicine also recognizes registered dietitians as the single identifiable group of health care professionals with standardized education, clinical training, continuing education, and national credentialing requirements necessary to be a provider of secondary and tertiary nutrition therapy (http://www.nap.edu/catalog.php?record_id=9741, p. 313). Utilization of this professional resource can greatly aid in determining individual recommendations, education, and implementation; and also demonstrates the complexity in nutritional status when disease states are compounding the aging process. The tools used for assessment of nutritional status have been discussed in the previous section. The next section focuses briefly on selected disease states and nutrition recommendations.

Cardiovascular Diseases

Cardiovascular diseases include atherosclerotic heart disease, hypertension, stroke, and chronic heart failure (previously known as congestive heart failure). In 2006, 34.2% of all deaths were attributed to cardiovascular disease and more than 80 million adults (one in three) have one or more cardiovascular disease symptoms (http://americanheart.org/downloadable/heart/1240250946756LS-1982%20Heart%20and%20Stroke%20Update.042009.pdf). Metabolic syndrome, a clustering of factors including hypertension, hyperglycemia, dyslipidemia, and prothrombotic and proinflammatory state, is also included in this disease arena and has been found to affect over 40% of those aged 60 and older (Ford, Giles, & Dietz, 2002). Healthy older adults can benefit from preventative lifestyle modifications recommended for all individuals over the age of two years barring that they do not limit the provision of adequate nutrients, demonstrated by unintentional weight loss over time. Modifiable risks in this population include the lowering of elevated low-density lipoprotein cholesterol (LDL); increasing depressed levels of high-density lipoprotein cholesterol (HDL), prevention or control of hypertension, avoiding obesity, and not smoking. Lifestyle changes to promote healthy blood lipids are listed in Table 14.7. For those with symptoms or previous surgical interventions, medication and more stringent nutrition guidelines may be recommended.

Hypertension

In the United States, 90% of the 55-year-old normotensive individuals will have hypertension by the age of 75 (Vasan et al., 2002). Over time the elevated pressure in the arteries can harm organs such as the heart, kidneys, brain, and eyes. The Dietary Approaches to Stop Hypertension (DASH) diet has

Table 14.7 Lifestyle Changes to Reduce the Risk of Cardiovascular Disease

To lower LDL and triglycerides:

- Keep the intake of saturated fat and cholesterol low
- Consume foods high in dietary fiber, especially soluble fiber in particular
- Include monounsaturated fats (olive and canola oil)
- Include omega 3 fatty acids (salmon, tuna, mackerel)
- Eliminate alcohol
- Lose weight if overweight

To raise HDL:

- Use monounsaturated fat in place of polyunsaturated fat
- Lose weight if overweight
- Limit trans fatty acid intake
- Avoid high carbohydrate diets
- Increase physical activity

been shown effective in the control of hypertension in the elderly (Appel et al., 2001; Padiyar, 2009) and is strongly recommended in the reduction of overall cardiovascular disease risk (Bazzano et al., 2002; Levitan, Wolk, & Mittleman, 2009). The eating plan is low in saturated fat, cholesterol, total fat, and sodium and rich in potassium, magnesium, and calcium (DHHS, 2006). The DASH diet includes eight to ten servings of fruits and vegetables, two to three servings of low-fat dairy, limited amounts of lean meats, and whole grains and nuts. The complexity and lower energy density of this diet may not be appropriate for some older adults.

Diabetes Mellitus

One of the major chronic diseases in the United States is diabetes mellitus (DM). In people aged 65 and older, the self-reported percentages of individuals with this diagnosis are 19% male and 17% female (http://www.agingstats.gov/agingstatsdotnet/Main_Site/Data/Data_2008.aspx). The hyperglycemia seen in individuals with DM causes many macro- and microvascular changes. As a result of poorly controlled blood glucose levels, DM is the leading cause of blindness, chronic renal insufficiency, peripheral neuropathy, and non-traumatic limb amputations. In the elderly, DM diminishes quality of life by further exaggerating the symptoms of aging. The first of the two major forms of DM is termed type I DM. Type 1 DM is an autoimmune disorder resulting from cell-mediated and antibody-mediated destruction of the beta-cells (insulin producing cells) in the pancreas. Insulin is required for the lifelong management of type 1 DM and while not typical, can develop in older adults. Type 2 DM, characterized by insulin resistance and defective insulin secretion, affects the majority of older adults with DM. While obesity is a prevalent co-occurring factor in individuals with type 2 DM, the high rates in the elderly (~45% with impaired glucose tolerance and type 2 DM combined) (Harris et al., 1998) are not fully explained by weight. Diagnoses of type 2 DM in the older population with BMI in the normal range or even underweight categories may indicate the importance of body fat distribution and the impact of aging *per se* on the body (Goodpaster et al., 2003).

The current criteria of diagnosis of diabetes in older adults are the same as those for younger adults, as determined by the American Diabetes Association (American Diabetes Association, 2009). Diagnosis in older adults can be more challenging due to the normal physiologic changes associated with aging. Changes such as confusion or incontinence and complications relating to diabetes are frequently the presenting symptoms instead of the more typical clinical symptoms such as polydipsia and glucosuria (Reed & Mooradian, 1990). Proper nutrition is critical in the management of DM with emphasis on liberalization of the diet as individuals age. Carbohydrate controlled diets are prominent in this age group. The goals of nutrition therapy for older adults with diabetes are the following (Mooradian, McLaughlin, Boyer, & Winter, 1999):

- Provide adequate calories and nutrient intake;
- Assist in the maintenance of blood glucose levels within the target range;
- Facilitate effective management of coexisting morbidities;
- Prevent, delay, or treat nutrition-related complications;
- Promote quality of life, safety, and overall well-being.

Pulmonary Diseases

Chronic obstructive pulmonary diseases (COPD), asthma, and pneumonia comprise the majority of pulmonary diseases in the elderly. The airflow obstruction that is symptomatic of COPD range from chronic bronchitis to emphysema, with emphysema sufferers more likely to present thin and wasted in appearance. Nutrition needs should focus on the provision of protein and calories. For the malnourished, a high-calorie, high-protein, moderate carbohydrate diet is indicated. Individuals with asthma, mainly facing exacerbations from cold air, exercise or infection, benefit from diets that provide adequate hydration and include small, balanced meals.

Cancer

The American Cancer Society predicts that the lifetime risk for developing any types of cancer in the United States is slightly less than one in two for men and a little more than one in three for women (http://www.cancer.org/docroot/STT/stt_0_2008.asp?sitearea=STT&level=1). The goals of proper individualized nutrition during cancer treatment or remission are: (1) to prevent or reverse nutrient deficiencies; (2) to preserve lean body mass; (3) to minimize nutrition-related side effects; and (4) to maximize the quality of life (Brown et al., 2003). Since elderly individuals are at greater risk of malnutrition due to aging, special attention should be given to the following recommendations made by the American Institute for Cancer Research (AICR): AICR's Nutrition of the Cancer Patient (http://www.aicr.org/site/DocServer/Nov2007_Nut_of_Can_Patient.pdf?docID=1567) (Table 14.8). The nutrition and weight management strategies for cancer survivors have also been documented by Uhley and Jen (2007).

Table 14.8 Recommendations for Treatment of Nutrition Problems during Cancer: AICR Nutrition of the Cancer Patient

Loss of weight and appetite
• Eat several small meals a day instead of three large meals. • When eating a meal, eat high-protein foods first, when your appetite is strongest. • Eat the most when you feel hungriest. • If the odors of food bother you, try eating your food cold or at room temperature. • Drink beverages between meals instead of with meals: drinking a beverage while you eat can make you feel full faster. • Add protein and calories to favorite foods. • Sip on high-calorie beverages during the day, such as juice, nectar, milk or a fruit and yogurt smoothie.
Diarrhea
• Try to drink at least 8 glasses of liquids each day. Drinking enough is especially important while you have diarrhea to prevent dehydration. • Good choices of fluids include water, diluted juices, broth or decaffeinated coffee or tea. • Caffeine in large amounts (regular coffee and tea or caffeinated soft drinks) may make diarrhea worse in some people. • Liquids at room temperature are easier to tolerate than those that are hot or cold. • Eat small amounts of food throughout the day instead of three large meals. • Include soluble fiber periodically throughout the day.
Constipation
• Drink more liquids, aiming for 8 to 10 glasses a day. Good choices are water, fruit juice (especially prune juice), and tea. • Have a hot drink such as tea, broth, hot lemonade, hot apple cider or hot prune juice about 30 minutes before your usual time for a bowel movement. • Eat a large breakfast, including a hot drink and high-fiber foods such as hot or cold bran cereal, whole wheat toast and fruit. • Try to get some exercise, such as taking a walk, every day. Talk to your doctor before starting a new exercise program.

Table 14.8 Recommendations for Treatment of Nutrition Problems during Cancer: AICR Nutrition of the Cancer Patient *Continued*

Nausea
• Eat six or more small meals during the day rather than three large meals. Eat slowly. • Keep the room well ventilated; some patients find that certain food odors produce nausea. • Drink beverages between meals rather than with meals. • Drink beverages cool or chilled and sip through a straw. • If nausea in the morning is a problem, keep crackers at your bedside to nibble on before you get up. • Rinse out your mouth before and after eating. If there is a bad taste in your mouth, suck on hard candy such as peppermint or lemon. • Avoid lying down for about an hour after eating.

Alzheimer's Disease (AD)

Causes of weight loss during AD include loss of appetite secondary to deterioration of brain regions associated with feeding behavior and function. Additionally, behavioral problems associated with AD make it difficult for individuals to consume adequate energy. The most common weight management strategy is to provide high-energy nutritional supplements to individuals at risk. Environmental and social interventions related to mealtimes and feedings are also important (Smith & Greenwood, 2008). The majority of studies relating nutrition to AD focused on prevention. Preventive nutrition strategies for AD include the "Mediterranean diet" focusing on unsaturated fatty acids (vascular mechanism) (Luchsinger & Mayeux, 2004) and other eating patterns that are high in vitamin B12 and folate (to lower circulating homocyteine levels) (Mohajeri & Leuba, 2009). However, the data on the effect of dietary management of AD are inconclusive.

MEDICATIONS THAT AFFECT APPETITE AND FOOD INTAKE

The incidences of many chronic diseases rise with age (Gilford, 1988). As a result, the majority of the elderly are suffering from polypharmacy. Major concerns about the multiple medications that the elderly are taking are the drug/drug and drug/nutrient interactions. Some drugs may affect nutrient absorption or distribution, while others may affect their excretion. In addition, some medications affect food intake (Gazewood & Mehr, 1998). Gazewood and Mehr (1998) proposed four mechanisms by which drugs may reduce appetite and cause weight loss: nausea or vomiting; anorexia; alteration of smell/taste; and hyper- or hypophagia. Some medications influencing nutrition and their effects on food intake are listed in Table 14.9.

DIVERSITY ISSUES THAT IMPACT THE NUTRITION STATUS

The aging population will grow more diverse in direct reflection of the demographic changes in the United States. The Federal Interagency Forum on Aging Related Statistics published the following information in the Older Americans 2008: Key Indicators of Well-Being report (http://www.agingstats.gov/agingstatsdotnet/Main_Site/Data/2008_Documents/tables/Tables.aspx): Non-Hispanic Whites, which represented 81% of the 65 and over population, are projected to drop to 61% in 2050. African Americans, Asians, and Hispanics are projected to increase from 9% to 12%, 3% to 8%, and 6% to

Table 14.9 Effects of Selected Medications on Appetite and Food Intake

Medication			Effects			
Category	**Treatment for**	**Example**	**Nausea/ Dysgeusia**	**Dysphagia**	**Anorexia**	**Vomiting**
ACE inhibitors	Hypertension, congestive heart failure	Captopril	X			
Antibiotics	Bacterial infection	Cefditoren Azithromycin Amoxicillin Nitrofurantoin	X	X	X	X
Anticholinergic agents	Gastritis Diverticulitis Asthma Parkinson's disease	Benzhexol Benapryzine Atropine		X	X	
Antiepileptic agents	Convulsion, epilepsy	Neurontin Lamictal, Cerebyx	X	X		X
Dilantin						
Antihistamines	Allergies	Zyrtec, Allegra Claritin, Tavist		X		
Benzodiazepines	Panic/anxiety disorder, insomnia, seizure	Valium Librium Xanax Ativan	X			X
Bisphosphonates	Osteoporosis	Fosamax Boniva	X		X	
Bronchodilators	Asthma	Ventolin	X	X		
Calcium channel blocker	Hypertension, angina	Dilacor Tiazac	X	X		
Corticosteroids	Rheumatoid arthritis IBS Scleroderma	Celestone Cortone Deltasone			X	
Decongestants	Sinus and head Congestion	Afrin, Sudafed	X			X

		Actifed				
Digoxin	Heart failure	Lanoxin	X			X
Dopamine agonists	Parkinson's disease	Apokyn	X	X	X	X
		Larodopa				
		Mirapex				
		Requip				
Hormonal agents	Menopausal symptoms	Estrogen/	X			
		Progesterone				
Hypoglycemic agents	Type 2 diabetes	Metformin	X	X	X	
HMG-CoA reductase	Hypercholesterolemia	Lipitore	X	X		
Inhibitors		Crestor				
		Zocor				
Iron supplement	Iron deficiency anemia	Fermiron	X	X	X	
		Feosol				
Nitroglycerin	Angina	Nitrolingual	X	X		
		Nitrostat				
NSAIDs	Pain, inflammation	Aspirin	X		X	
Opioid analgesics	Pain	Codeine,	X			X
		Morphine				
		Demerol				
		Anexsia				
SSRIs	Depression	Prozac	X	X		X
		Paxil				
		Zoloft				
Tricyclic antidepressant	Depression	Elavil	X	X		
		Anafranil				
		Norpramin				
		Sinequan				
Xanthine oxidase	Gout, kidney stones	Zyloprim	X	X		
Inhibitors						

ACE: Angiotensin-converting enzyme
IBS: Irritable bowel syndrome
HMG-CoA; hydroxy-methylglutaryl-coenzyme A
NSAID: Nonsteroidal anti-inflammatory drugs
SSRI: Selective serotonin reuptake inhibitors
Adapted from Huffman (2002), with permission

18%, respectively by 2050 for the 65 and over age group. These projections highlight a need for support and health systems to address more culturally diverse needs in the elderly.

Differences in education and income level by ethnicity also exist. Non-Hispanic Whites and Asians attained higher levels of high school and college than African Americans and Hispanics. In 2005, the median net worth of White households with individuals aged 65 and older ($226,900) was six times that of older African American households ($37,800). In 2007, it was estimated that 9.7% of the elderly live below the poverty level. However, the minority population is disproportionally affected. While 7.4% of elderly Whites are living under the poverty level, minority populations including 23.2% of the African American elderly, 11.3% of the Asian elderly, and 17.1% of the Hispanic elderly are living under the poverty level (http://www.census.gov/prod/2008pubs/p60-235.pdf). Income levels affect the individual's nutritional status (Drewnowski & Shultz, 2001; Jetter & Cassady, 2006). Financial hardship may impact the ability of the elderly to obtain adequate foods and nutrients, and this affects the minority population more than Whites (Klesges et al., 2001). Therefore, the minority elderly suffer more from malnutrition and morbidity and mortality associated with malnutrition. Even though there are federal programs aimed at reducing the health disparity among the different ethnic populations, the minority elderly population has a lower rate of receiving these aids due to lack of knowledge or other assistance (http://www.cdc.gov/aging/pdf/saha_2007.pdf).

There are also race differences in chronic disease prevalence. In 2005–2006, African Americans reported higher levels of hypertension and type 2 diabetes than non-Hispanic Whites (70% compared with 51% for HTN, and 29% compared with 16% for DM). Hispanics also report higher levels of diabetes than non-Hispanic Whites (25% compared to 16%), but similar levels of HTN (54% and 51%, respectively) and lower levels of arthritis (40% compared with 50%) (http://www.agingstats.gov/agingstatsdotnet/Main_Site/Data/2008_Documents/tables/Tables.aspx). Another study reported that Hispanic and African American older respondents had poorer glycemic control than non-Hispanic Whites. The modifiable factor of medication adherence showed racial disparities and indicated a need for programs to be adapted for language and education levels (Heisler et al., 2007). Specifically, there is an urgent need for good training of health care workers caring for the elderly to recognize and provide for their special needs and problems.

Living Arrangement

Older adults who have family support, even if they live alone, have better health and nutrition status than those without support. Payette and Shatenstein (2005) have reported that social isolation and perceived loneliness have negative impact on nutrition status. Also, those elderly who live in rural areas are more likely to experience nutritional risks due to isolation and transportation issues (McLaughlin & Jensen, 1998).

Table 14.10 The Basis for Educational and Care Activities for the Elderly: Report of the IDECG Working Group (Roubenoff, Scrimshaw, Shetty, & Woo, 2000)

- Consuming foods with high nutrient density but also meet the energy needs
- Due to higher protein needs, diets should contain sufficient protein
- Keep physically active
- Any unintentional weight loss should be evaluated and treated appropriately
- Avoid alcohol and tobacco abuse
- In addition to adequate diets, use fortified foods and supplements to prevent vitamin and mineral deficiencies
- If weight loss is indicated, reduce the intake of dietary fat and energy but maintain adequate protein intake
- Maintaining social networks and activities

CONCLUSION

Nutrition plays a vital role in health maintenance and disease prevention. With the U.S. population aging rapidly, it is critical that adequate nutrition support is provided for the elderly who are at risk of under- or malnutrition. On the other hand, many of the preventable chronic diseases originate at a much younger age. To ensure better chances of a quality life in older years, a healthy, physically active lifestyle beginning during childhood and including diets that are low in saturated fat, high in fruits and vegetables is vital. Consistency in maintaining a healthy lifestyle should be maintained from youth through the aging years. Table 14.10 summarizes educational and care activities recommended for maintaining health in older years (Roubenoff, Scrimshaw, Shetty, & Woo, 2000).

REFERENCES

Akner, G., & Cederholm, T. (2001). Treatment of protein-energy malnutrition in chronic nonmalignant disorders. *Am. J. Clin. Nutr.*, *76*, 6–24.

American Dietetic Association. (2005). Position of the American Dietetic Association: liberalization of the diet prescription improves the quality of life for older adults in long-term care. *J. Am. Diet Assoc.*, *105*, 1955–1965.

American Diabetes Association. (2009). Summary of Revision of the 2009 Clinical Practice Recommendations. *Diabetes Care*, *32*, S1–S5.

Appel, L., Espeland, M., Easter, L., Wilson, S., Folmar, S., & Lacy, C. (2001). Effects of reduced sodium intake on hypertension control in older individuals: results from the Trial of Nonpharmacologic Interventions in the Elderly (TONE). *Arch. Intern. Med.*, *161*, 685–693.

Bazzano, L. A., He, J., Ogden, L., Loria, C., Vupputuri, S., Myers, L., et al. (2002). Fruit and vegetable intake and risk of cardiovascular disease in US adults: the first National Health and Nutrition Examination Survey Epidemiologic Follow-up Study. *Am. J. Clin. Nutr.*, *76*, 93–99.

Bouillanne, O., Dupont-Belmont, C., Hay, P., Hamon-Vilcot, B., Cynober, L., & Aussel, C. (2009). Fat mass protects hospitalized elderly persons against morbidity and mortality. *Am. J. Clin. Nutr.*, *90*, 505–510.

Bouillanne, O., Morineau, G., Depont, C., Coulombel, I., Vincent, J.-P., Nicolis, I., et al. (2005). Geriatric Nutritional Risk Index: a new index for evaluating at-risk elderly medical patients. *Am. J. Clin. Nutr.*, *82*, 777–783.

Brown, J., Byers, T., Doyle, C., Coumeya, K., Demark-Wahnefried, W., Kushi, L., et al. (2003). Nutrition and physical activity during and after cancer treatment: an American Cancer Society guide for informed choices. *CA Cancer J. Clin.*, *53*, 268–291.

Brownie, S. (2006). Why are elderly individuals at risk of nutritional deficiency? *Int. J. Nurs. Practice*, *12*, 110–118.

Buzby, G., Knox, L., Crosby, L., Eisenberg, J., Haakenson, C., McNeal, G., et al. (1988a). Study protocol: a randomized clinical trial of total parenteral nutrition in malnourished surgical patients. *Am. J. Clin. Nutr.*, *47*(Suppl. 2), 366–391.

Buzby, G., Williford, W., Peterson, O., Crosby, L., Page, C., Reinhardt, G., et al. (1988b). A randomized clinical trial of total parenteral nutrition in malnourished surgical patients: the rationale and impact of previous clinical trials and pilot study on protocol design. *Am. J. Clin. Nutr.*, *47*(Suppl. 2), 357–365.

Chumlea, W. (2006). Is the MNA valid in different populations and across practice settings? *J. Nutr. Health Aging*, *10*, 524–527.

Chumlea, W., & Guo, S. (1992). Equations for predicting stature in white and black elderly individuals. *J. Geront.*, *47*, M197–M203.

Cornoni-Huntley, J., Harris, T., Everett, D., Albanes, D., Micozzi, M., Miles, T., et al. (1991). An overview of body weight of older persons, including the impact on mortality. *J. Clin. Epidemiol.*, *44*, 743–753.

DHHS. (2006). DASH eating plan. In *Lower Your Blood*. Washington, DC: National Institutes of Health.

Donini, L., Savina, C., & Cannella, C. (2003). Eating habits and appetite control in the elderly: the anorexia of aging. *Int. Psychogeriatr.*, *15*, 73–87.

Drewnowski, A., & Shultz, J. (2001). Impact of aging on eating behaviors, food choices, nutrition, and health status. *J. Nutr. Health Aging*, *5*, 75–79.

Easterling, C., & Robbins, E. (2008). Dementia and dysphagia. *Geriatric Nursing*, *29*, 275–285.

Ensrud, K., Ewing, S., Stone, K., Cauley, J., Bowman, P., & Cummings, S. (2003). Intentional and unintentional weight loss increase bone loss and hip fracture risk in older women. *J. Am. Geriatr. Soc.*, *51*, 1740–1747.

Feldblum, I., German, L., Castel, H., Harman-Boehm, I., Bilenko, N., Eisinger, M., et al. (2007). Characteristics of undernourished older medical patients and the identification of predictors for undernutrition status. *Nutr. J.*, *6*, 37.

Felson, D., Zhang, Y., Hannan, M., & Anderson, J. (1993). Effects of weight and body mass index on bone mineral density in men and women: the Framingham study. *J. Bone Miner. Res.*, *8*, 567–573.

Firth, M., & Prather, C. (2002). Gastrointestinal motility problems in the elderly patient. *Gastroenterology*, *122*, 1688–1700.

Fischer, J., & Johnson, M. (1990). Low body weight and weight loss in the aged. *J. Am. Diet. Assoc.*, *90*, 1697–1706.

Ford, E. S., Giles, W., & Dietz, W. (2002). Prevalence of the metabolic syndrome among US adults: findings from the Third National Health and Nutrition Examination Survey. *JAMA*, *287*, 356–359.

Furman, E. (2006). Undernutrition in older adults across the continuum of care: nutritional assessment, barriers, and interventions. *J. Gerontol. Nurs.*, *32*, 22–27.

Gazewood, J., & Mehr, D. (1998). Diagnosis and management of weight loss in the elderly. *J. Fam. Pract.*, *47*, 19–25.

Gilford, D. (Ed.), (1988). *The Aging Population in the Twenty-first Century: Statistics for Health Policy.* Washington, DC: National Academy Press.

Goodpaster, B., Krishnaswami, S., Resnick, H., Kelley, D., Haggerty, C., Harris, T., et al. (2003). Association between regional adipose tissue distribution and both type 2 diabetes and impaired glucose tolerance in elderly men and women. *Diabetes Care*, *26*, 372–379.

Goulding, M., Rogers, M., & Smith, S. (2003). Public health and aging: trends in aging–United States and worldwide. *MMWR*, *52*, 101–106.

Guigoz, Y. (2006). The Mini Nutritional Assessment (MNA®) review of the literature—what does it tell us? *J. Nutr. Health Aging*, *10*, 466–487.

Guigoz, Y., Vellas, B., & Garry, P. (1994). Mini nutritional assessment: a practical assessment tool for grading the nutritional state of elderly patients. *Fact. Res. in Gerontol.*, *4*(Suppl. 2), 15–59.

Harris, M., Flegal, K., Cowie, C., Eberhardt, M., Goldstein, D., Wiedmeyer, H., et al. (1998). Prevalence of diabetes, impaired fasting glucose, and impaired glucose tolerance in U.S. adults: the Third National Health and Nutrition Examination Survey, 1988–1994. *Diabetes Care*, *21*, 518–524.

Heisler, M., Faul, J., Hayward, R., Langa, K., Blaum, C., & Weir, D. (2007). Mechanisms for racial and ethnic disparities in glycemic control in middle-aged and older Americans in the health and retirement study. *Arch. Intern. Med.*, *167*, 1853–1860.

Huffman, G. (2002). Evaluating and treating unintentional weight loss in the elderly. *Am. Fam. Physician*, *65*, 640–650.

Jetter, K., & Cassady, D. (2006). The availability and cost of healthier food alternatives. *Am. J. Prev. Med.*, *30*, 38–44.

Kayser-Jones, J. (2000). Improving the nutritional care of nursing home residents. *Nursing Homes Long Term Care Management*, *49*, 56–59.

Klesges, L., Pahor, M., Shorr, R., Wan, J., Williamson, J., & Guralnik, J. (2001). Financial difficulty in acquiring food among elderly disabled women: results from the Women's Health and Aging study. *Am. J. Public Health*, *91*, 68–75.

Kumanyika, S. K., & Krebs-Smith, S. M (2000). Preventive nutrition issues in ethnic and socioeconomic groups in the United States. In A. Bendich, & R. J. Deckelbaum (Eds.), *Preventive Nutrition, Volume II: Primary and Secondary Prevention*. Totowa, NJ: Humana Press Inc.

Levitan, E. B., Wolk, A., & Mittleman, M. (2009). Consistency with the DASH diet and incidence of heart failure. *Arch. Intern. Med.*, *169*, 851–857.

Lichtenstein, A., Rasmussen, H., Yu, W., Epstein, A., & Russell, R. (2008). Modified MyPyramid for older adults. *J. Nutr.*, *138*, 5–11.

Luchsinger, J., & Mayeux, R. (2004). Dietary factors and Alzheimer's disease. *The Lancet Neurology*, *3*, 579–587.

MacIntosh, C., Morley, J., Wishart, J., Morris, H., Jansen, J., Horowitz, M., et al. (2001). Effect of exogenous cholecystokinin (CCK)-8 on food intake and plasma CCK, leptin, and insulin concentrations in older and young adults: evidence for increased CCK activity as a cause of the anorexia of aging. *J. Clin. Endocrinol. Metab.*, *86*, 5830–5837.

Mathey, M. (2001). Assessing appetite in Dutch elderly with the Appetite, Hunger and Sensory Perception (AHSP) questionnaire. *J. Nutr. Health Aging*, *5*, 22–28.

McCullough, G., Pelletier, C., & Steele, C. (2003). National dysphagia diet: what to swallow? *The ASHA Leader*, 16–27.

McGee, M., & Jensen, G. L. (2000). Nutrition in the elderly. *J. Clin. Gastroenterol.*, *30*, 372–380.

McLaughlin, D., & Jensen, L. (1998). The rural elderly: a demographic portrait. In R. Coward, & J. Krout (Eds.), *Aging in Rural Settings: Life Circumstances and Distinctive Features* (pp. 15–43). New York, NY: Springer.

Mohajeri, M., & Leuba, G. (2009). Prevention of age-associated dementia. *Brain Res. Bull.*, *80*, 315–325.

Mooradian, A., McLaughlin, S., Boyer, C., & Winter, J. (1999). Diabetes care of older adults. *Diabetes Spectrum*, *12*, 70–77.

Morley, J. (2001). Decreased food intake with aging. *J. Gerontol. Med. Sci.*, *56A*, 81–88.

Morley, J., & Thomas, D. (1999). Anorexia and aging: pathophysiology. *Nutrition*, *15*, 499–503.

National Dysphagia Diet Task Force. (2002). *National Dysphagia Diet: Standardization for Optimal Care*. Chicago, IL: American Dietetic Association.

Newman, A., Yanez, D., Harris, T., Duxbury, A., Enright, P., & Firied, L. (2001). Weight change in old age and its association with mortality. *J. Am. Geriatr. Soc.*, *59*, 1309–1318.

Ogden, C., Carroll, M., Curtin, L., McDowell, M., Tabak, C., & Flegal, K. (2006). Prevalence of overweight and obesity in the United States, 1999–2004. *JAMA*, *295*, 1549–1555.

Padiyar, A. (2009). Nonpharmacologic management of hypertension in the elderly. *Clin. Geriatr. Med.*, *25*, 213–219.

Park, S., & Johnson, M. (2006). What is an adequate dose of oral vitamin B in older people with poor vitamin B status? *Nutrition Reviews*, *64*, 373–378.

Payette, H., & Shatenstein, B. (2005). Determinants of healthy eating in community-dwelling elderly people. *Can. J. Public Health*, *2005*, S27–S31.

Reed, R., & Mooradian, A. (1990). Nutritional status and dietary management of elderly diabetic patients. *Clin. Geriatr. Med.*, *6*, 883–901.

Rolland, Y., Kim, M.-J., Gammack, J., Wilson, M.-M., Thomas, D., & Morley, J. (2006). Office management of weight loss in older persons. *Am. J. Med.*, *119*, 1019–1026.

Roubenoff, R., Scrimshaw, N., Shetty, P., & Woo, J. (2000). Report of the IDECG Working Group on the role of lifestyle including nutrition for the health of the elderly. *Eur. J. Clin. Nutr.*, *54*(Suppl. 3), S164–S165.

Rubenstein, L., Harker, J., Salva, A., Guigoz, Y., & Vellas, B. (2001). Screening for undernutrition in geriatric practice; developing the short-form Mini Nutritional Assessment (MNA-SF). *J. Geront.*, *56A*, M366–M377.

Schiffman, S., & Graham, B. (2000). Taste and smell perception affect appetite and immunity in the elderly. *Eur. J. Clin. Nutr.*, *54*, S54–S63.

Seidell, J., & Visscher, T. (2000). Body weight and weight change and their health implications for the elderly. *Eur. J. Clin. Nutr.*, *54*, S33–S39.

Smith, K., & Greenwood, C. (2008). Weight loss and nutritional considerations in Alzheimer disease. *J. Nutr. Elder*, *27*, 381–403.

Sullivan, D. (2000). Undernutrition in older adults. *Annals of Long-Term Care*, *8*, 41–46.

Uhley, V., & Jen, K.-L. C. (2007). Nutrition and weight management in cancer survivors. In M. Feuerstein (Ed.), *Handbook of Cancer Survivorship* (pp. 269–285). New York, NY: Springer.

Vasan, R. S., Beiser, A., Seshadri, S., Larson, M., Kannel, W., D'Agostino, R., et al. (2002). Residual lifetime risk for developing hypertension in middle-aged women and men: the Framingham Heart Study. *JAMA*, *287*, 1003–1010.

Vellas, B., Villars, H., Abellan, G., Soto, M., Rolland, Y., Guigoz, Y., et al. (2006). Overview of the MNA®—its history and challenges. *J. Nutr. Health Aging*, *10*, 456–465.

Villareal, D., Apovian, C., Kushner, R., & Klein, S. (2005). Obesity in older adults: technical review and position statement of the American Society for Nutrition and NAASO, the Obesity Society. *Obesity*, *13*, 1849–1863.

White, H., Pieper, C., & Schmader, K. (1998). The association of weight change in Alzheimer's disease with severity of disease and mortality: a longitudinal analysis. *J. Am. Geriatr. Soc.*, *46*, 1223–1227.

Wilson, M.-M., Thomas, D., Rubenstein, L., Chibnall, J., Anderson, S., Baxi, A., et al. (2005). Appetite assessment: simple appetite questionnaire predicts weight loss in community-dwelling adults and nursing home residents. *Am. J. Clin. Nutr.*, *82*, 1074–1081.

Wilson, M.-M., Vaswani, S., Liu, D., Morley, J., & Miller, D. (1998). Prevalence and causes of undernutrition in medical outpatients. *Am. J. Med.*, *104*, 56–63.

Yan, L., Daviglus, M., Liu, K., Pirzada, A., Garside, D., Schiffer, L., et al. (2004). BMI and health-related quality of life in adults 65 years and older. *Obesity*, *12*, 69–76.

CHAPTER 15

Assessment of Agitation in Older Adults

Jiska Cohen-Mansfield[1], Lori Schindel Martin[2]

[1] *George Washington University Medical Center, Washington, DC, USA, and Tel Aviv University Herczeg Institute on Aging and Sackler Faculty of Medicine, Tel-Aviv, Israel*

[2] *Daphne Cockwell School of Nursing, Ryerson University, Toronto, Ontario, Canada*

INTRODUCTION

Agitation has been defined as, "inappropriate verbal, vocal, or motor activity that is not judged by an outside observer to result directly from the needs or confusion of the agitated individual" (Cohen-Mansfield, 2008a). The *range of behaviors* included under this definition encompasses *repetitive acts* such as walking back and forth or repetition of words, *behaviors inappropriate to the social norms*, such as going into someone else's room and handling their belongings, or unbuttoning a blouse in public, and *aggressive behaviors* toward oneself or others. Those behaviors have been labeled problem behaviors, disruptive behaviors, disturbing behaviors, inappropriate behaviors, and agitation, terms which are generally used interchangeably. The analysis of agitation is based on the following assumptions:

1. **Who determines if this is a problem behavior?** The behavior is in the eyes of the beholder; in other words, it is determined on the basis of who perceives it as inappropriate. It may or may not be inappropriate from the point of view of the older person. The behavior may represent an underlying need that is not obvious to the observer, and the older person may not be consciously aware of this need or be able to express it because of dementia.
2. **The behavior is not necessarily disruptive.** Problem behaviors are not always disruptive. However, it is important to observe these behaviors because they can teach us about the internal state of the older person, particularly those residents who are withdrawn and may not, at first glance, appear agitated.
3. **The behavior is not necessarily dementia related.** Although agitated behaviors are more common among those suffering from dementia, some of them are also manifested by persons who are not cognitively impaired (Koss et al., 1997).

   When occurring with dementia, the behavior is not *a necessary outcome of dementia*. Problem behaviors do not refer to those behaviors which represent the actual deterioration involved with dementia, such as memory problems or incontinence at later stages of the disease. Whereas many of those suffering from dementia manifest problem behaviors, not all do.
4. **The problem behavior is an observable behavior and the definition does not assume any underlying emotional state to cause the behavior.** Despite the label "agitation," the behavior does not depend on the assumption of a state of anxiety. Such a state or other affective states are inferred from additional information.

Handbook of Assessment in Clinical Gerontology. DOI: 10.1016/B978-0-12-374961-1.10015-6

Staff care providers frequently feel helpless and anxious about managing agitation because of its ambiguous cause and lack of knowledge concerning effective methods of treatment. A first step in ameliorating this state of events is a systematic assessment of the behavior.

Subtypes of Problem Behaviors

Based on factor analyses in both a senior daycare population (Cohen-Mansfield, Werner, Watson, & Pasis, 1995) and in a nursing home population (Cohen-Mansfield, Marx, & Rosenthal, 1989), as well as validation from various international samples (Rabinowitz et al., 2005), we found problem behaviors to consist of four subtypes: physically aggressive behaviors; physically non-aggressive behaviors; verbally aggressive behaviors; and verbally non-aggressive behaviors. Although the behaviors are more likely to occur within each subtype than across subtypes, the subtypes are not independent (Cohen-Mansfield & Werner, 1998). They can be described as occurring on two dimensions: aggressive/non-aggressive and physical/verbal, as delineated in Figure 15.1.

CMAI – List of Behaviors

Rating Scale for Agitated Behaviors

never	less than once a week but still occurring	once or twice a week	several times a week	once or twice a day	several times a day	a few times an hour

verbal/vocal

verbally non-aggressive

complaining
negativism
repetitive sentences or questions
constant, unwarranted requests for attention or help

verbally aggressive

cursing and verbal aggression
making strange noises
verbal sexual advances
screaming

non-aggressive — aggressive

physically non-aggressive

performing repetitious mannerisms
inappropriate robing and disrobing
eating inappropriate substances
handling things inappropriately
trying to get to a different place
pacing, aimless wandering
intentional falling
general restlessness
hoarding things
hiding things

physically aggressive

physical sexual advances
hurting self or others
throwing things
tearing things
scratching
grabbing
pushing
spitting
kicking
biting
hitting

physical

FIGURE 15.1

Behaviors in the CMAI Organized by Dimensions.

WHY ASSESS AGITATION?

A clinician would want to assess agitation for a variety of reasons: to determine whether the older person is in need of intervention or alternative placement; to ascertain whether the caregivers' level of distress with the behavior is appropriate to the level of agitation exhibited; to determine whether a treatment is effective (or, conversely, how withdrawal of treatment affects agitation), and to assist in the choice of treatment. Obviously, for maximal utilization of the assessment, a better understanding of agitation, as well as its etiology and treatment than can be offered in this chapter, is necessary. That can be found in Cohen-Mansfield and Deutsch (1996), Cohen-Mansfield (2000b, 2005) and Cohen-Mansfield, Libin, and Marx (2007).

Often, staff members who work with cognitively impaired persons who display agitation substitute immediate psychotropic interventions for systematic investigation, analysis, planning, and evaluation problem behaviors. Assessment is crucial for all these stages of intervention. It is also important for monitoring quality of care. In institutional settings, it is therefore a fundamental component in the process of continuous quality improvement. Measurement is critical because it provides objective data, which focus attention on important clinical issues and replace opinion with data. Provision of excellence in care for the cognitively impaired individual who is agitated must be based on measurement so that clinical decisions are based on evidence rather than impressions or speculation.

AVAILABLE METHODOLOGIES FOR THE ASSESSMENT OF AGITATION

Three general methodologies have been used to assess agitation:

- **Informant ratings**, in which a caregiver rates the frequency or severity of the behaviors that constitute agitation. This is the most commonly used method and the one most likely to be used in clinical settings.
- **Observational methods** are systematic observations of the older person in his or her natural setting, e.g., home, hospital, nursing home, adult day care setting, etc. A trained research assistant observes the older person for a given time period, examines the behaviors and rates them on a standardized printed instrument or on a portable computer. Alternatively, the behaviors can be videotaped and then rated by a trained research assistant who views the videotapes in a manner similar to that of direct *in vivo* observations.
- **Technological devices** can automatically measure an aspect of the older person's behavior, such as level of activity at the ankle, or level of noise emitted.

Some practices represent a combination of methods, such as when a nursing staff member rates the behavior of the resident at the end of each hour or at the end of a nursing shift. Although commonly referred to as an observational method, this combination method does not involve the nursing staff member observing the older person for the complete hour or nursing shift. In fact, it is a summary of those behaviors observed via clinical work during the hour or the shift. From this point of view, it is a caregiver rating of behavior occurring over a short timeframe.

Informant Rating Methods

Many informant rating instruments have been used with community-dwelling elderly persons, hospital patients, and nursing home residents. A list of available assessments is included in Table 15.1.

Table 15.1 Informant Ratings for Assessing Agitation

Assessment	# Items (estimated # tapping behavior problems)	Scale
Dementia Behavior Disturbance Scale (DBD) (Baumgarten, Becker, & Gauthier 1990)	28 (19)	5-pt frequency
Disruptive Behavior Scale (DBS) (Beck, 1997); (Chafetz et al., 1987)	45 (all)	presence/absence 9-point severity
	29 (21)	7-pt frequency
Cohen-Mansfield Agitation Inventory—nursing home version (CMAI) (Cohen-Mansfield, Marx, & Rosenthal, 1989)	29 (all)	7-pt frequency
Cohen-Mansfield Agitation Inventory—Community (CMAI-C) (Cohen-Mansfield et al., 1995)	36 (all)	7-pt frequency 7-pt disruptiveness
Cohen-Mansfield Agitation Inventory — Short form (CMAI-S) (Werner, Cohen-Mansfield, Koroknay, & Braun, 1994)	14 (all)	5-pt frequency
The Neuropsychiatric Inventory (NPI) (Leuchter et al., 1994)	83 (62)	4-pt frequency 3-pt severity 6-pt disruptiveness
Behavioral Syndromes Scale for Dementia (Devanand et al., 1992)	33 (all)	varies accd to item: 6 point severity, yes/no occurrence
Columbia University Scale for Psychopathology in Alzheimer's Disease (Devanand et al., 1992)	26 (5)	varies accd to item: yes/no, 2-pt severity 4-pt severity
Care Taker Obstreperous-Behavior Rating Scale (COBRA) (Drachman et al., 1992)	30 (all)	5-pt frequency 5-pt severity
Brief Agitation Rating Scale for Nursing Home Elderly (BARS) (Finkel, 1993)	10 (all)	7-pt frequency 7-point disruptiveness
Gottfries-Brane-Steen Scale (GBS) (Gottfries, Brane, Gullberg, & Steen, 1982)	29 (4)	7-pt severity
Behavior and Mood Disturbance Scale (BMD) (Greene, Smith, Gardiner, & Timbury, 1982)	34 (10)	5-pt frequency or severity
Cornell Scale for Depression in Dementia (Alexopoulos, Abrams, Young, & Shamoian, 1988)	19 (2)	3-pt severity
Dementia Behavior Scale (DBS) (Reding, Haycox, Wigforss, Brush, & Blass, 1984)	8 (1)	7-pt frequency
Multidimensional Observation Scale for Elderly Subjects (MOSES) (Fisman, Gordon, Feleki, Helmes, McDonald, & Dupre, 1988)	40 (10)	5-pt frequency
Neurobehavioral Rating Scale (NRS) (Levin, et al., 1987)	27 (4)	7-pt severity
Dementia Signs and Symptoms Scale (DSSS) (Loreck, Bylsma, & Folstein, 1994)	43 (29)	4-pt severity 4-pt frequency
Stockton Geriatric Rating Scale (SGRS) (Meer & Baker, 1966)	33 (8)	3-pt frequency

Table 15.1 Informant Ratings for Assessing Agitation *Continued*

Assessment	# Items (estimated # tapping behavior problems)	Scale
Dysfunctional Behavior Rating Instrument (DBRI) (Molloy, McIlroy, Guyatt, & Lever, 1991)	25 (19)	6-pt frequency
Functional Dementia Scale (FDS) (Moore, Bobula, Short, & Mischel, 1983)	20 (8)	4-pt frequency
Disruptive Behavior Rating Scale (DBRS) (Mungas, Weiler, Franzi, & Henry, 1989)	21 (all)	5-pt severity 3-pt distress to staff
Behavior Problem Checklist (BPC) (Niederehe, 1988)	52 (16)	5-pt frequency; 5-pt duration; 5-pt reaction
Brief Psychiatric Rating Scale (Overall & Gorham, 1962)	16 (5)	7-pt frequency
Rating Scale for Aggressive Behavior in the Elderly (Patel & Hope, 1992)	21 (19)	4-pt frequency
Global Assessment of Psychiatric Symptoms (GAPS) (Raskin & Crook, 1988)	19 (3)	5-pt severity
The Nursing Home Behavior Problem Scale (Ray, Taylor, Lichtenstein, & Meador, 1992)	29 (23)	5-pt frequency
Behavioral Pathology in Alzheimer's Disease Rating Scale (BEHAVE-AD) (Reisberg et al., 1987)	25 (18)	4-pt severity
Pittsburgh Agitation Scale (PAS) (Rosen et al., 1994)	4 (all)	varies; 5-pt severity for most
The Alzheimer's Disease Assessment Scale (ADAS) (Mohs, 1996)	21 (4)	5-pt severity
Ryden Aggression Scale (RAS) (Ryden, 1988)	25 (all aggression)	6-pt frequency
Sandoz Clinical Assessment-Geriatric (SCAG) (Shader, Harmatz, & Salzman, 1974)	19 (4)	7-pt severity
Overt Aggression Scale (OAS) (Silver & Yudofsky, 1991)	16 (all)	presence/absence (also, duration, timing and intervention items)
Behavioral and Emotional Activities Manifested in Dementia (BEAM-D) (Sinha et al., 1992)	16 (9)	5-pt combined severity and frequency
Dementia Mood Assessment Scale (DMAS) (Sunderland, Hill, Lawlor, & Molchan, 1988)	24 (2)	7-pt severity
Behavior Rating Scale for Dementia of CERAD (Tariot et al., 1995)	51 (17)	3-pt frequency
Revised Memory and Behavioral Problems Checklist (RMBPC) (Teri et al., 1992)	24 (10)	5-pt frequency 5-pt reaction
GIP: Observational Ward Behavioral Scale (Verstraten, 1988)	82 (about half)	4-pt frequency
Psychogeriatric Dependency Rating Scales (PGDRS) (Wilkinson & Graham-White, 1980)	26 (15)	3-pt frequency
Memory and Behavior Problems Checklist (MBPC) (Zarit & Zarit, 1983)	29 (11)	6-pt frequency 5-pt caregiver distress

One example of an informant rating instrument is the Cohen-Mansfield Agitation Inventory (CMAI; Cohen-Mansfield, Marx, & Rosenthal, 1989). In the nursing home version, a nursing staff member who knows the resident well rates the frequency at which the resident manifested 29 behaviors, such as pacing, spitting, grabbing, pushing, biting, or complaining during the previous two weeks; rating is performed on a 7-point scale ranging from "never" to "a few times an hour." Most of the terms in this instrument are based on reports by nursing staff, and are therefore usually well understood. Another form of the CMAI includes both frequency and disruptiveness of each of the behaviors. Again, the frequency is rated on a 7-point scale, and subjective disruptiveness is rated on a 5-point scale. We do not expect to achieve a high inter-rater agreement on disruptiveness, because some caregivers are bothered by agitated behaviors and others are not. However, sometimes change in subjective perception of disruptiveness of behavior is the main purpose of treatment, rather than change in the behavior itself. Furthermore, despite its subjective nature, disruptiveness is related to both type of behavior and its frequency (Cohen-Mansfield, 2008a).

The final score of the CMAI is usually summarized as four scores based on the typology described above. Therefore the mean frequency for each of the syndromes, physically aggressive behaviors, physically non-aggressive behaviors, verbally aggressive behaviors and verbally agitated behaviors, is used. (In some analyses all aggressive behaviors cluster together, or all verbal behaviors correlate and we get three rather than four factors; see Cohen-Mansfield et al., 1995). Our findings indicate that these syndromes occur at different stages of dementia, and are correlated with different environmental conditions and different psycho-social characteristics (e.g., Cohen-Mansfield, Marx, & Werner, 1992; Cohen-Mansfield & Werner, 1995; Cohen-Mansfield, Culpepper, & Werner, 1995; Cohen-Mansfield & Libin, 2005). Lumping all the behaviors together can mask the significance of the findings.

Another example of an informant rating scale is the Pittsburgh Agitation Scale (Rosen et al., 1994). It rates agitated behaviors in four general behavior groups: Aberrant Vocalization, Motor Agitation, Aggressiveness, and Resisting Care, on a scale ranging from 0 to 4. The behaviors are assigned according to intensity, disruptiveness, and the ease with which the patient's behavior can be redirected. The brevity of the PAS makes it useful for repeated measurement such as for monitoring behavioral progression.

The Behavioral Pathology in Alzheimer's Disease Rating Scale (BEHAVE-AD; Reisberg et al., 1987) is yet another informant rating instrument, with 25 items, assessing paranoid/delusional ideation, hallucinations, activity disturbance (e.g., wandering, purposeless activity, inappropriate activity), aggressiveness, diurnal rhythm disturbance, affective disturbance, and anxieties and phobias. Items are rated on a severity scale ranging from 0 = "not present" to 3 = "present generally with an emotional and physical component." Additionally, the BEHAVE-AD has a 4-point scale of the global danger/disruptiveness of the behaviors for both the patient and caregivers.

It should be noted that the three examples are not based on superior attributes of these scales over others, but on the need to present a sample of the range of existing assessments.

Comparing Among *Informant Rating* Instruments

It has already been stated that there are many informant rating instruments (Table 15.1) which share many items and are generally very similar. They differ on several dimensions: the domains described, the type of scale used—and in consequence sensitivity, ceiling and floor effects; setting and informant used; content and length used; and the timeframe considered.

Domains

Table 15.1 estimates the number of items that focus on agitated behaviors in each of the instruments. Some of those instruments assess cognitive functioning, affect, and other constructs, in addition to agitation. For example, the NPI evaluates ten behavioral domains, including delusions/hallucinations, agitation/aggression, dysphoria, anxiety, apathy, disinhibition, irritability/lability, and aberrant motor activity. Those assessments that specifically assess inappropriate behaviors and do not mix different constructs in the same assessment instrument assist in guarding against an inappropriate mixing of different constructs. Some of the instruments are geared to a specific behavioral syndrome, such as the Ryden Aggression Scale (Ryden,1988); others are more global.

Informants

Another difference among instruments lies in the identity of the informant used. Should one interview nursing assistants, charge nurses, or family members? Obviously, since the assessments inquire about the frequency at which the behaviors occurred, the crucial point is the amount of contact the informant had with the older person during the period to be rated, and the informant's ability to observe and report the behavior. Some assessments are used with several types of informants.

Informant-based data reflect the perceptions of the informant. It may be affected by the informant's level of stress, such as a nursing staff member who has to assess residents when many on the unit have an acute illness, or, conversely, it may be affected by habituation to the behavior through long exposure. At times, informants may under-report behavior because of concern that high levels of inappropriate behavior may reflect negatively either on the quality of care they provide, or on the elderly person.

Content and Length

Content and length also differ among instruments. Scales vary from three items to approximately 40, although the content of many items can overlap. Frequently, three items do not capture the variability among inappropriate behaviors and do not remind the informant of the full range of behaviors which need to be rated. Detailed and focused instruments are important when it is unknown which behaviors are most crucial for any specific purpose in a given population. At other times a very short instrument is needed, such as when behaviors need to be continuously monitored to assess fluctuation or responsiveness to treatment in a clinical setting. For certain purposes not all items on the longer instruments are useful. Therefore, a shorter form of the CMAI has been developed, and has been used for clinical studies which lack funding, and therefore need to be conducted with minimal requirements of staff members. Furthermore, some projects concentrate on specific behaviors, such as pacing and wandering, or verbally disruptive behaviors, and thus may use shorter assessments which focus only on the behavior under study.

Related to the issue of length is content. Generally, short instruments either concentrate on a subset of the behaviors or lump some of them into somewhat larger categories. Depending on the population treated, indicators that collapse behaviors (e.g., all physical aggression is one item on the MDS) may be particularly useful, or may be too broad for the designation of treatment and monitoring of its effects.

Scales

Another difference among the assessments involves the scales used, including various frequency and disruptiveness scales. Points on the scale should be well defined; for example, the frequency of a number of times in a specified period is more precise and less open to interpretation than general terms like "a lot" or "frequently." Scales that emphasize the impact of the behavior generally focus on the disruptiveness of the behavior or on reactions to the behavior. The scale may also be responsible for a ceiling effect. When the population exhibits behaviors that occur much more frequently than once per day, instruments where the highest frequency noted is "daily" may not be sufficiently sensitive.

This is particularly important when a scale is being used to make decisions about the human resources necessary to manage behaviors.

Time Frames

Time frames on which the older person is rated depend on the study and on the scale used; some studies use the last nursing shift, i.e., the previous eight hours; others use the last month, or a time frame in between. The period chosen can vary according to the nature of the behaviors to be rated, and according to the memory which can be expected of caregivers. If the behavior is hitting or biting, raters usually remember such high-impact behaviors, even if they occurred a month prior to rating. If, on the other hand, the behavior is one with a low impact, such as repetitious mannerisms, it is less likely to be remembered for long periods of time.

Scoring

Last, there are various ways to score these assessments: the items can be summed by their frequency or by their disruptive impact, or by frequency weighted by disruptive impact. They can also be scored by syndromes; one can look at the most frequently occurring behavior, or at the most disruptive. Obviously these different methods will yield different rates and results. As mentioned before, we found meaningful differences between the syndromes of agitation, e.g., verbal behaviors, physically non-aggressive, and physically aggressive behaviors, and therefore for most purposes these should be scored separately. The final choice obviously depends, however, on the purpose of the assessment.

Observational Methods

Observational methods involve a person watching specified behaviors and rating them as they occur. There are several ways in which these can be performed. A research assistant can view the older person in his or her natural environment and check categories on a printed (i.e., paper and pencil) instrument each time a behavior occurs. If a mechanical device is used, the research assistant presses a button on the handheld computer—a personal digital assistant (PDA)—or scans a bar code from a list. Alternatively, the older person can be videotaped, which is then rated by a research assistant.

One major difficulty with the use of observational methods for assessing agitation is that many behaviors do not occur most of the time, so extensive periods of observation or a large quantity of observations may be needed in order to detect behaviors. That is especially true for rarer behaviors such as aggressive behavior, which are among the most important in terms of impact on others, but are infrequent.

A number of observational tools exist, including the Agitation Behavior Mapping Instrument (Cohen-Mansfield, Werner, & Marx, 1989) in which several aspects of agitation are examined: the frequency of occurrence of the agitated behaviors; the social environment, i.e., the identity of those in close proximity; the activity in which they are engaged, who initiated the activity; the location of the resident on the unit; environment characteristics; and body position. Proper use of the ABMI requires thorough training of the observers. The types of agitated behaviors observed are very similar to those found in informant ratings assessments.

Mechanical Devices

Mechanical devices have been used for assessing wandering, with instruments such as a pedometer, an actigraph, and a step sensor. These are typically attached at the ankle of the person, and measure the amount of walking performed by the older person. Most of these devices have a demonstrated validity against an observational criterion (Cohen-Mansfield, 1997). They vary in the degree to which they bother the older persons, the extent to which the older persons fidget with the devices, difficulty of putting the device on the older persons, and difficulty of transferring data from the device to workable data for the research (Cohen-Mansfield, 1997).

Use of technical devices has been very limited, and was generally confined to ambulatory behavior, with some trials of use of devices to analyze vocal (Cohen-Mansfield, Werner, Hammerschmidt, & Newman, 2003) and aggressive (Chen et al., 2008) behavior.

Comparing Methods of Assessment

Given the various methods available, including informant ratings, observational methods, and mechanical devices, how do we decide which methods to use? The decision will be based on the understanding of their differences on dimensions such as: *time sampling*, *objectivity*, and *cost*. In terms of *length of the period that is sampled* by the instrument, the time frame is longer for informant ratings, as you can ask about a period such as the last two weeks or a month. Very short periods are covered by live observations, and the same is true for videotapes, because it takes as long to code them as *in vivo* observations. Longer periods can be covered with technological devices. Similarly, observations are performed utilizing time sampling, i.e., specific time-limited periods are chosen for observation, such as observing a three-minute observation hourly for six hours a day for a week. No such planned time sampling takes place in informant raters; however, informant ratings sample the behavior by the contact of informant with the rated person. Following this is the decision concerning the appropriateness of each of these methods for assessing low-frequency behaviors, such as aggressive behavior. Informant ratings are usually reasonably appropriate for such behaviors, although it depends on salience of the behavior. Observations are, however, quite inappropriate for detection of low-frequency behaviors.

In terms of *objectivity*, informant ratings can be biased by the relationship between the informant and the person who is rated. That is sometimes a problem, depending on the purpose of assessment. If the ability of the caregiver to take care of the person is the focal point, then their perception of the behavior is likely to be the target behavior, whether objective or biased. If the focus is the behavior *per se*, then the bias is a source of concern, and other methods should be considered.

In terms of *cost*, caregiver ratings are relatively inexpensive, whereas observations are very costly. The cost of mechanical devices depends not only on the price of the device, but also on the costs mentioned before: patient handling of device; ease of use of device; costs of transferring data from device to workable data; etc. Finally, the actual choice of an assessment method will depend on the goals and resources of the user, and how they match the strengths and weaknesses of each method.

Treatment Model for Agitation and its Implications for Assessment

Although a complete discussion of the theoretical understanding of agitation and the ensuing treatment implications is beyond the scope of this chapter, a short discussion is necessary for an understanding of the assessment needs. Many of the agitated behaviors are conceptualized as resulting from unmet needs (Cohen-Mansfield, 2000a). An imbalance in the interaction between lifelong habits and personality, current physical and mental states, and less than optimal environmental conditions results in unmet needs. The dementia process itself poses an obstacle for appropriate need fulfillment because of impairments in both communication and in the ability to utilize the environment appropriately. The unmet need, as well as limitations in the ability to fulfill their own needs, result in frustration. Agitated behaviors can be an expression of this frustration, or of the discomfort of having an unmet need, such as physical pain. Alternatively, the behaviors may be instrumental, such as trying to solicit help or alleviate a need to be occupied via self-stimulation.

The different syndromes of agitation, physically aggressive, physically non-aggressive, verbally non-aggressive, and verbally aggressive behaviors are related to different needs. Based on correlational studies, we have found verbal behaviors to be related to physical pain, discomfort, loneliness, and depression. Physically non-aggressive behaviors are usually not related to suffering, occur under normal conditions, and appear to be adaptive in providing stimulation. Aggressive behaviors are those least explained by the unmet needs model, but some behaviors appear to be the result of discomfort, invasion of personal space, or an effort to communicate. Some may have a more direct neurobiological etiology.

Based on this conceptualization, we have developed an approach to treatment, which we have termed "Treatment Routes for Exploring Agitation" (TREA). TREA intervention emphasizes an individualized approach to treatment, based on the conclusion that different syndromes of disruptive behaviors have different etiologies, different meanings, and therefore require different approaches to treatment. Given that we assume that many of the behaviors result from unmet needs, the first step is to identify the need. Therefore, non-pharmacological approaches of identifying the need and aiming to fulfill it precede pharmacological approaches. Research has demonstrated the efficacy of this and other non-pharmacological approaches that are based on fulfilling both physiological and psychological needs (Cohen-Mansfield et al., 2007; Baker et al., 2003). It is suggested that non-pharmacological interventions can serve to delay institutionalization (Spijker et al., 2008). In developing a treatment plan, the remaining abilities, strengths, memories, and needs should be utilized, as well as recognition of disabilities, especially those in sensory perception and mobility. Unique characteristics of the individual such as past work, hobbies, important relationships, and sense of identity need to be explored to best match current activities to the person's abilities. Examples of the range of possible activities to use as stimulation can be found in Baker et al., 2003; Bowlby, 1993; Halpern, Bartlett, & Dowling, 1995; Russen-Rondinone & DesRoberts, 1996; Teri & Logsdon, 1991; Zgola, 1987.

The TREA approach is utilized to recognize needs by providing a series of questions for verbally disruptive behaviors, physically non-aggressive behaviors, and physically aggressive behaviors. The steps to be explored for verbally and vocally agitated behaviors include examination of potential physical pain, depressed affect, hallucinations/delusions, need for social contact (loneliness, fears), and understimulation. For physically non-aggressive behaviors, the main issues to be determined include: the possibility that it involves akathisia as an adverse side effect of medication, determination of whether the behavior represents discontent on the part of the older person, whether it poses a danger to the older person, and whether those in proximity to the older person or those caring for him or her are bothered by it. For aggressive behaviors, etiologies concerning physical discomfort, invasion of personal space, delusions/hallucinations, and triggering by an ADL event or by another person are explored. Once an etiology is established as a possible cause, a matching treatment approach is utilized.

Some of the etiologies to be uncovered are but a first step in further assessment. For example, if depressed affect is detected via self-report, observation of facial expression (see Lawton, Parmelee, Katz, & Nesselroade, 1996), or by informant rating, the reason for that affect needs to be ascertained. Indeed, social isolation is a common etiology for verbal agitation and may be related to the manifestation of depression as well.

Further details on the conceptualization of agitation and of the TREA approach can be found in Cohen-Mansfield and Deutsch (1996), Cohen-Mansfield, Libin, and Marx (2007), and in Cohen-Mansfield (2000b). Even from this brief summary, it should be evident that the assessment of the frequency and disruptiveness of agitation represents only a portion of the assessment needed to treat agitation. The specific etiology for the agitated behavior should be assessed when possible. At times, however, only an intervention trial may clarify whether a specific etiology is a likely one.

Clinically, the assessment needs to start with a *specific* description of the agitated behavior. It must be well defined. In order to determine the etiology of the behavior, several approaches can be taken.

1. According to the TREA approach a systematic investigation of the most common etiologies of the main syndromes is undertaken via current tools for those assessments. One example of an etiology, especially for verbal/vocal agitation is undiagnosed or inadequately treated pain. A complete description of the antecedents of the behavior can assist in the identification of its cause, such as when vocal behavior increases when the person is transferred. For cognitively impaired individuals it is useful to speak directly with as many care providers as possible about how the patient reacts to handling during personal care, range of motion, positioning, transferring and seating. A pain assessment for this population (Cohen-Mansfield & Lipson, 2007) should be utilized. The assessing clinician should observe personal care and handling activities to determine if agitated behaviors are related to these triggers. In addition to the examination of specific etiologies, the following are frequently used to assist in the determination of the reason for the agitated behavior.
2. In some clinical situations it is useful to define the frequency, intensity, and duration of the behavior via a behavioral "mapping" system that allows the clinician to answer the question: "What is the rhythm of this person's day?" This includes measurement of activity patterns that allow for an analysis of sleep/wake patterns, periods of calmness, periods of normal psychomotor activity, and periods of agitated behavior that are difficult or perceived as "impossible" to address. An example of this is found in the Q 30 minute Observation Record. This dementia mapping system allows the clinician to track sleep/wake, movement patterns, or periods of verbal or physical agitation in 30-minute segments through the 24-hour cycle. The behaviors can be color coded, and then improvements or other pattern changes over time after initiation of behavioral interventions can be determined. Once such a tool has been implemented, staff members are often surprised to discover that what they thought was unrelenting agitation is really episodic and time limited. In this way, staff can be assisted in recognizing patterns that will facilitate the placement of additional staffing resources or behavioral/environmental interventions that would reduce the overall level of agitation. Such a tool can be used to make clinical decisions, evaluate client outcomes of interventions, and educate/inform families about the outcomes of treatments being offered.
3. An examination of the stimulus/response relationship a person has with the environment. The clinical question driving measurement is: "What are the triggers which elicit behaviors in this person?" This form of measurement is often coined "Antecedent–Behavior–Consequence" (ABC) documentation. This type of documentation can assist the interdisciplinary team to identify those agitated behaviors that occur as a result of direct environmental influences that can be modified to prevent occurrence. ABC documentation can take the form of an interdisciplinary progress note where the following variables are present. These variables can be termed the five "Ws" of behavior:
   a. What is the specific behavior?
   b. Why does this need to be addressed?
   c. Where does it occur?
   d. When does it occur?
   e. Who is around when it happens?

   Typically, one may add: what has preceded the behavior or what may have triggered it? Who responded to the behavior and how?

All disciplines in an agency working with agitated persons should be familiar with these variables and know how to include them in a progress note describing an incident of behavioral agitation. It is critical for the holistic interdisciplinary team to be interested both in those triggers that elicit a stress response and those that elicit pleasure, happiness, and contentment. One form that ABC documentation can take is the initiation of a "behavioral *monitoring record*" whereby team members are asked to describe the observed behavior, and the possible variables that triggered the event, as well as the interventions selected to manage the event and the impact of the interventions selected.

A complete assessment of agitated behavior also includes the determination of a level of risk to oneself and others associated with the behavior. A determination of risk for the agitated behavior is conducted within the context of the organizational philosophy, the family philosophy, the impact on interdisciplinary resources, and the total environment, including co-patients. Behaviors can then be identified as low or high risk.

In order to develop an appropriate intervention, the assessment should also include remaining functional/cognitive abilities. At times the unmet needs causing agitation relate to excess disability and to the perpetual frustration of unobtainable mastery of previous skills (Bell & Troxell, 1997; Dawson, Wells, & Kline, 1993; Hall & Buckwalter, 1987; Jones, 1996; Lawton, 1970). If the person's remaining strengths are well understood by the direct care provider, they can be incorporated into the care plan so that the patient has opportunity to participate directly and has a sense of mastery. Disruptive behaviors are thereby eliminated or reduced in frequency. As previously mentioned, most agitated dementia behaviors are related to understimulation, due to little or no opportunity to engage in meaningful activity. Agitation is seen as the direct result of either under- or inappropriate stimulation within the environment and the demands that the resident responds to as a result of this. In order to promote a sense of mastery, control, and stimulation, care providers may use the Abilities Assessment Instrument (Dawson et al., 1993). In it care providers score patients on four subscales: (1) Self-care Abilities; (2) Social Abilities; (3) Interactional Abilities; and (4) Interpretive Abilities. Each of the subscales assists the care provider to understand those functional skills that remain and develop a care planning approach that supports enablement. The clinical team then documents activities for the person that are either *Abilities Enhancing* or *Abilities Compensating*. For example, under Self-care Abilities, the care provider assesses the spatial skills of the patient, thereby determining right/left orientation. If it is determined that the patient can distinguish the right arm from the left, all verbal cueing instructions can be given as follows: "George, please give me your *right* hand. Please, put your *right* hand in the sleeve of your sweater." This is also very helpful in the care of severely impaired patients who appear to be uncooperative with personal care. For example, "Helen, please relax your *left* hand. Helen, please open your *left* hand so that I can place your splint." Directions that take advantage of the remaining ability of spatial orientation can assist the care provider in helping the patient participate directly. This can also be quite helpful in reducing the number of catastrophic reactions and displays of agitated behavior because the patient simply did not understand the full extent of the simple instructions.

In order to tailor an intervention to prevent agitation in an older person, caregivers need to understand the abilities, preferences, needs, and identity of the person. Some useful assessments in this process include the following: the self-identity questionnaire (Cohen-Mansfield, Parpura-Gill, & Golander, 2006a, 2006b); the Self-maintenance Habits and Preferences in Elderly (SHAPE; Cohen-Mansfield & Jensen, 2007), and Pain Assessment In Noncommunicative Elderly persons (PAINE; Cohen-Mansfield, 2006).

In summary, the complete assessment of agitation involves, in addition to the direct assessment of agitation, a systematic examination of the likely etiologies of the behaviors, as well as identification of remaining functional/cognitive skill so that these can be utilized during everyday experiences.

UTILIZING ASSESSMENTS IN CLINICAL SITUATIONS

Placement/Admission/Screening

Appropriate Placement

In the province of Ontario, the CMAI is used to assist clinical teams to match clinical needs of the client with available resources. The Community Care Access Centers (CCACs) complete the CMAI on a client being recommended for admission to a long-term care facility or transfer from one facility to another. The clinical team uses the completed CMAI together with a demographic survey to identify client fit for admission and programming purposes. The CMAI assists the interdisciplinary team with identifying suitability for admission, and drafting a preliminary behavioral care plan based on their cognitive/functional skills, as well as the frequency, severity, and disruptiveness of their behavioral profiles. In this way clinical and adjunct care resources can be anticipated and put in place prior to the arrival of the client. For example, one-on-one behavioral supervision and extra environmental supports to enhance adjustment to the transition from home to the facility. This is particularly helpful in the case of the client with a volatile behavioral profile.

Admission

Assessment of agitation is helpful if included as part of a screening process whereby prospective clients are reviewed for suitability for admission. CMAI-disruptive is completed by care providers from the referring agency, and then is used as baseline data for consideration for eligibility for admission. It assists in identifying those patients who have behaviors that require assessment by an interdisciplinary team. If the behaviors described in written documentation are benign, or infrequent, the patient is not considered suitable for admission to a behavioral rehabilitation and monitoring unit. Instead a program of on-site education and support is recommended through the community psychogeriatric outreach team. In order to screen outpatients, the admission team looks for behaviors related to overt physical aggression that occur at a frequency of 2, or "less than once a week." If this is the rate of occurrence for a case, then the team immediately questions the suitability for admission. The "Disruptiveness" column often helps the team to determine how much the behavior is a nuisance for staff, and the degree to which the staff require supportive interventions so that they can learn to accommodate and cope with the behavior. For example, often it is the case that the patient exhibits benign behaviors such as disrobing or aimless wandering that in themselves are not of a high risk, but are seen as very disruptive to the routines and acceptable social behaviors with which nursing home staff feel comfortable. This type of problem behavior requires education and support rather than an admission to an acute behavioral unit. If the CMAI indicates that physically aggressive behaviors are occurring with a frequency of 5 through 7, meaning that behaviors are occurring frequently during a shift, or several times an hour, then it is determined that the patient requires admission for in-depth interdisciplinary assessment, and detailed behavioral observation and analysis. The CMAI can then be completed within 14 days of admission to correspond to the indicators found in the "Mood and Behavior Patterns" section of the Minimum Data Set. Scores on the CMAI in the category of physical aggression that indicate a frequency of less than daily have been used to consider transfer of the more stable patient to a step-down unit to await transfer back to the referring agency.

The CMAI-disruptive is also part of a provincial geriatric mental health training initiative to assist most skilled long-term care facilities use the tool as part of a standardized assessment protocol for referral to community psychogeriatric outreach teams. As a result of this initiative, smaller long-term care facilities who have no in-house mental health resources will have common data collection tools that will assist the out-of-house consultants make more accurate behavioral diagnoses when they receive a referral.

Staff Communication

Advanced practitioners in clinical teams can use the CMAI as a means to summarize and interpret the behavioral profile of a client, and as an outcome measure to planned behavioral interventions. The practitioner can read the progress notes, analyze the 24-hour dementia mapping sheet, fill out the CMAI as a "draft," discuss the frequency of disruptive categories with staff familiar with the patient, coming to a consensus about the responses and comparing and contrasting this with the previously documented behavioral profile. The advanced practitioner should include in their responsibilities directions to evening and night staff to complete the CMAI for their shift using the same process. Collaboration and discussion should occur between RNs, LPNs, Health Care Aides, and other team members. The completed forms can then be used to discuss the patient's behavioral profile at a preliminary care planning conference or an admission conference. During the admission conference the CMAI results should be compared to the pre-admission baseline form that was received from the referring agency. The completed CMAIs can also be used as a teaching tool to educate families about the frequency with which behaviors of interest are occurring. Families report that they find this discussion reassuring because the behavior is being discussed in objective, sensitive terms. The CMAI should also be completed quarterly in conjunction with the Minimum Data Set (MDS) quarterly assessments. When the behavioral profile appears to be more stable, decisions can be made about the suitability of transfer back to the referring agency or discharge to another facility. It is important to note that the interdisciplinary team should never consider the CMAI agitation data in isolation of other clinical data. It is helpful, however, to facilitate objective discussion about patient behavior and the frequency with which it occurs, rather than make clinical decisions based on opinion or impressions. Quantifying data on agitation helps the team focus on those behaviors that represent a risk and those behaviors that can and should be accommodated.

Treatment: Evaluation, Staff Communication, Patient Monitoring, and Treatment Selection

Mr Z is an 83-year-old patient admitted to a cognitive assessment unit (CAU) because he has frequently displayed overt physical aggression and erratic behavior toward his wife while living at home. He has been married for 50 years and has a son and a daughter, both of whom live considerable distances away. His wife has cared for him by herself for several years. He was admitted to the CAU through the local hospital's Emergency Room because he impulsively climbed a tree in the backyard, lost his balance and fell, fracturing his right wrist and clavicle. The admission took place because the description of the behavioral profile, the functional history, and the assessment of caregiver burden indicated that further review would be necessary. His behavior has been relatively stable since admission to the CAU, therefore he is being recommended for discharge to a local long-term care facility, because it has been determined that his wife is not capable of safely managing him any longer at home. The referring clinicians of the CAU indicated that Mr Z has been agitated, particularly at night, shouting out and banging on the bedrails. In addition, he is "resistive" to bathing and grooming activities. The clinical team at the LTC facility request that the CCAC complete and attach a CMAI to their transfer request. The behavioral profiles indicate that the frequency and level of disruptiveness of non-physical and physical aggressive behaviors are considered acceptable parameters to meet the admission criteria of the Dementia Support Unit at their facility. The level of calling out behaviors helps them plan for a room location that will not be disruptive to other residents. Upon admission a Q 30 Minute Dementia Observation Record is recorded for the first 14 days of admission. This document, in addition to others, is used to form an assessment by the interdisciplinary team and this is discussed at a clinical case review held within the third week of admission. During the review meeting, the team examines Mr Z's behavioral profile prior to and since admission, including a careful review of categories within the Cohen-Mansfield Agitation Inventory, behavioral mapping within each 24-hour cycle, and the circumstances surrounding events of catastrophic behavior. An Abilities Assessment Instrument (Dawson et al., 1993) is also completed and discussed.

Patterns of behavior cannot be completely understood without considering the full history of the patient's life experiences, and relating those to the present behavioral profile. The following therefore represents the details of the assessments that contributed to a full discussion of Mr Z's agitation.

Personhood

Mr Z was employed as a mechanical maintenance shift worker in the local steel mills. He emigrated to a large, industrial city in Ontario, Canada, from Italy in 1952. He met and married his wife in 1954. He has two children; a daughter and a son. His wife reports that he has always had a temper that flared easily. Irritability was a real problem just prior to retirement, especially since his ability to perform on the equipment was questioned by a foreman, and he was relegated to janitorial service. He felt this was insulting, and was finally offered early retirement. Since retirement he has become progressively more difficult to live with. Mr Z was diagnosed with dementia of the Alzheimer type in 2004. His wife has cared for him at home until this admission. The need for admission was facilitated by the fracture incident, but also Mr Z's night-time behavior. He would awaken at night, and then try to exit the house so that he could get to work. He has struck his wife several times in the last few months, particularly if he was thwarted from leaving the house at night. She is at the end of her rope and has become physically ill, requiring hospitalization.

Cohen-Mansfield Agitation Inventory

It is determined from reviewing the CMAI that Mr Z displays *physically aggressive behavior* several times a day. Specifically, the patient stations himself at the door to his room in order to prevent others from entering. He hits, kicks, pushes, and grabs when he perceives that his room is about to be entered. He displays *no physically non-aggressive behavior*. He does display *verbally agitated behavior* in that he frequently asks to call his wife on the telephone several times an hour, particularly between the hours of 7 and 9 pm before he settles for the evening. He will insist on calling his wife, even though he has talked to her several times in the preceding hour.

Behavioral Documentation

The Q 30 minute Dementia Observation Record behavioral documentation supports that the recorded incidents of aggression require several staff members to intervene to de-escalate the patient's behavior. From a risk perspective, he does not actively seek out other patients or exit the door to his room to hit patients who are walking in the hallway. His hitting out is limited to those people who actively turn, and attempt to pass him in the doorway to enter his room. The behavior is more likely to occur in the evening just after dinner, most frequently between 7 and 9 pm. The behavior can be prevented if a member of staff or volunteer monitor walks in the hallway with the patients who wander into his space, and by giving him activities of interest that occupy him.

Abilities Assessment

The patient requires assistance with grooming and dressing in that he needs to have his clothing laid out for him in sequence and be given verbal instruction regarding what to do. Sometimes he needs the activity demonstrated, and he will mimic what he has seen. He can appreciate humor, and can accurately label the emotions behind graphic depictions of faces demonstrating sadness, anger, and happiness. Staff can use this to assist him to calm himself when he becomes agitated when others enter his personal space. He can describe the structural components of a room, but cannot describe what the items in the room are for. Similarly he can describe objects, and name them, but cannot describe their purpose. He can, however, demonstrate their purpose and can mimic their use when he is shown a visual cue. The patient has very intact social skills, so every opportunity is given to have the hall monitors mimic appropriate social behaviors when other patients are in his vicinity. The context of the movement is that the other patients are "strolling" in their neighborhood and this is seen as less threatening to Mr Z. He will greet them appropriately in that context, rather than become suspicious that they will enter his "home."

The team uses the Cohen-Mansfield Agitation Inventory as a baseline measure to track the progression of behavioral stability after instituting a care plan that allows for the maintenance of remaining strengths. The care plan also puts in place a structure for the evenings that will encourage staff members to facilitate positive social interactions between Mr Z and other residents, so that his anger and aggression can be prevented.

Approximately six weeks after the first case conference, the behavioral documentation, including the Cohen-Mansfield Agitation Inventory, were reviewed and it was determined that the patient's behavior had stabilized. Fewer incidents of agitation were present in the patient, and a decision was made to plan discharge to a long-term care facility.

Treatment Continuation Evaluation—Case Studies

The CMAI can be used to facilitate discussion around initiation and titration of psychoactive medications. For example, an inventory can be taken of all psychoactive medications used for the purposes of behavioral control, and a comparison can be made of these with the scores on the CMAI. For patients who show behavioral indicators of overt physical aggression present at a frequency of 4 (a few times a week) or less, walking rounds can be conducted between the responsible family physician, advanced care practitioner and/or nurse practitioner, and the direct-care providers, so that plans can be made to titrate the medication to progressively lower doses until either the medication is discontinued, or behavioral occurrences increase in frequency. The CMAI should then be repeatedly completed (quarterly, for example) and used in conjunction with behavioral mapping observation sheets completed by the direct-care providers, in order to track each patient's behavioral response to the reduction of psychoactive medications.

The CMAI can also be used as an educational tool for families. An example occurred in a nursing home, where the family wanted to discontinue haloperidol use with their mother, whereas staff members considered it necessary to assist with keeping her behavioral profile stable. The staff agreed, however, to a discontinuation trial in which her behavior would be monitored daily with the CMAI (changing the period of rating to one day). After several weeks of such monitoring, staff were convinced that it was safe to continue the medication reduction trial. Alternatively, the CMAI can be useful to provide families with evidence that a particular pharmacological regimen is not necessary. For example, one family demanded that the patient of concern be medicated with larger doses of medication because they perceived the behavior while at home to be dangerous and they did not wish any staff members to be injured. The clinical team believed that the behaviors manifested while at home might not necessarily continue in the Dementia Support Unit, and indeed the CMAI revealed this to be the case. The admission conference included showing and explaining the results of the behavioral assessment using the CMAI, and the family subsequently felt confident in the team's decision to lower the dose of antipsychotic medication and eventually discontinue it.

Applied Clinical Research: Treatment Utility Evaluation of a New Bathing Intervention—Trial Case Study

Catastrophic responses to bathing and personal care activities are often a dilemma for direct-care providers. The behavioral descriptors contained in the CMAI can be used as outcome measures to evaluate specialized care plan interventions. For example, in the case of Mrs M, a 76-year-old obese patient with diabetes mellitus and concurrent cognitive impairment, the CMAI was used as an instrument to measure the impact of a bathing intervention. Mrs M became quite upset with any attempts to bathe her. Unfortunately, she experienced discomfort from several areas of excoriation of tissues under the breasts and skinfolds on her abdomen. The care staff were very concerned about her extremely physical response during bathing, which was manifested by kicking, biting, punching, and scratching. A towel bath procedure was customized for Mrs M, and the impact of this was evaluated using the CMAI as the baseline for making observations about Mrs M's physical and emotional responses to being handled. The CMAI behavioral indicators were used as descriptive anchors to compare Mrs M's responses to the towel bathing technique with her responses to a standard tub bath or bed bath using a basin. These data were recorded by the clinical team on the "Bathing Evaluation Form," which was the main outcome measure for the intervention of interest. The tool was developed to record the frequencies with which Mrs M hit, kicked, spit, yelled, etc., during personal care. The evaluation demonstrated a positive treatment effect in support of the use of therapeutic towel bathing for Mrs M's care. The CMAI can therefore be useful to promote practice change at the bedside.

INFLUENCE OF SETTING ON AGITATION AND ITS ASSESSMENT

The settings in which agitation can occur span the complete range of the geriatric landscape, ranging from home, congregate housing, adult day care, sheltered housing, assisted living, hospital, and nursing home. In terms of agitation, factors which determine the expected level of agitation and explanatory variables are levels of cognitive function, and familiarity with the setting. From this point of view, very low levels of dementia are present among community-dwelling elderly persons, whereas the nursing home environment, and the geriatric psychiatric hospital will have the highest rates. In addition to cognitive levels, selection factors play a role in allowing certain levels of agitation to occur only in some settings. In our studies we found the population of adult day care participants to manifest levels of cognitive decline similar to those in the nursing home. Nevertheless, levels of aggressive behaviors were considerably lower, presumably because they could not be tolerated in the adult day care setting. Familiarity with the setting is an important explanatory variable in that the period of adjustment to a new setting is likely to be accompanied by greater frustration and confusion, thereby resulting in increased levels of agitation. Finally, the hospital deserves special attention, because it frequently combines a completely new environment with physical pain or discomfort, and, at times, intrusive procedures. All of these are likely to elicit higher levels of agitation.

A complete assessment of agitated behaviors should include an assessment of the environment within which the resident is living. All aspects of the environment impact directly on the agitation level manifested by the resident. The structural environment considerations include such questions as location where the agitation is occurring, square footage of private space, furniture, wayfinding cues, seating, building materials, equipment availability, staffing ratios, etc. The sensory environment should be assessed for such features as noise levels, light quality, use of color, odor, and homelike atmosphere. The organizational environment should be evaluated for philosophy, model of care, practice standards, actual staff practice patterns, operationalization of supportive programming, and overall design and structure (Duffin, 2008; Morgan, Stewart, D'arcy, & Werezak, 2004; Mountain & Bowie, 1995;

Reimer, Slaughter, Donaldson, Currie, & Eliasziw, 2004; Slaughter, Calkins, Eliasziw, & Reimer, 2006). Staff attitudes and responses to resident needs and requests are particularly important in affecting agitation, as is the support, both physical and emotional, of the staff by the administration (Cohen-Mansfield & Parpura-Gill, 2007a). The appropriateness of the environment includes the preparedness of the clinical staff to meet the needs of older adults who become agitated. The staff should have educational and mentoring opportunities available to them so that they understand the principles of communication, person-centered care, customized bathing approaches, and behavioral management principles (Ayalon, Arean, Bornfeld, & Beard, 2009; Cohen-Mansfield & Parpura-Gill, 2007b; Cohen-Mansfield, 2008b; Finnema et al., 2005; Schindel-Martin et al., 2003; Sloane et al., 2004). It has been suggested that properly trained staff can reduce the incidence of physically aggressive episodes (Speziale, Black, Coatsworth-Puspoky, Ross, & O'Reagan, 2009). The impact of the environment on the fundamental experience of the resident in long-term care must be fully evaluated as part of the complete behavioral assessment of the resident who is agitated.

A major influence of a setting on agitation lies in staff members' understanding of the problem and its treatment, as well as the setting's ability to accommodate the behavior. If a setting allows safe access to the outside, pacing and wandering are likely to be perceived as less disruptive than in locations where no area for wandering is provided. Understanding of these factors is important for tailoring an assessment for a specific setting, and for evaluating an assessment across settings.

MULTICULTURAL ISSUES

Whereas no research specifically addressing multicultural issues in the assessment of agitation was found, some indirect findings may provide initial information on this topic. The CMAI has been translated to many languages, including French, German, Austrian, Chinese, Dutch, Swedish, Italian, Canadian English, Czech, Japanese, Korean, Belgian, Spanish, UK English, U.S. Spanish, etc. It has therefore been used in many cultures. Various reports support the notion that at least some features of agitation are similar across cultures. A summary of factor analyses of the CMAI based on previous reports from United States, Japan, Hong Kong, and the Netherlands, as well as analysis of other data from Australia, Europe, and Canada, and from the United States, shows that the factor structure is robust and therefore similar among these different national cultures (Rabinowitz et al., 2005). A French study examining the relationship between the syndromes of agitation and cognitive functioning also revealed relationships very similar to those discovered in the United States (Micas, Ousset, & Vellas, 1995). Mintzer, Nietert, Costa, and Waid (1996) compared the syndromes of agitation in African American and White elderly persons living in two settings: the nursing home and a selected community group. They concluded that agitation factors reported mainly in White populations apply to African American populations, and that level of agitation is predicted more by demographic variables and settings than by ethnic identity. In agreement with this conclusion is a discussion summary presented in the same volume of *International Psychogeriatrics*, 8 (Suppl. 3, 1996) describing low levels of agitation and violence among patients in psychiatric hospitals in India, but attributing those to the type of care received in these institutions.

SUMMARY

The assessment of agitation is crucial for clinical, administrative, and research purposes with a population suffering from dementia. Clinical issues include selection of treatment, monitoring effects of treatment, decisions concerning treatment discontinuation, and proper placement of elderly persons;

administrative issues include unit composition decisions, staff communication, and quality control and improvement processes. There are several approaches to the assessment of agitation, with informant ratings being the most practical for many clinical situations. A multitude of informant ratings exist, and the selection of the appropriate one would depend on the match between the assessment properties and the specific use required, including the expected rates of agitation and the resources to complete the assessments. Assessment for the purpose of treatment selection cannot be confined to the frequency and disruptiveness of the behavior, but has to examine the context of the behavior and likely etiologies, as well as a general understanding of the specific person's ability, preferences, and identity. The development of systematic approaches to such holistic assessment is currently under way.

REFERENCES

Alexopoulos, G. S., Abrams, R. C., Young, R. C., & Shamoian, C. A. (1988). Cornell scale for depression in dementia. *Society of Biological Psychiatry, 23*, 271–284.

Ayalon, L., Arean, P., Bornfeld, H., & Beard, R. (2009). Long term care staff beliefs about evidence based practices for the management of dementia and agitation. *Int. J. Geriatric Psych., 24*(2), 118–124.

Baker, R., Holloway, J., Holtkamp, C. C. M., Larsson, A., Hartman, L. C., Pearce, R., et al. (2003). Effects of multi-sensory stimulation for people with dementia. *Journal of Advanced Nursing, 43*(5), 465–477.

Baumgarten, M., Becker, R., & Gauthier, S. (1990). Validity and reliability of the dementia behavior disturbance scale. *Journal of the American Geriatrics Society, 38*(3), 221–226.

Beck, J. G. (1997). Mental health in the elderly—challenges for behavior therapy: introduction the special series. *Behavior Therapy, Winter, 28*(1), 1–2.

Bell, V., & Troxell, D. (1997). *The Best Friends Approach to Alzheimer's Care*. Baltimore, MD: Health Professions Press, Inc.

Bowlby, C. (1993). *Therapeutic Activities with Persons Disabled by Alzheimer's Disease and Related Disorders*. Gaithersberg, MD: Aspen.

Chafetz, P. K., West, H. L., Lindesay, J., Briggs, K., Lawes, M., MacDonald, A., & Herzberg, J. (1987). *Longitudinal Control Group Evaluation of a Special Care Unit for Dementia Patients: Initial Findings*.

Chen, D., Wactlar, H., Chen, M. Y., Gao, C., Bharucha, A., & Hauptmann, A. (2008). Recognition of aggressive human behavior using binary local motion descriptors. *Conf. Proc. IEEE Eng. Med. Biol. Soc., 2008*, 5238–5241.

Cohen-Mansfield, J. (1997). Turnover among nursing home staff. *Nursing Management, 28*(5), 59–64.

Cohen-Mansfield, J. (2000a). Theoretical frameworks for behavioral problems in dementia. *Alzheimer's Care Quarterly, 1*(4), 8–21.

Cohen-Mansfield, J. (2000b). Non-pharmacological management of behavioral problems in persons with dementia: the TREA model. *Alzheimer's Care Quarterly, 1*(4), 22–34.

Cohen-Mansfield, J. (2005). Non-pharmacological interventions for persons with dementia. *Alzheimer's Care Quarterly, 6*(2), 129–145.

Cohen-Mansfield, J. (2006). Pain Assessment in Noncommunicative Elderly Persons—PAINE. *Clinical Journal of Pain, 22*(6), 569–575, Erratum in: *Clin. J. Pain* (2007), 23(4), 381.

Cohen-Mansfield, J. (2007). Temporal patterns of agitation in dementia. *American Journal of Geriatric Psychiatry, 15*(5), 395–405, May.

Cohen-Mansfield, J. (2008a). Agitated behavior in persons with dementia: the relationship between type of behavior, its frequency, and its disruptiveness. *Journal of Psychiatric Research, 43*(1), 64–69, Nov.

Cohen-Mansfield, J. (2008b). The language of behaviour. In M. Downs, & B. Bowsers (Eds.), *Excellence in Dementia Care, Research into Practice* (pp. 187–211). McGraw Hill.

Cohen-Mansfield, J., & Billig, N. (1986). Agitated behaviors in the elderly: I. A conceptual review. *Journal of the American Geriatrics Society, 34*(10), 711–721.

Cohen-Mansfield, J., & Deutsch, L. (1996). Agitation: Subtypes and their mechanisms. *Seminars in Clinical Neurophysiology, 1*(4), 325–329.

Cohen-Mansfield, J., & Jensen, B. (2007). Self-maintenance Habits and Preferences in Elderly (SHAPE): reliability of reports of self-care preferences in older persons. *Aging: Clinical and Experimental Research, 19*(1), 61–68.

Cohen-Mansfield, J., & Libin, A. (2004). Assessment of agitation in elderly patients with dementia: correlations between informant rating and direct observation. *International Journal of Geriatric Psychiatry, 19*(9), 881–891, Sep.

Cohen-Mansfield, J., & Libin, A. (2005). Verbal and physical agitation in cognitively impaired elderly with dementia: robustness of syndromes. *Journal of Psychiatric Research, 39*, 325–332.

Cohen-Mansfield, J., & Lipson, S. (2007). The utility of pain assessment for analgesic use in persons with dementia. *PAIN, 134*(1–2), 16–23.

Cohen-Mansfield, J., & Parpura-Gill, A. (2007a). Practice style in the nursing home: dimensions for assessment and quality improvement. *International Journal of Geriatric Psychiatry, 23*(4), 376–386.

Cohen-Mansfield, J., & Parpura-Gill, A. (2007b). Bathing: a framework for intervention focusing on psychosocial, architectural and human factors considerations. *The Archives of Gerontology and Geriatrics, 45*(2), 121–135.

Cohen-Mansfield, J., & Werner, P. (1995). Environmental influences on agitation: an integrative summary of an observational study. *The American Journal of Alzheimer's Care and Related Disorders and Research, 10*(1), 32–37.

Cohen-Mansfield, J., & Werner, P. (1998). Longitudinal changes in behavioral problems in old age: a study in an adult day care population. *Journal of Gerontology: Medical Sciences, 53A*(1), M65–M71.

Cohen-Mansfield, J., Culpepper, W. J., & Werner, P. (1995). The relationship between cognitive function and agitation in senior day care participants. *International Journal of Geriatric Psychiatry, 10*, 585–595.

Cohen-Mansfield, J., Libin, A., & Marx, M. S. (2007). Non-pharmacological treatment of agitation: a controlled trial of systematic individualized intervention. *Journals of Gerontology: Medical Sciences, 62*(8), 908–916.

Cohen-Mansfield, J., Marx, M. S., & Rosenthal, A. S. (1989). A description of agitation in a nursing home. *The Journals of Gerontology, 44*(3), M77–M84.

Cohen-Mansfield, J., Marx, M. S., & Werner, P. (1992). Agitation in elderly persons: an integrative report of findings in a nursing home. *International Psychogeriatrics, 4*(Suppl. 2), 221–241.

Cohen-Mansfield, J., Parpura-Gill, A., & Golander, H. (2006a). Utilization of self-identity roles for designing interventions for persons with dementia. *Journals of Gerontology: Psychological Sciences, 61*(4), 202–212.

Cohen-Mansfield, J., Parpura-Gill., A., & Golander, H. (2006b). Salience of self-identity roles in persons with dementia: differences in perceptions among elderly persons, family members and caregivers. *Social Science & Medicine, 62*(3), 745–757.

Cohen-Mansfield, J., Werner, P., & Marx, M. S. (1989). An observational study of agitation in agitated nursing home residents. *International Psychogeriatrics, 1*(2), 153–165.

Cohen-Mansfield, J., Werner, P., Hammerschmidt, K., & Newman, J. (2003). Acoustic properties of vocally disruptive behaviors in the nursing home. *Gerontology, 49*(3), 161–167.

Cohen-Mansfield, J., Werner, P., Watson, V., & Pasis, S. (1995). Agitation among elderly persons at adult daycare centers: the experiences of relatives and staff members. *International Psychogeriatrics, 7*(3), 447–458.

Dawson, P., Wells, D., & Kline, K. (1993). *Enhancing the Abilities of Persons with Alzheimers and Related Dementias*. New York, NY: Springer.

Devanand, D. P., Brockington, C. D., Moody, B. J., Brown, R. P., Mayeux, R., Endicott, J., & Sackeim, H. A. (1992). Behavioral syndromes in Alzheimer's disease. *International Psychogeriatrics, 4*(Suppl. 2), 161–185.

Drachman, D. A., Swearer, J. M., O'Donnell, B. F., Mitchell, A. L., & Maloon, A. (1992). The Caretaker Obstreperous-Behavior Rating Assessment (COBRA) scale. *Journal of the American Geriatrics Society, 40*, 463–470.

Duffin, C. (2008). Designing care homes for people with dementia. *Nursing Older People, 20*(4), 22–24.

Finkel, S. I. (1993). Mental health and aging: a decade of progress. *Generations, 25*.

Finnema, E., Droes, R., Ettema, T., Ooms, M., Ader, H., Ribbe, M., & Van Tilburg, W. (2005). The effect of integrated emotion-oriented care versus usual care on elderly persons with dementia in the nursing home and on nursing assistants: a randomized clinical trial. *Int. J. Geriatric Psych., 20*(4), 330–343.

Fisman, M., Gordon, B., Feleki, V., Helmes, E., McDonald, T., & Dupre, J. (1988). Metabolic changes in Alzheimer's disease. *Journal of the American Geriatrics Society*, *36*(4), 298–300.

Gottfries, C.-G., Brane, G., Gullberg, B., & Steen, G. (1982). A new rating scale for dementia syndromes. *Archives of Gerontology and Geriatrics* 311–330.

Greene, J. G., Smith, R., Gardiner, M., & Timbury, G. C. (1982). Measuring behavioural disturbance of elderly demented patients in the community and its effects on relatives: a factor analytic study. *Age and Ageing*, *11*, 121–126.

Hall, G. R., & Buckwalter, K. C. (1987). Progressively lowered stress threshold: a conceptual model for care of adults with Alzheimer's disease. *Archives of Psychiatric Nursing*, *1*(6), 399–405.

Halpern, A. R., Bartlett, J. C., & Dowling, W. J. (1995). Aging and experience in the recognition of musical transpositions. *Psychology and Aging*, *10*(3), 325–342.

Jones, M. J. (1996). *Gentlecare: changing the experience of Alzheimers disease in a positive way.* Burnaby, BC: Moyra Jones Resources.

Koss, E., Weiner, M., Ernesto, C., Cohen-Mansfield, J., Ferris, S., Grundman, M., Schafer, K., Sano, M., Thal, L. J., Thomas, R., Whitehouse, P. J., & the Alzheimers Disease Cooperative Study. (1997). Assessing patterns of agitation in Alzheimers disease patients with Cohen-Mansfield Agitation Inventory. *Alzheimer Disease and Associated Disorders—An International Journal*, *11*(Suppl. 2), S45–S50.

Lawton, M. P. (1970). Assessment, integration and environments for older people. *The Geronotologist*, *10*, 38–46.

Lawton, M. P., Parmelee, P. A., Katz, I. R., & Nesselroade, J. (1996). Affective states in normal and depressed older people. *The Journals of Gerontology: Psychological Sciences and Social Sciences*, *51B*(6), P309–P316.

Leuchter, A., Simon, S. L., Daly, K. A., Rosenberg-Thompson, S., Abrams, M., Dunkin, J. J., et al. (1994). Quantitative EEG correlates of outcome in older psychiatric patients. *The American Journal of Geriatric Psychiatry*, *2*(3), 200–209.

Levin, H. S., High, W. M., Goethe, K. E., Sisson, R. A., Overall, J. E., Rhoades, H. M., et al. (1987). The neurobehavioral rating scale: assessment of the behavioral sequelae of head injury by clinician. *J. Neurol. Neurosurg. Psychiatry*, *50*, 183–193.

Loreck, D. J., Bylsma, F. W., & Folstein, M. F. (1994). The Dementia Signs and Symptoms Scale. *The American Journal of Geriatric Psychiatry*, *2*(1), 60–74, Winter.

Meer, B., & Baker, J. A. (1966). The Stockton geriatric rating scale. *Journal of Gerontology*, *21*, 392–403.

Micas, M., Ousset, P. J., & Vellas, B. (1995). Evaluation des troubles dur comportement. Presentation de Lechelle de Cohen-Mansfield. *La Revue Francaise De Psychiatrie Et De Psychologie Medicale*, *7*, 151–154.

Mintzer, J. E., Nietert, P., Costa, K., & Waid, L. R. (1996). Cross-cultural perspectives: agitation in demented patients in the United States. *Int. Psychogeriatr.*, *8*(Suppl. 3), 487–490.

Mohs, R. C. (1996). The Alzheimer's disease assessment scale. *International Psychogeriatrics*, *8*(2), 195–203.

Molloy, D. W., McIlroy, W. E., Guyatt, G. H., & Lever, J. A. (1991). Validity and reliability of the dysfunctional behaviour rating instrument. *Acta Psychiatr. Scand.*, *84*, 103–106.

Moore, J. T., Bobula, J. A., Short, T. B., & Mischel, M. (1983). A functional dementia scale. *The Journal of Family Practice*, *16*(3), 499–503.

Morgan, D., Stewart, N., D'arcy, C., & Werezak, L. (2004). Evaluating rural nursing home environments: dementia special care units versus integrated facilities. *Aging & Mental Health*, *8*(3), 256–265.

Mountain, G., & Bowie, P. (1995). The quality of long-term care for dementia: a survey of ward environments. *Int. J. Geriatric. Psych.*, *10*(12), 1029–1035.

Mungas, D., Weiler, P., Franzi, C., & Henry, R. (1989). Assessment of disruptive behavior associated with dementia: the disruptive behavior rating scales. *Journal of Geriatric Psychiatry and Neurology*, *2*(4), 196–202.

Niederehe, G. (1988). Assessments of the aged by relatives or significant others. *Psychopharmacology Bulletin*, *24*(4), 595–600.

Overall, J. E., & Gorham, D. R. (1962). The brief psychiatric rating scale. *Psychological Reports*, *10*, 799–812.

Patel, V., & Hope, R. A. (1992). A rating scale for aggressive behaviour in the elderly—the RAGE. *Psychological Medicine*, *22*, 211–221.

Rabinowitz, J., Davidson, M., De Deyn, P. P., Katz, I., Brodaty, H., & Cohen-Mansfield, J. (2005). Factor analysis of the Cohen-Mansfield Agitation Inventory in three large samples of nursing home patients with dementia and behavioral disturbance. *American Journal of Geriatric Psychiatry, 13*(11), 991–998.

Raskin, A., & Crook, T. (1988). Global Assessment of Psychiatric Symptoms (GAPS). *Psychopharmacology Bulletin, 24*(4), 721–725.

Ray, W. A., Taylor, J. A., Lichtenstein, M. J., & Meador, K. G. (1992). The nursing home behavior problem scale. *Journal of Gerontology, 47*(1), M9–M16.

Reding, M. J., Haycox, J., Wigforss, K., Brush, D., & Blass, J. P. (1984). Follow up of patients referred to a dementia service. *Journal of the American Geriatrics Society, 32*(4), 265–268.

Reimer, M., Slaughter, S., Donaldson, C., Currie, G., & Eliasziw, M. (2004). Special care facility compared with traditional environments for dementia care; a longitudinal study of quality of life. *JAGS, 52*(7), 1085–1092.

Reisberg, B., Borenstein, J., Salob, S. P., Ferris, S. H., Franssen, E., & Georgotas, A. (1987). Behavioral symptoms in Alzheimer's disease: phenomenology and treatment. *J. Clin. Psychiatry, 48*(5), (Suppl.), 9–15.

Rosen, J., Burgio, L., Kollar, M., et al. (1994). The Pittsburgh Agitation Scale. *The American Journal of Geriatric Psychiatry, 2*(1), 52–59.

Russen-Rondinone, T., & DesRoberts, A. M. (1996). Success through individual recreation: working with the low-functioning resident with dementia or Alzheimer's disease. *The American Journal of Alzheimer's Disease, 11*(1), 32–35.

Ryden, M. B. (1988). Aggressive behavior in persons with dementia who live in the community. *Alzheimer Disease and Associated Disorders, 2*(4), 342–355.

Schindel-Martin, L., Morden, P., Cetinski, G., Lasky, N., McDowell, C., & Roberts, J. (2003). Teaching staff to respond effectively to cognitively impaired residents who display self-protective behaviors. *American Journal of Alzheimer's Disease and Other Dementias, 18*(5), 273–281.

Shader, R. I., Harmatz, A. B., & Salzman, C. S. (1974). A new scale for clinical assessment in geriatric populations: Sandoz Clinical Assessment—Geriatric (SCAG). *Journal of the American Geriatrics Society, 22*(3), 107–113.

Silver, J. M., & Yudofsky, S. C. (1991). The overt aggression scale: overview and guiding principles. *Journal of Neuropsychiatry, 3*(2), S22–S29.

Sinha, D., Zemlan, F. P., Nelson, S., Bienenfeld, D., Thienhaus, O., Ramaswamy, G., & Hamilton, S. (1992). A new scale for assessing behavioral agitation in dementia. *Psychiatry Research, 41*, 73–88.

Slaughter, S., Calkins, M., Eliasziw, M., & Reimer, M. (2006). Measuring physical and social environments in nursing homes for people with middle- to late-stage dementia. *JAGS, 54*(9), 1436–1441.

Sloane, P., Hoeffer, B., Mitchell, C. M., McKenzie, D., Barrick, A. L., Rader, J., et al. (2004). Effect of person-centred showering and the towel bath on bathing-associated aggression, agitation, and discomfort in nursing home residents with dementia: a randomized, controlled trial. *JAGS, 52*(11), 1795–1804.

Speziale, J., Black, E., Coatsworth-Puspoky, R., Ross, T., & O'Reagan, T. (2009). Moving forward: evaluating a curriculum for managing responsive behaviours in a geriatric psychiatry inpatient population. *The Gerontologist, 49*(4), 570–576.

Spijker, A., Vernooij-Dassen, M., Vasse, E., Adang, E., Wollershiem, H., Grol, R., & Verhey, F. (2008). Effectiveness of non-pharmacological interventions in delaying the institutionalization of patients with dementia: a meta-analysis. *JAGS, 56*(6), 1116–1128.

Sunderland, T., Hill, J. L., Lawlor, B. A., & Molchan, S. E. (1988). NIMH Dementia Mood Assessment Scale (DMAS). *Psychopharmacology Bulletin, 24*(4), 747–753.

Tariot, P. N., Mack, J. L., Patterson, M. B., Edland, S. D., Weiner, M. F., Fillenbaum, G., et al. (1995). The behavior rating scale for dementia of the consortium to establish a registry for Alzheimer's disease. *American Journal Psychiatry, 152*(9), 1349–1357.

Teri, L., & Logsdon, R. G. (1991). Identifying pleasant activities for Alzheimer's disease patients: the pleasant events schedule-AD. *The Gerontologist, 31*(1), 124–127.

Teri, L., Truax, P., Logsdon, R., Uomoto, J., Zarit, S., & Vitaliano, P. P. (1992). Assessment of behavioral problems in dementia: the revised memory and behavioral problems checklist. *Psychology and Aging, 7*(4), 622–631.

Verstraten, P. F. J. (1988). The GIP: an observational ward behavior scale. *Psychopharmacology Bulletin*, *24*(4), 717.

Werner, P., Cohen-Mansfield, J., Koroknay, V., & Braun, J. (1994). The impact of a restraint-reduction program on nursing home residents. *Geriatric Nursing*, *15*(3), 142–146, May.

Wilkinson, I. M., & Graham-White, J. (1980). Psychogeriatric dependency rating scales (PGDRS): a method of assessment for use by nurses. *British Journal of Psychiatry*, *137*, 558–565.

Zarit, S. H., & Zarit, J. M. (1983). Cognitive impairment. In P. M. Lewinsohn, & L. Teri (Eds.), *Clinical Geropsychology* (pp. 38–81). New York, NY: Pergammon Press.

Zgola, J. M. L. (1987). *Doing Things: A Guide to Programming Activities for Persons with Alzheimers Disease and Related Disorders*. Baltimore, MD: The Johns Hopkins University Press.

CHAPTER

Assessing Sleep Problems of Older Adults

16

Tracy Trevorrow

Chaminade University of Honolul Honolulu, Hawaii, USA

INTRODUCTION

Experiencing poor sleep appears inevitable with advanced age, and sleep problems tend to compromise a person's quality of life more when they occur in the last decades of life. In a study of 9000 participants over age 65, 80% reported having sleep complaints and more than half reported that they had chronic sleep difficulties (Foley et al., 1995). Such high rates of sleep problems appear to reflect physical ailments and psychopathology more than aging *per se* (Bliwise, 1993; Foley, Ancoli-Israel, & Britz, 2004; Miles & Dement, 1980). As such, the development of a sleep problem for an older adult may signal the need for medical and psychological treatment. Insomnia, which is reported to be experienced by 20–40% of older adults, is associated with shorter survival (Gooneratne et al., 2006). Mortality due to common causes of death (e.g., heart disease, stroke, and cancer) is up to two times higher for older adults with sleep disorders compared to those who sleep well (Ancoli-Israel & Cooke, 2005; Morgan, Healey, & Healey, 1989; van Diest, 1990; Wingard & Berkman, 1983).

Dismissing, underestimating or mismanaging sleep disorder in older adults can lead to serious consequences. For example, a physician misinterpreting symptoms of sleep apnea as insomnia may choose to treat a patient with sedative medications, such as a benzodiazepine, which can lead to memory problems, disorientation, and falls resulting in hip fracture (Cumming & Le Couteur, 2003; Maher, 2004; Mejo, 1992). Failure to detect sleep apnea could be fatal (Gooneratne et al., 2006). Given the prevalence and significance of sleep-related disorders for older adults it is important that health care professionals appreciate the vital role of sleep in maintaining good physical and psychological health and to be able to identify, assess, and treat sleep pathology.

This chapter briefly reviews the process of age associated changes in sleep and the multiple causes of sleep disorders in older adults. It examines causal factors of sleep problems and then outlines assessment strategies and specific approaches and measures used to assess sleep. Case examples illustrate how various issues manifest in clinical practice. The chapter ends with a discussion of trends in the assessment of sleep problems in the context of demographic changes, such as age shifts in the population and increased ethnic diversity, as well as economic factors and technological advances. For readers interested in a review of treatment considerations for sleep disorder for older adults, see Ancoli-Israel and Ayalon (2006).

THE STRUCTURE OF SLEEP FOR OLDER ADULTS

The electroencephalographic (EEG) record, along with other physiological parameters, such as respiration, eye movement, and muscle tension, reflect the stages of sleep. Sleep stages typically occur in

Handbook of Assessment in Clinical Gerontology. DOI: 10.1016/B978-0-12-374961-1.10016-8

sequence, passing between lighter stages (1 and 2) and deeper stages (3 and 4). Arousal thresholds are lower during lighter stages, and deeper stages of sleep are associated with restorative bodily processes and a greater sense of wakefulness following sleep (Hauri, 1982). Deep stages of sleep often precede periods of rapid eye motion (REM) that are associated with dreaming and appear related to the consolidation of memory, particularly of complex information (Lader, Cardinali, & Pandi-Perumal, 2006).

As can be seen in Figure 16.1, the sleep of an older adult contrasts in predictable and significant ways from that of younger adults. Older adults tend to have slightly longer time for sleep onset and significantly less time in deeper sleep stages, particularly during the second half of the sleep period. The lack of deep sleep stages is accompanied by fewer episodes of REM sleep. Older adults are more likely to have multiple awakenings and tend to establish a polyphasic pattern of sleep with daytime napping (Picarsic et al., 2008). Many older adults experience a circadian rhythm shift, specifically an advance in sleep phase, resulting in their night's sleep starting early (around 7 or 8 pm) and ending early (around 3 or 4 am) (Monk, Reynolds, Machen, & Kupfer, 1992). Sleep changes associated with aging are summarized in Table 16.1. While substantial sleep changes are associated with aging, and decreased sleep quality and sleep time is associated with disease and psychological disorder, it should be noted that sleep changes do not always result in a subjective experience of disturbance (Engle-Friedman & Bootzin, 1991).

Sleep problems may be exacerbated by an older person's expectation regarding sleep. Lichstein (1988) observed that older adults, who are uninformed as to age-related sleep changes, may have the expectation that their sleep should remain as it was in middle age. This unrealistic expectation may result in distress. The following example illustrates such a circumstance.

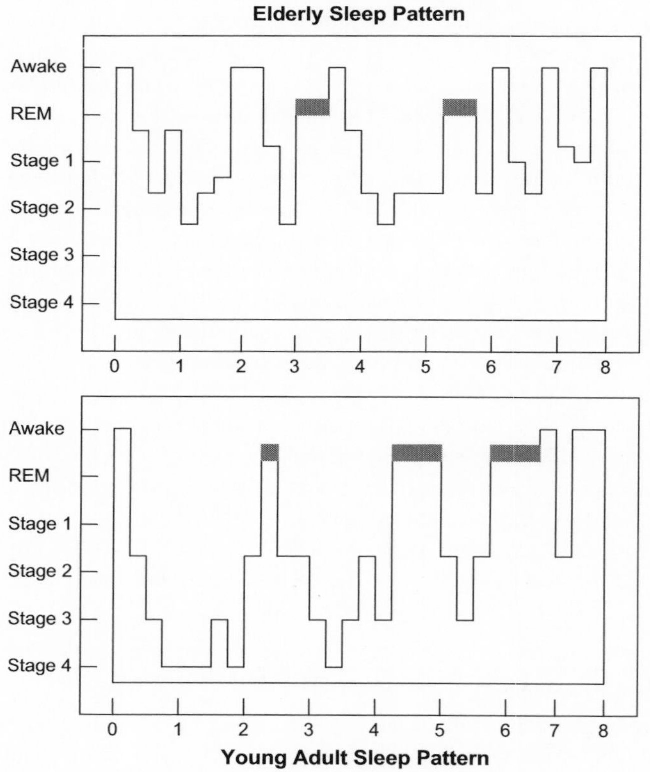

FIGURE 16.1

Sleep Patterns in Young and Older Adults.

Table 16.1 Sleep Changes Associated with Aging for Older Adults

Sleep Changes Associated with Aging for Older Adults
Retiring to bed earlier in the evening and arising earlier in the morning (phase advance)
Increased time to fall asleep (sleep latency)
Increased fluctuations between stages of sleep
Increased time to return to sleep once awoken
Decreased sleep efficiency (time in bed versus time asleep)
Decreased amount of deep sleep (stages 3 and 4)
Decreased REM sleep
REM sleep is more distributed across the night, rather than being mostly in the second half of sleep
Increased nap taking

Case Study 1—A patient distressed by changes in sleep due to aging

Mrs T was 67 years old when referred to a clinical psychologist by her family physician. The physician had determined that Mrs T had no significant medical conditions but may have an anxiety disorder. Initial screening measures did in fact reveal clinical levels of anxiety and depression. In addition to her psychological problems, Mrs T reported difficulties with her sleep. She complained that it was increasingly necessary to go to bed early in the evening, which was a marked departure from her life history of being a "night owl." She also woke frequently during her night's sleep, seldom slept past 5 am and started to take daily naps. She feared that these sleep changes, which had occurred over the past few years, were symptoms of dementia. Mrs T's anxiety and depression decreased when the psychologist reassured her that her sleep changes reflected normal aging and that the assessment of her memory ability was within normal limits. While Mrs T's pattern of sleep remained relatively unchanged during psychological treatment, she reported that she was less distressed about her quality of sleep.

CAUSES OF SLEEP DISTURBANCE

Illness and Sleep

Older adults suffer from a greater proportion of chronic disabling health problems than the general population, and these disabilities last longer and are more severe (Ancoli-Israel, 2000; Foley et al., 1995; Foley, Monjan, Simonsick, Wallace, & Blazer, 1999; Miles & Dement, 1980). Medical disease and chronic illness, rather than maturation *per se*, accounts for much of sleep disorder in older adults (Bliwise, 1993; Gislason & Almqvist, 1987).

Almost any illness has the capacity to disturb sleep, especially when the central nervous system is affected. The following is a non-exhaustive list of medical conditions more common in older adults that typically impair sleep:

1. Sleep apnea (Malholtra & White, 2002)
2. Periodic leg movements, restless legs (Barthlen, 2002)
3. Dementia (Alzheimer's) (Vitiello & Borson, 2001)
4. Cardiovascular disease (Hyyppa & Kronholm, 1989)
5. Diabetes (Resnick et al., 2003)
6. Menopause (Polo-Kantola, Saaresranta, & Polo, 2001)
7. Incontinence, nocturia (Coyne, 2003)
8. Alcohol dependency (Landolt & Gillin, 2001)
9. Nocturnal asthma (Kiyokawa et al., 1999)
10. Chronic pain (Cole, Dubois, & Kosinski, 2007)

Treating comorbid medical problems may reduce their effects on sleep, but is not likely to cure sleep problems entirely. It is important to note that sleep disorders and related medical problems must both be addressed (Ancoli-Israel & Cooke, 2005). Of the medical conditions that affect sleep of older adults, sleep disordered breathing demands particular attention because of its prevalence and the severity of its impact on sleep.

Sleep Apnea and Other Sleep-Related Respiratory Disturbances

Sleep-disordered breathing is the most common physical disorder that affects sleep, affecting nearly one-quarter of all older persons (Ancoli-Israel, 1989; Barthlen, 2002; Morin, 1993). Sleep-disordered breathing is more common in older men than older women (Ancoli-Israel & Coy, 1994) and more common in persons with diabetes (Strohl, 1996). Sleep apnea is the most common diagnosis of patients seen in sleep disorder clinics, accounting for 39% of older patients (Coleman et al., 1981). Ancoli-Israel and colleagues (1991, 1996) found that 24% of apparently healthy older adults living in the community, 33% of similarly aged inpatients, and 42% of nursing home residents met criteria for apnea.

Sleep apnea is characterized by brief cessation of airflow and hypopnea refers to a reduced airflow. Snoring is often associated with both of these ailments. As demonstrated in a prospective study, apnea increases with an individual's age (Bliwise, Carskadon, Carey, & Dement, 1984) and is associated with anatomical changes and diminished functioning of muscles around the pharyngeal airway (Malhotra, Crowley, Pillar, Kikinis, & White, 2000).

Researchers associate apnea with numerous medical problems, such as hypertension, obesity, and cardiac arrhythmias, as well as death. It results in the greatest functional impairment of all sleep disorders in older adults (Gooneratne et al., 2006; Lavie, Ben-Yosef, & Rubin, 1984; Wittels, 1985). Participants with a respiratory distress index (RDI) of greater than 30 episodes per hour had significantly shorter survival than participants with mild or no sleep-related breathing disorder, and died as much as two years earlier (Ancoli-Israel et al., 1996). Similarly, snoring may not be a benign "habit," as it is associated with death during sleep and in the early morning (Seppala et al., 1991). Failure to identify and treat sleep-disordered breathing results in a higher mortality rate (Partinen, Jamieson, & Guilleminault, 1988). Consider this example.

Case Study 2—A patient with obstructive sleep apnea

Mrs M was a 61-year-old, obese woman transferred to inpatient rehabilitation after having suffered a stroke. For the first few days of her rehabilitation, nurses reported Mrs M had difficulty waking, participating in self-care, breakfast, and morning therapies. Mrs M's physiatrist ordered a pulse oxymeter (a device that measures blood oxygen) to be worn throughout the night and for nurses to watch and record her sleep behavior. After a single night of assessment there were clear signs of obstructive sleep apnea, indicated by decreased blood oxygen, multiple arousal and post-resuscitative snorts. Rather than wait for more comprehensive evaluation from a sleep disorders center, a continuous positive air-pressure device (CPAP) was administered. Mrs M's sleep immediately improved, although CPAP was poorly tolerated at first. Her therapist noted that Mrs M's participation in early morning activities improved greatly.

The Impact of Medications on Sleep

In addition to illness, medications can compromise sleep. Older adults are prescribed a disproportionately high amount of drugs, particularly in the United States (van derHooft et al., 2005). Numerous medications alter sleep by either stimulating or depressing the central nervous system. For example, allergy medications and cold remedies may have caffeine which can promote insomnia. Psychotropic medications (antidepressants, anxiolytics) and those prescribed for physical illnesses (e.g., beta-blockers, bronchodilators, antihypertensives, and steroids) can also disrupt sleep (Ancoli-Israel & Cooke, 2005).

Older adults consume sleep medications about four times the rate of middle-age persons. Ironically, such medications may not be helpful and may even make sleep worse. There is little evidence that over-the-counter remedies improve sleep parameters, and the long-term use of prescribed sedative-hypnotics can perpetuate insomnia (Morin, 1993). Consider the next example.

Case Study 3—A patient dependent on alcohol and sleep medications

Mr B was a 65-year-old man referred to a sleep disorders center after reporting that he slept very little and sometimes not at all. This was particularly distressing to him because he found that even very heavy doses of prescribed medications and over-the-counter sleep remedies were of little help. A review of Mr B's medication use revealed that he had relied on sleeping medications and alcohol to get to sleep for over 40 years! After admission to inpatient treatment he was withdrawn from all sedative hypnotics. Mr B was instructed in relaxation techniques, sleep hygiene principles, and referred to a clinical psychologist for follow-up treatment regarding sleep management and alcohol dependence.

Psychological and Psychiatric Factors and Sleep

Psychological maladies and sleep problems can overlap and potentiate each other. Indeed, many psychiatric disorders have impaired sleep as part of their diagnostic criteria. Differentiating a sleep problem from a mental health problem can be difficult and yet essential in determining the appropriate course of therapy. Poor sleep often results in fatigue, poor concentration, decreased motivation, dysphoria, and a reduced sense of well-being (Spielman, 1986; Totterdell, Reynolds, Parkinson, & Briner, 1994). Major depression typically manifests with middle or terminal insomnia (American Psychiatric Association, 2000). It is a diagnostic challenge to differentiate whether the client has poor sleep due to being depressed, presents as depressed due to poor sleep, or has some combination of the two. Similarly, anxiety can result in insomnia and sleepless nights can contribute to being anxious (Lichstein & Riedel, 1994). Hauri (1982) notes that maladaptive conditioning can result from a person lying in bed being unable to sleep because of stress. The bed and bedroom become associated with arousal rather than sleep. Lichstein and Fanning (1990) found that subjects who had insomnia were more prone to cognitive arousal than those without insomnia, although others did not find such a relationship (Haynes, Adams, & Franzen, 1981; Sanavio, 1988).

Some sleep problems are distinctly related to a psychiatric condition and are, therefore, less likely to be confused as a consequence of aging. For example, delayed sleep onset is typical of almost all anxiety conditions (sans phobias) (Rosa, Bonnet, & Kramer, 1983), but is not a typical consequence of aging (Hauri, 1982). Night terrors or nightmares are the hallmark of PTSD and are also not associated with aging. In bipolar disorder there can be a cycling of sleep complaints. Insomnia is part of the manic phase; whereas hypersomnia is more frequent during the depressive cycle (Morin, 1993). Between mood swings, patients with bipolar mood disorder tend to experience circadian rhythm instability (Jones, Hare, & Evershed, 2005). Adults with schizophrenia often experience frequent awakenings thought to be the consequence of abnormal circadian temperature regulation (Morgan & Cheadle, 1976; Zarcone, 1989).

While there is a high prevalence of psychopathology among those with sleep disorders (Morin, 1993), it should be noted that older adults with sleep problems generally appear less depressed and anxious than their younger sleep-disordered counterparts (Roehrs, Zorick, Sicklesteel, Wittig, & Roth, 1983). In addition, not all people with sleep complaints are psychologically distressed (Zorick, Roth, Hartse, Piccione, & Stepanski, 1981). When an older person's psychological problems do accompany sleep disturbance, improvements in one will not automatically produce improvements in the other (Ancoli-Israel & Cooke, 2005). It is recommended, however, that when these problems are associated with a sleep complaint, the psychological issues are addressed first (Hauri, 1982). Consider the following case.

Case Study 4—A patient with major depression

Mr E was a 65-year-old retired school principal, who was referred by his physician to a sleep disorders center for chronic insomnia of approximately two years' duration. The physician noted that sedative hypnotics had proved ineffective, as was providing him with sleep hygiene guidelines. Mr E expressed reluctance to seek professional help and stated that his wife considered his sleep more of a problem than he did. Psychotherapeutic evaluation was not initially considered, perhaps due to Mr E's denials to his physician of having anything significantly wrong with his life or lifestyle. Ostensibly, Mr E appeared to be enjoying a relaxing, stress-free retirement.

Polysomnographic findings for two overnight observations indicated that Mr E was experiencing multiple awakenings, with decreased total sleep time (TST). REM latencies for both nights were around 20 minutes, and the first REM episodes were unusually long. In short, Mr E's sleep architecture was typical of major depression.

Referral to a clinical psychologist was suggested, but Mr E refused to attend sessions. Mr E was agreeable to a trial of sedating antidepressants which he reported improved his sleep almost immediately. Mr E later agreed to a trial of activating antidepressants (taken in the morning) with the understanding that it might promote his activity level during the day. This also appeared beneficial. On six month follow-up, Mr E reported maintaining improvements in sleep and also having made significant changes in lifestyle, taking up golf and serving as a consultant to the local school council.

Lifestyle, Environmental Factors, and Sleep

Sleep is affected by health practices, habits, and environmental influences, the so-called "sleep hygiene" factors (Maher, 2004). While it is rare for such factors to be the primary cause of insomnia (Fichten et al., 1995; Morgan, Healey, & Healey, 1989; Morin & Gramling, 1989; Zarcone, 1989), sleep hygiene factors should be evaluated in respect of their ability to complicate or exacerbate an existing sleep problem. Table 16.2 presents a list of lifestyle and environmental factors that have been found to disturb sleep.

SLEEP ASSESSMENT: MEASURES, METHODS, AND STRATEGY

In assessing sleep problems, health care providers must decide upon the method of assessment, such as whether to employ interviewing, self-monitoring, monitoring by bedpartner, observation, and/or physiologic assessment. Care providers typically make a choice between instruments, formats for interviews, or observations. Finally, a strategy may be determined that may provide a rationale for how to combine and coordinate methods and measures, addressing such issues as the frequency of assessment. Such a strategy may be dictated by the resources available to the provider and circumstances regarding reimbursement for services. For example, is a sleep laboratory available? Is this assessment covered by insurance?

While there are well-established ideals regarding the psychometric properties of measures such as high levels of sensitivity, reliability, validity, and utility, guidelines in the sleep literature regarding the

Table 16.2 Potential Lifestyle and Environmental Challenges to Sleep
Noise
Light
Inactivity
Prolonged naps
Alcohol, caffeine, smoking/tobacco products
Large meals and fluid intake immediately prior to bedtime
Conditioned arousal of sleep setting by behavior incompatible with sleep, e.g., eating in bed, watching TV, talking with bedpartner
Arousal from sexual activity
Fear of insomnia and arousal from effort to fall asleep
Stressful events and rumination about them
Reinforcement from others for having sleep problems
Circadian rhythm disruption from "jet lag" or shift work

selection of methods is less clear. Lichstein, Durrence, Riedel, Taylor, and Bush (2004) note that available sleep measures can rightfully claim some of the above psychometric qualities, but none can claim all.

Specific to strategy, Haynes and O'Brien (1990) advocate a multi-method assessment approach because identifying important functional relationships (i.e., between the sleeper and the environment) requires diverse methods. Haynes (1983) and Lichstein and Riedel (1994) recommend taking repeated measures so that causal relationships between variables may be explored through time-series analysis. Also, the factors that cause sleep disorders may themselves be in flux. Ongoing assessment may include periodic sleep diaries and a review of daytime habits, daytime functioning, and attitudes about sleep. Others have found regularly repeated assessments less useful for clinical work, given the expenditure of time and the lack of financial reimbursement for such efforts (Barlow, 1980; Emmelcamp, 1981). Finally, it should be noted that patients be educated regarding the need for follow-up assessments should sleep problems fail to improve or relapse. It is particularly important to reach bed partners and family members for patients who are limited in their ability to be aware of their sleep quality, such as patients with apnea or those with cognitive impairments.

The Sleep Assessment Interview

Interviewing is clearly the health care provider's most direct means of assessing the client's phenomenological experience regarding their sleep experience. The sleep assessment interview is typically semi-structured and a number of guides are available as to what to include in such an interview, depending on the particular agenda of the assessment (see, for example, Quan & Zee, 2004). Table 16.3 presents a compilation of areas to cover when conducting a sleep assessment interview. An initial questionnaire may be mailed to the client and returned prior to the initial interview. This allows the clinician the opportunity to tailor the interview to suit the need for gathering more specific information.

Table 16.3 Areas to Consider in a Sleep Assessment Interview

Nature of the complaint—what the problem is and when it occurs (i.e., sleep onset, sleep maintenance, early morning wake-up, daytime fatigue, nightmares, other?)
History of sleep complaint—(transient disturbance, longstanding complaint)
Current sleep/wake schedule
Symptoms of sleep disorders that may not be initially volunteered (restless legs, periodic limb movements, narcolepsy, gastro-esophageal reflux, parasomnias, sleep/wake schedule disruption)
Symptoms of sleep disordered breathing (disturbed breathing at night, observed snoring or post-resuscitative snorts, headache upon waking, partner sleeps in another room)
Daytime states, routines, activities (sleepiness, fatigue, functioning, mood, activities, satisfaction with daily routines)
Naps: frequency, time of day, length
Sleep hygiene (daytime activity, exercise, sleep environment, activity in bed, diet, use of stimulants/depressants)
History of professional treatment of the sleep complaint and a review of what the client has tried to remedy his or her sleep problem
Medical/physical problems
Use of prescription and non-prescription drugs
Psychiatric history and mental status review (symptoms of depression, anxiety, thought disorder, other psychological maladjustment)
Stressful circumstances (currently, when sleep problems began)
Information regarding antecedents, consequences, secondary gains, precipitating factors, perpetuating factors

Interview With the Bed Partner and Family

It is almost always helpful to include the patient's bed partner and/or members of the household in a sleep assessment, most obviously in cases where the client's memories may be poor or compromised through illness. However, even when the client proves to be a reliable historian, getting a bed partner's perspective is helpful. Bed partners may have witnessed snoring, apnic episodes, restless legs, and other pathonomonic behaviors of which the patient is unaware. Bed partners or household members may provide useful information regarding lifestyle factors that may be affecting sleep, such as daily activities, stressors, and substance use.

Sleep Diaries

Sleep diaries are daily logs of sleeping and waking activities and are the most practical, economical, and widely used method for assessing sleep (Bootzin & Engle-Friedman, 1981; Douglass, Carskadon, & Houser, 1990). Diaries can be used to establish baselines, provide valuable feedback to clients, monitor fluctuations in behavior, and provide data that serves as an outcome measure for treatment efficacy. They are particularly appropriate for assessing sleep/wake patterns of large samples (when physiological monitoring or observation is impractical), for measuring sleep events that are not easily assessed in the sleep laboratory, and for measuring infrequent sleep events (Rogers, Caruso, & Aldrich, 1993). Patients with insomnia should be encouraged to keep a sleep diary for two weeks or longer (Schneider, 2002).

Sleep diaries come in numerous formats, although most have similar features. (For examples see Barthlen, 2002; Morin, 1993.) Diaries may be customized to meet a clinical or research need. In these diaries, clients are asked to record the following daily information regarding their sleep and related behavior: bedtime; sleep onset; number and times of awakening; duration of each awakening; time of last awakening; naps; medications taken; reason for awakening; and rating of sleep quality. Clients should monitor factors suspected of compromising their sleep, such as smoking, caffeine intake, or anxious thoughts.

Sleep diaries have generally been found to be reliable, and to have acceptable sensitivity and specificity (Rogers, Caruso, & Aldrich, 1993). However, there are several significant limitations to diary monitoring. Data from sleep diaries tend to lack convergent validity. When compared with polysomnography, client's diary reports tend to overestimate sleep-onset time and underestimate sleep duration (Carskadon et al., 1976; Coates et al., 1982). Clients using diaries have also had difficulty estimating the number of awakenings and the depth of sleep (Browman & Tepas, 1976; Carskadon et al., 1976).

Not all subjects can effectively use diaries. There are obvious limits when assessing children or individuals with cognitive impairments. Rogers et al. (1993) found that subjects who took frequent naps and narcoleptic subjects made significantly more errors than control subjects when documenting their sleep/wake patterns. The decision to use sleep diaries with older adults should involve careful consideration, given their higher incidence of cognitive impairments, frequent daytime napping, and decreased daytime vigilance.

As with all self-monitoring tasks, sleep diaries tend to produce reactivity. People monitoring their sleep for the first time tend to act differently. This problem is usually resolved by having clients monitor themselves for periods long enough so that the process is no longer novel. This adjustment usually takes only a few days. Because compliance with self-monitoring can also be a problem, it is important to make the monitoring task easy and convenient. Even when the task is minimal, a clinician or researcher may never be sure that the week's diary entries were appropriately completed over time or just before they were turned in! One strategy used to guarantee that entries were prospectively entered is to have clients or research participants call or mail their information on a daily basis.

In the last decade developments in technology have made it easier to employ cell phones, handheld computers, and other portable devices for prospective monitoring. As suggested by Shiffman (1998), assessing a client's experience "on-the-fly" during their regular routines promotes the ecological validity of the measure. Devices may be programmed to cue the client at a specific time, on a time schedule, or randomly and they have a built-in date and clock record so it is known when clients make their entries. Despite these features, there is little indication in the professional literature that there is widespread adoption of such technology to assess sleep or daytime sleepiness.

Sleep Questionnaires and Rating Scales

Sleep questionnaires and rating scales are available to help the clinician assess a broad spectrum of sleeping behaviors and issues. While some measures assist the health care provider in efficiently and systematically reviewing multiple aspects of the client's sleep, others are more focused on a specific aspect of a sleep-related behavior or cognition. Several measures are available that assess a consequence of sleep disorder, such as sleepiness. Table 16.4 lists several of the more frequently used sleep and sleepiness questionnaires and rating scales, and provides a brief description of their features and suggested use.

Observational Measures of Sleep

The opportunity to observe a client's sleeping is perhaps the most significant advantage in assessing older adults' sleep in inpatient and convalescent settings. This is helpful as older patients or residents are likely to have a polyphasic distribution of sleep, napping throughout the day. Also, older patients or residents may be limited in their ability to provide information about their sleep experience due to medical problems or cognitive impairment.

An observational approach can be done simply by periodically observing whether the patient is awake, as defined by immobility of limbs and eyelids and being unresponsive when approached. Such observational rating correlated highly with polysomnography (Manabe et al., 2000). Cohen-Mansfield and colleagues developed an observational measure of sleep for use in nursing home settings (Cohen-Mansfield, Waldhorn, Werner, & Billig, 1990). The Observational Sleep Assessment Inventory (OSAI) consists of a checklist of sleep behaviors that may be completed by night-shift staff. The checklist includes observations of breathing and movement during sleep. The OSAI has been demonstrated to be a reliable and valid tool for assessing sleep and sleep pathology in nursing home residents. It has also been used effectively in assessing the sleep of stroke inpatients in a rehabilitation hospital (Trevorrow & Fast, 1998).

Sleep Assessment Technologies

Most health care providers do not perform physiological assessments of sleep parameters. However, knowledge of such approaches is likely to be helpful in determining whether to make a referral to a sleep disorders center and in understanding assessment results from such centers. Table 16.5 lists a number of more commonly used assessments, as well as some recent innovative approaches in sleep assessment.

Psychological Measures

Psychological distress or dysfunction may well be the appropriate focus of treatment to improve sleep. Clinicians or researchers interested in the psychological correlates of sleep disorder may use measures of global psychological functioning, such as the Brief Symptom Inventory (Derogatis, 1993). Measures of a specific psychological disorder, such as anxiety or depression, can be used such as the

Table 16.4 Sleep-related Questionnaires and Rating Scales

Questionnaire & Authors	Description	Comments/Suggested Use
Sleep Disorders Questionnaire (Douglass et al., 1994)	175 items; scales for sleep disorders, apnea, narcolepsy, psychiatric disorder, and periodic leg movements	Apnea and narcolepsy scales most discriminating, helps determine if sleep disorders center assessment is indicated
Pittsburgh Sleep Quality Index (PSQI) (Buysse, Reynolds, Monk, Berman, & Kupfer, 1989)	19-item 7 "component" scores; e.g., subjective sleep quality, 1 global score. Assesses sleep quality over past month	Distinguishes "good" versus "bad" sleepers and patients with significant sleep disturbance. Good psychometrics
St. Mary's Sleep Questionnaire (Leigh, Hindmarch, Bird, & Wright, 1988)	14 questions on sleep and early morning behavior. Sleep diary format	Assesses the sleep of hospital patients. Good test–retest reliability, 2 factors sleep latency and sleep quality
Leeds Sleep Evaluation Questionnaire (Parrot & Hindmarch, 1980)	10 self-rating VAS re: sleep and early morning behavior	Good psychometrics, frequently used for assessing medication effects
VSH Sleep Scale (Snyder-Hapern & Verran, 1987)	VAS for 7 sleep properties, 3 scales: sleep disturbance, efficiency, and supplementation	Simple to use, has been used with critically ill and disabled
Sleep Impairment Index (Morin, 1993)	11 items assessing degree of impairment. Yields a total score of perceived sleep impairment	Useful for assessing treatment outcome. Correlates with diary. Parallel version for bedpartner
Karolinska Sleepiness Scale (Gillberg, Kecklund, & Akerstedt, 1994)	9-point scale ranging from "very alert" to "very sleepy, fighting sleep, an effort to remain awake"	Clearer than the Stanford Sleepiness Scale. Correlates with EEG and reaction time
Epworth Sleepiness Scale (Johns, 1991)	8-items. Subjects rate their propensity to doze in common situations, e.g., while reading	Correlates with objective measures of sleepiness, differentiates both sleep disorder and sleep deprivation
Sleep Hygiene Index (Mastin, Bryson, & Corwyn, 2006)	13 statements of sleep hygiene. Likert scale re: frequency engaged	Correlates with sleep quality and sleepiness
Social Rhythm Metric (Monk, Flaherty, Frank, Hoskinson, Kupfer, 1990)	17 items of typical daily activity. Client endorses and notes time	Quantifies and compares client's daily rhythms of activity

Beck Depression Inventory (Beck, Ward, Mendelson, Mock, & Erbaugh, 1961), or the State Trait Anxiety Inventory (Spielberger, Gorsuch, & Lushene, 1970). Finally, health care providers may choose to assess cognitive functioning, with a brief questionnaire, such as the Short Portable Mental Status questionnaire (Pfieffer, 1975). Such measures are used to gain a snapshot of a patient's psychological status and to determine if a more comprehensive psychological evaluation is warranted. Unless severe cognitive deficit, psychopathology or personality disorder is suspected, lengthy and costly measures such as neuropsychological assessment batteries or comprehensive personality assessments are typically not warranted.

When to Refer to a Sleep Disorders Center

Referral to a sleep disorders center is warranted if sleep apnea is suspected. As previously stated, failure to treat sleep apnea can be fatal. Sleep disorders centers should also be consulted or referred to

Table 16.5 Sleep Assessment Technologies

Assessment	Description
Polysomnography	Conducted typically in a sleep disorders center but more recently approximated by home assessment systems. Simultaneous recording of EEG, eye movements, muscle tension, and, at times, respiration, blood oxygen, electrocardiogram, and heart rate. Typically done overnight to assess apnea/breathing-related sleep disorder, and restless legs. Provides information regarding sleep stages, depth of sleep, and REM sleep. Well-established reliability and validity. Recording may be affected by the discomfort and novelty of the procedure (i.e., high reactivity).
Multiple sleep latency test	Polysomnographic approach to assessing daytime sleepiness. Patients are placed in a dark, quiet, cool room to attempt sleep. Each segment lasts 20 minutes or until patient falls asleep. Assesses narcolepsy. Excellent reliability and validity, reactivity may be high.
Ambulatory monitoring	Typically small, lightweight devices worn by the patient for extended periods to monitor multiple physiological parameters, including EEG.
Actigraphy	A patient wears a device typically like a wristwatch that mechanically and electronically records movement and sometimes noise and light. Low movement is considered as sleep. This approach measures circadian behavior in the patient's natural environment. It typically overestimates sleep time and sleep efficiency and does not provide information regarding sleep quality.
Home sleep recording devices	In-home, bedside, recording units may be practical and inexpensive alternatives to polysomnography. The REMview™ (Respironics, Inc., Pittsburgh, Pennsylvania) records eyelid and head movements, via a headband-mounted movement detector. The "Limited Sleep-Recording Device" (Golpe, Jiménez, & Carpizo, 2002) assesses nasal airflow, body position, movement, pulse rate, and blood oxygen to determine sleep stages. The Zeo™ (Newton, Massachusetts), a commercial product sold directly to the public, uses a headband device with wireless transmission to a bedside unit to reportedly record sleep stages. The physiological parameter it is measuring is not specified.

in suspected cases of cataplexy (sudden loss of muscle tone) and restless legs syndrome. Polysomnographic evaluation for insomnia is not typically recommended. However, if a client is not responding to standard behavioral, environmental, and psychological approaches to managing sleep, referral may be warranted. A referral to a sleep disorders center for insomnia is only warranted after at least six months of comprehensive psychological and behavioral treatment. If a sleep disorders center is not available, clinicians should consult or refer to a neurologist.

Trends and Challenges in the Assessment of Sleep in Older Adults

Demographic, economic, technological, and cultural trends need to be considered in deciding how best to meet the needs of older adults with sleep disorders. The most obvious trend is the tremendous increase in the demand from older adults for clinical services for sleep disorders. In 2005, 12% of all Americans were 65 and older, and it is projected that this age group will comprise 21% of the population by 2025 (U.S. Bureau of the Census, 2009). The "graying" of America, as well as many other countries, will continue in absolute and relative terms well into the 21st century. This demographic shift presents many challenges to health care professionals who serve older adults. Training in medical schools and fields that service health care needs of older adults, such as clinical psychology, will need to develop the curriculum devoted to the prevention and treatment of sleep disorders. While the United States is advanced compared to many other countries in having over 15 university programs providing comprehensive training in the practice of sleep medicine, typically only two hours of teaching time is devoted to sleep and sleep disorders in medical school (Moldofsky, 2000).

There is a serious need for increased assessment of sleep apnea and related breathing-related sleep disorders. Largely due to an epidemic of obesity, 12 million Americans are thought to have sleep apnea; many of them are older adults (National Institutes of Health, 2009). One out of ten people over 65 has sleep apnea and most of these people are unaware that they have the condition (National Institutes of Health, 2009). The rates of apnea will likely increase with the relative and absolute increase of older Americans. Many lives can be saved and much reduction in suffering achieved by developing more systematic and effective means of screening for the disorder.

A promising area of sleep assessment is the development and application of devices used for physiological sleep measures. Physiological sleep assessments may be done increasingly outside the sleep laboratory, i.e., in the clinician's practice or as in-home assessments. This is particularly important when considering the trends regarding the incidence of apnea. Sleep apnea and hypopnea have been reliably assessed by devices set up by a technician in a patient's home (Golpe, Jiménez, & Carpizo, 2002). It is timely that new ways are being developed to detect apnea that are accurate and cost effective, particularly when compared to the expense of polysomnography done at sleep disorder centers.

There are several areas of research regarding the sleep of older adults that appear under-studied. Until quite recently, sleep research has not investigated the psychosocial context of older persons' sleep complaints. Many factors that contribute to whether an older adult seeks professional attention for sleep problems are not specific to the quality of their sleep. Further investigations of sleep relative to variables such as lifestyle, employment and relationship status, personality, and psychological adjustment appear warranted.

The U.S. society is increasingly heterogeneous in race and culture. Little is known about how cultural and racial factors impact sleep, sleep disorders, and health care utilization for sleep problems. Only one study appears to have investigated the sleep of specific ethnic groups of older adults in the United States in a literature search using Academic Search Premier. Sok (2006) found that first generation Korean American women have similar kinds and rates of sleep problems as the general population, but prefer Korean traditional health care practices to treat insomnia, such as acupuncture. Finally, as the number of older adults living in residential treatment, convalescent, and assisted-living environments increases it will be necessary for studies to address the assessment and promotion of sleep quality in such settings.

APPENDIX A

Epworth Sleepiness Scale

Rate the chance of dozing during the following situations.
"0" = never "1" = moderate chance "3" = high chance

1. sitting and reading
2. watching TV
3. sitting inactive in a public place, such as a theater or meeting
4. as a passenger in a car
5. lying down to rest in the afternoon
6. sitting or talking to someone
7. sitting quietly after lunch without alcohol
8. a car while stopped for a few minutes in traffic

Scoring: The numbers of the eight situations are added to give a global score from 0 to 24, with the higher rating relating to pathological sleepiness.

APPENDIX B

Pittsburgh Sleep Quality Index (PSQI)

Subject's Initials ________ ID# ________ Date ________ Time ____ AM/PM

PITTSBURGH SLEEP QUALITY INDEX

INSTRUCTIONS:
The following questions relate to your usual sleep habits during the past month only. Your answers should indicate the most accurate reply for the majority of days and nights in the past month. Please answer all questions.

1. During the past month, what time have you usually gone to bed at night?

   BED TIME ________

2. During the past month, how long (in minutes) has it usually taken you to fall asleep each night?

   NUMBER OF MINUTES ________

3. During the past month, what time have you usually gotten up in the morning?

   GETTING UP TIME ________

4. During the past month, how many hours of actual sleep did you get at night? (This may be different than the number of hours you spent in bed.)

   HOURS OF SLEEP PER NIGHT ________

For each of the remaining questions, check the one best response. Please answer all questions.

5. During the past month, how often have you had trouble sleeping because you...

a) Cannot get to sleep within 30 minutes

Not during the past month ____ Less than once a week ____ Once or twice a week ____ Three or more times a week ____

b) Wake up in the middle of the night or early morning

Not during the past month ____ Less than once a week ____ Once or twice a week ____ Three or more times a week ____

c) Have to get up to use the bathroom

Not during the past month ____ Less than once a week ____ Once or twice a week ____ Three or more times a week ____

d) Cannot breathe comfortably

Not during the past month ____ Less than once a week ____ Once or twice a week ____ Three or more times a week ____

e) Cough or snore loudly

Not during the past month ____ Less than once a week ____ Once or twice a week ____ Three or more times a week ____

f) Feel too cold

Not during the past month ____ Less than once a week ____ Once or twice a week ____ Three or more times a week ____

g) Feel too hot

Not during the past month ____ Less than once a week ____ Once or twice a week ____ Three or more times a week ____

h) Had bad dreams

Not during the past month ____ Less than once a week ____ Once or twice a week ____ Three or more times a week ____

i) Have pain

Not during the past month ____ Less than once a week ____ Once or twice a week ____ Three or more times a week ____

j) Other reason(s), please describe ____________________

____

How often during the past month have you had trouble sleeping because of this?

Not during the past month ____ Less than once a week ____ Once or twice a week ____ Three or more times a week ____

6. During the past month, how would you rate your sleep quality overall?

Very good ____

Fairly good ____

Fairly bad ____

Very bad ____

7. During the past month, how often have you taken medicine to help you sleep (prescribed or "over the counter")?

Not during the past month ____ Less than once a week ____ Once or twice a week ____ Three or more times a week ____

8. During the past month, how often have you had trouble staying awake while driving, eating meals, or engaging in social activity?

Not during the past month ____ Less than once a week ____ Once or twice a week ____ Three or more times a week ____

9. During the past month, how much of a problem has it been for you to keep up enough enthusiasm to get things done?

No problem at all ____

Only a very slight problem ____

Somewhat of a problem ____

A very big problem ____

10. Do you have a bed partner or room mate?

No bed partner or room mate ____

Partner/room mate in other room ____

Partner in same room, but not same bed ____

Partner in same bed ____

If you have a room mate or bed partner, ask him/her how often in the past month you have had . . .

a) Loud snoring

Not during the past month ____	Less than once a week ____	Once or twice a week ____	Three or more times a week ____

b) Long pauses between breaths while asleep

Not during the past month ____	Less than once a week ____	Once or twice a week ____	Three or more times a week ____

c) Legs twitching or jerking while you sleep

Not during the past month ____	Less than once a week ____	Once or twice a week ____	Three or more times a week ____

d) Episodes of disorientation or confusion during sleep

Not during the past month ____	Less than once a week ____	Once or twice a week ____	Three or more times a week ____

e) Other restlessness while you sleep; please describe ________________________________

____

Not during the past month ____	Less than once a week ____	Once or twice a week ____	Three or more times a week ____

Buysse DJ, Reynolds CF, Monk TH, Berman SR, Kupfer DJ: Psychiatry Research, 28:193-213, 1989.

lmw:F5.PSQ (4/2002)

References and Scoring

1 Reference

Buysse, D.J., Reynolds, C.F., Monk, T.H., Berman, S.R., & Kupfer, D.J. (1989). The Pittsburgh Sleep Quality Index: a new instrument for psychiatric practice and research. *Psychiatry Research*, 28:193–213.

Notes on data entry

The range of values for questions 5 through 10 are all 0 to 3.

Questions 1 through 9 are not allowed to be missing except as noted below. If these questions are missing then any scores calculated using missing questions are also missing. Thus it is important to make sure that all questions 1 through 9 have been answered.

In the event that a range is given for an answer (for example, "30 to 60" is written as the answer to Q2, minutes to fall asleep), split the difference and enter 45.

2 Scores—reportable in publications

On May 20, 2005, on the instruction of Dr Daniel J. Buysse, the scoring of the PSQI was changed to set the score for Q5J to 0 if either the comment or the value was missing. This may reduce the DURAT score by 1 point and the PSQI Total Score by 1 point.

PSQIDURAT	**DURATION OF SLEEP** IF Q4 ≥ 7, THEN set value to 0 IF Q4 < 7 and ≥6, THEN set value to 1 IF Q4 < 6 and ≥5, THEN set value to 2 IF Q4 < 5, THEN set value to 3 *Minimum Score = 0 (better); Maximum Score = 3 (worse)*

PSQIDISTB	**SLEEP DISTURBANCE**
	IF Q5b + Q5c + Q5d + Q5e + Q5f + Q5g + Q5h + Q5i + Q5j (IF Q5JCOM is null or Q5j is null, set the value of Q5j to 0) = 0, THEN set value to 0
	IF Q5b + Q5c + Q5d + Q5e + Q5f + Q5g + Q5h + Q5i + Q5j (IF Q5JCOM is null or Q5j is null, set the value of Q5j to 0) ≥ 1 and ≤9, THEN set value to 1
	IF Q5b + Q5c + Q5d + Q5e + Q5f + Q5g + Q5h + Q5i + Q5j (IF Q5JCOM is null or Q5j is null, set the value of Q5j to 0) > 9 and ≤18, THEN set value to 2
	IF Q5b + Q5c + Q5d + Q5e + Q5f + Q5g + Q5h + Q5i + Q5j (IF Q5JCOM is null or Q5j is null, set the value of Q5j to 0) > 18, THEN set value to 3
	Minimum Score = 0 (better); Maximum Score = 3 (worse)

PSQILATEN	**SLEEP LATENCY**
	IF Q5a + Q2 = 0, THEN set value to 0
Field recoded:	IF Q2 ≥ 0 and ≤15, THEN set value to 0
	IF Q2 > 15 and ≤30, THEN set value to 1
	IF Q2 > 30 and ≤60, THEN set value to 2
	IF Q2 > 60, THEN set value to 3)
	IF Q5a + Q2 ≥ 1 and ≤2, THEN set value to 1
Field recoded:	IF Q2 ≥ 0 and ≤15, THEN set value to 0
	IF Q2 > 15 and ≤30, THEN set value to 1
	IF Q2 > 30 and ≤60, THEN set value to 2
	IF Q2 > 60, THEN set value to 3)
	IF Q5a + Q2 ≥ 3 and ≤4, THEN set value to 2
Field recoded:	IF Q2 ≥ 0 and ≤15, THEN set value to 0
	IF Q2 > 5 and ≤30, THEN set value to 1
	IF Q2 > 30 and ≤60, THEN set value to 2
	IF Q2 > 60, THEN set value to 3)
	IF Q5a + Q2 ≥ 5 and ≤6, THEN set value to 3
Field recoded:	IF Q2 ≥ 0 and ≤15, THEN set value to 0
	IF Q2 > 15 and ≤30, THEN set value to 1
	IF Q2 > 30 and ≤60, THEN set value to 2
	IF Q2 > 60, THEN set value to 3)
	Minimum Score = 0 (better); Maximum Score = 3 (worse)

PSQIDAYDYS	**DAY DYSFUNCTION DUE TO SLEEPINESS**
	IF Q8 + Q9 = 0, THEN set value to 0
	IF Q8 + Q9 ≥ 1 and ≤2, THEN set value to 1
	IF Q8 + Q9 ≥ 3 and ≤4, THEN set value to 2
	IF Q8 + Q9 ≥ 5 and ≤6, THEN set value to 3
	Minimum Score = 0 (better); Maximum Score = 3 (worse)

PSQIHSE	**SLEEP EFFICIENCY**
	Diffsec = Difference in seconds between day and time of day Q1 and day Q3
	Diffhour = Absolute value of diffsec/3600
	newtib = IF diffhour ≥ 24, then newtib = diffhour – 24
	IF diffhour ≤ 24, THEN newtib = diffhour (NOTE, THE ABOVE JUST CALCULATES THE HOURS BETWEEN GNT (Q1) AND GMT (Q3))
	tmphse = (Q4/newtib) * 100
	IF tmphse ≥ 85, THEN set value to 0
	IF tmphse < 85 and ≥75, THEN set value to 1
	IF tmphse < 75 and ≥65, THEN set value to 2
	IF tmphse < 65, THEN set value to 3
	Minimum Score = 0 (better); Maximum Score = 3 (worse)

PSQISLPQUAL	**OVERALL SLEEP QUALITY**
	Q6
	Minimum Score = 0 (better); Maximum Score = 3 (worse)

PSQIMEDS	**NEED MEDS TO SLEEP**
	Q7
	Minimum Score = 0 (better); Maximum Score = 3 (worse)

PSQI	**TOTAL**
	DURAT + DISTB + LATEN + DAYDYS + HSE + SLPQUAL + MEDS
	Minimum Score = 0 (better); Maximum Score = 21 (worse)

APPENDIX C

Sleep Hygiene Index

Rating scale: Never = 0; Rarely = 1; Sometimes = 2; Frequently = 3; Always = 4

1. I take daytime naps lasting two or more hours.
2. I go to bed at different times from day to day.
3. I get out of bed at different times from day to day.
4. I exercise to the point of sweating within one hour of going to bed.
5. I stay in bed longer than I should two or three times a week.
6. I use alcohol, tobacco, or caffeine within four hours of going to bed.
7. I do something that may wake me up before bedtime (e.g., play videogames, use the internet, or clean).
8. I go to bed feeling stressed, angry, upset, or nervous.
9. I use my bed for things other than sleeping or sex (e.g., watch TV, read, eat, or study).
10. I sleep on an uncomfortable bed (e.g., poor mattress or pillow, too much or not enough blankets).
11. I sleep in an uncomfortable bedroom (e.g., too bright, too stuffy, too hot, too cold, or too noisy).
12. I do important work before bedtime (e.g., pay bills, schedule, or study).
13. I think, plan, or worry when I am in bed.

Scoring: Item scores are summed providing a global assessment of sleep hygiene.

References

American Psychiatric Association. (2000). *Diagnostic and Statistical Manual of Mental Disorders* (4th ed., text revision). Washington, DC: Author.

Ancoli-Israel, S. (1989). Epidemiology of sleep disorders. In T. Roth, & T. A. Roehrs (Eds.), *Clinics in Geriatric Medicine* (pp. 347–362). Philadelphia, PA: Saunders.

Ancoli-Israel, S. (2000). Insomnia in the elderly: a review for primary care practitioner. *Sleep*, *23*(1), S23–S30.

Ancoli-Israel, S., & Ayalon, L. (2006). Diagnosis and treatment of sleep disorders in older adults. *American Journal of Geriatric Psychiatry*, *14*, 95–103.

Ancoli-Israel, S., & Cooke, J. R. (2005). Prevalence and comorbidity of insomnia and effect on functioning in elderly populations. *Jags*, *53*, S264–S271.

Ancoli-Israel, S., & Coy, T. (1994). Are breathing disturbances in elderly equivalent to sleep apnea syndrome? *Sleep*, *17*(1), 77–83.

Ancoli-Israel, S., Kripke, D. F., Klauber, M. R., Mason, W. J., Fell, R., & Kaplan, O. (1991). Sleep disordered breathing in community-dwelling elderly. *Sleep*, *14*, 486–495.

Ancoli-Israel, S., Kripke, D. F., Klauber, M. R., Fell, R., Stepnowsky, C., Estline, E., Khazeni, N., & Chinn, A. (1996). Morbidity, mortality and sleep-disordered breathing in community dwelling elderly. *Sleep*, *19*, 277–282.

Barlow, D. H. (1980). Behavior therapy: the next decade. *Behavior Therapy*, *11*, 315–328.

Barthlen, G. M. (2002). Obstructive sleep apnea syndrome, restless legs syndrome, and insomnia in geriatric patients. *Geriatrics*, *57*(11), 34–39.

Beck, A. T., Ward, C. H., Mendelson, M., Mock, J., & Erbaugh, J. (1961). An inventory for measuring depression. *Archives of General Psychiatry*, *4*, 561–571.

Bliwise, D. L. (1993). Sleep in normal aging and dementia. *Sleep*, *16*, 40–81.

Bliwise, D. L., Carskadon, M., Carey, E., & Dement, W. (1984). Longitudinal development of sleep related respiratory disturbance in adult humans. *Journal of Gerontology*, *39*, 290–293.

Bootzin, R. R., & Engle-Friedman, M. (1981). The assessment of insomnia. *Behavioral Assessment*, *3*, 107–126.

Browman, C. P., & Tepas, D. I. (1976). The effects of presleep activity on all-night sleep. *Psychophysiology*, *13*, 536–540.

Buysse, D. J., Reynolds, C. F., Monk, T. H., Berman, S. R., & Kupfer, D. J. (1989). The Pittsburg sleep quality index: a new instrument for psychiatric practice and research. *Psychiatry Res.*, *28*(2), 193–213.

Carskadon, M. A., Dement, W. C., Mitler, M. M., Guilleminault, C., Zarcone, V., & Spiegel, R. (1976). Self-report versus sleep laboratory findings in 122 drug-free subjects with complaints of insomnia. *American Journal of Psychiatry*, *133*, 1382–1388.

Coates, T. J., Killen, J. D., George, J., Marchini, E., Silverman, S., & Thoresen, C. E. (1982). Estimating sleep parameters: a multitrait-multimethod analysis. *Journal of Consulting and Clinical Psychology*, *50*, 345–352.

Cohen-Mansfield, J., Waldhorn, R., Werner, P., & Billig, N. (1990). Validation of sleep observations in a nursing home. *Sleep*, *13*, 512–525.

Cole, J. C., Dubois, D., & Kosinski, M. (2007). Use of patient-reported sleep measures in clinical trials of pain treatment: a literature review and synthesis of current sleep measures and a conceptual model of sleep disturbance in pain. *Clinical Therapeutics*, *29*(11), 2580–2588.

Coleman, R. M., Miles, L. E., Guilleminault, C. C., Zarcone, V. P., van den Hoed, J., & Dement, W. C. (1981). Sleep-wake disorders in the elderly: a polysomnographic analysis. *Journal of the American Geriatric Society*, *29*, 289–296.

Coyne, K. S. (2003). The prevalence of nocturia and its effect on health-related quality of life and sleep in a community sample in the USA. *Journal of Urology International*, *92*(9), 948–954.

Cumming, R. G., & Le Couteur, D. G. (2003). Benzodiazepines and risk of hip fractures in older people: a review of the evidence. *Central Nervous System Drugs*, *17*(11), 825–837.

Derogatis, L. R. (1993). Brief symptom inventory. In *Administration, Scoring, & Procedures Manual*. Minneapolis, MS: National Computer Systems.

Douglass, A. B., Bornstein, R., Nino-Murcia, G., Keenan, S., Miles, L., Zarcone, V. P., Guilleminault, C., & Dement, W. (1994). The Sleep Disorders Questionnaire I: creation and multivariate structure of the SDQ. *Sleep*, *17*, 160–167.

Douglass, A. B., Carskadon, M. A., & Houser, R. (1990). Historical data base, questionnaires, sleep and life cycle diaries. In L. E. Miles, & R. Broughton (Eds.), *Medical Monitoring in the Home and Work Environment* (pp. 17–28). New York, NY: Raven Press.

Emmelcamp, P. M. (1981). The current and future status of clinical research. *Behavioral Assessment*, *3*, 249–253.

Engle-Friedman, M., & Bootzin, R. R. (1991). Insomnia as a problem for the elderly. In P. A. Wisoki (Ed.), *Handbook of Clinical Behavior Therapy with the Elderly Client* (pp. 273–298). New York, NY: Plenum Press.

Fichten, C. S., Creti, L., Amsel, R., Brender, W., Weinstein, N., & Libman, E. (1995). Poor sleepers who do not complain of insomnia: myths and realities about psychological and lifestyle characteristics of older good and poor sleepers. *Journal of Behavioral Medicine*, *18*, 189–223.

Foley, D., Ancoli-Israel, S., & Britz, P. (2004). Sleep disturbances and chronic disease in older adults: results of the 2003 National Sleep Foundation Sleep in America Survey. *J. Psychosom. Res.*, *56*, 497–502.

Foley, D. J., Monjan, A. A., Brown, S. L., Simonsick, E. M., Wallace, R. B., & Blazer, D. G. (1995). Sleep complaints among elderly persons: an epidemiologic study of three communities. *Sleep*, *18*, 425–432.

Foley, D. J., Monjan, A. A., Simonsick, E. M., Wallace, R. B., & Blazer, D. G. (1999). Incidence and remission of insomnia among elderly adults: an epidemiologic study of 6,800 persons over three years. *Sleep*, *22*(2), S366–S372.

Gillberg, M., Kecklund, G., & Akerstedt, T. (1994). Relations between performance and subjective ratings of sleepiness during a night awake. *Sleep*, *17*(3), 236–241.

Gislason, T., & Almqvist, M. (1987). Somatic diseases and sleep complaints: an epidemiological study of 3201 Swedish men. *Acta Medica Scandinavica*, *221*, 475–481.

Golpe, R., Jiménez, A., & Carpizo, R. (2002). Home sleep studies in the assessment of sleep apnea/hypopnea syndrome. *Chest*, *122*(4), 1156–1161.

Gooneratne, N. S., Gehrman, P. R., Nkwuo, E., Bellamy, S. L., Schutte-Rodin, S., Dinges, D. F., & Pack, A. I. (2006). Consequences of comorbid insomnia symptoms and sleep-related breathing disorder in elderly subjects. *Arch. Intern. Medicine*, *166*, 1732–1738.

Hauri, P. (1982). *The Sleep Disorders*. Kalamazoo, MI: Upjohn.

Haynes, S. (1983). Behavioral assessment. In M. Hersen, A. E. Kazdin, & A. S. Bellack (Eds.), *The Clinical Psychology Handbook* (pp. 397–425). New York, NY: Pergamon.

Haynes, S. N., Adams, A., & Franzen, M. (1981). The effects of pre-sleep stress on sleep-onset insomnia. *Journal of Abnormal Psychology*, *90*, 601–606.

Haynes, S. N., & O'Brien, W. H. (1990). Functional analysis in behavior therapy. *Clinical Psychology Review*, *10*, 649–668.

Hyyppa, M. T., & Kronholm, E. (1989). Quality of sleep and chronic illness. *Journal of Clinical Epidemiology*, *42*, 633–638.

Johns, M. W. (1991). A new method for measuring daytime sleepiness: the Epworth sleepiness scale. *Sleep*, *14*(6), 540–545.

Jones, S. H., Hare, D. J., & Evershed, K. (2005). Actigraphic assessment of circadian activity and sleep patterns in bipolar disorder. *Bipolar Disorder*, *7*(2), 176–186.

Kiyokawa, H., Yonemaru, M., Horie, S., Kasuga, I., Ichinose, Y., & Toyama, K. (1999). Detection of nocturnal wheezing in bronchial asthma using intermittent sleep tracheal sounds recording. *Respirology*, *4*(1), 37–45.

Lader, D., Cardinali, D. P., & Pandi-Perumal, S. R. (Eds.) (2006). *Sleep and Sleep Disorders: A Neuropsychopharmachological Approach*. New York, NY: Springer Science + Business Media.

Landolt, H.-P., & Gillin, J. C. (2001). Sleep abnormalities during abstinence in alcohol-dependent patients: aetiology and management. *CNS Drugs*, *15*(5), 413–425.

Lavie, P., Ben-Yosef, R., & Rubin, A. E. (1984). Prevalence of sleep apnea syndrome among patients with essential hypertension. *American Heart Journal*, *108*, 373.

Leigh, T. J., Hindmarch, I., Bird, H. A., & Wright, V. (1988). Comparison of sleep in osteoarthritic patients and age and sex matched healthy controls. *Annals of the Rheumatic Diseases*, *47*, 40–42.

Lichstein, K. L. (1988). Sleep compression treatment of an insomnoid. *Behaviour Therapy*, *19*(4), 625–632.

Lichstein, K. L., Durrence, H. H., Riedel, B. W., Taylor, D. J., & Bush, A. J. (2004). *Epidemiology of Sleep*. Mahwah, NJ: Lawrence Erlbaum.

Lichstein, K. L., & Fanning, J. (1990). Cognitive anxiety in insomnia: an analogue test. *Stress Medicine*, *6*, 47–51.

Lichstein, K. L., & Riedel, B. W. (1994). Behavioral assessment and treatment of insomnia: a review with an emphasis on clinical application. *Behavior Therapy*, *25*, 659–688.

Maher, S. (2004). Sleep in the older adult. *Nursing Older People*, *16*(9), 30–35.

Malhotra, A., Crowley, S., Pillar, G., Kikinis, R., & White, D. P. (2000). Aging-related changes in the pharyngeal structure and function in normal subjects. *Sleep*, *23*, A42.

Malhotra, A., & White, D. (2002). Obstructive sleep apnea. *The Lancet*, *360*(9328), 237–245.

Manabe, K., Matsui, T., Yamaya, M., Sato-Nakagawa, T., Okamura, N., Arai, H., & Sasaki, H. (2000). Sleep patterns and mortality among elderly patients in a geriatric hospital. *Gerontology*, *46*, 318–322.

Mastin, D. F., Bryson, J., & Corwyn, R. (2006). Assessment of sleep hygiene using the sleep hygiene index. *Journal of Behavioral Medicine*, *29*(3), 223–227.

Mejo, S. (1992). Anterograde amnesia linked to benzodiazepines. *Nurse Practitioner*, *17*(10), 44–50.

Miles, L. E., & Dement, W. C. (1980). Sleep and aging. *Sleep*, *3*, 119–120.

Moldofsky, H. (2000). The contribution of sleep medicine to the assessment of the tired patient. *Can. J. Psychiatry*, *45*(9), 798–802.

Monk, T. H., Flaherty, J. F., Frank, E., Hoskinson, K., & Kupfer, D. J. (1990). The Social Rhythmn Metric: An instrument to quantify the daily rhythmns of life. *Journal of Neurons Mental Disorders*, *178*(2), 120–126.

Monk, T. H., Reynolds, C. F., Machen, M. A., & Kupfer, D. J. (1992). Daily social rhythmns in the elderly and their relation to objectively recorded sleep. *Sleep*, *15*, 322–329.

Morgan, R., & Cheadle, A. J. (1976). Circadian body temperature in chronic schizophrenia. *British Journal of Psychiatry*, *129*, 350–354.

Morgan, K., Healey, D. W., & Healey, P. J. (1989). Factors influencing persistent subjective insomnia in old age: a follow-up study of good and poor sleepers aged 65–74. *Age and Aging*, *18*, 117–122.

Morin, C. M. (1993). *Insomnia: Psychological Assessment and Management*. New York, NY: Guilford.

Morin, C. M., & Gramling, S. E. (1989). Sleep patterns and aging: comparison of older adults with and without insomnia complaints. *Psychology and Aging*, *4*, 290–294.

National Institutes of Health. (2009). Retrieved from http://www.nih.gov/

Parrott, A. C., & Hindmarch, I. (1980). The Leeds sleep evaluation questionnaire in psychological investigations: a review. *Psychopharmacology*, *71*, 173–179.

Partinen, M., Jamieson, A., & Guilleminault, C. (1988). Long-term outcome for obstructive sleep apnea syndrome patients—mortality. *Chest*, *94*, 1200–1204.

Pfeiffer, E. (1975). A short portable mental status questionnaire for the assessment of organic brain deficit in elderly patients. *J. Am. Geriatr. Soc.*, *23*, 433–441.

Picarsic, J. L., Glynn, N. W., Taylor, C. A., Katula, J. A., Goldman, S. E., Studenski, S. A., & Newman, A. B. (2008). Self-reported napping and duration and quality of sleep in the lifestyle interventions and independence for elders pilot study. *Journal of the American Geriatrics Society*, *56*(9), 1674–1680.

Polo-Kantola, P., Saaresranta, T., & Polo, O. (2001). Aetiology and treatment of sleep disturbances during perimenopause and postmenopause. *CNS Drugs*, *15*(6), 445–452.

Quan, S. F., & Zee, P. (2004). Evaluating the effects of medical disorders on sleep in the older patient. *Geriatrics*, *59*(3), 37–42.

Resnick, H. E., Redline, S., Shahar, E., Gilpin, A., Newman, A., Walter, R., Ewy, G. A., et al. (2003). Diabetes and sleep disturbances. *Diabetes Care*, *26*(3), 702–709.

Roehrs, T., Zorick, F., Sicklesteel, J., Wittig, R., & Roth, T. (1983). Age-related sleep–wake disorders at a sleep disorders center. *Journal of American Geriatric Society*, *31*, 364–370.

Rogers, A. E., Caruso, C. C., & Aldrich, M. (1993). Reliability of sleep diaries for assessment of sleep/wake patterns. *Nursing Research*, *42*, 368–372.

Rosa, R., Bonnet, M. H., & Kramer, M. (1983). The relationship of sleep and anxiety in anxious subjects. *Biological Psychology*, *16*, 119–126.

Sanavio, E. (1988). Pre-sleep cognitive intrusions and treatment of onset-insomnia. *Behaviour Research and Therapy*, *26*, 451–459.

Schneider, D. L. (2002). Safe and effective therapy for sleep problems in the older patient. *Geriatrics*, *57*(5), 24–35.

Seppala, T., Partinen, M., Penttila, A., Aspholm, R., Tiainen, E., & Kaukianen, A. (1991). Sudden death and sleeping history among Finnish men. *Journal of Internal Medicine*, *229*, 23–28.

Shiffman, S. (1998). Ecological momentary assessment: health behavior in the field. *Annals of Behavioral Medicine*, *20*, S011.

Snyder-Halpern, R., & Verran, J. A. (1987). Instrumentation to describe subjective sleep characteristics in healthy subjects. *Res. Nurs. Health*, *10*, 155–163.

Sok, S. R. (2006). Sleep patterns and insomnia management in Korean-American older adult immigrants. *Journal of Clinical Nursing* 135–143.

Spielberger, C. D., Gorsuch, R. L., & Lushene, R. E. (1970). *Manual for the State-Trait Anxiety Inventory.* Palo Alto, CA: Consulting Psychologists Press.

Spielman, A. J. (1986). Assessment of insomnia. *Clinical Psychology Review*, *6*, 11–25.

Strohl, K. P. (1996). Diabetes and sleep apnea. *Sleep*, *19*, S225–S228.

Totterdell, P., Reynolds, S., Parkinson, B., & Briner, R. B. (1994). Associations of sleep with everyday mood, minor symptoms and social interaction experience. *Sleep*, *17*, 466–475.

Trevorrow, T., & Fast, K. (1998). Does sleep affect inpatient stroke rehabilitation? *Annals of Behavioral Medicine*, *20*, S103.

U.S. Bureau of Census (2009). Retrieved from http://www.census.gov/

van derHooft, C. S., Jong, G. W., Dieleman, J. P., Verhamme, K. M., van der Cammen, T. J., Stricker, B. H., & Sturkenboom, M. C. (2005). Inappropriate drug prescribing in older adults: the update 2002 Beers criteria—a population-based cohort study. *British Journal of Clinical Pharmacology*, *60*(2), 137–144.

van Diest, R. (1990). Subjective sleep characteristics as coronary risk factors, their association with type A behavior and vital exhaustion. *J. Psychosom. Res.*, *34*, 415–426.

Vitiello, M. V., & Borson, S. (2001). Sleep disturbances in patients with Alzheimer's disease: epidemiology pathophysiology and treatment. *CNS Drugs*, *15*(10), 777–796.

Wingard, D. L., & Berkman, P. T. (1983). Mortality risk associated with sleeping patterns among adults. *Sleep*, *6*, 102–107.

Wittels, E. H. (1985). Obesity and hormonal factors in sleep and sleep apnea. *Medical Clinician of North America*, *69*, 1265–1280.

Zarcone, V. P. (1989). Sleep hygeine. In M. Kryger, T. Roth, & W. Dement (Eds.), *Principles and Practice of Sleep Medicine* (pp. 490–493). Philadelphia, PA: Saunders.

Zorick, F. J., Roth, T., Hartse, K. M., Piccione, P., & Stepanski, E. (1981). Evaluation and diagnosis of persistent insomnia. *American Journal of Psychiatry*, *138*, 769–773.

CHAPTER

Treatment Adherence in Late-Life 17

Erin E. Emery[1], Erin L. Woodhead[1], Victor Molinari[2], Marcia G. Hunt[3]

[1] *Department of Behavioral Sciences, Rush University Medical Center, Chicago, IL, USA,*
[2] *Department of Aging and Mental Health Disparities, College of Behavioral and Community Sciences, Louis de la Parte Florida Mental Health Institute, University of South Florida, Tampa, FL, USA,*
[3] *VA Connecticut Healthcare System, Department of Psychiatry, Yale University School of Medicine, New Haven, CT, USA*

INTRODUCTION

In the United States in the last century, human life expectancy increased from 47 years to 77 years (CDC & MCF, 2007), partly due to improvements in health care and managing chronic health conditions. Eighty percent of older adults have at least one chronic illness, and 50% have two or more (NCHS, 2006). Managing these illnesses can be extremely difficult for older adults. According to the World Health Organization (WHO, 2003), treatment adherence rates are approximately 50%, with some variation by illness, treatment regimen, and adherence criteria.

The variability in reported rates of adherence to treatment plans is due, in part, to the development of a precise definition of adherence. "Compliance" has been used interchangeably with "adherence," although researchers have suggested that the term "compliance" minimizes the patient's role and reflects an overly authoritarian view, whereas "adherence" denotes a more collaborative patient/physician relationship (Eisenthal, Emery, Lazare, & Udin, 1979; Lutfey & Wishner, 1999). Christensen (2004, p. 3) provides a working definition of patient adherence: "the extent to which a person's actions or behavior coincides with advice or instruction from a health care provider intended to prevent, monitor, or ameliorate a disorder." This definition, however, remains focused on the health care provider's determination of the treatment plan. Since health care in general, and mental health treatment specifically, has an often disagreeable history of forcing or mandating treatment, particularly for marginalized groups, stressing that adherence incorporates a sense of partnership between patient and health care provider is critical.

RATES OF TREATMENT ADHERENCE

Treatment adherence rates vary by medical condition and measurement method. Rates of adherence are lowest for preventive regimens (20–50%) and highest for acute treatment regimens (60–80%); chronic condition adherence rates range from 40 to 70% (Christensen, 2004). A range of factors may also impact adherence in any individual. For example, among those with diabetes mellitus, adherence rates are poorest among females, those with comorbid depression, and those with negative attitudes

Handbook of Assessment in Clinical Gerontology. DOI: 10.1016/B978-0-12-374961-1.10017-X toward insulin, especially for those with limited general education and limited diabetic education (Lerman et al., 2009).

According to the National Council on Patient Information and Education (2007), at any given time, regardless of age group, up to 59% of those on five or more medications are taking them improperly. This group also reported that 12% of Americans do not fill their prescription at all, 22% take less of the medication than is prescribed on the label, and more than half of all Americans with chronic diseases do not follow their physician's medication and lifestyle guidance. Given that adults over the age of 65 are prescribed an average of seven to eight daily medications (Orwig, Brandt, & Gruber-Baldini, 2006; Steinman et al., 2006), it is highly likely that most older adult patients do not take their medications as indicated by their physicians.

The impact of treatment non-adherence is significant. Ten percent of all hospital admissions and 23% of all nursing home admissions are the result of patients failing to take prescription medications correctly (National Council on Patient Information and Education, 2007). Further, poor medication adherence cost has been estimated to range from $177 billion (Ernst & Grizzle, 2001) to $300 billion annually (DiMatteo, 2004) in total direct and indirect health care costs.

FACTORS INFLUENCING ADHERENCE

In light of the high rates of non-adherence across age groups and treatment regimens, researchers have focused efforts on determining what factors influence adherence. For clinicians who routinely work with older adults, it is important to understand how various factors influence adherence, in order to better understand the likely adherence pattern of any given patient.

Sociodemographic Variables

Researchers have posited that sociodemographic characteristics may impact adherence by influencing an individual's ability to acquire knowledge, communicate effectively with their health care providers, and to obtain effective social support around their diagnosis (e.g., Apter et al., 2003). Age has been examined as one predictor of adherence, with mixed results. Among adults with HIV/AIDS between the ages of 25 and 69, older adults were three times more likely than younger adults to be at least 95% adherent, as assessed by an electronic monitoring device (Hinkin et al., 2004; see discussion of assessment devices below). This and other research has suggested that older adults are generally more adherent than younger adults (e.g., Monane et al., 1996; Siegel, Lopez, & Meier, 2007). However, discontinuation of medication has been associated with older age among patients on cardiovascular drug regimens (e.g., Kulkarni, Alexander, Lytle, Heiss, & Peterson, 2006). In light of the mixed results of these studies, drawing conclusions about the influence of age on adherence is difficult, as it is likely a variable that interacts with other factors to predict adherence.

Cognitive Functioning

As the complexity of older adults' treatment regimens increase, the cognitive demands required for adequate adherence may also increase. Older adults with cognitive impairment may lack the memory function or organizational ability to create a schedule around taking medication, engage in self-care behaviors, or keep appointments. In fact, patients with cognitive impairment have been found to have a 2.3 times greater risk of adherence failure, as compared to patients without cognitive impairment (Hinkin et al., 2002). This difference may be primarily due to differences in executive functioning and verbal memory (Stoehr et al., 2008). Cognitive status has also been found to be an independent predictor of missed primary care appointments (Mackin & Arean, 2007). Thus, assessment of multiple cognitive domains is helpful for understanding adherence.

Health Literacy and Numeracy

Even for older adults who are cognitively intact, deciphering health-related information can be difficult. Health literacy is defined as one's ability to "obtain, process, and understand basic health information and services needed to make appropriate health decisions" (Institute of Medicine, 2004, p. 4). Results of the 2003 National Assessment of Adult Literacy indicated that adults over the age of 65 had the lowest health literacy compared to other sampled aged groups (Kutner, Greenberg, Jin, & Paulsen, 2006). Of those over age 65, 29% achieved a "below basic" level of health literacy, 30% achieved a "basic" level, 38% achieved an "intermediate" level, and only 3% achieved a "proficient" level (Kutner et al., 2006). Thus, the majority of older adults have difficulty summarizing and making simple inferences from prose text, locating information in complex documents, and completing arithmetic operations that require more than one step. Many of these processes are needed to understand medication instructions, dosing schedules, and the risk of potential side effects.

The concept of numeracy has also recently been discussed by several researchers (e.g., Peters, 2008) as being different from health literacy. Numeracy has been defined as "the degree to which individuals have the capacity to access, process, interpret, communicate, and act on numerical, quantitative, graphical, biostatistical, and probabilistic health information needed to make effective health decisions" (Golbeck, Ahlers-Schmidt, Paschal, & Dismuke 2005, p. 375). Due to the potentially risky nature of some medical decisions, the idea of numeracy has been examined in relation to one's ability to understand the risks inherent in a decision. In a study among community-dwelling older adults, the majority of participants were able to assess the magnitude of risk properly and to respond correctly to health-based calculations of probabilities, proportions, and percentages (Donelle, Hoffman-Goetz, & Arocha, 2007). However, when asked questions about broad numerical concepts, the majority of participants had difficulty comprehending the concept of probability, converting a percentage value to a proportion and converting a proportion to a percentage. Increased age was associated with decreased general numeracy skills, particularly among older adults age 80 to 90.

In light of these findings, health care providers should not assume that a patient's level of health literacy and numeracy is adequate to comprehend medication instructions, or to understand the specific symptoms or medical terms related to their disease. Davis and colleagues (1993) created the *Rapid Estimate of Adult Literacy in Medicine* (*REALM*) to identify patients with low literacy in medical settings. To maximize utility, a 7-item short form (*REALM-SF*) was created, as seen in Figure 17.1 (Arozullah et al., 2007). The *REALM-SF* was found to have adequate concurrent validity ($r = 0.88 - 0.97$, $p < 0.0001$) with the *Peabody Individual Achievement Test-Revised* (Markwardt, 1998), the *Wide Range Achievement Test* (Wilkinson, 1993), and the *Slosson Oral Reading Test-Revised* (Slosson, 1990); test–retest reliability was found to be excellent ($r = 0.99$, $p < 0.001$). Shea and colleagues (2004) found that REALM-SF scores were significantly related to education, age, and race, but not gender. When stratified by education, differences between African Americans and Caucasians remained significant.

Recently, a numeracy scale has been developed that is specific to numeracy skills used in diabetes management (Figure 17.2; Huizinga et al., 2008). *The Diabetes Numeracy Test* (*DNT*) is available in a full 43-item version and a shortened 15-item version. The DNT was validated on a sample of patients with type 1 and type 2 diabetes (average age approximately 55 years). Approximately 69% of participants had greater than 9th grade literacy as assessed by the *REALM*

Rapid Estimate of Adult Literacy in Medicine Short Form

(REALM-SF)

Suggested introduction: "We are studying medical word reading in order to improve communication between healthcare providers and patients. Here is a list of medical words that may be difficult to read."

Interviewer: Show the participant the Word List.

Then say, "Starting at the top of the list, please read each word aloud to me. If you don't recognize a word, you can say 'pass' and move on to the next word. Your results will be kept strictly confidential and will not be included in your other official medical records."

Interviewer: If the participant takes more than 5 seconds on a word, say "pass" and point to the next word. Hold this sheet so that it is not visible to the participant.

Fat	Not scored		
Flu	Not scored		
1. Behavior	1☐Correct	2☐ Mispronounced	3☐ Not attempted
2. Exercise	1☐Correct	2☐ Mispronounced	3☐ Not attempted
3. Menopause	1☐Correct	2☐ Mispronounced	3☐ Not attempted
4. Rectal	1☐Correct	2☐ Mispronounced	3☐ Not attempted
5. Antibiotics	1☐Correct	2☐ Mispronounced	3☐ Not attempted
6. Anemia	1☐Correct	2☐ Mispronounced	3☐ Not attempted
7. Jaundice	1☐Correct	2☐ Mispronounced	3☐ Not attempted

REALM-SF Scoring

Total Score (0—7)	Grade
0	≤ 3rd grade
1-3	4th-6th grade
4-6	7th-8th grade
7	≥ 9th grade

Fat
Flu
Behavior
Exercise
Menopause
Rectal
Antibiotics
Anemia
Jaundice

FIGURE 17.1

Rapid Estimate of Adult Literacy in Medicine Short Form.

(REALM-SF: Arozullah et al., 2007)

and 31% had greater than 9th grade numeracy as assessed by the *Wide Range Achievement Test* (Wilkinson, 1993). With this population, both the full and shortened versions of the DNT had acceptable internal consistency and construct validity. The DNT is publicly available through the Vanderbilt Diabetes Research and Training Center (http://www.mc.vanderbilt.edu/diabetes/drtc/preventionandcontrol/tools.php).

Question 1

You are told to follow the sliding scale shown here. The sliding scale indicates the amount of insulin you take based upon your blood sugar levels.

If Blood sugar is:	Units of Insulin
130-180	0
181-230	1
231-280	2
281-330	3
331-380	4

How much insulin would you take for a blood sugar of 295?

ANSWER ____ units

Correct answer: 3 units

Percent answered correctly 85%

Question 2

After seeing the Doctor, you are given the following instruction to lower a high blood sugar level before a meal:

"Starting with a blood sugar of 120, take 1 unit of Humalog insulin for each 50 points of blood sugar."

How much insulin should you take for a blood sugar of 375?

ANSWER ____ units

Correct: 5 units

Percent answered correctly 37%

FIGURE 17.2

Sample Items from the Diabetes Numeracy Test.

(Huizinga et al., 2008)

Patient Beliefs About the Illness or Disability

In a recent meta-analysis of the impact of patient beliefs on adherence, DiMatteo and her colleagues (2007) found that the odds of adherence were 2.5 times greater in those patients who believed that the disease to be treated was severe and a potential threat. Many theories have been developed about the role of patient beliefs about illness. Attribution theory examines the extent to which one believes an illness is related to internal causes, such as one's own behavior, or external causes, such as one's fate or genetics (cf., Horne, Weinman, & Hankins 1999). These attributions are related to beliefs about cure, and can influence one's adherence to treatment. Health locus of control (HLOC) theory also examines beliefs about the controllability of health and illness. Internal HLOC (believing one can control one's own health) may encourage more health promotion behaviors and may be linked to better adherence to treatment regimens than external HLOC (believing that factors outside of individual control are responsible for health outcomes). However, as discussed by Horne and Weinman (1998), a global measure of health locus of control such as the *Multidimensional Health Locus of Control Scales* (Wallston, Wallston, & Peabody, 1978) has little utility for predicting adherence behavior. Disease-specific perceived control scales, such as the *Perceived Control of Diabetes Scales*, have been shown to be more useful in predicting health behavior for specific chronic illnesses (Bradley, 1994).

Cultural Factors

Attitudes about illness may also be impacted by ethnicity, culture, or religion. In a review of literature on hypertension among older adults, Ontiveros and colleagues (1999) found that African American older adults were more likely to view hypertension as related to stress and health behavior, while Caucasians attributed the disease to genetic or mechanistic factors, and Latino older adults viewed hypertension as a normal part of aging, thus less treatable. It is highly likely that these beliefs would impact adherence to a treatment plan that was not consistent with these beliefs. In fact, the review

This questionnaire describes situations related to health. Please read each situation and imagine that it is happening to you. Use the following scale to indicate how similar the thought is to how you would think in that situation:

Not at all like I would think	*Only a little like I would think*	*Moderately like I would think*	*Quite a bit like I would think*	*Almost exactly like I would think*
1	2	3	4	5

1. Several of your coworkers have come down with the flu. You hear on the news that there is a flu outbreak and that people who are in contact with infected individuals should get immunizations to reduce their chances of getting ill. You find yourself thinking, "I had a flu vaccination last year and got sick anyway, immunizations never do me any good."

2. During a routine physical examination, your doctor notices a mole on your hand and suggests that you see a specialist to have it examined further. You recall that a friend of yours had a similar mole for years and it never caused her any problems. You think, "I'm sure it won't ever cause me a problem either."

3. During your last checkup, your cholesterol level was high, and your doctor recommended that you reduce the fat in your diet. Today at lunch you notice that all of your coworkers were eating hamburgers and french fries. You think, "If everybody eats like this, it can't be that bad for you."

4. Your doctor prescribes a medication for an illness and instructs you to finish the entire bottle of pills. After taking half of the medication, you notice that your symptoms have cleared up. You find yourself thinking, "If I don't feel sick anymore, the medicine is unnecessary."

5. Your doctor recommends a new medication for an ongoing health problem and indicates that about 10% of patients experience unpleasant side effects from the medicine. You think to yourself, "If anyone is going to have side effects, it's going to be me."

6. You have experienced an injury that has left you unable to work. Your doctor recommends a treatment that should allow you to return to work but only on a part-time basis. You find yourself thinking, "If the treatment can't cure me completely, it is not really worthwhile."

7. You have recently undergone surgery to correct a health problem. Your doctor informs you that the surgery was not successful and will need to be repeated. You find yourself thinking, "If it didn't work the first time, it probably never will in my case."

8. During a routine check-up, your doctor emphasizes the importance of exercise and eating right to prevent health problems. You notice that the doctor is quite overweight. You think to yourself, "If good eating habits and exercise were really important, he would lose weight himself."

9. Your doctor is instructing you in how to take a new medication. In the middle of the discussion, the doctor is called out of the room and says that a nurse will finish explaining how to use the medication. You find yourself thinking, "If this new treatment was really important, the doctor would finish giving me the instructions himself."

10. Because both of your parents had heart disease, you know that your risk for this illness is much greater than it is for most people. At a recent checkup, your doctor emphasizes that by making certain changes in your lifestyle, you would reduce your risk of heart disease by 50%. You find yourself thinking, "If heart disease runs in my family, whether or not I get it is really beyond my control."

11. You have been following a specific nutritional plan prescribed by your doctor for an ongoing health problem. This plan requires you to avoid desserts and other high-sugar foods. At a birthday party, everyone is eating cake. You think to yourself, "If I don't eat a piece of cake too, I'll spoil the party."

12. You have been taking a medication for six months and your medical problem has not improved. Your doctor has suggested a new drug. You think to yourself, "If the last medication didn't help, a new one won't do any good."

13. You were injured in a car accident two months ago and have been in physical therapy since then. Your doctor had predicted that you would be fully recovered by now, but you have only partially recovered. You think to yourself, "These past two months have been a complete waste."

14. You smoke and are overweight but have never had a major health problem. At a recent checkup, your doctor tells you that these habits put you at risk for health problems down the road. Both of your parents have similar habits and have lived long healthy lives. You find yourself thinking, "Smoking and eating too much just aren't a problem in my case."

FIGURE 17.3

Irrational Health Belief Scale.

(Christensen, Moran, & Wiebe, 1999)

indicated that older Caucasians were more likely to have a primary care physician and have had a blood pressure check than were African Americans or Latinos, while emergency room use was higher among African Americans. African Americans have also been found to be more likely to use home remedies than Caucasians (Brown & Segal, 1996).

15. You have been feeling generally fatigued since you started a new medication last month. Your doctor told you that the medication is extremely effective but that fatigue is a common side effect. You think to yourself, "Something that makes me feel this tired can't be any good for me."

16. You see a report in the media that suggests the majority of people still do not wear seat belts when they drive. You find yourself thinking, "There are so many people driving without using seatbelts, it can't be that dangerous."

17. You are planning an overseas trip, and your doctor recommends you receive a set of immunizations before you leave. You visited this same place last year without receiving any immunizations and did not become ill. You think to yourself, "If I didn't get ill last time, I'm sure I won't on this trip."

18. You are scheduled to undergo a medical test at the end of the day, and your doctor has instructed you not to eat any lunch before the procedure. That same day you are asked to attend a lunch meeting at work. You think to yourself, "I can't attend the meeting if I don't eat like everyone else."

19. You learn that you have a mild medical condition that causes you no discomfort but requires lifetime treatment with medication. Your doctor assures you that you will not experience any significant side effects from the medication and the condition is not likely to interfere with your functioning in a noticeable way. You find yourself thinking, "If I have to take this medication, my life will never be the same."

20. All of your family members (or roommates) have come down with a bad case of the flu in the past week, but so far you feel fine. You receive a message from their doctor that you should take special precautions to avoid becoming ill as well. You think to yourself, "If I'm not sick yet, I am probably immune."

FIGURE 17.3

Irrational Health Belief Scale (Cont'd).

Other cultural norms may also impact treatment adherence. For example, Japanese older adults have been found to be more likely to follow physicians' orders (Iihara, et al., 2004). This may be related to the culture dictating that physicians play a more authoritative role, and to Japan's universal health care system, which allows for access to health services. In contrast, older African Americans have been found to experience distrust of the American medical system, and thus are less likely to adhere to a treatment plan dictated by their physician (Siegal et al., 2007). Older Russian immigrants to the United States have expressed similar distrust of the American health care system, as well as the media, regarding health information (Benisovich & King, 2003).

Religious and spiritual beliefs warrant consideration when examining predictors of adherence, particularly among older adults. Some treatments are inconsistent with religious values, and some cultures are less likely to communicate this to providers unless directly asked. Further, patients may have specific beliefs, such as that an illness is a punishment from God, which may act as a barrier to treatment adherence. Although the relation between religious beliefs and adherence has not been well explored empirically among older adults, health care providers are encouraged to be sensitive to beliefs and practices that may impact adherence (Zivin & Kales, 2008).

Case Study

Mr Williams, a 72-year-old African American man, was hospitalized following a heart attack. His cardiologist, who had prescribed an ACE inhibitor, and recommended a specific diet and exercise plan a month prior, was perplexed by Mr Williams' choice not to fill the prescription or make any changes in his health behaviors. As the physician considered the lecture she was about to give the patient about his non-adherence, she noticed the Bible at his bedside. She asked Mr Williams if prayer was helping him cope with his health event. Mr Williams indicated that he was praying for forgiveness, but felt that the hypertension and heart attack were appropriate penance for misdeeds in his past. With some discussion, he indicated that he intentionally disregarded the physician's recommendations because he felt that he deserved God's punishment of cardiac disease. The physician consulted the chaplain, who administered the *Brief RCOPE*. Mr Williams' scores indicated a very high level of negative religious coping and minimal positive religious coping. The chaplain was able to discuss Mr Williams' experience of guilt and ways that he may be able to explore treatment plan options to preserve his cardiac health and spiritual well-being.

For the following questions, please circle the number that best corresponds to your views:

How much does your illness affect your life?

0 1 2 3 4 5 6 7 8 9 10

No affect at all — Severely affects my life

How long do you think your illness will continue?

0 1 2 3 4 5 6 7 8 9 10

A very short time — Forever

How much control do you feel you have over your illness?

0 1 2 3 4 5 6 7 8 9 10

Absolutely no control — Extreme amount of control

How much do you think your treatment can help with your illness?

0 1 2 3 4 5 6 7 8 9 10

Not at all — Extremely helpful

How much do you experience symptoms from your illness?

0 1 2 3 4 5 6 7 8 9 10

No symptoms at all — Many severe symptoms

How concerned are you about your illness?

0 1 2 3 4 5 6 7 8 9 10

Not at all concerned — Extremely concerned

How well do you feel you understand your illness?

0 1 2 3 4 5 6 7 8 9 10

Don't understand at all — Understand very clearly

How much does your illness affect you emotionally? (e.g., does it make you angry, scared, upset or depressed?

0 1 2 3 4 5 6 7 8 9 10

Not at all affected emotionally — Extremely affected emotionally

Please rank in rank-order the three most important factors that you believe caused your illness.

The most important causes for me:

1. ______________________

2. ______________________

3. ______________________

FIGURE 17.4

Brief Illness Perception Scale.

(Broadbent, Petrie, Main, & Weinman, 2006)

This example highlights not only the importance of assessing religious beliefs related to treatment adherence, but also the importance of a health care team working together to identify agreed-upon treatment goals and plans that fit with the patient's beliefs. The original *RCOPE*, a 17 factor measure of religious coping, with reliability coefficients ranging from 0.67 to 0.94, can also help to elucidate these beliefs (Pargament, Smith, Koenig, & Nielsen, 1998). A 14-item version (*Brief RCOPE*) measuring positive and negative religious coping has been used with older adult hospital patients with strong internal consistency (0.81–0.90) and good discriminant validity (Pargament, Smith, Koenig, & Perez, 1998; Pargament, Koenig, & Perez, 2000). Positive coping items in

BMQ-Specific

Your views about medicines prescribed for you*

- **We would like to ask you about your personal views about medicines prescribed for you.**
- **These are statements that other people have made about their medicines.**
- **Please indicate the extent to which you agree or disagree with them by ticking the appropriate box.**
- **There are no right or wrong answers. We are interested in your personal views.**

Rated: strongly agree, agree, uncertain, disagree, strongly disagree

My health, at present, depends on my medicines

Having to take medicines worries me

My life would be impossible without my medicines

Without my medicines I would be very ill

I sometimes worry about long-term effects of my medicines

My medicines are a mystery to me

My health in the future will depend on my medicines

My medicines disrupt my life

I sometimes worry about becoming too dependent on my medicines

My medicines protect me from becoming worse

*Note: To elicit beliefs about individual components of the treatment regimen the reference statement should refer to the medicine by name. e.g., *Your views about aspirin prescribed for you.* Additionally, items can refer to a named illness e.g., *Your views about medicines prescribed for your asthma.*

BMQ-General

Your views about medicines in general

- **We would like to ask you about your personal views about medicines in general.**
- **These are statements that other people have made about medicines in general.**
- **Please indicate the extent to which you agree or disagree with them by ticking the appropriate box.**
- **There are no right or wrong answers. We are interested in your personal views.**

Rated: strongly agree, agree, uncertain, disagree, strongly disagree

Doctors use too many medicines

People who take medicines should stop their treatment for a while every now and again

Most medicines are addictive

Natural remedies are safer than medicines

Medicines do more harm than good

All medicines are poisons

Doctors place too much trust on medicines

If doctors had more time with patients they would prescribe fewer medicines

FIGURE 17.5

The Beliefs About Medicines Questionnaire.

(Horne, Weinman, & Hankins, 1999)

response to a specific stressor include, "looked for a stronger connection with God" and "tried to see how God might be trying to strengthen me in this situation"; negative coping items include, "felt punished by God for my lack of devotion" and "questioned the power of God" (Pargament, Smith, Koenig, & Perez, 1998). Both measures employ a 4-point Likert scale reflecting the degree to which each mode of coping was employed in dealing with a stressor, with response options ranging from "not at all" to "a great deal."

Social Support

In addition to spiritual support, social support may encourage optimism and increase self-esteem related to management of the illness. Family members and friends may provide practical assistance and may buffer the stress of a chronic illness. DiMatteo's (2004) meta-analysis of the role of social support in adherence to medical treatment plans indicated that practical support, cohesive families, and living with a spouse were associated with improved treatment adherence. The same review suggests that attention also needs to be paid to the potential negative influence of social support, both intentional and unintentional (DiMatteo, 2004; Gallant, 2003). Facilitating discussion between a patient and family about the specific type of help they desire in their treatment regimen is recommended. Measures such as the *Interpersonal Support Evaluation List* (Cohen & Hoberman, 1983) or the *Diabetes Social Support Questionnaire* (Schlenk & Hart, 1984) may also be considered.

Personality/Psychopathology

Unützer and colleagues (2009) found that over the course of one year, older adults presenting in primary care with depression incurred total health care costs that were almost double those of individuals presenting without depression. This relationship is speculated to be partially related to the impact of mental health on treatment adherence (DiMatteo, Lepper, & Croghan, 2000). Researchers hypothesize that the presence of a mood disorder may impact patients' ability to follow through on a treatment regimen, potentially due to the impaired attention, energy, initiation, and motivation, along with feelings of helplessness, hopelessness, and worthlessness that are often experienced by patients with depression. Cognitive dysfunction associated with late-life depression may impair the ability of older adults to organize and implement an agreed-upon treatment plan, particularly for those with existing cognitive impairment (Hughes & Ganguli, 2009). Depression may also impact other measures related to adherence, such as irrational health beliefs ($r = 0.28$, $p < 0.001$; Christensen et al., 1999), some aspects of illness perception (e.g., illness coherence: $r = 0.21$, $p < 0.001$; Figueiras & Alves, 2007), beliefs about medicines (see Brown et al., 2005), and religious coping ($r = 0.31$, $p < 0.001$; Pargament et al., 1998).

Depressed patients of all ages have been found to be three times less likely to be adherent to a medical treatment plan than those not experiencing depression (DiMatteo et al., 2000). Bell and colleagues (2010) found that rural older adults ($n = 696$) with higher depression scores were less likely to engage in recommended exercise and diet plans, or follow recommendations for increased frequency of foot checks. Depression has also been found to be an independent predictor of missed primary care appointments (Mackin & Arean, 2007). DiMatteo and colleagues' (2000) meta-analysis indicated that anxiety had a less clear relation to adherence, though warrants further study.

The fact that depressed patients may have lower adherence to treatments for their other chronic diseases makes depression assessment and intervention important. There are several quick screening instruments for depressive symptoms that are validated for use among older adults and work well in a busy medical clinic, such as the *Geriatric Depression Scale* (GDS; Yesavage et al., 1982) and the *Patient Health Questionnaire-9* (PHQ-9; Spitzer, Kroenke, & Williams, 1999). Administering a quick screening instrument for depressive symptoms may aid in the assessment of adherence factors. There are also empirically supported treatments for depression which, when delivered successfully, may minimize some barriers to treatment adherence (e.g., cognitive behavioral therapy, interpersonal psychotherapy for depression, problem-solving therapy).

Personality characteristics have also been examined as predictors of treatment adherence. Researchers have used the Five-Factor Personality Model (Costa & McCrae, 1992) to study how various dimensions of neuroticism, extraversion, openness to experience, agreeableness, and conscientiousness relate to adherence behaviors. Broadly, individuals higher in neuroticism may engage in fewer positive health practices, whereas those high in conscientiousness may engage in more positive health practices and less risk-taking behavior (cf., Christensen, 2004). When examining older adults' adherence to general health behaviors (e.g., social activities, relaxation), Marks and Lutgendorf (1999) found that high levels of conscientiousness and low levels of neuroticism (as measured by the *Big Five Inventory*; John, Donahue, & Kentle, 1991) were associated with a greater likelihood of engaging in the behavior, further supporting the importance of personality characteristics in late-life health behavior. Among older adults, Insel and colleagues (2006) found that higher levels of independence, as assessed by the *Six-Factor Personality Questionnaire*, were associated with lower adherence to prescribed medication. There is relatively little examination of the impact of personality characteristics on adherence among older adults, although one might presume that the associations should be similar across the lifespan due to the proposed stability of personality traits. Christensen (2004) provides a comprehensive review of the literature on personality traits and adherence, concluding that higher levels of conscientiousness may distinguish between patients who are adherent versus non-adherent. Further research is needed to clarify the relationship between neuroticism and adherence, and to further explore the emerging relation between the "Type A" behavior pattern, characterized by cynicism, mistrust of others, and a generally oppositional style, and adherence to medication and treatment regimens (e.g., Rhodewalt & Fairfield, 1990).

Case Study

Ms Williams is an 82-year-old divorced African American woman with diabetes, hypertension, hypercholesterolemia; she had difficulty organizing her medications, and as a result, all three of these illnesses were not well controlled. Her cardiologist had recommended neuropsychological evaluation, but Ms Williams refused. Ms Williams also had a history of depression beginning at age 12, for which she had been in psychotherapy for the last year. Although her symptoms were still significantly distressing (PHQ-9 = 17/30), she was able to re-engage relationships with her estranged children, resume the daily exercise regimen recommended by her cardiologist, and began to utilize a pill box effectively for her medications. Ms Williams' psychologist repeatedly recommended antidepressant medication for her ongoing depressive symptoms, but Ms Williams was adamant that she would not allow anyone else to "control her mind" with medications. Extensive evaluation of her concerns about the medications yielded the finding that Ms Williams believed that psychiatric medications taken by her African American neighbors in Alabama made them "crazy," which led to involuntary hospitalization by the White doctors. She refused to allow herself to be degraded that way.

This case study highlights the cultural and historical experience factors that can lead to beliefs about illness and treatments, as well as the impact that depression can have on treatment adherence for other illnesses.

Serious Mental Illness

Adherence to medication regimens is particularly important for older adults with serious mental illness (SMI, e.g., schizophrenia, bipolar disorder). It is well known that psychiatric medication compliance is a major factor in relapse for those with SMI, and that late-life presents a unique set of challenges for this population with regard to adhering to proper medication schedules. Deliberate medication non-adherence may be less of a problem for older adults with SMI; unintentional non-adherence may be more of a problem (Depp & Lebowitz, 2007). That said, the mental health care system has a history of being less than collaborative in treatment planning and implementation, with forced or mandated treatment for many with serious mental illness. Partnership in treatment planning may be far more effective in increasing treatment adherence.

The Recovery movement in mental health is an excellent example of how this partnership can be conceptualized. Mental health recovery has been defined by the Substance Abuse and Mental Health Services Administration (SAMHSA, 2004) of the United States in their consensus statement as "...a journey of healing and transformation enabling a person with a mental health problem to live a meaningful life in a community of his or her choice while striving to achieve his or her full potential." The components of Recovery are applicable to all age groups and thought to drive overarching themes such as motivation and a sense of agency and autonomy which are likely to directly impact treatment adherence. That is, if a consumer of health services is able to direct their own treatment in concert with a treatment provider as a means to meet self-defined goals, it is very likely to increase a sense of ownership, partnering, and investment in self-care and, from a behavioral point of view, increase treatment adherence so that goals are reached.

The following is an example of how utilizing Recovery components can help specifically with treatment adherence for medication management:

Case Study

Mr Juarez is a 68-year-old man who has late-onset schizophrenia and who was very reluctant to take medication or see his therapist. Many supports were put in place by his treatment team, including visiting nurses for medication management to assist with any forgetfulness or confusion with medication, and reminder calls for therapy appointments. While these supports seemed to help for short periods of time, Mr Juarez would often stop his medication long enough that hospitalization was required for his symptoms to remit. Mr Juarez's new treatment provider utilized a Recovery approach that was holistic, included self-direction and individualization, and increased his sense of empowerment. Assessment was focused on identifying Mr Juarez's goals, which included finding a new apartment and getting a dog. Mr Juarez began to understand that maintaining his mental health would allow him to care for a dog and new apartment, thereby changing his life in a direction he very much desired. He also saw that committing to taking his medication regularly would be the quickest and most direct path to attaining his goals. After some months, he was managing his medication much more effectively, was looking for a new apartment, and started saving money for a dog.

As discussed above, working within the Recovery model may be instrumental in increasing adherence to a collaboratively developed treatment plan—for serious mental illness or any illness requiring a treatment plan. There are many measures that are "Recovery oriented" or that are designed to measure aspects of Recovery, including the *Illness Management and Recovery Scales* (Salyers, Godfrey, Mueser, & Labriola, 2007), *Recovery Self Assessment* (O'Connell, Tondora, Croog, Evans, & Davidson, 2005), and the *Recovery Oriented Systems Indicators Measure* (Onken, Dumont, Ridgway, Dornan, & Ralph, 2005), all of which have at least preliminary psychometrics. These measures are largely systems- and/or provider-focused. Measures of provider/patient communication and shared decision making, discussed in this chapter, may also be helpful in this regard.

MEASURING MEDICATION ADHERENCE

The most common method of assessing medication adherence is patient self-report (Gao & Nau, 2000), which may consist of simple questions asked by the provider or more complex questionnaires. Self-report has generally been found to be acceptably reliable and valid (Morisky, Green, & Levine, 1986; Rudd, 1993; Straka, Fish, Benson, & Suh, 1997), including in comparison to gold standard physical measures such as blood tests (Graham et al., 1994). Recall is a significant disadvantage for this form of measurement, however, particularly for older adults (see Ecological Momentary Assessment below for options to minimize this concern). In this section, we will review common methods and measures for assessing medication adherence.

Self-Report Measures of Adherence

Morisky Scales

Perhaps the most commonly used self-report measure of medication adherence in the last 20 years is the original *Morisky Scale* (Morisky, Green, & Levine, 1986), a four-item measure that assesses likelihood of medication adherence. The four items are: (1) Do you ever forget to take your medicine? (2) Are you careless at times about taking your medicine? (3) When you feel better, do you sometimes stop taking your medicine? (4) Sometimes if you feel worse when you take the medicine, do you stop taking it? The measure has been found to have adequate internal consistency ($\alpha = 0.61$), sensitivity (0.81), and specificity (0.44) (Morisky, Green, & Levine, 1986). Morisky and his colleagues (2008) created an expanded version (eight items) of this measure called the *Medication Adherence Scale* (Table 17.1), which is correlated with the original version ($r = 0.64$; $p < 0.05$). In the validation sample of 1367 predominantly low-socioeconomic status minority participants with hypertension (age mean 52.5, $SD = 12.2$ years), the scale was reliable ($\alpha = 0.83$), sensitive (93%), and specific (53%). Adherence scores were divided into high (8+), medium (6 to <8), and low (<6). Factors related to higher levels of adherence included better knowledge of the medical plan, more satisfaction with their care, family support, and better coping behavior. Poor adherence was related to higher stress, more complex treatment plans, and lower perceived health status.

Table 17.1 Medication Adherence Scale

1. Do you sometimes forget to take your high blood pressure pills?
2. Over the past two weeks, were there any days when you did not take your high blood pressure medicine?
3. Have you ever cut back or stopped taking your medication without telling your doctor because you felt worse when you took it?
4. When you travel or leave home, do you sometimes forget to bring along your medications?
5. Did you take your high blood pressure medicine yesterday?
6. When you feel like your blood pressure is under control, do you sometimes stop taking your medicine?
7. Taking medication every day is a real inconvenience for some people. Do you ever feel hassled about sticking to your blood pressure treatment plan?
8. How often do you have difficulty remembering to take all your blood pressure medication?

(Morisky, Ang, Krousel-Wood, & Ward, 2008)

Helpful Questions for Health Care Professionals

Often, health care professionals do not use a structured form to assess medication adherence. As summarized by MacLaughlin and colleagues (2005), many health care providers may ask a single, closed-ended question about adherence, such as, "Do you take your medications as prescribed?" This direct method of questioning has proved to be unreliable and runs the risk of alienating patients due to a fear of upsetting the provider with their response. In Table 17.2, we have included several questions suggested by MacLaughlin and colleagues (2005) that are designed to encourage an open discussion about adherence behavior.

Self-Report Measures of Adherence Beliefs

As discussed earlier in this chapter, when patients believe that their illness is severe and is a potential threat, adherence behavior increases (DiMatteo et al., 2007). Therefore, we have included several measures of patient beliefs about adherence and health behavior that health care professionals may find useful in their discussions with patients about treatment planning.

Irrational Health Belief Scale

The *Irrational Health Belief Scale* (Christensen, Moran, & Wiebe, 1999) was created in response to the assumptions of the Health Belief Model (HBM; Janz & Becker, 1984) that patients are rational when faced with decisions about their health. Health decisions, however, are often based on somewhat ambiguous information and may have to be made under less than ideal situations. Thus, Christensen (2004) argued that it is difficult to assume rational decision-making behavior in such an environment. Although not a direct measure of adherence, the *Irrational Health Belief Scale* (Christensen et al., 1999) assesses individual differences in the tendency of patients to engage in cognitive distortion or irrational appraisal around health decisions. On this measure, respondents indicate their level of agreement with patient thoughts presented in 20 health scenarios, on a scale ranging from 1 (not at all like I would think) to 5 (almost exactly like I would think). The measure has strong reliability ($\alpha = 0.84$), acceptable test–retest reliability after 18 months ($r = 0.57$), and acceptable construct validity in relation to several other measures [PANAS, Big Five Inventory, Personal Lifestyle Questionnaire (health practices score), Health Locus of Control].

Illness Perception Questionnaire

The Illness Perception Questionnaire (IPQ; Weinman, Petrie, Moss-Morris, & Horne, 1996) is a 57-item, Likert-type measure that assesses five components of illness representations, including Illness

Table 17.2 Helpful Questions for Providers

Medication Adherence Inquiries
Tell me how you take your medicines
How do you schedule your meal and medication times?
Do you use a pill box or organizer to help you take your medicines?
How do you manage to pay for your medicines?
If possible, would you like me to simplify your medication regimen?
If possible, would you like to explore some options for reducing your out-of-pocket medication expenses?
Show me how you use your inhaler
(taken from MacLaughlin et al., 2005)

Identity, Cause, Timeline, Consequences, and Control/Cure. The notion of illness representations is based on the Self-Regulatory Model (SRM; Leventhal, Leventhal, & Contrada, 1998), which proposes that a patient's representation of their illness is critical in determining how the patient copes with an illness (including adherence to treatment plans), regardless of whether coping involves doing something or delaying action. The SRM sees the patient as an active problem solver who has several processes occurring in parallel, as opposed to occurring in stages. Thus, a patient perceives a health threat, forms a representation of the threat (e.g., "this symptom isn't related to my diabetes"), develops an action plan, then re-evaluates that plan, and may go back to repeat other steps in the model based on a new representation of the threat (Horne & Weinman, 1998).

Internal consistency for the four subscales of the Illness Perception Questionnaire (excluding Cause) ranges from 0.73 to 0.82. Adequate concurrent validity was demonstrated with measures of perceived health and disability, recent doctor visits, and beliefs about recovery. The IPQ was found to discriminate between individuals with insulin dependent diabetes, rheumatoid arthritis, chronic fatigue syndrome, and chronic idiopathic pain. In terms of predictive validity, the Identity subscale predicted self-rated health at three months, and the Timeline subscale predicted three and six month ratings of the likelihood of further heart problems. The Control/Cure subscale scores were significantly related to patients' three and six month ratings of control over their heart problem and were negatively related to perceived likelihood of future heart problems at both time points.

The IPQ has several different versions that assess representations of different chronic illnesses and has been translated to multiple languages. There is also a version of the IPQ available for significant others (Weinman et al., 1996). A revised version of the IPQ (IPQ-R; Moss-Morris et al., 2002) has demonstrated adequate psychometric properties. Many IPQ versions are available online at http://www.uib.no/ipq/.

Beliefs About Medicines Questionnaire

Phatak and Thomas (2006) found that medication beliefs alone, as assessed by the *Beliefs about Medicines Questionnaire* (BMQ; Horne, Weinman, & Hankins, 1999), explained 22.4% of variation in non-adherence to chronic drug therapy. The BMQ was developed to assess commonly held beliefs about medicines, and was validated on several medical samples. The scale is comprised of 19 five-point Likert-style items about specific and general beliefs about medications. Items fall into four subscales: specific—necessity, specific—concerns, general—overuse, and general—harm. Internal consistency of the BMQ among several chronic-illness groups (e.g., asthmatic, diabetic, renal, cardiac) for the subscales of the BMQ ranged from 0.47 to 0.86. Test—retest reliability was conducted with the asthmatic group and was found to range from 0.60 to 0.78. Both criterion-related validity and discriminant validity was acceptable for all subscales of the BMQ. The chronic-illness groups used for validation of the BMQ had an average age of approximately 45 years, thus suggesting that further validation studies with an older adult sample may be needed to confirm the validity of this measure with older adult patients.

Assessing Stages of Change in Relation to Adherence

Stage models of health behavior posit that cognitions and behavior change over time, such that perceived susceptibility, threat, benefits, and barriers may reflect more of a dynamic rather than a static process (e.g., Horne & Weinman, 1998). The most commonly cited stage model is the Transtheoretical Model, also known as the Stages of Change Model, in which maintenance of health behavior occurs in five stages: pre-contemplation, contemplation, preparation, action, and maintenance (Prochaska & DiClemente, 1983). The stage that a patient is in for a particular illness may impact whether they are adherent to a treatment plan addressing that illness. Assessment measures have been developed to identify stages of change, such as those for individuals with addictive behaviors (see DiClemente, Schlundt, & Gemmell, 2004) and pain (*Multidimensional Pain Readiness to Change Questionnaire 2*; Nielsen, Jensen, Ehde, Kerns, & Molton, 2008). These scales have been used with older adults, but age-specific normative data are limited. The *Stages of Change Questionnaire in Osteoarthritis* is comprised of 15 items that correspond to the pre-contemplation stage, contemplation stage, and action stage (Heuts et al., 2005). Reliability for the three subscales in a sample of adults in primary care, aged 40–60, was good ($\alpha = 0.72$ to 0.79).

Ecological Momentary Assessment (EMA)

EMA is a method that can be used to measure many individual adherence factors (Table 17.3). EMA is designed to minimize the problems associated with retrospective recall, retrospective bias including emotional valence, and to maximize the ecological validity of measurement by monitoring events (behaviors, thoughts, emotions, experiences) at the time and place in which they occur. EMA can also account for diurnal variation in targets of measurement and can be used to compare behaviors, psychological states, and physiological data (e.g., mood assessment and physical activity concurrent with cortisol collection OR mood assessment concurrent with each episode of eating or smoking). Three general categories of EMA are most common: (1) diaries; (2) experience sampling; and (3) event-based sampling (Moskowitz & Young, 2006). Diaries typically assess experience in fixed intervals, most often daily, and involve retrospective recall. Experience sampling frequently uses a device [e.g., pager, cell phone, personal digital assistant (PDA)] to signal the respondent to report on experience at random times during the day. Event-based sampling elicits reports at the time of a particular event (e.g., meal times, after interpersonal conflict, before exercise). Although EMA provides information with great utility, it can also be very expensive (depending on the type of technology utilized), require a great deal of training of participants and management of problems with technology in the field, and be complicated to analyze the mass of time-dependent data (data representing both a strength and a challenge of the technique).

Cain and colleagues' (2009) review of 40 studies of EMA use with adults over the age of 50 indicated that healthy and clinical populations had similar strong adherence rates with EMA. Data collection frequency ranged from every 45 minutes to weekly, and duration ranged from one day to 168 days using both clinical and non-clinical samples. The 15% of studies that reported less than 80% adherence had more complex or demanding requirements, such as recording every 45 minutes

Table 17.3 Sample EMA Diary for Medication, Exercise, and Diet Adherence

Hour	Medication	Exercise	Food Intake	
6:00a–7:00a	Medication: ____________ Dose: ____________	Activity ____________ #Minutes ____________	Food:	Amount:
7:00a–8:00a	Medication: ____________ Dose: ____________	Activity ____________ #Minutes ____________	Food:	Amount:
8:00a–9:00a	Medication: ____________ Dose: ____________	Activity ____________ #Minutes ____________	Food:	Amount:

(Kamarck et al., 2002) or recording every time a high-frequency activity was performed (Johnson & Bytheway, 2001). Dropout was primarily associated with a lack of understanding of procedures by participants (Hnatiuk, 1991), which is a factor for consideration among older adults with cognitive decline, or if considering the use of technology among older adults with little experience using such devices. In addition to PDA-type devices, paper diaries have been enhanced with computers to determine when diaries were opened and written on, with adherence rates of 94% (Stone, Schwartz, Broderick, & Hufford, 2002). Researchers in the Longitudinal Aging Study Amsterdam (LASA; Jacelon & Imperio, 2005; Johnson & Bytheway, 2001) compared diaries of medication use and global self-report measures, and concluded that EMA can be considered the "gold standard" of adherence measurement, or can be used to identify participant reporting discrepancies.

Composition and format of EMA instruments vary widely. In a study of older adults' physical activity, Cartmel and Moon (1992) compared the format and length of two diary instruments and found that a longer, more detailed diary was the more accurate assessment tool for physical activity, while a shorter instrument was better for assessing sitting time. EMA instruments also frequently include state measures and items later independently rated by researchers. For example, Katz and colleagues (2005) studied side effects of two medications commonly used by older adults (metoclopramide and naproxen), and whether or not the side effects impacted adherence. Along with documenting medication adherence, participants completed the *Positive and Negative Affect Scale* (Lawton, Kleban, Dean, Rajagopal, & Parmelee, 1992) and a report on "daily events that were outside of their usual day-to-day routines" (p. 72) at the end of each day. Events were later rated by two independent raters as positive, negative, or neutral. Participants were trained in the use of daily diaries prior to data collection. Medication adherence was 97%. Similarly, Miaskowski and colleagues (2001) studied adults with cancer (mean age = 59) using EMA and found overall adherence rates that ranged from 85 to 91% for scheduled medications and 22 to 27% for as-needed (PRN) medications. Lower rates of PRN medication usage were related to worse pain control. Given that these rates are higher than general studies of adherence, it is possible that the EMA assessment itself increased adherence.

Visual Analog Scales (VAS)

VAS have also been utilized in EMA research. VAS are measures of subjective or behavioral experience (e.g., pain, physical exercise). They are typically presented as a 10 cm line with descriptive anchors at each end, such as "completed all prescribed activities today" to "completed none of the prescribed activities today." Respondents place a vertical line through the point on the scale that best fits their experience with that construct at that moment. The placement of that mark is measured and then used as either a continuous variable or the line is broken into segments to create a discrete variable; the latter is often for comparison with Likert-type scales. Studies of medication adherence for adults taking medication for diabetes and hypercholesterolemia using VAS have found moderate correlations between VAS and prescription claims databases (Nau et al., 2007).

Performance-Based Measures of Adherence

Drug Regimen Unassisted Grading Scale

The *Drug Regimen Unassisted Grading Scale* (*DRUGS*; Edelberg, Shallenberger, & Wei, 1999) is an individual performance-based measure assessing respondents' ability to identify medications, access them, take the appropriate dosage, and take it at the correct time (Table 17.4). Respondents or caregivers provide their own medication list and dosing schedule to the administrator of the measure. The respondent then identifies each of the medications, opens the appropriate container, removes the appropriate dose, and indicates appropriate times to take the medication on a daily calendar.

Table 17.4 Drug Regimen Unassisted Grading Scale

TABLE–Drug Regimen Unassisted Grading Scale									
Medication List (container or chart)	**Medication List (self-report)**	**Identification**		**Access**		**Dosage**		**Timing**	
		Able	**Unable**	**Able**	**Unable**	**Able**	**Unable**	**Able**	**Unable**
Maximum Score:		Total Score:				Summary Score:		%	
Total Medications:				Total Doses:					
Time:									

(DRUGS; Edelberg, Shallenberger, & Wei, 1999)

Successful performance yields one point for each of these four actions. The number of medications is multiplied by four to obtain a maximum score; correct responses are added and then divided by the number of medications and multiplied by 100 to obtain a percentage of correct responses (0–100).

In a sample of 59 adults over the age of 70 living in continuing care retirement facilities, the mean summary score on DRUGS was 93.2 ± 11.25 (range 50 to 100; higher scores indicate better accuracy). Interrater reliability and test–retest reliability were greater than 0.90. Increasing age was associated with lower DRUGS scores ($r = -0.41$, $p = 0.001$). DRUGS score was not related to gender, education, or living arrangement. Residents in assisted-living facilities had lower DRUGS tool scores compared with those living independently (82.0% vs. 93.8%, $p = 0.009$). In a prospective follow-up study of the same participants 12 months later, declines in DRUGS scores were associated with score declines on the Mini-Mental State Exam (MMSE) and the timed "Up and Go" test (Edelberg, Shallenberger, Hausdorff, & Wei, 2000).

Medication Management Ability Assessment

Another performance-based measure, the *Medication Management Ability Assessment* (*MMAA*) is a structured role-play measure designed to functionally assess the respondent's ability to follow a prescribed medication regimen, including the ability to hear instructions and read labels (Patterson et al., 2002). While this measure is strongly predictive of actual medication management, it is complex and time-intensive to administer. See Chapter 5 for a more detailed description of this measure.

Hopkins Medication Schedule

The Hopkins Medication Schedule (Carlson, Fried, Xue, Tekwe, & Brandt, 2005) was created to objectively assess one's ability to understand and implement a routine prescription medication. The measure presents a hypothetical physician's prescription for antibiotics and aspirin. As part of the performance-based assessment, individuals are asked to fill in a daily schedule for taking the medication and to fill in the compartments of a pill box. The measure was validated on older adult women ranging in age from 70 to 79. In this sample, 22% were completely unable to complete the schedule, fill the pill box, or both. Performance on the schedule was positively associated with scores on a backward digit-span task and on a memory recall task. Performance with the pill box was associated with measures of executive functioning.

Medication Management Instrument for Deficiencies in the Elderly

The Medication Management Instrument for Deficiencies in the Elderly (MedMaIDE; Orwig, Brandt, & Gruber-Baldini, 2006) was designed to provide a comprehensive, standardized assessment of older adults' ability to self-medicate in the home environment (Figure 17.6). The MedMaIDE can be administered by untrained care providers, including family members. The measure consists of 20 items that assess what a person knows about the medication they are taking, how to take their medication, and how to get their medication from a doctor or pharmacy. The MedMaIDE was validated on a sample of 50 community-dwelling adults over the age of 65. Internal consistency of the measure was

Medication Management Instrument for Deficiencies in the Elderly (MedMaIDE)

What a Person Knows About Their Medications
Have the individual... **YES**

**1. Name all the medications taken each day, including prescription and over-the-counter medications (including milk magnesia, nutritional supplements, herbs, vitamins, Tylenol, etc.).
**2. State the time of day that each prescription medication is to be taken.
**3. Tell how the medications should be taken (by mouth, with water, on skin, etc.)
**4. State why he/she is taking each medication.
**5. State the amount of each medication to be taken at each time during the day.
6. Identify if there are problems after taking the medication (i.e., dizziness, upset stomach, constipation, loose stool, frequent urination, etc.).
7. Do you get medication help from anyone?
If YES, from whom? Type of help?
8. What other medications do you have on hand or available (i.e., eye drops, creams, lotions, or nasal sprays that are outdated, unused or discontinued)?

If a Person Knows How to Take Their Medications
Ask the individual to... ***YES***

**1. Demonstrate filling a glass with water.
**2. Remove top from medication container (vial, bubble pack, pill box, etc.).
**3. Demonstrate counting out required number of pills into hand or cup.
**4. Demonstrate administering the medication (e.g., put hand with medication in it to open mouth; put hand to eye for eye drops; hand to mouth for inhaler; draw up insulin; or place a topical patch).
**5. Sip enough water to swallow medication.
Record how the medications are currently being stored.

If a Person Knows How to Get Their Medications
Have the individual... ***YES***

**1. Identify if a refill exists on a prescription.
**2. Identify whom to contact to get a prescription refilled.
**3. Explain resources to obtain the medication (can arrange transportation to pharmacy, pharmacy delivers, family picks it up, etc.).
4. After getting a new refill, do you look at the medication before you take it to make sure it is the same as the one you finished?
5. Do you have a prescription card? YES NO
Do you use your prescription card? YES NO
If YES, specify type:
6. Are there medications that you need that you cannot obtain? YES NO
If YES, ask person to explain.

** If NO, it is counted as a 1 in the Deficiency Score.

TOTAL DEFICIENCY SCORE:_________ (sum of the three deficiency scores: maximum total score = 13)

FIGURE 17.6

Medication Management Instrument for Deficiencies in the Elderly.

(MedMaIDE; Orwig, Brandt, & Gruber-Baldini, 2006)

acceptable at 0.71. Test—retest reliability and inter-rater reliability was also acceptable at 0.93 and 0.74, respectively. Concurrent validity was modest, at −0.52, when examining the association between the MedMaIDE score and pill count compliance.

Electronic Measurement of Adherence

Electronic devices have been developed for measuring and increasing medication adherence and physical activity, among other behaviors.

Electronic Pill Bottle Cap/Pill Box

The most common electronic device for measuring medication adherence is the electronic pill bottle cap or pill box such as the *Medication Event Monitoring System* (*MEMS*; Aardex, Switzerland) or *Maya* (MedMinder; Newton, MA). Such devices have a microchip embedded in the cap or box to record the time and date when the container is opened (these devices cannot determine whether or not a pill was actually taken or in what dose), and some can also provide a visual (flashing light) and/or audio cue (beep or song) to remind the individual to take the medication. Some companies also provide internet linkage to record the container being opened, and can send email, phone, or text message reminders to the patient, family, or physician if doses are missed, as well as reminders to refill prescriptions at appropriate times. Such pill containers range in price from $30 to $250 or more, based on the type of data recorded and associated data collection service. Some insurance companies have linked with manufacturers to pay for these products and services if adherence rates are over 80%.

Research with such devices (without cues provided) suggests that patients' self-report of adherence is significantly higher (71%) than pill cap monitoring (55%; Bond et al., 2005). Additionally, clinicians' estimates of adherence are not significantly correlated with electronic cap data (Parker et al., 2007). Electronic pill dispensers result in fewer missed doses (1.7 missed doses) than manually filled pill boxes (15.1 missed doses), and control group (19.7 missed doses; Bond et al., 2005). Significant problems have been noted related to incorrect usage of the devices (e.g., Matsui et al., 1994), so extensive training and/or assistance with such devices may be considered, particularly for older adults with cognitive impairment.

Accelerometers

Accelerometry-based activity monitors are typically small battery-operated devices worn on a belt or waistline, or on the wrist. They measure acceleration in three planes: anterior-posterior; vertical; and medial-lateral. Trost and colleagues' review (2005) suggests that three to five days of assessment is required to accurately assess regular physical activity. Accelerometers provide more objective measures of activity that provide "real-time" assessment of intensity, duration, and frequency of activity. They are low burden and remove the barrier of impaired cognitive status. However, the devices do not provide context for the activity (e.g., cannot differentiate between housekeeping and gardening), do not measure energy expenditure, can miss upper body movement with typical placement at the waist (thus not helpful for those in wheelchairs), cannot determine load-bearing vs. non-load-bearing activities, and can be expensive. Multiple researchers caution that, while newer technology minimizes user error, researchers must be well trained in using the equipment, rationale for placement, and calibration issues (Lyons, Culhane, Hilton, Grace, & Lyons, 2009; Murphy, 2009).

Accelerometers have been used to measure sleep (e.g., Sivertson et al., 2006), exercise, and activities of daily living (e.g., Farran et al., 2008; Welk, Blair, Wood, Jones, & Thompson, 2000). Use of these devices has been growing in research with older adults (e.g., Focht, Sanders, Brubaker, & Rejeski, 2003). In a study of 34 older adults with primary insomnia, actigraphy was highly sensitive to detect sleep (95.2%), but poor in detecting wakefulness (specificity = 36.3%) (Sivertson et al., 2006).

Farran and colleagues (2008) used an accelerometer (*Mini Mitter*: Model #GT7164, Mini Mitter, Bend, OR) along with the 41-item *Community Healthy Activities Model Program for Seniors (CHAMPS) Questionnaire* (Stewart et al., 2001; measure is available online: http://sbs.ucsf.edu/iha/champs/resources/qxn/download.html) to assess adherence to a home-based physical activity intervention with older adult caregivers of individuals with dementia. Accelerometer-measured activity was associated with CHAMPS total physical activity minutes ($r = 0.70$; $p < 0.01$) and total moderate activity minutes ($r = 0.72$; $p < 0.01$). Another study reported correlations of CHAMPS and the *Mini Mitter* ranging from 0.36 to 0.59 for ankle placement and 0.42 to 0.61 for waist placement (Harada, Chiu, King, & Stewart, 2001).

Provider Factors

Several researchers (Bakken et al., 2000; Heisler, Bouknight, Hayward, Smith, & Kerr, 2002; Heisler, Cole, Weir, Kerr, & Hayward, 2007; Schneider, Kaplan, Greenfield, Li, & Wilson, 2004) have examined whether specific characteristics of the provider/patient relationship impact whether a patient is more or less adherent to a treatment plan.

When examining predictors of diabetes self-management behaviors (e.g., taking medications, exercising, following a diet, checking blood glucose levels, and checking feet for sores) among patients at a Veterans' Affairs hospital (mean age = 67 years), Heisler and colleagues (2002) found that patients' ratings of physician communication (5 item scale, $\alpha = 0.93$) and level of participatory decision-making (4-item scale; $\alpha = 0.96$) were predictive of patients' self-reported diabetes management (5-item scale; $\alpha = 0.68$), even after controlling for sociodemographic and health variables. These researchers used subscales from a measure created and validated by the Veterans Administration as part of the Diabetes Quality Improvement Project (Krein, Hayward, Pogach, & Boots Miller, 2000).

Heisler and colleagues (2007) expanded this line of research to a national study of 1588 community-dwelling older adults with diabetes. Physician communication style was associated with medication taking and foot care, but not other self-management behaviors, whereas participatory decision-making style was significantly associated with only exercise and blood glucose monitoring. Both communication style and decision-making style were associated with following a diabetic diet, although decision-making style was more significantly associated with diet than communication style. Consistent with the Recovery model, these results suggest that participatory decision-making may be critical for changing complex behaviors such as exercise, diet, and monitoring of blood glucose levels.

Patients with diabetes (mean age = 65) who reported low levels of physician trust (five items from the Primary Care Assessment Survey; Safran et al., 1998) have been found to be at significantly higher risk of underutilizing medications in response to medication cost pressures than patients with similar cost pressures but greater trust in their physicians (Piette, Heisler, Krein, & Kerr, 2005). Cost pressures were assessed with two items: "In the past 12 months, have you ever taken less of any medication than prescribed by your doctor because of the cost?" and "Other than the cost, have you ever taken less medication than prescribed for any other reason?" (p. 1750). Low income was a risk factor for cost-related underuse among low-trust patients but not among high-trust patients with similar incomes. Thus the patient/provider relationship itself may mitigate adherence barriers. Medication cost is discussed further below.

System-Level Factors

System-level factors can act as barriers to obtaining appropriate treatment and to adhering to a treatment plan. The cost of medications and the availability of medical care are two system factors that may have direct and significant effects on medication adherence. In 2001, approximately ten million

Medicare beneficiaries had no prescription drug coverage (Poisal & Murray, 2001). In a 2003 study examining health outcomes of Medicare beneficiaries, 13% had full prescription coverage, 61% had partial coverage, and 27% had no coverage (Mojtabai & Olfson, 2003). Seven percent reported cost-related poor adherence, which translates to approximately two million Medicare beneficiaries.

Cost

Although we might expect a larger number of older adults to have prescription coverage following the introduction of Medicare Part D in 2006, payment for prescriptions remains a significant problem, particularly for those with fixed income and those without Medicare. In fact, even in Canada, with its universal health care, cost-associated non-adherence was found to be 5.1%, in contrast to the U.S. rate of 9.9% ($p < 0.001$) (Kennedy & Morgan, 2006). Those with insurance in both countries (6.2%) were significantly less likely to report non-adherence related to cost than Americans without insurance (28.2%) and Americans and Canadians without specific coverage for prescriptions (16.2%).

In a study of older adults with diabetes, 19% of participants reported cutting back on medication use in the prior year, 11% reported cutting back on their diabetes medications, and 7% reported cutting back on their diabetes medications at least once per month, all due to cost of the medications (Piette, Heisler, & Wagner, 2004). In order to cover the costs of medications, 28% reported forgoing food or other essentials to pay for medications, 14% added to their existing credit card debt in order to pay for medication, and 10% borrowed money from family or friends to pay for their prescriptions. Although many health care providers are sensitive to the fact that cost is a barrier to treatment, this study found that few participants were offered information about managing the costs of medications. As can be seen from the results of this study, the impact of medication cost can have a direct effect on whether patients achieve adequate treatment adherence. Assessment of the impact of cost on medication adherence has typically been measured with a few specific questions, such as "In the past 12 months, have you ever taken less of any medications than prescribed by your doctor because of the cost?" and "Other than the cost, have you ever taken less medication than prescribed for any other reason?" (Piette et al., 2005, p. 1750).

Availability of Health Care

Recent national initiatives have worked to increase the availability of medical care. However, real and perceived barriers to care persist, which directly impact treatment availability and adherence. Previous research has documented that U.S. adults receive about half of recommended health care services (McGlynn et al., 2003). In a study of characteristics of patients who received recommended care, women were found to receive a higher proportion of recommended care than men, quality-of-care scores declined with age, and those with a household income over $50,000 had better quality-of-care scores than those with incomes under $15,000 (Asch et al., 2006). When examining differences in quality-of-care scores related to ethnic minority status, African American patients had higher scores than Caucasian patients, even when other sociodemographic characteristics, health status, and use of inpatient and outpatient services were controlled for, a finding which is contrary to many other studies. This study concludes that, although there may be small differences in quality-of-care scores between individuals who have various combinations of the factors examined (e.g., African American females with high household income vs. Caucasian males with low household income), the greatest disparity for all groups is the gap between recommended care and actual care.

Perceived barriers in access to care can also impact treatment adherence. In a study of perceived discrimination among African American and Caucasian adults, African American participants with more than two lifetime discrimination experiences (in any context) were 2.6 times more likely to delay seeking medical treatment and evidence non-adherence to treatment regimens (Casagrande, Gary,

LaVeist, Gaskin, & Cooper, 2007). Caucasians with more than two lifetime discrimination experiences were 3.3 times more likely to evidence delay or non-adherence behaviors.

INTERVENTIONS

While a complete review of interventions is beyond the scope of this chapter, it is important to note that multiple interventions have been developed to increase adherence to health treatment plans. At the most basic level, merely tracking behavior can significantly increase adherence to plans. In the last few years a number of researchers have developed modules to increase medication compliance in older adults, particularly for those with mental illness. Most of these are nestled within broad cognitively-based skills training models and psychosocial rehabilitation health management approaches (Pratt, Van Citters, Mueser, & Bartels, 2008) for those with bipolar disorder or schizophrenia. For example, Depp, Lebowitz, Patterson, Lacro, and Jeste (2007) developed and pilot tested a "Medication Adherence Skills Training" (MAST-BD) manual to improve compliance for older adults with bipolar disorder which includes didactic, motivational, medication management, and symptom management components. Pilot results suggest middle-aged and older adults with bipolar disorder accept the programs and self-report more medication adherence and management ability, fewer depressive symptoms, and improvements on some health-related quality of life domains.

Using a biopsychosocial approach targeting older adults with schizophrenia, Liberman (2003) described a VA Medical Center medication management program which teaches how to obtain information about medications, to identify side effects, and to "negotiate medication issues with health care providers." The author lists a variety of patient characteristics that reflect barriers against effective clinician/older patient collaboration and makes recommendations on how to overcome them. These include cognitive impairment, lack of understanding of the illness, and not seeing a connection between medication administration and positive effects of maintaining their remission. Interestingly, the author notes that some provider and clinic setting characteristics can also be obstacles towards treatment progress. Mental health professionals who are paternalistic and negativistic, and clinics that are difficult to access by public transportation with long waiting times and unresponsive staff members disrupt the therapeutic alliance. The author suggests that perhaps there is too much focus on symptoms and not enough emphasis on quality-of-life issues. Indeed, a recent study suggests that older adults prefer a collaborative role with psychiatrists and as much involvement in decision-making as do younger adults with SMI (O'Neal et al., 2008).

Other programs are geared to address the therapeutic management of older adults which have modules that specifically target management of health and medication compliance including the Functional Adaptation Skills Training (FAST; Patterson et al., 2003), Cognitive-Behavioral Skills Training (CBSST; McQuaid et al., 2000), and Skills Training + Health Management (ST+HM) intervention (Bartels et al., 2004), and the Helping Older People Experience Success (HOPES; McCarthy, Mueser, & Pratt, 2008) program.

Shared Decision-Making in Treatment Planning

As discussed above, one intervention to improve adherence may be to involve older adults in the decision-making process around the proposed treatment plan. Consistent with the Recovery model, the concept of shared decision-making has received increased attention, with its focus on a decision-making process jointly shared by patients and their health care providers (e.g., Gravel, Légaré, & Graham, 2006). Shared decision-making was born out of a movement to find a compromise between a paternalistic model of medical decision-making, where the physician provides "expert" advice to a passive patient, and the informed choice model of decision-making, where a patient is provided with all the information to make a decision, but is not guided as to which direction is best matched to their particular symptoms, preferences, and values (Elwyn, Edwards, & Kinnersley, 1999).

Researchers examining older adults' views on shared decision-making have found that some older adult patients do not have a desire to be involved in decision-making (Belcher, Fried, Agostini, & Tinetti, 2006), or have a lower preference for involvement, as compared to younger adults (Schneider et al., 2006). Belcher and colleagues (2006) developed a semi-structured interview to assess decision-making preferences, using questions such as:

- "Each person is different in how they talk to, and interact with, their doctor about medicine. How do you talk to your doctor about medicine?
- What do you talk about?
- When making decisions about what medicine to give a patient, it helps doctors to know the patient's feelings and concerns about the medicine. What things can you think of that might help people be a part of making decisions about their medicine?
- What things keep people from being a part of making decisions about medicine with their doctor?" (p. 299).

Schneider and colleagues (2006) measured shared decision-making using the *Autonomy Preference Index* (*API*; Ende, Razis, Ash, & Moskowitz, 1989), a 14-item, 5-point Likert scale measure of preferences for involvement in decision-making (six items) and obtaining comprehensive information from one's health care provider (eight items). Scores are adjusted to obtain overall range of 0 (lack of desire to participate) to 100 (strongest desire to participate). Test–retest reliability (0.83) and internal consistency ($\alpha = 0.82$) for the measure were found to be excellent (Schneider et al., 2006). The API has also been validated in German (Giersdorf, Loh, & Harter, 2004).

CONCLUSIONS

With life expectancy and chronic illness prevalence increasing, understanding treatment adherence becomes paramount to improving health outcomes and quality of life for older adults, and health care costs for all. Treatment adherence is multi-faceted and not comprehensively conceptualized by any single model. Multiple individual, provider, and systems-level factors must be taken into account to fully understand why older adults may or may not adhere to a treatment plan. Many assessments are available to measure these factors, including those that measure attitudes, beliefs, performance, or behavior, using self-report, observational, electronic, or physiological methods. As with most treatment modalities, however, the relationship between patient and provider appears to be key in maximizing treatment adherence. Consistent with the Recovery model, identifying and working within the patient's goals for treatment and for life, which may reflect their socioeconomic status, culture, education, health literacy, cognitive status, and personality, is most likely to lead to adherence to an agreed upon plan.

References

Apter, A. J., Boston, R. C., George, M., Norfleet, A. L., Tenhave, T., Coyne, J. C., et al. (2003). Modifiable barriers to adherence to inhaled steroids among adults with asthma: it's not just black and white. *J. Allergy Clin. Immunol.*, *111*, 1219–1226.

Arozullah, A. M., Yarnold, P. R., Bennett, C. L., Soltysik, R. C., Wolf, M. S., Ferreira, R. M., et al. (2007). Development and validation of a short-form, rapid estimate of adult literacy in medicine. *Medical Care*, *45*, 1026–1033.

Asch, S. M., Kerr, E. A., Keesey, J., Adams, J. L., Setodji, C. M., Malik, S., & McGlynn, E. A. (2006). Who is at greatest risk for receiving poor-quality health care? *N. Engl. J. Med.*, *354*, 1147–1156.

Bakken, S., Holzemer, W. L., Brown, M., Gail, M., Powell-Cope, G. M., Turner, J. G., et al. (2000). Relationships between perception of engagement with health care provider and demographic characteristics, health status, and adherence to therapeutic regimen in persons with HIV/AIDS. *AIDS Patient Care STDs*, *14*, 189–197.

Bartels, S. J., Forrester, B., Mueser, K. T., Miles, K. M., Dums, A. R., Pratt, S. I., et al. (2004). Enhanced skills training and health care management for older persons with severe mental illness. *Community Mental Health Journal*, *40*, 75–90.

Belcher, V. N., Fried, T. R., Agostini, J. V., & Tinetti, M. E. (2006). Views of older adults on patient participation in medication-related decision making. *J. Gen. Intern. Med.*, *21*, 298–303.

Bell, R. A., Andrews, J. S., Arcury, T. A., Snively, B. M., Golden, S. L., & Quandt, S. A. (2010). Depressive symptoms and diabetes self-management among rural older adults. *Am. J. Health Behav.*, *34*(1), 36–44.

Benisovich, S. V., & King, A. C. (2003). Meaning and knowledge of health among older adult immigrants from Russia: a phenomenological study. *Health Educ. Res.*, *18*, 135–144.

Bond, C. A., MacLaughlin, E. J., Raehl, C. L., Treadway, A. K., Sterling, T. L., & Zoller, D. P. (2005). Assessing medication adherence in the elderly. *Drugs & Aging*, *22*(3), 231–255.

Bradley, C. (1994). Measures of perceived control in diabetes. In C. Bradley (Ed.), *Handbook of Psychology and Diabetes* (pp. 291–331). London, UK: Harwood Academic Publishers.

Brown, C., Battista, D. R., Bruehlman, R., Sereika, S. S., Thase, M. F., & Dunbar-Jacob, J. (2005). Beliefs about antidepressant medications in primary care patients: relationship to self-reported adherence. *Med. Care*, *43*, 1203–1207.

Brown, C. M., & Segal, R. (1996). The effects of health and treatment perceptions on the use of prescribed medication and home remedies among African American and white American hypertensives. *Soc. Sci. Med.*, *43*, 903–917.

Cain, A. E., Depp, C. A., & Jeste, D. V. (2009). Ecological momentary assessment in aging research: a critical review. *Journal of Psychiatric Research*, *43*, 987–996.

Carlson, M. C., Fried, L. P., Xue, Q., Tekwe, C., & Brandt, J. (2005). Validation of the Hopkins Medication Schedule to identify difficulties in taking medications. *J. Gerontol. A Biol. Sci. Med. Sci.*, *60*, 217–223.

Cartmel, B., & Moon, T. E. (1992). Comparison of two physical activity questionnaires, with a diary, for assessing physical activity in an elderly population. *Journal of Clinical Epidemiology*, *45*, 877.

Casagrande, S. S., Gary, T. L., LaVeist, T. A., Gaskin, D. J., & Cooper, L. A. (2007). Perceived discrimination and adherence to medical care in a racially integrated community. *J. Gen. Intern. Med*, *22*, 389–395.

Centers for Disease Control and Prevention and the Merck Company Foundation. (2007). *The State of Aging and Health in America*. Whitehouse Station, NJ: Merck Company Foundation.

Christensen, A. (2004). *Patient Adherence to Medical Treatment Regimens: Bridging the Gap Between Behavioral Science and Biomedicine*. New Haven, CT: Yale University Press.

Christensen, A. J., Moran, P. J., & Wiebe, J. S. (1999). Assessment of irrational health beliefs: relation to health practices and medical regimen adherence. *Health Psychology*, *18*, 256–262.

Cohen, S., & Hoberman, H. M. (1983). Positive events and social supports as buffers of life change stress. *Journal of Applied Social Psychology*, *13*, 99–125.

Costa, P. T., & McCrae, R. R. (1992). *NEO PI-R Professional Manual*. Odessa, FL: Psychological Assessment Resources Inc.

Davis, T. C., Long, S. W., Jackson, R. H., Mayeaux, E. J., George, R. B., Murphy, P. W., & Crouch, M. A. (1993). Rapid estimate of adult literacy in medicine: a shortened screening instrument. *Fam. Med.*, *25*, 391–395.

Depp, C. A., & Lebowitz, B. D. (June 2007). Enhancing medication adherence in older adults with bipolar disorder. http://www.psychiatrymmc.com/enhancing-medication-adherence-in-older-adults-with-bipolar-disorder/#more-31. Accessed 7/30/09.

Depp, C. A., Lebowitz, B. D., Patterson, T. L., Lacro, J. P., & Jeste, D. V. (2007). Medication adherence skills training for middle-aged and elderly adults with bipolar disorder: development and pilot study. *Bipolar Disorder*, *9*, 636–645.

DiClemente, C. C., Schlundt, D., & Gemmell, L. (2004). Readiness and stages of change in addiction treatment. *American Journal on Addictions, 13*, 103–119.

DiMatteo, M. R., Lepper, H. S., & Croghan, T. W. (2000). Depression is a risk factor for noncompliance with medical treatment: meta-analysis of the effects of anxiety and depression on patient adherence. *Arch. Intern. Med., 160*, 2101–2107.

DiMatteo, M. R. (2004). Social support and patient adherence to medical treatment: a meta-analysis. *Health Psychology, 23*, 207–218.

DiMatteo, M. R. (2004). Variations in patients' adherence to medical recommendations: a quantitative review of 50 years of research. *Medical Care, 42*, 200–209.

DiMatteo, M. R., Haskard, K. B., & Williams, S. L. (2007). Health beliefs, disease severity, and patient adherence: a meta-analysis. *Medical Care, 45*, 521–528.

Donelle, L., Hoffman-Goetz, L., & Arocha, J. F. (2007). Assessing health numeracy among community-dwelling older adults. *Journal of Health Communication, 12*(7), 651–665.

Edelberg, H. K., Shallenberger, E., & Wei, J. Y. (1999). Medication management capacity in highly functioning community-living older adults: detection of early deficits. *Journal of the American Geriatrics Society, 47*, 592–596.

Edelberg, H. K., Shallenberger, E., Hausdorff, J. M., & Wei, J. Y. (2000). One-year follow-up of medication management capacity in highly functioning older adults. *The Journals of Gerontology. Series A, Biological Sciences and Medical Sciences, 55*, M550–M553.

Eisenthal, S., Emery, R., Lazare, A., & Udin, H. (1979). "Adherence" and the negotiated approach to patienthood. *Archives of General Psychiatry, 36*, 393–398.

Elwyn, G., Edwards, A., & Kinnersley, P. (1999). Shared decision-making in primary care: the neglected second half of the consultation. *British Journal of General Practice, 49*, 477–482.

Ende, J., Kazis, L., Ash, A., & Moskowitz, M. A. (1989). Measuring patients' desire for autonomy: decision making and information-seeking preferences among medical patients. *J. Gen. Intern. Med., 4*, 23–30.

Ernst, F. R., & Grizzle, A. J. (2001). Drug-related morbidity and mortality: updating the cost-of-illness model. *J. Am. Pharm. Assoc., 41*, 192–199.

Farran, C. J., Staffileno, B. A., Gilley, D. W., McCann, J. J., Li, Y., Castro, C. M., & King, A. C. (2008). A lifestyle physical activity intervention for caregivers of persons with alzheimer's disease. *American Journal of Alzheimer's Disease and Other Dementias, 23*, 132–142.

Figueiras, M. J., & Alves, N. C. (2007). Lay perceptions of serious illnesses: an adapted version of the Revised Illness Perception Questionnaire (IPQ-R) for healthy people. *Psychology and Health, 22*(2), 143–158.

Focht, B. C., Sanders, W. M., Brubaker, P., & Rejeski, W. J. (2003). Validity of the CSA accelerometer for the measurement of physical activity in older adults with chronic disease. *Journal of Physical Activity and Aging, 11*, 293–304.

Gallant, M. P. (2003). The influence of social support on chronic illness self-management: a review and directions for research. *Health Educ. Behav., 30*, 170–195.

Gao, X., & Nau, D. P. (2000). Congruence of three self-report measures of medication adherence among HIV patients. *Annals of Pharmacotherapy, 34*, 1117–1122.

Giersdorf, N., Loh, A., & Harter, M. (2004). Measuring shared decision making. *Z. Arztl. Fortbild., 98*, 135–141.

Golbeck, A. L., Ahlers-Schmidt, C. R., Paschal, A. M., & Dismuke, S. E. (2005). A definition and operational framework for health numeracy. *American Journal of Preventive Medicine, 29*, 375–376.

Graham, N. M., Jacobson, L. P., Kuo, V., Chmiel, J. S., Morgenstern, H., & Zucconi, S. L. (1994). Access to therapy in the multicenter AIDS cohort study, 1989–1992. *J. Clin. Epidemiol., 47*, 1003–1012.

Gravel, K., Légaré, F., & Graham, I. D. (2006). Barriers and facilitators to implementing shared decision-making in clinical practice: a systematic review of health professionals' perceptions. *Implementation Science, 1*, 16.

Harada, N. D., Chiu, V., King, A. C., & Stewart, A. L. (2001). An evaluation of three self-report physical activity instruments for older adults. *Medicine and Science in Sports and Exercise, 33*(6), 962–970.

Heisler, M., Bouknight, R. R., Hayward, R. A., Smith, D. M., & Kerr, E. A. (2002). The relative importance of physician communication, participatory decision making, and patient understanding in diabetes self-management. *J. Gen. Intern. Med., 17*, 243–252.

Heisler, M., Cole, I., Weir, D., Kerr, E. A., & Hayward, R. A. (2007). Does physician communication influence older patients' diabetes self-management and glycemic control? Results from the Health and Retirement Study (HRS). *Journal of Gerontology, 62A*, 1435–1442.

Heuts, P. H., de Bie, R. A., Dijkstra, A., Aretz, K., Vlaeyen, J. W., Schouten, H. J., et al. (2005). Assessment of readiness to change in patients with osteoarthritis: development and application of a new questionnaire. *Clinical Rehabilitation, 19*, 290–299.

Hinkin, C. H., Castellon, S. A., Durvasula, R. S., Hardy, D. J., Lam, M. N., Mason, K. I., et al. (2002). Medication adherence among HIV+ adults: effects of cognitive function and regimen complexity. *Neurology, 59*, 1944–1950.

Hinkin, C. H., Hardy, D. J., Mason, K. I., Castellon, S. A., Durvasula, R. S., Lam, M. N., & Stefaniak, M. (2004). Medication adherence in HIV-infected adults: effect of patient age, cognitive status, and substance abuse. *AIDS, 18*, 19–25.

Hnatiuk, S. H. (1991). Experience sampling with elderly persons: an exploration of the method. *International Journal of Aging and Human Development, 33*, 45.

Horne, R., & Weinman, J. (1998). Predicting treatment adherence: an overview of theoretical models. In L. B. Myers, & K. Medence (Eds.), *Adherence to Treatment in Medical Conditions* (pp. 25–50). Amsterdam: Harwood Academic Publishers.

Horne, R., Weinman, J., & Hankins, M. (1999). The Beliefs about Medicines Questionnaire: the development and evaluation of a new method for assessing the cognitive representation of medication. *Psychology and Health, 14*, 1–24.

Hughes, T. F., & Ganguli, M. (2009). Modifiable midlife risk factors for late-life cognitive impairment and dementia. *Curr. Psychiatry Rev., 5*(2), 73–92.

Huizinga, M. M., Elasy, T. A., Wallston, K. A., Cavanaugh, K., Davis, D., Gregory, R. P., et al. (2008). Development and validation of the Diabetes Numeracy Test (DNT). *BMC Health Serv. Res., 8*, 96.

Iihara, N., Tsukmoto, T., Morita, S., Miyoshi, C., Takabatake, K., & Kurosaki, Y. (2004). Beliefs of chronically ill Japanese patients that lead to intentional non-adherence to medication. *J. Cardiovasc. Nurs., 29*, 417–424.

Insel, K. C., Reminger, S. L., & Hsiao, C. (2006). The negative association of independent personality and medication adherence. *Journal of Aging and Health, 18*, 407–418.

Institute of Medicine. (2004). *Health Literacy: A Prescription to End Confusion*. Washington, DC: Institute of Medicine, Board on Neuroscience and Behavioral Health, Committee on Health Literacy.

Jacelon, C. S., & Imperio, K. (2005). Participant diaries as a source of data in research with older adults. *Qualitative Health Research, 15*, 991–997.

Janz, N. K., & Becker, M. H. (1984). The health belief model: a decade later. *Health Education Quarterly, 11*, 1–47.

John, O. P., Donahue, E. M., & Kentle, R. L. (1991). *The "big five" inventory—versions 4a and5a (technical report)*. Berkeley, CA: Institute of Personality Assessment and Research.

Johnson, J., & Bytheway, B. (2001). An evaluation of the use of diaries in a study of medication in later life. *International Journal of Social Research Methodology, 4*, 183–204.

Kamarck, T. W., Janicki, D. L., Shiffman, S., Polk, D. E., Muldoon, M. F., Liebenauer, L. L., & Schwartz, J. E. (2002). Psychosocial demands and ambulatory blood pressure: a field assessment approach. *Physiology and Behavior, 77*, 699–704.

Katz, I. R., Morales, K., Datto, C., Streim, J., Oslin, D., DiFilippo, S., & Have, T. T. (2005). Probing for affective side effects of drugs used in geriatric practice: use of daily diaries to test for effects of metoclopramide and naproxen. *Neuropsychopharmacology, 30*, 1568–1575.

Kennedy, J., & Morgan, S. (2006). A cross-national study of prescription nonadherence due to cost: data from the joint Canada–United States survey of health. *Clinical Therapeutics, 28*, 1217–1224.

Krein, S. L., Hayward, R. A., Pogach, L., & Boots Miller, B. J. (2000). Department of Veterans Affairs' quality enhancement research initiative for diabetes mellitus. *Med. Care, 38*, I38–I48.

Kulkarni, S., Alexander, K., Lytle, B., Heiss, G., & Peterson, E. (2006). Long-term adherence with cardiovascular drug regimens. *American Heart Journal, 151*, 185–191.

Kutner, M., Greenberg, E., Jin, Y., & Paulsen, C. (2006). *The health literacy of America's adults: results from the 2003 National Assessment of Adult Literacy (NCES 2006–483). US Department of Education*. Washington, DC: National Center for Education Statistics.

Lawton, M. P., Kleban, M. H., Dean, J., Rajagopal, D., & Parmelee, P. A. (1992). The factorial generality of brief positive and negative affect measures. *Journal of Gerontology*, *47*, 228–237.

Lerman, I., Díaz., J. P., Ibarguengoitia, M. E., Pérez, F. J., Villa, A. R., Velasco, M. L., et al. (2009). Nonadherence to insulin therapy in low-income, type 2 diabetic patients. *Endocrine Practice*, *15*, 41–46.

Leventhal, H., Leventhal, E. A., & Contrada, R. J. (1998). Self-regulation, health, and behavior: a perceptual-cognitive approach. *Psychology and Health*, *13*, 717–733.

Liberman, R. P. (2003). Biobehavioral treatment and rehabilitation for older adults with schizophrenia. In C. I. Cohen (Ed.), *Schizophrenia into Later Life: Treatment, Research and Policy*. Washington, DC: American Psychiatric Publishing Inc.

Lutfey, K. E., & Wishner, W. J. (1999). Beyond "compliance" is "adherence": improving the prospect of diabetes care. *Diabetes Care*, *22*, 635–639.

Lyons, G., Culhane, K., Hilton, D., Grace, P., & Lyons, D. (2009). A description of an accelerometer-based mobility monitoring technique. *Medical Engineering & Physics*, *27*, 497–504.

Mackin, R. S., & Arean, P. A. (2007). Cognitive and psychiatric predictors of medical treatment adherence among older adults in primary care clinics. *International Journal of Geriatric Psychiatry*, *22*(1), 55–60.

MacLaughlin, E. J., Raehl, C. L., Treadway, A. K., Sterling, T. L., Zoller, D. P., & Bond, C. A. (2005). Assessing medication adherence in the elderly: which tools to use in clinical practice? *Drugs Aging*, *22*, 231–255.

Marks, G. R., & Lutgendorf, S. K. (1999). Perceived health competence and personality factors differentially predict health behaviors in older adults. *Journal of Aging and Health*, *11*, 221–239.

Markwardt, F. C. (1998). *Peabody Individual Achievement Test-Revised: Manual*. Circle Pines, MN: American Guidance Service.

Matsui, D., Hermann, C., Klein, J., Berkovitch, M., Olivieri, N., & Koren, G. (1994). Critical comparison of novel and existing methods of compliance assessment during a clinical trial of an oral iron chelator. *Journal of Clinical Pharmacology*, *34*, 944–949.

McCarthy, M., Mueser, K. T., & Pratt, S. I. (2008). Integrated psychosocial rehabilitation and health care for older people with serious mental illness. In D. Gallagher-Thompson, A. M. Steffen, & L. W. Thompson (Eds.), *Handbook of Behavioral and Cognitive Therapies with Older Adults*. New York, NY: Springer.

McGlynn, E. A., Asch, S. M., Adams, J., Keesey, J., Hicks, J., DeCristofaro, A., & Kerr, E. A. (2003). The quality of health care delivered to adults in the United States. *N. Engl. J. Med.*, *348*, 2635–2645.

McQuaid, J. R., Granholm, E., McClure, F. S., Roepke, S., Pedrelli, P., Patterson, T. L., & Jeste, D. V. (2000). Development of an integrated cognitive-behavioral and social skills training intervention for older adults with schizophrenia. *Journal of Psychotherapy Practice and Research*, *9*, 149–156.

Miaskowski, C., Dodd, M. J., West, C., Paul, S. M., Tripathy, D., Koo, P., & Schumacher, K. (2001). Lack of adherence with the analgesic regimen: a significant barrier to effective cancer pain management. *Journal of Clinical Oncology*, *19*(23), 4275–4279.

Mojtabai, R., & Olfson, M. (2003). Medication costs, adherence, and outcomes among Medicare beneficiaries. *Health Affairs*, *22*, 220–229.

Monane, M., Bohn, R. L., Gurwitz, J. H., Glynn, R. J., Levin, R., & Avorn, J. (1996). Compliance with antihypertensive therapy among elderly Medicaid enrollees: the roles of age, gender, and race. *American Journal of Public Health*, *86*, 1805–1808.

Morisky, D. E., Ang, A., Krousel-Wood, M., & Ward, H. J. (2008). Predictive validity of a medication adherence measure in an outpatient setting. *Journal of Clinical Hypertension*, *10*, 348–354.

Morisky, D. E., Green, L. W., & Levine, D. M. (1986). Concurrent and predictive validity of a self-reported measure of medication adherence. *Medical Care*, *24*, 67–74.

Moskowitz, D. S., & Young, S. N. (2006). Ecological momentary assessment: what it is and why it is a method of the future in clinical psychopharmacology. *Journal of Psychiatry and Neuroscience*, *31*, 13–20.

Moss-Morris, R., Weinman, J., Petrie, K. J., Horne, R., Cameron, L. D., & Buick, D. (2002). The revised illness perception questionnaire (IPQ-R). *Psychology and Health*, *17*, 1–16.

Murphy, S. L. (2009). Review of physical activity measurement using accelerometers in older adults: considerations for research design and conduct. *Preventive Medicine*, *48*, 108–114.

National Center for Health Statistics. (2006). *Health, United States with Chart Books for Trends in the Health of Americans*. Washington, DC: US Government Printing Office.

National Council on Patient Information and Education (2007). *Enhancing Prescription Medication Adherence: A National Action Plan*. Bethesda, MD.

Nau, D. P., Steinke, D. T., Williams, L. K., Austin, R., Lafata, J. E., Divine, G., & Pladevall, M. (2007). Adherence analysis using visual analog scale versus claims-based estimation. *Annals of Pharmacotherapy*, *41*, 1792–1797.

Nielson, W. R., Jensen, M. P., Ehde, D. M., Kerns, R. D., & Molton, I. R. (2008). Further development of the Multidimensional Pain Readiness to Change Questionnaire: the MPRCQ2. *The Journal of Pain*, *9*(6), 552–565.

O'Connell, M., Tondora, J., Croog, G., Evans, A., & Davidson, L. (2005). From rhetoric to routine: assessing perceptions of recovery-oriented practices in a state mental health and addiction system. *Psychiatr. Rehabil. J.*, *28*, 378–386.

O'Neal, E. L., Adams, J. R., McHugo, G. J., Van Citters, A. D., Drake, R. D., & Bartels, S. J. (2008). Preferences of older and younger adults with serious mental illness for involvement in decision-making in medical and psychiatric settings. *American Journal of Geriatric Psychiatry*, *16*, 826–833.

Onken, S., Dumont, J., Ridgway, P., Dornan, D., & Ralph, R. (2005). *Mental health recovery: what helps and what hinders? A national research project for the development of recovery facilitating system performance indicators*. Alexandria, VA: NASMHPD, National Technical Assistance Center for State Mental Health Planning. Located on 7/15/2009 at http://128.197.26.34/cpr/repository/documents/pdf/rosireportjointconf2004.pdf.

Ontiveros, J. A., Black, S. A., Jakobi, P. L., & Goodwin, J. S. (1999). Ethnic variation in attitudes toward hypertension in adults ages 75 and older. *Prev. Med.*, *29*, 443–449.

Orwig, D., Brandt, N., & Gruber-Baldini, A. L. (2006). Medication management assessment for older adults in the community. *The Gerontologist*, *46*, 661–668.

Pargament, K. I., Koenig, H. G., & Perez, L. M. (2000). The many methods of religious coping: development and initial validation of the RCOPE. *Journal of Clinical Psychology*, *56*, 519–543.

Pargament, K. I., Smith, B. W., Koenig, H. G., & Nielsen, J. (1998). Religious coping and health status in medically ill hospitalized older adults. *Journal of Nervous and Mental Disease*, *186*, 513–521.

Pargament, K. I., Smith, B. W., Koenig, H. G., & Perez, L. (1998). Patterns of positive and negative religious coping with major life stressors. *Journal for the Scientific Study of Religion*, *37*, 710–724.

Parker, C. S., Chen, Z., Price, M., Gross, R., Metlay, J. P., Christie, J. D., et al. (2007). Adherence to warfarin assessed by electronic pill caps, clinician assessment, and patient reports: results from the IN-RANGE study. *Journal of General Internal Medicine*, *22*, 1254–1259.

Patterson, T. L., Lacro, J., McKibbin, C. L., Moscona, S., Hughs, T., & Jeste, D. V. (2002). Medication Management Ability Assessment: results from a performance-based measure in older outpatients with schizophrenia. *Journal of Clinical Psychopharmacology*, *22*, 11–19.

Patterson, T. L., McKibbin, C., Taylor, M., Goldman, S., Davila-Fraga, W., Bucardo, J., & Jeste, D. V. (2003). Functional Adaption Skills Training (FAST): a pilot psychosocial intervention study in middle-aged and older patients with chronic psychotic disorders. *American Journal of Geriatric Psychiatry*, *11*, 17–23.

Peters, E. (2008). Numeracy and the perception and communication of risk. *Annal. NY Acad. Sci.*, *1128*, 1–7.

Phatak, H. M., & Thomas, J., III. (2006). Relationships between beliefs about medications and nonadherence to prescribed chronic medications. *Annals of Pharmacotherapy*, *40*, 1737–1742.

Piette, J. D., Heisler, M., & Wagner, T. H. (2004). Problems paying out-of-pocket medication costs among older adults with diabetes. *Diabetes Care*, *27*, 384–391.

Piette, J. D., Heisler, M., Krein, S., & Kerr, E. A. (2005). The role of patient-physician trust in moderating medication nonadherence due to cost pressures. *Arch. Intern. Med*, *165*, 1749–1755.

Poisal, J. A., & Murray, L. (2001). Growing differences between Medicare beneficiaries with and without drug coverage. *Health Affairs*, *20*, 74–85.

Pratt, S. I., Van Citters, A. D., Mueser, K. T., & Bartels, S. J. (2008). Psychosocial rehabilitation in older adults with serious mental illness: a review of the research literature and recommendations for development of rehabilitation approaches. *American Journal of Psychiatric Rehabilitation*, *11*, 7–40.

Prochaska, J. O., & DiClemente, C. C. (1983). Stages and processes of self-change of smoking: toward an integrative model of change. *Journal of Consulting and Clinical Psychology*, *51*, 390–395.

Rhodewalt, F., & Fairfield, M. (1990). An alternative approach to Type A behavior and health: psychological reactance and medical noncompliance. *Journal of Social Behavior and Personality*, *5*, 323–342.

Rudd, P. (1993). The measurement of compliance: medication taking. In N. A. Krasnegor, L. Epstein, S. B. Johnson, & S. J. Yaffe (Eds.), *Developmental Aspects of Health Compliance Behavior* (pp. 185–213). Hillsdale, NJ: Lawrence Erlbaum Associates.

Safran, D. G., Kosinski, M., Tarlov, A. R., Rogers, W. H., Taira, D. H., Lieberman, N., & Ware, J. E. (1998). The Primary Care Assessment Survey: tests of data quality and measurement performance. *Med. Care*, *36*, 728–739.

Salyers, M. P., Godfrey, J. L., Mueser, K. T., & Labriola, S. (2007). Measuring illness management outcomes: a psychometric study of clinician and consumer rating scales for illness self management and recovery. *Community Mental Health Journal*, *43*, 459–480.

Schlenk, E. A., & Hart, L. K. (1984). Relationship between health locus of control, health value, and social support and compliance of persons with diabetes mellitus. *Diabetes Care*, *7*, 566–574.

Schneider, A., Körner, T., Mehring, M., Wensing, M., Elwyn, G., & Szecsenyi, J. (2006). Impact of age, health locus of control and psychological co-morbidity on patients' preferences for share decision making in general practice. *Patient Education and Counseling*, *61*, 292–298.

Schneider, J., Kaplan, S. H., Greenfield, S., Li, W., & Wilson, I. B. (2004). Better physician-patient relationships are associated with higher reported adherence to antiretroviral therapy in patients with HIV infection. *J. Gen. Intern. Med.*, *19*, 1096–1103.

Shea, J. A., Beers, B. B., McDonald, V. J., Quistberg, D. A., Ravenell, K. L., & Asch, D. A. (2004). Assessing health literacy in African American and Caucasian adults: disparities in rapid estimate of adult literacy in medicine (REALM) scores. *Family Medicine*, *36*, 575–581.

Siegel, D., Lopez, J., & Meier, J. (2007). Antihypertensive medication adherence in the Department of Veterans Affairs. *The American Journal of Medicine*, *120*, 26–32.

Sivertsen, B., Omvik, S., Pallesen, S., Bjorvatn, B., Havik, O. E., Kvale, G., et al. (2006). Cognitive behavioral therapy vs zopiclone for treatment of chronic primary insomnia in older adults. A randomized controlled trail. *JAMA*, *295*, 2851–2858.

Slosson, R. J. L. (1990). *Slosson Oral Reading Test-Revised*. East Aurora, NY: Slosson Educational Publishers.

Spitzer, R. L., Kroenke, K., & Williams, J. B. W. (1999). Validation and utility of a self-report version of PRIME-MD: the PHQ primary care study. *JAMA*, *282*, 1737–1744.

Steinman, M. A., Landefeld, C. S., Rosenthal, G. E., Berthenthal, D., Sen, S., & Kaboli, P. J. (2006). Polypharmacy and prescribing quality in older people. *Journal of the American Geriatrics Society*, *54*, 1516–1523.

Stewart, A. L., Mills, K. M., King, A. C., Haskell, W. L., Gillis, D., & Ritter, P. L. (2001). CHAMPS physical activity questionnaire for older adults: outcomes for interventions. *Medicine & Science in Sports & Exercise*, *33*, 1126–1141.

Stoehr, G. P., Lu, S., Lavery, L., Vander Bilt, J., Saxton, J. A., Chang, C. H., & Ganguli, M. (2008). Factors associated with adherence to medication regimens in older primary care patients: the steel valley seniors survey. *The American Journal of Geriatric Pharmacotherapy*, *6*, 255–263.

Stone, A. A., Schwartz, J. E., Broderick, J. E., & Hufford, M. R. (2002). Patient non-compliance with paper diaries. *BMJ*, *324*, 1193–1194.

Straka, R. J., Fish, J. T., Benson, S. R., & Suh, J. T. (1997). Patient self-reporting of compliance does not correspond with electronic monitoring: an evaluation using isosorbide dinitrate as a model drug. *Pharmacotherapy*, *17*, 126–132.

Substance Abuse and Mental Health Services Administration. (2004). *National Consensus Conference on Mental Health Recovery and Mental Health Systems Transformation.*

Trost, S. G., McIver, K. L., & Pate, R. R. (2005). Conducting accelerometer-based activity assessments in field-based research. *Medicine & Science in Sports & Exercise*, *37*, S531–S543.

Unützer, J., Schoenbaum, M., Katon, W. J., Fan, M. Y., Pincus, H. A., Hogan, D., & Taylor, J. (2009). Healthcare costs associated with depression in medically ill fee-for-service Medicare participants. *Journal of the American Geriatrics Society*, *57*, 506–510.

Wallston, K. A., Wallston, B. S., & Peabody, G. (1978). Development of the Multidimensional Health Locus of Control (MHLC) scales. *Health Education & Behavior*, *6*, 160–170.

Weinman, J., Petrie, K. J., Moss-Morris, R., & Horne, R. (1996). The Illness Perception Questionnaire: a new method for assessing the cognitive representation of illness. *Psychology & Health*, *11*, 431–445.

Welk, G. J., Blair, S. N., Wood, K., Jones, S., & Thompson, R. W. (2000). A comparative evaluation of three accelerometry-based physical activity monitors. *Medicine & Science in Sports & Exercise*, *32*, S489–S497.

Wilkinson, G. S. (1993). *Wide Range Achievement Test* (3rd ed.). Wilmington, DE: Wide Range.

World Health Organization. (2003). *Adherence to Long Term Therapies—Evidence for Action*. Geneva: WHO Publications.

Yesavage, J. A., Brink, T. L., Rose, T. L., Lum, O., Huang, V., Adey, M., & Leirer, V. O. (1982). Development and validation of a geriatric depression screening scale: a preliminary report. *Journal of Psychiatric Research*, *17*, 37–49.

Zivin, K., & Kales, H. C. (2008). Adherence to depression treatment in older adults: a narrative review. *Drugs and Aging*, *25*, 559–571.

PART 3

Cognition

CHAPTER

18

Geriatric Neuropsychological Assessment

John L. Woodard

Department of Psychology, Wayne State University, Detroit, MI, USA

INTRODUCTION

Neuropsychological assessment of older adults has assumed a prominent role in a variety of contexts. For example, neuropsychological assessment plays a critical role in evaluations for dementia and for tracking dementia-related changes. Neuropsychologists also use assessment results to tailor specific rehabilitation strategies for older adults based on their individual patterns of strengths and weaknesses, thereby maximizing treatment outcomes. Pre- and post-surgical neuropsychological assessment has been successful in identifying particular pre-surgical or post-surgical risk factors for complications, and it can generate strategies for treating or rehabilitating adverse post-surgical outcomes, should they occur. Results of neuropsychological evaluation are also essential for monitoring outcomes of pharmacologic and behavioral treatments and appropriateness of specific placements.

Advances in the field of geriatric neuropsychology have been able to confront a variety of challenges, including the lack of availability of normative data, circumventing sensory and motor limitations, reducing the amount of time required to administer and score instruments, and improving the reliability and validity of new measures. In addition, streamlining of assessment procedures, sometimes dictated by third-party payers, often requires neuropsychologists to gather more data using fewer instruments. Thus, focused and efficient batteries are assuming greater importance.

The purposes of this chapter are to establish a variety of contexts and purposes of geriatric neuropsychological assessment, to describe contemporary issues associated with neuropsychological assessment of older adults, and to review recent empirical literature associated with the use of newly developed and commonly used cognitive and mood assessment instruments with older adults. Empirical studies describing the use of these measures with diverse populations will be covered where possible. The chapter will conclude with a case study illustrating some of the principles discussed in this chapter.

CONTEXTS AND PURPOSES OF GERIATRIC NEUROPSYCHOLOGICAL ASSESSMENT

Dementia Evaluation

Neuropsychological assessment has assumed a central place in the detection and tracking of dementia, particularly Alzheimer's disease (AD). Neuropsychological testing is required for the diagnosis of AD using NINCDS-ADRDA criteria (McKhann et al., 1984), and it has been endorsed by the American Academy of Neurology (AAN, 1996). In addition, it has been included as an evaluation component for

Handbook of Assessment in Clinical Gerontology. DOI: 10.1016/B978-0-12-374961-1.10018-1

the diagnosis of dementia (Knopman et al., 2001) and mild cognitive impairment (MCI; Petersen et al., 2001b) practice parameters for the American Academy of Neurology. With novel pharmacologic treatments becoming available for AD, early detection of cognitive changes is becoming increasingly critical. Cognitive assessment is an important component in the evaluation of pharmacologic management of dementia (Doody et al., 2001). Neuropsychological measures, particularly of memory, have shown promise for predicting future cognitive change in cognitively healthy persons (Blacker et al., 2007; Guarch, Marcos, Salamero, & Blesa, 2004; Kluger, Ferris, Golomb, Mittelman, & Reisberg, 1999; Marquis et al., 2002; Masur, Fuld, Blau, Crystal, & Aronson, 1990; Masur, Sliwinski, Lipton, Blau, & Crystal, 1994). These findings have been particularly strong for carriers of the apolipoprotein E (APOE) ϵ4 allele (Caselli et al., 2007). Although they show a strong propensity for identifying the likelihood of future cognitive change, neuropsychological measures may provide less information regarding the regional location and biochemical changes associated with AD-related progression relative to other biomarkers, such as cerebrospinal fluid (CSF) and structural and functional imaging biomarkers. Among persons with existing mild cognitive impairment (MCI), neuropsychological assessment has shown promise for identifying those persons who will likely progress to AD (Albert, Moss, Tanzi, & Jones, 2001; De Jager, Hogervorst, Combrinck, & Budge, 2003; DeCarli et al., 2004; Nestor, Scheltens, & Hodges, 2004).

A recent study of skilled nursing facility patients revealed that 84.2% of individuals carrying a "suspected" dementia diagnosis in their chart actually did not meet criteria for dementia when objective neuropsychological measures were administered (Mansdorf, Harrington, Lund, & Wohl, 2008). The majority of these individuals met DSM-IV Axis I criteria (75%) or MCI criteria (25%) instead. This study illustrates the importance of administering appropriate objective neuropsychological measures, rather than relying on subjective impressions, in generating accurate diagnoses for facilitating treatment planning.

Neuropsychologists are also frequently called on to evaluate risks of more complex outcomes or behaviors that are frequently associated with dementia. For example, neuropsychological evaluation has been useful in the assessment of fall risk (Thurman, Stevens, & Rao, 2008) and evaluating driving risk among AD patients (Dubinsky, Stein, & Lyons, 2000) and non-demented older adults (Bieliauskas, 2005).

Neuropsychological measures have also been used to predict the ability to perform basic and instrumental activities of daily living (BADL and IADL, respectively). Because impairment in daily living skills is a necessary component of dementia, this domain is particularly important to assess. Several studies have used subscales from the Mattis Dementia Rating Scale (MDRS) to predict BADL and IADL skills. For example, the cognitive domains of executive functioning and memory were found to be predictive of IADL, but not BADL, competence among AD patients (Vitaliano, Breen, Albert, Russo, & Printz, 1984). Executive functioning and memory were also shown to predict everyday functioning in a psychogeriatric sample (Nadler, Richardson, Malloy, Marran, & Brinson, 1993). Visuospatial functioning and memory were the two strongest cognitive predictors of IADL competency in a sample of 108 psychogeriatric inpatients (Richardson, Nadler, & Malloy, 1995). A number of other studies have highlighted the importance of executive functioning measures in predicting ability to perform daily living skills (Baird, Podell, Lovell, & McGinty, 2001; Bell-McGinty, Podell, Franzen, Baird, & Williams, 2002; Cahn et al., 1998; Grigsby, Kaye, Baxter, Shetterly, & Hamman, 1998; Jefferson, Barakat, Giovannetti, Paul, & Glosser, 2006). Royall and colleagues have published a thorough review of the current state of the field with respect to what is known about cognitive correlates of functional capacity (Royall et al., 2007).

Cross-culturally, cognitive functioning (particularly executive attentional processes) plays a significant role in the prediction of self-reported measures of BADL and IADL skills. Using survey data obtained in Taiwan and the United States, Ofstedal and colleagues found that cognitive functions are strong predictors of IADL skills in both countries (Ofstedal, Zimmer, & Lin, 1999). Executive attention has been shown to be more associated with IADL than BADL (Carlson et al., 1999). A study from France replicated the association between cognitive functioning and IADL skills among non-demented older adults, suggesting that different neuropsychological components are associated with different IADL tasks (Barberger-Gateau et al., 1992). Finally, Loewenstein and colleagues have found measures of executive functioning, memory, and visuospatial functioning to account for unique variance over and above that of global cognitive status (measured by the MMSE) when predicting IADL performance that has been directly observed (rather than relying on self-report) in both English speaking and Hispanic dementia patients (Loewenstein et al., 1992; Loewenstein, Argüelles, Argüelles, & Linn-Fuentes, 1994; Loewenstein, Argüelles, Barker, & Duara, 1993).

Treatment Planning

Neuropsychological assessment can play a critical role in adding useful information for treatment planning. A target of this type of evaluation would be the identification of specific strengths and weaknesses in order to tailor a patient's treatment to maximize adherence to the treatment plan. Identification of post-surgical cognitive or psychological concerns can also target specific patients for interventions that can enhance subsequent quality of life. For example, a thorough assessment of psychosocial and personality functioning has been shown to identify important predictors of compliance and morbidity in transplant patients (Bernazzali et al., 2005; Chacko, Harper, Gotto, & Young, 1996; Chacko, Harper, Kunik, & Young, 1996). In fact, even situationally defined distress observed pre-surgically has been shown to predict survival time following cardiac transplant (Chacko, Harper, Gotto & Young 1996). Pre-surgical assessment of cognitive appraisals and coping styles has also been shown to be effective for identifying post-transplant patients who could benefit from counseling and psychological intervention (Burker, Evon, Sedway, & Egan, 2004). Cognitive functioning is also important to monitor, both pre- and post-surgically, as cognitive complaints are often associated with decreased quality of life after transplantation (Harder et al., 2002).

Neuropsychological assessment plays a critical role in the pre-surgical evaluation of candidates for surgical treatment of Parkinson's disease (Baron et al., 1996; Bronte-Stewart, 2003), particularly to rule out dementia, which is a contraindication for this type of intervention. Finally, neuropsychological assessment has also been used in rehabilitation settings as a predictor of post-surgical complications, as well as treatment outcome. For example, cognitive impairment has been shown to be a significant predictor of post-operative delirium following orthopedic surgery for hip fracture in older adults (Juliebo et al., 2009). Older hip fracture patients with cognitive impairment have been shown to demonstrate significant functional improvement following intensive post-fracture rehabilitation, and the majority of patients avoided subsequent discharge to a skilled nursing facility (Goldstein, Strasser, Woodard, & Roberts, 1997). In short, neuropsychological assessment is an important component of care that can enhance the quality of treatment of a number of medical conditions frequently seen in late life.

Outcome Monitoring

Neuropsychological assessment can play a significant role in the monitoring of critical clinical or research outcomes. As noted above, neuropsychological evaluation can identify important pre-surgical or post-surgical issues that can guide post-surgical treatment decisions. From a clinical standpoint, assessing the presence of adverse cognitive or emotional changes following surgery can be an important end-point to monitor. For instance, coronary artery bypass graft (CABG) surgery is sometimes associated with post-surgical cognitive changes. In one recent study, pre-surgical subjective memory complaints, presence of mild cognitive impairment, and type of cardiac surgery (e.g., valve replacement) were risk factors for post-operative delirium (Veliz-Reissmuller, Aguero Torres, van der Linden, Lindblom, & Eriksdotter Jonhagen, 2007). Gottesman and colleagues successfully used several brief cognitive measures to monitor for cognitive changes following CABG (Gottesman et al., 2007). Finally, the time course of cognitive changes following CABG has recently been examined in a three-year longitudinal study (Knipp et al., 2008); cognitive changes followed a two-stage course characterized by an early improvement followed by later decline. Early post-surgical cognitive changes were associated with long-term cognitive impairment.

In light of its standardized and relatively objective nature, it is not surprising that neuropsychological evaluation is frequently used as a critical outcome measure for pharmacologic intervention studies. For example, neuropsychological testing has been used as a critical outcome measure in a number of clinical trials of pharmacologic interventions for Alzheimer's disease (Almkvist, Darreh-Shori, Stefanova, Spiegel, & Nordberg, 2004; Farlow & Lilly, 2005; Goekoop, Scheltens, Barkhof, & Rombouts, 2006; Hashimoto et al., 2005; Krishnan et al., 2003; Sobow & Kloszewska, 2007; Visser, Scheltens, Pelgrim, & Verhey, 2005) among other treatments for neurological disorders. Given the availability of alternate forms of neuropsychological instruments, changes due to practice effects can be minimized, enabling one to focus on aspects of true cognitive change. Furthermore, age-related cognitive changes are well characterized for a number of cognitive domains. However, some domains of cognition are relatively poorly understood, and cognitive measures have differential sensitivity to change in a given domain. Finally, some aspects of cognition may be more malleable in response to a pharmacologic intervention than others. Each of these issues makes the selection of a neuropsychological outcome battery a task that must be carried out with considerable care and forethought.

PRACTICAL CONSIDERATIONS IN THE ASSESSMENT OF OLDER ADULTS

As discussed above, neuropsychological assessment requires the placement of test results into a particular context. Assessment of older adults has a set of unique considerations that must be taken into account in understanding a particular pattern of cognitive test results. Because polypharmacy is frequently increased among older adults, medication use must be carefully considered when examining the neuropsychological profile. In addition, chronic health conditions that can produce prolonged or transient changes in neuropsychological functioning are common among older adults. Physical and sensory limitations can also influence cognitive performance on neuropsychological measures. Careful screening for these limitations is relatively easy to implement and can make significant contributions toward interpretation of neuropsychological test results. Finally, social supports are an important influence on emotional functioning in late-life. The availability of social networks and supports for older adults can dramatically influence aspects of mental and cognitive health. In the subsequent sections, these issues will be considered in turn.

Medication Use

Patterns of medication use among older adults may complicate the interpretation of neuropsychological assessment results in a variety of ways. For instance, age-related changes in organ function may lead to altered pharmacokinetics of many medications, which may, in turn, result in adverse drug reactions. In addition, some medications can precipitate cognitive impairment or an acute confusional state. Forty-four percent of men and 57% of women aged 65 years or older take five or more medications per day, and 3% of men and 12% of women in this age group take ten or more medications per day (Kaufman, Kelly, Rosenberg, Anderson, & Mitchell, 2002) This pattern of polypharmacy leads to greater risk for drug interactions and poorer health outcomes (Fick et al., 2003; Hajjar, Cafiero, & Hanlon, 2007; Hanlon et al., 2009; Steinman et al., 2006). Given this extremely high frequency of medication use in the elderly, it is perhaps not surprising that 50% of accidental drug-related deaths occur in geriatric patients (Preston, O'Neal, & Talaga, 1997). Several age-related conditions could be contributing factors, including impaired or variable organ function, presence of comorbid diseases, and visual or other cognitive impairment that could lead to medication non-compliance, confusion of directions, or possible overdose. Medication non-compliance among older adults can often be attributed to complicated directions for medication use, sensory impairment, cognitive and memory deficits, child-resistant packaging, and cost (Preston et al., 1997).

Although medication side effects are frequently observed among older adults, effects associated with medication overuse or underuse can also be problematic. In these cases, identification and termination of the offending medication(s) can potentially reverse these symptoms. Cardiovascular drugs are associated with the greatest number of adverse drug reactions in older adults, followed by central nervous system agents, non-steroidal anti-inflammatory drugs, endocrine agents, antibiotics, GI agents, respiratory agents, and blood formation and coagulation agents (Cooper, 1996). Use of some medications, such as sedatives, antidepressants, and neuroleptics can elevate the risk of falls among older adults (Hanlon et al., 2009; Thurman et al., 2008). Given these numerous factors, both number and type of medications used are important to consider as both predisposing and complicating factors when evaluating older adults (Cumming et al., 1991).

Comorbid Chronic Health Conditions

Several chronic health conditions increase in prevalence in late-life, including arthritis, cancer, diabetes, heart disease, hypertension, stroke, thyroid disease, and pulmonary disease. Each of these conditions can produce transient cognitive fluctuation or physical/sensory impairment. These conditions co-occur in late-life neurological conditions, such as Alzheimer's disease and Parkinson's disease, making it challenging to attribute cognitive change to a particular etiology. In a sample of dementia patients, cognitively impaired patients without dementia, and cognitively intact community-dwelling older adults, approximately 27% of these individuals had been hospitalized on at least one occasion in the prior year (Schmader et al., 1998). The most common chronic medical condition across all of the groups was arthritis, followed by hypertension, and heart disease. Among the cognitively intact and cognitively impaired groups, diabetes was the fourth most common medical condition, whereas for dementia patients, stroke was fourth most common, followed by diabetes.

Physical, Sensory, and Cognitive Limitations

Intact physical and sensory skills are essential for maintaining independence with respect to activities of daily living in older adults (Myers, Young, & Langlois, 1996). In a sample of community-dwelling persons over 85 years of age, difficulty executing both basic activities of daily living (BADL) and instrumental activities of daily living (IADL) were reported in 78% of respondents (Krach, DeVaney, DeTurk, & Zink, 1996). This study also noted that ability to perform activities of daily living was related most strongly to ratings of both physical and mental functioning, and least strongly to social and economic functioning on the Older American Resources Survey (OARS; Fillenbaum, 1988). In addition, several studies have shown a relationship between sensory loss and decreased functional ability among older adults (Colsher & Wallace, 1993; Oster, 1976; Ravaglia et al., 1997). In one of these studies (Ravaglia et al., 1997), 81% of participants over 90 years of age demonstrated either partial or total dependence for performing BADL using the Katz ADL scale (Katz, Downs, Cash, & Grotz, 1970). However, only 7% of women maintained complete ADL independence, versus 34% of men. Bathing, dressing, toileting, and transfer were the most difficult BADLs for both men and women, while continence and eating posed the least difficulties. Functional blindness and reduced visual acuity are also prevalent in late-life (Salive et al., 1992). In short, physical/sensory compromises in the elderly may produce decreased strength and mobility, difficulty seeing obstacles and hazards, and reduced ability to use hearing in order to avoid potential hazards. These limitations place older adults at extremely high risk of experiencing an injury, typically a fall (Benson & Lusardi, 1995; Salgado, Lord, Packer, & Ehrlich, 1994; Tinetti, Doucette, Claus, & Marottoli, 1995).

Sensory impairment across multiple domains is particularly problematic. The combination of visual and hearing impairment impacts functional capacity substantially more than sensory impairment in a single domain (Keller, Morton, Thomas, & Potter, 1999). In addition, multiple domain sensory impairment affected functional status independently of mental status and comorbid illness (Keller et al., 1999).

In addition to age-related changes in physical and sensory functioning, ability to perform daily living skills is dependent upon a complex interplay between numerous cognitive abilities in the elderly, and compromises in cognitive functioning can elevate the risk of injury (Myers et al., 1996). For example, the prominent decline in visuospatial ability with increasing age (Flicker, Ferris, Crook, Bartus, & Reisberg, 1986; Howieson, Holm, Kaye, Oken, & Howieson, 1993), as well as age-related changes in executive functioning (Axelrod, Goldman, & Henry, 1992; Carlson et al., 1999; Grigsby et al., 1998; Mittenberg, Seidenberg, O'Leary, & DiGiulio, 1989) and memory (Albert, 1988; Baddeley, 1986; Botwinick & Storandt, 1974; Craik, 1986, 1990; Hultsch & Dixon, 1990; Swihart & Pirozzolo, 1988; Talland, 1965), place older adults at high risk of experiencing an injury (Nyberg & Gustafson, 1997; Rapport, Hanks, Millis, & Deshpande, 1998). Measures of visuospatial ability, executive functioning, and memory have been shown to account for unique variance over and above that of global cognitive status when predicting IADL performance in healthy and demented elderly persons (Benedict, Goldstein, Dobraski, & Tannenhaus, 1997; Loewenstein et al., 1993; Loewenstein, Rubert et al., 1992; Mahurin, DeBettignies, & Pirozzolo, 1991; Nadler et al., 1993; Richardson et al., 1995; Vitaliano et al., 1984), and when predicting positive rehabilitation outcomes and discharge destination in cognitively impaired elderly hip fracture patients (Goldstein et al., 1997). There are several excellent textbooks that cover these issues in greater detail that should be consulted by the interested reader (La Rue, 1992; Lezak, 1995; Spreen & Strauss, 1998).

Social Supports

The extent of perceived social support in one's life has been shown to predict numerous health outcomes, including survival, particularly among older women (Lyyra & Heikkinen, 2006). Older adults are faced with a number of challenges, including loss of peer supports due to death and illness, as well as limited mobility, which reduces opportunities to engage in pleasurable social activities. A number of studies have found a positive relationship between social incentives (Langer et al., 1979), having a socially engaging lifestyle (Yeh & Liu, 2003) and cognitive functioning, and having an extensive social network has even been proposed to protect against dementia (Fratiglioni, Wang, Ericsson, Maytan, & Winblad, 2000). However, it has been unclear whether loss of social supports is a consequence or a cause of cognitive decline. There is still much to be learned about the impact of social supports on cognitive functioning and functional status, and these issues are particularly important to consider and address during neuropsychological evaluations with older adults.

AVAILABILITY OF NORMATIVE DATA FOR OLDER ADULTS

A particular challenge facing the geriatric neuropsychologist is the relative dearth of normative data for older adults. Fortunately, a number of contemporary measures now have normative data through approximately age 90. However, until relatively recently, normative data for some of the most common neuropsychological and intellectual functioning measures extended only to age 74 at most, leading some researchers to develop their own normative data (Ryan, Paolo, & Brungardt, 1992). Heaton and colleagues (Heaton, Grant, & Matthews, 1991) developed extensive normative data for the Wechsler Adult Intelligence Scale-Revised (WAIS-R; Wechsler, 1981) and for measures from an expanded Halstead-Reitan neuropsychological battery, creating demographic adjustments for age, sex, and education. However, the normative data extended only to 74 years of age, making them of limited use with a substantial proportion of the older adult population.

Mayo Older American Normative Studies

The Mayo Older American Normative Studies (MOANS) have made significant contributions to providing normative data for a number of measures for older adults. The first normative data from this series of studies were published in 1992 in a supplemental issue of *The Clinical Neuropsychologist*. Using a large sample of 526 predominantly Caucasian participants between the ages of 55 and 97, the authors presented age- and education-corrected normative data for the WAIS-R (Ivnik et al., 1992a). Although normative data existed for the Wechsler Memory Scale-Revised (WMS-R; Wechsler, 1987), and the Rey Auditory Verbal Learning Test (RAVLT; Rey, 1958; Schmidt, 1996), MOANS data were subsequently presented for the WMS-R (Ivnik et al., 1992b) and the RAVLT (Ivnik et al., 1992c), extending the age norms for these measures upwards. The rationale for computing age and education corrections in their normative sample was also described (Malec et al., 1992). The MOANS normative data use the concept of finding the closest "midpoint age" to the examinee's chronological age to serve as the normative reference, which helps to characterize more accurately the expected level of performance for a given age. Rather than relying on average performance within a specific decade, age peer groups can be reduced to as close as within two years of the examinee's chronological age.

Since the introduction of the initial MOANS studies, normative data have been presented for the Free and Cued Selective Reminding Test (Ivnik et al., 1997), verbal category fluency (Lucas et al., 1998a), the Mattis Dementia Rating Scale (Lucas et al., 1998b), Rey Auditory Verbal Learning Test Recognition Trial (Harris, Ivnik, & Smith, 2002), and Visual Form Discrimination Test and copy trial for the Rey-Osterrieth Complex Figure (Machulda et al., 2007). Given that educational opportunities and experiences can vary considerably across individuals, a focus on including IQ as a normative variable has been introduced for many neuropsychological measures using the MOANS sample. Age- and IQ-adjusted normative data using the MOANS sample have been published for the Boston Naming Test, Multilingual Aphasia Examination (MAE) Token Test and Judgment of Line Orientation (Steinberg, Bieliauskas, Smith, Langellotti, & Ivnik, 2005d), the Trail-Making Test, Stroop Test and MAE Controlled Oral Word Association Test (Steinberg, Bieliauskas, Smith, & Ivnik, 2005a), the Wechsler Memory Scale-Revised (Steinberg, Bieliauskas, Smith, & Ivnik, 2005b), and the Rey Auditory Verbal Learning Test and Visual Spatial Learning Test (Steinberg, Bieliauskas, Smith, Ivnik, & Malec, 2005c). Using a "Core Battery" consisting of the WAIS-R, WMS-R, and Rey AVLT, factor analyses have identified a five factor structure, consisting of Verbal Comprehension (WAIS-R Information, Vocabulary, Comprehension, and Similarities), Perceptual Organization (WAIS-R Picture Completion, Picture Arrangement, Block Design, Object Assembly, and Digit Symbol), Attention (WAIS-R Digit Span and Arithmetic, WMS-R Mental Control, Visual Span, and Logical Memory I), Learning (AVLT Learning Over Trials, WMS-R Figural Memory, Logical Memory I, Visual Associates I & II, Verbal Associates I & II, and Visual

Reproduction I), and Retention (AVLT percent retention, WMS-R Logical Memory percent retention, WMS-R Visual Reproduction percent retention) (Smith et al., 1992). This factor structure has been replicated in a clinical sample (Smith, Ivnik, Malec, & Tangalos, 1993).

Given that the MOANS data were collected on a very ethnically homogeneous sample residing in the upper Midwestern United States, separate normative data have been published for the Mayo Older African American Normative Studies (MOAANS). This sample of over 300 African American participants between the ages of 56 and 94 residing in Jacksonville, Florida, was administered most of the neuropsychological measures that were administered to the original Caucasian sample (Lucas et al., 2005d). Normative data for African Americans is available for the WMS-R (Lucas et al., 2005c), the Rey Auditory Verbal Learning Test (Ferman et al., 2005), the Mattis Dementia Rating Scale (Rilling et al., 2005), and the Boston Naming Test, Controlled Oral Word Association Test, Verbal Category Fluency, Animal Naming, MAE Token Test, Wide Range Achievement Test-3 Reading Subtest, Trail Making Test, Stroop Test, and Judgment of Line Orientation (Lucas et al., 2005b). The authors collected data for the WAIS-R, but given that the WAIS-III was released during data collection, the authors did not publish the WAIS-R data. However, the data are available from the authors upon request (Lucas et al., 2005a). Using the Core Battery described earlier, a five-factor structure has been replicated using the African American normative data (Pedraza et al., 2005).

Normative Data for the Oldest Old

As will be described in subsequent sections, revisions of existing cognitive and neuropsychological instruments are extending the age range of normative data through 90 years of age. Given the growing older adult population over 75 years of age, these extended normative data are of obvious clinical utility. However, few normative data exist for persons over 90 years of age. Although these individuals comprise a relatively small proportion of the population, there are still situations in which they could benefit from neuropsychological evaluation. However, without satisfactory normative data to compare their performance against, it is difficult to make confident clinical decisions.

Among the oldest old, it is unclear just what constitutes normal aging, as dementia, sensory impairment, and physical limitations have an extremely high prevalence in this group. If normative data are to be collected in this age group, a decision must be made as to whether to include a random sample of persons in this age group (to characterize cognitive performance in the "typical" older adult) or whether to exclude persons with physical, sensory, or cognitive limitations (which could result in a very small sample).

Although persons over 100 years of age have been followed in a number of studies, cognitive functioning has not been a typical focus of investigation. Miller and colleagues studied a population-based sample of 244 centenarians and near-centenarians, aged 98 to 108 years of age, and contrasted their performance with a random sample of octogenarians (Miller et al., in press). This sample was drawn from a 44 county region in northern Georgia in the United States and included persons in skilled nursing facilities as well as older adults living in the community. In this study, normative data were presented for the Mini-Mental State Examination (Folstein, Folstein, & McHugh, 1975), the Behavioral Dyscontrol Scale (Grigsby, Kaye, & Robbins, 1992; Kaye, Grigsby, Robbins, & Korzun, 1990), and the Severe Impairment Battery (Saxton, McGonigle-Gibson, Swihart, Miller, & Boller, 1990; Saxton & Swihart, 1989). Data are presented for two age cohorts in the octogenarian group (80–84 and 85–89) and four age cohorts (98–99, 100–101, 102–103, and 104+) in the centenarian group. Cognitive performance on each of these broad measures in centenarians and near-centenarians was substantially below that of octogenarians. The substantial difference between these two extreme age groups indicate that normative data for centenarians have value for characterizing the "typical" mean and range of cognitive performance among persons in this age group.

CLINICAL CONSIDERATIONS IN ASSESSING THE OLDER ADULT

Perhaps the most important consideration in neuropsychological assessment of older adults is to encourage their maximal level of performance. It is critical that the examinee understand the reasons for the assessment, as well as what will be expected of them during the evaluation. Adequate notification and preparation prior to the assessment can pay significant dividends in the establishment of rapport from the beginning of the evaluation. Furthermore, personal contact with the examinee on the day prior to the assessment can be used to ensure that appropriate corrective devices (glasses, hearing aids) and collateral informants are brought to the evaluation, if needed.

Establishing rapport through a friendly and supportive relationship is critical in the assessment of older adults. Some examinees may be extremely self-conscious of their cognitive limitations and may be intimidated by the testing session itself. Other examinees may have limited awareness of their deficits and become somewhat resistant to the evaluation of cognitive domains that reveal specific shortcomings. Finally, many patients have not been suitably prepared for what to expect of the neuropsychological evaluation.

It is often helpful to begin the evaluation with a relaxed discussion of the purpose of the assessment. The examinee should be reassured that the evaluation will not only examine particular areas that are challenging, but it will also thoroughly study abilities that are being performed well. The examinee should be supported for their successes and supported in the event of failures. Periodic breaks may be helpful in managing episodic frustration or fatigue. In some cases, multiple brief testing sessions across separate days may minimize fatigue. If this procedure is used, scheduling the examinee at the same time of day may help to minimize diurnal fluctuations in cognitive status.

Considerations regarding the testing environment itself are also important. Adequate lighting (preferably using full spectrum light) is extremely important. One may wish to have an additional desk lamp or floor lamp in case additional lighting may be required. Adequate ventilation and a reasonable degree of soundproofing and separation from nearby rooms are also essential. While testing rooms can vary from medical examination rooms to standard office settings, every effort should be paid to minimizing significant distractions and clutter in the room. Testing should take place at a standard office desk, if possible, in order to provide enough room to perform various tasks during the evaluation. The examinee's chair is also a critical consideration. An ergonomic chair, with sufficient lumbar support and adjustable controls, will help ensure that the examinee may remain in a comfortable posture during the evaluation.

As noted earlier, physical and sensory limitations are common among older adults. These challenges can complicate the interpretation of test results, and they can also make testing somewhat more difficult for the examinee. Simple screening of vision and hearing at the outset of any evaluation should be an essential and routine component of all assessments. Relatively gross screening of vision may be undertaken prior to the evaluation, using a near-card screener (available in most medical bookstores) to assess the examinee's ability to read accurately. Alternatively, the examinee can be asked to simply read a short paragraph from a book or magazine. Hearing can be grossly screened by standing behind the examinee and lightly rubbing the fingers together, alternating between each ear. The examinee can be asked to identify the side of the sound source. Sometimes a snap of the fingers might be required, or even louder stimuli may be necessary. By documenting the level of stimuli needed to elicit a response prior to neuropsychological testing, subsequent test results can be placed in the context of the degree of sensory impairment, if present. It is clearly much better to identify vision or hearing limitations prior to undertaking the evaluation than after the evaluation has been completed.

Because arthritis is extremely common among older adults (Schmader et al., 1998), it should be routinely evaluated as a contributing factor to slow or inefficient motor performance. For instance, an examinee with arthritis may have difficulty holding a pencil adequately, and may have particular difficulty with tasks requiring significant manual manipulation. Standardized stimulus materials should always be used when possible, although patients with visual impairment can sometimes benefit from presentation of stimulus material that has been enlarged on a photocopier. As an alternative, a magnifying glass can be kept in the testing room in case magnification of stimuli is necessary. For examinees with diminished auditory acuity, small audio amplifiers that are often available at local drug stores may be helpful adjuncts during the assessment. Importantly, the presence of any sensory deficit that may affect performance and deviations from standardized procedures must be documented by the examiner in the clinical report. Storandt has presented an extremely helpful chapter describing additional principles and recommendations for assessment of older adults (Storandt, 1994).

MEASURES FOR ASSESSING NEUROPSYCHOLOGICAL FUNCTIONING IN OLDER ADULTS

In the following section, measures for assessing intellectual, memory, and executive functioning, along with dementia screening measures and brief measures of anxiety and depressive symptoms, will be described, with a focus on their application to older adults. Measures such as the Wechsler Adult Intelligence Scale-IV (WAIS-IV; Wechsler, 2008) and Wechsler Memory Scale-IV (WMS-IV; Wechsler, 2009) are relatively new, whereas others are well established (e.g., RAVLT; Rey, 1958). Each of these tests has its own set of strengths and weaknesses, although each also has unique features that can be useful in both clinical and research contexts.

Intellectual Functioning Measures

Wechsler Adult Intelligence Scale-III (WAIS-III; Wechsler, 1997)

There has been a steady progression of improvements with new revisions of the Wechsler Adult Intelligence Scale over the years. The third edition of the Wechsler Adult Intelligence Scale (WAIS-III) improved upon its predecessor, the Wechsler Adult Intelligence Scale-Revised (WAIS-R; Wechsler, 1981) in a number of ways. A significant enhancement provided by the WAIS-III was the upward extension of age-based normative data from the previous upper limit of 75 years of age to a new upper limit of 89 years of age. At the time of the WAIS-III revision, the population of adults aged 75 years and over constituted 5.5% of the total population of the United States (U.S. Bureau of the Census, 1995). Estimates as of July 2008 suggest that this figure has grown slightly to approximately 6.2% (U.S. Bureau of the Census, 2008), or approximately 1.24 out of every 20 U.S. citizens. This growing segment of the population indicates the striking need for extended age-based normative data. The WAIS-III did not provide age-based normative data for persons aged 90 years and older. Although this age group constitutes a smaller proportion of the population as of July 2008 (0.71%), census estimates suggest considerable growth, having risen from 0.52% in July 2000 (U.S. Bureau of the Census, 2008).

Several other structural and cosmetic changes were also introduced with the WAIS-III that were helpful in facilitating the performance of older adults. For example, the WAIS-III updated a number of items to make them more contemporary for both older and younger persons alike. The artwork on several subtests was also made more contemporary, colorful, and larger (e.g., Picture Completion) to help with visual acuity difficulties, and some manipulanda (e.g., Picture Arrangement cards) were made sturdier. The WAIS-III also introduced a different structure in which four index scores (corresponding to independent factors derived from WAIS-III subtests) could be used independently of or to supplement three IQ scores. However, the structure of the index scores was observed to be different for persons 75 years of age and over relative to younger adults. Although the Verbal Comprehension

Index (Vocabulary, Information, and Similarities subtests) and the Working Memory Index (Digit Span, Arithmetic, and Letter-Number Sequencing subtests) were stable across the ages covered by the WAIS-III, the Perceptual Organization and Processing Speed factors reflected different subtest loadings for older and younger persons. For persons under 75 years of age, the Perceptual Organization factor included the Picture Completion, Block Design, Matrix Reasoning, and Picture Arrangement subtests, while the Processing Speed factor was made up of the Digit Symbol-Coding and Symbol Search subtests. In contrast, for persons between 75 and 89 years of age, the Perceptual Organization factor consisted solely of the Matrix Reasoning subtest, while the three remaining timed subtests (Picture Completion, Picture Arrangement, Block Design) loaded on the Processing Speed factor along with Digit Symbol-Coding and Symbol Search. Despite these age-related structural differences in the structure of cognition, the publisher recommended that the structure seen for younger adults be applied to older adults in light of results of confirmatory factor analyses and clinical validity studies.

Wechsler Adult Intelligence Scale (WAIS-IV; Wechsler, 2008)

The WAIS-IV was released in 2008. The WAIS-IV extended the age range beyond that of the WAIS-III by one year (from 89 years, 11 months to 90 years, 11 months). The WAIS-III normative group included 200 participants in each of 11 age groups (from 16 years through 79 years), 150 participants in the 80—84 year age group, and 100 participants in the 85—89 year age group. In contrast, the WAIS-IV included 100 fewer participants than the WAIS-III in each of the 70—74 year and 75—79 year groups, and 50 fewer participants in the 80—84 year groups. Thus, the WAIS-IV normative data are based on a smaller sample for three of the four older age groups, as compared with the WAIS-III. Nevertheless, for older adults, the standard errors of measurement are generally smaller for the WAIS-IV subtests that are shared in common with the WAIS-III, as well as for the index scores and Full Scale IQ.

Several structural changes were made to the WAIS-IV. The Verbal IQ and Performance IQ were eliminated. Currently, the principal index scores include the Full Scale IQ, the Verbal Comprehension Index, the Perceptual Reasoning Index, the Working Memory Index, and the Processing Speed Index. The WAIS-IV no longer includes the Picture Arrangement and Object Assembly subtests, nor are two previously optional procedures for Digit Symbol (Incidental Learning and Copy) used in the current version. Three new subtests were added to the WAIS-IV. In Visual Puzzles, a timed subtest, the examinee is asked to reconstruct a completed puzzle using three, and only three, response options. Figure Weights presents the examinee with a scale that has missing weights and selects a response that will balance the scale. Figure Weights is not administered to persons who are 70 years of age or over. Cancellation requires the examinee to view a structured arrangement of shapes and mark target shapes as quickly as possible. Cancellation is also not administered to persons who are 70 years of age or over. Comprehension, Picture Completion, Figure Weights, Cancellation, and Letter—Number Sequencing are supplemental subtests that may be substituted for other subtests that are spoiled or unable to be administered. However, normative data for the latter three subtests (Figure Weights, Cancellation, and Letter—Number Sequencing) are not available for persons who are 70 years of age or older, and thus they are not used as supplemental subtests for older adults. These three subtests were omitted for older adults in order to reduce possible fatigue effects during standardization. Therefore, for persons 70 years of age and older, only Picture Completion and Comprehension may be used as supplemental subtests for their respective index scores. However, if an older adult spoils a subtest from either the Working Memory Index or Processing Speed Index, the index score cannot be computed, but proration of the Full Scale IQ can be performed.

The core subtests for the Verbal Comprehension Index include Similarities, Vocabulary, and Information. Core subtests for the Perceptual Reasoning Index include Block Design, Matrix

Reasoning, and Visual Puzzles. The Working Memory Index uses Digit Span and Arithmetic as its core subtests. Finally, the core subtests for the Processing Speed Index include Symbol Search and Coding. According to the WAIS-IV Technical and Interpretive Manual (Wechsler, 2008), the average time required to administer the ten core subtests is 67 minutes, a reduction of approximately 13 minutes over the WAIS-III.

Several changes to the WAIS-IV focused on addressing sensory and psychomotor speed limitations for older adults. For example, subtest instructions are now made explicit on sample items, regardless of performance accuracy. That is, the problem-solving approach that should be used is described for the examinee regardless of whether they perform a sample item correctly. In addition, the number of items with time bonus points was reduced for Block Design and completely eliminated for Arithmetic. The inclusion of phonetically similar numbers (e.g., 5 and 9) and letters has been eliminated on Digit Span and Letter–Number Sequencing, in order to minimize the influence of reduced auditory acuity. In like manner, visual stimuli and artwork have been made larger to compensate for reduced visual acuity. Finally, motor demands have also been minimized by eliminating motor-dependent subtests, such as Picture Arrangement and Object Assembly. These latter subtests have been replaced with subtests that have relatively few motor demands, such as Figure Weights and Visual Puzzles.

The WAIS-IV includes clinical validity studies that were performed with a number of clinical groups, and persons with mild cognitive impairment (MCI) and Alzheimer's disease (AD) were included among these groups. The MCI sample included 53 persons between the ages of 59 and 90 years with clinically defined MCI (Petersen et al., 2001a, 2001b). Relative to a matched control group, significant reductions on FSIQ and all four index scores were observed for the MCI group. Significant reductions across all subtests except Vocabulary, Symbol Search, Letter–Number Sequencing, Figure Weights, and Cancellation were observed (Wechsler, 2008). The AD group included 44 individuals between 58 and 90 years of age who were identified with mild AD according to diagnostic criteria (McKhann et al., 1984). FSIQ and all index scores and subtests were significantly reduced compared to a matched control group. These reductions associated with mild AD were particularly noteworthy for the Processing Speed Index and its core subtests, as well as for Information and Arithmetic (Wechsler, 2008).

Kaufman Adolescent and Adult Intelligence Test (KAIT; Kaufman & Kaufman, 1993, 1997)

The KAIT was developed as an individually administered intelligence test for persons between the ages of 11 and 85 years and older. It was based on an integration of the fluid and crystallized intelligence model (Horn & Cattell, 1966, 1967; Horn, 1985, 1989), as well as aspects of Piaget's theory of formal operations (Piaget, 1972) and Luria's neuropsychological concepts of planning ability (Luria, 1980). The integration of multiple theories of intelligence and cognitive processing lends considerable appeal to this measure.

The KAIT yields Fluid, Crystallized, and Composite IQs with a mean of 100 and standard deviation of 15. A 60-minute Core Battery may be administered, or additional data (including delayed recall) may be obtained by administering a 90-minute Expanded Battery. The Expanded Battery is typically recommended for use with older adults, given the presence of the additional neuropsychological components in the battery. The normative sample consisted of 2000 adolescents and adults between the ages of 11 and 94 years. The upper age group includes 100 persons between the ages of 75 and 94 years (65 females and 35 males), a group that spans nearly two decades. The lack of more age-specific normative data in the upper end of the age spectrum is potentially problematic. Nevertheless, age-related differences in fluid and crystallized intelligence across the lifespan are observed in the normative data for the KAIT (Kaufman & Kaufman, 1997). Crystallized intelligence abilities increased or remained the same through 50 years of age and did not begin to decline until ages 75 and older. Fluid intelligence abilities reached a peak around 20 years of age followed by a plateau between 20 and 50 years of age, and ending with a drop in ability after 55 years of age.

The subtests of the KAIT are generally quite novel and are unlike many cognitive measures routinely used in clinical practice. The Crystallized IQ scale is made up of four subtests: Definitions; Auditory Comprehension; Double Meanings; and Famous Faces. The Definitions subtest assesses knowledge of word meanings. It presents several letters of the target word, along with blanks indicating several other missing letters. In addition, a clue about the word's meaning is presented, and the examinee must use the configuration of the word along with the clue to identify the target word. Auditory Comprehension requires listening to a recording of a news story and then answering questions about the story. Double Meanings presents two sets of word clues, and the examinee must find a word that is closely related to both word clues. Famous Faces, an alternate subtest, involves identifying the names of famous individuals based on a photograph and a verbal clue.

The Fluid Scale includes four subtests. Rebus Learning requires the examinee to associate a word or concept with various rebus drawings. "Sentences" of rebuses are then presented, and the examinee must interpret the sentence using only the rebuses. Logical Steps involves logical reasoning skills based on visual and auditory premises. Based on the premises given, the examinee must respond to a series of questions by applying logical reasoning skills. Mystery Codes requires the examinee to identify specific codes associated with a picture and then deduce a code for a novel picture based on the preceding codes and pictures. This task involves a timed component. Memory for Block Designs is an alternate subtest for the Fluid Scale. An abstract design is briefly presented to the examinee and subsequently removed. The examinee must recall the design and reproduce it using six cubes. This measure is also timed.

Additional subtests include Rebus Delay Recall and Auditory Delayed Recall. These measures assess the ability to recall the previously learned rebuses after 45 minutes and the ability to recall the previously presented news story after 25 minutes, respectively.

Despite its excellent initial normative data, there do not appear to be revised normative data available to reflect changing census demographics. The measure consists of a number of novel, theoretically based tests, but unfortunately, relatively few research studies have employed the KAIT. The integration between assessment of both intellectual and neuropsychological abilities is highly appealing, particularly for older adults. Updated normative data and/or a revised version of the KAIT may enhance its utility in the future. Nevertheless, consideration should be given to the KAIT in research settings where assessment of fluid and crystallized intellectual skills are of interest.

Woodcock-Johnson Tests of Cognitive Ability (WJ III COG; Woodcock, McGrew, & Mather, 2001b)

Although it is often considered for use with younger individuals in the context of a psychoeducational battery, the WJ III COG might be considered for use with older adults. The WJ III COG is a third-generation measure that originated with the Woodcock-Johnson Psycho-Educational Battery (Woodcock & Johnson, 1977). It is made up of 20 subtests that assess different aspects of cognitive functioning. It may be divided into two sections: the Standard Battery (tests 1–10) and the Extended Battery (tests 11–20). The administration of this battery extends considerable flexibility to the examiner to choose combinations of test score clusters of clinical interest, depending on the purpose of the evaluation. Therefore, one need not administer all tasks comprising either battery. The examiner is free to select and administer subtests that are tailored to answering the referral question. Each subtest takes approximately five minutes, and seven standard subtests that make up the Cognitive Battery typically take 35 to 45 minutes to administer.

The test is rooted in the Cattell-Horn-Carroll (CHC; Carroll, 1993, 1997, 1998; Horn & Cattell, 1966, 1967; Horn, 1985; Horn & Noll, 1997) theory of cognitive abilities. Although it provides a broad index of general intellectual ability (Stratum III) and 20 indexes of narrow cognitive abilities (Stratum I), its primary purpose is to assess broad factor scores based on CHC theory (Stratum II).

The broad factors scores include Comprehension-Knowledge (Gc), Long-Term Retrieval (Glr), Visual-Spatial Thinking (Gv), Auditory Processing (Ga), Fluid Reasoning (Gf), Processing Speed (Gs), and Short-Term Memory (Gsm). The WJ III COG Technical Manual illustrates hypothesized changes in each of these Stratum II abilities over the lifespan. The different developmental trajectories of each of these abilities provide evidence that they represent unique constructs associated with cognitive functioning.

The WJ III COG was standardized on a representative sample of the U.S. population, including 8818 individuals between the ages of 24 months and 90 years of age and older. The adult sample included 1843 subjects. The original normative data were based on the final 2000 U.S. Census statistics. A normative update was released in 2007 (WJ III NU; McGrew, Schrank, & Woodcock, 2007), which updated U.S. Census projections and applied a bootstrapping approach for estimating sample statistics and computing revised normative data. The bootstrapping approach is a state-of-the-art statistical approach for generating more precise sample estimates for a given age group. It is important to note that no new normative data were collected. The Normative Update simply applied updated census statistics to existing data to generate more accurate normative information.

The Woodcock Johnson-III Achievement Battery (WJ III ACH; Woodcock, McGrew, & Mather, 2001a) is also available, with normative data extending through 90 years of age. This battery is typically administered as a supplement to the WJ III COG. It includes 22 subtests designed to sample aspects of oral language and academic achievement. Consistent with CHC theory, several additional cognitive domains are assessed by the WJ III COG. The domains include Reading−Writing (Grw), Mathematics (Gq), and Oral Language and Knowledge. This latter domain includes a Story Recall test that assesses recall of a prose passage, together with a delayed recall component that requires reconstructive memory. The Understanding Directions subtest assesses aspects of working memory, including the ability to learn specific instructions and maintain them in awareness until a new command changes the directions. Oral comprehension is a listening comprehension task requiring several aspects of complex cognitive processing. Picture Vocabulary may also be a useful adjunct to a neuropsychological battery to evaluate object recognition and semantic retrieval.

The Woodcock Johnson-III Cognitive and Achievement test batteries are frequently used for the assessment of learning disabilities and general psychoeducational evaluation. They appear to be less often used for the assessment of older adults, which is somewhat puzzling given its excellent standardization data and assessment of specific broad cognitive abilities that show differing developmental trajectories across the age span. It is noteworthy that the recent revisions of the Wechsler Adult Intelligence Scale (WAIS-III and WAIS-IV) have attempted to align themselves more consistently with CHC theory. The recent abandonment of the Verbal IQ and Performance IQ in favor of emphasizing the four index scores (which have direct correlates with CHC theory Stratum II factors) is similar in many respects to the structure of the WJ III COG battery. Unfortunately, despite its relatively long history (since at least 1977), there is very little research that investigates the use of the Woodcock-Johnson measures with older adults. Future research applying the WJ-III Cognitive and Achievement batteries to older adults could refine and extend our current understanding of the nature and pattern of age-related cognitive changes.

Memory Assessment Measures

Wechsler Memory Scale-IV (WMS-IV; Wechsler, 2009)

The WMS-IV was released in early 2009. As with the WAIS-IV, particular attention was paid to revising the battery with older adults in mind. For example, the WMS-IV includes a brief cognitive screening tool that may help identify persons with dementia. In addition, during standardization, most older adults received the WMS-IV first, followed by the WAIS-IV on next day in order to minimize fatigue. The number of subtests administered in the older age range is also reduced.

The standardization sample for the WMS-IV included 1400 adults; 900 adults between the ages of 16 and 69 were included in the standardization sample for the Adult Battery and 500 adults between 65 and 90 years of age were included in the standardization sample for the Older Adult Battery. The WMS-IV contains the following subtests: Logical Memory; Verbal Paired Associates; Designs; Visual Reproduction; Spatial Addition; Symbol Span; and Brief Cognitive Status Exam. The Adult Battery is designed to yield five memory index scores, including the Auditory Memory Index (includes Logical Memory I & II and Verbal Paired Associates I & II), the Visual Memory Index (includes Visual Reproduction I & II and Designs I & II), the Visual Working Memory Index (includes Spatial Addition & Symbol Span), the Immediate Memory Index (includes Logical Memory I, Verbal Paired Associates I, Designs I, and Visual Reproduction I), and the Delayed Memory Index (includes Logical Memory II, Verbal Paired Associates II, Designs II, and Visual Reproduction II). New subtests to this edition of the WMS-IV include Designs, Spatial Addition, Symbol Span, and Brief Cognitive Status exam.

The Older Adult Battery, for persons who are between 65 and 90 years of age, includes Logical Memory, Verbal Paired Associates, and Visual Reproduction. This battery yields only four index scores, including the Auditory Memory Index (includes Logical Memory I & II and Verbal Paired Associates I & II), the Visual Memory Index (includes Visual Reproduction I & II), the Immediate Memory Index (includes Logical Memory I, Verbal Paired Associates I, and Visual Reproduction I), and the Delayed Memory Index (includes Logical Memory II, Verbal Paired Associates II, and Visual Reproduction II). The Symbol Span subtest may also be administered, although a Visual Working Memory Index is not obtainable.

Unlike its predecessor, the WMS-IV permits one to substitute scores from the California Verbal Learning Test-II (Trials 1−5 Free Recall T score and Long-Delay Free Recall z score) for the immediate and delayed Verbal Paired Associates scaled scores, in order to form an alternate Auditory Memory Index. In addition, it should be noted that for persons between 65 and 70 years of age, the examiner has a choice of administering the Standard Adult Battery or the Older Adult Battery.

During its standardization, the WMS-IV Older Adult Battery was administered to multiple clinical groups, three of which have direct relevance to aging: mild AD; MCI; and Major Depressive Disorder (Wechsler, 2009). In the mild AD clinical validity study, 48 patients with mild AD between the ages of 65 and 89 years were administered the Older Adult Battery. All mean index scores and subtest scores were significantly lower than a matched control group, although the General Ability Index (GAI) of the mild AD group was nearly 2½ standard deviations below that of the control group. Effect sizes were 2.0 or larger for all comparisons. Logical Memory II and Verbal Paired Associates I had the lowest subtest scores.

Examinees identified with MCI according to specific criteria who were between the ages of 55 and 84 were administered either the Adult Battery ($n = 14$) or the Older Adult Battery ($n = 36$). The GAIs for the MCI participants were slightly lower than the matched control group, but both groups performed in the average range. All index scores were significantly below those of the matched control group, although the biggest disparity was on the Visual Working Memory Index. For the MCI group, all memory index scores were one-third to one-half a standard deviation below the GAI, while memory index scores were more consistent with the GAI for the matched controls. Logical Memory I and II, Designs I, and Spatial Addition produced the largest disparities between MCI participants and matched controls.

The WMS-IV Older Adult Battery was administered to a small sample of examinees ($n = 10$) between the ages of 65 and 81 years who were diagnosed with Major Depressive Disorder (MDD) according to DSM-IV-TR criteria. Index scores for the MDD group were solidly in the average range, although effect sizes in the 0.7 to 0.8 range suggested lower performance for the MDD group. The only statistically significant difference between controls and the MDD group was on the Auditory Memory Index (uncorrected for multiple comparisons). The greatest subtest difference between the MDD group and matched controls was on Logical Memory I. Given the relatively small sample size in the MDD group, additional studies using larger samples are needed to understand more thoroughly the influence of MDD on WMS-IV subtest performance.

Rey Auditory Verbal Learning Test (AVLT; Rey, 1958)

This test was first described as a five-trial study-test word list learning procedure with a delayed recognition testing procedure designed to study characteristics of verbal learning and recall. Although over 20 different administration procedures have been described for the AVLT over the years (Schmidt, 1996), Muriel Lezak has been perhaps the most instrumental in introducing a relatively uniform AVLT administration technique to clinical neuropsychology (Lezak, 1976, 1983, 1995). The AVLT involves five sequential presentations of a 15-word list (List A, Trials 1 through 5). Each word is presented at the rate of one word per second. Following the first presentation of all 15 words, the examinee is asked to recall verbally as many words as possible. After the fifth attempt to recall List A words, a new 15-word list (List B) is presented to the examinee. After the examinee has recalled as many words as possible from List B (interference list recall trial, or Trial 6), he or she is asked again to recall as many words as possible from List A (post-interference recall trial, or Trial 7). After approximately 30 minutes, the examinee is again asked to recall as many words from List A as possible (Delayed Recall Trial). Finally, if the examinee generates only 13 words or fewer following the delayed recall trial, a recognition trial ensues, in which the 15 words from List A are interspersed with List B words and 20 distractor words that were not on either List A or List B. The examinee is asked to indicate whether the word presented was from List A. As noted earlier, there are a number of administration modifications that have been reported for the AVLT, which use various combinations of recognition testing formats, as well as inclusion or exclusion of the interference list or delayed recall (Schmidt, 1996). Normative data can be found in several excellent sources as well (Mitrushina, Boone, & D'Elia, 1998; Schmidt, 1996; Spreen & Strauss, 1998).

The AVLT can be a challenging task for many older adults. However, it provides a wealth of data for characterizing several aspects of memory functioning, and it can be particularly valuable in assessing suspected early dementia. Among healthy participants, the total number of words recalled across List A, Trials 1–5 has been shown to decrease with increasing age (Geffen, Moar, O'Hanlon, Clark, & Geffen, 1990), as persons over 70 years of age recalled at least ten fewer words than participants between the ages of 16 and 59. Persons between the ages of 60 and 69 recalled at least eight fewer words than participants under 40 years of age. Another study of memory functioning in 161 healthy older participants between the ages of 62 and 100 years demonstrated that the total number of words recalled across all trials of the AVLT decreased significantly with age and was also positively related to education (Petersen, Smith, Kokmen, Ivnik, & Tangalos, 1992). Similar findings have been reported when comparing the delayed recall trial with Trial 5 (Vakil & Agmon-Ashkenazi, 1997). Older participants recalled fewer words overall than younger participants. However, a significant age by trial interaction was observed, reflecting a somewhat steeper forgetting rate for the older group relative to the younger group (Vakil & Agmon-Ashkenazi, 1997).

Among healthy participants between the ages of 16 and 86, primacy and recency serial position effects have been demonstrated, with younger participants and females tending to recall more words at a given serial position (Geffen et al., 1990). In a sample of older participants between the ages of 57 and 85, similar primacy and recency serial position effects were demonstrated, with younger participants again tending to recall more words at a given serial position than older participants (Mitrushina, Satz, Chervinsky, & D'Elia, 1991).

Component analyses of multi-trial list learning tasks have demonstrated gains of new words across adjacent trials, as well as the omission of previously recalled words on subsequent trials (Tulving, 1964). Examination of the number of new words recalled on a given trial that were not recalled on the immediately preceding trial reflects gained access (intertrial learning). Gained access reflects the ability to profit from repeated presentations of the word list and is an important aspect of the learning curve. The number of words recalled on a given trial that were not recalled on the immediately succeeding trial reflects lost access or intertrial forgetting, and reflects another aspect of the learning curve. The concepts of gained and lost access have been investigated across the age span (Dunlosky & Salthouse, 1996). Relative to younger participants, no significant differences between older and younger participants were observed with respect to lost access, although older participants demonstrated significantly less gained access than younger participants. These findings suggest that age-related declines in trial-to-trial acquisition may affect list learning more than trial-to-trial forgetting over the age span (Dunlosky & Salthouse, 1996). Gained and lost access components in Alzheimer's patients and healthy controls, matched on age, education, and gender, have also been compared (Woodard, Dunlosky, & Salthouse, 1999). The component analyses revealed significantly decreased gained access and significantly greater lost access from trial-to-trial in the Alzheimer's patients relative to matched controls (Woodard, Dunlosky et al., 1999). More importantly, Woodard et al. noted that gained access and lost access were uncorrelated, suggesting that these two performance indexes are independent and separable. The concept of gained and lost access was investigated more recently (Moulin, James, Freeman, & Jones, 2004), and the results of Woodard et al. (1999) were replicated in a larger sample of AD, MCI, and healthy elderly participants using the CERAD Word List Learning measure. Finally, gained and lost access scores have been investigated in four age groups, using healthy participants (Davis et al., 2003). Increasing age was associated with increases in lost access. In contrast to the findings presented by Dunlosky and Salthouse (1996), gained access was observed to be the greatest between Trials 1 and 2, whereas Dunlosky and Salthouse (1996) demonstrated the lowest gained access between Trials 1 and 2. Nevertheless, age differences were minimal for measures of gained access.

California Verbal Learning Test-II (CVLT-II; Delis, Kramer, Kaplan, & Ober, 2000)

The CVLT-II is a 16-item word list-learning task that permits the analysis of a number of aspects of immediate and delayed auditory-verbal memory. In many respects, the administration and interpretation of the CVLT-II is similar to that of the AVLT. However, the words on the CVLT-II are drawn from several semantic categories. There are five study-test learning trials, followed by presentation of a distractor list. After recall of the distractor list has been attempted, the examinee is asked to recall the original list (Short-Delay Free Recall). Next, each of the semantic category cues is presented in an attempt to facilitate recall (Short-Delay Cued Recall). Thirty minutes later, the examinee is again asked to recall the original word list (Long-Delay Free Recall) and then is provided with the semantic category cues once more (Long-Delay Cued Recall). Finally, recognition testing may be performed using a "yes-no" format and a forced choice format.

The 16-item version may be too overwhelming and stressful for persons with even mild memory impairment. Therefore, a 9-item "dementia version" of the CVLT (Kaplan, 1995; Libon et al., 1996; Woodard, Goldstein, Roberts, & McGuire, 1999) was created to lower the floor of the memory test. It is administered in largely the same way as the parent instrument, although it consists of only three words from each of three semantic categories.

Fuld Object Memory Evaluation (FOME; Fuld, 1981; Fuld, Maser, Blau, Crystal, & Aronson, 1990)

The (FOME 1990) was developed for testing learning and memory in elderly persons, and has been standardized on both nursing home residents and community-dwelling people. In addition to assessing components of immediate and delayed memory performance, it also yields indexes of right-left discrimination, object naming accuracy, and semantic verbal fluency. Ten common objects are presented in a black cloth bag (bottle, ball, key, nail, matchbook, ring, button, playing card, cup, and scissors) and the examinee is asked to identify each of the objects, first by touch, and then by vision. Thus, multiple sensory modalities are used to maximize the acquisition of the to-be-learned material. Left and right hands are systematically alternated in order to provide information regarding right-left discrimination. After identifying all objects by touch and pulling each object out of the bag to see if the examinee was right, the objects are replaced in the bag, and a 60-second verbal category generation task (First Names) is used as a distractor task. The examinee is then asked to recall the objects from the bag during a 60-second recall period. Four more recall trials then follow in which the examinee is reminded of the omitted items at the end of each 60-second recall period and distracted using 30-second verbal category generation tasks (foods, things that make people happy, vegetables, things that make people sad). Because it uses a selective reminding paradigm (Buschke, 1973; Buschke & Fuld, 1974), the examinee's storage efficiency (number of items recalled after the distractor task, presumed to be recalled from long-term storage) and retrieval efficiency (number of words recalled on each trial) may be assessed. Retrieval efficiency may further be broken down into repeated retrieval (the number of items recalled on successive trials without reminding), which is presumed to reflect normal memory, and ineffective reminders (the number of failures to recall an item on two successive trials), interpreted as a sign of impaired memory.

The FOME has been used in a number of studies of aging, dementia, and therapeutic trials. Excellent psychometric and normative data are available for use of the FOME (Fuld, 1981; Marcopulos, McLain, & Giuliano, 1997). The FOME has been used in a number of studies to predict development of dementia (Fuld et al., 1990; Masur et al., 1994) and it has shown significant correlations with neuropathological markers of dementia at autopsy (Dickson et al., 1995). It has also shown excellent cross-cultural applicability in both Hispanic (Loewenstein, Rubert, Argüelles, & Duara, 1995) and Japanese (Fuld, Muramoto, Blau, Westbrook, & Katzman, 1988) populations. It has also been shown to be remarkably insensitive to the effects of education (Marcopulos & McLain, 2003; Marcopulos, Gripshover, Broshek, McLain, & Brashear, 1999; Marcopulos et al., 1997).

Measures of Executive Functioning

Assessment of executive functioning skills is critically important when evaluating older adults. Although there are several different aspects and definitions of executive functioning, this set of skills involves the capacity to modulate one's behavior in response to environmental demands. Skills subsumed within this domain include behavioral regulation of motor functioning, working memory, capacity for inhibition, and simple and divided attention abilities. Executive functioning skills are among the earliest to decline with advancing age (Axelrod, Goldman, & Henry, 1992; Boone, Miller, & Lesser, 1993; Chao & Knight, 1997; Moscouitch & Winocur, 1995). There is a strong relationship between the capacity for independent living and the integrity of executive functioning abilities (Baird et al., 2001; Bell-McGinty et al., 2002; Cahn et al., 1998; Grigsby et al., 1998; Jefferson, Paul, Ozonoff, & Cohen, 2006). Ability to engage in instrumental activities of daily living appears to be directly tied to intact executive functioning skills (Jefferson, Paul et al., 2006; Royall et al., 2007). Careful assessment of these skills in older adults can reveal patterns of strengths and weaknesses that may be amenable to environmental supports and interventions.

Numerous measures of executive functioning have been well-studied in the literature, including the Wisconsin Card Sorting Test (Grant & Berg, 1948), Halstead Category Test (Reitan & Wolfson, 1985), Tower of Hanoi and Tower of London Tests, Trail Making Test (Reitan, 1958), and Stroop Test (Golden, 1978). However, the following section will cover three broad measures of executive functioning skills that are fairly brief and can be implemented easily with older adults.

Behavioral Dyscontrol Scale (BDS; Grigsby, Kaye, & Robbins, 1992; Kaye, Grigsby, Robbins, & Korzun, 1990)

The BDS evaluates the ability to regulate motor control, inhibition, and intentional guidance of behavior. A number of items are based on procedures developed by Luria (Luria, 1980) and are administered in standardized fashion. BDS scores have been shown to be superior to the MMSE as a unique predictor of functional autonomy in several studies (Kaye et al., 1990; Suchy, Blint, & Osmon, 1997). Four items assess simple and complex motor sequencing skills. Three items assess capacity for inhibition and suppression of a dominant response tendency. One item assesses verbal alphanumeric sequencing ability. The final item is the examiner's assessment of the examinee's insight into their performance. The first eight items are scored on a 0 (failure), 1 (impaired performance), 2 (normal performance) scale, while the last item is scored on a 0 (complete absence of ability to judge one's own performance) to 3 (intact insight) scale. This scoring methodology yields a maximum score of 19, with cognitively normal older persons scoring a mean of 12.8 ($SD = 3.9$) (Grigsby et al., 1992). There is an alternative scoring system in which the variance can be increased. In the alternative system, the first eight items are scored on a 0 through 3 scale, and the final item is scored on a 0 through 4 scale.

BDS scores have been shown to be predictive of mortality in older adults, independently of comorbid illnesses and demographics (Amirian et al., 2009). Assessment of executive functioning with the BDS was also found to be useful for informing nurses' admission prognoses for rehabilitation potential in a geriatric rehabilitation facility (Myers, Grigsby, Teel, & Kramer, 2009). Components of the BDS have been helpful for predicting aggression in psychogeriatric patients (Suchy & Bolger, 1999), with performance on the two go-no go tasks being more impaired in aggressive patients than in non-aggressive patients. A fluid intelligence factor derived from three BDS items was also more impaired in aggressive patients than in non-aggressive patients. An electronic version of the BDS has also been developed and successfully validated (Suchy, Derbidge, & Cope, 2005).

Delis-Kaplan Executive Functioning System (D-KEFS; Delis, Kaplan, & Kramer, 2001)

The D-KEFS consists of a collection of nine executive functioning measures that can be administered collectively or in a stand-alone fashion, and they can be administered in a group setting or individually. Normative data for each of these measures were collected on over 1750 (Homack, Lee, & Riccio, 2005) persons between the ages of 8 and 89, matched to United States Census Data, and all of the tests are co-normed. Most of these measures are familiar to neuropsychologists and are variants of measures that have a longstanding history of use in clinical neuropsychology. The following measures comprise the D-KEFS: Verbal Fluency Test; Design Fluency Test; Tower Test; Color-Word Interference Test; Sorting Test; Trail Making Test; Twenty Questions Test; Word Context Test; and Proverbs Test. The Proverbs Test can be used with persons between ages 16 and 89, although the remaining tests can be administered to persons between 8 and 89 years of age.

A thorough test review of the D-KEFS has been presented recently (Homack et al., 2005). As noted earlier, a particular advantage of this measure is that the individual tests in the battery can be administered as a whole, individually, or in specific groups designed to evaluate a particular aspect of executive functioning under different conditions. Interestingly, the authors state that most currently used measures of executive functions were developed in the 1940s, and the D-KEFS was designed to serve as a way to expand our knowledge regarding executive functions by implementing novel approaches to their assessment. The measure uses a cognitive process approach to evaluating performance, in order to characterize the unique methods used by a patient to obtain a particular score.

D-KEFS measures have been used as predictors of a variety of outcomes in a number of studies. For example, by comparing performance on the switching conditions of the Verbal Fluency and Design

Fluency tests in a sample of older adults, non-demented carriers of the APOE ε4 allele demonstrated a greater asymmetry in performance between the two tests than cognitively intact persons who did not carry the APOE ε4 allele (Houston et al., 2005). In another study of older adults between 65 and 92 years of age, a composite executive functioning measure made up of a scaled score average of the Trail Making Test, the Tower Test, the Verbal Fluency (Letter Fluency) Test, and the Design Fluency Test from the D-KEFS was shown to be positively related to performance on the Direct Assessment of Functional Status-Revised (DAFS-R; Loewenstein et al., 1989), a directly observed measure of instrumental and basic activities of daily living skills (Mitchell & Miller, 2008). Using a self-report measure of instrumental activities of daily living (Lawton & Brody, 1969), Jefferson and colleagues reported that the D-KEFS Color-Word Interference test, a measure of behavioral inhibition, was a significant predictor of multiple instrumental activities of daily living (Jefferson, Paul et al., 2006).

One limitation to the D-KEFS that has recently been proposed in the literature concerns the low reliability of D-KEFS contrast scores. The availability of contrast scores would theoretically permit neuropsychologists to interpret discrepancies in performance between different measures or different aspects of executive functioning. However, using test–retest and internal consistency reliability data from the D-KEFS manual, Crawford and colleagues (Crawford, Sutherland, & Garthwaite, 2008) have recently noted that the median reliability of D-KEFS contrast scores is only 0.30, and their associated standard errors of measurement were relatively large. As a result of this study, the authors recommend against using the D-KEFS contrast scores for clinical interpretation of an examinee's strengths and weaknesses.

Executive Interview (EXIT-25; Royall, Mahurin, & Gray, 1992)

The EXIT-25 is a 25-item measure designed to assess executive functioning. Taking approximately 10–15 minutes, the measure assesses domains such as verbal and design fluency, alphanumeric sequencing, spontaneous verbal description of a picture, memory, motor sequencing, and frontal lobe reflexes. The measure can easily be administered at the bedside and is highly portable.

EXIT-25 scores have been demonstrated to distinguish between possible AD patients with depression and patients with depression alone (Royall, Mahurin, & Cornell, 1995), and they are an important determinant of the level of care received by older retirees (Royall, Chiodo, & Polk, 2005). EXIT-25 scores also have been helpful in distinguishing between AD and frontal-type dementia (Royall, Mahurin, & Cornell, 1994). EXIT-25 scores are also associated with resistiveness to physical care in dementia patients (Stewart, Gonzalez-Perez, Zhu, & Robinson, 1999), and a substantial negative correlation ($r = -0.872$) has been reported between the EXIT-25 and the DAFS-R (Pereira, Yassuda, Oliveira, & Forlenza, 2008). Using an abbreviated EXIT (EXIT-15), an association was observed between gait speed decline and executive functioning (Atkinson et al., 2007). The EXIT-25 has also been used as an outcome measure in a pharmacologic intervention study for vascular dementia, and treatment with galantamine improved executive functioning after 26 weeks relative to placebo (Auchus et al., 2007).

Brief Measures of Mood

Assessment of Depression and Anxiety

The prevalence of clinically significant symptoms of anxiety and depression is relatively high among older individuals as compared with younger adults. Among community-dwelling elders, the prevalence of significant depressive symptoms has been estimated to range between 3 and 26% (Beekman, Copeland, & Prince, 1999; Beekman et al., 1995; Blazer, Burchett, Service, & George, 1991; Copeland et al., 1999; Hybels & Blazer, 2003). Anxiety disorders are also highly prevalent in late life. The National Institute of Mental Health Epidemiological Catchment Area (NIMH-ECA) studies

(Regier et al., 1988; Weissman, Leaf, Holzer, & Merikangas, 1985), based only on assessment of community-dwelling adults, revealed that anxiety disorders occur four to eight times more frequently than major depression among individuals aged 65 and older. A point prevalence rate for anxiety disorders of 7.3% in older adults was reported in the NIMH-ECA study (Regier et al., 1988). A point prevalence rate of 3.5% for community-dwelling elders was reported in a Canadian survey, but the rate was higher (5%) for elders living in institutional settings (Bland, Newman, & Orn, 1988). Indeed, Juninger et al. (1993) reported anxiety disorder rates nearly three times higher among nursing home residents relative to a community-dwelling sample. Differences between older adults residing independently and those residing in assisted living facilities suggest that some anxiety disorders may be significantly more prevalent among older adults living in supported environments (Calamari, Janeck, & Deer, 2002).

Evaluation of depression and anxiety disorders in older adults should be performed cautiously (Kogan, Edelstein, & McKee, 2000; Stanley & Beck, 1997). For example, detection and diagnosis of depression and anxiety in older adults may be complicated by the use of assessment instruments that have not been validated with elders (Fuentes & Cox, 1997), by older adults' reluctance to report psychological problems (Lasoski, 1986), or by their tendency to attribute psychological symptoms to physical conditions (Gurian & Miner, 1991). Furthermore, symptoms of depression and anxiety among older adults may differ from those expressed by younger adults (Stanley & Beck, 2000). Older adults may experience increased concern for cognitive functioning that may be associated with subtle cognitive changes associated with normal aging or to more significant changes associated with neurological disorders (Calamari et al., 2002). This concern may lead to a hypervigilance for cognitive changes, in addition to distress over perceived dysfunction. In addition, unique stressors emerging in later life (e.g., health concerns, loss of social supports, decreased financial resources, reduced mobility) may exacerbate life-long vulnerabilities and/or chronic symptoms, thereby producing significant anxiety pathology.

A number of brief self-report inventories and behavioral rating scales have been developed in order to assess the presence of anxiety and depressive symptoms and their change with treatment. For depression, these measures include the Geriatric Depression Scale (Yesavage, Brink, Rose, & Adey, 1986; Yesavage et al., 1983), the Hamilton Depression Rating Scale (HDRS-17; Hamilton, 1960), the Beck Depression Inventory-II (BDI-II; Beck, Steer, & Brown, 1996), and the Center for Epidemiological Screening-Depression (CES-D; Radloff, 1977). Brief measures for assessing anxiety include the Hamilton Anxiety Rating Scale (HARS; Hamilton, 1959), the Beck Anxiety Inventory (BAI; Beck, Epstein, Brown, & Steer, 1988), and the State-Trait Anxiety Inventory (STAI; Spielberger, Gorsuch, & Lushene, 1970).

CONTEMPORARY ISSUES IN GERIATRIC NEUROPSYCHOLOGY

Computer-Based Testing

Because most traditional cognitive measures involve a paper and pencil format or tangible manipulanda, they are likely to have some degree of familiarity with most examinees. However, a new generation of computer-based instruments has been introduced in recent years. Given that many older individuals have had little experience with computers, these instruments should be used carefully with older adults, taking into account each individual's familiarity with computer technology. For some persons, increased anxiety or confusion may result from using a computer or sophisticated stimulus recording materials or manipulanda during cognitive assessment.

Despite these caveats, there are a number of advantages of computer-based assessment instruments. For example, measures can be administered in a standardized fashion, and scoring can be virtually error free each time the instrument is used. Instructions can be presented in the auditory and/ or visual modalities, and the need for reading ability can be de-emphasized. This advantage also means that even persons with visual or hearing impairments can be administered the same computer battery in many cases. Examinees can have instructions repeated as often as needed. Subjectivity in scoring can be virtually eliminated via computer scoring algorithms. Finally, a given cognitive measure can be administered in exactly the same way during repeated assessments.

Reaction times to various stimuli can also be measured to the nearest millisecond. However, the actual timing accuracy is dependent on simultaneously running processes as well as the operating system. Any programs that have been started by the user, programs typically loaded during start-up, and internet access and Wi-Fi or Bluetooth service should be terminated prior to using a computer-based test. Computer-based tests can also be administered in groups (e.g., in a computer laboratory) or individually. Computer-based tasks are also portable and readily available to be implemented on smaller handheld devices or laptop computers. Typically, no data entry is required for computer-based testing. Data collected on a given subject can be imported to a database, thereby minimizing the impact of data entry errors. No administration or scoring expertise is often needed. Computer-based testing also enables neuropsychologists to assess persons in distant locations. For example, a computer battery could be administered in a remote location, and the data can be subsequently transmitted by fax or internet to the neuropsychologist for interpretation. Web-based delivery of a battery of computer tests is also possible, eliminating the need for complicated installation procedures and the use of a dedicated computer for the evaluation.

Although these many advantages of computer-based assessment are alluring, several disadvantages of computer-based assessment must also be considered. Many computer-based measures are platform dependent and cannot be administered on computers using different operating systems. However, web-based delivery of computer-based measures is helping to minimize the impact of this limitation. It is important to consider the technology associated with a given computer, as hardware issues could potentially produce timing differences across machines. It is important to calibrate the accuracy of a given computer before implementing it for clinical purposes, because computers with faster processors may yield different timing accuracy compared to those with slower processors. Other factors, such as the amount of video memory, whether the computer is a desktop or laptop, and the screen size and luminescence must all be taken into account in order to assess the absolute accuracy of the to-be-used computer. Input devices, such as keyboards, mice, or button boxes also have different latencies that could affect timing. Because one of the principal advantages of computer-based tests is timing accuracy, it is important for a developer of a computer-based test to include a calibration routine that can be used to calibrate a given machine using internal timing algorithms prior to its implementation for research or clinical use. Response boxes with virtually no timing delay are available and should also be implemented with computer-based cognitive assessments.

Subtest paradigms are currently somewhat limited in computer-based assessment. For example, most memory tasks are in a recognition-testing format. Recall testing is somewhat difficult to implement for a computer-based platform. Attention measures are typically limited to either simple or choice reaction time types of measures. Computer-based measures can also be costly. Although there are a few exceptions, many computer-based assessment battery's require yearly licensing fees or per use charges.

There are also human factors to take into account that could produce interindividual differences in task performance. The relative distribution of left and right mouse button presses must be taken into account for a given task, because the index and middle fingers may have different reaction times for a particular task. These differences can be magnified if serial administrations of a measure have differing numbers of right and left mouse button presses. Further, the way in which one uses an input device (e.g., resting a finger on a mouse button versus striking the mouse button with a finger) may also produce error variance unless controlled.

A final disadvantage related to computer-based assessment is that it is difficult to know when an individual is not putting forth good effort. Unless the examinee is monitored throughout the administration of the computer-based tasks, the extent to which they put forth consistent effort is an unknown. It is possible to build in algorithms to facilitate a "smart" administration that is sensitive to the examinee's level of performance. If accuracy or reaction time falls outside of a predetermined level, the program can prompt for the intervention of the test administrator. Continuous prompts can also be built into a program to encourage more diligent effort. Strategies designed to enhance the reliability of computer-based assessments, particularly when they are associated with greater task complexity, are essential for the success of this particular assessment approach. It is important to remain mindful of the fact that, in general, the only behavior that is actually measured in computer-based tests is the pressing of a button or key or the movement of the mouse.

Each of the above limitations has obvious technological solutions. Perhaps the most important issue involved with computer-based assessment is ensuring that timing on a given computer is accurate and reproducible, as well as comparable across different machines. Standardization of computers, operating systems, and input devices would have a significant effect on enhancing the reliability and validity of computer-based assessment of cognitive functioning.

There are a variety of computer-based cognitive assessment instruments currently available for research and clinical use. Some of the more prominent computer-based cognitive assessment measures include the HeadMinder Cognitive Screening Test (HeadMinder, Inc., New York, NY), CogState (CogState, Ltd., Melbourne, Australia), Automated Neuropsychological Assessment Metrics (ANAM; Center for the Study of Human Operator Performance, University of Oklahoma, Norman, OK), and Mindstreams (NeuroTrax Corp., Newark, NJ). An excellent review of the current status of the use of computer-based testing with older adults has been presented by Wild and colleagues (Wild, Howieson, Webbe, Seelye, & Kaye, 2008) but also see (Doniger & Simon, 2009; Wild & Kaye, 2009).

Research using computer-based cognitive measures with older adults is still in its infancy. Nevertheless, research with a number of these computer-based approaches has demonstrated that they show promise for screening and early detection of cognitive impairment, and they can be used for tracking dementia progression and as outcome measures in interventional trials. For example, ANAM has demonstrated efficacy as a screening tool for mild cognitive impairment (Kane, Roebuck-Spencer, Short, Kabat, & Wilken, 2007), and AD patients have been shown to be reliably impaired on several working memory measures from ANAM (Levinson, Reeves, Watson, & Harrison, 2005). ANAM has also been used as an outcome measure for an interventional trial of a transdermal nicotine patch for treatment of AD (White & Levin, 2004). In this latter study, decision reaction time from ANAM demonstrated improvement following patch administration. Using four administrations of CogState within a three-hour period, CogState demonstrated promise for detecting patients with MCI by virtue of diminished learning performance over the repeated trials (Darby, Maruff, Collie, & McStephen, 2002). CogState was also more sensitive to subtle memory change than a word list learning test or computer-based paired associate learning task after eight repeat administrations over 12 months (Maruff et al., 2004). In another study, while the Hopkins Verbal Learning Test (Brandt, 1991) was shown to detect MCI more accurately than CogState, CogState demonstrated stronger relationships with subjective memory complaints and competence in performing activities of daily living (de Jager, Schrijnemaekers, Honey, & Budge, 2009).

Perhaps some of the most extensive research on computer-based testing with older adults has been done with the Mindstreams computerized cognitive test battery. Initial validation studies found that the computer-based measures of memory, executive functioning, visuospatial ability and verbal fluency were particularly effective for differentiating healthy older adults from persons with MCI (Dwolatzky et al., 2003, 2004). Mindstreams has also been validated for differentiating participants with MCI from healthy older adults in urban African Americans (Doniger, Jo, Simon, & Crystal, 2009). This computer battery demonstrated efficacy for detecting cognitive impairment, even in the presence of depressive symptoms (Doniger et al., 2006), and it has been used as an outcome measure for assessing the effects of pharmacologic intervention in older adults with depression (Paleacu et al., 2007). No differences in cognitive performance on Mindstreams computer-based measures have been noted between post-menopausal short- and long-term users and non-users of hormone replacement therapy (Lavi et al., 2007). In an 11-center trial of the feasibility of implementing Mindstreams in an office-based setting, 83% of 2888 older adult patients rated the battery as easy to use (Fillit, Simon, Doniger, & Cummings, 2008). In addition, 73% of persons who do not use a computer, 70% of patients older than 75 years of age, and 69% of poor performing patients rated the tests as easy to use. Mindstreams also has a recently described co-normed estimate of premorbid intelligence that can be used to enhance classification of performance of persons with low or high levels of intellectual functioning (Doniger, Simon, & Schweiger, 2008).

Multicultural Neuropsychology

Within recent years, increasing attention has been focused on multicultural issues in clinical neuropsychology. Although a number of major tests have attempted to develop normative data based on a sample that is ethnically representative of the United States population, the issue of whether or to what extent normative standards should be developed for ethnic minorities is controversial (Manly, 2005, 2008; Manly & Echemendia, 2007). Corrections designed to be applied to specific ethnic minorities that adjust for age, sex, and number of years of education are intended to improve diagnostic sensitivity and specificity. However, these types of corrections have the potential to be particularly misleading when applied to test performance of older adults. Educational corrections can be particularly misleading, because of differential educational opportunities and qualities across majority and minority groups. In addition, given the relative lack of normative data for older adults in general, application of such corrections would be based on a small number of individuals, raising the potential for inaccuracies. Cultural differences between African American and Caucasian individuals have also been suggested to influence informant-based reports, leading to a reduced likelihood of diagnosing cognitive impairment, no dementia (CIND) in African Americans based on informant report relative to objective cognitive evaluation (Potter et al., 2009).

The intent of many measures that rely on an ethnically representative standardization sample appears to be portraying an examinee's performance relative to an average person of a given age from the United States. However, more specific normative data are sometimes needed to enhance diagnostic accuracy (Manly & Echemendia, 2007). A major issue that must be weighed in the decision to use or not use culturally based performance corrections rests with the question to be answered. For example, is the critical question one of diagnosis or a placement into a particular program? Alternatively, will a person's level of performance be used to qualify them for a particular service? Finally, one may be interested in whether a repeat evaluation shows a significant change from an earlier baseline level of performance. An argument for the use of culturally specific normative data could be put forth for the first two questions, although the issue of normative data becomes perhaps less important when an individual serves as their own clinical control.

The Hispanic population is currently the largest and fastest growing racial/ethnic group in the United States (U.S. Census Bureau, 2007), with the African American population constituting the second largest segment. While the following references are far from comprehensive, a considerable amount of ethical and normative research has been published for use with Hispanic individuals (Acevedo et al., 2009; Ardila, Rodriguez-Menendez, & Rosselli, 2002; Ardila, Rosselli, & Puente, 1994; Artiola i Fortuny, Heaton, & Hermosillo, 1998; Artiola i Fortuny & Mullaney, 1997; Ostrosky-Solis, Quintanar, & Ardila, 1989; Ponton & Ardila, 1999; Rey et al., 2001; Rey, Feldman, Rivas-Vazquez, Levin, & Benton, 1999;

Rosselli, Ardila, Florez, & Castro, 1990; Rosselli, Ardila, Salvatierra et al., 2002; Rosselli, Ardila, Santisi et al., 2002) and for African American individuals (Ferman et al., 2005; Hendrie et al., 1995; Lucas et al., 2005a, 2005b, 2005c, 2005d; Marcopulos & McLain, 2003; Pedraza et al., 2009, 2005; Rilling et al., 2005; Unverzagt et al., 1996, 1995; Welsh et al., 1995; Woodard, Auchus, Godsall, & Green, 1998; Yochim, Bank, Mast, MacNeill, & Lichtenberg, 2003).

There is clearly much research that still needs to be done in order to determine whether the diagnostic accuracy of many commonly used neuropsychological measures might be improved by inclusion of corrections for ethnicity (Romero et al., 2009). Along these lines it would appear to be critically important to take into account the degree of acculturation that has taken place for a given individual (Artiola i Fortuny et al., 1998; Manly, 2006; Manly, Byrd, Touradji, & Stern, 2004; Manly et al., 1998; Ponton & Ardila, 1999). It would be hard to argue that the same standards for performance should be applied to an individual who has resided in the United States for only six months compared to an individual who has lived in the country for 25 years. It is somewhat striking that many neuropsychological performance corrections for ethnic minorities have focused principally on demographic variables, rather than taking into account known base rates of diseases in specific ethnic groups, in specific geographic regions, at specific ages, etc.

Because of the significant impact of culture on many neuropsychological tests, it may be extremely difficult to develop versions of currently used measures that could be equally applied across ethnic majority and minority groups alike. We will likely have to tailor our evaluations to focus on assessing relatively basic neuropsychological functions. This type of problem is certainly not new. Howard Andrew Knox was faced with the same dilemma when attempting to assess non-English-speaking immigrants who arrived at Ellis Island between 1912 and 1916, just prior to World War I (Boake, 2002; Richardson, 2003; Vecchi & Richardson, 2001). Knox was faced with the task of developing creative measures that assessed important cognitive constructs, but which could be applied across cultures. A similar degree of creativity will likely be required in meeting contemporary challenges to multicultural neuropsychology.

Report Writing

A number of important texts and papers have been written on the topic of report writing. Although general practical and ethical principles would certainly apply in generating a neuropsychological report for an older individual, a number of specific recommendations can be offered. First, test results should be communicated to the referral source (and to the patient) as quickly as is feasible. This guideline is especially important for inpatient settings in order to permit a patient's test results to have a maximum impact on their treatment. This type of communication may take the form of a brief phone call with the referral source, or a brief and written or typewritten note in the client's chart.

Psychological reports should also make sure that the referral question is thoroughly answered. At times, ancillary issues and findings may arise during the course of an assessment, and these new issues may take the focus off the referral question. Nevertheless, every effort should be made to address the specific referral question(s) in the test results and subsequent recommendations. With respect to recommendations, the more specific the recommendation, the more likely the patient will be to actually act on that recommendation. Therefore, if the patient is being referred for psychotherapy, for example, listing two or three specific referral sources with telephone numbers will greatly enhance the likelihood that the client will follow up with that suggestion.

There are a number of different ways to organize a neuropsychological report. Some reports organize findings in a test-by-test format, whereas other reports may present test results based on specific themes or organized by cognitive domain. The inclusion of technical language or jargon also varies from report to report. In a recent study of report writing styles, a theme-based organization was preferred to a test-by-test organization by a group of experienced and inexperienced teachers alike

(Pelco, Ward, Coleman, & Young, 2009). Such an organization likely increases comprehension and retention of the information, because it is placed in a specific context. This format underlined the first sentence of a paragraph, and subsequently provided supporting information: "*Mary demonstrated a significantly greater weakness in auditory-verbal memory functioning relative to visual memory functioning*." Interestingly, there were few preference differences between a theme-based technical report (12th grade reading level) and a theme-based non-technical (8th grade reading level) report. The authors suggest that because little information is lost by presenting the results in a non-technical format, such an approach can be used to generate a report that would be equally understandable for a referral source or for the client and their family.

Serial Testing

Assessment of cognitive change over time frequently plays a major role in geriatric neuropsychology. Because diagnoses, such as dementia, require evidence of cognitive change over time, the ability to unequivocally document such a change becomes a significant clinical issue. Clearly, not all cognitive change among older adults is related to dementia, and it is important to be able to identify possible reasons for change on neuropsychological measures among older adults. Assessment of clinical change is also important in evaluating effectiveness of interventions for a variety of neurological and psychological conditions. A number of factors related to measurement of cognitive abilities make detection of actual change somewhat difficult. For example, measurement error due to less than perfect reliability of measures may obscure cognitive change over time. The effects of practice, particularly due to previous exposure to various cognitive measures, may also mask subtle cognitive change. Finally, the statistical phenomenon of regression to the mean can potentially magnify test–retest changes among persons who perform at the upper or lower limits of a given cognitive measure.

A variety of approaches have been used to address this clinical issue (Frerichs & Tuokko, 2005). One popular approach considers significant cognitive change to have occurred if test–retest performance differs by at least one standard deviation or more. However, this approach does not take into account absolute level of performance or the inherent unreliability of cognitive measures. One of the earliest approaches to this problem proposed a formula that takes into account the reliability of a given measure in assessing test–retest differences (Jacobson & Truax, 1991) and was among the first to suggest adoption of a so-called "reliable change index (RCI)." The RCI was computed according to the following formula:

$$RCI = \frac{x_2 - x_1}{SE_{diff}}; SE_{diff} = \sqrt{2(SD_x\sqrt{1 - r_{xx}})^2}$$

Thus, the standard error of the difference score is a function of the measure's standard deviation and the test–retest reliability of the measure of interest. The RCI is in z-score units, so RCI exceeding 1.96 would be associated with significant change ($p < 0.05$).

Other approaches simultaneously consider measurement error and practice effects (Chelune, Naugle, Luders, Sedlak, & Awad, 1993). Here, the practice effect can be defined by the mean difference between the baseline and follow-up administrations of the measure in a normative sample. Thus, the anticipated difference between an individual's follow-up score and their pretest score plus expected practice effect would be 0. Thus, a 90% confidence interval can be formed around the difference between follow-up and baseline score, corrected for expected practice effect.

$$[(x_2 - x_1) - (\overline{X}_2 - \overline{X}_1)] \pm SE_{diff} \times 1.645$$

Another approach advocated a standardized regression-based approach to evaluating change (McSweeny, Naugle, Chelune, & Luders, 1993). The advantage of this approach is that it takes into account both practice effects and regression to the mean by using a regression formula derived on a healthy control sample. This regression formula defines the expected change on a particular measure and can be applied at the individual level for each measure of interest. In this approach, post-test scores are simply predicted from pretest scores in the normative sample using standard multiple regression. If desired, entry of a second block of predictors including demographic variables, such as age, sex, and education, can be added. The weights associated with pretest score and demographic predictors can then be applied to an individual's data. Standardized regression-based scores exceeding 1.96 indicate significant cognitive change at the $p < 0.05$ level. Sawrie and colleagues demonstrated the application of this approach to assessing clinically relevant change among older adults (Sawrie, Marson, Boothe, & Harrell, 1999). The obvious drawback to the above procedures is the need to have access to a large normative population to derive the standardized regression-based formulas.

Case Study

Background

Ms J is a 75-year-old, Caucasian female with 12 years of education. Ms J and her family reported concerns about memory changes in which she sometimes repeated questions that she asked moments earlier. She has a paternal family history of Alzheimer's disease (AD), and, given her age, was appropriately concerned about development of AD herself. She even requested APOE genotyping, which revealed that she was a heterozygous carrier of the APOE ε4 allele. She stated that she has been quite healthy throughout her life and currently takes no medications. She rated her current subjective health as "Good." She has a 30 pack-year history of smoking and consumes one alcoholic beverage per day. Despite her subjective concern with memory functioning, she lives independently in the community and reported no difficulty carrying out activities of daily living.

Test results

Laboratory data revealed normal vitamin B12, folate, creatinine, and thyroid stimulating hormone, although homocysteine was slightly elevated at 19.0 mg/dl. Ms J was administered a brief neuropsychological battery as an initial screening. Her word recognition ability from the Reading subtest on the Wide Range Achievement Test-IV was 105, suggesting that her global premorbid skills are solidly in the average range. She denied significant depressive symptoms, obtaining scores of 2 on the Geriatric Depression Scale, 3 on the Center for Epidemiological Screening-Depression Scale, and 7 on the Beck Depression Inventory-II. Her score on the Mini-Mental State Examination (MMSE) was 30/30, and she also obtained a perfect total score (144/144; age and education corrected MOANS scaled score of 17) on the Mattis Dementia Rating Scale-2 (DRS-2; Form 1). She demonstrated an uneven performance on the learning trials of the RAVLT, recalling 8, 11, 8, 13, and 14 words across the five learning trials (Trials 1–5 score = 54). She recalled 7 words from List B and 13 words from List A on Trial 6, suggesting no compelling susceptibility to proactive or retroactive interference. She recalled 13 words after a 20-minute delay and demonstrated a long-term percent retention score of 93%. During recognition testing, she correctly recognized all 15 words and committed only one false positive error. She reported no impairment of instrumental or basic activities of daily living on the Lawton Personal Self-Maintaining Scale. She was asked to return in 18 months for a follow-up evaluation, given her family history and subjective concerns.

Follow-up evaluation

Ms J was still living independently but reported that her memory concerns were increasing. She continued to deny depressive symptoms on the Geriatric Depression Scale, as she endorsed only one item. Although she obtained a perfect 30/30 on the MMSE, her DRS-2 (Form 2) total score declined to 135. On this latter measure, she demonstrated declines on the Conceptualization and Memory subtests. Her age and education corrected MOANS scaled score was 10, demonstrating a drop of over two standard deviations. On an alternate form of the RAVLT, her immediate learning performance declined substantially. She recalled 6, 8, 10, 9, and 9 words across the five learning trials (Trials 1–5 score = 42). She recalled 7/15 words from List B and recalled 9/15 words on Trial 6, again suggesting no compelling susceptibility to proactive or retroactive interference. After 30 minutes, she recalled 8/15 words, with a long-term percent retention score of 89%. She correctly recognized 11/15 words, but committed two false positive errors during delayed recognition testing. She again reported that she was able to perform basic and instrumental activities of daily living without assistance on the Lawton Personal Self-Maintaining Scale.

Comment

Although Ms J's MMSE score remained stable after 18 months, she demonstrated a significant decline on the DRS-2. Her raw score change (144 to 135) of −9 points after 18 months is beyond the 90% reliable change boundaries corrected for practice effects that have been advocated by Pedraza and colleagues (Pedraza et al., 2007), suggesting significant cognitive change. Even after correcting for age and education, the drop in her overall MOANS scaled score was substantial (17 to 10). Although her absolute scores on these measures would be considered within normal limits, the degree of change over this short period of time is concerning.

Similarly, Ms J's 12-word decline on the Rey AVLT on the number of words recalled on Trials 1 through 5 (54 to 42) exceeds the 12-month reliable change boundary proposed by Knight and colleagues (Knight, McMahon, Skeaff, & Green, 2007). Although her long-term percent retention was not substantially different across evaluations (93% vs. 89%), her 5-word decline in the number of words recalled after 30 minutes and 4-word decline during delayed recognition testing also exceeded 12-month 90% reliable change boundaries (Knight et al., 2007). Although Ms J's test–retest interval was slightly longer than the 12-month interval utilized by Knight and colleagues, her substantial decline on the DRS-2, genetic risk for AD (positive family history and presence of the APOE ϵ4 allele), and a vascular risk factor (elevated homocysteine), coupled with the changes observed on the Rey AVLT, suggest a strong likelihood of progressive cognitive decline.

SUMMARY

In this chapter, several diverse roles played by neuropsychological assessment of older adults have been reviewed. Practical considerations that should be taken into account when evaluating older individuals, such as medication use, presence of comorbid chronic diseases, sensory and physical limitations, and availability of social supports, have also been addressed. These issues can potentially impact assessment results, and should be considered first when interpreting assessment data. The relative dearth of normative data for adults in late-life has been addressed to a large degree by studies, such as the Mayo Older American Normative Study and the Georgia Centenarian Study. However, obtaining representative samples of older adults for normative studies can still be a substantial challenge, and it is likely that future normative studies will need to characterize more precisely basic health status of a sample, such as number and type of medications used and presence and severity of chronic medical illnesses. For example, given the high prevalence of medical illness in late-life, it will be important to consider how the presence of particular diseases impacts cognition in late-life, rather than using the presence of a particular disease as an exclusion criterion.

Several basic clinical strategies for assessing older adults were presented. Next, an overview of several cognitive domains (intellectual functioning, memory functioning, executive functioning, and mood status) that are important to assess in late-life, along with a discussion of representative measures of these domains, were presented. Issues related to computer-based testing in older adults were also presented. Finally, broad topics of increasing interest to geriatric neuropsychology were briefly covered, including report writing, multicultural neuropsychology, and serial assessment.

Despite the significant advances that have been achieved in the field of geriatric neuropsychology, there are still a number of gaps in our knowledge of neuropsychological functioning in late-life. Much research on cognitive aging is focused on specific problems, such as identification of cognitive decline. Fewer studies have focused on positive aspects of aging, including the growth of wisdom, creativity, and aspects of life satisfaction among older adults. In addition, there have been relatively few novel clinical instruments developed for use with older adults within the last five years. A number of traditional paper and pencil measures commonly used for assessing cognitive, psychosocial, and personality functioning, as well as for assessing ability to perform daily living skills, are decades old. Even relatively new measures, such as the D-KEFS, use new strategies for interpreting performance on existing, older tests. Revisions of older instruments, such as the WAIS-IV and the WMS-IV have made some important modifications to address physical and sensory limitations seen in late-life, although few new procedures for assessing cognitive functioning have been implemented. The field of geriatric neuropsychology could benefit substantially from progress in using technology effectively for enhancing clinical and research assessment tools. Growth in these broad areas over the next decade would be a welcome addition to the field.

References

AAN. (1996). Assessment: Neuropsychological testing of adults. Considerations for neurologists. Report of the Therapeutics and Technology Assessment Subcommittee of the American Academy of Neurology. *Neurology, 47*(2), 592–599.

Acevedo, A., Krueger, K. R., Navarro, E., Ortiz, F., Manly, J. J., Padilla-Velez, M. M., et al. (2009). The Spanish translation and adaptation of the Uniform Data Set of the National Institute on Aging Alzheimer's Disease Centers. *Alzheimer Dis. Assoc. Disord., 23*(2), 102–109.

Albert, M. S. (1988). Cognitive function. In M. S. Albert, & M. B. Moss (Eds.), *Geriatric Neuropsychology* (pp. 33–53). New York, NY: Guilford.

Albert, M. S., Moss, M. B., Tanzi, R., & Jones, K. (2001). Preclinical prediction of AD using neuropsychological tests. *J. Int. Neuropsychol. Soc., 7*(5), 631–639.

Almkvist, O., Darreh-Shori, T., Stefanova, E., Spiegel, R., & Nordberg, A. (2004). Preserved cognitive function after 12 months of treatment with rivastigmine in mild Alzheimer's disease in comparison with untreated AD and MCI patients. *Eur. J. Neurol., 11*(4), 253–261.

Amirian, E., Baxter, J., Grigsby, J., Curran-Everett, D., Hokanson, J. E., & Bryant, L. L. (2009). Executive function (capacity for behavioral self-regulation) and decline predicted mortality in a longitudinal study in Southern Colorado. *J. Clin. Epidemiol, 63*(3), 307–314.

Ardila, A., Rodriguez-Menendez, G., & Rosselli, M. (2002). Current issues in neuropsychological assessment with Hispanics/Latinos. In F. R. Ferraro (Ed.), *Minority and Cross-cultural Aspects of Neuropsychological Assessment* (pp. 161–179). Lisse, Netherlands: Swets & Zeitlinger.

Ardila, A., Rosselli, M., & Puente, A. E. (1994). *Neuropsychological Evaluation of the Spanish Speaker.* New York, NY: Plenum.

Artiola i Fortuny, L., Heaton, R. K., & Hermosillo, D. (1998). Neuropsychological comparisons of Spanish-speaking participants from the U.S.-Mexico border region versus Spain. *J. Int. Neuropsychol. Soc., 4*(4), 363–379.

Artiola i Fortuny, L., & Mullaney, H. A. (1997). Neuropsychology with Spanish speakers: Language use and proficiency issues for test development. *J. Clin. Exp. Neuropsychol., 19*(4), 615–622.

Atkinson, H. H., Rosano, C., Simonsick, E. M., Williamson, J. D., Davis, C., Ambrosius, W. T., et al. (2007). Cognitive function, gait speed decline, and comorbidities: The health, aging and body composition study. *J. Gerontol. A Biol. Sci. Med. Sci., 62*(8), 844–850.

Auchus, A. P., Brashear, H. R., Salloway, S., Korczyn, A. D., De Deyn, P. P., & Gassmann-Mayer, C. (2007). Galantamine treatment of vascular dementia: A randomized trial. *Neurology, 69*(5), 448–458.

Axelrod, B. N., Goldman, R. S., & Henry, R. R. (1992). Sensitivity of the Mini-Mental State Examination to frontal lobe dysfunction in normal aging. *J. Clin. Psychol., 48*(1), 68–71.

Baddeley, A. D. (1986). *Working Memory.* Oxford, UK: Oxford University Press.

Baird, A., Podell, K., Lovell, M., & McGinty, S. B. (2001). Complex real-world functioning and neuropsychological test performance in older adults. *Clin. Neuropsychol., 15*(3), 369–379.

Barberger-Gateau, P., Commenges, D., Gagnon, M., Letenneur, L., Sauvel, C., & Dartigues, J. F. (1992). Instrumental activities of daily living as a screening tool for cognitive impairment and dementia in elderly community dwellers. *J. Am. Geriatr. Soc., 40*(11), 1129–1134.

Baron, M. S., Vitek, J. L., Bakay, R. A., Green, J., Kaneoke, Y., Hashimoto, T., et al. (1996). Treatment of advanced Parkinson's disease by posterior GPi pallidotomy: 1-year results of a pilot study. *Ann. Neurol., 40*(3), 355–366.

Beck, A. T., Epstein, N., Brown, G., & Steer, R. A. (1988). An inventory for measuring clinical anxiety: Psychometric properties. *J. Consult. Clin. Psychology, 56*, 893–897.

Beck, A. T., Steer, R. A., & Brown, G. K. (1996). *Beck Depression Inventory-Second Edition Manual*. San Antonio, TX: Psychological Corporation.

Beekman, A. T., Copeland, J. R., & Prince, M. J. (1999). Review of community prevalence of depression in later life. *Br. J. Psychiatry, 174*, 307–311.

Beekman, A. T., Deeg, D. J., van Tilburg, T., Smit, J. H., Hooijer, C., & van Tilburg, W. (1995). Major and minor depression in later life: A study of prevalence and risk factors. *J. Affect. Disord., 36*(1–2), 65–75.

Bell-McGinty, S., Podell, K., Franzen, M., Baird, A. D., & Williams, M. J. (2002). Standard measures of executive function in predicting instrumental activities of daily living in older adults. *Int. J. Geriatr. Psychiatry, 17*(9), 828–834.

Benedict, R. H., Goldstein, M. Z., Dobraski, M., & Tannenhaus, J. (1997). Neuropsychological predictors of adaptive kitchen behavior in geriatric psychiatry inpatients. *J. Geriatr. Psychiatry Neurol., 10*(4), 146–153.

Benson, C., & Lusardi, P. (1995). Neurologic antecedents to patient falls. *J. Neurosci. Nurs., 27*(6), 331–337.

Bernazzali, S., Basile, A., Balistreri, A., Carmellini, M., Cevenini, G., Lovera, G., et al. (2005). Standardized psychological evaluation pre- and posttransplantation: A new option. *Transplant Proc., 37*(2), 669–671.

Bieliauskas, L. A. (2005). Neuropsychological assessment of geriatric driving competence. *Brain Inj., 19*(3), 221–226.

Blacker, D., Lee, H., Muzikansky, A., Martin, E. C., Tanzi, R., McArdle, J. J., et al. (2007). Neuropsychological measures in normal individuals that predict subsequent cognitive decline. *Arch. Neurol., 64*(6), 862–871.

Bland, R. C., Newman, S. C., & Orn, H. (1988). Period prevalence of psychiatric disorders in Edmonton. *Acta Psychiatr. Scand. Suppl., 338*, 33–42.

Blazer, D., Burchett, B., Service, C., & George, L. K. (1991). The association of age and depression among the elderly: An epidemiologic exploration. *J. Gerontol., 46*(6), M210–M215.

Boake, C. (2002). From the Binet-Simon to the Wechsler-Bellevue: Tracing the history of intelligence testing. *J. Clin. Exp. Neuropsychol., 24*(3), 383–405.

Boone, K. B., Miller, B. L., & Lesser, I. M. (1993). Frontal lobe cognitive functions in aging: Methodologic considerations. *Dementia, 4*(3–4), 232–236.

Botwinick, J., & Storandt, M. (1974). *Memory Related Functions and Age*. Springfield, IL: Charles C. Thomas.

Brandt, J. (1991). The Hopkins Verbal Learning Test: Development of a new memory test with six equivalent forms. *The Clinical Neuropsychologist, 5*(2), 125–142.

Bronte-Stewart, H. (2003). Parkinson's disease: Surgical options. *Curr. Treat. Options Neurol., 5*(2), 131–147.

Burker, E. J., Evon, D. M., Sedway, J. A., & Egan, T. (2004). Appraisal and coping as predictors of psychological distress and self-reported physical disability before lung transplantation. *Prog. Transplant, 14*(3), 222–232.

Buschke, H. (1973). Selective reminding for analysis of memory and learning. *J. Verb. Learn. Verb. Behav., 12*, 543–550.

Buschke, H., & Fuld, P. A. (1974). Evaluating storage, retention and retrieval in disordered memory and learning. *Neurology, 24*, 1019–1025.

Cahn, D. A., Sullivan, E. V., Shear, P. K., Pfefferbaum, A., Heit, G., & Silverberg, G. (1998). Differential contributions of cognitive and motor component processes to physical and instrumental activities of daily living in Parkinson's disease. *Arch. Clin. Neuropsychol., 13*(7), 575–583.

Calamari, J. E., Janeck, A. S., & Deer, T. M. (2002). Cognitive processes and obsessive compulsive disorder in older adults. In R. O. Frost, & G. Steketee (Eds.), *Cognitive Approaches to Obsessions and Compulsions: Theory, Assessment, and Treatment* (pp. 315–335). Amsterdam, Netherlands: Pergamon/Elsevier Science Inc.

Carlson, M. C., Fried, L. P., Xue, Q. L., Bandeen-Roche, K., Zeger, S. L., & Brandt, J. (1999). Association between executive attention and physical functional performance in community-dwelling older women. *J. Gerontol. B Psychol. Sci. Soc. Sci., 54*(5), S262–S270.

Carroll, J. B. (1993). *Human Cognitive Abilities: A Survey of Factor-Analytic Studies*. New York, NY: Cambridge University Press.

Carroll, J. B. (1997). The three-stratum theory of cognitive abilities. In D. P. Flanagan, J. L. Genshaft, & P. L. Harrison (Eds.), *Contemporary Intellectual Assessment: Theories, Tests, and Issues* (pp. 122–130). New York, NY: Guilford.

Carroll, J. B. (1998). Human cognitive abilities: A critique. In J. J. McArdle, & R. W. Woodcock (Eds.), *Human Cognitive Abilities in Theory and Practice* (pp. 5–24). Mahwah, NJ: Erlbaum.

Caselli, R. J., Reiman, E. M., Locke, D. E., Hutton, M. L., Hentz, J. G., Hoffman-Snyder, C., et al. (2007). Cognitive domain decline in healthy apolipoprotein E epsilon4 homozygotes before the diagnosis of mild cognitive impairment. *Arch. Neurol.*, *64*(9), 1306–1311.

Chacko, R. C., Harper, R. G., Gotto, J., & Young, J. (1996). Psychiatric interview and psychometric predictors of cardiac transplant survival. *Am. J. Psychiatry*, *153*(12), 1607–1612.

Chacko, R. C., Harper, R. G., Kunik, M., & Young, J. (1996). Relationship of psychiatric morbidity and psychosocial factors in organ transplant candidates. *Psychosomatics*, *37*(2), 100–107.

Chao, L. L., & Knight, R. T. (1997). Prefrontal deficits in attention and inhibitory control with aging. *Cereb. Cortex*, *7*(1), 63–69.

Chelune, G. J., Naugle, R. I., Luders, H., Sedlak, J., & Awad, I. A. (1993). Individual change after epilepsy surgery: Practice effects and base-rate information. *Neuropsychology*, *7*, 41–52.

Colsher, P. L., & Wallace, R. B. (1993). Geriatric assessment and driver functioning. *Clin. Geriatr. Med.*, *9*(2), 365–375.

Cooper, J. W. (1996). Probable adverse drug reactions in a rural geriatric nursing home population: A four-year study. *J. Am. Geriatr. Soc.*, *44*(2), 194–197.

Copeland, J. R., Beekman, A. T., Dewey, M. E., Hooijer, C., Jordan, A., Lawlor, B. A., et al. (1999). Depression in Europe. Geographical distribution among older people. *Br. J. Psychiatry*, *174*, 312–321.

Craik, F. I. M. (1986). A functional account of age differences in memory. In F. Kliz, & H. Hagendorf (Eds.), *Human Memory and Cognitive Capabilities: Mechanisms and Performances*. Amsterdam, Netherlands: Elsevier.

Craik, F. I. M. (1990). Changes in memory with normal aging: A functional view. In R. J. Wurtman (Ed.), *Advances in Neurology* (Vol. 51: Alzheimer's disease). New York, NY: Raven Press.

Crawford, J. R., Sutherland, D., & Garthwaite, P. H. (2008). On the reliability and standard errors of measurement of contrast measures from the D-KEFS. *J. Int. Neuropsychol. Soc.*, *14*(6), 1069–1073.

Cumming, R. G., Miller, J. P., Kelsey, J. L., Davis, P., Arfken, C. L., Birge, S. J., et al. (1991). Medications and multiple falls in elderly people: The St Louis OASIS study. *Age Ageing*, *20*(6), 455–461.

Darby, D., Maruff, P., Collie, A., & McStephen, M. (2002). Mild cognitive impairment can be detected by multiple assessments in a single day. *Neurology*, *59*(7), 1042–1046.

Davis, H. P., Small, S. A., Stern, Y., Mayeux, R., Feldstein, S. N., & Keller, F. R. (2003). Acquisition, recall, and forgetting of verbal information in long-term memory by young, middle-aged, and elderly individuals. *Cortex*, *39*(4–5), 1063–1091.

De Jager, C. A., Hogervorst, E., Combrinck, M., & Budge, M. M. (2003). Sensitivity and specificity of neuropsychological tests for mild cognitive impairment, vascular cognitive impairment and Alzheimer's disease. *Psychol. Med.*, *33*(6), 1039–1050.

De Jager, C. A., Schrijnemaekers, A. C., Honey, T. E., & Budge, M. M. (2009). Detection of MCI in the clinic: Evaluation of the sensitivity and specificity of a computerised test battery, the Hopkins Verbal Learning Test and the MMSE. *Age Ageing*, *38*(4), 455–460.

DeCarli, C., Mungas, D., Harvey, D., Reed, B., Weiner, M., Chui, H., et al. (2004). Memory impairment, but not cerebrovascular disease, predicts progression of MCI to dementia. *Neurology*, *63*(2), 220–227.

Delis, D. C., Kaplan, E., & Kramer, J. H. (2001). *Delis-Kaplan Executive Function System (D-KEFS) Technical Manual*. San Antonio, TX: The Psychological Corporation.

Delis, D. C., Kramer, J. H., Kaplan, E., & Ober, B. A. (2000). *CVLT-II: California Verbal Learning Test Second Edition Adult Version Manual*. San Antonio, TX: The Psychological Corporation.

Dickson, D. W., Crystal, H. A., Bevona, C., Honer, W., Vincent, I., & Davies, P. (1995). Correlations of synaptic and pathological markers with cognition of the elderly. *Neurobiol Aging*, *16*(3), 285–298, discussion 298–304.

Doniger, G. M., Dwolatzky, T., Zucker, D. M., Chertkow, H., Crystal, H., Schweiger, A., et al. (2006). Computerized cognitive testing battery identifies mild cognitive impairment and mild dementia even in the presence of depressive symptoms. *Am. J. Alzheimers Dis. Other Demen.*, *21*(1), 28–36.

Doniger, G. M., Jo, M. Y., Simon, E. S., & Crystal, H. A. (2009). Computerized cognitive assessment of mild cognitive impairment in urban African Americans. *Am. J. Alzheimers Dis. Other Demen.*, *24*(5), 396–403.

Doniger, G. M., & Simon, E. S. (2009). Computerized cognitive testing in aging. *Alzheimers Dement.*, *5*(5), 439–440.

Doniger, G. M., Simon, E. S., & Schweiger, A. (2008). Adjustment of cognitive scores with a co-normed estimate of premorbid intelligence: Implementation using Mindstreams computerized testing. *Appl. Neuropsychol.*, *15*(4), 250–263.

Doody, R. S., Stevens, J. C., Beck, C., Dubinsky, R. M., Kaye, J. A., Gwyther, L., et al. (2001). Practice parameter: Management of dementia (an evidence-based review). Report of the Quality Standards Subcommittee of the American Academy of Neurology. *Neurology*, *56*(9), 1154–1166.

Dubinsky, R. M., Stein, A. C., & Lyons, K. (2000). Practice parameter: risk of driving and Alzheimer's disease (an evidence-based review): Report of the Quality Standards Subcommittee of the American Academy of Neurology. *Neurology*, *54*(12), 2205–2211.

Dunlosky, J., & Salthouse, T. A. (1996). A decomposition of age-related differences in multi-trial free recall. *Aging, Neuropsychology, & Cognition*, *3*, 2–14.

Dwolatzky, T., Whitehead, V., Doniger, G. M., Simon, E. S., Schweiger, A., Jaffe, D., et al. (2003). Validity of a novel computerized cognitive battery for mild cognitive impairment. *BMC Geriatr.*, *3*, 4.

Dwolatzky, T., Whitehead, V., Doniger, G. M., Simon, E. S., Schweiger, A., Jaffe, D., et al. (2004). Validity of the Mindstreams computerized cognitive battery for mild cognitive impairment. *J. Mol. Neurosci.*, *24*(1), 33–44.

Farlow, M. R., & Lilly, M. L. (2005). Rivastigmine: An open-label, observational study of safety and effectiveness in treating patients with Alzheimer's disease for up to 5 years. *BMC Geriatr.*, *5*, 3.

Ferman, T. J., Lucas, J. A., Ivnik, R. J., Smith, G. E., Willis, F. B., Petersen, R. C., et al. (2005). Mayo's Older African American Normative Studies: Auditory Verbal Learning Test norms for African American elders. *Clin. Neuropsychol.*, *19*(2), 214–228.

Fick, D. M., Cooper, J. W., Wade, W. E., Waller, J. L., Maclean, J. R., & Beers, M. H. (2003). Updating the Beers criteria for potentially inappropriate medication use in older adults: Results of a US consensus panel of experts. *Arch. Intern. Med.*, *163*(22), 2716–2724.

Fillenbaum, G. G. (1988). *Multidimensional Functional Assessment of Older Adults*. Hillsdale, NJ: Lawrence Erlbaum Publishing.

Fillit, H. M., Simon, E. S., Doniger, G. M., & Cummings, J. L. (2008). Practicality of a computerized system for cognitive assessment in the elderly. *Alzheimers Dement.*, *4*(1), 14–21.

Flicker, C., Ferris, S. H., Crook, T., Bartus, R. T., & Reisberg, B. (1986). Cognitive decline in advanced age: Future directions for the psychometric differentiation of normal and pathological age changes in cognitive function. *Developmental Neuropsychology*, *2*(4), 309–322.

Folstein, M. F., Folstein, S. E., & McHugh, P. R. (1975). "Mini-Mental State:" A practical method for grading the cognitive state of patients for the clinician. *J Psychiatr Res.*, *12*, 189–198.

Fratiglioni, L., Wang, H. X., Ericsson, K., Maytan, M., & Winblad, B. (2000). Influence of social network on occurrence of dementia: A community-based longitudinal study. *Lancet*, *355*(9212), 1315–1319.

Frerichs, R. J., & Tuokko, H. A. (2005). A comparison of methods for measuring cognitive change in older adults. *Arch. Clin. Neuropsychol.*, *20*(3), 321–333.

Fuentes, K., & Cox, B. J. (1997). Prevalence of anxiety disorders in elderly adults: a critical analysis. *Journal of Behavior Therapy and Experimental Psychiatry*, *28*(4), 269–279.

Fuld, P. A. (1981). *The Fuld Object-Memory Evaluation*. Chicago, IL: Stoelting Instrument Company.

Fuld, P. A., Masur, D. M., Blau, A. D., Crystal, H., & Aronson, M. K. (1990). Object-memory evaluation for prospective detection of dementia in normal-functioning elderly: Predictive and normative data. *J. Clin. Exp. Neuropsych.*, *12*, 520–528.

Fuld, P. A., Muramoto, O., Blau, A., Westbrook, L., & Katzman, R. (1988). Cross-cultural and multi-ethnic dementia evaluation by mental status and memory testing. *Cortex*, *24*(4), 511–519.

Geffen, G., Moar, K. J., O'Hanlon, A. P., Clark, C. R., & Geffen, L. B. (1990). Performance measures of 16- to 86-year old males and females on the Auditory Verbal Learning Test. *The Clinical Neuropsychologist*, *4*(1), 45–63.

Goekoop, R., Scheltens, P., Barkhof, F., & Rombouts, S. A. (2006). Cholinergic challenge in Alzheimer patients and mild cognitive impairment differentially affects hippocampal activation—a pharmacological fMRI study. *Brain*, *129*(Pt 1), 141–157.

Golden, J. C. (1978). *Stroop Color and Word Test*. Chicago, IL: Stoelting.

Goldstein, F. C., Strasser, D. C., Woodard, J. L., & Roberts, V. J. (1997). Functional outcome of cognitively impaired hip fracture patients on a geriatric rehabilitation unit. *J. Am. Geriatr. Soc.*, *45*(1), 35–42.

Gottesman, R. F., Hillis, A. E., Grega, M. A., Borowicz, L. M., Jr., Selnes, O. A., Baumgartner, W. A., et al. (2007). Early postoperative cognitive dysfunction and blood pressure during coronary artery bypass graft operation. *Arch. Neurol.*, *64*(8), 1111–1114.

Grant, D. A., & Berg, E. A. (1948). A behavioral analysis of degree of reinforcement and ease of shifting to new responses in a Weigl-type card-sorting problem. *J. Exp. Psychol.*, *38*, 404.

Grigsby, J., Kaye, K., Baxter, J., Shetterly, S. M., & Hamman, R. F. (1998). Executive cognitive abilities and functional status among community-dwelling older persons in the San Luis Valley Health and Aging Study. *J. Am. Geriatr. Soc.*, *46*(5), 590–596.

Grigsby, J., Kaye, K., & Robbins, L. J. (1992). Reliabilities, norms and factor structure of the Behavioral Dyscontrol Scale. *Percept. Mot. Skills*, *74*(3 Pt 1), 883–892.

Guarch, J., Marcos, T., Salamero, M., & Blesa, R. (2004). Neuropsychological markers of dementia in patients with memory complaints. *Int. J. Geriatr. Psychiatry*, *19*(4), 352–358.

Gurian, B. S., & Miner, J. H. (1991). Clinical presentation of anxiety in the elderly. In C. Salzman, & B. D. Lebowitz (Eds.), *Anxiety in the Elderly: Treatment and Research* (pp. 31–44). New York, NY: Springer.

Hajjar, E. R., Cafiero, A. C., & Hanlon, J. T. (2007). Polypharmacy in elderly patients. *Am. J. Geriatr. Pharmacother.*, *5*(4), 345–351.

Hamilton, M. (1959). The assessment of anxiety states by rating. *British Journal of Medical Psychology*, *32*, 50–55.

Hamilton, M. (1960). A rating scale for depression. *J. Neurol. Neurosurg. Psychiatry*, *23*, 56–61.

Hanlon, J. T., Boudreau, R. M., Roumani, Y. F., Newman, A. B., Ruby, C. M., Wright, R. M., et al. (2009). Number and dosage of central nervous system medications on recurrent falls in community elders: The Health, Aging and Body Composition study. *J. Gerontol. A Biol. Sci. Med. Sci.*, *64*(4), 492–498.

Harder, H., Cornelissen, J. J., Van Gool, A. R., Duivenvoorden, H. J., Eijkenboom, W. M., & van den Bent, M. J. (2002). Cognitive functioning and quality of life in long-term adult survivors of bone marrow transplantation. *Cancer*, *95*(1), 183–192.

Harris, M. E., Ivnik, R. J., & Smith, G. E. (2002). Mayo's Older Americans Normative Studies: Expanded AVLT Recognition Trial norms for ages 57 to 98. *J. Clin. Exp. Neuropsychol.*, *24*(2), 214–220.

Hashimoto, M., Kazui, H., Matsumoto, K., Nakano, Y., Yasuda, M., & Mori, E. (2005). Does donepezil treatment slow the progression of hippocampal atrophy in patients with Alzheimer's disease? *Am. J. Psychiatry*, *162*(4), 676–682.

Heaton, R. K., Grant, I., & Matthews, C. G. (1991). *Comprehensive Norms for an Expanded Halstead-Reitan Battery: Demographic Corrections, Research Findings, and Clinical Applications*. Odessa, FL: Psychological Assessment Resources.

Hendrie, H. C., Hall, K. S., Hui, S., Unverzagt, F. W., Yu, C. E., Lahiri, D. K., et al. (1995). Apolipoprotein E genotypes and Alzheimer's disease in a community study of elderly African Americans. *Ann. Neurol.*, *37*, 118–120.

Homack, S., Lee, D., & Riccio, C. A. (2005). Test review: Delis-Kaplan executive function system. *J. Clin. Exp. Neuropsychol*, *27*(5), 599–609.

Horn, J. L. (1985). Remodeling old models of intelligence. In B. B. Wolman (Ed.), *Handbook of Intelligence: Theories, Measurements, and Applications* (pp. 237–278). New York, NY: Wiley.

Horn, J. L. (1989). Cognitive diversity: A framework of learning. In P. L. Ackerman, R. J. Sternberg, & R. Glaser (Eds.), *Learning and Individual Differences: Advances in Theory and Research* (pp. 61–116). New York, NY: W.H. Freeman.

Horn, J., & Cattell, R. (1967). Age differences in fluid and crystallized intelligence. *Acta Psychol.*, *26*(2), 107–129.

Horn, J. L., & Cattell, R. B. (1966). Refinement and test of the theory of fluid and crystallized general intelligences. *Journal of Educational Psychology*, *57*, 253–270.

Horn, J. L., & Noll, J. (1997). Human cognitive capabilities: Gf-Gc theory. In D. P. Flanagan, J. L. Genshaft, & P. L. Harrison (Eds.), *Contemporary Intellectual Assessment: Theories, Tests, and Issues* (pp. 53–91). New York, NY: Guilford.

Houston, W. S., Delis, D. C., Lansing, A., Jacobson, M. W., Cobell, K. R., Salmon, D. P., et al. (2005). Executive function asymmetry in older adults genetically at-risk for Alzheimer's disease: verbal versus design fluency. *J. Int. Neuropsychol. Soc.*, *11*(7), 863–870.

Howieson, D. B., Holm, L. A., Kaye, J. A., Oken, B. S., & Howieson, J. (1993). Neurologic function in the optimally healthy oldest old: Neuropsychological evaluation. *Neurology*, *43*, 1882–1886.

Hultsch, D. F., & Dixon, R. A. (1990). Learning and memory in aging. In J. E. Birren, & K. W. Shaie (Eds.), *Handbook of the Psychology of Aging* (pp. 259–274). New York, NY: Academic Press.

Hybels, C. F., & Blazer, D. G. (2003). Epidemiology of late-life mental disorders. *Clin. Geriatr. Med.*, *19*(4), 663–696.

Ivnik, R., Malec, J., Smith, G., Tangalos, E., Petersen, R., Kokmen, E., et al. (1992a). Mayo's older Americans normative studies: WAIS-R norms for ages 56 to 97. *The Clinical Neuropsychologist*, *6*(Suppl.), 1–30.

Ivnik, R., Malec, J., Smith, G., Tangalos, E., Petersen, R., Kokmen, E., et al. (1992b). Mayo's older Americans normative studies: WMS-R Norms for ages 56 to 94. *The Clinical Neuropsychologist*, *6*(Suppl.), 49–82.

Ivnik, R. J., Malec, J. F., Smith, G., Tangalos, E., Petersen, R., Kokmen, E., et al. (1992c). Mayo's older Americans normative studies: Updated AVLT norms for ages 56 to 97. *The Clinical Neuropsychologist*, *6* (Suppl.), 83–104.

Ivnik, R. J., Smith, G. E., Lucas, J. A., Tangalos, E. G., Kokmen, E., & Petersen, R. C. (1997). Free and cued selective reminding test: MOANS norms. *J. Clin. Exp. Neuropsychol*, *19*(5), 676–691.

Jacobson, N. S., & Truax, P. (1991). Clinical significance: A statistical approach to defining meaningful change in psychotherapy research. *J. Consult. Clin. Psychol*, *59*(1), 12–19.

Jefferson, A. L., Barakat, L. P., Giovannetti, T., Paul, R. H., & Glosser, G. (2006). Object perception impairments predict instrumental activities of daily living dependence in Alzheimer's disease. *J. Clin. Exp. Neuropsychol.*, *28*(6), 884–897.

Jefferson, A. L., Paul, R. H., Ozonoff, A., & Cohen, R. A. (2006). Evaluating elements of executive functioning as predictors of instrumental activities of daily living (IADLs). *Arch. Clin. Neuropsychol.*, *21*(4), 311–320.

Juliebo, V., Bjoro, K., Krogseth, M., Skovlund, E., Ranhoff, A. H., & Wyller, T. B. (2009). Risk factors for preoperative and postoperative delirium in elderly patients with hip fracture. *J. Am. Geriatr. Soc.*, *57*(8), 1354–1361.

Juninger, J., Phelan, E., Cherry, K., & Levy, J. (1993). Prevalence of psychopathology in elderly persons in nursing homes and in the community. *Hospital and Community Psychiatry*, *44*, 381–383.

Kane, R. L., Roebuck-Spencer, T., Short, P., Kabat, M., & Wilken, J. (2007). Identifying and monitoring cognitive deficits in clinical populations using Automated Neuropsychological Assessment Metrics (ANAM) tests. *Arch. Clin. Neuropsychol.*, *22*(Suppl. 1), S115–S126.

Kaplan, E. (1995). California Verbal Learning Test (dementia version). In M. D. Lezak (Ed.), *(personal communication) in Neuropsychological Assessment*. New York, NY: Oxford.

Katz, S., Downs, T. D., Cash, H. R., & Grotz, R. C. (1970). Progress in development of the index of ADL. *Gerontologist*, *10*(1), 20–30.

Kaufman, A. S., & Kaufman, N. L. (1993). *Kaufman Adolescent and Adult Intelligence Test (KAIT) Manual*. Circle Pines, MN: American Guidance Service.

Kaufman, A. S., & Kaufman, N. L. (1997). The Kaufman Adolescent and Adult Intelligence Test (KAIT). In D. P. Flanagan, J. L. Genshaft, & P. L. Harrison (Eds.), *Contemporary Intellectual Assessment: Theories, Tests, and Issues* (pp. 209–229). New York, NY: Guilford.

Kaufman, D. W., Kelly, J. P., Rosenberg, L., Anderson, T. E., & Mitchell, A. A. (2002). Recent patterns of medication use in the ambulatory adult population of the United States: the Slone survey. *JAMA*, *287*(3), 337–344.

Kaye, K., Grigsby, J., Robbins, L. J., & Korzun, B. (1990). Prediction of independent functioning and behavior problems in geriatric patients. *J. Am. Geriatr. Soc.*, *38*(12), 1304–1310.

Keller, B. K., Morton, J. L., Thomas, V. S., & Potter, J. F. (1999). The effect of visual and hearing impairments on functional status. *J. Am. Geriatr. Soc.*, *47*(11), 1319–1325.

Kluger, A., Ferris, S. H., Golomb, J., Mittelman, M. S., & Reisberg, B. (1999). Neuropsychological prediction of decline to dementia in nondemented elderly. *J. Geriatr. Psychiatry Neurol.*, *12*(4), 168–179.

Knight, R. G., McMahon, J., Skeaff, C. M., & Green, T. J. (2007). Reliable Change Index scores for persons over the age of 65 tested on alternate forms of the Rey AVLT. *Arch. Clin. Neuropsychol.*, *22*(4), 513–518.

Knipp, S. C., Matatko, N., Wilhelm, H., Schlamann, M., Thielmann, M., Losch, C., et al. (2008). Cognitive outcomes three years after coronary artery bypass surgery: Relation to diffusion-weighted magnetic resonance imaging. *Ann. Thorac. Surg.*, *85*(3), 872–879.

Knopman, D. S., DeKosky, S. T., Cummings, J. L., Chui, H., Corey-Bloom, J., Relkin, N., et al. (2001). Practice parameter: Diagnosis of dementia (an evidence-based review). Report of the Quality Standards Subcommittee of the American Academy of Neurology. *Neurology*, *56*(9), 1143–1153.

Kogan, J. N., Edelstein, B. A., & McKee, D. R. (2000). Assessment of anxiety in older adults: Current status. *J. Anxiety Disord.*, *14*(2), 109–132.

Krach, P., DeVaney, S., DeTurk, C., & Zink, M. H. (1996). Functional status of the oldest-old in a home setting. *J. Adv. Nurs.*, *24*(3), 456–464.

Krishnan, K. R., Charles, H. C., Doraiswamy, P. M., Mintzer, J., Weisler, R., Yu, X., et al. (2003). Randomized, placebo-controlled trial of the effects of donepezil on neuronal markers and hippocampal volumes in Alzheimer's disease. *Am. J. Psychiatry*, *160*(11), 2003–2011.

Langer, E. J., Rodin, J., Beck, P., Weinman, C., & Spitzer, L. (1979). Environmental determinants of memory improvement in late adulthood. *J Pers Soc Psychol.*, *37*(11), 2003–2013.

La Rue, A. (1992). *Aging and Neuropsychological Assessment*. New York, NY: Plenum.

Lasoski, M. C. (1986). Reasons for low utilization of mental health services by the elderly. *Clinical Gerontologist: The Journal of Aging and Mental Health*, *5*(1–2), 1–18.

Lavi, R., Doniger, G. M., Simon, E., Hochner-Celnikier, D., Zimran, A., & Elstein, D. (2007). The effect of hormone replacement therapy on cognitive function in post-menopausal women. *QJM*, *100*(9), 567–573.

Lawton, M. P., & Brody, E. M. (1969). Assessment of older people: Self-maintaining and instrumental activities of daily living. *Gerontologist*, *9*(3), 179–186.

Levinson, D., Reeves, D., Watson, J., & Harrison, M. (2005). Automated neuropsychological assessment metrics (ANAM) measures of cognitive effects of Alzheimer's disease. *Arch. Clin. Neuropsychol.*, *20*(3), 403–408.

Lezak, M. D. (1976). *Neuropsychological Assessment*. New York, NY: Oxford University Press.

Lezak, M. D. (1983). *Neuropsychological Assessment* (2nd ed.). New York, NY: Oxford University Press.

Lezak, M. D. (1995). *Neuropsychological Assessment* (3rd ed.). New York, NY: Oxford University Press.

Libon, D. J., Mattson, R. E., Blosser, G., Kaplan, E., Malamut, B. L., Sands, L. P., et al. (1996). A nine-word dementia version of the California Verbal Learning Test. *Clin. Neuropsychol.*, *10*, 237–244.

Loewenstein, D. A., Amigo, E., Duara, R., Guterman, A., Hurwitz, D., Berkowitz, N., et al. (1989). A new scale for the assessment of functional status in Alzheimer's disease and related disorders. *Journal of Gerontology*, *4*, 114–121.

Loewenstein, D. A., Ardila, A., Rosselli, M., Hayden, S., Duara, R., Berkowitz, N., et al. (1992). A comparative analysis of functional status among Spanish- and English-speaking patients with dementia. *J. Gerontol.*, *47*(6), P389–P394.

Loewenstein, D. A., Argüelles, T., Argüelles, S., & Linn-Fuentes, P. (1994). Potential cultural bias in the neuropsychological assessment of the older adult. *J. Clin. Exp. Neuropsychol.*, *16*, 623–629.

Loewenstein, D. A., Argüelles, T., Barker, W. W., & Duara, R. (1993). A comparative analysis of neuropsychological test performance of Spanish-speaking and English-speaking patients with Alzheimer's disease. *Journal of Gerontology*, *48*, P142–P149.

Loewenstein, D. A., Rubert, M. P., Argüelles, T., & Duara, R. (1995). Neuropsychological test performance and prediction of functional capacities among Spanish-speaking and English-speaking patients with dementia. *Archives of Clinical Neuropsychology*, *10*, 75–88.

Loewenstein, D. A., Rubert, M. P., Berkowitz-Zimmer, N., Guterman, A., Morgan, R., & Hayden, S. (1992). Neuropsychological test performance and prediction of functional capacities in dementia. *Behavior, Health, and Aging*, *2*, 149–158.

Lucas, J. A., Ivnik, R. J., Smith, G. E., Bohac, D. L., Tangalos, E. G., Graff-Radford, N. R., et al. (1998a). Mayo's older Americans normative studies: Category fluency norms. *J. Clin. Exp. Neuropsychol.*, *20*(2), 194–200.

Lucas, J. A., Ivnik, R. J., Smith, G. E., Bohac, D. L., Tangalos, E. G., Kokmen, E., et al. (1998b). Normative data for the Mattis Dementia Rating Scale. *Journal of Clinical & Experimental Neuropsychology*, *20*, 536–547.

Lucas, J. A., Ivnik, R. J., Smith, G. E., Ferman, T. J., Willis, F. B., Petersen, R. C., et al. (2005a). A brief report on WAIS-R normative data collection in Mayo's Older African Americans Normative Studies. *Clin. Neuropsychol.*, *19*(2), 184–188.

Lucas, J. A., Ivnik, R. J., Smith, G. E., Ferman, T. J., Willis, F. B., Petersen, R. C., et al. (2005b). Mayo's Older African Americans Normative Studies: Norms for Boston Naming Test, Controlled Oral Word Association, Category Fluency, Animal Naming, Token Test, WRAT-3 Reading, Trail Making Test, Stroop Test, and Judgment of Line Orientation. *Clin. Neuropsychol.*, *19*(2), 43–269.

Lucas, J. A., Ivnik, R. J., Smith, G. E., Ferman, T. J., Willis, F. B., Petersen, R. C., et al. (2005c). Mayo's Older African Americans Normative Studies: WMS-R norms for African American elders. *Clin. Neuropsychol.*, *19*(2), 189–213.

Lucas, J. A., Ivnik, R. J., Willis, F. B., Ferman, T. J., Smith, G. E., Parfitt, F. C., et al. (2005d). Mayo's Older African Americans Normative Studies: Normative data for commonly used clinical neuropsychological measures. *Clin. Neuropsychol.*, *19*(2), 162–183.

Luria, A. R. (1980). *Higher Cortical Functions in Man*. New York, NY: Basic Books, Inc.

Lyyra, T. M., & Heikkinen, R. L. (2006). Perceived social support and mortality in older people. *J Gerontol B Psychol Sci Soc Sci.*, *61*(3), S147–S152.

Machulda, M. M., Ivnik, R. J., Smith, G. E., Ferman, T. J., Boeve, B. F., Knopman, D., et al. (2007). Mayo's Older Americans Normative Studies: Visual Form Discrimination and copy trial of the Rey-Osterrieth Complex Figure. *J. Clin. Exp. Neuropsychol.*, *29*(4), 377–384.

Mahurin, R. K., DeBettignies, B. H., & Pirozzolo, F. J. (1991). Structured assessment of independent living skills: Preliminary report of a performance measure of functional abilities in dementia. *Journal of Gerontology*, *46*, 58–66.

Malec, J. F., Ivnik, R. J., Smith, G. E., Tangalos, E. G., Petersen, R. C., Kokmen, E., et al. (1992). Mayo's Older Americans Normative Studies: Utility of corrections for age and education for the WAIS-R. *The Clinical Neuropsychologist*, *6*(S1), 31–47.

Manly, J. J. (2005). Advantages and disadvantages of separate norms for African Americans. *Clin. Neuropsychol.*, *19*(2), 270–275.

Manly, J. J. (2006). Deconstructing race and ethnicity: Implications for measurement of health outcomes. *Med. Care*, *44*(11 Suppl. 3), S10–S16.

Manly, J. J. (2008). Critical issues in cultural neuropsychology: Profit from diversity. *Neuropsychol. Rev.*, *18*(3), 179–183.

Manly, J. J., Byrd, D. A., Touradji, P., & Stern, Y. (2004). Acculturation, reading level, and neuropsychological test performance among African American elders. *Appl. Neuropsychol.*, *11*(1), 37–46.

Manly, J. J., & Echemendia, R. J. (2007). Race-specific norms: Using the model of hypertension to understand issues of race, culture, and education in neuropsychology. *Arch. Clin. Neuropsychol.*, *22*(3), 319–325.

Manly, J. J., Miller, S. W., Heaton, R. K., Byrd, D., Reilly, J., Velasquez, R. J., et al. (1998). The effect of African-American acculturation on neuropsychological test performance in normal and HIV-positive individuals. The HIV Neurobehavioral Research Center (HNRC) Group. *J. Int. Neuropsychol. Soc.*, *4*(3), 291–302.

Mansdorf, I. J., Harrington, M., Lund, J., & Wohl, N. (2008). Neuropsychological testing in skilled nursing facilities: The failure to confirm diagnoses of dementia. *J. Am. Med. Dir. Assoc.*, *9*(4), 271–274.

Marcopulos, B., & McLain, C. (2003). Are our norms "normal"? A 4-year follow-up study of a biracial sample of rural elders with low education. *Clin. Neuropsychol.*, *17*(1), 19–33.

Marcopulos, B. A., Gripshover, D. L., Broshek, D. K., McLain, C. A., & Brashear, H. R. (1999). Neuropsychological assessment of psychogeriatric patients with limited education. *Clin. Neuropsychol.*, *13*(2), 147–156.

Marcopulos, B. A., McLain, C. A., & Giuliano, A. J. (1997). Cognitive impairment or inadequate norms? A study of healthy, rural, older adults with limited education. *Clin. Neuropsychol.*, *11*(2), 111–131.

Marquis, S., Moore, M. M., Howieson, D. B., Sexton, G., Payami, H., Kaye, J. A., et al. (2002). Independent predictors of cognitive decline in healthy elderly persons. *Arch. Neurol.*, *59*(4), 601–606.

Maruff, P., Collie, A., Darby, D., Weaver-Cargin, J., Masters, C., & Currie, J. (2004). Subtle memory decline over 12 months in mild cognitive impairment. *Dement. Geriatr. Cogn. Disord.*, *18*(3–4), 342–348.

Masur, D. M., Fuld, P. A., Blau, A. D., Crystal, H., & Aronson, M. K. (1990). Predicting development of dementia in the elderly with the Selective Reminding Test. *J. Clin. Exp. Neuropsych.*, *12*, 529–538.

Masur, D. M., Sliwinski, M., Lipton, R. B., Blau, A. D., & Crystal, H. A. (1994). Neuropsychological prediction of dementia and the absence of dementia in healthy elderly persons. *Neurology*, *44*, 1427–1432.

McGrew, K. S., Schrank, F. A., & Woodcock, R. W. (2007). *Technical Manual. Woodcock-Johnson III Normative Update*. Itasca, IL: Riverside.

McKhann, G. M., Drachman, D., Folstein, M. F., Katzman, R., Price, D., & Stadlan, E. M. (1984). Clinical diagnosis of Alzheimer's disease: Report of the NINCDS-ADRDA work group. *Neurology, 34*, 939–944.

McSweeny, A. J., Naugle, R. I., Chelune, G. J., & Luders, H. (1993). "T scores for change": An illustration of a regression approach to depicting change in clinical neuropsychology. *The Clinical Neuropsychologist, 7*, 300–312.

Miller, L. S., Mitchell, M., Woodard, J. L., Davey, A., Martin, P., & Poon, L. W. (in press). Normative data for centenarians. *Aging, Neuropsychology, and Cognition.*

Mitchell, M., & Miller, L. S. (2008). Prediction of functional status in older adults: The ecological validity of four Delis-Kaplan Executive Function System tests. *J. Clin. Exp. Neuropsychol.*, *30*(6), 683–690.

Mitrushina, M., Satz, P., Chervinsky, A., & D'Elia, L. (1991). Performance of four age groups of normal elderly on the Rey Auditory-Verbal Learning Test. *J. Clin. Psychol.*, *47*(3), 351–357.

Mitrushina, M. N., Boone, K. B., & D'Elia, L. F. (1998). *Handbook of Normative Data for Neuropsychological Assessment*. New York, NY: Oxford.

Mittenberg, W., Seidenberg, M., O'Leary, D. S., & DiGiulio, D. V. (1989). Changes in cerebral functioning associated with normal aging. *J. Clin. Exp. Neuropsychol.*, *11*(6), 918–932.

Moscovitch, M., & Winocur, G. (1995). Frontal lobes, memory, and aging. *Annals of the New York Academy of Sciences*, *769*, 119–150.

Moulin, C. J. A., James, N., Freeman, J. E., & Jones, R. W. (2004). Deficient acquisition and consolidation: Intertrial free recall performance in Alzheimer's disease and mild cognitive impairment. *J. Clin. Exp. Neuropsychol.*, *26*(1), 1–10.

Myers, A. H., Young, Y., & Langlois, J. A. (1996). Prevention of falls in the elderly. *Bone*, *18*(1 Suppl.), 87S–101S.

Myers, J. S., Grigsby, J., Teel, C. S., & Kramer, A. M. (2009). Nurses' assessment of rehabilitation potential and prediction of functional status at discharge from inpatient rehabilitation. *Int. J. Rehabil. Res.*, *32*(3), 264–266.

Nadler, J. D., Richardson, E. D., Malloy, P. F., Marran, M. E., & Brinson, M. E. H. (1993). The ability of the Dementia Rating Scale to predict everyday functioning. *Archives of Clinical Neuropsychology*, *8*, 449–460.

Nestor, P. J., Scheltens, P., & Hodges, J. R. (2004). Advances in the early detection of Alzheimer's disease. *Nat. Med.*, *10*(Suppl.), S34–S41.

Nyberg, L., & Gustafson, Y. (1997). Fall prediction index for patients in stroke rehabilitation. *Stroke*, *28*(4), 716–721.

Ofstedal, M. B., Zimmer, Z. S., & Lin, H. S. (1999). A comparison of correlates of cognitive functioning in older persons in Taiwan and the United States. *J. Gerontol. B Psychol. Sci. Soc. Sci.*, *54*(5), S291–S301.

Oster, C. (1976). Sensory deprivation in geriatric patients. *J. Am. Geriatr. Soc.*, *24*(10), 461–464.

Ostrosky-Solis, F., Quintanar, L., & Ardila, A. (1989). Detection of brain damage: Neuropsychological assessment in a Spanish speaking population. *Int. J. Neurosci.*, *49*(3–4), 141–149.

Paleacu, D., Shutzman, A., Giladi, N., Herman, T., Simon, E. S., & Hausdorff, J. M. (2007). Effects of pharmacological therapy on gait and cognitive function in depressed patients. *Clin. Neuropharmacol.*, *30*(2), 63–71.

Pedraza, O., Graff-Radford, N. R., Smith, G. E., Ivnik, R. J., Willis, F. B., Petersen, R. C., et al. (2009). Differential item functioning of the Boston Naming Test in cognitively normal African American and Caucasian older adults. *J. Int. Neuropsychol. Soc.*, *15*(5), 758–768.

Pedraza, O., Lucas, J. A., Smith, G. E., Willis, F. B., Graff-Radford, N. R., Ferman, T. J., et al. (2005). Mayo's older African American normative studies: Confirmatory factor analysis of a core battery. *J. Int. Neuropsychol. Soc.*, *11*(2), 184–191.

Pedraza, O., Smith, G. E., Ivnik, R. J., Willis, F. B., Ferman, T. J., Petersen, R. C., et al. (2007). Reliable change on the Dementia Rating Scale. *J. Int. Neuropsychol. Soc.*, *13*(4), 716–720.

Pelco, L. E., Ward, S. B., Coleman, L., & Young, J. (2009). Teacher ratings of three psychological report styles. *Training and Education in Professional Psychology*, *3*(1), 19–27.

Pereira, F. S., Yassuda, M. S., Oliveira, A. M., & Forlenza, O. V. (2008). Executive dysfunction correlates with impaired functional status in older adults with varying degrees of cognitive impairment. *Int. Psychogeriatr.*, *20*(6), 1104–1115.

Petersen, R., Smith, G., Kokmen, E., Ivnik, R., & Tangalos, E. (1992). Memory function in normal aging. *Neurology, 42*, 396–401.

Petersen, R. C., Doody, R., Kurz, A., Mohs, R. C., Morris, J. C., Rabins, P. V., et al. (2001a). Current concepts in mild cognitive impairment. *Archives of Neurology, 58*, 1985–1992.

Petersen, R. C., Stevens, J. C., Ganguli, M., Tangalos, E. G., Cummings, J. L., & DeKosky, S. T. (2001b). Practice parameter: early detection of dementia: Mild cognitive impairment (an evidence-based review). Report of the Quality Standards Subcommittee of the American Academy of Neurology. *Neurology, 56*(9), 133–1142.

Piaget, J. (1972). Intellectual evolution from adolescence to adulthood. *Human Development, 15*, 1–12.

Ponton, M. O., & Ardila, A. (1999). The future of neuropsychology with Hispanic populations in the United States. *Arch. Clin. Neuropsychol., 14*(7), 565–580.

Potter, G. G., Plassman, B. L., Burke, J. R., Kabeto, M. U., Langa, K. M., Llewellyn, D. J., et al. (2009). Cognitive performance and informant reports in the diagnosis of cognitive impairment and dementia in African Americans and whites. *Alzheimers Dement., 5*(6), 445–453.

Preston, J. D., O'Neal, J. H., & Talaga, M. C. (1997). *Handbook of Clinical Psychopharmacology for Therapists* (2nd ed.). Oakland, CA: New Harbinger Publications.

Radloff, L. (1977). The CES-D scale: a new self report depression scale for research in the general population. *Appl. Psychol. Meas., 1*, 385–401.

Rapport, L. J., Hanks, R. A., Millis, S. R., & Deshpande, S. A. (1998). Executive functioning and predictors of falls in the rehabilitation setting. *Arch. Phys. Med. Rehabil., 79*(6), 629–633.

Ravaglia, G., Forti, P., Maioli, F., Boschi, F., Cicognani, A., Bernardi, M., et al. (1997). Determinants of functional status in healthy Italian nonagenarians and centenarians: A comprehensive functional assessment by the instruments of geriatric practice. *J. Am. Geriatr. Soc., 45*(10), 1196–1202.

Regier, D. A., Boyd, J. H., Burke, J. D., Jr., Rae, D. S., Myers, J. K., Kramer, M., et al. (1988). One-month prevalence of mental disorders in the United States. Based on five Epidemiologic Catchment Area sites. *Arch. Gen. Psychiatry, 45*(11), 977–986.

Reitan, R. M. (1958). Validity of the Trail Making test as an indication of organic brain damage. *Perceptual and Motor Skills, 8*, 271–276.

Reitan, R. M., & Wolfson, D. (1985). *The Halstead-Reitan Neuropsychological Test*. Tucson, AZ: Neuropsychology Press.

Rey, A. (1958). *L'examen clinique en psychologie*. Paris, France: Presses Universitaires de France.

Rey, G. J., Feldman, E., Hernandez, D., Levin, B. E., Rivas-Vazquez, R., Nedd, K. J., et al. (2001). Application of the multilingual aphasia examination—Spanish in the evaluation of Hispanic patients post closed-head trauma. *Clin. Neuropsychol., 15*(1), 13–18.

Rey, G. J., Feldman, E., Rivas-Vazquez, R., Levin, B. E., & Benton, A. (1999). Neuropsychological test development and normative data on Hispanics. *Arch. Clin. Neuropsychol., 14*(7), 593–601.

Richardson, E. D., Nadler, J. D., & Malloy, P. F. (1995). Neuropsychologic prediction of performance measures of daily living skills in geriatric patients. *Neuropsychology, 9*, 565–572.

Richardson, J. T. (2003). Howard Andrew Knox and the origins of performance testing on Ellis Island, 1912–1916. *Hist. Psychol., 6*(2), 143–170.

Rilling, L. M., Lucas, J. A., Ivnik, R. J., Smith, G. E., Willis, F. B., Ferman, T. J., et al. (2005). Mayo's Older African American Normative Studies: Norms for the Mattis Dementia Rating Scale. *Clin. Neuropsychol., 19*(2), 229–242.

Romero, H. R., Lageman, S. K., Kamath, V. V., Irani, F., Sim, A., Suarez, P., et al. (2009). Challenges in the neuropsychological assessment of ethnic minorities: Summit proceedings. *Clin. Neuropsychol., 23*(5), 761–779.

Rosselli, M., Ardila, A., Florez, A., & Castro, C. (1990). Normative data on the Boston Diagnostic Aphasia Examination in a Spanish-speaking population. *J. Clin. Exp. Neuropsychol., 12*(2), 313–322.

Rosselli, M., Ardila, A., Salvatierra, J., Marquez, M., Matos, L., & Weekes, V. A. (2002). A cross-linguistic comparison of verbal fluency tests. *Int. J. Neurosci., 112*(6), 759–776.

Rosselli, M., Ardila, A., Santisi, M. N., Arecco Mdel, R., Salvatierra, J., Conde, A., et al. (2002). Stroop effect in Spanish-English bilinguals. *J. Int. Neuropsychol. Soc., 8*(6), 819–827.

Royall, D. R., Chiodo, L. K., & Polk, M. J. (2005). An empiric approach to level of care determinations: The importance of executive measures. *J. Gerontol. A Biol. Sci. Med. Sci.*, *60*(8), 1059–1064.

Royall, D. R., Lauterbach, E. C., Kaufer, D., Malloy, P., Coburn, K. L., & Black, K. J. (2007). The cognitive correlates of functional status: A review from the Committee on Research of the American Neuropsychiatric Association. *J. Neuropsychiatry Clin. Neurosci.*, *19*(3), 249–265.

Royall, D. R., Mahurin, R. K., & Cornell, J. (1994). Bedside assessment of frontal degeneration: distinguishing Alzheimer's disease from non-Alzheimer's cortical dementia. *Exp. Aging Res.*, *20*(2), 95–103.

Royall, D. R., Mahurin, R. K., & Cornell, J. (1995). Effect of depression on dementia presentation: Qualitative assessment with the Qualitative Evaluation of Dementia (QED). *J. Geriatr. Psychiatry Neurol.*, *8*(1), 4–11.

Royall, D. R., Mahurin, R. K., & Gray, K. F. (1992). Bedside assessment of executive cognitive impairment: The Executive Interview. *J. Am. Geriatr. Soc.*, *40*, 1221–1226.

Ryan, J. J., Paolo, A. M., & Brungardt, T. M. (1992). WAIS-R test-retest stability in normal persons 75 years and older. *Clin. Neuropsychologist*, *6*, 3–8.

Salgado, R., Lord, S. R., Packer, J., & Ehrlich, F. (1994). Factors associated with falling in elderly hospital patients. *Gerontology*, *40*(6), 325–331.

Salive, M. E., Guralnik, J., Christen, W., Glynn, R. J., Colsher, P., & Ostfeld, A. M. (1992). Functional blindness and visual impairment in older adults from three communities. *Ophthalmology*, *99*(12), 1840–1847.

Sawrie, S. M., Marson, D. C., Boothe, A. L., & Harrell, L. E. (1999). A method for assessing clinically relevant individual cognitive change in older adult populations. *J. Gerontol. B Psychol. Sci. Soc. Sci.*, *54*(2), P116–P124.

Saxton, J., & Swihart, A. A. (1989). Neuropsychological assessment of the severely impaired elderly patient. *Clin Geriatr Med.*, *5*, 531–543.

Saxton, J., McGonigle-Gibson, K. L., Swihart, A. A., Miller, V. J., & Boller, F. (1990). Assessment of the severely impaired patient: description and validation of a new neuropsychological test battery. *Psychological Assessment*, *2*, 298–303.

Schmader, K. E., Hanlon, J. T., Fillenbaum, G. G., Huber, M., Pieper, C., & Horner, R. (1998). Medication use patterns among demented, cognitively impaired and cognitively intact community-dwelling elderly people. *Age Ageing*, *27*(4), 493–501.

Schmidt, M. (1996). *Rey Auditory and Verbal Learning Test: A Handbook.* Los Angeles, CA: Western Psychological Services.

Smith, G. E., Ivnik, R. J., Malec, J. F., Kokmen, E., Tangalos, E. G., & Kurland, L. T. (1992). Mayo's Older Americans Normative Studies (MOANS): factor structure of a core battery. *Psychol. Assess.*, *4*(3), 382–390.

Smith, G. E., Ivnik, R. J., Malec, J. F., & Tangalos, E. G. (1993). Factor structure of the Mayo Older Americans Normative Sample (MOANS) core battery: Replication in a clinical sample. *Psychol. Assess.*, *5*(1), 121–124.

Sobow, T., & Kloszewska, I. (2007). Cholinesterase inhibitors in mild cognitive impairment: A meta-analysis of randomized controlled trials. *Neurol. Neurochir. Pol.*, *41*(1), 13–21.

Spielberger, C. D., Gorsuch, R. C., & Lushene, R. E. (1970). *Manual for the State-Trait Anxiety Inventory.* Palo Alto, CA: Consulting Psychologists Press.

Spreen, O., & Strauss, E. (1998). *A Compendium of Neuropsychological Tests: Administration, Norms, and Commentary* (2nd ed.). New York, NY: Oxford University Press.

Stanley, M. A., & Beck, J. G. (1997). Anxiety disorders in the elderly: The emerging role of behavior therapy. *Behavior Therapy*, *28*(1), 83–100.

Stanley, M. A., & Beck, J. G. (2000). Anxiety disorders. *Clin. Psychol. Rev*, *20*(6), 731–754.

Steinberg, B. A., Bieliauskas, L. A., Smith, G. E., & Ivnik, R. J. (2005a). Mayo's Older Americans Normative Studies: Age- and IQ-Adjusted Norms for the Trail-Making Test, the Stroop Test, and MAE Controlled Oral Word Association Test. *Clin. Neuropsychol.*, *19*(3–4), 329–377.

Steinberg, B. A., Bieliauskas, L. A., Smith, G. E., & Ivnik, R. J. (2005b). Mayo's Older Americans Normative Studies: Age- and IQ-Adjusted Norms for the Wechsler Memory Scale—Revised. *Clin. Neuropsychol.*, *19*(3–4), 378–463.

Steinberg, B. A., Bieliauskas, L. A., Smith, G. E., Ivnik, R. J., & Malec, J. F. (2005c). Mayo's Older Americans Normative Studies: Age- and IQ-Adjusted Norms for the Auditory Verbal Learning Test and the Visual Spatial Learning Test. *Clin. Neuropsychol.*, *19*(3–4), 464–523.

Steinberg, B. A., Bieliauskas, L. A., Smith, G. E., Langellotti, C., & Ivnik, R. J. (2005d). Mayo's Older Americans Normative Studies: Age- and IQ-Adjusted Norms for the Boston Naming Test, the MAE Token Test, and the Judgment of Line Orientation Test. *Clin. Neuropsychol.*, *19*(3–4), 280–328.

Steinman, M. A., Landefeld, C. S., Rosenthal, G. E., Berthenthal, D., Sen, S., & Kaboli, P. J. (2006). Polypharmacy and prescribing quality in older people. *J. Am. Geriatr. Soc.*, *54*(10), 1516–1523.

Stewart, J. T., Gonzalez-Perez, E., Zhu, Y., & Robinson, B. E. (1999). Cognitive predictors of resistiveness in dementia patients. *Am. J. Geriatr. Psychiatry*, *7*(3), 259–263.

Storandt, M. (1994). General principles of assessment of older adults. In M. Storandt, & G. R. VandenBos (Eds.), *Neuropsychological Assessment of Dementia and Depression in Older Adults: A Clinician's Guide* (pp. 7–32). Washington, DC: American Psychological Association.

Suchy, Y., Blint, A., & Osmon, D. C. (1997). Behavioral Dyscontrol Scale: Criterion and predictive validity in an inpatient rehabilitation unit population. *Clin. Neuropsychol.*, *11*(3), 258–265.

Suchy, Y., & Bolger, J. (1999). The Behavioral Dyscontrol Scale as a predictor of aggression against self or others in psychogeriatric inpatients. *Clin. Neuropsychol.*, *13*(4), 487–494.

Suchy, Y., Derbidge, C., & Cope, C. (2005). Behavioral Dyscontrol Scale-Electronic Version: First examination of reliability, validity, and incremental utility. *Clin. Neuropsychol.*, *19*(1), 4–26.

Swihart, A. A., & Pirozzolo, F. J. (1988). The neuropsychology of aging and dementia: Clinical issues. In H. A. Whitaker (Ed.), *Neuropsychological Studies of Nonfocal Brain Damage*. New York, NY: Springer-Verlag.

Talland, G. A. (1965). Three estimates of work span and their stability over the adult years. *Quart. J. Exp. Psychol.*, *17*, 301–307.

Thurman, D. J., Stevens, J. A., & Rao, J. K. (2008). Practice parameter: Assessing patients in a neurology practice for risk of falls (an evidence-based review): Report of the Quality Standards Subcommittee of the American Academy of Neurology. *Neurology*, *70*(6), 473–479.

Tinetti, M. E., Doucette, J., Claus, E., & Marottoli, R. (1995). Risk factors for serious injury during falls by older persons in the community. *J. Am. Geriatr. Soc.*, *43*(11), 1214–1221.

Tulving, E. (1964). Intratrial and intertrial retention: notes towards a theory of free recall verbal learning. *Psychol. Review*, *71*, 219–237.

U.S. Bureau of the Census. (1995, July). Current population reports, national and state population estimates: 1990 to 1994. Report Number P25–1127.

U.S. Census Bureau. (2007). Minority Population Tops 100 Million. Retrieved November 30, 2009, from http://www.census.gov/Press-Release/www/releases/archives/population/010048.html

U.S. Bureau of the Census (2008). Annual Estimates of the Resident Population by Sex and Five-Year Age Groups for the United States: April 1, 2000 to July 1, 2008 (NC-EST2008–01).

Unverzagt, F., Hall, K., Torke, A., Rediger, J., Mercado, N., Gureje, O., et al. (1996). Effects of age, education, and gender on CERAD neuropsychological test performance in an African-American sample. *Clin. Neuropsychol.*, *10*, 180–190.

Unverzagt, F. W., Hall, K. S., Torke, A. M., Rediger, J. D., Mercado, N., & Hendrie, H. C. (1995). The CERAD neuropsychological test battery: Norms from an African-American sample. *Journal of the International Neuropsychological Society*, *1*.

Vakil, E., & Agmon-Ashkenazi, D. (1997). Baseline performance and learning rate of procedural and declarative memory tasks: Younger versus older adults. *J. Gerontol. B Psychol. Sci. Soc. Sci.*, *52*(5), P229–P234.

Vecchi, T., & Richardson, J. T. (2001). Measures of visuospatial short-term memory: The Knox Cube Imitation Test and the Corsi Blocks Test compared. *Brain Cogn.*, *46*(1–2), 291–295.

Veliz-Reissmuller, G., Aguero Torres, H., van der Linden, J., Lindblom, D., & Eriksdotter Jonhagen, M. (2007). Pre-operative mild cognitive dysfunction predicts risk for post-operative delirium after elective cardiac surgery. *Aging Clin. Exp. Res.*, *19*(3), 172–177.

Visser, P. J., Scheltens, P., Pelgrim, E., & Verhey, F. R. (2005). Medial temporal lobe atrophy and APOE genotype do not predict cognitive improvement upon treatment with rivastigmine in Alzheimer's disease patients. *Dement. Geriatr. Cogn. Disord.*, *19*(2–3), 126–133.

Vitaliano, P. P., Breen, A. R., Albert, M. S., Russo, J., & Printz, P. N. (1984). Memory, attention, and functional status in community residing Alzheimer type dementia patients and optimally healthy aged individuals. *Journal of Gerontology*, *39*(58–64), 58–64.

Wechsler, D. (1981). *Wechsler Adult Intelligence Scale-Revised*. San Antonio, TX: Psychological Corporation.

Wechsler, D. (1987). *Wechsler Memory Scale-Revised*. San Antonio, TX: Psychological Corporation.

Wechsler, D. (1997). *WAIS-III/WMS-III Technical Manual*. San Antonio, TX: Psychological Corporation.

Wechsler, D. (2008). *Wechsler Adult Intelligence Scale-Fourth Edition (WAIS-IV) Technical and Interpretive Manual*. San Antonio, TX: Pearson.

Wechsler, D. (2009). *WMS-IV Technical and Interpretive Manual*. San Antonio, TX: Pearson.

Weissman, M. M., Leaf, P. J., Holzer, C. E., 3rd, & Merikangas, K. R. (1985). The epidemiology of anxiety disorders: A highlight of recent evidence. *Psychopharmacol. Bull.*, *21*(3), 538–541.

Welsh, K. A., Fillenbaum, G., Wilkinson, W., Heyman, A., Mohs, R. C., Stern, Y., et al. (1995). Neuropsychological test performance in African-American and white patients with Alzheimer's disease. *Neurology*, *45*, 2207–2211.

White, H. K., & Levin, E. D. (2004). Chronic transdermal nicotine patch treatment effects on cognitive performance in age-associated memory impairment. *Psychopharmacology (Berl.)*, *171*(4), 465–471.

Wild, K., Howieson, D., Webbe, F., Seelye, A., & Kaye, J. (2008). Status of computerized cognitive testing in aging: A systematic review. *Alzheimers Dement.*, *4*(6), 428–437.

Wild, K. V., & Kaye, J. (2009). Response to Doniger. *Alzheimers Dement.*, *5*(5), 441.

Woodard, J. L., Auchus, A. P., Godsall, R. E., & Green, R. C. (1998). An analysis of test bias and differential item functioning due to race on the Mattis Dementia Rating Scale. *J. Gerontol. B Psychol. Sci. Soc. Sci*, *53* (6), 370–374.

Woodard, J. L., Dunlosky, J. A., & Salthouse, T. A. (1999). Task decomposition analysis of intertrial free recall performance on the Rey Auditory Verbal Learning Test in normal aging and Alzheimer's disease. *J. Clin. Exp. Neuropsychol.*, *21*(5), 666–676.

Woodard, J. L., Goldstein, F. C., Roberts, V. J., & McGuire, C. (1999). Convergent and discriminant validity of the CVLT (Dementia Version). *J. Clin. Exp. Neuropsychol.*, *21*(4), 553–558.

Woodcock, R. W., & Johnson, M. B. (1977). *Woodcock-Johnson Psycho-Educational Battery*. Itasca, IL: Riverside.

Woodcock, R. W., McGrew, K. S., & Mather, N. (2001a). *Woodcock-Johnson III Tests of Achievement*. Itasca, IL: Riverside.

Woodcock, R. W., McGrew, K. S., & Mather, N. (2001b). *Woodcock-Johnson-III Tests of Cognitive Abilities*. Itasca, IL: Riverside.

Yeh, S. C., & Liu, Y. Y. (2003). Influence of social support on cognitive function in the elderly. *BMC Health Serv Res.*, *3*(1), 9.

Yesavage, J. A., Brink, T. L., Rose, T. L., & Adey, M. (1986). The Geriatric Depression Rating Scale: Comparison with other self-report and psychiatric rating scales. In L. Poon (Ed.), *Handbook for Clinical Memory Assessment of Older Adults* (pp. 153–167). Washington, DC: American Psychological Association.

Yesavage, J. A., Brink, T. L., Rose, T. L., Lum, O., Huang, V., Adey, M., et al. (1983). Development and validation of a geriatric depression screening scale: a preliminary report. *J. Psychiatr. Res.*, *17*, 37–49.

Yochim, B. P., Bank, A. L., Mast, B. T., MacNeill, S. E., & Lichtenberg, P. A. (2003). Clinical utility of the Mattis Dementia Rating Scale in older, urban medical patients: An expanded study. *Aging, Neuropsychology, and Cognition*, *10*(3), 230–237.

CHAPTER

19 Screening Instruments and Brief Batteries for Dementia

Benjamin T. Mast, Adam Gerstenecker
Department of Psychological and Brain Sciences, University of Louisville, KT, USA

INTRODUCTION

Cognitive impairment is the most frequent mental health syndrome affecting older adults and is a leading cause of disability, psychological distress, and health care expenditures. Dementia syndromes such as Alzheimer's disease (AD) have grown in prevalence as advances in medical care have increased longevity. As many as one in seven adults over the age of 71 have dementia (Plassman et al., 2007) and some have predicted that the number of individuals with dementia will triple by the year 2050 with the greatest increase among those over the age of 85 (Hebert, Scherr, Bienias, Bennett, & Evans, 2003). Moreover, many older adults who do not have dementia nonetheless have some milder form of cognitive impairment that affects their ability to function and which may signal higher risk for developing dementia than those who do not have similar impairment (Plassman et al., 2008; Petersen et al., 2001). Considerable attention has been given to developing pharmacological and psychosocial interventions aimed at reducing or reversing cognitive impairment and dementia, but many of these have fallen short of expectations. At best pharmacological approaches slow the progression of symptoms for a short period of time for some but not all individuals (Birks, 2006; Raschetti, Albanese, Vanacore, & Maggini, 2007; Rodda & Walker, 2009; Trinh, 2003). Some have hypothesized that these medications would be more effective if initiated earlier in the dementia syndrome, leading to a renewed emphasis on earlier detection of cognitive impairment.

Early identification of cognitive impairment may also lead to empowerment of the cognitively impaired person and their family by giving them the opportunity to become more educated regarding the illness, which can lead to better decision-making and less stress. On the other hand, ruling out cognitive impairment can lead elders complaining of memory loss to look for other explanations (depression, illness, normal age-related change, etc.). As dementia becomes more advanced the purposes of brief batteries shift toward evaluating the impact of cognitive impairment on daily functioning, the need for environmental support to ensure safety, and a variety of clinical situations such as treatment and discharge planning (e.g., can the person live alone safely?). Although all instruments require evidence of clinical utility and validity, additional psychometric features may be emphasized depending upon the purpose of the assessment. Whereas instruments used for earlier detection of dementia syndromes require high levels of sensitivity, instruments used for the purpose of predicting functioning have greater requirements for predictive validity.

In this chapter we review commonly used cognitive screening instruments and brief batteries for dementia. This chapter builds upon the work of MacNeill & Lichtenberg (1999) from the previous edition of this Handbook. We have included those that have received the most empirical investigation

Handbook of Assessment in Clinical Gerontology. DOI: 10.1016/B978-0-12-374961-1.10019-3

over the past ten years. In some cases this required updating the evidence concerning previously reviewed instruments (e.g., CERAD, 7 minute screen, Mattis Dementia Rating Scale) and in other cases evaluating new instruments which were not available at the time of the first edition (e.g., RBANS, Mini-Cog, GP-COG). Each instrument was evaluated for evidence concerning: (1) clinical utility including sensitivity, specificity, and area under the curve (AUC) in receiver operating characteristics (ROC) analyses; (2) administration features including brevity, standardization, and ease of administration; (3) availability of normative data applicable to diverse patient populations; and (4) the extent to which the measures tap into key cognitive abilities that are most affected by aging and dementia (e.g., memory and executive functioning).

As screening measures are increasingly relied upon to detect dementia in its earliest stages, consideration should be given to whether they measure domains that are often the first signs of a clinical problem. The literatures describing normal aging, AD, and vascular cognitive impairment highlight common underlying brain changes and their cognitive correlates. First, volumetric brain changes accompanying the normal aging process appear to differentially affect brain regions, with most evidence indicating that the prefrontal cortex and its subcortical connections in the striatum (caudate, putamen) experience the earliest and most severe changes (Raz, 2005; Raz & Rodrigue, 2006). Second, cerebrovascular risk factors such as hypertension and diabetes grow increasingly common with advancing age and appear to exacerbate these frontal-subcortical changes (Gunning-Dixon & Raz, 2003; O'Brien, 2006; Raz, Rodrigue, & Acker, 2003). Third, early AD changes preferentially affect medial temporal lobe structures such as the hippocampus and entorhinal cortex, perhaps even prior to the development of clinically significant dementia (Bennett et al., 2006; Bondi, Salmon, Galasko, Thomas, & Thal, 1999; Collie & Maruff, 2000; Schmitt et al., 2000; Galvin et al., 2005). Finally, emerging evidence suggests that executive dysfunction may develop even earlier than memory impairment, and that both precede observable decline on global measures of cognition such as the MMSE (Carlson, Xue, Zhou, & Fried, 2009). The practical implication is that screening measures and brief batteries will most effectively detect these early changes when they are focused on the cognitive domains most affected: learning and memory (particularly delayed recall) and executive functioning (Backman, Jones, Berger, Laukka, & Small, 2005; Bondi et al., 1999; Collie & Maruff, 2000; Grober & Kawas, 1997; Gunning-Dixon & Raz, 2000; Gunning-Dixon & Raz, 2003; Stout et al., 1999; West, 1996). In this review, we evaluate the extent to which these measures tap into these critical cognitive abilities in addition to the traditional psychometric criteria.

We also evaluate these measures in light of their applicability to diverse populations, both in terms of English speaking minority elders in the United States and whether the measures have been translated and tested in non-English speaking samples. These data are becoming increasingly relied upon as the aging population continues to grow more diverse and empirical data often show group level differences on many cognitive screening tests (Manly, 2008). Although age, education, and even race stratified norms are available for some screens and neuropsychological measures (Lucas et al., 2005; Patton et al., 2003; Rilling et al., 2005), these may not fully capture the underlying variability of interest when considering diverse samples (Manly & Echemendia, 2007). The nature and quality of educational experiences have proven to significantly impact cognitive test scores in later life (Allaire & Whitfield, 2004; Manly, Byrd, Touradji, & Stern, 2004). Manly and colleagues have demonstrated that controlling for quality of education, as approximated by WRAT Reading scores, significantly reduces or eliminates differences between African American and White samples, and that the reading scores were a better predictor of cognitive performance than years of formal education (Manly, Jacobs, Touradji, Small, & Stern, 2002; Manly et al., 2004). With regard to language, most cognitive tests were developed and validated on English speaking samples, but the practice of geriatric neuropsychology has grown more diverse over time, both in relation to the assessment of elders who do not speak English or are bilingual within North American clinics (Mindt et al., 2008) and in relation to the detection of dementia worldwide (Sosa et al., 2009).

Table 19.1 Screening Measures for Dementia

Measure	Authors/Reference	Domains Tested	Studied in Diverse Samples and/or Multiple Translations
MMSE	Folstein, Folstein, & McHugh, 1975	orientation memory attention constructional praxis	Yes
Mini-Cog	Borson, Scanlan, Brush, Vitaliano & Dokmak, 2000	memory constructional praxis executive function	Yes
MIS	Buschke et al., 1999	memory	Yes
GPCOG	Brodaty et al., 2002	orientation memory constructional praxis executive function	Yes
7MS	Solomon et al., 1998	orientation memory verbal fluency constructional praxis executive function	Yes
MoCA	Nasreddine et al., 2005	executive function constructional praxis memory orientation naming attention language abstraction	Yes
Clock Drawing Test CLOX	See Shulman, 2000 Royall, Cordes, & Polk, 1998	constructional praxis executive function	Yes

SCREENING FOR DEMENTIA—THE LEGACY OF THE MMSE

The majority of screening research has focused upon community and primary care settings. Boustani and colleagues (2003) note that 50–66% of all cases of dementia are missed in primary care and that most of these are individuals with mild to moderate dementia. This statistic suggests that there is a great opportunity for screening measures to improve upon the care being offered to these individuals, and that there is likely a discrepancy between the plethora of available screening tools and what is actually being utilized in these settings. Boise et al. (1999) found that general practitioners view the Mini-Mental State Examination (MMSE; Folstein et al., 1975) as impractical for use in a primary care setting due to the duration of its administration. This observation is bolstered by the fact that the average length of time a patient is seen in a primary care setting in the United States is 19 minutes (Flocke, Frank, & Wenger, 2001) and 8–11 minutes in Europe (Deveugele, Derese, van den Brink-Muinen, De Maeseneer, & Bensing, 2002).

Nonetheless, the MMSE is the most widely recognized and utilized screening measure for dementia and other cognitive impairment. It was originally developed to assess global cognitive

Table 19.2 Brief Batteries for Dementia

Measure	Author/reference	Domains Tested	Studied in Diverse Samples
CERAD	Morris et al., 1989 Welsh, Butters, Hughes, Mohs & Heyman, 1992	orientation memory verbal fluency attention constructional praxis	Yes
RBANS	Randolph, Tierney, Mohr, & Chase, 1998	immediate memory delayed memory visual-spatial/construction attention language	Limited
Elements of NSRP and other batteries			
DRS DRS-2	Mattis, 1988 Jurica et al., 2001	attention initiation/perseveration construction conceptualization memory	Yes
FOME	Fuld, 1981	memory	Yes

functioning by testing orientation, registration, short-term recall, attention, calculation, visuo-constructional skills, and praxis. The MMSE has a number of limitations including a ceiling effect rendering it less sensitive to early dementia, limited focus on memory (3 points out of 30) and the lack of an executive functioning component (Brodaty, Fay, Gibson, & Burns, 2006; Kahokehr, Siegert, & Weatherall, 2004; Lorentz, Scanlan, & Borson, 2002; Tombaugh & Mcintyre, 1992). Scores are significantly influenced by age and education, but the availability of corrected norms mitigates this limitation to the extent that they are utilized over the traditional cut-score method (Tombaugh, McDowell, Kristjansson, & Hubley, 1996). Despite these limitations 51% of general practitioners who screen older patients for dementia use the MMSE (Brodaty et al., 2006). This statistic may contribute to large numbers of missed dementia diagnoses in the primary care setting, particularly in the early stages when the MMSE is less sensitive. As Zarit and colleagues (2008) noted, "The MMSE has become like a somewhat embarrassing member of the family; we all know Uncle Henry's flaws, but we continue to invite him to holiday dinner, because we cannot imagine the alternative" (p. 411). Yet, despite the limitations of the MMSE, its broad application with a common metric makes it the instrument against which other screening instruments are compared.

In the sections that follow we review alternative dementia screening measures that may be more applicable to detection of mild to moderate dementia in primary care settings. We begin with three screens (Mini-Cog, MIS, GP-COG) that have been singled out as particularly promising by separate reviews focused on primary care. The first review evaluated whether these possess characteristics appropriate for application to the primary care setting: validation in a community, population, or general practice setting; ease and length of administration; and demonstration of a misclassification rate less than the MMSE and an NPV greater than the MMSE (Brodaty et al., 2006). The second review (Lorentz et al., 2002) evaluated the face validity, sensitivity, specificity, vulnerability to bias, acceptability to patients and doctors, ease of administration and scoring, and the practicality of interpretation by a non-specialist for screeners that had administration time of 10 minutes or less and validation in a community or clinical sample. Finally, Milne and colleagues (2008) used 16 selection criteria under four key domains: practicality; feasibility; range of applicability; and psychometric properties. Convergent evidence from these three reviews highlights the utility and applicability of these three measures. Below we describe each of these measures in detail followed by three additional screening measures which have received considerable attention (7 minute screen, MoCA, and Clock Drawing Tests). The dementia screening measures described below are by no means exhaustive. An attempt was made to include measures that are currently receiving the most empirical attention. A number of other measures (i.e., ABCS, NUCOG, CAST, ADSPC) have not yet received as much attention in research studies and are therefore not discussed, but could prove to be quite effective with additional research.

Mini-Cog

The Mini-Cog combines two simple cognitive tasks: clock drawing and delayed recall of three words (Borson, Scanlan, Chen, & Ganguli, 2003). First, the examiner asks the person being tested to listen to and then repeat three unrelated words. Next, the tested person is instructed to draw a circle and the face of a clock within the circle and to set the hands of the clock to reflect 11:10. After completion of the clock drawing, the person is asked to recall the three words. (If the three words are not able to be recalled upon the initial recall trial, this portion may be skipped.) The Mini-Cog takes approximately three minutes to administer and was developed to be free of bias effects from race, culture, education, and language while at the same time enhancing the operating characteristics of the clock drawing test (CDT) as a dementia screening tool (Borson et al., 2000).

One point is given for each correctly recalled word; two points for a "normal" clock drawing; and zero points for an "abnormal" clock drawing. Mini-Cog scores from 0 to 2 lie in the "probably impaired" range while scores from 3 to 5 lie in the "probably not impaired" range (Borson, Scanlan, Watanabe, Tu, & Lessig, 2006). In the original validation sample of 249 ethnically diverse older adults (dementia base rate of 50%), the Mini-Cog significantly outperformed the MMSE by achieving sensitivity of 99% and specificity of 93% (Borson et al., 2000). In a second population-based study (Borson et al., 2003) of 1179 older adults from the MoVIES project (6.4% dementia prevalence) the Mini-Cog achieved a sensitivity of 76% and specificity of 89%. Although lower than the validation sample, these properties were not unexpected, due to the low base rate of dementia in the sample, and still outperformed the MMSE (Borson et al., 2003).

In light of its short duration, ease of administration, and utility in samples of varying dementia base rates and demographics, the Mini-Cog appears to be an attractive option for use in primary care. The Mini-Cog has been shown to demonstrate significantly better sensitivity than primary care physicians in the detection of cognitive impairment in a predominantly ethnic minority sample (84% to 41%, respectively) with the discrepancy being most apparent in the early stages of dementia (58% vs. 6% at CDR 0.5; and 92% vs. 6% at CDR 1.0, respectively) (Borson et al., 2006). The Mini-Cog has also been shown to be equally effective when administered by expert or naïve raters (Scanlan & Borson, 2001) further demonstrating its potential utility in primary care settings.

Nonetheless, the Mini-Cog suffers from many of the same limitations as other clock drawing tests: lack of sensitivity to mild cognitive impairment and differing operating characteristics based upon CDT scoring methods. Lessig, Scanlan, Nazemi, & Borson, (2007) suggested that substituting a new algorithm based upon a simplified CDT scoring system examining six critical errors—wrong time setting, number substitution, number repetition, missing numbers, no hands, and refusal—could increase the utility of the Mini-Cog.

Memory Impairment Screen (MIS)

The Memory Impairment Screen (MIS; Buschke et al., 1999) is a four-word delayed recall memory test that was developed to be a simple yet accurate dementia screen that can be administered in approximately four minutes (Kuslansky, Buschke, Katz, Sliwinski, & Lipton, 2002). The person is presented with four flashcards each containing one word that belongs to a distinct semantic category. The person is asked to read the word (e.g., New York) on the flashcard and associate the word with its appropriate semantic category (e.g., city). Once all four flashcards have been read and the associated semantic category given, the tested person is then asked to engage in a distracter task for approximately 2–3 minutes (counting from 1 to 20 forwards and backwards) and then recall as many words from the flashcards as they can remember. If a word is not recalled, the examiner verbally presents the semantic category associated with the unretrieved word and gives a second opportunity to recall the word. A total of eight points is possible: two points for each word recalled without semantic cues and one point for each word recalled with the aid of semantic cues. Scores of four or less are considered indicative of cognitive impairment and a more comprehensive dementia assessment is warranted, although the authors also recommend selecting optimal cutscores based upon the intended clinical or research application (Buschke et al., 1999).

The authors of the MIS originally studied the instrument in a sample of 483 community volunteers, 10% of whom had dementia. AUC was 0.94, and no significant effects of education were reported. Using a cutscore of 4, the MIS achieved sensitivity of 80%, specificity of 96%, PPV of 69%, and NPV of 98% when screening for all dementia and demonstrated a higher (87%) sensitivity when the evaluation was restricted to Alzheimer's disease (Buschke et al., 1999). In comparing the MIS to a conventional three-word memory test in a sample of 240 community-dwelling elders with a 12% dementia prevalence, Kuslansky et al. (2002) reported no effects of education and determined the MIS to be superior to a conventional three-word memory test as a dementia screen. Kuslansky and colleagues (2002) reported clinical utility estimates similar to the original sample—86% sensitivity, 97% specificity, 80% PPV, 96% overall correct classification rate and 93% AUC.

Many researchers view the MIS as having the potential for broad utility in a primary care setting because of its ease of administration and short duration (Holsinger, Deveau, Boustani, & Williams, 2007), and have continued to conduct research on ways to improve its operating characteristics. For instance, Chopard et al. (2007) demonstrated that the operating characteristics of the MIS could be increased to significantly outperform the MMSE by combining it with the Isaacs Set Test (IST; Issacs & Kennie, 1973). Rotrou et al. (2007) observed that the operating characteristics of the MIS could be increased by making the distracter task 10 minutes as opposed to 2–3 minutes, and Grober et al. (2008) presented evidence that the addition of a short verbal fluency test such as animal naming (potentially administered during the distracter phase) may improve detection of early-stage dementia. The MIS has been also shown to be an effective screening measure when administered by telephone (Lipton et al., 2003), and Cherbuin, Anstey, & Lipnicki, (2007) recommended the MIS be validated in a self-administered electronic format.

General Practitioners Assessment of Cognition (GP-COG)

The General Practitioners Assessment of Cognition (GPCOG; Brodaty et al., 2002) was developed to be used by general practitioners in primary care settings and combines cognitive and informant data into a 4–5 minute, two-stage dementia screening instrument. Nine total points are available on the cognitive portion: 1 point for orientation to time; 1 point for knowledge of a high-profile news story; 1 point for providing correct numbering and spacing; and 1 point for placing the time as "ten minutes past eleven" on a clock drawing task; and five points for recalling "John, Brown, 42, West Street, Kensington" (one point for each unit). Scores of nine (indicative of no cognitive impairment) or less than five (indicative of cognitive impairment) do not require an informant portion. For scores of 5 through 8, the informant is asked six questions comparing the patient's present functioning to that observed "a few years ago." If the informant indicates that the evaluated person has more current difficulty with three or more of the six tasks in question, including memory of recent conversations, misplacing items, word finding difficulties, money management, medication management, and need for travel assistance (Brodaty, Kemp, & Low, 2004), the evaluated person is considered cognitively impaired and in need of a more comprehensive dementia assessment.

In the original validation study the GPCOG was as effective as or better than the MMSE, demonstrating 85% sensitivity, 86% specificity, PPV of 71%, and an overall misclassification rate of 14% in a general practitioner recruited sample of 283 community-dwelling elders with a dementia base rate of 29%. In a second study using the same sample, the authors of the GPCOG examined demographic influence and found the GPCOG to be susceptible to age effects but free of effects due to education, gender, or the presence of depression (Brodaty et al., 2004). A later study by Basic et al. (2009) found the GPCOG to be more sensitive, but also more apt to exhibit lower specificity, PPV, and NPV than the MMSE in a sample with a dementia prevalence of 38%. Moreover, although the GPCOG patient and informant sections may be used in the absence of the other, the combination of the two sections outperformed each section used alone.

Nonetheless, the GPCOP has notable limitations. Although inclusion of an informant section adds useful information and strengthens the operating characteristics of the GPCOG, these benefits will be excluded for those who do not have access to an informant with knowledge of their functioning over a number of years. A limited number of studies examining the operating characteristics of the GPCOG are available, with most of these being conducted by the authors of the measure and in samples with a high prevalence of dementia. Further studies examining the GPCOG in samples of different demographics and dementia base rates are recommended. See Appendix for GP-COG test.

Seven-Minute Screen

The Seven-Minute Screen (7MS; Solomon et al., 1998) was designed to be used in a primary care setting and to meet the following criteria: can be administered by a medical technician; requires no clinical judgment to score and minimal training to administer; takes into consideration the latest research on the differences between normal aging and AD; and demonstrates a high ability to discriminate between people with AD and those experiencing normal aging. The four subtests are based upon existing dementia screens assessing different domains: orientation for time, based on the Benton Temporal Orientation Test (Benton, 1983); memory, based on the Enhanced Cued Recall Test (Grober, Buschke, Crystal, Bang, & Dresner, 1988) in which 16 pictures are visually presented and the tested person is instructed to recall the pictures with semantic cues given if necessary; clock drawing based on the seven-item Clock Drawing Test developed by Freedman et al. (1994); and verbal fluency in which the tested person is instructed to name as many animals as possible in one minute.

Scoring of the 7MS is achieved via a weighted scoring mechanism based upon the logistic regression model derived by the authors. A hand-held calculator—included with the test materials—returns an indicator variable that denotes the probability of dementia (Lawrence, Davidoff, Katt-Lloyd, Auerbach, & Hennen, 2001). A high probability (>0.9) is indicative of cognitive impairment with a more comprehensive cognitive assessment recommended; a low probability (<0.1) is not indicative of cognitive impairment and no further testing is recommended; and a "Retest/Deferred" function (between 0.1 and 0.9) is seen as ambiguous with a second testing session to be done within 6–9 months (Solomon & Pendlebury, 1998).

The original validation sample of the 7MS (Solomon et al., 1998) included 120 people living in the Vermont area, half of whom had a known dementia diagnosis. Sensitivity and specificity were both determined to be 100% with no effect of age or education on 7MS scores. One thousand repeated random samples of 30 people from the AD group and 30 people from the non-AD group were then calculated with sensitivity observed to be 92% and specificity observed to be 96%. Meulen et al. (2004) found similar results in a Dutch sample of 587 elders with a 58% dementia base rate. Average 7MS administration time reached 13 minutes, yielded an area under the ROC curve of 0.989, a sensitivity of 92.9%, specificity of 93.5%, PPV of 98%, and NPV of 75% which significantly outperformed the MMSE, especially in the detection of mild dementia. Ijuin et al. (2008) studied the 7MS in a sample of 154 community-dwelling elders with no cognitive impairment or early stage AD (CDR of 0.5−1) and determined the 7MS to have significantly better clinical utility (90.5% sensitivity and 92.3% specificity) than both the MMSE and MIS. In a sample of 66 Norwegian community-dwelling elders without cognitive impairment (Skjerve et al., 2007), the average duration of administration of the 7MS was approximately 12 minutes as opposed to the administration duration of 7 minutes and 42 seconds reported in the original sample. Age and education effects were present for the Verbal Fluency subtest. The 7MS has been administered in many countries and has been translated into and validated in Greek (Tsolaki et al., 2002), Dutch (Meulen et al., 2004), German (Reischies & Kühl, 2005), Spanish (Del Ser, Sánchez-Sánchez, de Yébenes, Munoz, & Otero, 2006), Norwegian (Skjerve et al., 2007), and Japanese (Ijuin et al., 2008).

Despite its excellent operating characteristics and the inclusion of a scoring calculator and training video in the testing packet, both Lorentz et al. (2002) and Brodaty, Fay, Gibson, & Burns, (2006) view the 7MS as being too difficult and requiring too much training for widespread application in a primary care setting. Another factor limiting the 7MS's applicability as a dementia screen in the primary care setting is that it took approximately 12 minutes to administer in a majority of studies. However, this may be less of a barrier for mass community screening events. Lawrence et al. (2001) and Lawrence et al. (2003) trained volunteers to administer the 7MS to large groups of elders during a community screening day. The volunteers reported little to no problems administering the measure, and it was well accepted by the people being assessed. Moreover Ijuin et al. (2008) modified the 7MS into a paper-and-pencil form so it could be administered to large groups at one time without changing its underlying operating characteristics.

Montreal Cognitive Assessment (MoCA)

The Montreal Cognitive Assessment (MoCA; Nasreddine et al., 2005) takes approximately 10 minutes to administer and was designed to detect mild cognitive impairment in elders scoring in the normal range on the MMSE. Thirty items assessing multiple cognitive domains are contained in the MoCA: short-term memory (5 points); visuospatial abilities via clock drawing (3 points), and a cube copy task (1 point); executive functioning via an adaptation of Trail Making Test Part B (1 point), phonemic fluency (1 point), and verbal abstraction (2 points); attention, concentration, and working memory via target detection (1 point), serial subtraction (3 points), digits forward (1 point), and digits backward (1 point); language via confrontation naming with low-familiarity animals (3 points), and repetition of complex sentences (2 points); and orientation to time and place (6 points) (Nasreddine et al., 2005). The MoCA is scored by obtaining an item total and the authors recommend a clinical cutoff score of 26. The measure is available in 27 languages along with instructions and normative data at http://www.mocatest.org/.

In the original validation study, the MoCA was administered to 277 elders—93 AD, 94 MCI, and 90 NC—recruited from the Jewish General Hospital Memory Clinic in Montreal, Quebec (Nasreddine et al., 2005). Both English and French versions were used so the measure could be administered according to language preference. The MoCA outperformed the MMSE across both MCI and AD groups (MoCA sensitivity 0.90 and 1.00, respectively), but its specificity was observed to be lower than that of the MMSE (although still high at 0.87). PPV for the MoCA was 0.89 for both groups and

NPV of 0.91 and 1.00 for the MCI and AD groups, respectively. The MoCA was influenced by education, prompting the authors to recommend adding one point to the cutscore for elders with over 12 years of education.

Subsequent studies have demonstrated a trend characterized by high sensitivity and low specificity for the MoCA. In a study by Smith and colleagues (2007), the utility estimates of the MoCA and MMSE were compared in a sample of 67 elders (32 AD, 23 MCI, and 12 NC). Sensitivity of the MoCA and MMSE (using a cutscore of 26) were observed to be 0.83 and 0.17, respectively, for the MCI group and 0.94 and 0.25, respectively, for the AD group. These sensitivities were comparable to those of the validation study, but the obtained specificity of 0.50 was significantly lower. In a later study by Luis, Keegan, and Mullan, (2009) the recommended cutscore was re-evaluated. At a cutoff of 26, the MoCA yielded high sensitivity but low specificity, but when a cutscore of 23 was used, both sensitivity and specificity were excellent (0.96 and 0.95, respectively).

The MoCA has also received empirical attention for its ability to detect cognitive impairment in people with Parkinson's disease. In a study of 100 patients diagnosed with PD and scoring in the normal range on the MMSE, Nazem et al. (2009) found that 52% of the sample scored below the MoCA's recommended cutoff. Zadikoff et al. (2008) also found that a sample of PD patients performed significantly worse on the MoCA than the MMSE—32% scoring below the cutoff on the MoCA compared to only 11% on the MMSE. A caveat does exist, however, for both the previously mentioned studies. The number of Parkinson's patients scoring below the cutoff score on the MoCA and MMSE were compared, but not the overall operating characteristics of the two measures.

The MoCA is a promising alternative to the MMSE because of its sensitivity to early detection of dementia and MCI. Although Holsinger et al. (2007) recommended the MoCA for use by primary care physicians with "plenty of time available" (p. 2401), further empirical attention is needed. The MoCA's range of specificity is wide across the few studies that have examined its clinical utility, and it has not been compared to screens other than the MMSE. Therefore, comparisons across cutscores and CDR rating to other recently developed dementia screens requiring less time to administer is recommended. See Appendix for MOCA test.

Clock Drawing Tests

The drawing and/or copying of clocks is a widely used approach to dementia screening and also serves as a component of numerous other screening measures described above (Mini-Cog, GPCOG, 7MS, MoCA). Clock Drawing Tests (CDTs) are brief, easy to administer, and generally well accepted by test administrators and the individuals being tested. Typically the tested person is asked to "draw a circle and place the numbers in the circle to make it look like a clock" and to "draw the hands on the clock to make the time read 10 minutes past 11 o'clock." Even though most CDTs follow a similar format, over a dozen CDT systems exist and may yield differing operational characteristics. In the most comprehensive review of CDTs to date, Shulman (2000) found the mean sensitivity and specificity to be approximately 85%, but more recent studies have brought this finding into question (Seigerschmidt et al., 2002). He also observed that lengthy CDT scoring systems do not significantly outperform shorter versions.

The AUC of five frequently used CDT scoring systems—the Shulman method (Shulman, Shedletsky & Silver, 1986), the Sunderland method (Sunderland et al., 1989), the Wolf-Klein method (Wolf-Klein, Silverstone, Levy, & Brod, 1989), the Mendez method (Mendez, Ala, & Underwood, 1992), and the Watson method (Watson, Arfken, & Birge, 1993)—were compared in a sample of 127 consecutive referrals to a clinic in Sydney, Australia (Storey, Rowland, Basic, & Conforti, 2001). High inter- and intra-rater correlation coefficients were observed on all scoring methods, but the Shulman and Mendez methods demonstrated the largest observed areas under the ROC curve at 0.79 and 0.78, respectively. The Shulman (93% sensitivity and 55% specificity) and Mendez (96% sensitivity and

26% specificity) methods significantly outperformed the Sunderland and Watson methods in the detection of dementia, but the authors of the study still caution in the use of any CDT method as a stand-alone dementia screen, presumably due to low specificity. In a study of the ability of CDT to detect questionable or early stage dementia, Seigerschmidt et al. (2002) found four scoring methods to be more appropriate for the detection of clear dementia rather than for questionable or mild dementia (CDR = 0.5) in which the tests yield a high number of false positives.

Although the drawing component relies to some extent upon visual-spatial abilities, Royall has argued that CDTs also assess executive control functions that govern performance on this visual-spatial task, and accounts for a large proportion of variance in low clock drawing scores. He developed a two-stage clock drawing task (CLOX; Royall, Cordes & Polk, 1998) in an attempt to separate the executive control needed to complete a clock drawing task from the task itself. In the first stage (CLOX1) the tested person is instructed to "Draw me a clock that says 1:45. Set the hands and numbers on the face so that a child could read them." In the second stage (CLOX2) the tested person is instructed to copy a clock that was drawn by the test administrator. CLOX1 was observed as being highly correlated with an independent measure of executive control while CLOX2 was found to be highly correlated with the MMSE. In addition, the CLOX measures have demonstrated the ability to predict IADL functioning and level of care more effectively than the MMSE (Lavery et al., 2005; Royall, Chiodo, & Polk, 2000; Royall, Chiodo, & Polk, 2005).

Summary of Screening Instruments

Several of the measures described above demonstrate excellent utility, brevity, standardization, and application in diverse samples. In consideration of the key cognitive domains, most contain an emphasis on memory, particularly delayed recall (with the exception of the GP-COG and CDT). The Mini-Cog and GP-COG include a delayed recall component, albeit a somewhat limited one, and similar to the MMSE. The MoCA, MIS, and 7MS have slightly more demanding memory tasks and appear to be more effective in detecting mild dementia. The Mini-Cog, 7MS, and GP-COG may detect executive dysfunction via the Clock Drawing component, although the extent to which CDTs measure executive functioning vs. visual-spatial and general cognitive functioning is still uncertain. The MoCA screen is somewhat unique in that it seeks to evaluate executive functioning with multiple items (trail making, clock drawing, abstraction), and has a more detailed focus on memory. Like the MMSE, the MIS does not have an executive functioning component, although as indicated by Grober and colleagues (2008) a verbal fluency measure could be included in the delay which could aid in the evaluation of executive functioning similar to the 7MS.

BRIEF BATTERIES

Often a positive dementia screen will trigger a more in-depth evaluation of cognitive functioning using a brief neuropsychological battery. As noted by MacNeill and Lichtenberg (1999), longer test batteries used with other neuropsychological populations (e.g., traumatic brain injury, seizure disorders) can lead to frustration, fatigue, and fear among older patients who may not be able to tolerate lengthy procedures due to greater medical comorbidity and physical changes. Therefore, an emphasis on brief batteries has been welcome within geriatric neuropsychology. As with the screening review, we focus our attention upon updating research either on batteries reviewed in the previous edition or on batteries which have emerged since that publication.

Consortium to Establish a Registry for Alzheimer's Disease (CERAD) Battery

The CERAD neuropsychological battery contains five subtests including an abbreviated (15 item) Boston Naming Test, Animal Naming, the MMSE, constructional praxis (copying line drawings), and a word list memory task with immediate and delayed recall and recognition components (Morris et al., 1989; Welsh, et al., 1992). Since the review by MacNeill and Lichtenberg (1999), this battery has received considerable attention in the psychometric literature and has been studied extensively in diverse samples over the past 10 years including African Americans, Japanese Americans, Native Americans, and samples from Australia, Brazil, Jamaica, Finland, and Korea (Bertolucci et al., 2001; Collie, Shafiq-Antonacci, Maruff, Tyler, & Currie, 1999; Fillenbaum et al., 2005; Fillenbaum, Peterson, Welsh-Bohmer, Kukull, & Heyman, 1998; Karrasch, Sinerva, Gronholm, Rinne, & Laine, 2005; Lee et al., 2004, 2002; Whyte et al., 2005; Unverzagt et al., 1999, 1996;). Moreover, the several CERAD subtests including verbal fluency and the word list memory tasks have been included for analysis in the 10/66 Dementia Research Groups study of population norms in urban and rural regions across the globe including communities in Latin America (Cuba, Dominican Republic, Venezuela, Peru, and Mexico), China, and India (Sosa et al., 2009). All sample sites, with the exception of India, demonstrated normative data that was similar to norms obtained using American and European samples. Age and education effects were observed on all examined CERAD subtests across all sample sites. Effects of region (rural scoring lower than urban) were present with word list memory and word list recall being less affected than verbal fluency. This difference appeared to be related more to quality of education than to differences in language or culture.

Although originally designed to tap into several domains relevant to dementia assessment, recent psychometric work suggests that the battery measures overall dementia severity more effectively than separate abilities. A principal components analysis by Straus and Fritsch (2004) indicated that a single latent variable accounted for a majority of variance contained in the CERAD battery, suggesting that investigators use caution in using the CERAD battery to evaluate patterns of cognitive impairment in AD (Strauss & Fritsch, 2004). Further reflecting the recent evidence of a single factor structure of the CERAD battery, Chandler et al. (2005) developed a summary CERAD total score that effectively differentiated among mild AD from normal controls, MCI from normal controls, and MCI from AD—93.7% sensitivity, 92.6% specificity; 81.4% sensitivity, and 72.6% specificity; and 80% sensitivity and 81.4% specificity, respectively (Chandler et al., 2005). Good convergent validity was also shown by significant correlations between the newly proposed CERAD total score with other indices such as the Clinical Dementia Rating (CDR) scale and Blessed Dementia Rating Scale (BDRS).

Repeatable Battery for the Assessment of Neuropsychological Status (RBANS)

The RBANS is a relatively new battery designed to: (1) be administered in under 30 minutes; (2) tap into a variety of functions affected by dementia; (3) with alternate forms that can be utilized upon retest occasions; and (4) include a range of difficulty with applicability for use in normal aging and dementia (Randolph et al., 1998). It yields a total score and five index scores (Immediate Memory, Delayed Memory, Visual-Spatial/Constructional Ability, Attention, and Language) from 12 subtests. The original norms spanned ages 20–89 and the test has seen widespread application in a number of clinical populations including dementia, stroke, schizophrenia, and traumatic brain injury. The test has received considerable psychometric evaluation from the OKLAHOMA studies (Oklahoma Longitudinal Assessment of Health Outcomes in Mature Adults) which include 824 community-dwelling older adults between the ages of 65 and 94 recruited from primary care settings. The prevalence of dementia in this sample is unclear although 166 patients "judged to lack the cognitive capacity to make informed decisions" (p. 1066) were excluded (Beatty, Mold, & Gontkovsky, 2003). No other exclusion criteria were used in most studies using these data; however, 106 were appropriately excluded due to neurological compromise (e.g., stroke, Parkinson's disease, head injury) in the papers providing new normative data (Duff et al., 2003; Patton et al., 2003). Data from this study suggest that age and education significantly impact RBANS scores (Beatty et al., 2003; Gontkovsky, Mold, & Beatty, 2002), and therefore age and education corrected normative tables have been produced from the OKLAHOMA data (Duff et al., 2003). The RBANS has demonstrated excellent internal consistency (Gontkovsky, Beatty, & Mold, 2004) and one-year test–retest reliability for the Total Score (>0.8) (Duff et al., 2005). Although the test has five index scores, factor analyses of the RBANS subtest scores support a two factor solution reflecting verbal memory and visual processing factors (Duff et al., 2006).

The original validation study by Randolph and colleagues focused on differentiating 20 patients with Alzheimer's disease and 20 patients with Huntington's disease from 40 age and education matched controls. Both clinical groups (AD and HD) differed from controls on all index scores, with the exception that AD patients were not significantly different on the visual-spatial/construction index. AD and HD patients yielded similar Total Scores, but demonstrated differences from each other across index scores leading to the calculation of a Cortical/Subcortical Index (CSI). AD patients (cortical dementia) scored lower on the Delayed Memory and Language indices, whereas HD patients (subcortical dementia) scored lower on the Attention and Visual-Spatial/Construction indices. The CSI is calculated by subtracting the average of the Delayed Memory and Language indices from the average of the Attention and Visual-Spatial/Construction indices. Scores less than zero suggest a subcortical profile and scores greater than zero a cortical profile (Randolph et al., 1998). In the validation study this yielded 93% correct classification of AD and HD. Age and education corrected norms for CSI scores have been provided by Duff and colleagues (2007) from the OKLAHOMA study, which aids in the interpretation of obtained CSI scores (e.g., scores ranging from −3 to 12.5 are relatively common). However, data from this study also suggest that the classification of cortical vs. subcortical may not be highly stable over time (one and two year follow-up), suggesting that further empirical validation of the CSI is needed (Duff, Schoenberg, Mold, Scott, & Adams, 2007).

In the original validation study, the RBANS was able to effectively discriminate dementia from normal controls with 90% sensitivity and 90% specificity; however, these were based upon a median split of raw scores, rather than incorporating standard scores which would aid in their clinical use. A follow-up study by Duff and colleagues (2008) evaluated the clinical utility of RBANS standard scores (Total and Index Scores; mean of 100, SD of 15) using 69 patients with AD (consensus panel diagnosis according to NINCDS-ADRDA criteria) and 69 age, education, and gender matched controls. The memory index scores (Immediate and Delayed) demonstrated the best utility (AUC of 0.96 and 0.98), and most of the index scores demonstrated very good clinical utility using cutscores of 1.0 to 1.5 standard deviations below the mean (equivalent to standard scores of 85 and 77) (Duff et al., 2008). Although these results are quite promising, one caveat is that the clinicians involved in the consensus diagnosis for AD were not blind to RBANS scores suggesting a lack of independence. On the other hand, the authors report that the clinicians making the diagnosis utilized multiple sources of information consistent with standard guidelines including patient history, laboratory tests, neuroimaging, CDR scores, and other well-validated neuropsychological measures such as the MMSE and Logical Memory II subtest of the WMS-III. Thus, although the RBANS is a promising brief battery for detecting dementia, it requires further empirical study in relation to its clinical utility for this purpose.

Although the test is available in multiple translations, there has been little empirical study of the RBANS in diverse samples. The majority of the OKLAHOMA sample is described as "largely Caucasian, well-educated, and regular attendees of primary care" (p. 858; Duff et al., 2007). One study utilized 50 African American elders from the OKLAHOMA study in comparison to matched Caucasian elders to determine whether RBANS scores differed between these groups. African American elders demonstrated statistically lower on the Total RBANS score, 3 of the 5 index scores (Delayed Memory, Visual-Spatial/Construction, and Language), and 10 of the 12 subtests (all except List Learning and Digit Span). The effect sizes ranged from small to large (Total Score, Delayed

Memory, and Language). In light of these differences the authors calculated separate RBANS norms for use with older African Americans.

Mattis Dementia Rating Scale and Fuld Object Memory Evaluation

The DRS and FOME have been included in a number of brief batteries, including the Normative Studies Research Project (Lichtenberg, Ross, Youngblade, & Vangel, 1998; Mast, MacNeill, & Lichtenberg, 2000), and continue to receive considerable empirical attention.

Mattis Dementia Rating Scale

The Dementia Rating Scale (DRS; Mattis, 1988) is a measure of general cognitive abilities that takes 15–30 minutes to administer and can be used as part of a brief assessment battery. In designing the DRS, the authors wanted to address floor effects they perceived as weakening the effectiveness of other measures when assessing elders' cognitive functioning, particularly when evaluating dementia severity over time. The DRS is comprised of 32 stimulus cards and 36 tasks that measure cognitive functioning across 6 subscales: attention (8 items); initiation/perseveration (11 items); construction (6 items); conceptualization (6 items); and memory (5 items). Total scores of 123 or less are identified by the authors as indicative of cognitive impairment, and similar numbers have been confirmed in subsequent research (Yochim, Bank, Mast, MacNeill, & Lichtenberg, 2003). For the detection of early stage dementia, a total score of 131 or memory subscale score of less than 20 was recommended by Shay et al. (1991).

Minor scoring refinements have been included in an updated version of the DRS (DRS-2; Jurica et al., 2001). Age and education norms are expanded in the DRS-2 without altering test administration, items, or materials. Since the DRS is currently distributed with the updated scoring refinements, the following review will contain references to the DRS-2 wherever possible.

The DRS-2 normative sample included 623 predominately well-educated, Caucasian elders aged 56–105 from the Mayo Older Adult Normative Study (MOANS; Lucas et al., 1998). Caution has been urged when interpreting the scores of ethnic minorities or those with less than eight years of education (Mattis et al., 2002), although additional normative data from a sample of 307 African American elders aged 55 and older have been developed from the Mayo Older African American Normative Studies (MOAANS) data (Rilling et al., 2005).

An alternate form of the DRS-2 is also available (DRS-2AF; Schmidt, 2004) which adds to its clinical utility by controlling for practice effects when tracking changes in cognitive functioning over time. Schmidt et al. (2005) demonstrated adequate reliability for DRS-2AF total score and across subscales over a 60 minute retest interval (Total Score 0.82, Attention 0.77, Initiation/Perseveration 0.66, Conceptualization 0.70, Memory 0.80; Construction subscale was not included due to significant kurtosis) in a sample of 52 community-dwelling non-demented elders. Schmidt et al. (2005) also demonstrated construct validity for the DRS-2AF through significant correlations with related measures (MMSE with DRS-2AF total score; WAIS-III Digit Span with DRS-2AF Attention subscale; Animal Fluency with DRS-2AF Initiation/Perseveration, Attention, and Memory subscales; WAIS-III similarities with DRS-2AF Conceptualization subscale; and HVLT-R delayed recall with DRS-2AF Memory subscale). Furthermore, a sensitivity of 90%, specificity of 96%, and correct classification rate of 94% was obtained using the DRS-2AF in a sample of 65 elders aged 60 and older with a 46% dementia prevalence (Schmidt et al., 2006).

Changes in cognition over time were examined using the DRS-2 by Miller and Pliskin (2006) in a sample of 63 elders meeting diagnostic criteria for AD. The entire sample was administered using the DRS-2 during initial evaluation and follow-up (M = 11.11 months) with 33 of the elders receiving a second follow-up (M = 12.42 months) administration. Baseline scores did not differ from initial follow-up, while Total Score, Attention, Initiation/Perseveration, and Memory were found to be significantly lower at second follow-up.

One aspect of the DRS that makes it a useful part of a brief battery is its ability to distinguish among different forms of dementia. For example, autopsy confirmed that frontotemporal dementia (FTD) was found to differ from autopsy confirmed AD in DRS presentation in a study by Rascovsky et al. (2008). The FTD group performed significantly worse on the Initiation/Perseveration and Conceptualization subscales than the AD group, but better on the Memory and Construction subscales. Using this pattern, the study's authors were able to correctly classify 82% of all elders in the FTD and AD groups, and 89% of elders in the mild to moderate FTD and AD groups. In an earlier study, Aarsland et al. (2003) examined the differences in scores on the DRS among four groups of elders including those diagnosed with Parkinson's disease with dementia (PDD), dementia with Lewy bodies (DLB), progressive supranuclear palsy (PSP), and AD. The PDD and DLB groups exhibited better performance on the Memory subscale than the AD group, but worse performance on the Initiation/Perseveration and Construction scales.

Fuld Object Memory Evaluation

The Fuld Object Memory Evaluation (FOME) is a neuropsychological test that was originally developed to assess episodic memory function in an elderly population (Fuld, 1981). The FOME is unique from most other instruments used as dementia screens due to its multi-modal process of encoding: tactile; auditory; and visual. The tested person is initially instructed to place their hand into a bag that contains ten common objects (e.g., key, mug, playing card) and asked to name the object using only their sense of touch. The tested person then removes the object from the bag, visually confirms the selection, and verbally names the object with mistakes being corrected by the test administrator. This process is repeated one by one until all ten objects have been identified and removed from the bag. The objects are then removed from sight, and a verbal fluency distracter task is initiated for approximately 60 seconds. Next, the tested person is given 60 seconds to name as many objects as they can remember that were initially contained in the bag. This is followed by a selective reminding procedure and the process is repeated four more times for a total of five trials. A total of 50 points is possible on the FOME (one point for each correctly recalled item during each trial) with scores of 30 or lower deemed indicative of cognitive impairment.

Operating characteristics of the FOME are relatively unaffected by education or ethnicity and have demonstrated excellent utility in detecting dementia (Chung, 2009; La Rue, 1989; Loewenstein, Duara, Arguelles, & Arguelles, 1995; Marcopulos, Gripshover, Broshek, McLain, & Brashear, 1999; Mast, Fitzgerald, Steinberg, MacNeill, & Lichtenberg, 2001; Wall, Deshpande, MacNeill & Lichtenberg, 1998;). The FOME has demonstrated excellent utility in detecting mild dementia (sensitivity and specificity >0.95) in both English and Spanish speaking elders (Loewenstein et al., 1995) and has also demonstrated high sensitivity (0.98) in detecting dementia among older African Americans using the retrieval cutscore of 30 (Mast et al., 2001). The slope of learning over five trials has been associated with daily functioning (IADLs) (Mast & Allaire, 2006). The FOME places fewer demands on processing speed than other list learning measures such as the California Verbal Learning Test (CVLT) or the Hopkins Verbal Learning Test (HVLT). Because the learning and encoding of words occurs at a slower pace on the FOME, it may be a purer measure of memory function than other measures which may partially confound memory and processing speed, which is the ability most affected by normal aging (Salthouse, 1993, 1994).

Due to the time and materials needed to administer the FOME it is usually administered as part of a brief battery rather than a stand-alone screener. The FOME is, however, a useful dementia screen and a viable alternative for screening elders with hearing and/or visual impairment (Chung & Ho, 2009). The development of a shorter, three-trial version of the FOME may increase its use as a screener.

However, when combined with other measures such as the DRS-2, the FOME can be very effective in evaluating dementia (Mast, MacNeill, & Lichtenberg, 2000).

Because the brief batteries reviewed lack a strong emphasis on executive functioning, supplemental tests of this construct should be included (e.g., Trail Making Test, Controlled Oral Word Association Test). The use of both screening measures and brief batteries is demonstrated in the case study below, along with supplementation with measures that are sensitive to executive dysfunction.

Case Study

Ms P is a 90-year-old woman whose son and primary care physician requested an evaluation of her memory and cognitive functioning. She had been living independently until a year ago when she fell and fractured her leg. Although she was reportedly living independently, medical records indicate that she has had some difficulty with balance, repetitive language, and forgetfulness over the past two to three years. Her primary care physician screened her with the MMSE two years ago and she received a score of 27 out of 30. More recently she was given the Mini-Cog. She initially recalled 3 of 3 words but could not recall any after a short delay. Her clock drawing test score was 2 out of 4. She had previously been diagnosed as having Mild Cognitive Impairment by her PCP, but the recent failure on the Mini-Cog screener prompted further testing with a brief battery.

Test results

Ms P's performance on a test of reading ability (an indicator of premorbid functioning) was average (post-high school level; Scaled Score = 110). Her general cognitive functioning was in the low average range (DRS-2 Total = 120). Her performance on the Attention subscale of the DRS-2 was high average (72nd–81st percentile) and the Construction and Conceptualization subscales were average (41st–59th percentile). Her DRS-2 Memory (3rd–5th percentile) and Initiation/Perseveration (6th–10th percentile) scores were in the moderately and mildly impaired ranges, respectively. On the FOME Ms P retrieved 24 over five trials (out of 50) which was significantly impaired. In terms of language abilities, she demonstrated average performance on tests of verbal comprehension (71st percentile), category fluency (Animal Naming 25th percentile), and lexical fluency (40th–50th percentile). Her performance on the Trail Making Test was low average (14th percentile) on Part A and mildly impaired (8th percentile) on Part B. She did not endorse any of the items on the Geriatric Depression Scale.

Conclusions

Ms P demonstrated significant cognitive strengths in several areas of functioning, but also demonstrated significant impairment in memory and executive functioning. Moreover her low average general cognitive functioning likely represents a slight decline from premorbid levels of functioning, which taken together with impairment in memory and executive functioning is consistent with a mild dementia syndrome.

CHALLENGES TO THE STANDARD APPROACH

Intra-individual variability on cognitive measures

An underlying assumption of cognitive screening and evaluation using brief batteries has been that the one-time test administration provides a reliable estimate of the person's general level of cognitive functioning. It is not typically assumed that the person would perform better (or worse) on another occasion and the testing results are used as an estimate of functioning which we believe to be stable over the short term. Although this may be a reasonable assumption based upon classical test theory, particularly when the test has high levels of reliability, research from the cognitive aging literature challenges this assumption by demonstrating that both normally functioning older adults and those with cognitive impairment can demonstrate considerable variability over relatively brief periods of time (Allaire & Marsiske, 2005; Strauss, MacDonald, Hunter, Moll, & Hultsch, 2002). Moreover, intra-individual variability in performance on cognitive measures increases in the context of dementia and cognitive impairment (Hultsch, MacDonald, Hunter, Levy-Bencheton, & Strauss, 2000). Although this has not been studied specifically in relation to cognitive screening the implication is that intra-individual variability on cognitive measures such as that observed in the Hultsch and Allaire studies could impact the result of cognitive screening efforts, particularly when scores fall near established cutscores. The development of alternate forms on two of these batteries (DRS-2 and RBANS) allows for repeat administration without significant practice effects; however, the extent to which short-term variability might be present has not been studied. As we learn more about the short-term stability of cognitive functioning among people with suspected dementia, the field may need to respond by specifically evaluating the extent to which screening measures and brief batteries are affected.

Technology and Screening

Testing in the context of dementia can be accomplished through a number of means and in a number of different settings. Brief batteries and screens have traditionally been administered by paper and pencil in a community setting or clinic offices, but advances in technology and changes in our health care system have led to increasing use of automated testing systems in both telephone and computerized formats. Screening instruments designed to be administered by telephone or computer may serve an important role in the screening process and be a candidate for more widespread application in the future. Many elders living in a rural region often find it difficult to receive cognitive impairment screening due to transportation issues or lack of proximity to a specialist. People living in underserved regions have limited access to general practitioners, psychiatrists, and psychologists who could potentially administer a dementia screening instrument. For people with limited access to health care, an alternative to dementia screening measures that require in-person administration is therefore needed. Dementia screening measures administered by telephone or computer may fill a void left by a lack of available resources to a segment of the population.

Two of the most widely used and researched telephone screening measures are the Memory Impairment Screen by Telephone (MIS-T; Lipton et al., 2003) and the Telephone Instrument for Cognitive Status (TICS; Brandt, Spencer, & Folstein, 1988). The TICS is a mental status screen that was developed using the MMSE as a model and takes approximately 10 minutes to administer. TICS total score has been highly correlated with the MMSE (Brandt et al., 1988). The TICS has been translated into and validated in several foreign languages, including Spanish (Desmond, Tatemichi, & Hanzawa, 1994; Gude Ruiz, Calvo Mauri & Carrasco Lopez, 1994), Italian (Ferruccil et al., 1998), Finnish (Jarvenpaa et al., 2002), and Japanese (Konagaya et al., 2007). A shorter version of the TICS (TICS-m) is also available, has been validated in Hebrew (Beeri, Werner, Davidson, Silverman, & Schmidler, 2003), and slightly outperforms the TICS in the detection of mild cognitive impairment (Welsh, Breitner & Magruder-Habib, 1993).

For the telephone version of the MIS, the person being tested is presented with two words and asked to repeat them. The test administrator then presents a category cue that is associated with one of the two initially presented words and instructs the person to choose which word forms the proper association. Next, the administrator presents the category cue for the remaining word and repeats the process using different words and associated category cues. Following a 2–3 minute distracter task, the person is instructed to recall as many of the words as possible. If a word is not recalled, the examiner verbally presents the semantic category associated with the unretrieved word and gives a second opportunity to recall the word. Scoring is done in the same manner as for the in-person MIS.

In the original validation study of the MIS-T (Lipton et al., 2003), the TICS and MIS-T were compared in a sample of 300 elders (9% had dementia) and demonstrated AUC estimates of 0.92 and 0.86, respectively. Using the best performing cutscores for the sample, the MIS-T had a sensitivity of 78%, specificity of 93%, and PPV of 52% compared to the TICS's sensitivity of 74%, specificity of 86%, and PPV of 34% for the detection of all dementias. This pattern was also evident for the detection of AD with the MIS-T yielding a sensitivity of 89%, specificity of 93%, and PPV of 45% compared to the TICS's sensitivity of 83%, specificity of 86%, and PPV of 27%. Sensitivity of the MIS-T for the detection of AD was improved when a category fluency task was administered during the distracter phase (89%) but still did not reach the sensitivity of the in-person MIS (93%).

Dementia screening instruments administered by computer have not been as well validated as those administered by telephone. There are a number of challenges when validating or administering a computer screening measure that are not present when validating or administering a telephone screening measure. Familiarity with keyboards and computers in general may affect scores on computerized screening measures, and touch screens (a viable alternative that can help alleviate some of this effect) are expensive. Many computer screening instruments require reading and writing so they cannot be administered to those with poor reading skills, and computer screens that utilize reaction time in their scores may be affected by fatigue, frustration, or motor deficits not associated with dementia. There is, however, promise for the future application of computer screening measures. Several systems are under development (Headminder Cognitive Screening Test, Mindstreams) and await peer reviewed validation studies.

APPENDIX

Patient name:__________________________ **Date:**_____________

GPCOG Screening Test

Step 1: Patient Examination

Unless specified, each question should only be asked once

Name and Address for subsequent recall test

1. "*I am going to give you a name and address. After I have said it, I want you to repeat it. Remember this name and address because I am going to ask you to tell it to me again in a few minutes: John Brown, 42 West Street, Kensington.*" (Allow a maximum of 4 attempts).

	Correct	Incorrect
Time Orientation		
2. *What is the date?* (exact only)	☐	☐
Clock Drawing – use blank page		
3. *Please mark in all the numbers to indicate the hours of a clock* (correct spacing required)	☐	☐
4. *Please mark in hands to show 10 minutes past eleven o'clock* (11.10)	☐	☐
Information		
5. *Can you tell me something that happened in the news recently?* (Recently = in the last week. If a general answer is given, eg "war", "lot of rain", ask for details. Only specific answer scores).	☐	☐
Recall		
6. *What was the name and address I asked you to remember*		
John	☐	☐
Brown	☐	☐
42	☐	☐
West (St)	☐	☐
Kensington	☐	☐

(*To get a total score, add the number of items answered correctly*
Total correct (score out of 9) **/9**

If patient scores 9, no significant cognitive impairment and further testing not necessary.
If patient scores 5-8, more information required. Proceed with Step 2, informant section.
If patient scores 0-4, cognitive impairment is indicated. Conduct standard investigations.

Informant Interview

Date: ____________

Informant's name: ______________________________

Informant's relationship to patient, i.e. informant is the patient's: ____________

These six questions ask how the patient is compared to when s/he was well, say 5 – 10 years ago

Compared to a few years ago:

	Yes	No	Don't Know	N/A
▪ Does the patient have more trouble remembering things that have happened recently than s/he used to?	☐	☐	☐	
▪ Does he or she have more trouble recalling conversations a few days later?	☐	☐	☐	
▪ When speaking, does the patient have more difficulty in finding the right word or tend to use the wrong words more often?	☐	☐	☐	
▪ Is the patient less able to manage money and financial affairs (e.g. paying bills, budgeting)?	☐	☐	☐	☐
▪ Is the patient less able to manage his or her medication independently?	☐	☐	☐	☐
▪ Does the patient need more assistance with transport (either private or public)? (If the patient has difficulties due only to physical problems, e.g bad leg, tick 'no')	☐	☐	☐	☐

(To get a total score, add the number of items answered 'no', 'don't know' or 'N/A')

Total score (out of 6) ☐

If patient scores 0-3, cognitive impairment is indicated. Conduct standard investigations.

Brodaty et al, *JAGS* 2002; 50:530-534

Web site: http://www.gpcog.com.au

MONTREAL COGNITIVE ASSESSMENT (MOCA)

NAME :
Education :
Sex :
Date of birth :
DATE :

VISUOSPATIAL / EXECUTIVE

E End, A, 5, B, 2, 1 Begin, D, 4, 3, C

[ ]

Copy cube

[ ]

Draw CLOCK (Ten past eleven) (3 points)

[ ] Contour [ ] Numbers [ ] Hands

POINTS ___/5

NAMING

[ ] [ ] [ ] ___/3

MEMORY Read list of words, subject must repeat them. Do 2 trials, even if 1st trial is successful. Do a recall after 5 minutes.

	FACE	VELVET	CHURCH	DAISY	RED
1st trial					
2nd trial					

No points

ATTENTION Read list of digits (1 digit/ sec.).
Subject has to repeat them in the forward order [ ] 2 1 8 5 4
Subject has to repeat them in the backward order [ ] 7 4 2 ___/2

Read list of letters. The subject must tap with his hand at each letter A. No points if ≥ 2 errors
[ ] FBACMNAAJKLBAFAKDEAAAJAMOFAAB ___/1

Serial 7 subtraction starting at 100 [ ] 93 [ ] 86 [ ] 79 [ ] 72 [ ] 65
4 or 5 correct subtractions: **3 pts**, 2 or 3 correct: **2 pts**, 1 correct: **1 pt**, 0 correct: **0 pt** ___/3

LANGUAGE Repeat : I only know that John is the one to help today. [ ]
The cat always hid under the couch when dogs were in the room. [ ] ___/2

Fluency / Name maximum number of words in one minute that begin with the letter F [ ] _____ (N ≥ 11 words) ___/1

ABSTRACTION Similarity between e.g. banana - orange = fruit [ ] train – bicycle [ ] watch - ruler ___/2

DELAYED RECALL

		FACE	VELVET	CHURCH	DAISY	RED	
	Has to recall words **WITH NO CUE**	[ ]	[ ]	[ ]	[ ]	[ ]	Points for UNCUED recall only
Optional	Category cue						
	Multiple choice cue						

___/5

ORIENTATION [ ] Date [ ] Month [ ] Year [ ] Day [ ] Place [ ] City ___/6

 Version 7.1 **www.mocatest.org** Normal ≥26 / 30

TOTAL ___/30
Add 1 point if ≤ 12 yr edu

Administered by: ______________________

REFERENCES

Aarsland, D., Litvan, I., Salmon, D., Galasko, D., Wentzel-Larsen, T., & Larsen, J. P. (2003). Performance on the dementia rating scale in Parkinson's disease with dementia and dementia with Lewy bodies: Comparison with progressive supranuclear palsy and Alzheimer's disease. *Journal of Neurology, Neurosurgery & Psychiatry, 74*(9), 1215–1220.

Allaire, J. C., & Marsiske, M. (2005). Intraindividual variability may not always indicate vulnerability in elders' cognitive performance. *Psychology and Aging*, 390–401.

Allaire, J. C., & Whitfield, K. E. (2004). Relationships among education, age, and cognitive functioning in older African Americans: the impact of desegregation. *Aging Neuropsychology and Cognition, 11*, 443–449.

Backman, L., Jones, S., Berger, A. K., Laukka, E. J., & Small, B. J. (2005). Cognitive impairment in preclinical Alzheimer's disease: a meta-analysis. *Neuropsychology, 19*, 520–531.

Basic, D., Khoo, A., Conforti, D., Rowland, J., Vrantsidis, F., Logiudice, D., et al. (2009). Rowland Universal Dementia Assessment Scale, Mini-Mental State Examination and General Practitioner Assessment of Cognition in a multicultural cohort of community-dwelling older persons with early dementia. *Australian Psychologist, 44*(1), 40–53.

Beatty, W. W., Mold, J. W., & Gontkovsky, S. T. (2003). RBANS performance: influences of sex and education. *Journal of Clinical and Experimental Neuropsychology, 25*, 1065–1069.

Beeri, M. S., Werner, P., Davidson, M., Silverman, J., & Schmidler, J. (2003). Validation of the modified Telephone Interview for Cognitive Status (TICS-m) in Hebrew. *International Journal of Geriatric Psychiatry, 18*(5), 381–386.

Bennett, D. A., Schneider, J. A., Arvanitakis, Z., Kelly, J. F., Aggarwal, N. T., Shah, R. C., et al. (2006). Neuropathology of older persons without cognitive impairment from two community-based studies. *Neurology, 66*, 1837–1844.

Benton, A. L. (1983). *Contributions to Neuropsychological Assessment*. New York, NY: Oxford University Press Inc.

Bertolucci, P. H. F., Okamoto, I. H., Brucki, S. M. D., Siviero, M. O., Toniolo Neto, J., & Ramos, L. R. (2001). Applicability of the CERAD neuropsychological battery to Brazilian elderly. *Arquivos de Neuro-Psiquiatria, 59*, 532–536.

Birks, J. (2006). Cholinesterase inhibitors for Alzheimer's disease. *Cochrane Database of Systematic Reviews, 25* (1), CD005593.

Boise, L., Camicioli, R., Morgan, D. L., Rose, J. H., & Congleton, L. (1999). Diagnosing dementia: Perspectives of primary care physicians. *Gerontologist, 39*, 457–464.

Bondi, M. W., Salmon, D. P., Galasko, D., Thomas, R. G., & Thal, L. J. (1999). Neuropsychological function and apolipoprotein E genotype in the preclinical detection of Alzheimer's disease. *Psychology and Aging, 14*, 295–303.

Borson, S., Scanlan, J. M., Chen, P., & Ganguli, M. (2003). The Mini-Cog as a screen for dementia: validation in a population-based sample. *Journal of the American Geriatric Society, 51*, 1452–1454.

Borson, S., Scanlan, J. M., Watanabe, J., Tu, S. P., & Lessig, M. (2006). Improving identification of cognitive impairment in primary care. *International Journal of Geriatric Psychiatry, 21*, 349–355.

Borson, S., Scanlan, J., Brush, M., Vitaliano, P., & Dokmak, A. (2000). The mini-cog: a cognitive "vital signs" measure for dementia screening in multi-lingual elderly. *International Journal of Geriatric Psychiatry, 15*, 1021–1027.

Boustani, M., Peterson, B., Hanson, L., Harris, R., & Lohr, K. N. (2003). Screening for dementia in primary care: a summary of the evidence for the U.S. Preventive Services Task Force. *Annals of Internal Medicine, 138*, 927–937.

Brandt, J., Spencer, M., & Folstein, M. (1988). Telephone Interview for Cognitive Status. *Neuropsychiatry, Neuropsychology, & Behavioral Neurology, 1*, 111–117.

Brodaty, H., Fay, L. L., Gibson, L., & Burns, K. (2006). What is the best dementia screening instrument for general practitioners to use? *American Journal of Geriatric Psychiatry, 14*, 391–400.

Brodaty, H., Kemp, N. M., & Low, L. F. (2004). Characteristics of the GPCOG, a screening tool for cognitive impairment. *International Journal of Geriatric Psychiatry, 19*, 870–874.

Brodaty, H., Pond, D., Kemp, N. M., Luscombe, G., Berman, K., Harding, L., & Huppert, F. (2002). The GPCOG: a new screening test for dementia designed for general practice. *Journal of the American Geriatric Society*, *50*, 530–534.

Buschke, H., Kuslansky, G., Katz, M., Stewart, W. F., Sliwinski, M. J., Eckholdt, H. M., & Lipton, R. B. (1999). Screening for dementia with the Memory Impairment Screen (MIS). *Neurology*, *52*, 231–237.

Carlson, M. C., Xue, Q., Zhou, J., & Fried, L. P. (2009). Executive decline and dysfunction precedes declines in memory: The Women's Health and Aging Study II. *The Journals of Gerontology: Series A: Biological Sciences and Medical Sciences*, *64*(1), 110–117.

Chandler, M. J., Lacritz, L. H., Hynan, L. S., Barnard, H. D., Allen, G., Deschner, M., et al. (2005). A total score for the CERAD neuropsychological battery. *Neurology*, *65*, 102–106.

Cherbuin, N., Anstey, K. J., & Lipnicki, D. M. (2008). Screening for dementia: a review of self- and informant-assessment instruments. *International Psychogeriatrics*, *20*(Suppl. 3), 431–458.

Chopard, G., Pitard, A., Ferriera, S., Vanholsbeeck, G., Rumbach, L., & Galmiche, J. (2007). Combining the Memory Impairment Screen and the Isaacs Set Test: a practical tool for screening dementias. *Journal of the American Geriatric Society*, *55*, 1426–1430.

Chung, J. C. C. (2009). Clinical validity of Fuld Object Memory Evaluation to screen for dementia in a Chinese society. *International Journal of Geriatric Psychiatry*, *24*, 156–162.

Chung, J. C. C., & Ho, W. S. K. (2009). Validation of Fuld Object Memory Evaluation for the detection of dementia in nursing home residents. *Aging & Mental Health*, *13*, 274–279.

Collie, A., & Maruff, P. (2000). The neuropsychology of preclinical Alzheimer's disease and mild cognitive impairment. *Neuroscience and Biobehavioral Reviews*, *24*, 365–374.

Collie, A., Shafiq-Antonacci, R., Maruff, P., Tyler, P., & Currie, J. (1999). Norms and the effects of demographic variables on a neuropsychological battery for use in healthy ageing Australian populations. *Australian and New Zealand Journal of Psychiatry*, *33*, 568–575.

Del Ser, T., Sánchez-Sánchez, F., de Yébenes, M. J. G., Munoz, D. G., & Otero, A. (2006). Validation of the Seven-Minute Screen Neurocognitive Battery for the diagnosis of dementia in a Spanish population-based sample. *Dementia and Geriatric Cognitive Disorders*, *22*(5–6), 454–464.

Desmond, D. W., Tatemichi, T. K., & Hanzawa, L. (1994). The Telephone Interview for Cognitive Status (TICS): reliability and validity in a stroke sample. *International Journal of Geriatric Psychiatry*, *9*, 803–807.

Deveugele, M., Derese, A., van den Brink-Muinen, A., De Maeseneer, J., & Bensing, J. (2002). Consultation length in general practice: cross sectional study in six European countries. *British Medical Journal*, *325* (7362), 472–477.

Duff, K., Beglinger, L. J., Schoenberg, M. R., Patton, D. E., Mold, J., Scott, J. G., et al. (2005). Test–retest stability and practice effects of the RBANS in a community dwelling elderly sample. *Journal of Clinical and Experimental Neuropsychology*, *27*, 565–575.

Duff, K., Humphreys Clark, J. D., O'Bryant, S. E., Mold, J. W., Schiffer, R. B., & Sutker, P. B. (2008). Utility of the RBANS in detecting cognitive impairment associated with Alzheimer's disease: sensitivity, specificity, and positive and negative predictive powers. *Archives of Clinical Neuropsychology*, *23*, 603–612.

Duff, K., Langbehn, D. R., Schoenberg, M. R., Moser, D. J., Baade, L. E., Mold, J., et al. (2006). Examining the repeatable battery for the assessment of neuropsychological status: factor analytic studies in an elderly sample. *American Journal of Geriatric Psychiatry*, *14*, 976–979.

Duff, K., Pattern, D., Schoenberg, M. R., Mold, J., Scott, J. G., & Adams, R. L. (2003). Age- and education-corrected independent normative data for the RBANS in a community dwelling elderly sample. *Clinical Neuropsychologist*, *17*, 351–366.

Duff, K., Schoenberg, M. R., Mold, J. W., Scott, J. G., & Adams, R. L. (2007). Normative and retest data on the RBANS cortical/subcortical index in older adults. *Journal of Clinical and Experimental Neuropsychology*, *29*, 854–859.

Ferruccil, L., Del Lungo, I., Guranlnik, J. M., Bandinelli, S., Benvenuti, E., Salani, B., et al. (1998). Is the Telephone Interview for Cognitive Status a valid alternative in persons who cannot be evaluated by the Mini Mental State Examination? *Aging Clinical and Experimental Research*, *10*, 332–338.

Fillenbaum, G. G., McCurry, S. M., Kuchibhatla, M., Masaki, K. H., Borenstein, A. R., Foley, D. J., et al. (2005). Performance on the CERAD neuropsychology battery of two samples of Japanese-American elders: norms for persons with and without dementia. *Journal of the International Neuropsychological Society, 11*, 192–201.

Fillenbaum, G. G., Peterson, B., Welsh-Bohmer, K. A., Kukull, W. A., & Heyman, A. (1998). Progression of Alzheimer's disease in black and white patients: the CERAD experience, part XVI. Consortium to Establish a Registry for Alzheimer's Disease. *Neurology, 51*, 154–158.

Flocke, S. A., Frank, S. H., & Wenger, D. A. (2001). Addressing multiple problems in the family practice office visit. *The Journal of Family Practice, 50*(3), 211–216.

Folstein, M. F., Folstein, S. E., & McHugh, P. R. (1975). Mini Mental State: a practical method for grading the cognitive state of patients for the clinician. *Journals of Gerontology: Series B: Psychological Sciences & Social Sciences, 12*, 189–198.

Freedman, M., Leach, L., Kaplan, E., Winocur, G., Shulman, K. I., & Delis, D. C. (1994). *Clock Drawing: A Neuropsychological Analysis*. New York, NY: Oxford University Press Inc.

Fuld, P. A. (1981). *Fuld Object Memory Evaluation Instruction Manual*. Wood Dale, IL: Stoelting.

Galvin, J. E., Powlishta, K. K., Wilkins, K., McKeel, D. W. J., Xiong, C., Grant, E., et al. (2005). Predictors of preclinical Alzheimer disease and dementia: a clinicopathologic study. *Archives of Neurology, 62*(5), 758–765.

Gontkovsky, S. T., Beatty, W. W., & Mold, J. W. (2004). Repeatable battery for the assessment of neuropsychological status in a normal, geriatric sample. *Clinical Gerontologist, 27*, 79–86.

Gontkovsky, S. T., Mold, J. W., & Beatty, W. W. (2002). Age and educational influences on RBANS index scores in a nondemented geriatric sample. *Clinical Neuropsychologist, 16*, 258–263.

Grober, E., & Kawas, C. (1997). Learning and retention in preclinical and early Alzheimer's disease. *Psychology and Aging, 12*, 183–188.

Grober, E., Buschke, H., Crystal, H., Bang, S., & Dresner, R. (1988). Screening for dementia by memory testing. *Neurology, 38*(6), 900–903.

Grober, E., Hall, C., McGinn, M., Nicholls, T., Stanford, S., Ehrlich, A., et al. (2008). Neuropsychological strategies for detecting early dementia. *Journal of the International Neuropsychological Society, 14*, 130–142.

Gude Ruiz, R., Calvo Mauri, J. F., & Carrasco Lopez, F. J. (1994). The Spanish version and pilot study of a telephone test of cognitive status for evaluation and screening in dementia assessment and follow-up. *Aten Primaria, 15*, 61–66.

Gunning-Dixon, F. M., & Raz, N. (2000). The cognitive correlates of white matter abnormalities in normal aging: a quantitative review. *Neuropsychology, 14*, 224–232.

Gunning-Dixon, F. M., & Raz, N. (2003). Neuroanatomical correlates of selected executive functions in middle-aged and older adults: a prospective MRI study. *Neuropsychologia, 41*, 1929–1941.

Hebert, L. E., Scherr, P. A., Bienias, J. L., Bennett, D. A., & Evans, D. A. (2003). Alzheimer disease in the US population: prevalence estimates using the 2000 census. *Archives of Neurology, 60*, 1119–1122.

Holsinger, T., Deveau, J., Boustani, M., & Williams, J. W. (2007). Does this patient have dementia? *The Journal of the American Medical Association, 297*, 2391–2404.

Hultsch, D. F., MacDonald, S. W. S., Hunter, M. A., Levy-Bencheton, J., & Strauss, E. (2000). Intraindividual variability in cognitive performance in older adults: comparison of adults with mild dementia, adults with arthritis, and healthy adults. *Neuropsychology*, 588–598.

Ijuin, M., Homma, A., Mimura, M., Kawai, Y., Gondo, Y., Imai, Y., & Kitamura, S. (2008). Validation of the 7-minute screen for the detection of early-stage Alzheimer's disease. *Dementia and Geriatric Cognitive Disorders, 25*(3), 248–255.

Isaacs, B., & Kennie, A. T. (1973). The Set Test as an aid to the detection of dementia in old people. *British Journal of Psychiatry, 123*, 467–470.

Jarvenpaa, T., Rinne, J. O., Raiha, I., Lopponen, M., Kaprio, J., Hinkka, S., & Koskenvuo, M. (2002). Characteristics of two telephone screens for cognitive impairment. *Dementia and Geriatric Cognitive Disorders, 13*(3), 149–155.

Jurica, P. J., Leitten, C. L., & Mattis, S. (2001). *Dementia Rating Scale-2: Professional manual*. Lutz, FL: Psychological Assessment Resources.

Kahokehr, A., Siegert, R. J., & Weatherall, M. (2004). The frequency of executive cognitive impairment in elderly rehabilitation inpatients. *Journal of Geriatric Psychiatry and Neurology, 17*(2), 68–72.

Karrasch, M., Sinerva, E., Gronholm, P., Rinne, J., & Laine, M. (2005). CERAD test performances in amnestic mild cognitive impairment and Alzheimer's disease. *Acta Neurologica Scandinavica, 111*, 172–179.

Konagaya, Y., Washimi, Y., Hattori, H., Watanabe, T., Ohta, T., & Takeda, A. (2007). Validation of the Telephone Interview for Cognitive Status (TICS) in Japanese. *International Journal of Geriatric Psychiatry, 22*(7), 695–700.

Kuslansky, G., Buschke, H., Katz, M., Sliwinski, M., & Lipton, R. B. (2002). Screening for Alzheimer's disease: the Memory Impairment Screen versus the conventional three-word memory test. *Journal of the American Geriatric Society, 50*, 1086–1091.

La Rue, A. (1989). Patterns of performance on the Fuld Object Memory Evaluation in elderly inpatients with depression or dementia. *Journal of Clinical and Experimental Neuropsychology, 11*, 409–422.

Lavery, L. L., Starenchak, S. M., Flynn, W. B., Stoeff, M. A., Schaffner, R., & Newman, A. B. (2005). The clock drawing test is an independent predictor of incident use of 24-hour care in a retirement community. *Journals of Gerontology Series A-Biological Sciences and Medical Sciences, 60*, 928–932.

Lawrence, J. M., Davidoff, D. A., Katt-Lloyd, D., Berlow, Y. A., Savoie, J. A., & Connell, A. (2003). Is large-scale community memory screening feasible? Experience from a regional memory-screening day. *Journal of the American Geriatrics Society, 51*(8), 1072–1078.

Lawrence, J. M., Davidoff, D., Katt-Lloyd, D., Auerbach, M., & Hennen, J. (2001). A pilot program of improved methods for community-based screening for dementia. *American Journal of Geriatric Psychiatry, 9*(3), 205–211.

Lee, D. Y., Lee, K. U., Lee, J. H., Kim, K. W., Jhoo, J. H., Kim, S. Y., et al. (2004). A normative study of the CERAD neuropsychological assessment battery in the Korean elderly. *Journal of the International Neuropsychological Society, 10*, 72–81.

Lee, J. H., Lee, K. U., Lee, D. Y., Kim, K. W., Jhoo, J. H., Kim, J. H., et al. (2002). Development of the Korean version of the Consortium to Establish a Registry for Alzheimer's Disease Assessment Packet (CERAD-K): clinical and neuropsychological assessment batteries. *Journals of Gerontology Series B-Psychological Sciences & Social Sciences, 57*, 47–53.

Lessig, M. C., Scanlan, J. M., Nazemi, H., & Borson, S. (2007). Time that tells: critical clock-drawing errors for dementia screening. *International Psychogeriatrics, 20*(3), 459–470.

Lichtenberg, P. A., Ross, T. P., Youngblade, L., & Vangel, S. J. (1998). Normative studies research project test battery: detection of dementia in African American and European American urban elderly patients. *Clinical Neuropsychologist, 12*, 146–154.

Lipton, R. B., Katz, M. J., Kuslansky, G., Sliwinski, M. J., Stewart, W. F., Verghese, J., Crystal, H. A., & Buschke, H. (2003). Screening for dementia by telephone using the Memory Impairment Screen. *Journal of the American Geriatric Society, 51*, 1382–1390.

Loewenstein, D. A., Duara, R., Arguelles, T., & Arguelles, S. (1995). Use of the Fuld Object-Memory Evaluation in the Detection of Mild Dementia Among Spanish-Speaking and English-Speaking Groups. *American Journal of Geriatric Psychiatry, 3*, 300–307.

Lorentz, W. J., Scanlan, J. M., & Borson, S. (2002). Brief screening tests for dementia. *Canadian Journal of Psychiatry, 47*, 723–733.

Lucas, J. A., Ivnik, R. J., Smith, G. E., Ferman, T. J., Willis, F. B., Petersen, R. C., et al. (2005). Mayo's Older African Americans Normative Studies: norms for Boston Naming Test, Controlled Oral Word Association, Category Fluency, Animal Naming, Token Test, Wrat-3 Reading, Trail Making Test, Stroop Test, and Judgment of Line Orientation. *Clinical Neuropsychologist, 19*, 243–269.

Lucas, J. A., Ivnik, R. J., Smith, G. E., Bohac, D. L., Tangalos, E. G., Kokmen, E., et al. (1998). Normative data for the Mattis Dementia Rating Scale. *Journal of Clinical and Experimental Neuropsychology, 20*(4), 536–547.

Luis, C. A., Keegan, A. P., & Mullan, M. (2009). Cross validation of the Montreal Cognitive Assessment in community dwelling older adults residing in the southeastern US. *International Journal of Geriatric Psychiatry,* 24:197–201.

MacNeill, S. E., & Lichtenberg, P. A. (1999). Screening instruments and brief batteries for assessment of dementia. In P. A. Lichtenberg (Ed.), *Handbook of assessment in clinical gerontology* (pp. 417–441). New York, NY: Wiley.

Manly, J. J., & Echemendia, R. J. (2007). Race-specific norms: using the model of hypertension to understand issues of race, culture, and education in neuropsychology. *Archives of Clinical Neuropsychology, 22*, 319–325.

Manly, J. J. (2008). Race, culture, education, and cognitive test performance among older adults. In S. M. Hofer, & D. F. Alwin (Eds.), *Handbook of Cognitive Aging: Interdisciplinary Perspectives*. Thousand Oaks, CA, US: Sage Publications, Inc.

Manly, J. J., Byrd, D. A., Touradji, P., & Stern, Y. (2004). Acculturation, reading level, and neuropsychological test performance among African American elders. *Applied Neuropsychology, 11*, 37–46.

Manly, J. J., Jacobs, D. M., Touradji, P., Small, S. A., & Stern, Y. (2002). Reading level attenuates differences in neuropsychological test performance between African American and White elders. *Journal of the International Neuropsychological Society, 8*, 341–348.

Marcopulos, B. A., Gripshover, D. L., Broshek, D. K., McLain, C. A., & Brashear, H. R. (1999). Neuropsychological assessment of psychogeriatric patients with limited education. *The Clinical Neuropsychologist, 13*, 147–156.

Mast, B. T., & Allaire, J. C. (2006). Verbal learning and everyday functioning in dementia: an application of latent variable growth curve modeling. *Journal of Gerontology. Behavioral Psychological Science and Social Science, 61*, 167–173.

Mast, B. T., Fitzgerald, J., Steinberg, J., MacNeill, S. E., & Lichtenberg, P. A. (2001). Effective screening for Alzheimer's disease among older African Americans. *Clinical Neuropsychology, 15*, 196–202.

Mast, B. T., MacNeill, S. E., & Lichtenberg, P. A. (2000). Clinical utility of the Normative Studies Research Project test battery among vascular dementia patients. *Clinical Neuropsychology, 14*, 173–180.

Mattis, S. (1988). *Dementia Rating Scale: Professional manual*. Odessa, FL: Psychological Assessment Resources.

Mattis, S., Jurica, P., & Leitten, C. (2002). *Dementia Rating Scale-2 Professional Manual*. Odessa, FL: Psychological Assessment Resources.

Mendez, M. F., Ala, T., & Underwood, K. L. (1992). Development of scoring criteria for the clock drawing task in Alzheimer's disease. *Journal of the American Geriatrics Society, 40*, 1095–1099.

Meulen, E. F. J., Schmand, B., van Campen, J. P., Ponds, R. W., Verhey, F. R., Scheltens, P., & de Koning, S. J. (2004). The 7 Minute Screen: a neurocognitive screening test highly sensitive to various types of dementia. *Journal of Neurology, Neurosurgery & Psychiatry, 75*(5), 700–705.

Miller, J. M., & Pliskin, N. H. (2006). The clinical utility of the Mattis Dementia Rating Scale in assessing cognitive decline in Alzheimer's disease. *International Journal of Neuroscience*, *5*, 613–627.

Milne, A., Culverwell, A., Guss, R., Tuppen, J., & Whelton, R. (2008). Screening for dementia in primary care: a review of the use, efficacy and quality of measures. *International Psychogeriatrics, 20*(5), 911–926.

Mindt, M. R., Arentoft, A., Germano, K. K., D'Aquila, E., Scheiner, D., Pizzirusso, M., et al. (2008). Neuropsychological, cognitive, and theoretical considerations for evaluation of bilingual individuals. *Neuropsychology Review, 18*, 255–268.

Morris, J. C., Heyman, A., Mohs, R. C., Hughes, J. P., van Belle, G., Fillenbaum, G., et al. (1989). The Consortium to Establish a Registry for Alzheimer's Disease (CERAD). Part I. Clinical and neuropsychological assessment of Alzheimer's disease. *Neurology, 39*, 1159–1165.

Nasreddine, Z. S., Phillips, N. A., Bedirian, V., Charbonneau, S., Whitehead, V., Collin, I., et al. (2005). The Montreal Cognitive Assessment, MoCA: a brief screening tool for mild cognitive impairment. *Journal of the American Geriatric Society, 53*, 695–699.

Nazem, S., Siderowf, A. D., Duda, J. E., Have, T. T., Colcher, A., Horn, S. S., et al. (2009). Montreal cognitive assessment performance in patients with Parkinson's disease with "normal" global cognition according to mini-mental state examination score. *Journal of the American Geriatrics Society, 57*(2), 304–308.

O'Brien, J. T. (2006). Vascular cognitive impairment. *American Journal of Geriatric Psychiatry, 14*, 724–733.

Patton, D. E., Duff, K., Schoenberg, M. R., Mold, J., Scott, J. G., & Adams, R. L. (2003). Performance of cognitively normal African Americans on the RBANS in community dwelling older adults. *Clinical Neuropsychologist*, *17*, 515–530.

Petersen, R. C., Doody, R., Kurz, A., Mohs, R. C., Morris, J. C., Rabins, P. V., et al. (2001). Current concepts in mild cognitive impairment. *Archives of Neurology*, *58*, 1985–1992.

Plassman, B. L., Langa, K. M., Fisher, G. G., Heeringa, S. G., Weir, D. R., Ofstedal, M. B., et al. (2008). Prevalence of cognitive impairment without dementia in the United States. *Annals of International Medicine*, *148*, 427–434.

Plassman, B. L., Langa, K. M., Fisher, G. G., Heeringa, S. G., Weir, D. R., Ofstedal, M. B., et al. (2007). Prevalence of dementia in the United States: the aging, demographics, and memory study. *Neuroepidemiology*, *29*, 125–132.

Randolph, C., Tierney, M. C., Mohr, E., & Chase, T. N. (1998). The Repeatable Battery for the Assessment of Neuropsychological Status (RBANS): preliminary clinical validity. *Journal of Clinical and Experimental Neuropsychology*, *20*, 310–319.

Raschetti, R., Albanese, E., Vanacore, N., & Maggini, M. (2007). Cholinesterase inhibitors in mild cognitive impairment: a systematic review of randomised trials. *PLoS Medicine*, *4*, e338.

Rascovsky, K., Salmon, D. P., Hansen, L. A., & Galasko, D. (2008). Distinct cognitive profiles and rates of decline on the Mattis Dementia Rating Scale in autopsy-confirmed frontotemporal dementia and Alzheimer's disease. *Journal of the International Neuropsychological Society*, *14*(3), 373–383.

Raz, N., & Rodrigue, K. M. (2006). Differential aging of the brain: patterns, cognitive correlates and modifiers. *Neuroscience and Biobehavioral Reviews*, *30*, 730–748.

Raz, N. (2005). The aging brain observed in vivo: differential changes and their modifiers. In R. Cabeza, L. Nyberg, & D. Park (Eds.), *Cognitive Neuroscience of Aging: Linking Cognitive and Cerebral Aging* (pp. 19–57). New York, NY: Oxford University Press.

Raz, N., Rodrigue, K. M., & Acker, J. D. (2003). Hypertension and the brain: vulnerability of the prefrontal regions and executive functions. *Behavioral Neuroscience*, *117*, 1169–1180.

Reischies, F. M., & Kühl, K.-P. (2005). Seven-Minute-Screen (7MS) in der ambulanten und klinischen Demenzdiagnostik. *Zeitschrift für Gerontopsychologie & -psychiatrie*, *18*, 143–154.

Rilling, L. M., Lucas, J. A., Ivnik, R. J., Smith, G. E., Willis, F. B., Ferman, T. J., et al. (2005). Mayo's Older African American Normative Studies: norms for the Mattis Dementia Rating Scale. *Clinical Neuropsychology*, *19*, 229–242.

Rodda, J., & Walker, Z. (2009). Ten years of cholinesterase inhibitors. *International Journal of Geriatric Psychiatry*, *24*, 437–442.

Rotrou, J., Battal-Merlet, L., Wenisch, E., Chausson, C., Bizet, E., Dray, F., et al. (2007). Relevance of 10-min. delayed recall in dementia screening. *European Journal of Neurology*, *14*, 144–149.

Royall, D. R., Chiodo, L. K., & Polk, M. J. (2000). Correlates of disability among elderly retirees with "subclinical" cognitive impairment. *Journals of Gerontology Series A-Biological Sciences and Medical Sciences*, *55*, M541–M546.

Royall, D. R., Chiodo, L. K., & Polk, M. J. (2005). An empiric approach to level of care determinations: the importance of executive measures. *Journals of Gerontology Series A-Biological Sciences and Medical Sciences*, *60*, 1059–1064.

Royall, D. R., Cordes, J. A., & Polk, M. (1998). CLOX: an executive clock drawing task. *Journal of Neurology, Neurosurgery & Psychiatry*, *64*(5), 588–594.

Salthouse, T. A. (1993). Speed mediation of adult age-differences in cognition. *Developmental Psychology*, *29*, 722–738.

Salthouse, T. A. (1994). The nature of the influence of speed on adult age-differences in cognition. *Developmental Psychology*, *30*, 240–259.

Scanlan, J., & Borson, S. (2001). The mini-cog: receiver operating characteristics with expert and naive raters. *International Journal Geriatric Psychiatry*, *16*, 216–222.

Schmidt, K. S. (2004). *Dementia Rating Scale-2 Alternate Form: Manual supplement*. Lutz, FL: Psychological Assessment Resources.

Schmidt, K. S., Mattis, P., Adams, J., & Nestor, P. (2005). Alternate-form reliability of the Dementia Rating Scale-2. *Archives of Clinical Neuropsychology, 20*(4), 436–441.

Schmitt, F. A., Davis, D. G., Wekstein, D. R., Smith, C. D., Ashford, J. W., & Markesbery, W. R. (2000). "Preclinical" AD revisited: neuropathology of cognitively normal older adults. *Neurology, 55*, 370–376.

Schmidt, K. S., Lieto, J. M., Kiryankova, E., & Salvucci, A. (2006). Construct and concurrent validity of the Dementia Rating Scale-2 Alternate Form. *Journal of Clinical and Experimental Neuropsychology, 28*(5), 646–654.

Seigerschmidt, E., Mosch, E., Siemen, M., Förstl, H., & Bickel, H. (2002). The clock drawing test and questionable dementia: reliability and validity. *International Journal of Geriatric Psychiatry, 17*, 1048–1054.

Shay, K. A., Duke, L. W., Conboy, T., Harrell, L. E., Callaway, R., & Folks, D. G. (1991). The clinical validity of the Mattis Dementia Rating Scale in staging Alzheimer's dementia. *Journal of Geriatric Psychiatry and Neurology, 4*, 18–25.

Shulman, K. I. (2000). Clock-drawing: is it the ideal cognitive screening test? *International Journal of Geriatric Psychiatry, 15*(6), 548–561.

Shulman, K. I., Shedletsky, R., & Silver, I. L. (1986). The challenge of time: clock-drawing and cognitive function in the elderly. *International Journal of Geriatric Psychiatry, 1*, 135–140.

Skjerve, A., Nordhus, I. H., Engedal, K., Braekhus, A., Nygaard, H. A., & Pallesen, S. (2007). Seven-Minute Screen performance in a normal elderly sample. *International Journal of Geriatric Psychiatry, 22*(8), 764–769.

Smith, T., Gildeh, N., & Holmes, C. (2007). The Montreal Cognitive Assessment: validity and utility in a memory clinic setting. *The Canadian Journal of Psychiatry, 52*(5), 329–332.

Solomon, P. R., & Pendlebury, W. W. (1998). Recognition of Alzheimer's disease: the 7 Minute Screen. *Family Medicine, 30*(4), 65–271.

Solomon, P. R., Hirschoff, A., Kelly, B., Relin, M., Brush, M., DeVeaux, R. D., & Pendlebury, W. W. (1998). A 7-minute neurocognitive screening battery highly sensitive to Alzheimer's disease. *Archives of Neurology, 55*(3), 349–355.

Sosa, A., Albanese, E., Prince, M., Acosta, D., Ferri, C., Guerra, M., et al. (2009). Population normative data for the 10/66 Dementia Research Group cognitive test battery from Latin America, India and China: a cross-sectional survey. *BMC Neurology, 9*, 48.

Storey, J. E., Rowland, J. T. J., Basic, D., & Conforti, D. B. (2001). A comparison of five clock scoring methods using ROC (receiver operating characteristics) curve analysis. *International Journal of Geriatric Psychiatry, 16*(4), 394–399.

Stout, J. C., Bondi, M. W., Jernigan, T. L., Archibald, S. L., Delis, D. C., & Salmon, D. P. (1999). Regional cerebral volume loss associated with verbal learning and memory in dementia of the Alzheimer type. *Neuropsychology, 13*, 188–197.

Strauss, E., MacDonald, S. W. S., Hunter, M., Moll, A., & Hultsch, D. F. (2002). Intraindividual variability in cognitive performance in three groups of older adults: cross-domain links to physical status and self-perceived affect and beliefs. *Journal of the International Neuropsychological Society,* 893–906.

Strauss, M. E., & Fritsch, T. (2004). Factor structure of the CERAD neuropsychological battery. *Journal of the International Neuropsychological Society, 10*, 559–565.

Sunderland, T., Hill, J. L., Mellow, A. M., Lawlor, B. A., Gundersheimer, J., Newhouse, P. A., & Grafman, J. H. (1989). Clock drawing in Alzheimer's disease: a novel measure of dementia severity. *Journal of the American Geriatric Society, 37*, 725–729.

Tombaugh, T. N., & Mcintyre, N. J. (1992). The Mini-Mental-State-Examination—a comprehensive review. *Journal of the American Geriatrics Society, 40*, 922–935.

Tombaugh, T. N., McDowell, I., Kristjansson, B., & Hubley, A. M. (1996). Mini-Mental State Examination (MMSE) and the modified MMSE (3MS): a psychometric comparison and normative data. *Psychological Assessment, 8*, 48–59.

Trinh, N. H., Hoblyn, J., Mohanty, S., & Yaffe, K. (2003). Efficacy of cholinesterase inhibitors in the treatment of neuropsychiatric symptoms and functional impairment in Alzheimer's disease. *JAMA: Journal of the American Medical Association, 289*, 210–216.

Tsolaki, M., Iakovidou, V., Papadopoulou, E., Aminta, M., Nakopoulou, E., Pantazi, T., & Kazis, A. (2002). Greek validation of the Seven-Minute Screening Battery for Alzheimer's disease in the elderly. *American Journal of Alzheimer's Disease and Other Dementias*, *17*(3). 139–148.

Unverzagt, F. W., Hall, K. S., Torke, A. M., Rediger, J. D., Mercado, N., Gureje, O., et al. (1996). Effects of age, education, and gender on CERAD neuropsychological test performance in an African American sample. *Clinical Neuropsychologist*, *10*, 180–190.

Unverzagt, F. W., Morgan, O. S., Thesiger, C. H., Eldemire, D. A., Luseko, J., Pokuri, S., et al. (1999). Clinical utility of CERAD neuropsychological battery in elderly Jamaicans. *Journal of the International Neuropsychological Society*, *5*, 255–259.

Wall, J. R., Deshpande, S. A., MacNeill, S. E., & Lichtenberg, P. A. (1998). The Fuld Object Memory Evaluation, a useful tool in the assessment of urban geriatric patients. *Clinical Gerontologist*, *19*, 39–49.

Watson, Y. I., Arfken, C. L., & Birge, S. J. (1993). Clock completion: an objective screening test for dementia. *Journal of the American Geriatric Society*, *41*, 235–1240.

Welsh, K. A., Butters, N., Hughes, J. P., Mohs, R. C., & Heyman, A. (1992). Detection and staging of dementia in Alzheimer's disease. Use of the neuropsychological measures developed for the Consortium to Establish a Registry for Alzheimer's Disease. *Archives of Neurology*, *49*, 448–452.

Welsh, K., Breitner, J., & Magruder-Habib, K. (1993). Detection of dementia in the elderly using Telephone Screening of Cognitive Status. *Neuropsychiatry, Neuropsychology, & Behavioral Neurology*, *6*, 103–111.

West, R. L. (1996). An application of prefrontal cortex function theory to cognitive aging. *Psychological Bulletin*, *120*, 272–292.

Whyte, S. R., Cullum, C. M., Hynan, L. S., Lacritz, L. H., Rosenberg, R. N., & Weiner, M. F. (2005). Performance of elderly Native Americans and Caucasians on the CERAD Neuropsychological Battery. *Alzheimer Disease & Associated Disorders*, *19*, 74–78.

Wolf-Klein, G. P., Silverstone, F. A., Levy, A. P., & Brod, M. S. (1989). Screening for Alzheimer's disease by clock drawing. *Journal of the American Geriatric Society*, *37*, 730–734.

Yochim, B. P., Bank, A. L., Mast, B. T., MacNeill, S. E., & Lichtenberg, P. A. (2003). Clinical utility of the Mattis dementia rating scale in older, urban medical patients: an expanded study. *Aging Neuropsychology and Cognition*, *10*, 230–237.

Zadikoff, C., Fox, S. H., Tang-Wai, D. F., Thomsen, T., de Bie, R. M., Wadia, P., et al. (2008). A comparison of the mini mental state exam to the Montreal cognitive assessment in identifying cognitive deficits in Parkinson's disease. *Movement Disorders: Official Journal of the Movement Disorder Society*, *23*(2), 297–299.

Zarit, S. H., Blazer, D., Orrell, M., & Woods, B. (2008). Throwing down the gauntlet: can we do better than the MMSE? *Aging & Mental Health*, *12*(4), 411–412.

CHAPTER

Cognitive Assessment in Late Stage Dementia

20

Cameron J. Camp[1], Michael J. Skrajner[2], Michelle M. Lee[3], Katherine S. Judge[4]

[1] *Hearthstone Alzheimer Care, Woburn, MA, USA,*

[2] *Hearthstone Alzheimer Care, Wiboughby, OH, USA,*

[3] *Department of Behavioral Medicine, Midwestern University, Downers Grove, IL, USA,*

[4] *Department of Psychology, Cleveland State University, Cleveland, OH, USA*

INTRODUCTION

The purpose of this chapter is not to provide an extensive overview of all or most of the instruments used to assess cognitive function in late stage dementia. Such compilations already exist, and their authors have done an excellent job of summarizing assessment instruments currently in use (e.g., Auer, Sclan, Yaffee, & Reisberg, 1994; Bellelli, Frisoni, Bianchetti, & Trabucci, 1997; Boller, Verny, Hugonot-Diener, & Saxton, 2002; Morris, 1997; Perlick & Mattis, 1994; Reisberg, Sclan, Franssen, Kluger, & Ferris, 1994, 1996; Saxton & Boller, 2006; Weiner et al., 1996). While we will review some of the instruments used for assessing cognition in late stage dementia, this will be done within a different context. The focus of this chapter is to encourage the development of new assessment instruments designed to assist in the development of new interventions for this population. Such assessments and interventions must map onto elements in the infrastructure of care delivery systems for persons with dementia, which in turn will enable assessment and intervention to be sustainable. Therefore, we will discuss not only the information that current instruments provide, but also what they do not provide. We will attempt to elaborate a framework or set of boundary conditions for a new generation of cognitive assessment measures, and discuss the uses of such measures. It is our hope that readers of this chapter will be encouraged to view cognitive assessment in late stage dementia as an integral part of an overall program for designing interventions (cf., Weaverdyck, 1990, 1991a, 1991b). We will offer examples of some initial efforts in this area to illustrate these points, and how intrinsic motivators within care delivery systems for persons with dementia can be related to assessment and intervention. We will also address multicultural diversity issues as they relate to these issues.

PROBLEMS IN ASSESSING COGNITION IN LATE STAGE DEMENTIA

If measures for assessing cognition in late stage dementia already exist, why should there be a call to develop new ones? A multitude of problems still challenge those who attempt to make such assessments. Most research on classification and test development in dementia has had two primary goals: (1) providing a diagnosis of dementia and (2) providing inclusion/exclusion criteria for clinical trials research. As a result, most research in test development has been conducted on persons with "pure" (or

Handbook of Assessment in Clinical Gerontology. DOI: 10.1016/B978-0-12-374961-1.10020-X probable) Alzheimer's disease (AD), with an emphasis on early to middle stages of AD. These individuals have been the primary targets for creating tests that can accurately diagnose AD at earlier and earlier points in its progression. More recently, this population has been targeted for testing the efficacy of pharmacological interventions.

This has been driven, to some (perhaps a large) extent, by the demands of the U.S. Food and Drug Administration that any drug designed to alleviate cognitive symptoms of dementia demonstrate a statistically significant effect using the cognitive subtest of the Alzheimer Disease Assessment Scale-Cognitive (ADAS-cog; Mohs & Cohen, 1988). The ADAS-cog has become, in essence, the gold standard by which any intervention for Alzheimer's and related disorders is determined to be effective or not, and as such this assessment has been translated into a number of languages. Of course, sensitivity to this measure generally is greater in persons with earlier stages of dementia compared to later stages of dementia, where floor effects are more likely to be obtained for this measure. [It is of interest to note that Namenda® (memantine HCl), the first drug developed to treat symptoms of more advanced dementia, was developed in Europe under a different regulatory system for drug development for dementia.] This has led some researchers and clinicians to refer to late stage or severe dementia as the "neglected half of Alzheimer disease" (Auer et al., 1994).

By contrast, in long-term care facilities, where most persons in late stage dementia reside, pure AD is rarely encountered. Comorbid conditions are the norm rather than the exception, and these may affect cognitive status, functional ability, and the expression of dementia's progression in significant but unknown ways (Lichtenberg, 1994, 1998). For example, declines in sensory and motor functioning that are generally present in persons with late stage dementia make it difficult to maintain standardized assessment protocols, and challenge the validity of many test scores. Many assessment tools that have traditionally been used with less impaired persons with dementia are limited by floor effects when used with persons with severe dementia. In addition, brevity of assessment is especially important in late stage dementia to guard against fatigue and frustration. Finally, it is important for instruments designed specifically to test cognitive performance in persons with late stage or severe dementia to be validated cross-culturally. For example, the Severe Impairment Battery (SIB; Saxton, McGonigle-Gibson, & Boller (1990) has translated versions that have been validated with individuals in several countries (see Saxton & Boller, 2006). As Boller et al. (2002) indicate, there is a high proportion of severe dementia among inpatients across countries. Thus, the ongoing development of cross-culturally valid assessment tools for severe dementia is especially important.

Problems in assessing cognitive status in late stage dementia extend beyond existing instruments themselves, for they involve more fundamental questions such as: How should late stage dementia be defined? Why should cognitive assessment be conducted for persons with late stage dementia? How should cognition in advanced dementia be assessed? Can cost-effective measures be developed that can be used on a large scale? Who should conduct these assessments? How should information obtained from these assessments be utilized? In this section we will discuss some of these problems, and review representative cognitive assessment measures within this general context.

Defining Late Stage Dementia

First and foremost, the definition of late stage dementia or "severe impairment" in dementia lacks precision, and varies according to the setting, the comparison group, the purpose, and the professional making this judgment. One way in which late stage dementia or severe impairment may be characterized is via global rating scales. Saxton and Boller (2006) discuss several global rating scales that have been used to define severe dementia. Severe dementia has been delineated by a "score of 6 or 7 on the Global Deterioration Scale (GDS)," or "a score of 3 or higher on the Clinical Dementia Rating (CDR) scale," or "categories 6a to 7f of the Functional Assessment Staging Test (FAST)" (Saxton &

Boller, 2006, p. 43). Saxton and Boller (2006) also point out that scores of <10 on the Mini-Mental State Exam (MMSE) are believed to signify the level of cognitive impairment seen in severe dementia. Thus, there appears to be no single "gold standard" criterion for determining when an individual has severe or late stage dementia.

Why Should we Assess Cognition in Advanced Dementia?

There are several interwoven rationales for such testing. With better medical management tools, it has become progressively clear that even very advanced dementia is amenable to observation, testing, management, and intervention. For example, Naomi Feil (e.g., Feil & de Klerk-Rubin, 2002), in her validation approach to communicating with persons with dementia, argues forcefully for the need to continue to work with persons with moderate to advanced dementia, and to their ability to respond to intervention.

One important role of testing would be to provide an indication of relatively spared abilities—areas of strengths in addition to weaknesses (Lichtenberg, 1994, 1998). Knowledge of a resident's cognitive status can provide relevant information regarding appropriate level of stimulation, the development of relevant management plans as well as possible cognitive and/or behavioral interventions, and adequacy of treatments (both psychological and pharmacological). But while there are benefits to cognitive assessment in advanced dementia, attempts to create assessment tools for this purpose have met with challenges.

Limited Sensitivity of Tests Used for Diagnosing Dementia

Most tests used for evaluating mild and moderate dementia have limited sensitivity (and thus limited usefulness) in more severely impaired individuals, in part because of the dissolution of language skills seen in late stage dementia. For example, the MMSE (Folstein, Folstein, & McHugh, 1975) is a standard industry tool used to validate new cognitive measures. It is widely considered to be one of the most reliable and valid screening tests for mild to moderate dementia. However, the MMSE has a heavy emphasis on verbally transmitted information and therefore exhibits floor effects when assessing persons with severe cognitive difficulties. As a result, the MMSE generates scores of questionable validity for more cognitively impaired individuals (Salmon, Thal, Butters, & Heindel, 1990), especially those with severe language impairments. This is only exacerbated if sensory deficits are present.

It is estimated that one-third of the residents in long-term care facilities in the U.S. obtain floor effect scores on traditional mental status assessments (Teresi, Lawton, Ory, & Holmes, 1994). The inability to measure cognitive changes has led to the hypothesis that progression might slow down in later stages of the disease (Yesavage & Brooks, 1991). Such a conclusion may be less than justified if standard cognitive assessment measures are simply insensitive to change in persons with advanced dementia. We will next review attempts to develop instruments specifically designed for this population in an effort to create measures that are more sensitive to individual variability.

Approaches to Cognitive Assessment in Late Stage Dementia

Three approaches have traditionally been followed to evaluate those persons unable to achieve minimal scores on standardized tests. One approach focuses on defining stages of dementia severity. Another approach is the evaluation of functional capabilities. The third approach considers the assessment of cognitive functions with tests developed for severely impaired individuals. The instruments we have selected to review within each of these three domains may not rely exclusively on a single approach, but have different emphases reflecting the predominance of a particular approach.

Defining Stages of Dementia Severity

An example of the first approach, the *Clinical Dementia Rating Scale* (CDR; Hughes, Berg, Danziger, Coben, & Martin, 1982), helps the clinician to rate severity of AD and related disorders on a 5-point scale from 0 (normal) to 3 (severe stage) based on clinical interviews with an informant and the person with dementia. Areas coded are memory, orientation, judgment, problem solving, community affairs, home and hobbies. The CDR is used internationally to determine stages of dementia severity (see Perneczyky et al., 2006). While the CDR is a valid and reliable instrument for rating dementia severity, it may be too burdensome to use in general practice and requires a reliable informant (Perneczyky et al., 2006). However, recent data indicate that the MMSE scores of 0–10 mapped onto CDR stage 3 for severe dementia in a sample of outpatients at a university clinic for cognitive disorders, suggesting that the MMSE may be substituted for the CDR when staging information needs to be gathered quickly and easily (Perneczyky et al., 2006). However, when substituting the MMSE for the CDR to obtain dementia staging, it is necessary to keep in mind the aforementioned general limitations in using the MMSE in persons with severe dementia and that the outpatient sample mentioned above may not be representative of persons with severe dementia in general (see Perneczyky et al., 2006).

The *Global Deterioration Scale* (GDS; Reisberg, 1988) is based on a hierarchical, generalized, downward progression scheme. This scale describes seven global stages of dementia, from normality to severe impairment. This scale assumes progressive deterioration across all cognitive domains, making it sometimes difficult to apply to atypical dementias, such as frontal lobe dementia. A companion scale, the *Functional Assessment Staging* (FAST; Reisberg, Ferris, de Leon, & Crook, 1982) assesses decline in ability to perform basic activities of daily life. Scores range from normality (stage 1) to severe dementia (stage 7). Items have been designed to correspond to the respective GDS stages.

The *Hierarchical Dementia Scale* (HDS; Cole & Dastoor, 1987) was developed as an extension of the Mattis Dementia Rating Scale (MDRS; Mattis, 1976). The HDS incorporates Piagetian concepts and assumes that declines in neuropsychological function follow a hierarchical pattern that reverses the order of normal cognitive development (see also Camp et al., 1997; Sclan, Foster, Reisberg, Franssen, & Welkowitz, 1990; Thornbury, 1992; Vance, Camp, Kabacoff, & Greenwalt, 1996). The HDS consists of 20 subscales covering a number of primarily cognitive functions. Items within each subscale are arranged hierarchically in order of difficulty. The examiner begins with items corresponding to the estimated overall level of functioning of the person with dementia, and then continues upward or downward based on the performance of the individual (i.e., using an adaptive testing approach). Testing time is 40–50 minutes, but less with increased familiarity. Several studies have found favorable results for the reliability and validity of the HDS when used over time. Bickel (1996) reported that the HDS had good test–retest reliability within different levels of dementia, and that the HDS generally correlated highly with the MMSE.

One strength of the HDS approach is its use of a hierarchical organization scheme that allows it to be quickly made more or less challenging according to the ability level of the individual being tested. A drawback to work done thus far with the HDS is that sample sizes used in research with this instrument have been small, especially with regard to persons with advanced dementia, although initial results are encouraging. Like Piagetian measures, the HDS is primarily descriptive rather than prescriptive. In other words, the HDS is a useful tool for describing current levels of functioning and for providing more fine-grained descriptions than many other measures. However, it does not prescribe methods for improving level of functioning. Boller et al. (2002) note that the HDS may be more useful in identifying and tracking moderately severe cognitive deficits than diagnosing and assessing severe dementia.

Auer et al. (1994) have taken a similar approach to assessment of dementia with the creation of the *Modified Ordinal Scales of Psychological Development* (M-OSPD). This represents a modification of an ordinal scale of development designed for assessment of children and based on Piagetian stages of development, and includes measures of constructs from Piagetian theory such as visual pursuit and object permanence, causality, and schemes. No language skills are necessary for assessment. The M-OSPD has good psychometric properties, and the authors make several important points about issues in advanced dementia that can critically affect attempts to assess cognitive performance, such as rigid limbs, lack of motivation/institutionalization, differential responses to strangers versus familiar persons administering tests, etc.

A general shortcoming of the aforementioned scales is that, like most stage scales, they often have difficulty accommodating variability in the progression of dementia across different cognitive (and behavioral) domains, i.e., problems with the issues of horizontal and vertical decalage, to use Piaget's term (see Ginsburg & Opper, 1988, for a discussion of these concepts). For example, communication skills and reading ability in persons with late stage dementia prove to be better than would be expected from staging descriptions used in the GDA and FAST (Bayles, Tomoeda, Cruz, & Mahendra, 2000). In addition, while good at providing descriptions of areas of cognitive deterioration, these measures do not focus on means of ameliorating problems caused by such deterioration. Lin et al. (2009), for example, found that both acupressure and the use of Montessori-based activities for dementia (which will be described in detail later in this chapter), were beneficial in reducing agitation in persons with advanced dementia in a sample of long-term care residents in Taiwan.

Evaluation of Functional Capabilities

The second approach to cognitive assessment in late stage dementia is to focus on evaluation of functional capabilities. Historically, nursing homes gathered only limited information on functional status and cognition. The 1987 Congressional mandate in the Omnibus Budget Reconciliation Act (OBRA) now requires facilities to complete a standardized assessment of each resident's functional, medical, psychosocial, and cognitive status, known as the Minimum Data Set (MDS; Morris et al., 1994). The MDS-based *Cognitive Performance Scale* (CPS) combines selected MDS items into a single, functional hierarchical cognitive performance scale and is modeled on the MMSE and the *Test for Severe Impairment* (TSI; Albert & Cohen, 1992), which we will describe shortly.

The CPS provides a functional view of cognitive performance, with a global and hierarchical decision tree, in five domains: coma status; "short-memory OK;" capacity to make daily decisions; ability to communicate requests; and eating independence. This nursing scale provides practical, but only global, impressions of functional status. Its relation to underlying cognitive mechanisms is not well established. The CPS primarily serves nurses' needs, as it focuses on ADL items and indirect measures of cognitive performance.

The *Bedford Alzheimer Nursing Severity Scale* (BANS-s; Volicer, Hurley, Lathi, & Kowall, 1994) comprises seven items evaluating functional (ambulating, dressing, eating) and cognitive (speech, eye contact) abilities, and pathological symptoms (sleep/wake cycle disturbance, muscle rigidity). The usefulness of this scale is restricted to descriptions of global performance with little sensitivity to changes in behavior. Bellelli et al. (1997) found that the BANS-s correlated well with other cognitive status measures (ranging from $r = 0.6$ to $r = 0.8$), and was least likely to show floor effects of all measures examined. The authors note that motor function and mobility were important discriminators among severely demented individuals.

The *Alzheimer Disease Cooperative Study Activities of Daily Living Scale for Severe Impairment* (ADCS-ADL-sev; Galasko et al., 2005) was specifically developed to assess daily functioning in persons with moderate to severe dementia. This 19-item scale assesses basic ADLs (e.g., eating, toileting) as well as instrumental ADLs (IADLs) that may continue to be meaningful in severe dementia (e. g., watching TV, using telephones and light-switches, being left alone). It can be administered by an interviewer to an informant in about 15 minutes. The ADACS-ADL-sev correlates well with measures of both cognitive (MMSE and the Severe Impairment Battery) and global (CDR and GDS) functioning (Galasko et al., 2005). In addition, the ADCS-ADL-sev is sensitive enough to detect decline over 6 and 12 months in moderate to severe community-dwelling individuals with AD and may be used to assess the impact of treatment interventions on daily functioning (Galasko et al., 2005). Consequently, the ADCS-ADL-sev may be particularly useful for gathering detailed information about ADLs as part of intervention studies, although briefer, more simplistic scales that can be administered by unskilled personnel may be a better choice for general clinical practice (Galasko et al., 2005).

Three important lessons come from studies using these measures: (1) standard measures of dementia assessment will indeed have floor effects if other factors such as motor functioning are not included in an assessment; (2) assessment in long-term care will be generally undertaken when it serves the (sometimes mandated) needs of a facility; (3) assessment in long-term care settings will be primarily conducted by facility staff who are not psychologists. It is simply too costly for nursing homes to use psychologists for large-scale and repetitive assessments. Since this is where many if not most persons with advanced dementia reside, this is a critical consideration in the development of cognitive assessment measures.

Multicultural Issues in Functional Capacity

Multicultural issues also impact the development of assessments designed to determine functional capacity and related interventions to enhance or maintain functional capacity in persons with dementia. For example, an important ability to be assessed with implications for care planning would be the ability to use tools, which involves eye/hand coordination, fine and gross motor skills, grip, along with range of motion. Tool usage also relates to self-care issues such as feeding oneself.

One intervention approach that will be discussed in more detail shortly, Montessori-based activity programming, highlights the importance of developing and implementing multicultural issues in assessment protocols and intervention programs. A particular activity, "hidden treasure," was developed for individuals with more advanced dementia. This activity involves tool use practice. A plastic tub is filled almost to the top with grains of rice. Under the surface of the rice is "hidden treasure" – eight objects to be found with the use of a long-handled slotted spoon. When participants dig into the rice and find an object, they are to lift the object in the spoon, and then gently move the spoon back and forth to sift out the grains of rice through the slots in the spoon. Next to the tub is a laminated template, with eight circles on it. Participants are to place each discovered object on a circle. Thus, participants with advanced dementia can know how many objects have been found and how many still are missing through the use of the template, rather than having to use short-term memory. All of the information needed to complete the task is contained in the materials themselves, which utilizes a Montessori education concept known as "control of error." In addition, the skills associated with the activity mentioned above receive practice through repetition, but within the context of a game rather than as drill.

However, when we presented this to the rabbi for inspection at our Orthodox Jewish facility, he commented that it was a fine activity with the exception that it could not be used during Passover, when Jewish residents were forbidden from touching uncooked grain. When a manual describing this activity was being translated into Japanese (Camp, 1999), our translator informed us that we would have to substitute something else for rice, such as lentils. She stated that the use of rice in this manner would be considered extremely inappropriate by elderly Japanese, who had suffered from hunger during war and to whom each grain of rice was precious. A visiting Fulbright scholar from India told us that for her residents, the hidden objects should be rocks, because this would simulate an activity of daily living in which rocks and other material needed to be extracted from home-grown rice before cooking. These examples illustrate the importance of any assessment tool and/or intervention for persons with dementia being translated culturally, as well as linguistically.

To further illustrate this point, our manual (Camp, 1999) was translated into Spanish by colleagues in Spain. However, we were told not to use the manual with older adults from Latin America. Some Spanish words that are innocuous when used on the Iberian Peninsula have a vulgar connotation when used in Latin America. Thus, it appears that our Spanish language manual needs to be translated from Iberian Spanish into Latin American Spanish.

Assessment of Cognitive Functions

The third approach primarily considers the assessment of cognitive function with tests that represent downward extensions of previously developed cognitive assessment measures for dementia. We will examine several such tests that have been developed.

The *Severe Impairment Battery* (SIB; Saxton et al., 1990) was specifically developed to evaluate the cognitive and behavioral symptoms of severe dementia. The SIB consists of 40 questions covering nine areas of cognition: social interaction; memory; orientation; language; attention; praxis; visuo-spatial ability; construction; and orientation to name. Items are presented as single verbal or one-step commands enhanced by gestural cues. The test is untimed and credit is given for partial and non-verbal responses. Testing time is approximately 20 minutes. SIB scores correlate well with the MMSE ($r = 0.74$) and has good test–retest reliability ($r = 0.85$). The SIB is sensitive enough to detect decline over time in individuals with severe AD and has been used in clinical trials (see Saxton & Boller, 2006). The SIB also is better than the Preliminary Neuropsychological Battery in differentiating performances among severely impaired older adults with MMSE scores between 5 and 10 (Barbarotto, Cerri, Acerbi, Molinari, & Capitani, 2000). In addition, the SIB has been used cross-culturally and has demonstrated validity in French, Italian, Spanish, and Korean populations (Ahn, Kim, Ku, Saxton, & Kim, 2006; see Saxton & Boller, 2006).

A key feature of the SIB is it assesses several remaining abilities in persons with severe dementia. For example, motor functioning and activities of daily living are assessed through demonstration. Reading ability and the ability to follow multi-step directions and auditory commands are also assessed at levels applicable to persons with severe dementia. Other important abilities that are assessed are color recognition and color naming, shape naming and shape matching, and the ability to count. The SIB assesses language production in a non-threatening manner by asking participants to name things they like to eat. Social skills are assessed by introducing oneself, shaking hands with the participant, and engaging in general conversation.

The memory sections of the SIB rely heavily on explicit memory processes that may be difficult and confusing for persons with severe cognitive impairment. These sections would not assess remaining abilities in memory and are likely to produce floor effects. Persons with severe dementia have limited attention spans and fatigue easily, thus using the SIB for assessment purposes may not produce optimal testing results. Also, the SIB can be tiring for a client who has additional impairments, such as sensory deficits, attention difficulties, brief sustained attention, extreme cognitive impairments (e.g., MMSE < 5), or agitation.

In response to such concerns, the SIB-Short Form (SIB-S) was developed based on data from individuals with severe dementia in the United States and France (Saxton et al., 2005). The SIB-S is psychometrically sound and retains many of the features of the SIB, but with an administration time of only 10–15 minutes (Saxton et al., 2005). The SIB-S also is reliable and valid for use with Korean persons with severe Alzheimer's disease (Ahn, Kim, Saxton, & Kim, 2007). The SIB-S is a better choice than the SIB for persons with very severe dementia (Saxton et al., 2005) and may be particularly helpful in evaluating those individuals with MMSE scores of 0. Subsequently, this may facilitate the inclusion of individuals with advanced symptoms of dementia in therapeutic trials (Saxton et al., 2005).

The *Test for Severe Impairment* (TSI; Albert & Cohen, 1992) addresses some of the concerns raised by the MMSE, as it minimizes reliance on language skills. The TSI was designed for persons with MMSE scores of 10 or less and assesses six areas: motor performance; language comprehension; language production; immediate and delayed memory; conceptualization; and general knowledge. This test was designed to take approximately 10 minutes, and test materials were selected on the basis of availability and portability (e.g., paper clips, a key, a spool of thread). TSI scores correlate well with the MMSE ($r = 0.83$), and test–retest reliability is high ($r = 0.96$). It is valid and sensitive to change in severely impaired persons with AD (Jacobs et al., 1999). A modified version of the TSI (m-TSI) has not found additional benefits above and beyond the original TSI in nursing home residents with moderate to end-stage dementia (Appollonio et al., 2001).

The TSI is short and does not rely heavily on verbal commands, multi-step commands, or higher-ordered cognitive processes. The motor performance section of the TSI assesses motor skills related to ADL functioning (combing one's hair) and fine motor skills (manipulating a pen cap and writing one's name). These brief motor assessments translate into functional capacities on a number of self-care activities. For example, if the resident can manipulate a pencil then they are probably capable of self-feeding. The language section of the TSI loads primarily on auditory commands through language comprehension and language production. In addition, useful information such as color recognition and naming are assessed, which can provide valuable information to clinicians, such as the level of anomia experienced by the person with dementia. The memory section of the TSI assesses participant's short-term memory capacity and understanding of object permanence. The general knowledge section of the TSI is a nice addition because it assesses long-term memory, specifically semantic knowledge, such as counting ability. The conceptualization section provides easy assessment of problem-solving skills and decision-making skills for persons with severe dementia. Last, the TSI allows for a brief look at social competence, for example, if the client shakes hands after prompting from the clinician.

Areas not assessed by the TSI include matching and/or recognizing and identifying different shapes and sizes, which are abilities many persons with severe dementia still retain. Also, the delayed memory section of the TSI would probably exhibit floor effects with persons with severe dementia. Other remaining abilities that are spared far into the course of dementia which are not assessed by the TSI include one-to-one number and object correspondence and the ability to read. These abilities can be useful when preparing appropriate programming for persons with severe dementia, as we will discuss in detail later.

The *Severe Cognitive Impairment Profile* (SCIP; Peavy et al., 1996) was designed to assess cognitive functioning in persons with advanced dementia who would generate floor effects with more standard assessment tools (e.g., MMSE scores of 0). The SCIP assesses a range of abilities, including overall behavior, attention, language, memory, motor functioning, arithmetic, visuospatial ability, and conceptualization. With only a 30-minute administration time and good psychometric qualities, it overcomes many of the problems encountered by other assessment tools focused on advanced dementia.

Finally, the MMSE has been modified to reduce floor effects in cases of severe dementia. The *Severe Mini-Mental State Examination* (SMMSE; Harrell, Marson, Chatterjee, & Parrish, 2000) is a 30-point scale that briefly assesses several abilities. These include overlearned information, executive skills, language, and simple visuospatial function.

Summary of Assessment Issues in Advanced Dementia

By the time a person has reached advanced stages of dementia, diagnosis is not a question and most drugs designed to influence cognitive functioning in dementia are not routinely tested (or prescribed if available, with some recent exceptions). Most cases of advanced dementia are seen within long-term care facilities. Within these settings, where regulations require documentation of change in functional and medical status, progression of dementia is documented via routine administration of the MDS, sometimes in conjunction with the MMSE. Documentation beyond this level is not required for advanced dementia, and thus other means of assessing cognitive status are not utilized. In settings such as assisted living apartments, private homes, etc., where regulations do not require extensive or periodic documentation of cognitive status compared to long-term care facilities, use of cognitive assessment in advanced dementia is more sporadic and less frequent.

Significant efforts have been made to create assessment tools sensitive to individual differences in late stage dementia. This line of research has produced measures indicating that even in late stage or severe dementia, variability among individuals exists, some cognitive abilities are relatively spared, and cognitive decline continues to progress (see Boller et al., 2002; Saxton & Boller, 2006). However, researchers interested in developing measures that will be used on a large scale must find a way of enabling persons working in long-term care settings to conduct these assessments, and provide a rationale for why it is in the best interest of both residents and staff to conduct them and repeat them over time. Further, researchers need to continue to develop measures that are valid and culturally appropriate for the individuals whom they are assessing. Efforts also need to be made to ensure that staff working in long-term care settings are sufficiently trained to administer such measures in a competent and multiculturally sensitive manner.

MEETING THE CHALLENGE: INTERVENTION MODELS

Where, then, is the impetus for cognitive assessments in advanced dementia? From the perspective that dementia in its advanced stages represents the effects of an intractable illness, and that dementia care should primarily be palliative, there is no real need to do more than a cursory assessment. However, an emerging alternative perspective of dementia, based on biopsychosocial models of disease, challenges this perception (e.g., Judge, Menne, & Whitlatch, 2009; Kitwood, 1997). Researchers taking this new perspective assume that interventions for dementia, even advanced dementia, have both practical and theoretical significance. A seminal model representing this perspective has been developed by Weaverdyck. She emphasizes the need to evaluate multiple factors within both the person with dementia and his or her physical environment, as well as the need for assessment to guide the intervention process.

Weaverdyck's Model

Weaverdyck (1990, 1991a, 1991b) has provided a compelling argument for the need to integrate assessment with intervention for persons with dementia. Weaverdyck (1990) states that the function of assessment in persons with dementia is to provide answers to two basic questions: "What is happening?" and "Why is it happening?" This information then facilitates the answer to a third question: "What are we going to do about it?" In other words, "…assessment is primarily for the purpose of intervention development…" (Weaverdyck, 1991a, p. 38). In her approach, there is an emphasis on identifying competencies as a basis for interventions. Weaverdyck (1990, 1991a, 1991b) emphasizes four primary targets for assessment: environment; task; caregiver; and person.

The first target for assessment, the environment, includes the physical, social, and emotional environment, as well as the cognitive environment, i.e., the extent to which an environment is intellectually stimulating. In Taiwan, for example, the first author visited a pilot adult day health center set up by the government. The nurses' station had many jars behind the desk, similar in appearance to an herbalist's shop. In one corner was a Christian chapel, and in another corner a Buddhist chapel. Additionally, stoves for cooking had been made to appear similar to brick ovens used in rural homes.

The second target for assessment is task—the activity that the person with dementia is performing or expected to perform. Weaverdyck provides a general model for analyzing task complexity for persons with dementia, and guidelines for simplifying tasks to the point that an individual with dementia will be able to complete them successfully.

The first author, for example, spoke recently with a nurse in Darwin, Australia. This woman worked at a long-term care facility that had several indigenous/aboriginal residents. A new female resident with dementia arrived, and when staff tried to give the resident a shower the older woman became hysterical. The nurse visited the resident's community, then returned and rearranged the shower experience. Now, the resident goes outside, sits on a rock (behind a screen), and washes off using a garden hose. In this case, the environment and the task were modified to allow the person with dementia to complete the bathing process successfully. This more familiar way of cleansing herself allowed the resident to independently bathe in the manner to which she was accustomed. Forcing a person with dementia from this culture to go into an enclosed room and be squirted with hot water from a pipe in a wall would be cruel.

The third target is the caregiver, with an emphasis on examining a caregiver's stressors, general caregiving competencies, and especially the quality and types of interactions between the caregiver and the person with dementia. The final target is the person with dementia. Thus, she places a strong emphasis on the use of activities as interventions for dementia, and provides a number of examples of activities that can reduce problem behaviors.

Weaverdyck's approach is commendable on several grounds. It emphasizes the need to link assessment and intervention for dementia populations. It also includes an emphasis on the person/environment interface—the need to analyze environments and tasks that persons with dementia encounter—and focuses on discovering strengths that could enable persons with dementia to interact more effectively with their environments. Her approach is soundly grounded in neuropsychological assessment practices and theory, and is extremely comprehensive.

This approach has two primary shortcomings, however. Because the model is so comprehensive, it may be difficult to implement for persons with advanced dementia. This is because such individuals are generally in long-term care facilities, many (often most) having their care costs paid by Medicaid. In most cases institutions providing care for such persons will not have the resources, personnel, or incentive to undertake such a comprehensive evaluation process. In addition, while her approach clearly emphasizes the need to use activities as therapeutic interventions and to link assessment with intervention, there is often a lack of detail in specifying the linkage between specific evaluation outcomes and corresponding recommendations for activity programming. To some extent, this is the result of the approach's comprehensive and generalized perspective. In addition, there are few comprehensive programs of activities onto which cognitive evaluation might be mapped.

The Healthcare Triangle

Within the United States, there are three key areas of interest to managers and administrators of facilities providing care to persons with advanced dementia (or to persons with moderate or early stage or no dementia). These are related to what can be called the *Healthcare Triangle Model* (Camp, 2006b; Camp & Brush, 2003), and involve *reimbursement/income*, *marketing*, and *surviving state inspections*. This is true whether or not a facility or company is a for-profit or not-for-profit entity (ask any administrator of a not-for-profit facility whether the balance sheet is important and this will be verified). Within skilled nursing facilities, income for providing care for persons with advanced dementia is generally determined by the services provided to these residents over and above standard care. For example, within the MDS system, there is a program known as *Restorative Nursing*.

Ray (2008) provides an excellent overview of this program. In essence, Restorative Nursing programs are designed to create interventions based on assessments of resident's needs to maintain or improve function, minimize complications, and prevent decline. Programs in Restorative Nursing involve an active or passive range of motion, and splint or brace assistance. In addition, there are several activities that require training and practice. These include: Bed Mobility; Walking; Eating/Swallowing; Communication; Transferring; Dressing or Grooming; Amputation/Prosthesis Care; and Other. In addition, scheduled toileting and bladder retraining often are included as Restorative Nursing Programs, as can be Activities of Daily Living (ADLs) and Dining Programs, Sensory Stimulation and Cognitive Orientation, Socialization Opportunities, and Integration of Religious/Spiritual Practices into Daily Routines (Ray, 2008). Provision of such programs, under the right circumstances, can result in additional revenues for a facility, in addition to improving the quality of life of residents. While there is no industry "standard" for assessment used for Restorative Nursing, the MDS also can be used as an initial place to examine potential areas of concern that can be targeted for interventions (Ray, 2008).

In addition, Restorative Nursing programs can address "flagged" or problematic areas known as "Quality Indicators" (QIs) within the MDS system. Inspectors look for flagged QIs as indicators of poor care, which can be the cause of citations if not addressed. The MDS also provides suggested action plans, or RAPs, to guide interventions when a QI flag has been discovered. Most nursing homes have a staff member or two, usually nurses, whose job is to monitor MDS data gathering and reporting. Nurses conduct assessments related to Restorative Nursing programs, create and monitor interventions, and report results (Ray, 2008).

We start with the assumption that for an intervention to be truly effective in long-term care facilities where dementia care is provided, any intervention must be demonstrated to positively impact at least one of the areas of the Healthcare Triangle. These are the areas paramount to chief executive officers, regardless of whether a facility is non-profit or for-profit. Interventions that do not positively address these areas are likely to disappear as soon as the psychologist responsible for introducing them leaves the building. As is readily apparent, Restorative Nursing programs impact at least two of the critical areas of the Healthcare Triangle. It is therefore critical that assessment and intervention, especially for persons with advanced dementia, must be made explicitly relevant to areas of the Healthcare Triangle. If not, no matter what their psychometric properties, assessments developed by psychologists outside of this system will be ignored, and as a result the quality of life of persons with dementia will not be influenced by the work of the psychologist.

It is important to note that the motivators of administrators can vary widely across different cultures. For example, in parts of Canada many nursing homes are administered by the government. A person seeking a nursing home for a relative may be given a list of state run facilities in the area where their relative lives and told to pick from among that short list. Marketing issues are much different in such a system compared to the United States. In another example, the first author was asked how to provide a cognitive intervention such as spaced retrieval (Camp, 2006b) to residents of nursing homes in Canada. [In the United States, rehabilitation professionals such as speech-language pathologists or occupational therapists have been trained to use this intervention to enable persons with dementia to achieve goals related to safety, personal care, decreased apathy, etc. (see Camp, 2006b for a detailed description of the intervention and its applications).] His response was, "First, rehabilitation staff are trained to apply the technique, as well as how to document and bill for the service. Then, they apply the technique in nursing homes, and train staff how to maintain the therapeutic goals achieved." His Canadian colleague responded, "What if there are no rehabilitation staff members in the facility? Can we train activity professionals to apply the intervention?" His response was, "How will an activity professional bill for the service?" His colleague's response was, "Why would they bill for the service?" Clearly, a different set of motivators had to be discerned to enable implementation of this intervention to be successful within the Canadian long-term care system.

Summary of Intervention Issues in Advanced Dementia

In summary, cognitive assessment for advanced dementia should be focused on intervention. In many cases, such intervention will take the form of therapeutic activities programming. The presence of recreational therapists in long-term care settings (in addition to volunteers, visiting family members, and nursing staff who have occasional opportunities to engage in activities with residents) provides an important avenue for implementing activity-based interventions. Cognitive assessment for this population should therefore be clearly linked to activity programming, and must be conducted and evaluated in such a manner that it can be implemented within long-term care settings and map on to the motivators of management within these settings. To the extent that motivators such as Restorative Nursing programs map onto activities, it is possible for staff other than recreational therapists to implement activities in ways that positively impact elements of the Healthcare Triangle Model. Recreational therapists and/or rehabilitation professionals such as occupational therapists, physical therapists, or speech-language pathologists can assist nursing staff with assessments, staff training, and implementation of such programs. We will next discuss an initial attempt to create such an approach to cognitive assessment.

Montessori-Based Intervention and Assessment

Initial pilot work on development of an assessment system for more advanced dementia using Montessori-based activities (Camp, Koss, & Judge, 1999) was expanded in a project funded by the National Institute on Aging (grant R01 AG021508-01A1; C. Camp, PI). This tool, the Montessori-Based Assessment System (MAS), is centered on activities based on Montessori teaching methods and materials. These activities are used to reduce the expression of disability associated with dementia. Further, the MAS has been designed to assist in developing restorative nursing programs within the context of the MDS.

Use of Montessori Activities for Persons with Dementia

Many researchers have suggested that during later stages of dementia, cognitive abilities may be lost in reverse developmental sequence, i.e., first-in/last-out—the reverse order in which cognitive abilities were developed in childhood (Auer et al., 1994; Biringer & Anderson, 1992; Camp et al., 1993; Lipinska, Bäckman, & Herlitz, 1992; [Nolen, 1988;] Reisberg, 1985, 1986; Sclan et al., 1990; Thornbury, 1992). If so, developmental sequencing of cognitive abilities may be a useful guide and the basis for creating interventions and programming for persons with AD (Camp et al., 1993; Vance et al., 1996). But the question then becomes one of selecting an approach on which to base a broad array of interventions that would be effective across a variety of individuals and levels of dementia. We decided to begin with an approach widely and effectively used to teach cognitive and functional skills to children—the Montessori Method developed by Maria Montessori.

The Montessori teaching method is developmentally and programmatically based and is used to train children in the areas of practical life (activities of daily living), sensorial experiences, language, math, engaging and maintaining the environment, science, and social skills. Montessori techniques seem well suited for persons with dementia. Each lesson is first presented at its simplest level and each subsequent lesson, increasing in complexity, is a variation of previously mastered skills or concepts.

For example, children first learn to distinguish a rough versus a smooth surface by touch, then they learn to discriminate between different levels of roughness through manipulating various grades of sandpaper. Later, children are shown a globe on which the continents are represented by sandpaper and the oceans by a smooth blue surface. This is their introduction to land and water as geologic forms. It is also their introduction to geography. Learning to distinguish and name the continents by their shape and location follows.

Materials are taken from the everyday environment and are designed not to be "toys," but tools to prepare the person for independent living. Persons with dementia need structure and order in their environment and activities, as changes in routine or physical surroundings may be upsetting and/or overwhelming (Vance et al., 1996). Maria Montessori said the same of her young students, and thus all activities involve a structure and order that both comforts and facilitates focused attention. Key elements of activities include immediate feedback, high probability of success, and repetition. Tasks are broken down into steps that can be mastered and then sequenced, an approach familiar to occupational and physical therapists. Finally, persons with dementia demonstrate the ability to learn through procedural or non-declarative memory [(Squire, 1992, 1994)], a phenomenon remarkably similar to what Montessori described as "unconscious learning" in children (Bäckman, 1992; Camp et al., 1993; Vance et al., 1996). For a much fuller description of the Montessori Method, the reader is referred to Chattin-McNichols (1992). Extensive discussion of the utility of this approach for cognitive rehabilitation in dementia is also available for those interested (e.g., Camp, 2001, 2006a; Camp et al., 1993, 1997; Dreher, 1997; Vance et al., 1996). Manuals for creating and presenting a variety of other Montessori-based activities for persons with dementia are commercially available (Camp, 1999; Camp et al., 2006; Joltin, Camp, Noble, & Antenucci, 2005), as well as short stories designed for individual or small group reading and discussion activities, or readers could contact the first author about these manuals and materials.

Montessori schools for children exist throughout the world, and curricula are designed to fit within local cultures and customs. In Hawaii, the first author visited a Montessori school and found a sorting activity designed to allow discrimination of different types of lava from volcanoes. Similarly, in Taiwan, a Mandarin language version of the first Montessori-based programming manual for persons with dementia has photos showing clients of adult day centers for dementia engaged in activities. One activity involves drawing words and other shapes in sand, and the participant in the photo is using a chopstick to make the drawings. When we provide training in implementing Montessori-based activities for dementia, we ask staff of facilities to redesign an ice-cream social so that residents or clients with dementia take ownership of the program, and can successfully fulfill social roles in that context. When the first author provided such training in Australia, the audience was unfamiliar with the concept of an ice-cream social, and so the target activity had to be changed to a "sausage sizzle." For caregivers of indigenous/aboriginal populations in Australia, the target activity had to be changed to a camp cook-out, which involved the preparation of kangaroo tails for the meal. In France, the target activity became an outing to gather chestnuts and then make and serve treats made from the chestnuts.

Montessori-Based Activities Used for Cognitive Assessment in Dementia

With regard to cognitive assessment in advanced dementia, we are primarily interested in documenting remaining abilities, and in finding ways in which these abilities can be expressed. As has been discussed elsewhere (Camp & Mattern, 1999), our intervention strategies have a rehabilitation orientation rather than just a focus on maintenance of remaining abilities. An underlying assumption of our work is that even in late stage dementia improvement in functional capacity is possible, especially as regards reduction of excess disability (Kitwood, 1997). Therefore, our assessment is designed to: (1) target abilities in which successful interventions can be developed and (2) document improvement in functioning.

Description of the MAS

The Montessori-Based Assessment System (MAS) has gone through several revisions. In its present and final form, the MAS consists of five Montessori-based activities, all of which tap into a variety of skills typically not addressed in other assessments. Below is a description of each activity, along with a summary of the skills being assessed.

Hand Washing

The resident is instructed to take a cloth out of a Wet Ones® container, wash their hands with the cloth, and throw away the cloth into a small paper bag, which acts as a waste basket.

Skills tested in this activity include:

1. the ability to use pincer grip (when the person takes the cloth out of the container);
2. range of motion (when the person throws away the cloth); and
3. the ability to follow directions (throughout this activity).

These skills relate to numerous Restorative Nursing elements such as Range of Motion, ADLs, Communication, etc. Also, the ability to follow directions is assessed, either from verbal prompts or by imitating the actions of the individual administering the test. This information can be translated into a variety of programs.

Short Story, Depth Perception, and Color Intensity

The resident is handed a seven page booklet. The booklet contains a title page, four pages of extremely large-print text (48 point Arial bold) about the invention of the cash register, a page with a reading comprehension question, and a page that tests depth perception and color intensity. The title page has a double purpose: it provides the title of the story contained in the booklet ("James Jacob Ritty: the Story of an Invention"), and it also acts as a vision test. The text "James Jacob Ritty" is 80 point type size; the phrase "The Story" is 48 point type size; the phrase "of an" is 24 point type size; the word "Invention" is 10 point type size. The client is instructed to turn to the first page and read it out loud. When the client reaches the bottom of the page, a stop sign is visible, which acts as a cue for the client to stop reading. The client is then asked to turn to page two and follow the person administering the test as they read it. The client reads page three; the person administering the test reads page four. Throughout, notes are taken on which words were misread and/or not read at all by the client. The participant is instructed to read and answer the reading comprehension question on the next page.

The next page is split into two parts. The top half of the page tests for depth perception: a blue square is printed to look like it is on top of a red square. The participant is asked to identify the square that looks farthest away and then to identify the square that looks nearest. The bottom half of the page tests for the ability to recognize color intensity: three reddish squares are included and the client must decide which one looks the darkest and which one looks the lightest.

Skills tested in this activity include:

1. the ability to read small phrases of text in varying sizes of font out loud (when the person reads the title page);
2. the ability to turn pages of a book (when the person is asked to turn to each page of the story);
3. the ability to read sentences of large print text out loud (when the person is asked to read each page of the story);
4. the ability to follow basic external cues (when the client is expected to stop reading as indicated by the stop sign at the bottom of the page);
5. the ability to comprehend written materials (when the client is asked to answer the reading comprehension question);

6. depth perception (when the client is administered the depth perception portion of the test);
7. color intensity (when the client is administered the color intensity portion of the test); and
8. the ability to follow directions (throughout this activity).

This set of abilities maps on to a wide range of possible Restorative Nursing programs. For example, the ability to read, take turns when reading, and listen to others as they read aloud indicates that the individual with dementia could benefit from taking part in a small reading group. As mentioned previously, short stories for persons with dementia are typically used for small groups. Within the Restorative Nursing regulations, small group activities can be included if there are no more than four persons in the group. In addition, restorative programs are presented to one person at a time for a maximum of 15 minutes per program. In this case, if four long-term care residents with dementia were in a reading group for one hour, then all four individuals would be receiving a restorative program for that day (e.g., language, socialization). Even persons with low vision or who are blind can take part in such programs by listening to the reading of the stories and then taking part in the discussions regarding the content.

Land/Water Sorting

A category sorting template is placed in front of the client, which is a large piece of paper (11" × 17") with black rectangles and squares printed on it. The template looks like this:

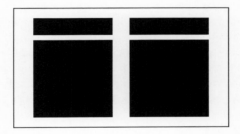

At the beginning of the activity, the client is asked to identify a rectangle and also to identify a square. A category label, which reads "Land" and is printed on a small sheet of paper the same size and shape as the black rectangles printed above, is presented to the client. The client is asked to read the word and place it on a rectangle that matches it. The same is done for the other category label, "Water."

If done correctly, the template looks like this:

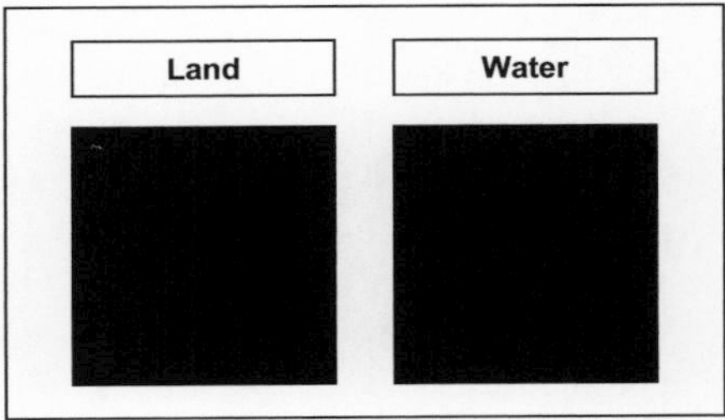

The client is then presented with a card which reads "Mountain." The card is a white piece of paper, which is the same size and shape as the black squares pictured above. The client is asked to read the card out loud, indicate whether it belongs to the category "Land" or "Water," and then place the card where it belongs, underneath the corresponding "Land" or "Water" label. The same procedure is followed for five other cards, each of which has a different word (i.e., lake, ocean, country, Pacific, and Austria) printed on it. For each card, it is separately noted whether the person could read the word, categorize it, and/or place it on the template.

Skills tested in this activity include:

1. the ability to identify shapes (when the person is asked to identify a rectangle and square);
2. the ability to read single words (when the person is asked to read the cards);
3. the ability to manipulate cards (when the person is asked to place the cards on the template);
4. the ability to categorize (when the person is asked to categorize words into one of two categories);
5. the ability to use different levels of abstraction in the representatives of categories (when the person is asked to match each card to the corresponding concept);
6. the ability to use a template (when the person is asked to place the cards on the template); and
7. the ability to follow directions (when the person is asked to read, place labels, match cards, etc. throughout the activity).

For Restorative Nursing Programs, knowing the level of abstraction available to the person with dementia provides clinicians and staff with a better understanding of the form of communication that is most effective in delivering such programs. In addition, the ability to use a template and manipulate objects has important implications. For example, if a resident loses their dentures because they have been mislaid and has forgotten where the dentures were placed, a template can be helpful. For example, the person with dementia can be trained to put their dentures on a template inside a container whenever the dentures are to be taken out. Templates also can be used to allow a resident to set their own place at a table for meals, to remind the resident where to put a fork down once it has been used to eat a bite of food, etc. Using templates enables individuals with dementia to engage in activities and perform at a higher level than without, and are related to key issues of Dining, ADLs, and other restorative programs.

In addition, there are many activities that can be created using categorization or matching abilities that build on an individual's current abilities. For example, the names of army bases can be matched with the cities in which they were located for a person with a military background. Names of children or grandchildren can be matched with photographs. Baseball teams can be categorized as belonging to the National League or the American League. Orchestral instruments can be categorized into woodwind or stringed instruments. The key issue is that once procedural memory processes are engaged and used for categorizing or matching, individualized activity content can be created. Further, more general content can be used in group activities, as well.

Fine Motor Skills and Color Matching

The client is presented with a rectangular tray, which is separated into three compartments, each of which is a primary color (i.e., red, yellow, or blue). The participant is asked to identify the red, yellow, and blue rectangles on the tray. The client is then asked to count how many colored rectangles they see. A plastic cereal bowl is then placed in front of the person, which contains three rubberized "spike" balls. Like the compartments on the tray, the balls are red, yellow, and blue. The participant is asked to use tweezers (or their hands, if they are unable to use the tweezers) to transfer the balls from the dish to the matching colored compartment on the tray. Once the person has finished this, they are asked to use an ice-cream scoop to transfer the balls from the tray back to the dish. Finally, the participant is instructed separately to hand back the tray, bowl, and ice-cream scoop.

Skills tested in this activity include:

1. the ability to identify the three primary colors (when the person is asked to identify the color of each rectangle on the tray);

2. the ability to count (when the person is asked to count the number of rectangles on the tray);
3. the ability to use pincer grip (when the person is asked to use the tweezers to transfer the balls from the bowl to the tray);
4. the ability to match colors (when the person is asked to transfer the balls to the matching color on the tray);
5. the ability to use gross motor skills (when the person is asked to use the ice-cream scoop to transfer the balls from the tray back to the bowl);
6. the ability to use range of motion (when the person is asked to transfer the balls using the tweezers and the ice-cream scoop);
7. the ability to recognize the names of objects typically used in the kitchen (when the participant is asked to hand back the bowl, tray, and ice-cream scoop); and
8. the ability to follow directions (throughout this activity).

Several key motor skills related to self-care and ADLs within Restorative Programs are assessed using this activity. The ability to color match relates to use of environmental cues. Recognition of object names and the ability to return such objects can allow receptive language skills to be assessed, which may be especially useful in the presence of expressive language difficulties.

Dressing Vest

The person is presented with a modified vest. This vest, which is made out of a synthetic, leather-like material, is made simply to rest on one's neck (there are no arm holes) and has just one button. Separate vests are available for men and women, since the placement of buttons differs for each gender. The person is asked to put the vest on (by putting it over their head), to button the vest, to unbutton it, to fold the vest, to place it into a bag (which has a zipper on it), and to zip the bag. This is done in a manner which allows assessment of the ability to do some of these steps in sequence, or if the task must be accomplished one step at a time.

Skills tested in this activity include:

1. range of motion (when the person is asked to put the vest on over their head);
2. pincer grip/the ability to button (when the person is asked to button and unbutton the vest);
3. the ability to fold clothes (when the person is asked to fold the vest);
4. the ability to transfer items to a bag (when the person is asked to put the vest into the bag);
5. the ability to use a zipper (when the person is asked to zip the bag); and
6. the ability to follow directions (throughout this activity).

Dressing and grooming restorative programs are addressed in this task. In addition, assessment of ability to sequence steps in a multi-step task is especially useful in designing restorative programs, which we will elaborate next.

How the MAS is Administered

A key feature of the MAS is the use of a multiple step-down procedure for administration, which ranges from multi-step instructions to physical demonstration and imitation, and which allows even individuals with severe dementia to participate. Additionally, and perhaps more importantly, is the use of this assessment information for developing and tailoring intervention programs for individuals with dementia that also are aligned with the goals of Restorative Nursing programs. The instructions for each activity are initially presented verbally to residents. Since persons with dementia have difficulty following multi-step directions, verbal instructions are provided for *no more than* two to three steps at a time. For example, as mentioned above, the vest activity consists of the resident putting on a vest, buttoning it, taking it off, unbuttoning it, folding it, and putting it away. So, for the vest activity, we first say, "Please put on the vest and button it." If the resident is successful with this, we next say, "Please take off the vest and unbutton it and fold it," and so on.

In keeping with the Montessori approach, if a resident is unable to follow the full multi-step verbal direction, verbal instructions are given one step at a time. For example, if a client is having trouble at the beginning of the vest activity in following a two-step verbal direction, a single verbal direction would be given, "Please put on the vest." Then, only after this task was completed would the resident be asked to "Please button the vest."

For individuals who find one-step instructions difficult, physical cues are provided. For instance, if after giving a resident one-step instructions, they do not seem to understand that we are asking them to put on the vest, we would physically cue the resident by making the motion of putting a vest around our neck. This gives the resident a more concrete idea of what is being asked of them and often provides enough help to get the resident started.

If this approach is unsuccessful, a full physical demonstration of the task is given. In each MAS kit, an extra vest is included for demonstrating the task. When necessary, the vest is taken out and the test administrator says "Watch me" and then puts the vest around their neck. Last, the administrator says, "Now its your turn."

When full physical demonstration of the task does not work, hand-over-hand guidance is provided. This is a common strategy in which one's hand is placed over the client's hand to help the person initiate the manipulation of the object. The person providing the guidance does not complete the task for the client; rather, the hope is that the initial guidance will act as a prompt for the client to take action.

By conducting the MAS, we do not merely want to find out whether a resident is capable of completing a given activity "perfectly" on the first try, though this certainly would provide us with useful information. It is equally important to find out whether a resident is capable of completing parts of an activity and/or whether a resident is capable of completing parts of an activity only after various levels of demonstration are used. An important feature of the MAS is that although the activities used in the assessment themselves assess certain strengths, appropriately administering the test (following the Montessori principles noted above) is of utmost importance for obtaining as much information from the test as possible, especially for individuals with severe or advanced dementia.

An Example of Using the MAS

The following example illustrates how data gathered from the MAS can be used to develop an effective intervention program tailored to the needs of individuals with dementia. A resident at a skilled nursing facility, Molly, exhibits problematic behavior when lunch begins. She is in the moderate to advanced stages of dementia, and, besides her obvious cognitive decline due to Alzheimer's, she is beginning to lose some fine and gross motor skills. She gets to the table at lunch before most of the other residents and struggles to use her utensils, which leads to agitation, aggressive verbal exchanges with other residents, reduced calorie intake, weight loss, and potential dehydration. Upon further examination, it is found that she has difficulty getting dressed in the morning, maintaining her personal appearance, and that she often stays in her room, refusing to take part in activities. Her verbalizations are very brief, and she becomes easily confused when staff give her verbal instructions. If this pattern continues, the MDS QI flags will begin to be seen (e.g., weight loss, dehydration, does not take part in activities, etc.).

After conducting the MAS with the resident, it is found that, among other things, she is capable of using a template for the Land/Water Sort (though she sometimes incorrectly categorizes the words). She was almost able to use the small tweezers (she could squeeze the tweezers, but her vision was not good enough to find the spikes on the ball), but was able without much trouble to use the ice-cream scoop during the Fine Motor Activity. She could name colors and match objects of the same color.

She was able to read and comprehend the Short Story, and take turns reading a page aloud, listening to the assessor read a page aloud, and then read a page aloud herself again. She could put on the vest, but had trouble with the buttons. She could follow one-step commands, and could imitate full physical demonstrations of tasks.

The MAS assessment has provided a wealth of information for developing a restorative nursing program to improve her ability to use utensils and to reduce her difficulties at meals. More than likely, this information would not have been gathered from other assessment approaches, as these approaches do not adequately evaluate the remaining cognitive, physical, social, and functional abilities in individuals with moderate to severe dementia. Assistive eating utensils with large handles could be provided, along with practice using these utensils to transfer objects. A nursing assistant could do this activity with Molly, while developing methods for customizing an activity that involves fine motor skills matched to Molly's interests. Therefore, engaging in therapeutic activities could serve a key purpose in motivating individuals while they practice important skills (i.e., pincer grip, eye/hand coordination, strengthening hand-grip) needed to successfully perform ADLs, such as eating. For instance, a template, used as a place mat, could be provided that outlined the location of the utensils, plate, and water glass. If she was interested in cooking, staff could ask Molly to help cut out recipes and paste them into a book for her grandchildren to use when they get older. Adaptive clothing could be acquired to make it easier for the resident to dress herself more independently. Additionally, Molly could participate in a small (four or less) reading group, in which participants take turns reading each page aloud, and then answering discussion and reminiscence questions.

The MAS also provides insight into how to deal with her difficult behavior that she experiences before lunch. For example, she could work with staff in practicing a specific task that fills a given social role and fits within her capabilities. When she gets to the lunchroom, it will be her job to turn on a CD player which has a specific "call to lunch" song. The play button will be a different color than the other buttons, with a bit of sandpaper on it as well (giving both a visual and a tactile cue as to which button to press). Once the song was started, Molly would go to a location at the entrance to the dining area (marked with an "X" or a colored area of a rug), where she would be the "hostess" in charge of greeting other residents as they came to lunch.

The MAS and Sensory Deficits

With regard to visual deficits, we have developed the MAS with input from specialists working with persons with low vision. However, if a person with dementia cannot see the materials well or is blind, the MAS still can provide useful information. For example, can the person with dementia follow verbal instructions? If so, can the person sequence steps? Can the person use tools? Does the person retain range of motion? How are their fine and/or gross motor skills? Can the person listen to a story read to them and comprehend the information? Can they answer questions about the story? Can the person put on a vest? Use buttons? Can the person categorize if the category labels and category items are read aloud? At what level of abstraction can they categorize concepts? Can the person follow and/or imitate hand-over-hand guided direction? Assessment of these abilities provides a wealth of information for designing restorative programs for individuals with dementia and visual deficits.

A similar process can be used for residents who are hard of hearing or cannot hear. For instance, is the person capable of following written instructions? Can the person imitate? Can the person categorize and/or use templates? Put on a vest? Sequence? It should come as no surprise that there are Montessori schools that exclusively serve children with severe hearing impairments. Using a Montessori approach to assessment and activity creation enables the strengths of the individual to become apparent, leading to the creation of activities and programming that is likely to be successful.

Multicultural Issues and the MAS

With regard to Hand Washing, Fine Motor Skills and Color Matching, and the Dressing Vest tasks on the MAS, these can be presented with little or no verbalization on the part of the examiner. It may be preferable to do so in cases of advanced dementia with extreme agitation and limited receptive language skills, as a slow and deliberate physical demonstration of the task with a non-verbal invitation to imitate what was done may reduce stress in these individuals. As such, these tasks also can be presented in a similar way to persons who do not speak English. With regard to the Land/Water Sorting task, this involves the translation of the verbal material into another language, although this is not a difficult task. The task still could be presented without verbal instructions if the person with dementia is not visually impaired. With regard to the Short Story, Depth Perception, and Color Intensity, verbal instructions would have to be given in the resident's language. In addition, a story with similar properties (length, type size and font, reading level) would have to be created in the resident's language and that was culturally relevant. For example, printed "English" materials from the United States are viewed as misspelled when read by residents with dementia in Australian facilities. Therefore, using UK English would be advisable in this case.

Training Long-Term Care Staff to Administer the MAS

As part of the work in developing the MAS, we have trained nursing staff at long-term care facilities to implement the MAS. In addition, we currently are training activity professionals within long-term care settings to administer and use the MAS. We are working with such staff to demonstrate how information from the MAS can be translated into plans of care that address Restorative Nursing and QIs within the MDS. We view this work as critical to the long-term success and widespread implementation of the measure. If these staff cannot map the use of the MAS on to the motivators of administrators, such as the elements of the Healthcare Triangle, then the MAS will not be an instrument for improving the quality of life of persons with advanced dementia.

SUMMARY AND CONCLUSIONS

Cognitive assessment for persons with late stage dementia, for the most part, will continue to be conducted in long-term care settings by non-psychologists. At present, long-term care staff such as nurses, social workers, etc., do this as part of their mandatory MDS surveys, occasionally supplemented by a measure such as the MMSE. For the foreseeable future, this will not change. Psychologists will not be provided sufficient incentives to conduct such assessments. At this point, there is sufficient evidence that cognitive assessment instruments provide valid information about persons with advanced dementia and are sensitive enough to detect change over time. Assessing individuals over time can provide important information about the nature of cognitive change in severe dementia, the effectiveness of a treatment intervention, and the evaluation and targeting of an individual's treatment needs and relative strengths. The central questions in this area are whether such assessments will be given, by whom, how often, and for what specific purpose. In addition, multicultural diversity issues need to be considered when conducting such assessments to ensure that they are being completed in a multiculturally competent manner.

The work we described regarding the MAS represents an attempt to address these issues and answer these latter questions. The MAS documents the remaining abilities of persons with severe dementia and is flexible enough to extend to lower levels of functional ability, regardless of the type of loss (cognitive, motor, sensory, or social). In addition, the assessment allows for differentiation between losses that may impact functional ability. By emphasizing ability rather than disability this assessment avoids many combative responses from participants that effect assessment. Also, it can be completed in a short period of time or split up into several sessions to ensure accurate assessment of abilities. It has the potential to elicit useful information for designing restorative programs in the presence of sensory deficits, lack of expressive language, and potentially across different languages and cultures. It can be administered by staff members of long-term care facilities, which not only makes it more likely to be used, but also addresses issues such as anxiety produced when a strange person attempts to give an assessment to a person with advanced dementia.

We envision the development of an assessment system that will be conducted by long-term care as an integral component of the development of activities for nursing home residents in their care. Use of the MAS can generate activities which can, in turn, map on to the reimbursement/income and surviving inspections areas of the Healthcare Triangle through implementation within Restorative Nursing programs. Furthermore, Montessori-based activities can address a wide range of issues related to CMS regulations and inspections (Camp, Breedlove, Malone, Skrajner, & McGowan, 2007). In addition, companies and facilities that have implemented Montessori-based programming have received awards for excellence on national (Camp, 2006a) and state levels. Winning such prestigious awards in activities programming/dementia care is an important marketing and selling point for marketing directors and facility administrators. This presents the opportunity to have events, press releases, etc., extolling the quality of care provided at facilities or companies receiving such awards. Marketing directors then become advocates for continuing and expanding such programs. (Think of a poster with Molly smiling and performing her hostess duties!) If the use of Montessori-based programming leads to successful marketing campaigns to maintain or increase census, then the final motivator of the Healthcare Triangle has been connected to such programming. Thus, the use of the MAS could be an entry into long-term care facilities for Montessori-based programming. Or, if such programming is in place, then it is a natural extension of such programming to start to include within Restorative Nursing. Either pathway leads to an increased quality of life for residents.

In conclusion, while it is important to continue the process we have begun in developing the MAS, and to further examine and refine the psychometric properties and validities (construct, concurrent, etc.), we would propose that the development of a good assessment instrument for late stage dementia is a necessary but not a sufficient condition. The instrument must also be designed so that it will be used on a large scale as part of an overall effort to create interventions. Given the current nature of care for late stage dementia in this country at this time, we believe that our approach is more likely to be used on a large scale than other instruments developed thus far. While our efforts, as reported here, are very much a work in progress, it is our purpose to provide readers with a new context for considering cognitive assessment for late stage dementia, and to inspire others to work along similar lines of thought.

ACKNOWLEDGMENTS

We wish to thank the following persons for their contributions to the grant project on which the MAS is based: Jeanne Mattern, Gregg Gorzelle, Sandra Stennis, Jessica Haberman, Marcia Neundorfer, Vince Antenucci, Adena McGowan, Cristina Frentiu, Christine Luci, Melanie Tusick, Susan Todd, Halle Rose, Sherri Fenda, Maura Rogers, and Carole Kalman. Inquiries regarding the contents of this chapter should be addressed to: Cameron J. Camp, PhD, Director of Research and Product Development, Hearthstone Alzheimer Care, 23 Warren Ave, Suite 140, Woburn, MA 01801; (440) 829-4927; camp@thehearth.org Preparation of this manuscript was supported, in part, by grant R01 AG021508-01A1 from the National Institute of Aging to the first author.

REFERENCES

Ahn, I. S., Kim, J. H., Ku, H. M., Saxton, J., & Kim, D. K. (2006). Reliability and validity of the Severe Impairment Battery (SIB) in Korean dementia patients. *Journal of Korean Medical Science*, *21*, 506–517.

Ahn, I. S., Kim, J. H., Saxton, J., & Kim, D. K. (2007). Reliability and validity of a short form of the Severe Impairment Battery in Korean Alzheimer's disease patients. *International Journal of Geriatric Psychiatry*, *22*, 682–687.

Albert, M., & Cohen, C. (1992). The test for severe impairment: An instrument for the assessment of patients with severe cognitive dysfunction. *Journal of the American Geriatric Society*, *40*, 449–453.

Appollonio, I., Gori, C., Riva, G. P., Spiga, D., Ferrari, A., Ferrarese, C., & Frattoloa, L. (2001). Cognitive assessment of severe dementia: The Test for Severe Impairment. *Archives of Gerontol. Geriatr.*, *S7*, 5–31.

Auer, S. R., Sclan, S. G., Yaffee, R. A., & Reisberg, B. (1994). The neglected half of Alzheimer's disease: Cognitive and functional concomitants of server dementia. *Journal of the American Geriatrics Society*, *42*, 1266–1272.

Bäckman, L. (1992). Memory training and memory improvement in Alzheimer's disease: Rules and exceptions. *Acta Neurologica Scandinavica*, *84*, 84–89.

Barbarotto, R., Cerri, M., Acerbi, C., Molinari, S., & Capitani, E. (2000). Is the SIB or the BNP better than MMSE in discriminating the cognitive performance of severely impaired elderly patients? *Archives of Clinical Neuropsychology*, *15*, 21–29.

Bayles, K. A., Tomoeda, C. K., Cruz, R. F., & Mahendra, N. (2000). Communication abilities of individuals with late-stage Alzheimer disease. *Alzheimer Disease and Associated Disorders*, *14*(3), 176–181.

Bellelli, G., Frisoni, G. B., Bianchetti, A., & Trabucchi, M. (1997). The Bedford Alzheimer Nursing Severity Scale for the severely demented: Validation study. *Alzheimer Disease and Related Disorders*, *11*(2), 71–77.

Bickel, H. (1996). The Hierarchic Dementia Scale: Usage. *International Psychogeriatrics*, *8*, 213–224.

Biringer, F., & Anderson, J. R. (1992). Self-recognition in Alzheimer's disease: a mirror and video study. *Journal of Gerontology*, *49*, 383–388.

Boller, F., Verny, M., Hugonot-Diener, L., & Saxton, J. (2002). Clinical features and assessment of severe dementia: A review. *European Journal of Neuorology*, *9*, 125–136.

Camp, C. J. (2006a). Montessori-Based Dementia Programming™ in long-term care: a case study of disseminating an intervention for persons with dementia. In R. C. Intrieri, & L. Hyer (Eds.), *Clinical Applied Gerontological Interventions in Long-term Care* (pp. 295–314). New York, NY: Springer.

Camp, C. J. (2006b). Spaced retrieval: a case study in dissemination of a cognitive intervention for persons with dementia. In D. Koltai Attix, & K. A. Welsch-Bohmner (Eds.), *Geriatric Neuropsychological Assessment and Intervention* (pp. 275–292). New York, NY: The Guilford Press.

Camp, C. J. (2001). From efficacy to effectiveness to diffusion: making the transitions in dementia intervention research. *Neuropsychological Rehabilitation*, *11*, 495–517.

Camp, C. J. (Ed.). (1999). *Montessori-based Activities for Persons with Dementia: Volume 1*. Beachwood, OH: Menorah Park Center for Senior Living.

Camp, C. J., Breedlove, J., Malone, M. L., Skrajner, M. J., & McGowan, A. (2007). Adjusting activities to meet CMS guidelines using Montessori-Based Dementia Programming®. *Activity Director's Quarterly*, *8*(1), 34–46.

Camp, C. J., & Brush, J. A. (January 2003). *Managing residents with dementia utilizing the success of the Healthcare Triangle Model*. Austin, TX: Symposium presented for Northern Speech Services.

Camp, C. J., Foss, J. W., Stevens, A. B., Reichard, C. C., McKitrick, L. A., & O'Hanlon, A. M. (1993). Memory training in normal and demented populations: The E-I-E-I-O model. *Experimental Aging Research*, *19*, 277–290.

Camp, C. J., Judge, K. S., Bye, C. A., Fox, K. M., Bowden, J., Bell, M., Valencic, K., & Mattern, J. M. (1997). An intergenerational program for persons with dementia using Montessori methods. *The Gerontologist*, *37*, 688–692.

Camp, C. J., Koss, E., & Judge, K. S. (1999). Cognitive assessment in late stage dementia. In P. A. Lichtenberg (Ed.), *Handbook of Assessment in Clinical Gerontology* (1st ed.) (pp. 442–467). New York, NY: John Wiley & Sons.

Camp, C. J., & Mattern, J. M. (1999). Innovations in managing Alzheimer's disease. In D. E. Biegel, & A. Blum (Eds.), *Innovations in Practice and Service Delivery Across the Lifespan* (pp. 276–294). New York, NY: Oxford University Press.

Camp, C. J., Schneider, N., Orsulic-Jeras, S., Mattern, J., McGowan, A., Antenucci, V. M., et al. (2006). *Montessori-based Activities for Persons with Dementia: Vol. 2*. Beachwood, OH: Menorah Park Center for Senior Living.

Chattin-McNichols, J. (1992). *The Montessori Controversy*. Albany, NY: Delmar.

Cole, M. G., & Dastoor, D. P. (1987). A new hierarchic approach to the measurement of dementia. *Psychosomatics*, *28*, 298–304.

Dreher, B. B. (1997). Montessori and Alzheimer's: A partnership that works. *American Journal of Alzheimer's Disease*, *12*, 138–140.

Feil, N., & de Klerk-Rubin, V. (2002). *The Validation Breakthrough: Simple Techniques for Communicating with People with "Alzheimer's-type Dementia."* Baltimore, MD: Health Professions Press.

Folstein, M. F., Folstein, S. E., & McHugh, P. R. (1975). Mini-Mental State: A practical method for grading the cognitive state of patients for the clinician. *Psychiatry Research*, *12*, 189–198.

Galasko, D., Schmitt, F., Thomas, R., Jin, S., Bennet, D., & Ferris, S. (2005). Detailed assessment of activities of daily living in moderate to severe Alzheimer's disease. For the Alzheimer's Disease Cooperative Study. *Journal of the International Neuropsychological Society*, *11*, 446–453.

Ginsburg, H., & Opper, S. (1988). *Piaget's Theory of Intellectual Development* (2nd ed.). Englewood Cliffs, NJ: Prentice-Hall.

Harrell, L. E., Marson, D., Chatterjee, A., & Parrish, J. A. (2000). The Severe Mini-Mental State Examination: a new neuropsychologic instrument for the bedside assessment of severely impaired patients with Alzheimer's disease. *Alzheimer Disease and Associated Disorders: An International Journal*, *14*(3), 168–175.

Hughes, C. P., Berg, L., Danzinger, W. L., Coben, L. A., & Martin, R. L. (1982). A new clinical scale for the staging of dementia. *British Journal of Psychiatry*, *140*, 566–572.

Jacobs, D. M., Albert, S. M., Sano, M., Del Castillo-Castanada, C., Paik, M. C., Marder, K., et al. (1999). Assessment of severe impairment in advanced AD: The Test for Severe Impairment. *Neurology*, *52*, 1689–1691.

Joltin, A., Camp, C. J., Noble, B. H., & Antenucci, V. M. (2005). *A Different Visit: Activities for Caregivers and their Loved Ones with Memory Impairment*. Beachwood, OH: Menorah Park Center for Senior Living.

Judge, K. S., Menne, H. L., & Whitlatch, C. J. (2009). The Stress Process Model for individuals with dementia. *The Gerontologist*; doi:10.1093/geront/gnp162.

Kitwood, T. (1997). *Dementia Reconsidered*. Buckingham, UK: Open University Press.

Lichtenberg, P. A. (1994). *A Guide to Psychological Practice in Geriatric Long-term Care*. New York, NY: The Haworth Press.

Lichtenberg, P. A. (1998). *Mental Health Practice in Geriatric Health Care Settings*. New York, NY: The Haworth Press.

Lin, L., Yang, M., Kao, C., Wu, S., Tang, S., & Lin, J. (2009). Using acupressure and Montessori-based activity to decrease agitation for residents with dementia: A cross-over trial. *Journal of the American Geriatrics Society*, *57*, 1022–1029.

Lipinska, B., Bäckman, L., & Herlitz, A. (1992). When Greta Garbo is easier to remember than Stefan Edberg: Influences of prior knowledge on recent memory in Alzheimer's disease. *Psychology and Aging*, *2*, 214–220.

Mattis, S. (1976). Dementia rating scale. In R. Bellack, & B. Karasu (Eds.), *Geriatric Psychiatry* (pp. 77–121). New York, NY: Grune and Stratton.

Morris, J. C. (1997). Alzheimer's disease: A review of clinical assessment and management issues. *Geriatrics*, *52* (Suppl. 2), S22–S25.

Morris, J. C., Brant, E. F., Mehr, D. R., Hawes, C., Phillips, C., Mor, V., & Lipsitz, L. A. (1994). MDS Cognitive Performance Scale. *Journal of Gerontology: Medical Sciences*, *49*, M174–M182.

Mohs, R. C., & Cohen, L. (1988). Alzheimer's Disease Assessment Scale (ADAS). *Psychopharmacologic Bulletin*, *24*, S627–S628.

Nolen, N. R. (1988). Functional skill regression in late-stage dementias. *The American Journal of Occupational Therapy, 42*, 666–669.

Peavy, G. M., Salmon, D. P., Rice, V. A., Galasko, D., Samuel, W., Taylor, K. I., et al. (1996). Neuropsychological assessment of severely demented elderly. *Archives of Neurology, 53*(4), 367–372.

Perlick, D., & Mattis, S. (1994). Neuropsychological assessment in chronic care settings: Potential utility and special considerations for evaluating dementia in the elderly. *Alzheimer Disease and Associated Disorders, 8* (Suppl. 1), S209–S213.

Perneczyky, R., Wagenpfeil, S., Komossa, K., Grimmer, T., Diehl, J., & Kurz, A. (2006). Mapping scores onto stages: Mini-Mental State Examination and Clinical Dementia Rating. *American Journal of Geriatric Psychiatry, 14*, 139–144.

Ray, M. (2008). Restorative nursing and the MDS. Accessed at: www.cdphe.state.co.us/hf/mdsoasis/RestorativeNursingAndMDS.pdf

Reisberg, B. (1985). Assessment tool for Alzheimer's type dementia. *Hospital and Community Psychiatry, 6*, 593–595.

Reisberg, B. (1986). Dementia: A systematic approach to identifying reversible cues. *Geriatrics, 4*, 30–46.

Reisberg, B. (1988). Functional assessment staging (FAST). *Psychopharmacological Bulletin, 24*, 53–659.

Reisberg, B., Ferris, S. H., de Leon, M. J., et al. (1982). The Global Deterioration scale for assessment of primary degenerative dementia. *American Journal of Psychiatry, 139*, 1136–1139.

Reisberg, B., Sclan, S. G., Franssen, E., Kluger, A., & Ferris, S. (1994). Dementia staging in chronic care populations. *Alzheimer Disease and Associated Disorders, 8*(Suppl. 1), S188–S205.

Reisberg, B., Franssen, E. H., Bobinski, M., Auer, S., Monteiro, I., Boksay, I., et al. (1996). Overview of methodologic issues for pharmacologic trials in mild, moderate, and severe Alzheimer's disease. *International Psychogeriatrics, 8*(2), 159–194.

Salmon, D. P., Thal, L. J., Butters, N., & Heindel, W. C. (1990). Longitudinal evaluations of dementia of the Alzheimer type. *Neurology, 40*, 1225–1230.

Saxton, J., & Boller, F. (2006). Cognitive functions in severe dementia. In A. Burns, & B. Winblad (Eds.), *Severe Dementia* (pp. 43–49). New York, NY: John Wiley & Sons.

Saxton, J., Kastengo, K. B., Hugonot-Diener, L., Boller, F., Verny, M., Sarles, C. E., et al. (2005). Development of a short form of the Severe Impairment Battery. *American Journal of Geriatric Psychiatry, 13*(11), 999–1005.

Saxton, J., McGonigle-Gibson, K., & Boller, F. (1990). Assessment of severely impaired patients: Description of a new neuropsychological test battery. *Psychological Assessment, 2*, 298–303.

Sclan, S. G., Foster, J. R., Reisberg, B., Franssen, E., & Welkowitz, J. (1990). Application of Piagetian measures of cognition in severe Alzheimer's disease. *Psychiatric Journal of the University of Ottawa, 15*(4), 221–226.

Squire, L. R. (1992). Memory and the hippocampus: A synthesis from findings with rats, monkeys, and humans. *Psychological Review, 99*, 195–231.

Squire, L. R. (1994). Declarative and nondeclarative memory: Multiple brain systems supporting learning and memory. In D. L. Schacter, & E. Tulving (Eds.), *Memory systems* (pp. 203–232). Cambridge, MA: MIT Press.

Teresi, J., Lawton, M. P., Ory, M., & Holmes. (1994). Measurement issues in chronic care populations: Dementia special care. *Alzheimer Disease and Associated Disorders, 8*(Suppl. 1), 144–183.

Thornbury, J. M. (1992). Cognitive performance on Piagetian tasks by Alzheimer's disease patients. *Research on Nursing and Health, 15*, 11–18.

Vance, D., Camp, C. J., Kabacoff, M., & Greenwalt, L. (1996). Montessori methods: Innovative interventions for adults with Alzheimer's disease. *Montessori Life, 8*, 10–12.

Volicer, L., Hurley, A. C., Lathi, D. C., & Kowall, N. W. (1994). Measurement of severity in advanced Alzheimer disease. *Journal of Gerontology: Medical Sciences, 49*, M223–M226.

Weaverdyck, S. E. (1990). Intervention-based neuropsychological assessment. In N. L. Mace (Ed.), *Dementia Care: Patient, Family, and Community* (pp. 32–73). Baltimore, MD: The Johns Hopkins University Press.

Weaverdyck, S. E. (1991a). Assessment as a basis for intervention. In D. H. Coons (Ed.), *Specialized Dementia Care Units* (pp. 205–223). Baltimore, MD: The Johns Hopkins University Press.

Weaverdyck, S. E. (1991b). Intervention to address dementia as a cognitive disorder. In D. H. Coons (Ed.), *Specialized Dementia Care Units* (pp. 224–244). Baltimore, MD: The Johns Hopkins University Press.

Weiner, M. F., Koss, E., Wild, K., Folks, D., Tariot, P., Luszczynska, H., & Whitehouse, P. (1996). Measures of psychiatric symptoms in Alzheimer's patients: A review. *Alzheimer Disease and Associated Disorders*, *10*(1), 20–30.

Yesavage, J. A., & Brooks, J. O. (1991). On the importance of longitudinal research in Alzheimer's disease. *Journal of the American Geriatric Society*, *39*, 942–944.

CHAPTER 21

Assessing the Personal Preferences of Persons with Dementia

Carol J. Whitlatch, PhD

Margaret Blenkner Research Institute, Benjamin Rose Institute, Cleveland, OH, USA

INTRODUCTION

For individuals with dementia and their family members the onset of symptoms of memory loss brings with it a host of changing emotions including fear, anxiety, depression, denial, and apprehension about the future (Aneshensel, Pearlin, Mullan, Zarit, & Whitlatch, 1995; Clare, Kinsella, Logsdon, Whitlatch, & Zarit, in press). These individuals and their families often attempt to hide the symptoms of memory loss or create elaborate strategies to compensate for failing memory. Over time, as cognitive functioning deteriorates, the ability of the individual to perform self-care activities and make decisions also declines. Often, there comes a time when families and professionals decide that their loved one or client (if no family are available) should not be making decisions alone. But when is it time to take away the decision-making role for individuals with dementia (IWDs)? When are individuals no longer able to voice accurately their preferences for the care they need now or will need in the future? What can be done to ensure that decisions made by or on behalf of IWDs accurately reflect their preferences?

This chapter provides guidance for understanding, assessing, respecting, and (when appropriate) carrying out the preferences of individuals with dementia. The chapter begins with a brief description of the demographic changes surrounding the incidence of dementia and the impact on the professionals and family members who provide care. Next, a discussion of the issues related to early diagnosis and the implications for individuals, families, and health care professionals facing the challenges of living with and/or assisting individuals with dementia. The chapter highlights: (1) the challenges of understanding the personal preferences and decision-making abilities of individuals with dementia; (2) the ability of IWDs to answer questions reliably and accurately; and (3) the various decisions that are made by IWDs, families, and the professionals who work with them. A variety of instruments will be described that assess the personal preferences of IWDs. As well, the importance of familial, cultural, and socioeconomic factors in addition to the level of cognitive ability will be discussed when assessing and reassessing care values and preferences. The chapter provides a description of a psychosocial intervention designed to assess and resolve discrepancies about care preferences, and ends with a look to the future of research and practice strategies for assessing personal preferences.

Handbook of Assessment in Clinical Gerontology. DOI: 10.1016/B978-0-12-374961-1.10021-1

INCIDENCE OF DEMENTIA AND OTHER COGNITIVE IMPAIRING CONDITIONS

The number of adults in the United States with chronic conditions that impair cognitive functioning (e.g., Alzheimer's disease, non-specific dementia, Parkinson's disease) is roughly estimated to be between 13 and 16 million (Family Caregiver Alliance, 2001). The annual number of incident cases of Alzheimer's disease specifically is expected to grow from between 3.5 and 5 million in 2009 to nearly 8 million in 2030 when the baby boomers will be over the age of 65 (Herbert, Beckett, Scherr, & Evans, 2001). Similar growth is expected throughout the world. Alzheimer's Disease International (ADI, 2008) estimates that in 2008 there were 30 million individuals with dementia worldwide, a number which is expected to grow to over 100 million in 2050. ADI also reports that the proportion of individuals with dementia in developing countries is difficult to estimate, because few persons live to age 65. Currently, however, it appears that the majority of individuals who have dementia live in developing countries. In 2001, ADI (2008) estimated that 60% of individuals with dementia lived in developing countries. This number is expected to increase to 71% by 2040 (ADI, 2008). The increase in the number of IWDs with dementia will likely be associated with a comparable increase in the number of families who will find themselves providing care and making decisions with or on behalf of their relatives. These numbers will likely increase further as a result of improvements in medical technologies that help diagnose cognitive conditions earlier in the disease progression and help individuals live longer even as their symptoms become more life threatening.

With IWDs being diagnosed earlier and more accurately, we can expect more and more families to enter the health and social service system earlier in the disease process. In California, for example, where families receive services through a statewide system of Caregiver Resource Centers (CRCs), the average onset of cognitive impairment decreased in 1996 to 4.8 years prior to initial intake, compared to the 1990 average of 6.0 years (Family Caregiver Alliance, 1996). Similarly, 26% of the families seeking help in 1996 from CRCs contacted the CRC within the first year following onset of their relative's illness, compared to 14% before 1990 (Family Caregiver Alliance, 1996). Unpublished data from the Alzheimer's Disease Research Center at the University Hospitals of Cleveland suggest that IWDs and their family caregivers are coming to the center one year earlier in the disease progression (4.5 years after onset in 1992 vs. 3.6 years in 1999; Smyth, 1999). These trends have created an opportunity for earlier and more consistent involvement of both the family caregiver and impaired adult in everyday care decisions. Taken together, it appears that there will be an increasing number of individuals and families living with dementia, aware of their condition in the early stages of the disease, living with the condition for a longer period of time, and facing challenges that previous cohorts of IWDs did not face. (For additional information on the incidence and prevalence of dementia, see Chapter 6: Dementia syndromes in the older adult.)

These changes have implications for IWDs, for the family caregivers who provide assistance, and for the health care systems that support the entire family. The onset of symptoms of dementia and the subsequent confirmation of diagnosis can have a profound effect on individuals as they try to adjust to their changing abilities and come to terms with their future cognitive losses. Relationships with loved ones often change, symptoms of depression and anxiety can surface, and social and professional interactions outside the family can become awkward. Likewise, family caregivers (CGs), whose responsibilities are often unpredictable and long-term, report that their care responsibilities affect relationships with family and friends, as well as their leisure time, social activities, financial security, and mental and physical health (Aneshensel et al., 1995; Vitaliano et al., 2002; Yee & Schulz, 2000). The increasing number of families affected by dementia will likely strain health care systems because these families will expect services and assistance starting at younger ages, and for longer periods of time. Health care systems and the public policies that fund aging services will need to develop and sustain training initiatives and programs for providers who support these families so that they will be prepared for the potentially stressful changes that lie ahead.

EARLY DIAGNOSIS OF DEMENTIA: CHALLENGES AND OPPORTUNITIES

Improvements in medical procedures and technologies have led to an increase in the number of individuals diagnosed, the accuracy of the diagnosis, and the timing of the diagnosis of dementia. These improvements have created opportunities and challenges for individuals and their families. One advantage of early and accurate diagnosis is that pharmacological interventions for dementia-related symptoms can be prescribed which can have the greatest benefit in the early stages of the disease (Chang & Silverman, 2004). On the other hand, the confirmation of a dementia diagnosis can challenge the IWD and their family members as they begin to learn about the illness that is responsible for current and future changes in memory, behavior, and mood. Individuals diagnosed in the early stages of dementia confront a variety of unique challenges that individuals with less awareness (e.g., in the later stages) do not face. Qualitative research describes the challenges facing early-stage IWDs (e.g., memory loss, difficulty following conversations, disorientation, and fluctuating awareness) that affect the individual's mood and well-being (Phinney, 1998). IWDs at this stage of awareness understand that their activities (social, professional, leisure) are changing, that the quality of relationships will change as they become increasingly dependent on others, and that they are at risk of losing their roles as contributing members of their families and society.

For family members of individuals with dementia, the months or years leading up to diagnosis can be a time of increasing stress and uncertainty. During this time, IWDs experience a range of memory, personality, and behavioral changes that can put into motion a cascading process of stress that unfolds over time and leads to negative physical and mental health consequences for their CGs. Caring for an older adult, especially one suffering from dementia, is associated with increased risk of adverse outcomes, including symptoms of depression and anxiety, poor health, and heightened rates of mortality (Aneshensel et al., 1995; Kiecolt-Glaser & Glaser, 2002; Schulz & Beach, 1999; Schulz, O'Brien, Bookwala, & Fleissner, 1995). Between 40 and 70% of CGs have clinically significant symptoms of depression, a prevalence rate that is higher than for age-matched controls (Anthony-Bergstone, Zarit, & Gatz, 1988) and for people caring for a family member with another type of chronic illness (Birkel, 1987; Ory, Hoffman, Yee, Tennstedt, & Schulz, 1999). The CG's depressive symptoms may emerge when the IWD's memory and behavior problems are mild, and before a formal diagnosis of dementia is made (Garand, Dew, Eazor, DeKosky, & Reynolds, 2005). Caregivers can experience other negative consequences such as anxiety, anger, and diminished physical health (Aneshensel et al., 1995; Anthony-Bergstone et al., 1988; Friss & Whitlatch, 1991; Gallagher, Rose, Rivera, Lovett, & Thompson, 1989a; Gallagher, Wrabetz, Lovett, DelMaestro, & Rose, 1989b; Pruchno, Kleban, Michaels, & Dempsey, 1990; Pruchno & Resch, 1989; Schulz et al., 1995, 2002; Whitlatch, Feinberg, & Sebesta, 1996). These findings illustrate the enduring impact of stressors on well-being, and highlight the need to intervene before the occurrence of long-term and irreversible damage.

Although the medical community has placed an emphasis on early detection and treatment of dementia, service providers and policy makers have not correspondingly emphasized early psychosocial intervention to address the various stressors and consequences experienced by both the early-stage IWD and their CG. Most current services and programs address needs of families in the later stages of dementia, when the IWD's awareness is significantly limited. As a result, IWDs in the later stages are often excluded from the decision-making process that focuses on everyday care or medical treatment. Instead, these later-stage interventions appropriately focus on improving the CG's well-being. During the earlier stages, however, the CG may already feel overwhelmed and overloaded by care responsibilities. As a result, later stage programs: (1) miss an opportunity for prevention of care-related stress; and (2) ignore the perspective of the IWD, who in the early stages of dementia has both the intellectual competence and the desire to participate actively in decisions about their care (Feinberg & Whitlatch, 2001). Early-stage IWDs often recognize that their CGs cannot by themselves provide all of the care that may be needed in the future, but will need some assistance (Whitlatch et al., 2006). Early-stage psychosocial interventions have the potential to help IWDs communicate their preferences, foster a partnership between the IWD and CG, and develop a plan that incorporates the IWD's preferences. These interventions can help empower IWDs to be involved in decision-making and CGs to make future care decisions that reflect the preferences of IWDs, as well as balance their own needs.

UNDERSTANDING PREFERENCES AND DECISION MAKING FOR EARLY-STAGE FAMILIES

As noted, the impact of the onset of dementia and the subsequent changes and stress that result affect IWDS and their families in profound ways. One challenge families often face surrounds the need for making everyday and health care decisions with or on behalf of a family member with impaired judgment and planning capacity (Whitlatch, 2006; Whitlatch & Feinberg, 2007). In an attempt to make decisions that reflect their relative's preferences, many families often try to strike a balance among conflicting preferences for care. Providing care can be additionally stressful as families try to separate the needs, preferences, and best interests of the chronically ill person from those of family members (Feinberg, Whitlatch, & Tucke, 2000). For example, a daughter caring for her father may be overwhelmed by the demands of his care needs. She may experience added stress when she is forced to choose between his desire that only *she* provide assistance and her desperate need for help in caring for him. Balancing IWD preferences with CG needs can be stressful for both individuals. This is especially noteworthy given findings that within family care dyads, each care partner (i.e., the IWD and the CG) reports being more concerned about the other person's well-being than they are about their own (Whitlatch & Feinberg, 2003).

Decision-Making Involvement of Individuals with Dementia

Understanding the personal care preferences of adults of any age, regardless of cognitive ability, is not without its challenges and uncertainties. First, it is useful to determine or feel confident that the IWD has the ability to make a decision or to be involved in decision-making on their behalf. It is possible to assess an IWD's ability or capacity to make decisions performing or managing IADLs or functional problems (also referred to as "everyday decision-making capacity"; Lai, Gill, Cooney, Hawkins, & Karlawish, 2008; Lai & Karlawish, 2007). This information can be used to provide useful information about an IWD's day-to-day problem-solving ability. By measuring four decision-making abilities that are highly related to executive functioning (i.e., understanding, appreciation, reasoning, and expressing a choice; Lai et al., 2008), the IWD and their family can more clearly understand the IWD's strengths, weaknesses, and changing circumstances that make living independently safe or unsafe. An IWDs involvement in decision-making can also be assessed (Menne, Tucke, Whitlatch, & Feinberg, 2008). Clinicians can compare the IWD's responses to questions about decision-making to the family caregiver's perception of the IWD's involvement. This comparison can help generate discussion about how to enhance appropriate IWD decision-making involvement. Interventions that enhance or preserve "everyday decision-making capacity" hold promise for early-stage individuals, who can be empowered to voice their preferences, and their caregivers who typically have their relative's best interests in mind (Whitlatch & Feinberg, 2003).

After decision-making capacity and involvement has been established, the IWD's preferences can be determined, including preferences about every day care, general health care, community-based and facility-based long-term care, life sustaining treatments, and end-of-life care (Carpenter, Kissel, & Lee, 2007; Degenholtz et al., 1997; Patrick, Starks, Cain, Uhlmann, & Pearlman, 1994; Van Haitsma, 2000; Wolff, Kasper, & Shore, 2008). Unfortunately, few studies have examined the daily care decisions that individuals with chronic illness and their family caregivers make together (Young, 1994), especially when cognitive impairment is involved. An exception is the work of Robinson and colleagues who interviewed couples with one partner in early-stage dementia (Robinson, Clare, & Evans, 2005). These authors suggest that care dyads may adjust to their changing roles by creating a shared understanding of dementia. Similarly, Sebern (2005, 2008) notes that a "shared care" perspective, an interpersonal process that includes aspects of communication, decision-making, and reciprocity, may be useful for understanding the support and exchange that occurs within care dyads regardless of diagnosis.

Do Families Know Their Relative's Personal and Care Preferences?

Many family members and service providers question the need for assessing an IWD's care preferences. Why not just ask family members about their relative's preferences for care? A slowly growing body of research indicates that family CGs have a general understanding of the importance of certain care values and preferences to their relatives with chronic conditions including dementia (Carpenter, Van Haitsma, Ruckdeschel, & Lawton, 2000; Feinberg & Whitlatch, 2001; Van Haitsma, 2000; Whitlatch, 2006; Whitlatch, Feinberg, & Tucke, 2005a). However, CGs are not completely certain of the preferences of IWDs and typically underestimate the importance of preferences with few exceptions (e.g., importance of living in one's own home, importance of having personal privacy; Whitlatch, Piiparinen, & Feinberg, 2009). Adult children have been found to be fairly accurate in predicting their parents' overall preferences for care, but overestimate their parents' desires for predictability, routine, and control, while underestimating their desires for enrichment and personal growth (Carpenter, Lee, Ruckdeschel, Van Haitsma, & Feldman, 2006). Compared to their family CGs, IWDs place greater emphasis on autonomy, safety, quality of care, and not being a burden (Whitlatch et al., 2009). The one exception is that CGs seem to understand that their relatives with dementia feel social interactions are less important than other care preferences. Overall, there are but a handful of research studies that examine the views and care preferences of people with dementia. As a result, the views of IWDs are neither uniformly considered nor incorporated in care planning (Cohen, 1991).

The lack of a clear understanding of a family member's values for care has implications for the provision of care. This is especially critical as the symptoms of dementia progress, because this "perception gap" (Whitlatch et al., 2009) seems to intensify over time, but not because of increasing cognitive impairment. Instead, research suggests that CGs increasingly misperceive their relative's preferences for care while the IWD's preferences remain surprisingly stable (Piiparinen & True, 2008). It appears that family caregivers are not the most reliable proxies for information about an IWD's preferences (Carpenter et al., 2007; Whitlatch & Feinberg, 2003). It may be possible, however, to adjust the misperceptions of family CGs so that they have a more accurate understanding of their relative's care preferences. Interventions and clinical protocols that incorporate these findings (see Whitlatch, Judge, Zarit, & Femia, 2006) may prove helpful to practitioners trying to help care dyads balance each other's preferences for care and develop a mutually acceptable plan of care (McCullough, Wilson, Teasdale, Koppakchi, & Skelly, 1993).

Are IWDs Able to Provide Reliable and Valid Responses?

Before we move to a description of a few promising assessment tools, it is important to acknowledge that there are only a handful of measures designed specifically to assess preferences for cognitively intact older adults. There are even fewer measures that have been tested with samples of IWDs. One reason for this shortage of measurement tools is that many practitioners and family members question the reliability and validity of responses of IWDs. Yet, there is mounting evidence that IWDs are able to provide accurate and consistent responses to a variety of types of questions. This evidence counters the firmly held beliefs of many family members and professionals who doubt the accuracy and consistency of an IWD's responses to factual questions and their ability to express care preferences (Woods, 1999). Moreover, research indicates that individuals with mild to moderate cognitive impairment (i.e., scores between 18 and 26 on the Mini-Mental State Examination; Folstein, Folstein, & McHugh, 1975) are able to state consistent choices, communicate preferences for daily care, make informed care decisions (Clark, 2004; Clark, Piiparinen, True, & Whitlatch, 2007), and choose someone, typically a family caregiver, to make decisions for them when they can no longer do so themselves (Feinberg & Whitlatch, 2001; Logsdon, Gibbons, McCurry, & Teri, 1999; Squillace, Mahoney, Shoop, Simon-Rusinowitz, & Desmond, 2002).

More recent research informs us that the type of information queried varies in its reliability and validity. Specifically, answers to static fact-based questions such as date of birth tend to be the most reliable as compared to dynamic fact-based questions (e.g., age) which tend to be least reliable. Answers to questions about preferences, while fairly reliable, are not as reliable as answers to questions about specific facts in general (with the exception of age), which is true for cognitively intact as well as mild to moderately cognitively impaired individuals (Whitlatch & Piiparinen, 2008). In other words, if we ask two older adults (one who is cognitively intact and the other who is mildly cognitively impaired) to answer a series of static fact-based questions, their answers will be consistent over a one-week period. On the other hand, if we ask them questions about their preferences for favorite colors or food, both older adults will be fairly reliable in their responses, but not as reliable as their answers to static fact-based questions.

Over time, as the symptoms of dementia become more severe, IWDs begin to lose the ability to answer factual questions (e.g., age or birth date). However, IWDs with moderate cognitive loss are still able to respond accurately 74% of the time as compared to 89% of the time for IWDs with mild impairment (Whitlatch, Piiparinen, & Clark, 2007). Moreover, and compared to responses to factual

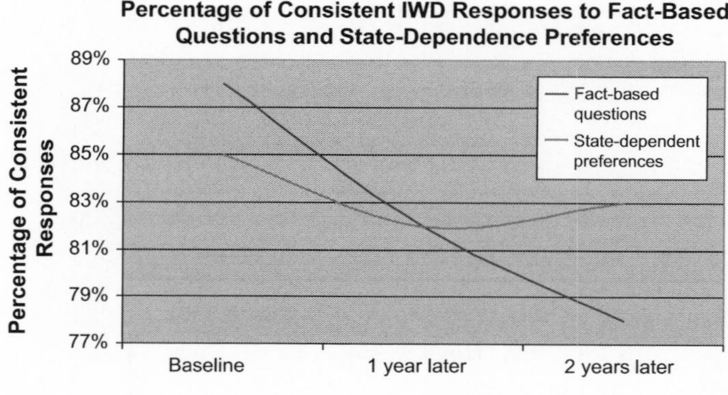

FIGURE 21.1

Percentage of Consistent IWD Responses to Fact-Based Questions and State-Dependence Preferences.

questions, an IWD's ability to answer questions about simple preferences remains relatively stable (see Figure 21.1; Clark et al., 2007). IWDs seem to be able to state consistently their care preferences even as their level of cognitive ability declines (Whitlatch et al., 2007). Stated another way, IWDs in the early stages of dementia are most reliable when they are responding to fact-based questions as compared to preference questions. Over time, their ability to answer fact-based questions declines, but their ability to answer preference questions remains relatively stable (Whitlatch et al., 2007). Thus, the presence of cognitive impairment does not translate into inability to articulate preferences or feelings, or answer questions reliably (Carpenter et al., 2007).

The Role of Practitioners in Helping Families Understand Personal and Care Preferences

Family members and friends are not the only people involved in discussions with IWDs about care and personal preferences. Nurses, case managers, social workers, physicians, and other professionals need to be aware of the potential and ability of IWDs to be involved in discussions about their care as long as possible. Unfortunately, even when clients are cognitively intact, case managers in community-based and long-term care settings are not uniformly willing to incorporate an assessment of care values and preferences into their care planning, even though clients are willing to discuss these issues (Degenholz, Kane, & Kivnick, 1997). Similar to communication and decision-making within families, communication with the patient—family caregiver—practitioner care triad is characterized by a lack of communication and a high rate of misunderstanding of diagnosis, prognosis, care decision-making, discharge planning, and home care follow-up (Beisecker, Chrisman, & Wright, 1997; Downs, Clibbens, Rae, Cook, & Woods, 2002; Fried, Bradley, & O'Leary, 2003; Hansen, Archbold, Stewart, Westfall, & Ganzini, 2005; Li, Stewart, Imle, Archbold, & Felver, 2000). Thus it appears that miscommunication and lack of communication about care preferences and decision-making may be fairly universal within caregiving families, and not uncommon in the interactions between providers and families (Whitlatch, 2008).

In addition to understanding IWDs' preferences for everyday care or decisions made in the early stages of dementia, it is also important to understand preferences for long-term, more intensive acute care, or end-of-life care that might be necessary in the later stages of dementia. The current literature on long-term care preferences indicates that older adults believe that in-home care (formal or informal) would be preferable when help is needed with instrumental and personal activities of daily living (IADs and PADLs; Wolff et al., 2008). On the other hand, many older adults believe that if an individual has dementia, it would be best if the individual had nursing home care (Wolff et al., 2008). Related research on health-state preferences and life-sustaining treatment decisions attempts to measure and/or balance quality of life and length of life. By measuring preferences for "health states worse than death," we are able to understand an individual's evaluation of their quality of life and potential preferences for life sustaining procedures (Patrick et al., 1994).

Practice Implications for IWDs, Families, and Providers

The growing literature indicating that IWDs are able to respond accurately to questions about preferences has significant practice implications. First, families and providers need to recognize that IWDs unable to state factual information accurately and reliably may be able to articulate preferences for their care. Stating preferences for care may be more critical to quality of life than the ability to remember certain facts such as age or current date. To ensure that family CGs can understand their relative's preferences it is important to discuss care values and preferences as early as possible in the course of the disease.

INSTRUMENTS THAT ASSESS PERSONAL PREFERENCES AND DESIRES

The development of measures to assess personal and care preferences has led to a small handful of tools that can be used in research and practice settings. These measures vary in the types of preferences assessed, the manner in which they have been developed and validated, and the settings in which they have been used.

Values and Preferences Scale (VPS)

The development of the Values and Preferences Scale (VPS) emphasized the exploration of aspects of everyday life that IWDs consider important and the need to understand better whether family caregivers were familiar with their relative's care-related values and preferences (Whitlatch et al., 2005a). Unlike the few studies that had previously assessed the values and preferences of older adults for everyday home- and community-based care, no prior studies had assessed the values and preferences for IWDs *and* their family caregivers. Consequently, items for the VPS were drawn from two previous exploratory studies with cognitively intact samples (Degenholtz et al., 1997; McCullough et al., 1993), with additional items generated in consultation with an advisory committee familiar with the care issues of this population. (For more information about the development and psychometric testing of the VPS see Whitlatch et al., 2005a and Whitlatch et al., 2009.) Thus, two forms of the VPS are available. One form assesses the importance of specific care values to the IWD (or other individuals with chronic conditions). A second form assesses the family caregiver's perceptions of the IWD's care values.

As seen in Appendix A, the most current version of the VPS (Whitlatch et al., 2009) contains 24 items that tap four domains of care values: Autonomy (7 items); Burden (5 items); Social Interactions (5 items); and Safety/Quality of Care (7 items). IWDs and family caregivers are interviewed separately in private, most typically by a trained interviewer, although we are currently testing a self-administered version for caregivers. IWDs are asked: "How important is it for you to...[have a say in who provides care], [keep your same doctors], [not be an emotional burden]" whereas family caregivers are asked: "How important is it for your relative to...[have a say in who provides care], [keep his/her same doctors], [not be an emotional burden]" and so on. The original 37-item version of the VPS used a Likert scale of seven values that was visually represented using a ladder. In addition, we required IWDs to rank the most important care value within the items that comprised each subdomain. In testing the VPS with our earliest sample of IWDs we quickly learned: (1) the ladder was disorienting and distracting; (2) having seven response choices was confusing; and (3) IWDs were unable to rank their preferences. As a result, we do not use a ladder for response categories, have moved to a three-level response option (very important, somewhat important, or not at all important), and do not ask IWDs to rank order their preferences. Overall, we have found that the 37 questions in the VPS are easily understood by IWDs and their family caregivers.

Psychometric testing of the VPS indicates that a number of items could be removed because of low variance or ambiguous factor loadings (see Appendix A and Whitlatch et al., 2009). These items, however, have important clinical relevance and can be asked of care partners as a way to prompt discussion of preferences that are critical to quality of care. For example, a large majority of IWDs report, and their CGs understand, that they would prefer not to move to a nursing home. What CGs do not understand is that many IWDs are open to discussing nursing home options and not completely against the possibility of moving to an assisted living or skilled nursing facility if care becomes too stressful for the CG. Including items about nursing home options or other sensitive issues can facilitate discussions that lead to increased understanding about and respect for the preferences of both care partners. Our research team has assessed 267 family care dyads (i.e., IWDs and their family CGs) using the VPS over the course of up to five years. Additionally, we have used the VPS with a sample of 324 older adults who are cognitively intact ($n = 220$) or cognitively impaired ($n = 104$) and have found responses to remain consistent over a one-week period regardless of presence of cognitive impairment (Whitlatch et al., 2008).

When we first introduced the VPS to care dyads, we found that many research participants told our interviewers that the questions made them wonder about their care partner's responses. Many IWDs and CGs indicated that they thought it would be helpful to discuss the questions with their care partner. As a result of these and other encouraging comments, we developed a protocol incorporating the VPS within a clinical intervention as a way to encourage discussion within care dyads about values for care. The Early Diagnosis Dyadic Intervention (EDDI), which is described more thoroughly in "Enhancing Decision-Making and Understanding of Personal Preferences in Dementia" on page 560, uses the VPS as a tool for helping care dyads discuss and realign values for care. The VPS can be used by social workers, nurses, and others who work with care dyads dealing with chronic illness, including cognitive impairment. Preliminary and anecdotal experience using the VPS suggests that it is useful for creating a dialog between care partners that can lead to a more congruent understanding of each person's care values.

Case Study 1—Using the Values and Preferences Scale—Mr and Mrs P

Mr P is a 72-year-old man recently diagnosed with early-stage dementia who is accompanied by Mrs P, his 69-year-old wife. Married nearly 50 years, the couple has a few chronic conditions (e.g., osteoarthritis, heart disease) in addition to Mr P's early-stage dementia. The couple has enrolled in a dyadic intervention trial (Early-stage Dementia Dyadic Intervention, described later in this chapter) which includes nine in-home sessions of dyadic counseling over the course of 13 weeks. They have been interviewed in person, but separately and have completed assessment tools to evaluate their care values and preferences, stress, depression, etc. In the first two sessions, the counselor provided education about dementia, gave guidance for improving communication, and established rapport with the couple. In this session (Session 3), the couple first meets together with the counselor who describes: (1) the primary goal of the session (i.e., help each care partner identify their perception of the IWD's care values); and (2) general session procedures (i.e., couple meets together and separately with the counselor to discuss their responses to the VPS). During the 20 minutes that Mr P meets with the counselor, Mrs P uses the time to catch up on housework and to bake cookies for their grandchildren.

The counselor begins by reviewing with Mr P his responses to the VPS. To facilitate this discussion, the counselor uses a specially designed magnet board that includes four laminated magnet pieces that represent the four subdomains of the VPS. Prior to the session, the counselor has reviewed Mr P's responses and determined the rank order of the care values by calculating the mean of the items within each subdomain. The counselor has arranged the four magnet pieces vertically so that the most important care value is in the highest position. In all, Mr. P's initial rankings from most important to least important are: Social Interactions; Autonomy; Safety/Quality of Care; and Burden. (For the actual session, the categories have been renamed so that the wording is more understandable to clients: Activities with others; Independence; Safety/Who helps out; and Family stress; respectively).

The counselor asks Mr P if the order of the four magnets reflects his views about which care values are most important to him. Mr P responds slowly, not because he does not understand the question, but, as he notes, because he is surprised that this is how the values come together. The counselor reminds him of the exact wording of a few of the questions within each category. Mr P persists and indicates that he feels that his safety and how he is cared for are most important to him and that his interactions with friends and family are least important. The counselor rearranges the magnet pieces to reflect Mr P's values and asks where Mr P would place Independence and Family Stress. Mr P agrees with the previous ranking where Independence is more important than Family Burden. Mr P's final ordering is: Safety/Who helps out; Independence; Family stress; and Activities with others.

The counselor next meets with Mrs P. During the 10 minutes that Mrs P meets with the counselor, Mr P uses the telephone to confirm a number of upcoming doctor appointments and to arrange for transportation. Similar to the procedure with Mr P, the counselor has rank ordered Mrs P's responses on her magnet board prior to the session. Recall that Mrs P's responses are to the question of her perception of her husband's care preferences and not her own preferences for his care. Mrs P's initial ranking is very similar to Mr P's with the exception of Safety/Who helps out being ranked last. Mrs P does not change her initial ranking.

Next, Mr and Mrs P meet together with the counselor who uses Mr P's magnet board and adds Mrs P's responses vertically and next to Mr P's responses. The counselor asks the couple if they notice any similarities or differences in their responses. Mr P responds immediately and with some frustration that his wife does not know his preferences better. Mrs P reacts to his frustration with defensiveness and anger accusing him of never talking about these specific care questions. The counselor quickly steps in and acknowledges that there are differences in their responses, but that the differences are very few, and that differences are very common in families. The counselor reminds the couple that their goal is not necessarily to agree, but to use the session time to discuss care issues so that Mrs P understands better her husband's preferences. With this improved understanding, she can make more informed care decisions that reflect Mr P's preferences rather than becoming distressed about being uncertain of his stated preferences. The couple agrees to this goal and the counselor encourages Mr P to clarify first why Activities with others is least important to him. Mr P next discusses why Safety/Who helps out is most important and so on. At one point, Mrs P acknowledges that some of her responses may reflect her own preferences rather than her perception of her husband's preferences. The counselor commends Mrs P on her honesty and ability to recognize how her own values affect her views of what her husband prefers. The session ends with the counselor writing down the final rank order within the couple's individual Care Notebooks so that they can each reflect on the final ordering.

Preferences for Everyday Living Inventory (PELI)

The Preferences for Everyday Living Inventory (PELI) was developed using concept mapping, a statistical and measurement method "that produces a pictorial representation—literally a map—of items" (p. 336; Carpenter et al., 2000). Mapping requires research participants to sort items into groups of perceived similarity. Items are generated by and are of interest to researchers, who, in this case, were interested in the psychosocial preferences of older adults. The research team generated 470 items based on literature review and focus group meetings with older adults from various social and living situations (e.g., senior centers, assisted living, and nursing home). The team divided the items into broad ("I enjoy reading") versus nested ("At what times of day do you enjoy reading") categories of items. This procedure generated 80 broad items such as "have weekly contact with family," "keep busy," "choose what to wear," "keep to regular routine," "have friends involved in my care." Next, 28 research participants sorted the items "into groups that reflected areas of preferences for everyday living" (p. 338; Carpenter et al., 2000). Results indicated that items sorted along two axes with clustering of six preference domains: social contact; growth activities; leisure activities; self-dominion; support aids; and caregivers and care. These domains show both convergence and divergence to the four care values domains of the VPS. [NOTE: one item (i.e., I like to keep in frequent contact with my friends) was eliminated due to a typographical error on the concept mapping questionnaire; Carpenter et al., 2000.]

Within the six preference domains there are between five and 22 items. Examples of specific items include: (1) Social Contact (13 items), have weekly contact with family, meet new people, be a group leader, participate in religious activities, be center of attention; (2) Growth Activities (14 items), read, be challenged, do new things, listen to music, keep busy, travel, shop for bargains, being in lively, noisy place; (3) Leisure Activities (9 items), get around town independently, eat at restaurants, watch TV, snack, stay around house, alcoholic beverages; (4) Self Dominion (22 items), feel in control of life, have privacy, choose what I wear, have a plan for my day, be where it is quiet, have carpeting around, keep regular routine, nap; (5) Support Aids (5 items), decide when to take medications, keep clean, use herbs, vitamins, supplements, use ramps, hand rails, etc.; (6) Caregiver and Care (16 items), know about medical condition/treatment, family members help with care, have friends involved in my care, discuss personal things with staff, caregivers have same background, help to get motivated. (For a complete list of all PELI items see Carpenter et al., 2000.)

The research team that has used the PELI most extensively notes that "older adults genuinely enjoyed completing the instrument" possibly because the content is "quite different from the questions they are used to being asked by home health nurses or other usual service providers" (Carpenter, personal communication, 2009). In addition, when adult children also completed the PELI to predict their parents' answers, "both generations found it very interesting—the parents because it gave them the chance to tell their children what was important to them, and the children because they learned how little they knew about their parent" (Carpenter, personal communication, 2009). A self-report version of the PELI has also been used with older adults who completed it independently by mail. While these adults had no difficulty completing the PELI, a few felt it was a little long (Van Haitsma, personal communication, 2009). Overall, this team of researchers agrees that respondents especially enjoy completing the PELI when it provides an opportunity for social interaction with an interviewer or family member, as compared to when it is used solely for information gathering (Carpenter personal communication, 2009; Van Haitsma personal communication, 2009).

SHAPE: Self-Maintenance Habits and Preferences in Elderly

The SHAPE questionnaire (Cohen-Mansfield & Jensen, 2007a, 2007b) assesses self-care preferences as a way to aid in the design of care plans that reflect the actual preferences of older adults. SHAPE was developed to fill a void in the assessment literature that has failed to document and provide tools to assess preferences for activities of daily living (ADLs; Cohen-Mansfield & Jensen, 2007a). SHAPE consists of 115 close-ended questions that assess the respondent's preferences for sleeping (29 items), eating (36 items), dressing and grooming (12 and 11 items, respectively) and hygiene (27 items). Items vary in their response options depending on the nature of the ADL. For example, questions about dressing include: "When do you dress? Immediately after rising, after taking a bath or shower, after breakfast, other, no preference;" "Do you have privacy while you dress? Yes, no, or no preference;" "Do you use ironed clothing? Yes, no, or no preference" and so on.

Cohen-Mansfield and Jensen (2007a, 2007b) report that over a two-week period, older adults respond to SHAPE questions with a high degree of reliability and high percentage agreement rates. Likewise, the authors found high levels of reliability for item importance. The authors report SHAPE interviews to last approximately 75 minutes and that differences exist in ratings of importance of certain items (Cohen-Mansfield & Jensen, 2007b). For example, women rated dressing and grooming as more important than men, and as level of education increases, so do importance ratings overall. Results of studies using SHAPE suggest: (1) interventions that attempt to align previous preferences with current practices have the potential to "enhance the quality of life" of older persons (Cohen-Mansfield & Jensen, 2007a, 2007b); (2) information gained from SHAPE assessments can be used to develop a plan of care that reflects a client's stated preferences as opposed to preferences reported by proxy informants; and (3) data gathered in the aggregate can be used to develop care plans, services, and interventions that correspond to the preferences and needs of a majority or largest number of older adults (Cohen-Mansfield & Jensen, 2007a, 2007b).

Decision-Making Involvement Scale (DMI)

The Decision-Making Involvement Scale (DMI; Menne et al., 2008) was developed based on earlier work of Conroy and Yuskauskas (1996) who created the Decision Control Inventory to measure quality of life outcomes among persons with mental retardation and developmental disabilities. Feinberg et al. (2000) adapted Conroy and Yuskauskas's inventory for use in their research with IWDs and family CGs. As shown in Appendix A, the 15 items of the DMI assess dimensions of IWD decision-making such as "what to spend money on," "what foods to buy," "what clothes to wear" and so on. IWDs are asked to describe their decision-making involvement on a four point scale: 0 = not at all involved; 1 = a little involved; 2 = fairly involved; 3 = very involved. A CG version of the DMI scale was also developed based on the idea that increasing IWD autonomy must involve, at a minimum, both care partners. When a CG does not know, agree with, or act in accordance with an IWD's preference for care there is the potential for added CG stress (Whitlatch, 2001). Therefore, the DMI scale asks CGs for their perceptions of how involved they think their relative is in decision-making for each of the items.

Psychometric analyses of the DMI scale indicate that it has good internal consistency, convergent and divergent validity, and functions adequately as a one-factor scale (Menne et al., 2008). IWD and CG responses are positively and significantly correlated, yet low values and mean comparisons indicate that CGs consistently report lower levels of IWD decision-making involvement than reported by IWDs (Menne et al., 2008). Analyses with both CG and IWD samples indicate that level of cognitive impairment is related to decision-making involvement: as level of impairment increases, decision-making involvement decreases. Lastly, findings suggest that decision-making involvement is "related to quality of life for CGs and IWDs," and that other areas of CG well-being such as depression, negative relationship strain, "may be enhanced when the IWD is more involved in decision-making" (Menne et al., 2008). Moreover, the DMI can be used to promote discussions within care dyads that clarify each person's role and lead to potential changes in the decision-making process.

DO PREFERENCES FOR CARE VARY ACROSS DIFFERENT POPULATIONS?

As described earlier, the current literature about and measures available to assess the personal and/or care preferences of adults with chronic illness including dementia is growing at a slow but encouraging pace. Yet, we know little at this time about the care preferences of adults with various cultural or ethnic backgrounds, or adults from different socioeconomic groups, or even differences between men and women or differences depending upon diagnosis, symptomatology, or living arrangement (Cohen-Mansfield & Jensen, 2007b). A few exceptions exist.

First, we know that compared to IWDs with higher socioeconomic resources, persons with lower socioeconomic resources report that living in their own home and having money to leave to family are less important (Whitlatch & Feinberg, 2003). It is possible that many of these IWDs who do not live in their own home, but in the homes of a family caregiver or in housing that they rent, have never placed importance on living in their own home. Likewise, these IWDs do not have extra money to leave to family so this is not a value that is highly rated. Unfortunately, because these findings are confounded with the cultural background of the two groups (i.e., the IWDs with lower socioeconomic status were African American whereas the higher socioeconomic group was predominantly Euro American), the specific source of the differences cannot be determined. Cohen-Mansfield & Jensen (2007b) report that in their sample of community-dwelling older adults, as level of education increased so did importance ratings overall. The authors suggest that this finding is also likely to be associated with socioeconomic status (SES) since education and SES are typically linked.

Second, although there is evidence that compared to Euro Americans, African Americans are more likely to prefer end-of-life care options that are more aggressive (Crawley et al., 2000; Hopp & Duffy, 2000), there is also evidence that an individual's health literacy is associated more with treatment choice than is their cultural background (Volandes et al., 2008). To date, no studies have examined these differences in older adults with dementia. However, these findings point to the importance of examining health literacy when studying health care decision-making regardless of the presence of cognitive loss.

Lastly, there are very few findings related to gender and kin group differences. In one of the few studies that examine gender differences in preferences, Cohen-Mansfield & Jensen (2007b) note that cognitively intact older women place greater importance on dressing and grooming habits than do their male peers. Clearly, there is much work to be done in the study of preferences for care among male and female IWDs, individuals and caregivers of diverse backgrounds, and IWDs depending upon their gender.

ENHANCING DECISION-MAKING AND UNDERSTANDING OF PERSONAL PREFERENCES IN DEMENTIA

One strategy for bridging the knowledge gap and improving IWD and caregiver outcomes is a dyadic approach that brings together the IWD and the family caregiver to discuss care needs (Whitlatch et al., 2006). This type of approach facilitates education on the illness, discussion of feelings and thoughts, and skill building for both care partners. Surprisingly few interventions include both the IWD and the family caregiver, although a few exist (see Clare, 2002) and show promise for improving IWD and CG outcomes. Dyadic interventions can have an individual focus or a group focus. Individually focused dyad interventions are designed for the IWD and family caregiver to meet with a trained counselor, while group-focused programs bring together groups of IWDs and family CGs. Group programs often have time for the IWDs to meet together, for CGs to meet together, and then to have both groups meet together.

One dyadic intervention in particular shows promise by addressing a number of issues, including everyday decision-making, relationship strain, and symptoms of depression. Early Diagnosis Dyadic Intervention (EDDI) provides care partners with information about the symptoms of dementia, and affords a structured exploration and discussion of care preferences and needs, including the importance of independence, social interactions, and quality care (Whitlatch et al., 2006). Dyads work with a trained EDDI counselor to learn about the illness progression, strategies for enhancing everyday decision making (for both the IWD and the family caregiver), and techniques for alleviating strain associated with the illness. These techniques help to reduce negative outcomes such as depression and negative mood, and enhance quality of life. EDDI employs interactive strategies with both care partners and includes exercises to promote dialog about care preferences.

The Values and Preferences Scale (VPS), described earlier in the chapter, is one tool used in EDDI. A second tool used as part of the EDDI program is the Preferences for Care Tasks measure (PCT; Whitlatch et al., 2006). As with the VPS, both care partners separately complete the PCT during an initial in-person intake or assessment interview. The PCT asks IWDs: "If there comes a time when you need help with day-to-day tasks, who would you prefer to help you with…" (specific care tasks). Examples of the 19 care tasks include help with: taking medications; housework; shopping; preparing meals; eating; bathing; finances; getting in/out of bed; dressing; toileting; and so on. The IWD is asked if he would prefer to have his care partner help, or other family/friends, or a paid provider help with these care tasks. The CG, on the other hand, is asked: "When the time comes for your [husband] to need help with day-to-day tasks, who do you think he will prefer to help him?"

Case Study 1(cont.)—Preferences for care tasks—Mr and Mrs P

After Mr and Mrs P have completed the PCT, they meet together with the practitioner who has arranged Mr P's responses on a specially designed magnet board that contains three circles ("Circles Diagram") and includes laminated magnetic strips corresponding to the care tasks (see Appendix B). The practitioner has arranged the IWD's magnets within each of the three circles representing Mr P's preferences for who would help with each care task. Prior to the session the practitioner has also arranged Mrs P's magnets within the three circles representing her perceptions of who Mr P would prefer to help him with care tasks. The clinician meets with the couple to: (1) encourage them to react to the placement of the magnets; (2) point out discrepancies and similarities; (3) help the couple realign or reorder the care tasks magnets if one circle is too full; and (4) discuss the final order of magnets for both Mr P's preferences and Mrs P's perceptions of Mr P's care preferences. This exercise is very useful for care partners regardless of initial level of agreement or understanding. We have found that nearly all dyads place the majority of their magnet care tasks within the CAREGIVER circle.

When the couple first views their PCT's Circles Diagrams they are both shocked at the disproportionate number of care tasks that Mrs P is expected to perform. Mrs P is extremely distressed: "This makes me feel completely overwhelmed. I know this is what we both want, but it's not going to be easy to do all of this." (Mrs P's reaction is similar to nearly all CGs. For example, a caregiving daughter voiced a comparable reaction: "I want to do all this, but with my own health problems, I'm not sure I will be able to.") For Mr P and nearly all other IWDs, the visual representation of his wife's circle overflowing with care tasks is critical to his understanding and accepting that his wife is expected to do too much. Nearly every IWD acknowledges, as does Mr P, that "this isn't fair" or "she can't do everything" or "I think we need to move some of those magnets." And indeed, this is the next step of the exercise: to work with Mr and Mrs P to move magnets/care tasks out of Mrs P's circle and into the PAID PROVIDERS and/or FAMILY AND FRIENDS circles. Mr and Mrs P agree that they would be willing to ask their daughter to prepare a few meals and take Mr P to the doctor. Disagreement occurs around tasks such as: (1) laundry: Mrs P is not willing to let outsiders work with their dirty clothes; (2) shopping: Mrs P admits being too picky about produce; and (3) finances: Mr P will only allow their own accountant to handle their bills and taxes. At the end of the session, the practitioner copies onto worksheets the final positioning of the care tasks so that both Mr and Mrs P have their own copy. It is our hope with Mr and Mrs P, and all the dyads we work with, that each care partner will return to these diagrams as they make decisions together and when the CG is required to make care decisions on their own.

Our work with approximately 50 dyads indicates that both care partners are typically willing and able to come to agreement about the moving of at least a few magnets/care tasks. This experience helps each care partner to understand better the perspective of their partner, and there is often a sense of relief and hope brought on by the knowledge that they understand each other. At the other extreme, dyads who share little understanding and agreement initially can come to an understanding of the other person's perspective. The goal of this exercise and the procedure with the Values and Preferences Scale is not to force care partners to come to an agreement about what care values and tasks are most important, because ultimately it is the IWD's preferences that are the point of interest and concern. These exercises are meant to provide a structured and safe forum, a starting point, for frank, open, and sometimes difficult discussions about current and future care preferences.

Group Approaches for Eliciting Preferences

Group approaches to intervening with both members of the care dyad show similarly promising results. In addition, group interventions are especially appealing because they tend to be more cost effective and serve larger numbers of care partners. Early-stage dyadic groups are typically short-term, structured, often include an educational component, and offer participants opportunity for socializing, support, and stress management (Clare et al., in press; Yale, 1995; [Zarit, Femia, Watson, Rise-Oeschger & Kakos, 2006]). Both individual and group interventions have the potential to improve communication and mutual decision-making for care partners facing the challenges of memory loss.

Self-Awareness of Cognitive Losses and Skills

When determining the ability of an IWD to participate in and experience gains from any psychosocial intervention, it is important to recognize the role of metacognition (i.e., self-awareness of cognitive skills) and the related condition of anosognosia (i.e., the denial of cognitive disabilities or lack of awareness of deficits related to memory and/or daily activities; Adair, Schwartz, & Barrett, 2003). Lack of metacongitive ability and/or the presence of anosognosia will likely have a significant impact on the success of interventions that rely on an IWD's input, feedback, and acknowledgment and attribution of cognitive loss as a result of a disease state. Zannetti et al. (1999 as cited by Adair et al., 2003) report that as cognitive ability declines so does an IWD's awareness of cognitive and functional deficits. These authors report that IWDs with MMSE scores (Folstein et al., 1975) greater than 24 were found to have metacognitive skills that were fairly intact, IWDs with MMSE scores between 23 and 12 had significant decline in cognitive awareness, and IWDs with MMSE scores less than 12 had very low levels of awareness. IWDs who lack self-awareness of cognitive skills (or deny their cognitive loss) may gain little from interventions designed to enhance cognitive functioning or improve communication and decision-making skills, because IWDs may misattribute their cognitive losses to other external or internal sources unrelated to their disease. Caregivers and IWDs who are more proactive and fully engaged in the intervention process, as compared to care partners who are in denial about the disease, may experience fewer gains and poorer outcomes. Likewise, care partners who are more reactive and focused on fulfilling basic needs such as food, housing, and employment (Whitlatch et al., 2006), may also be less invested and less actively involved in the intervention process, and in turn may experience fewer positive gains.

REASSESSMENT OF CARE VALUES AND PREFERENCES AND A LOOK TO THE FUTURE

Given the limited literature about assessing care and personal preferences, it is not surprising that information and guidance about reassessment of preferences is nearly non-existent. Assessing the care values and personal preferences of IWDs and family CGs throughout the course of the illness has the potential to enhance the well-being of both care partners (Whitlatch et al., 2009), although there is no published data that empirically supports this contention. As with any reassessment, it is important that the timing is based on evidence that an adequate amount of time has passed so that change can be captured. Again, there is no published evidence that supports a specific timeframe for capturing change in personal or care preferences. Carpenter and colleagues (2007) re-evaluated the personal preferences of IWDs and cognitively intact older adults with dementia one year after their initial assessment and found that these preferences remained relatively stable (i.e., moderate to good), but less so for IWDs. As noted earlier in the chapter, longitudinal work with care dyads supports this finding in part: IWDs were stable in their care values, whereas their family caregiver's perceptions of these values became less accurate (Piiparinen & True, 2008).

These findings are encouraging, but do not provide guidance about the timing or utility of reassessment for enhancing outcomes for IWDs and family CGs. Moreover, reassessment may be useful for gauging altered preferences that are a product of changing life experiences resulting from dementia or other chronic illnesses. For example, a daughter caring for her father may have an early memory of his dislike of nursing homes and that she promised that she would never move him to any long-term care facility. This promise, made when everyone was healthy and had few external stressors, may become irrelevant as her father's disease progresses and his care requirements become overwhelming. If the dyad is reassessed about their care values or personal preferences, they may learn that their preferences have changed as a result of: (1) the father's understanding that his increasing everyday and medical care needs are too much for his daughter; and (2) the daughter's acceptance that her lack of training in managing her father's medical care needs (e.g., intravenous medications) could be detrimental to her father's health and that he would be safer in a more supervised environment.

Indeed, this example of changed preferences is not unusual for care dyads facing the dynamic and long-term stress of living with dementia and other chronic conditions (Whitlatch et al., 2007). If both the IWD and CG are encouraged to work together with a well-trained practitioner to express their preferences and expectations they may be able to come to a new and more feasible understanding of the illness experience that has lasting benefits for both. It is important to remember, though, that empowering one care partner can have a tremendous impact, negative or positive, on the other care partner. For example, returning to Mr P who feels he is maintaining his independence by staying at home alone rather than attending an adult day program. Granting his preference to remain at home may end up burdening Mrs P, because Mr P calls and interrupts her many times at work throughout the day. If the couple were to engage in discussions with a trained practitioner about each care partner's expectations, preferences, and limitations, it is likely that the couple could come to an altered understanding and, in turn, adopt new strategy for meeting each of their needs.

WHERE DO WE GO FROM HERE?

One of the most difficult realizations that face nearly all individuals with dementia is the recognition and acceptance of their changing cognitive ability. These individuals experience a gradual transition as they move from making decisions either completely independently or in combination with family or professionals, to being totally dependent on family or practitioners who are expected to safeguard and act in accordance with their perceived best interests. For families, the transition parallels that of the IWD and is marked by significant changes in their relationship with their loved one with dementia. We know relatively little about the specific mechanisms underlying this process of change. Few theoretical models of an IWD's illness experience exist which can guide researchers and practitioners in determining how best to intervene to ameliorate stress for the IWD (for an exception see Menne et al., 2008), although models exist for family caregivers (Aneshensel et al., 1995). Thus, the first direction for future work is for researchers, practitioners, and family members to work together to develop a model or models that capture the experience of IWDs as they adjust to and cope with their changing circumstances over time. With this model practitioners and researchers can determine the most effective points for intervention where the evaluation of care and personal preferences has the greatest impact on well-being and other IWD outcomes.

But before points for and mechanisms of intervention can be established, there must be valid and reliable measures to assess and reassess the preferences of IWDs (and individuals with other chronic conditions) that can be used: (1) in a variety of settings (i.e., home and community-based, assisted living, long-term care); (2) by practitioners from different disciplines; and (3) on behalf of families of diverse backgrounds, geographies, situations, and economic circumstances. To meet this need, currently used measures could be adapted for use in diverse settings and on behalf of diverse client populations. No doubt, questions will need to be revised, added, deleted, and reconsidered. The process of measurement development will shed light on the larger process of decision-making and personal preferences for IWDs and individuals with other chronic conditions. The information gained will help practitioners to understand better the preferences of their clients, provide families with a clear understanding of their relatives' preferences, and give hope to individuals with dementia and other chronic conditions that their voices are heard and their preferences respected.

It is critical to understand that knowing an individual's personal and care preferences does not imply these preferences will be acted on or carried out. Circumstances change, family members encounter their own physical and emotional health conditions, and individuals with dementia reconsider the effect their illness has on those around them. Therefore, reassessment is critical and the timing of optimal reassessment needs to be determined, or at least guidelines established. In addition, practitioners need to recognize that there must be a balance between the preferences of IWDs and the ability of family members to carry out these preferences. An imbalance could lead to negative consequences for the IWD and/or family caregiver. Clearly, there is much to be done in both the research and practice communities regarding the ongoing assessment of personal and care preferences for individuals with dementia. Families and individuals with dementia will benefit greatly from these types of focused investigations, which have the potential to improve quality of life for all individuals touched by dementia.

ACKNOWLEDGMENTS

This research was supported by grants from the National Institute of Aging (P50 AG08012), the National Institute of Mental Health (R01070629), and grant 90CG2566 from the Administration on Aging, U.S. Department of Health and Human Services. I wish to thank Justin Johnson, BA, Research Assistant with the Benjamin Rose Institute, for his assistance with references and citations.

APPENDIX A: VALUES AND PREFERENCES SCALE (VPS)

Subdomain names in parentheses represent the wording that is used to refer to that domain when working with the care dyad.

Response options:

VERY IMPORTANT, SOMEWHAT IMPORTANT, NOT AT ALL IMPORTANT

Asked of the individual with dementia	Asked of the family caregiver
How important is it for you to:	How important is it for your relative to:

(INDEPENDENCE) AUTONOMY

- Do things for yourself
- Come/go as you please
- Organize daily routines in your own way
- Spend money how you want
- Have something to do
- Have time for yourself
- Make own financial decisions

(ACTIVITIES W/OTHERS) SOCIAL INTERACTIONS

- Do things with others
- Be with family/friends
- Be part of family celebrations
- Keep in touch with past
- Keep in touch with distant family and friends

BURDEN (FAMILY STRESS)

- Avoid being a physical burden
- Avoid being an emotional burden
- That CG not put his/her life on hold for you
- Avoid being a financial burden
- Have money to leave the family

SAFETY/QUALITY OF CARE (WHO HELPS OUT)

- Feel safe inside the home
- Be in touch with others in an emergency
- Be safe from crime
- Keep the same doctor
- Choose the family who helps
- Have reliable help
- Choose who is excluded from helping you

Examples of Items removed because of low variance or ambiguous factor loadings:

Have comfortable place to live, maintain dignity, live in own home, not to live in a nursing home, avoid family conflict, have personal privacy, feel useful.

Decision Making Involvement Scale (DMI)

Response options:

0 = Not at all involved; 1 = A little involved; 2 = Fairly involved; 3 = Very involved.

Asked of the individual with dementia

"How involved are you in making decisions about:"

Asked of the family caregiver

"How involved is your relative in making decisions about:"

IWD: What to spend your money on?

CG: What to spend money on?

Visiting with friends?
What foods to buy?
When to go to bed?
When to get up?
What to do in your spare time?
Being physically active?
Participating in religious/spiritual activities?
Expressing affection?
Having a pet?
What to eat at meals?
Choosing places to go?
What clothes to wear?
Choosing what to wear?
Choosing where to live?
Getting medical care?

APPENDIX B: PREFERENCES FOR CARE TASKS (PCT) WORKSHEET & MAGNET BOARD LAYOUT

Asked of the IWD: WHO WOULD YOU PREFER TO HELP YOU WITH…?
Asked of the CG: WHO DO YOU THINK YOUR [REL] WOULD PREFER TO HELP HIM/HER WITH…?

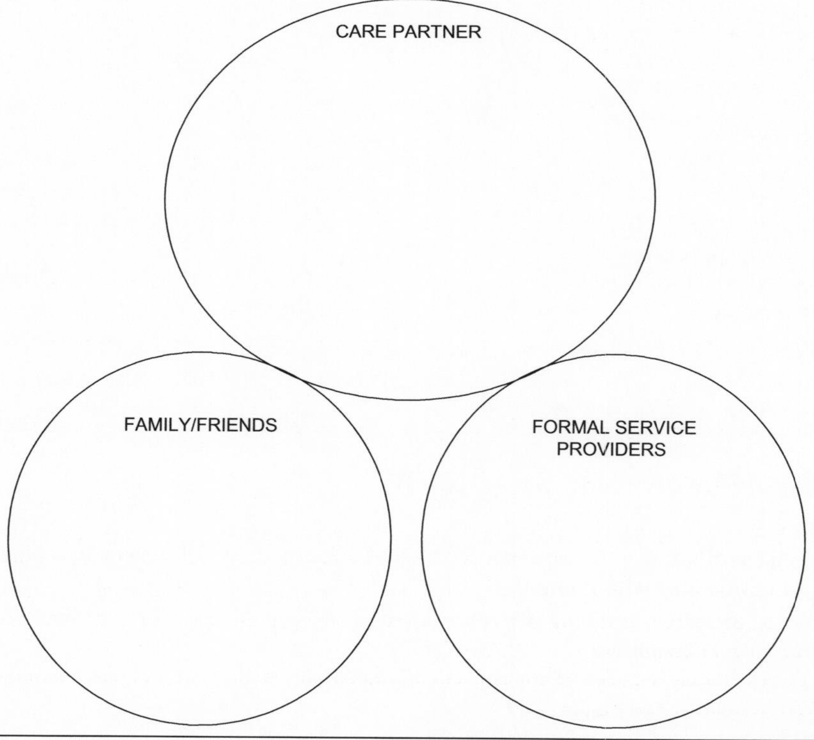

A. Taking medication
B. Housework
C. Shopping for food
D. Cooking
E. Laundry
F. Driving/Transportation
G. Financial/legal matters
H. Eating
K. Toileting
L. Help your care partner during the night
M. Doing things your care partner enjoys
N. When your care partner feels restless/bored
O. When your care partner feels sad/upset
P. Getting your care partner in/out of bed
Q. Making MD appointments for your care partner

References

Adair, J. C., Schwartz, R. L., & Barrett, A. M. (2003). Anosognosia. In K. M. Heilman, & E. Valenstein (Eds.), *Clinical Neuropsychology* (pp. 185–213). New York, NY: Oxford University Press.

Alzheimer's Disease International Fact Sheet (2008). The prevelance of dementia. http://www.alz.co.uk/adi/pdf/prevalence.pdf

Aneshensel, C. S., Pearlin, L. I., Mullan, J. T., Zarit, S. H., & Whitlatch, C. J. (1995). *Profiles in Caregiving: The Unexpected Career*. New York, NY: Academic Press.

Anthony-Bergstone, C. R., Zarit, S. H., & Gatz, M. (1988). Symptoms of psychological distress among caregivers of dementia patients. *Psychology and Aging*, *3*, 245–248.

Beisecker, A. E., Chrisman, S. K., & Wright, L. J. (1997). Perceptions of family caregivers of persons with Alzheimer's disease: communication with physicians. *American Journal of Alzheimer's Disease*, *12*, 11.

Birkel, R. C. (1987). Toward a social ecology of the home-care household. *Psychology & Aging*, *2*, 294–301.

Carpenter, B. D., Van Haitsma, K., Ruckdeschel, K., & Lawton, M. (2000). The psychological preferences of older adults: A pilot examination of content and structure. *The Gerontologist*, *3*, 335–348.

Carpenter, B. D., Kissel, E. C., & Lee, M. M. (2007). Preferences and life evaluations of older adults with and without dementia: reliability, stability, and proxy knowledge. *Psychology and Aging*, *22*(3), 650–655.

Carpenter, B. D., Lee, M., Ruckdeschel, K., Van Haitsma, K. S., & Feldman, P. H. (2006). Adult children as informants about parent's psychosocial preferences. *Family Relations*, *55*(5), 552–563.

Chang, C. Y., & Silverman, D. H. (2004). Accuracy of early diagnosis and its impact on the management and course of Alzheimer's disease. *Expert Review of Molecular Diagnosis*, *4*, 63–69.

Clare, L., Kinsella, G.J., Logsdon, R., Whitlatch, C., & Zarit, S. (in press). Building resilience in mild cognitive impairment and early-stage dementia: innovative approaches to intervention and outcome evaluation. In B. Resnick, K. Roberta, & L. Gwyther (Eds.), *The Handbook of Resilience in Aging: The Key to Successful Aging*. Springer Publishing.

Clare, L. (2002). We'll fight it as long as we can: coping with the onset of Alzheimer's disease. *Aging and Mental Health*, *6*, 139–148.

Clark, P.A. (2004). Accuracy and reliability of information from persons with dementia. Gerontological Society of America Annual Meeting; 2004 Nov: Washington, DC.

Clark, P.A., Piiparinen, R., True, S., & Whitlatch, C.J. (2007). Variation in consistency of information from individuals with dementia. Presented as part of the symposium "Longitudinal research with family caregiving dyads," Whitlatch, C.J. (organizer) at the 60th Annual Scientific Meeting of the Gerontological Society of America, San Francisco, CA.

Cohen, D. (1991). The subjective experience of Alzheimer's disease: the anatomy of an illness as perceived by patients and families. *American Journal of Alzheimers Disease and Other Dementias*, *6*(6), 6–11.

Cohen-Mansfield, J., & Jensen, B. (2007a). Self-maintenance habits and preferences in elderly (SHAPE): reliability of reports of self-care preferences on older persons. *Aging-Clinical and Experimental Research*, *19*, 61–68.

Cohen-Mansfield, J., & Jensen, B. (2007b). Dressing and grooming preferences of community-dwelling older adults. *Journal of Gerontological Nursing*, 31–39.

Conroy, J. W., & Yuskauskas, A. (1996). *Independent evaluation of the Monadnock Self-Determination Project*. Ardmore, PA: The Center for Outcomes Analysis.

Crawley, L., Payne, R., Bolden, J., Payne, T., Washington, P., & Williams, S. (2000). Palliative and end-of-life care in the African American community. *Journal of the American Medical Association, 284*, 2518–2521.

Degenholtz, H., Kane, R. A., & Kivnick, H. Q. (1997). Care-related preferences and values of elderly community-based LTC consumers: can case managers learn what's important to clients? *Gerontologist, 37* (6), 767–776.

Downs, M., Clibbens, R., Rae, C., Cook, A., & Woods, R. (2002). What do general practitioners tell people with dementia and their families about the condition? A survey of experience in Scotland. *Dementia: The International Journal of Social Research and Practice, 1*, 47–58.

Family Caregiver Alliance. (1996). *Incidence and Prevalence of the Major Causes of Adult-Onset Brain Impairment in the United States and California*. San Francisco, CA: Family Caregiver Alliance.

Family Caregiver Alliance (2001). *Incidence and Prevalence of the Major Causes of Brain Impairment*. San Francisco, CA. http://www.caregiver.org/caregiver/jsp/print_friendly.jsp?nodeid=438

Feinberg, L. F., & Whitlatch, C. J. (2001). Are cognitively impaired adults able to state consistent choices? *The Gerontologist, 41*(3), 374–382.

Feinberg, L. F., Whitlatch, C. J., & Tucke, S. S. (2000). *Making Hard Choices: Respecting both Voices*. San Francisco, CA: Family Caregiver Alliance.

Folstein, M. F., Folstein, S. E., & McHugh, P. R. (1975). "Mini-Mental State": a practical method for grading the cognitive state of patients for the clinician. *Journal of Psychiatric Research, 12*, 189–198.

Fried, T. R., Bradley, E. H., & O'Leary, J. (2003). Prognosis communication in serious illness: perceptions of older patients, caregivers, and clinicians. *Journal of American Geriatric Society, 51*, 1398–1403.

Friss, L. R., & Whitlatch, C. J. (1991). Who's taking care? A statewide study of family caregivers. *The American Journal of Alzheimer's Care and Related Disorders and Research, 6*, 16–26.

Gallagher, D., Rose, J., Rivera, P., Lovett, S., & Thompston, L. W. (1989a). Prevalence of depression in family caregivers. *The Gerontologist, 29*, 449–456.

Gallagher, D., Wrabetz, A., Lovett, S., DelMaestro, S., & Rose, J. (1989b). Depression and other negative effects in family caregivers. In E. Light, & B. Lebowitz (Eds.), *Alzheimer's Disease Treatment and Family Stress: Directions for Future Research* (pp. 218–244). Washington, DC: US Government Printing Office.

Garand, L., Dew, M. A., Eazor, L. R., DeKosky, S. T., & Reynolds, C. F. (2005). Caregiving burden and psychiatric morbidity in spouses of persons with mild cognitive impairment. *International Journal of Geriatric Psychiatry, 20*(6), 512–522.

Hansen, L., Archbold, P. G., Stewart, B., Westfall, U. B., & Ganzini, L. (2005). Family caregivers making life-sustaining treatment decisions. *Journal of Gerontological Nursing, Nov.* 28–35.

Herbert, L. E., Beckett, L. A., Scherr, P. A., & Evans, D. A. (2001). Annual incidence of Alzheimer's disease in the United States projected to the years 2000 through 2050. *Alzheimer Disease and Associated Disorders, 15* (4), 169–173.

Hopp, F. P., & Duffy, S. A. (2000). Racial variations in end-of-life care. *Journal of the American Geriatrics Society, 48*, 658–663.

Kiecolt-Glaser, J. K., & Glaser, R. (2002). Depression and immune function: central pathways to morbidity and mortality. *Journal of Psychosomatic Research, 53*, 873–876.

Lai, J. M., Gill, T. M., Cooney, L. M., Hawkins, K. A., & Karlawish, J. (2008). Everyday decision-making ability in older adults with cognitive impairments. *American Journal of Geriatric Psychiatry, 16*(8), 693–696.

Lai, J. M., & Karlawish, J. (2007). Assessing the capacity to make everyday decisions: a guide for clinicians and an agenda for future research. *American Journal of Geriatric Psychiatry, 15*, 101–111.

Li, H., Stewart, B. J., Imle, M. A., Archbold, P. G., & Felver, L. (2000). Families and hospitalized elders: a typology of family care actions. *Research in Nursing & Health, 23*, 3–16.

Logsdon, R. G., Gibbons, L. E., McCurry, S. M., & Teri, L. (1999). Quality of life in Alzheimer's disease: patient and caregiver reports. *Journal of Mental Health and Aging, 5*(1), 21–32.

McCullough, L. B., Wilson, N. L., Teasdale, T. A., Koppakchi, A. L., & Skelly, J. R. (1993). Mapping personal, familial, and professional values in long-term care decisions. *The Gerontologist, 33*(3), 324–332.

Menne, H. L., Tucke, S. S., Whitlatch, C. J., & Feinberg, L. F. (2008). Decision-making involvement scale for individuals with dementia and family caregivers. *American Journal of Alzheimers Disease and Other Dementias, 23*(1), 23–29.

Ory, M. G., Hoffman, R. R., Yee, J. L., Tennstedt, S., & Schulz, R. (1999). Prevalence and impact of caregiving: a detailed comparison between dementia and nondementia caregivers. *The Gerontologist*, *39*, 177–185.

Patrick, D. L., Starks, H. E., Cain, K. C., Uhlmann, R. F., & Pearlman, R. A. (1994). Measuring preferences for health states worse than death. *Medical Decision Making*, *14*, 9–18.

Phinney, A. (1998). Living with dementia from the patient's perspective. *Journal of Gerontological Nursing*, *24*, 8–15.

Piiparinen, R., & True, S. (2008). Everyday care values and preferences within care dyads: incongruence across time. 32nd Annual Ohio Professional and Student Conference on Aging. Cleveland, OH: Ohio Association of Gerontology and Education.

Pruchno, R. A., & Resch, N. L. (1989). Aberrant behaviors and Alzheimer's disease: mental health effects on spouse caregivers. *Journal of Gerontology: Social Sciences*, *44*, S177–S182.

Pruchno, R. A., Kleban, M. H., Michaels, J. E., & Dempsey, M. P. (1990). Mental and physical health of caregiving spouses: development of a causal model. *Journals of Gerontology: Psychological Sciences*, *45*, P192–P199.

Robinson, L., Clare, L., & Evans, K. (2005). Making sense of dementia and adjusting to loss: psychological reactions to a diagnosis of dementia in couples. *Aging & Mental Health*, *9*(4), 337–347.

Schulz, R., O'Brien, A. T., Bookwala, J., & Fleissner, K. (1995). Psychiatric and physical morbidity effects of Alzheimer's disease caregiving: prevalence, correlates, and causes. *The Gerontologist*, *35*, 771–791.

Schulz, R., & Beach, S. R. (1999). Caregiving as a risk factor for mortality: the caregiver health effects study. *Journal of the American Medical Association*, *282*, 2215–2219.

Schulz, R., O'Brien, A., Czaja, S., Ory, M., Norris, R., Martire, L. M., et al. (2002). Dementia caregiving research: in search of clinical significance. *The Gerontologist*, *42*, 589–602.

Sebern, M. D. (2008). Refinement of the Shared Care Instrument-revised: a measure of a family care interaction. *Journal of Nursing Measurement*, *16*(1), 43–60.

Sebern, M. D. (2005). Psychometric evaluation of the Shared Care Instrument in a sample of home health care family dyads. *Journal of Nursing Measurement*, *13*(3), 175–191.

Smyth, K. A. (1999). *Personal communication*. Cleveland, OH: Director, Caregiving Core, the University Hospitals Alzheimer Disease Research Center.

Squillace, M. R., Mahoney, K. J., Shoop, D. M., Simon-Rusinowitz, & Desmond, S. M. (2002). An exploratory study of personal assistance service choice and decision-making among persons with disabilities and surrogate representatives. *Journal of Mental Health and Aging*, *8*(3), 225–240.

Van Haitsma, K. (2000). The assessment and integration of preferences into care practices for persons with dementia residing in the nursing home. In R. Rubinstein, M. Moss, & M. Kleban (Eds.), *The Many Dimensions of Aging*. New York, NY: Springer.

Vitaliano, P. P., Scanlan, J. M., Jianping, Z., Savage, M. V., Hirsch, I. B., & Siegler, I. C. (2002). A path model of chronic stress, the metabolic syndrome, and coronary heart disease. *Psychosomatic Medicine*, *64*(3), 418–435.

Volandes, A. E., Paasche-Orlow, M., Gillick, M. R., Cook, E. F., Shaykevich, S., Abbo, E. D., & Lehmann, L. (2008). Health literacy not race predicts end-of-life care preferences. *Journal of Palliative Medicine*, *11*(5), 754–762.

Whitlatch, C. J. (2001). Including the person with dementia in family caregiving research and practice. *Aging and Mental Health*, 5 (Supplement), 72–74

Whitlatch, C. J. (2006). Older consumers and decision making: a look at family caregivers and care receivers. In S. Kunkel, & V. Wellin (Eds.), *Consumer Voice and Choice in Long-term Care* (pp. 3–20). New York, NY: Springer Publishing Company.

Whitlatch, C.J. (2008). Informal caregivers: communication and decision making. *American Journal of Nursing*, 108(9):73–77. This article was also published as a special supplement within the *Journal of Social Work Education, 44*(3) (Fall 2008), 89–95 as part of an agreement between the Council on Social Work Education and *AJN*.

Whitlatch, C. J., & Feinberg, L. F. (2003). Planning for the future together in culturally diverse families: making everyday care decisions. *Alzheimer's Care Quarterly*, *4*(1), 50–61.

Whitlatch, C. J., & Feinberg, L. F. (2007). Family care and decision making. In C. Cox (Ed.), *Handbook of Social Work Practice and Dementia* (pp. 129–147). New York, NY: Springer.

Whitlatch, C. J., Feinberg, L. F., & Sebesta, D. S. (1996). Depression in family caregivers: adaptation over time. *Journal of Health and Aging*, *9*, 222–243.

Whitlatch, C. J., Feinberg, L. F., & Tucke, S. S. (2005a). Accuracy and consistency of responses from persons with dementia. *Dementia: The International Journal of Social Research and Practice*, *4*(2), 171–183.

Whitlatch, C. J., Judge, K., Zarit, S. H., & Femia, E. E. (2006). A dyadic intervention for family caregivers and care receivers in early-stage dementia. *Gerontologist*, *46*, 688–694.

Whitlatch, C. J., & Piiparinen, R. (2008, December). *Enhancing the role of older adults in research and care planning*. Chicago, IL: Final report submitted to the Retirement Research Foundation.

Whitlatch, C. J., Piiparinen, R., & Clark, P. (2007, November). *Decision making and service use in caregiving families*. Bethseda, MD: Final report submitted to the National Institute on Aging.

Whitlatch, C. J., Piiparinen, R., & Feinberg, L. F. (2009). The perception gap in everyday long-term care: do family caregivers know their relatives values and preferences for care? *Dementia: The International Journal of Social Research and Practice*, *8*(2), 223–243.

Woods, B. (1999). The person in dementia care. *Generations*, *23*(3), 35–45.

Wolff, J. L., Kasper, J. D., & Shore, A. D. (2008). Long-term care preferences among older adults: a moving target? *Journal of Aging & Social Policy*, *20*(2), 182–200.

Yale, R. (1995). *Developing Support Groups for Individuals with Early-stage Alzheimer's Disease: Planning, Implementation, and Evaluation*. Baltimore, MD: Health Professionals Press.

Yee, J. L., & Schulz, R. (2000). Gender differences in psychiatric morbidity among family caregivers: a review and analysis. *The Gerontologist*, *40*(2), 147–164.

Young, R. F. (1994). Elders, families, and illness. *Journal of Aging Studies*, *8*(1), 1–15.

Zanneti, O., Valloti, B., Frisoni, G. B., Geroldi, C., Bianchetti, A., Pasqualetti, P., & Trabucchi, M. (1999). Insight in dementia: when does it occur? Evidence for a nonlinear relationship between insight and cognitive status. *Journal of Gerontology Series B: Psychological Sciences and Social Sciences*, *54B*, 100–106.

Zarit, S. H., Femia, E. E., Watson, J., Rice-Oeschger, L. & Kakos, B. (2004). Memory Club: A group intervention for people with early-stage dementia and their care partners. *The Gerontologist, 44*, 262–269.

PART

4

Everyday Functioning

CHAPTER

Assessment of Capacity

22

Jennifer Moye[1], Michelle Braun[2]

[1] *Department of Psychiatry, Harvard Medical School,*

[2] *Inpatient Mental Health, Boston VA Healthcane System, Harvard Medical School*

INTRODUCTION

This chapter provides an overview of the theory and practice of assessing civil capacities (e.g., health care, finances, independent living) in older adults who have neurological or psychiatric conditions—focusing specifically on the nature of capacity evaluation within usual health care settings. This chapter is not directed at clinicians who receive the majority of their capacity assessment referrals through the legal system (courts or attorneys), or for the practicing forensic psychologist, whose background and practice needs vary. This chapter concerns the prospective assessment of capacity, namely a patient in a health care setting who is experiencing an urgent problem where a decision is needed, and does not address retrospective assessment of capacity (which may arise in legal disputes when the evaluator is asked to consider whether an individual had the capacity to make a decision or complete a transaction at an earlier point, at times post-mortem).

WHAT IS CAPACITY?

"Decision-making capacity," "capacity," and "competency" are terms used in different settings and by different disciplines. It is important to understand how these terms have been defined in clinical and legal settings, and how those definitions are evolving. The terms may be misused in some clinical settings, leading to confusion about the assessment task and the implications of the outcome of a clinical assessment. An understanding of the use of these terms can help guide accurate and appropriate geriatric assessment.

Clinical Capacity

The term "capacity" when used in a clinical setting refers to a professional clinical judgment as to whether a specific individual has the requisite cognitive, decisional, affective, and practical abilities to be judged to have the ability to complete a specific task (e.g., drive a car) or make a specific decision (e.g., refuse a medical treatment). The term comes into use most frequently if an individual makes a decision that puts their health, assets, property, or self at significant risk—typically a risk that is new for the person, incongruent with behavior when stable, that is in the context of a neuropsychiatric condition. In these situations, clinicians or family members may raise the question: "Is this individual 'competent'?" and are usually seeking the authority to make, or have another person make, decisions for the identified patient. The term "capacity" is favored in clinical settings, and now also favored in legal settings, although the term "competency" is still encountered in clinical settings.

Handbook of Assessment in Clinical Gerontology. DOI: 10.1016/B978-0-12-374961-1.10022-3

Capacity Versus Competency

The term "capacity" is preferable to the term "competency." Historically, in the clinical setting, the use of the term capacity distinguishes a clinical judgment of capacity from a legal determination of competency. This distinction no longer holds, as legal professionals now prefer the term capacity. Another reason why capacity is preferred to competency is that the term capacity conveys the idea of functioning within a specific area, whereas competency can imply "all or nothing"—the person, as a whole, is competent or not. The use of the term capacity reflects an awareness by clinical and legal professionals that an individual may have capacity for one task but not another. Applying this change in terminology to the clinical setting, if a referral for question of competency is raised, it may be helpful to reframe the question for the referring party as "capacity" and further to ask "capacity for what," as there are many different types of capacity. In the health care setting, questions of capacity are most frequently encountered in regard to medical consent, sexual consent, financial management, independent living, and driving. In contrast, a host of specific financial capacities which are less likely to arise in health care settings may arise in court settings or private practices that work with attorneys, including testamentary capacity (capacity to execute a will), donative capacity, capacity to contract, and capacity to convey real property (Marson, Sawrie et al., 2000). In addition, there has been recent attention to capacity to vote (Hurme & Appelbaum, 2007) and capacity to consent to research (Jefferson et al., 2008; Kim, Caine, Currier, Lebouici, & Ryan 2001). These "civil" capacities are distinguished from "criminal" capacities that arise when an individual has been charged with a crime (e.g., capacity to stand trial, capacity for criminal responsibility, etc.).

Decisional Versus Executional Capacity

Some use the term "decision-making capacity" because it identifies that often what is in question is the individual's capacity to make a decision, and provides a useful distinction from the concept of executional capacity (Collopy, 1988). That is, a person may lack the capacity to execute a task (e.g., completing a check) but retain the ability to make decisions about a task (e.g., determining whether to send a check to a certain person or agency). This is an important reminder that physical disability in no way implies incapacity. However, it is also important to note that some capacities are more complex, and do require both decisional and performance skills (e.g., driving).

Actions That Follow Clinical Findings of Incapacity

Often, a clinical finding of incapacity is followed by an activation of a surrogate decision-maker. For example, if medical or financial actions are needed and there is a previously appointed decision-maker, such as an agent under a health care proxy or power of attorney document, the surrogate's authority springs into effect upon a clinical finding of incapacity. If there is no previously appointed decision-maker, and one is required, a guardianship may be needed (except in the area of medical consent, where law in some states may allow the consent of the next of kin without requiring a guardian). Also, in emergency situations where there is clear decisional incapacity and life threatening illness (e.g., such as a myocardial infarction needing intervention in an emergency room), the physician may act without the permission of a surrogate, depending on state law.

A clinical finding of incapacity does not provide authority for involuntary commitment, nor is an individual who is involuntarily committed presumed to lack decisional capacity. The legal standards for these two issues—incapacity versus danger to self/others (necessitating involuntary commitment)—are different, relying on different legal bases. Interventions to protect those who lack capacity (such as guardianship) come from the state's responsibility to protect vulnerable adults from harm. Interventions to protect those who are at risk of hurting themselves or others (such as involuntary commitment) come from the state's "police power."

Autonomy Versus Protection in Capacity Assessment

A professional finding of capacity involves weighing the obligation to promote autonomy versus protect from harm. Sometimes a clinical finding of incapacity may not lead to a specific surrogate appointment, but nevertheless result in a loss of autonomy because it compels actions by others. For example, a clinical finding that an adult lacks the capacity to drive may engage the health care provider or family action to restrict or remove driving formally (e.g., reporting to the DMV) or informally (e.g., taking the keys away) (state laws vary regarding whether clinicians can or must report driving incapacity to the state Department of Motor Vehicles). At times, when the decision to promote autonomy or protect from harm seems arduous, an ethics consultation to a hospital ethics committee is important to make sure the clinical actions are just.

Legal Capacity

All adults are presumed to have capacity in the eyes of the law unless otherwise determined in a court of law. Capacity, when used as a legal term, refers to a judicial finding regarding an individual, as raised in the context of a legal hearing or dispute, and in consideration of the legal standard. Of note, when a lawyer assesses capacity in the office (e.g., makes a determination of whether a person has the capacity to execute a will, etc.), this is also referred to as a legal determination of capacity.

A legal standard (sometimes called a legal test) refers to how capacity is defined in statute and case law. The legal standard for a capacity can be vague and general—and therefore usually does not make it obvious as to how the clinical capacity assessment should be carried out. However, a clinician must be familiar with the legal standard for any specific capacity being assessed, and ground the clinical assessment in the standard. Summaries of legal standards for common civil capacities can be found in new handbooks produced by the American Bar Association Commission on Law and Aging and the American Psychological Association (www.apa.org/pi/aging). However, to find the specific legal standard in a state it will be necessary to confer with an attorney—such as the legal counsel of a hospital or an attorney in private practice with expertise in matters of civil capacity.

Capacity as Defined in Guardianship Law

Questions of civil capacity of older adults come to the court most often in guardianship (in some states called conservatorship) proceedings. The legal process for guardianship begins when a family member or other interested party files a petition for guardianship of another individual, followed by a hearing to determine the legal capacity of the alleged incapacitated person. If incapacity is found by the judge, a guardian is appointed. In many states there is a distinction between a guardian of the person (e.g., responsible for day-to-day issues of care, residence, activities) versus guardian of estate (e.g., responsible for managing assets). Guardianship authority usually includes the right to make decisions about ordinary health care treatment, with exceptions specified in statutes for extraordinary medical treatment that require court permission, such as administration of psychotropic medication, involuntary commitment, sterilization, and ECT (Berg, Appelbaum, Lidz, & Parker, 2001). With increasingly blended families living at geographic distances, inter-jurisdictional matters of guardianship are arising. That is, because guardians are appointed in a court within a state, if the guardian wants to move the incapacitated person to a new jurisdiction or to another state, additional legal proceedings may be involved. Courts and legislatures are working to resolve such issues.

While guardianship may be necessary, concerns about the process of guardianship appointment have been evident since at least the 1970s, and often involve issues of limited due process, lack of protection of rights, poor interface between medical providers and the court, overly intrusive interventions, and the potential for guardianship to hasten institutionalization (Horstman, 1975; Mitchell, 1978).

In determining capacity in guardianship hearings, judges rely upon "medical evidence," usually in the form of a clinical report or certificate completed by a physician, psychologist or other qualified health care provider. Historically the basis for incapacity was the presence or absence of a medical diagnosis, and thus medical evidence was often provided by a physician who confirmed the diagnosis to the courts. Unfortunately, clinical evaluations for the purposes of guardianship have historically been, and for the most part remain to this date, very brief and conclusory (meaning the clinician offers a conclusion but does not describe the data that support the conclusion), not allowing for limitations to guardianship orders (Bulcroft, Kielkopf, & Tripp, 1991; Dudley & Goins, 2003; Keith & Wacker, 1992; Moye et al., 2007).

Recognizing these problems, state statutes for guardianship have undergone significant reform over the past 20 years to enhance due process protections, such as being certain the individual is notified of the guardianship hearing, making real accommodations to have the person present, and considering the individual's choice of a guardian. The new laws have also matched statutory definitions of decision-making capacity to more empirically grounded understandings of the brain. Legal definitions of incapacity under guardianship have shifted away from diagnosis-based definitions to "functional" definitions. In most states, a diagnosis is a necessary but not sufficient component of incapacity. Courts are interested in diagnoses and how the disorders or symptoms of the disorder affect "function" (e.g., decision-making, judgment, behavior, etc.). Note that the law's use of the word "functional" is different from psychology's and gerontology's use of the term. In the law, the term "functional abilities" is more general, referring to descriptions of the individual's strengths and weaknesses in cognition and behavior. In gerontology, the term "functional abilities" is narrower, typically used in reference to activities of daily living (ADLs) and independent activities of daily living (IADLs) (Lawton & Brody, 1969). When courts ask for medical evidence to focus on function, they mean they want more than just a diagnosis; they want to know about the individual's strengths and weaknesses in decision-making and judgment (e.g., neuropsychological test results), and everyday behavior (e.g., IADL or capacity instrument test results).

The American Bar Association Commission on Law and Aging keeps up-to-date, state-by-state charts of the legal definitions of incapacity in guardianship statutes, which are updated as they change. These tables (available at http://www.abanet.org/aging/guardianship/-lawandpractice/home.html) are a tremendous resource for clinicians who want to find the statutory citation for guardianship law in their state. In addition, by analyzing the different statutes across states, one can obtain a broad understanding of various legal standards for incapacity (although for any specific case the clinician must refer to the definition within the jurisdiction). Definitions of incapacity in guardianship laws tend to have one to four elements: the presence of a disabling condition; cognitive impairment; functional impairment; and a necessity element (degree of risk and failure of less restrictive alternatives that necessitates the guardianship intervention).

The Uniform Guardianship and Protective Proceedings Act (UGPPA) is a model guardianship law developed by a consensus body [the National Conference of Commissioners on Uniform State Laws (NCCUSL) http://www.nccusl.org] which for more than 100 years has worked to develop model laws that represent the most current legal thinking on a matter and may serve as models for states that are in the process of revising statutes. The UGPPA has been endorsed by leading elder law organizations. The definition of an incapacitated person in the Uniform Act is "an individual who, for reasons other than being a minor, is unable to receive and evaluate information or make or communicate decisions [cognitive component] to such an extent that the individual lacks the ability [functional component] to meet essential requirements for physical health, safety, or self-care [necessity component], even with appropriate technological assistance" [brackets added]. Although this definition does not have a diagnostic component, most states also require diagnostic information. An operationalized clinical example of the UGPPA definition might include the following information: an individual with

Alzheimer's dementia of moderate severity [disabling condition], who due to severe delayed memory and executive dysfunction [cognitive component] lacks the ability to make decisions regarding or independently manage personal care, health care, and finances [functional component] and, in the absence of close family, is at substantial danger of self-neglect and financial exploitation even when provided extensive in-home services and supports [necessity component].

Limited Guardianship

A key part of guardianship reform is a change in judicial practice to favor limited guardianship rather than full guardianship. Previously, courts found persons "incompetent" and appointed a plenary or full guardian—with the authority to make all decisions for the incapacitated person (except for those excluded by statute), and with the incapacitated person (formerly called "the ward") losing all decisional rights. Guardianship reform advocates assert that plenary appointments caused the individual to be "un-personed" in the eyes of the law, and have sought to emphasize the significant consequences of a plenary guardianship; namely, that the incapacitated individual was no longer a person in the eyes of the law due to a total loss of rights.

In recent years courts have moved away from the practice of full guardianship to favor (or in some states *require*) "limited" guardianship. Limited guardianship means that the judge's guardianship order (sometimes called a "letter") provides the guardian with limited authority to make decisions in only those areas where the individual requires assistance, and preserves rights in any area where the individual still has the capacity to make decisions. This practice is consistent with a contemporary scientific understanding of neurologic and psychiatric illness in which a person may have strengths and weaknesses in cognitive functioning translating to intact or impaired specific capacities. Admittedly the practice of limited guardianship is harder for everyone—the determination of the order is more nuanced and takes more time, the courts require more information from the clinician, and the clinician must take more time to provide detailed information. The push for limited guardianship is a matter of rights, attempting to balance the concerns of autonomy versus protection, and limit the removal of rights.

Capacity as Defined in Health Care Consent Law

Capacity to consent to medical treatment is a specific capacity rooted in the concept of informed consent, in which informed consent must be voluntary (the person must not be coerced), knowledgeable (the person must be informed about the condition, treatments, and alternatives), and the person must have the capacity to make the decision. The Uniform Health Decisions Act defines medical consent capacity as an individual's "ability to understand the significant benefits, risks, and alternatives to proposed health care and to make and communicate a health care decision." State-specific definitions regarding medical consent capacity are often located in advance directive statutes, durable power of attorney statutes, and in the body of case law. The capacity to consent to medical treatment is perhaps the most well-studied and discussed capacity.

In reviewing consent capacity law within the United States, various scholars have identified four discrete abilities that are often present in legal standards for medical consent capacity: the ability to understand diagnostic and treatment information; appreciate the significance of this information; reason about the risks and benefits of treatment alternatives; and evidence a choice (Grisso & Applebaum, 1998b). A problem in one or more of these areas, in concert with other factors, may lead to legal determinations of incapacity to make a medical decision. "Understanding" refers to the ability to comprehend diagnostic and treatment-related information. This concept includes not only the ability to remember newly presented words and phrases, but also the ability to comprehend the meaning of these words and phrases, and to exhibit that comprehension to the physician or evaluator. "Appreciation" refers to the ability to determine the significance of the treatment information relative to the individual's situation, focusing on the nature of the diagnosis and the possibility that treatment would be beneficial, and involves both cognitive and emotional appreciation. Thus, "understanding" refers to whether the individual can comprehend basic information about a condition and treatment, while "appreciation" refers to whether the individual believes that the information is accurate and applies to him or her. "Reasoning" is the process of deciding on treatment by comparing alternatives in light of consequences, and through integrating, analyzing, and manipulating information. Reasoning involves including drawing inferences about the impact of alternatives on everyday life considering one's own personal values and preferences. Although it is not usually explicitly stated, the verb "to make" in some health care capacity statutes may refer to the process of reasoning. "Expressing a choice" concerns the basic ability to communicate a decision about treatment, and applies to individuals who cannot or will not express a choice, or who are ambivalent. This legal framework for consent capacity translates fairly well into clinical assessments, as will be discussed later.

Capacity to Appoint a Durable Power of Attorney

In clinical settings it may become clear that an individual cannot make a health care decision, or manage home or finances any longer, and needs a surrogate decision-maker, but unfortunately has never completed a durable power of attorney document. A clinician may be asked, can that person now execute a durable power of attorney document to name a person to make health care or financial decisions. Can the person now execute a durable power of attorney document to name that person to make health care or financial decisions?

A durable power of attorney may be named for health care or finances. A similar document is an advance directive, which is a form of durable power of attorney for health care in which a person names an agent to make decisions in the event of their incapacity, and may instruct the individual on what to do in the event of an advanced terminal illness. Most states have statutes that define durable power of attorney and/or health care proxy laws and procedures. Typically these statutes offer little to define the capacity standard that must be present to execute such a document. Some mention the concepts of "sound mind" and being under no constraint or undue influence.

It is generally agreed that the standard is one of understanding such as in contractual capacity. That is, the durable power of attorney or health care proxy document may be seen as a type of contract; it is most important that the individual understands what they are doing in each section of the document.

The clinician evaluating capacity in this case may therefore wish to disclose each element of the document, and then ask questions to ascertain the degree of understanding. For example, the evaluator may explain: an advance directive is a legal form that states your preferences about your future care if you become too sick to speak for yourself. It is not required, but can be helpful. In the first section, you name a person to make health care decisions. It can be anyone, but should be someone you trust and who knows you. In the second section you state what kinds of treatments you want. It may help others to know what you would choose. Follow-up questions could include: What is an advance directive? What will your health care proxy do for you? Who would you choose as the person to make decisions for you? Why would you choose or trust this person? What is a living will? Why do you want to do it? What happens if you get worse and you are unable to speak for yourself?

One of the conundrums about advance directives is the general sentiment that we want to encourage people to complete these, and the risks of not completing these may be prolongation of care and a situation a person would not want. Therefore we do not want to create obstacles to their completion. On the other hand, the documents are complex, and if the evaluator carefully discloses every element on most forms, the individual will become quickly overwhelmed. How then to strike the balance between encouraging completion and valid and meaningful completion, particularly in a compromised individual. The risks of completing a durable power of attorney for finances appear to be greater and more complex in some cases, so the disclosure and inquiry may compel greater sensitivity to detail than does a durable power of attorney for health care.

CLINICAL EVALUATIONS OF CAPACITY

Settings for Clinical Assessment of Capacity

Concerns about capacity arise in the health care setting under several scenarios. Clinicians working with older adults may encounter questions of capacity in outpatient mental health practice, outpatient neuropsychological assessment practice, nursing homes or assisted living centers, home-based care settings, and inpatient psychiatry or medicine. Each of these settings shapes the context of the capacity evaluation, the implications of the outcome, and the urgency with which an answer may be needed. Concerns about capacity to make health care decisions generally arise when clinicians are recommending one treatment that the patient is refusing, and are concerned about the patient's reasoning through that decision. Concerns about capacity to care for self or property typically arise when the clinician comes into contact with an individual who is not adequately caring for self or property, and the clinician feels compelled to intervene (with an outpatient) or not to discharge back to home (with an inpatient). Concerns about capacity to manage their estate may arise when a patient reveals unusual financial expenditures or losses, or is feeling anxious or overwhelmed by the pressure of supporting the spending habits (including drug use) of another adult. Similarly, clinicians may become aware of difficulties with driving and be asked to perform a clinical assessment of the capacity to drive, or referring medical providers may question capacity to drive after an individual has been diagnosed with dementia.

Most clinicians working with older adults are likely to find their referrals for questions of legal capacity increasing. This is likely related to several factors including longer lifespan (often with more chronic or advanced illnesses), geographically distant support systems (versus family members who are present to assist), and concerns that others may be exploiting an older adult's impairments. Today an increasing proportion of elderly, and in particular "old-old" adults (75 and older), are encountered in clinical settings. Clear and obvious dementias often lead to concerns about legal capacities, and the prevalence of dementia increases with age (Alzheimer's Association, 2006). More frequent are older adults with multiple chronic health conditions, with some, such as vascular risk factors (e.g., coronary artery disease, diabetes, hypertension, hypercholesterolemia), presenting a risk for central nervous system (CNS) damage (as reviewed in Braun, 2008). The effect of these diseases on decision-making abilities varies between individuals; it may be subtle, and may affect some aspects of decision-making and not others.

Problems with Clinical Assessment of Capacity

In the past, evaluations of capacity were addressed to physicians, in part because statutes governing matters of capacity in guardianship and health care law required a medical opinion, and hospital policies and procedures followed suit. Thus, historically, clinical evaluations of the capacity of older adults were based on a physician's interview or the physician's knowledge of the patient. More recently, standardized cognitive and functional assessments by licensed psychologists are the norm, particularly for complex cases, where discrete cognitive and functional data are needed. Now, many state laws recognize psychologists and in some states other practitioners (advance practice nurses, social workers, occupational therapists) as experts who can provide evidence or testify about civil capacities, and hospital policies and procedures reflect this shift.

Clinical assessments of capacity require an astute professional clinical judgment. A comprehensive clinical interview is an essential component. However, there can be problems with capacity assessments that rely only upon interview and do not include standardized assessments of cognition and function. When individual expert assessments of competency in elderly persons have been compared to multidisciplinary panel assessments, there is lack of agreement (Kaplan, Strange, & Ahmed, 1988;

Rutman & Silberfeld, 1992). Furthermore, even when individual experts are consistent in their knowledge of legal standards for competency, they may apply them incorrectly and inconsistently (Markson, Kern, Annas, & Glantz, 1994). Low reliability of capacity evaluations is a particular concern for marginally demented patients, as physicians achieved only a 56% judgment agreement (kappa = 0.14) in evaluating capacity to consent in mildly demented patients (Marson, McInturff, Hawkins, Bartolucci, & Harrell, 1997) even when shown a structured assessment, although reliability improved when clinicians were trained to consider the four legal standards for consent capacity (Marson, Earnst, Jamil, Bartolucci, & Harell, 2000).

The low reliability of capacity evaluations may be exacerbated by factors such as dual roles, affective reactions, insensitivity to individual differences (e.g., the impact of race, culture, religion on decisions), lack of empirical models and measures, and confusion about the task. A national survey of 395 clinical practitioners found continuing confusion regarding the assessment of capacity (Ganzini, Volicer, Nelson, & Derse, 2003). Common pitfalls included confusion between clinical assessments of capacity and legal determinations of competency, the belief that actions against medical advice indicate incapacity, and the assumption that cognitive or psychiatric disorders necessarily imply incapacity. Clinicians vary in what they consider to be appropriate risks (Clemens & Hayes, 1997) and "safe-enough gambles" for older adults in discharge planning. Determining where to draw the line in promoting an individual's autonomy versus protecting the individual from harm can be extremely difficult.

Clinicians may zero in on different cognitive abilities in arriving at capacity conclusions (Marson, Hawkins, McInturff, & Harrell, 1997). Some clinicians may focus more on the patient's "rationality" whereas others may focus more on the extent to which choices are consistent with values (Braun, Gurrera, Karel, Armesto, & Moye, in press).

Differences between how professionals and patients view life and treatment decisions is one factor that may influence reliability. Professionals estimate a patient's quality of life differently, typically as less desirable, than does the patient (Starr, Pearlmann, & Uhlmann, 1986; Uhlmann & Pearlmann, 1991). In addition, family and physician proxies are poor at predicting patients' treatment preferences (Seckler, Meier, Mulvihill, & Cammer Paris, 1991). In evaluating the extent to which decisions are "rational," experts may have difficulty appreciating the elderly patient's perspective, given that the elderly individual's decision-making is informed by a lifetime of experience.

In fact, life experience may be an especially strong predictor of decision-making in older adults, who tend to focus more on interpersonal and experiential elements of problems than younger adults (Blanchard-Fields, 1996). Individual differences play a significant role in medical treatment decisions (Karel, 2000). For example, African Americans are more likely to choose life-sustaining medical treatments, with less concern about "quality of life," than Caucasian Americans who are more concerned about "quantity of life" (Caralis, Davis, Wright, & Marcial, 1993; Eleazer et al., 1996; Hopp & Duffy, 2000), and for these and other reasons could be judged incorrectly to have higher rates of incapacity (Cairns et al., 2005). In a similar vein, individuals from ethnic minority groups were less likely to endorse the appropriateness of allowing surrogates to consent for an incapacitated person to participate in research (Kim et al., 2009). Cultural and religious values and beliefs may be critical determinants of an individual's approach to medical decision-making (Garrett, Harris, Norburn, Patrick, & Danis, 1993; Klessig, 1992), as is an individual's experiences with illness or caregiving (Allen-Burge & Haley, 1997; Collopy, 1999; Karel, Powell, & Cantor, 2004). For example, dementia caregivers may be less likely than non-caregivers to endorse life-sustaining interventions when asked to consider hypothetical scenarios (Allen-Burge & Haley, 1997).

As adults age, they may become more proficient decision-makers, considering less information before making decisions (Johnson, 1990; Meyer, Russo, & Talbot, 1995; Streufert, Pogash, Piasecki, & Post, 1990) and make decisions more quickly (Meyer et al., 1995). This has been described as a shift from analytic or controlled processing (Yates & Patalano, 1999) to one that uses shortcuts in the complex decision-making process (Finucane, Alhakami, Slovic, & Johnson, 2000; Kahneman, Slovic, & Tversky, 1982) or is more automatic (Titov & Knight, 1997). Reliance upon rule-based or automatic processing (versus analytic processing) may enable adults with diminished cognitive resources to compensate for their cognitive deficits. But if the capacity evaluation emphasizes analytic and controlled decisional processes, it may misjudge equally valid but less explicitly analytic decision-making.

Cultural Considerations in Capacity Assessment

Underlying the comments in the five preceding paragraphs is the issue of individual differences and cultural considerations—that the reliability and validity of capacity judgments may be affected by a failure to appreciate the impact of age, gender, race, education, socioeconomic status, on the process by which others arrive at decisions, and a failure to be sensitive to those differences between the evaluator and the person being evaluated.

Often a first step in a capacity evaluation is one of disclosure—and disclosure can pre-date the capacity referral—meaning the capacity referral can be generated after a physician discloses a medical recommendation and the patient refuses treatment. Although it seems obvious, it is not uncommon to find a situation where the patient does not understand what is disclosed—*not* because the individual has a deficit in "understanding" but because the information was not disclosed in a manner the person could possibly understand because of language differences or diminished health literacy. When low English proficiency is noted, it is important to locate an examiner who speaks the patient's native language, and is familiar with their culture, using native language equivalent (e.g., among other measures, the WAIS-III and Geriatric Depression Scale have Spanish forms), and if a native language speaking evaluator is not available, to use a professional translator. In addition, the examiner should directly ask the patient and family members about cultural considerations and values (see values section later), and consult with practitioners familiar with multicultural assessment (APA, 2005; Virnig & Morgan, 2002).

ADVANCES IN CAPACITY ASSESSMENT

Capacity Assessment Instruments

One approach to improving the reliability and validity of capacity assessment has been the development of capacity assessment instruments, also called forensic assessment instruments (Grisso, 2003). These instruments attempt to operationalize the functional elements of capacity in reference to legal standards, enhancing the inter-rater reliability of capacity assessment and the validity of capacity assessment (i.e., directing the assessment towards the specific capacity rather than general mental status). Some key instruments are summarized in Appendix C, and are further reviewed in various sources (see American Bar Association and American Psychological Association, 2008; Grisso, 2003, Moye et al., 2007).

Capacity Assessment Handbooks

The American Bar Association (ABA) Commission on Law and Aging and the American Psychological Association (APA) sponsored an effort to provide guidance about capacity evaluation to members of their organizations—lawyers and judges (members of ABA), and psychologists (members of APA)—growing out of an existing inter-agency task force (American Bar Association and

American Psychological Association Assessment of Capacity in Older Adults Project Working Group, 2005, 2006, 2008). Similar efforts are under way for other disciplines such as physicians and financial professionals. The *ABA-APA Handbook for Psychologists* (American Bar Association and American Psychological Association, 2008; henceforth referred to as the *Handbook*) describes a nine part conceptual framework for capacity assessment, and a process for capacity assessment. The remainder of this chapter will summarize the framework and process, illustrate its use in a case, and summarize available capacity assessment tools.

Capacity Assessment Framework

The *Handbook* outlines nine components necessary for clinical capacity assessment of older adults: (1) Legal Standard; (2) Functional Elements; (3) Diagnosis; (4) Cognitive Underpinnings; (5) Psychiatric or Emotional Factors; (6) Values; (7) Risk Considerations; (8) Steps to Enhance Capacity; and (9) Clinical Judgment of Capacity. This framework represents an evolution of the seminal work by Tom Grisso (Grisso, 1986, 2003) to provide a framework for the evaluation of capacities. This framework differs from Dr Grisso's in that it is directed towards the psychologist practicing in a clinical setting with older adults, reflecting clinical considerations such as consideration of values, weighing of clinical risks, enhancing clinical functioning, and integrates the evolution of guardianship law (specifically the primary emphasis on an individual's functioning). Each of the components will be briefly described (for detailed review, refer to the *Handbook* available at http://www.apa.org/pi/aging/capacity_psychologist_handbook.pdf, or through request to the APA Office on Aging).

Legal Standard

As noted above, the clinician must begin with an understanding of the legal standard for the specific capacity in question, and have familiarity with the legal process being considered. Issues to clarify might include: Is guardianship being pursued? What is the definition of incapacity under guardianship in the older adult's state of residence? What is the legal procedure? What is required in the clinical evaluation? Or, if medical consent is the issue, what is the definition of medical consent capacity in the state in statutes (such as durable power of attorney or health care decision-making statutes) and how does case law refine that definition? Does the person have a surrogate appointed? If not, does the state have a default surrogate consent law? What sorts of decisions can a surrogate make versus which ones need to be reviewed by the court? As previously noted, answers to these questions can be found by accessing state-specific guardianship information on the ABA's Commission for Law and Aging website and/or by conferring with a lawyer who is familiar with legal issues in the patient's state.

Knowing this information will help the evaluator plan for the clinical assessment to ensure all components required by law are addressed, and so that the evaluator can work with the health care team to guide the approach to the case. It is possible that a request for a clinical evaluation of capacity may be made by an individual not familiar with the law or related practice. For example, a request may be made for a clinical evaluation of financial capacity to support an application for a guardian to complete paperwork necessary for nursing home admission. However, if the individual has a previously appointed health care proxy and a previously appointed durable power of attorney, and the nursing home will work with such surrogates who can support the older adult in navigating the transfer to the nursing facility, this process might be considered as an alternative to the potential loss of rights associated with a guardianship procedure.

Functional Elements

After clarifying the capacity issue in question, and becoming familiar with the legal standard, the evaluator can then discern the constituent functional elements of the capacity. Sometimes the legal standard will provide direction on the functional elements—for example, in medical consent the functional elements are "understanding, appreciation, reasoning, and expressing a choice" as defined in the law. At other times the evaluator will need to refer to existing resources or use their own judgment in outlining the key functional elements. For example, if independent living is in question, based on a review of the case, the referring party's functional concerns about the individual should become clear with a series of questions such as: Which tasks appear to be most challenging for the individual (managing medications, keeping the home clean, maintaining adequate hygiene, exercising judgment in staying safe in the community)? How have functional concerns caused problems? Are these problems new or longstanding? Have these problems happened or are others afraid they may happen? Clinical literature may provide a guide; for example, activities of daily living (ADLs) (e.g., grooming, toileting, eating, transferring, dressing) and instrumental activities of daily living (IADLs) (e.g., abilities to manage finances, health, and functioning in the home and community) may be areas to evaluate.

Diagnosis

Problems with capacity do not arise simply as a result of old age. It is important to determine the diagnosis driving the functional impairment, as such information will obviously define the likely course of the problem and interventions that may help.

Cognitive Underpinnings

What cognitive functions is the diagnosis likely to affect? What cognitive processes are necessary to support the functions in question? It is useful to go into a capacity evaluation with a list of cognitive tasks that are likely most relevant to the diagnosis or functional abilities, as this will direct the selection of the neuropsychological battery. Further, describing functional deficits alone is usually insufficient to come to an informed judgment about capacity. Knowing the cognitive underpinnings of a functional task, and assessing these, often leads to a more complete prediction of how the person might perform the task over time in an unsupervised setting. Assessment of cognition is also often necessary to provide information relevant to the legal standard. For example, cognition is a component of incapacity under guardianship statutes in most states. Assessment of cognition should of course consider the individual's educational, socioeconomic, and racial background in the interpretation of test data, as would occur in any sound neuropsychological assessment, and special attention should be paid to utilizing tests that have been adequately normed on older adults (Busch & Chapin, 2008).

Psychiatric or Emotional Factors

For some individuals, it is not so much the neurocognitive deficits that explain the functional impairment, but psychiatric or emotional factors (such as an individual who has bipolar disorder, lacks insight, is non-compliant with medications, and is frequently manic). Similarly, profound depression or significant delusional disorder may impair an individual's capacity.

Values and Preferences

Many general psychological or neuropsychological geriatric assessments may consider the person's functional, cognitive, and emotional abilities in the context of a diagnosis. The sixth component in the capacity framework presented in the *Handbook* further distinguishes how a capacity assessment may differ from a general geriatric assessment. Age, race, ethnicity, culture, gender, sexual orientation, and religion may impact a person's values and preferences for health care, where or how they live, how money is spent, with whom time is spent, and the level of risk or comfort that is desirable to make life good or meaningful, among other factors (Blackhall, Murphy, Frank, Michel, & Azen, 1995; Hornung et al., 1998). Such values lay the personal foundation for decisions. Consideration of values is one of the key areas where issues of diversity and individual differences enter into a capacity assessment. The extent to which an individual's current decisions are consistent with longstanding values may be an indicator of capacity (American Bar Association, 2002), although it should be noted that values may change with experience, so a change in values does not indicate a change in capacity. Capacity assessments often involve understanding the process by which a person came to a decision. The evaluator's job is to evaluate the decision-making *process*, but not the outcome. Thus, it is important to remember that an individual has the right to make a decision that the examiner may personally think is unwise for the individual, especially when those decisions are consistent with long-held values, preferences, and patterns. Questions to consider adding to a clinical interview to assess individual values are listed in Appendix A of this chapter.

Risk of Harm

Has the individual suffered significant harm in the past? For example, have they been found in grossly unsanitary conditions inconsistent with their values? Has the individual been duped out of a significant amount of money? What are the risks if the individual continues to retain decisional autonomy? If medical consent is in question, how risky is acceptance or refusal of treatment? Risk assessment plays a key role in capacity evaluation (Ruchinskas, 2005), which considers the seriousness of the risk and the likelihood of risk in the context of the supports available (or that could be made available) to minimize the risk. Although some degree of risk is present in making any decision or doing any task, the evaluator examines whether the risk facing the individual is significant, and more than their peers face in similar situations.

Means to Enhance Capacity

The eighth component of the capacity framework presented in the *Handbook* is a consideration of maximizing capacity both during the evaluation and in the future. At times, an older adult may be thought to lack capacity, when instead the issue is that accommodations are needed to enhance hearing or vision, or to break complex information down into smaller elements; or perhaps interventions can improve cognitive or psychiatric deficits. Like any geriatric assessment, capacity evaluation can provide an opportunity to outline interventions—and to determine whether capacity needs to be reconsidered after interventions have been given time to work. Familiarity with common interventions to help older adults compensate for sensory, cognitive, and physical deficits is therefore useful for those doing capacity evaluation. A list of such interventions is provided in Appendix B.

It is in this section that the clinician will wish to be clear about the need for re-evaluation. Repeat decisional capacity assessments can be important tools in measuring change over time; assisting with differential diagnosis; and determining when changes in medical, cognitive, or psychiatric status are likely to impact capacity. The clinician completing the initial assessment will recommend that a repeat assessment occur after a given amount of time, based on the estimated time it may take for a condition, such as delirium, to clear, treatment to work, or a situation to change. The process of decisional capacity reassessment should factor in all of the issues that are considered in any type of psychometrically based reassessment, including the potential impact of practice effects, the need to compare results against baseline measures, the determination of reliable change, and the need to determine what specific measures should be readministered (i.e., depending on the question, it may not be necessary to re administer the entire battery).

Clinical Judgment

Often, when new to the process of capacity evaluation, it is natural to feel "I've assessed the measurable things—functioning, cognition, psychiatric symptoms—I understand the diagnostic cause, and I have a good sense of what this person's values are and the risks facing this person, but how do I pull it all together to provide an answer?" What is often challenging about capacity assessment is that the evaluator is being asked to provide a clear, concise, clinical judgment—and quite often a dichotomous one (yes or no)—for a very complex situation with potentially agonizing ethical implications.

A professional clinical judgment is just that: it is the evaluator's opinion, bringing together all the data and weighing it in light of the person's values, risks, and interventions to maximize functioning. Like a neuropsychological report, a capacity report may elucidate the diagnosis and describe the cognitive strengths and weaknesses. However, the capacity report goes beyond this to offer an opinion about the capacity in question. Although coordinating the data and considerations can feel overwhelming at times, it is important to remember that a structured, well-planned, comprehensive evaluation is more likely to lead the evaluator to a conclusion than an informal subjective interview that does not assess the constituent functional elements or the cognitive and psychiatric impairments related to those. But that is not to say that a judgment will necessarily be easy to form or to offer. Clinical supervision and consultation are important in gaining clarity and confidence in offering clinical judgments about capacity, especially as the evaluator becomes familiar with the process, and when results of tests or procedures are inconsistent.

A PROCESS FOR CAPACITY ASSESSMENT

The *Handbook* describes in some detail a process for approaching capacity assessment. The process is then summarized in a worksheet, reprinted here in Appendix D. Following some general comments about the process, a case will be presented in order to illustrate the steps involved.

One thing that distinguishes capacity assessment from general geriatric assessments is the extent of work that typically occurs prior to the actual assessment. As outlined in the worksheet, the evaluator must first be an investigator to clarify the referral, namely what capacities are in question, the background to the referral, why the question is being raised, and where the outcome of the assessment may lead. Once the specific capacity in question is understood, the evaluator can define the relevant legal standard and functional elements to consider. As with any geriatric assessment, a review of the record, interviews with collaterals, and preparing for accommodations to maximize functioning during the standardized assessment often pre-date testing with the individual.

Informed consent must be obtained prior to completing a capacity assessment. Such consent should involve disclosure of the procedure, the associated risks and benefits, and assess the individual's understanding of these. The final report should describe in detail what was disclosed and how the person conveyed their consent or assent. The individual may lack the capacity to consent to the evaluation, but still assent (i.e., agree to participate without fully demonstrating an understanding of the risks and benefits), which should then be distinguished and detailed in the written report.

As described in the framework, the standardized assessment likely considers the functional elements relevant to the capacity, and includes a cognitive or neuropsychological battery, and a psychiatric evaluation. One of the most critical ways in which a capacity evaluation is distinguished from a neuropsychological evaluation is the focus on the functional assessment, ideally through the inclusion of standardized capacity instruments geared to assess the core functional elements. A number of these instruments are described or provided in Appendix C. It is beyond the scope of this chapter to describe general neuropsychological assessment. As a general rule it is helpful to evaluate the neuropsychological functioning of the individual, focusing on those neuropsychological tasks most relevant to the capacity in question. For example, if the capacity evaluation request is for an individual who is mildly delirious after one week of refusing dialysis, and the question surrounds the individual's capacity in continuing to refuse dialysis, it will be critical to evaluate mental status and determine the extent to which delirium is impacting the person's consent capacity. At the same time, the degree of delirium may make completion of a full neuropsychological battery impossible and invalid. Therefore, clinical judgment is always necessary in the selection of the neuropsychological battery. For a higher functioning person who is medically stable, and for whom the capacity issue is complex and high risk, a complete neuropsychological assessment can be invaluable. The assessment of values (see Appendix B) and risks is typically completed through a clinical interview with the older adult, as well as through interviews with collaterals and a review of history.

After all assessment data have been gathered, the clinician arrives at a clinical judgment. The worksheet from the *Handbook* suggests the clinical judgment has three components. First, the multi-axial diagnosis should be provided, with explicit discussion of prognoses and recommendations for re-evaluation. Second, the capacity conclusions are offered, integrating the functional findings with the cognitive and psychiatric assessment in view of the values and risks considerations. Finally, recommendations for treatment are offered. Each clinical evaluation of capacity and clinical judgment will be organized according to the training, preferences, and practice patterns of the clinician, and the demands of the case. While this process is one approach that evaluators may find useful, it is not the only approach.

SPECIAL ISSUES IN CAPACITY ASSESSMENT

Capacity assessment rarely occurs as described in a textbook. Evaluating capacities of older adults can be challenging, perplexing, and rife with ethical shades of gray, involving an older adult's personal decisions and the quality of life itself. These evaluations require astute selection and administration of appropriate assessment tests—but that is only the beginning—particularly when the case involves complex contextual, historical, personal, and situational variables. Team members may vary in whether they lead towards autonomy versus protection in the care of an older adult, and the capacity evaluator is often keenly aware of their own internal conflict in both those directions. What follows is a brief exposition of some of the "not in the textbook" questions that have been raised to the authors over the years.

Issues in Informed Consent

There are many complex issues that arise in the process of informed consent—beyond the not so simple matter of whether a person whose capacity you are evaluating has the capacity to consent to the evaluation. One of the challenges that clinicians have experienced is how to deal with concerns that the individual will refuse to consent to the evaluation after the clinician provides full disclosure of the risks of the capacity evaluation—i.e., a loss of rights. Occasionally we have observed students new to capacity assessment who skirt around or even avoid disclosing the risks of the evaluation because they recognize that "If I tell the patient the potential outcome they won't cooperate." But of course the risks of the evaluation must be disclosed to the person being evaluated.

We have addressed this question through both the content and process of informed consent. A subtle shift in discussing the risks of the evaluation can be helpful. For example, clarifying the issue of limited guardianship and comprehensive assessment (or limited interventions—if guardianship is not the issue) is often useful. That is, a comprehensive and complete evaluation may identify areas of weakness in which the evaluator may recommend an intervention or surrogate decision-maker, but can also identify areas of strength in which decision-making autonomy and rights should be preserved. Moreover (and while we recognize this is not always the case), patients know when the evaluator is "dancing around" an issue, and often respond well to direct, clear, and truthful explanations of the concerns that have been raised, and the procedures and outcomes. In our experience, honesty has, at times, laid the groundwork for trust in the working relationship, and that trust has helped to resolve issues collaboratively.

Others have raised the issue of the "slippery slope" of consent. This issue occurs when an individual consents to a "general" neuropsychological assessment and then later want to use the neuropsychological test findings in a capacity determination. This is indeed a significant concern, especially when it happens in complex clinical situations where the patient may have restricted choices in health care—such as patients residing in long-term care facilities or involved in home-based primary care interventions. One suggestion to approaching this problem is to clarify for the team that a neuropsychological evaluation is different from a capacity evaluation, which must involve separate consent, and must consider additional variables, namely functional evaluation and information on values and preferences.

We recognize this is not a fail-safe solution—for example, what to do when that sinking feeling arises while performing a cognitive evaluation: a capacity issue rises up, perhaps involving elder abuse, in the context of a routine cognitive evaluation. It seems unethical not to act on the risk issue and it seems unethical to convert the cognitive assessment into capacity commentary, when the patient did not consent to that purpose. If clinicians find they are working with a population at high risk for "slippery slope" consent problems, the clinician may need to make the initial consent process more robust. In the best of all worlds, the geriatric team is well integrated, aware of the tension between autonomy and protection and their own relative leanings, and are able to establish a productive and trusting relationship with the older adult and relevant community service providers. Consultation with others and experience working with older adults over time can make negotiating these dilemmas more familiar, if not more clear.

Issues of Limits in Test Data and Test Time

Another issue that has come to our attention is the pressure to offer capacity opinions in the absence of adequate data. One example of this is the emergency request that comes in at 4:00 pm on a Friday for a patient who wants to leave against medical advice and the team who feels the patient lacks the capacity to do so, but the patient does not meet criteria for civil commitment. The team wants the decision immediately and the patient does not comply with evaluation.

While time is tight, it is still crucial to approach every referral request as an investigation: ask, why now? Is this really a crisis? Who are the parties involved? It may be possible not to do the evaluation, but instead to do "systems" therapy. Occasionally a patient may want to leave because of anguish over a specific issue that can be mediated if only someone will sit and listen to the patient. Examples of this may be a conflict with a specific provider, having felt forced to undergo a procedure or having not been heard in the midst of a procedure gone awry, or procedures or decisions being repeatedly delayed. Sometimes the issue is pain, fear, loneliness, or something simpler such as a desire for some type of food or object from home.

On the other hand, sometimes the referral is valid—the patient wants to go, they are not in obvious medical distress (such as delirium), but are at risk to return home. The evaluator must obviously do their best, offer an opinion, and of course qualify the opinion in the context of the limitations of the data. In some cases, the individual may not meet criteria for civil commitment, but may be considered an "elder at risk" under adult protective statutes, so adult protective services or other visiting nurse or case management services may be enrolled to provide support after discharge. At the same time, while adult protective services are tremendous resources in supporting at risk elders, the availability of adult protective services does not substitute for a solid discharge plan.

These and other complex ethical issues demand more study and discussion in the literature. It will be useful to hear more from clinicians on the front lines about the dilemmas faced, and avenues for resolution. Determinations of the capacity of older adults who are noted to have cognitive and behavioral difficulties are serious ethical judgments, requiring the careful consideration of clinical data, values, and risks. The clinical evaluations of abilities for these determinations are complicated due to the complex presentation and psychosocial factors in most cases, and often the involvement of multiple comorbid conditions, psychosocial stressors, and systemic and environmental pressures and supports. Clinicians involved in these evaluations must be clear about the assessment task, how clinical concerns differ from legal processes, and how legal standards are evolving, even though there may be considerable confusion in their health care setting about these issues.

A comprehensive capacity assessment can significantly shape the care of the older adult, but is different from other assessments. Careful evaluation of the referral itself and thoughtful planning of the assessment will ensure that the assessment answers the referral question and is ethical in nature. An assessment should include a clinical interview with targeted questions regarding the situation in question and the person's values. Historical information, interview data, and test data must be integrated to arrive at conclusions in the context of a diagnosis and the functional considerations related to the capacity in question. Recommendations for intervention and follow-up should maximize autonomy of the patient and advocate for the use of all appropriate clinical services. The conclusion should be concise and decisive. The case described here illustrates the potential complexity of these evaluations, the care that must be taken in their completion, the importance of considering individual and cultural differences, and the imperative to enhance opportunities for autonomy through clinical interventions while also maximizing safety.

Case Study

Case introduction

Mrs G is an 82-year-old, recently widowed, Caucasian female with medical history significant for mild mixed dementia (symptoms of cortical/Alzheimer's pathology and subcortical/vascular pathology) since 2007, moderate bereavement-related depression (with no prior psychiatric history), congestive heart failure, high cholesterol, diabetes, peripheral neuropathy, recurrent urinary tract infections (UTI), and osteoarthritis. Her primary care physician, Dr B, has been her family physician for at least 20 years. She is currently under his care as a medical inpatient after being treated for delirium, with presumed etiology related to a recent UTI and labile blood sugar (resulting from medication non-compliance in the context of confusion). There is tension between her children, and disagreement about her ability to live independently. Dr B is concerned that she will continue to have repeated episodes of confusion that could compromise her health and safety, and wonders whether her dementia has impacted her independent living ability. He is requesting a decisional capacity evaluation to assess her independent living skills. The process for approaching the case is summarized in the ABA-APA Capacity Worksheet for Psychologists (American Bar Association and American Psychological Association, 2008), a blank form of which is presented in Appendix D.

Name: Mrs G Date(s) of Evaluation: 11/17, 11/19/2009

Psychologist: Dr A Place of Evaluation: Hospital X, Boston MA

A. Pre-Assessment Screening

Issue	Questions to Consider
What functional and decisional capacities are in question:	**What types of decisional or functional processes are in question?** **Independent living** *What data are needed?* ***Functional, cognitive, psychiatric, informant*** *Am I appropriately qualified to assess these?* ***As a doctoral psychologist with experience working with older adults, I feel qualified to assess psychiatric, informant-based, and functional test information. I have basic neuropsychology training, but depending on the complexity of the case, I may need to consult with a neuropsychologist to assist with test selection and interpretation.***

Issue	Questions to Consider
Who is involved in this case:	**Who is the client?** Because this evaluation is being requested by Mrs G's physician, Dr B, Mrs G is the client (if a lawyer were involved or the evaluation was being requested by the court, client information may or may not change). **Who are the interested parties?** Mrs G's three children (two daughters, one son). One of the daughters, Jane, is estranged, and the children disagree about her daily functional abilities. **Who is requesting the evaluation?** Mrs G's primary care physician, Dr B. **Who sees the report?** Dr B, Mrs G. **Is the court or litigants involved?** No, though one daughter, Jane, has remarked that she may wish to hire an attorney if the evaluation shows that Mrs G is able to live independently, given that Jane does not feel she is able to do so.
Who is the older adult:	**What is the person's history, age, cultural background, primary language, sensory functioning?** Mrs G, an 82-year-old recently widowed Caucasian English-speaking female with a high school education. She is hard of hearing.
When does this evaluation need to be completed:	**How urgent is the request?** Dr B would like the evaluation completed prior to Mrs G's projected discharge from the hospital in one week. **Is there a court date?** No. **What is the timeframe of interest?** Prediction of functioning post-discharge based on information from prior to and during admission.
Where and how will the evaluation take place:	**In what setting does the evaluation take place?** Inpatient medical hospital setting. **What accommodations are needed to maximize performance?** Quiet testing/interview room in hospital with no interruptions; examiner will speak loudly to accommodate Mrs G's hearing problems, and use a pocket talker.
Why is this question being raised:	**Why now?** Mrs G is hospitalized for recent heart palpitations and confusion, and her daughter Jane voiced concerns to Dr B about her ability to live independently. **What is the history of the case?** She has lived independently since her daughter Jane moved out three years ago. Her husband died four years ago, and she was diagnosed with mixed dementia two years ago. **Will a capacity evaluation resolve the problem?** Yes, it will provide information to answer the current question of independent living ability **Have all less restrictive alternatives and interventions been exhausted?** Not at this time, as the family and Dr B are unsure what types of interventions, if any, would be helpful.
Is the patient medically stable:	**Have all temporary and reversible causes of cognitive confusion been assessed and treated?** She exhibited delirium until three days into her hospitalization; etiology was presumed to relate to a urinary tract infection and labile blood sugar.

B. Informed Consent.

Understanding	Issues to Disclose
Why is the evaluation requested? Mrs G was informed that the evaluation was requested to assess whether she has the skills to return to live on her own given concerns about her "thinking skills" and "ability to manage daily tasks." **Procedures involved in evaluation?** Mrs G was informed that the evaluation would include an interview with her, as well as functional and neuropsychological testing; also, with her consent, an informant interview with her three children and a record review would be conducted.	

(*Continued*)

Understanding	Issues to Disclose

Potential risks? Mrs G was informed that the information gathered might reveal that she needs assistance living independently, or that she needs to live in a supervised setting to maximize her safety and functioning.
Potential benefits? Mrs G was informed that the information gathered might reveal that she does not need assistance to live independently.
Uses of the report? Mrs G was informed that the report would be reviewed by Dr B, and entered into her medical record. She was informed that she may request a copy for her records if she would like.
Limits on privacy and confidentiality? Mrs G was informed that the report, as a part of her medical record, would be available to staff within the hospital, but that it could not be released outside of the hospital or to her family without her consent unless there was a court order to obtain her records.
Mrs G understands and consents.

C. Setting up the Assessment: Legal Standard and Functional Elements.

What is the legal standard for the capacity in question?
Under Massachusetts guardianship law, the most relevant standard for capacity to live independently in this case, an "Incapacitated person" is an individual who has a clinically diagnosed condition that results in an inability to receive and evaluate information or make or communicate decisions to such an extent that the individual lacks the ability to meet essential requirements for physical health, safety, or self-care, even with appropriate technological assistance.
What are the functional elements to consider?
1. Performance of ADLs (activities of daily living) and IADLs (instrumental activities of daily living).
2. Cognitive capacity to reason about independent living (transportation, health, safety).

D. Record Review

Medical records	**Diagnoses:** Mild mixed dementia (symptoms of cortical/Alzheimer's pathology and subcortical/vascular pathology) since 2007, moderate bereavement-related depression (with no prior psychiatric history), medical history significant for congestive heart failure, high cholesterol, diabetes, peripheral neuropathy, recurrent urinary tract infections (UTI), and osteoarthritis. **Laboratory Tests:** Urinalyses showed evidence of UTI until 3 days post-admission; blood sugar elevated until 2 days post-admission; metabolic panel, thyroid, and B12 within normal limits. **Imaging:** 2006 Brain MRI showed evidence of mild small vessel ischemic disease, and no areas of focal abnormality and no acute changes. **Other Treatments:** Obtained copy of 2007 neuropsychological testing report. **Medications:** Glyburide, Aricept, Fosamax, Lipitor, Effexor, Lyrica, and Naproxen prn for arthritis pain.
Legal records	Documents filed in the court: Not applicable. Financial statements: Not applicable. HCP/POAHC documents: None
Other records	None

E. Collateral Interviews

Family (son John, daughter Jane, and daughter Mary were interviewed with Mrs G for 60 minutes on 11/15/08) Mrs G's daughter Jane, estranged from her two siblings, and with a historically strained relationship with Mrs G, is very distressed about Mrs G's functioning (in contrast, her siblings are not distressed, and feel that Mrs G is doing "fine," though they do not visit her often). Jane lives in a nearby state, visits her mother bimonthly, and notes that Mrs G has needed increased assistance with housecleaning, and has exhibited increased forgetfulness during conversations, as well as difficulty navigating to new locations while driving. Jane reports that she became concerned about these issues after Mrs G was first hospitalized two years ago for a urinary tract infection. Jane also feels that Mrs G's diagnosis of dementia should preclude her from living alone and driving. Jane's recent visit to Mrs G prompted Mrs G's current hospitalization last week after Jane observed her to be confused and sluggish. Mrs G had reportedly not taken her medications for a few days and her house was unkempt. Mrs G and her other children feel that Jane is overreacting to the situation. After heated discussion with her siblings and Mrs G, Jane abruptly left the interview. At that time, Mrs G's other children discussed their belief that Jane had been overly dependent on Mrs G, given that she reportedly had lived with Mrs G until three years ago (one year after Mrs G's husband died). At that time, Mrs G reports that she had asked Jane to leave because she felt that Jane was "borrowing too much money from me and not paying me back." At that time, Jane moved to a nearby state, and has been reportedly continuing to borrow money when she visits. Jane would like to move back in with Mrs G, reportedly to help her with her daily functioning, but Mrs G prefers to live alone. All of Mrs G's children are concerned that she has appeared increasingly depressed since her husband died four years ago, and has stopped asking about her grandchildren. Mrs G's other children feel that she has no difficulty with any aspects of daily functioning. They note that Mrs G has had periods of temporary confusion over the past several years during which she is non-compliant with medications and "doesn't make sense," but they feel that she quickly returns to her baseline level of functioning after she "sees her doctor to have her medications adjusted." They note that she manages her finances well, and that she has had no accidents or tickets while driving.

Staff/Professional caregivers Dr B reports that he has been Mrs G's family physician for the past 20 years, and that she had always been courteous and jovial until her husband's death four years ago. Since that time, he feels she has "given up." Although she has had chronic problems with congestive heart failure, high cholesterol, diabetes, and peripheral neuropathy, he felt that these issues were mild and well controlled. He became concerned about intermittent confusion about four years ago when she started to have regular UTIs. He feels her daughter, Jane, had been helpful to Mrs G at times, but also noted that there has been historic stress between Jane and Mrs G. He feels that Mrs G's dementia has mildly worsened over the past few years, but finds her to still be fairly intact.

Other

N/A

F. Accommodating and Enhancing Capacity during the Assessment

The following things were done to maximize functioning during testing:

Assess recent events and losses, such as bereavement
Explore medical factors such as nutrition, medications, hydration
Select tests in consideration of cultural and language issues; administer tests in primary language
Select tests that are validated for the age of the person
Assess ability to read and accommodate reading difficulties
Adjust seating, lighting; use visual and hearing aids
Consider fatigue; take breaks; use multiple testing sessions

G. Assessment Data

Functional Elements: Assessed via:	X Objective Assessment	X Clinical Interview

Tests administered:

Independent Living Scales (ILS)

Summary of results:

Level of impairment: Managing Money subscale = high/independent range; Management of Home and Transportation subscale = moderate/semi-independent range; Health and Safety = moderate/semi-independent range; Social Adjustment = high/independent range.

Describe: Results indicate that financial management and social functioning are intact, but that there may be some need for assistance in management of health, safety, transportation, and home.

Cognitive Underpinnings:	Assessed via:	X Objective Assessment	X Clinical Interview

Tests administered:

Mini-Mental Status Examination (MMSE)
Repeatable Battery for the Assessment of Neuropsychological Status (RBANS-A)
Wechsler Adult Intelligence Scale-III (WAIS-III): Letter-Number Sequencing, Vocabulary, Block Design, Arithmetic, Similarities subtests
Wide Range Achievement Test (WRAT-IV): Reading subtest
Boston Naming Test (BNT)
Delis Kaplan Executive Functioning System (D-KEFS): Phonemic, Semantic Fluency, and Sorting subtests
Trail Making Tests A and BClock Drawing
Finger Tapping
Grooved Pegboard

(*Continued*)

Cognitive Underpinnings:	Assessed via:	X Objective Assessment	X Clinical Interview

Summary of results:

1. Sensory Acuity: Visual and tactile processing intact; Auditory perception intact with combination of hearing aids and examiner speaking loudly
2. Motor Activity and Speed of processing: Finger Tapping and Grooved Pegboard = mildly impaired bilaterally; Processing speed, as assessed with Trails A and RBANS Coding subtest = mildly impaired
3. Attention and Concentration: RBANS Digit Span = average
4. Working memory: WAIS-III Letter-Number Sequencing = moderately impaired
5. Short term/recent memory and Learning: RBANS List Learning = low average; RBANS Story Learning = average
6. Long term memory/delayed memory: RBANS List Recall = mildly impaired; RBANS List Recognition = average; RBANS Story Recall = low average; RBANS Figure Recall = average
7. Understanding or Receptive Language: Within normal limits, as evidenced by intact comprehension throughout interview and testing
8. Communication or Expressive Language: Within normal limits, as evidenced by good articulation and prosody; no anomia in conversation, though mild impairment on BNT
9. Arithmetic: WAIS-III Arithmetic = mildly impaired
10. Verbal Reasoning: WAIS-III Similarities = low average
11. Visual-Spatial and Visuo-Constructional Reasoning: Visual perception is average (RBANS Figure Copy); Visual analysis and synthesis is low average (WAIS-III Block Design)
12. Executive Functioning: Trails B = mildly impaired; D-KEFS Phonemic and Semantic Fluency = mildly impaired; Clock Drawing = borderline impaired (8/10)
13. Other: Baseline verbal intellectual functioning, as measured via reading (WRAT-IV Reading) and Vocabulary (WAIS-III Vocabulary) = low average, consistent with reports that she obtained low average to average grades (C's and D's) throughout elementary school and high school

Psychiatric/Emotional Factors (possible domains):	X Objective Assessment	X Clinical Interview

1. Disorganized Thinking: N/A; thinking was generally linear and goal-directed, with mild tangentiality that may have related to previous diagnosis of mixed dementia versus psychiatric issues
2. Hallucinations: N/A; she denies any history of hallucinations, which is verified by her children and medical records
3. Delusions: N/A; she denies any history of delusions, which is verified by her children and medical records
4. Anxiety: she has no previous history of treatment for anxiety, though she appeared mildly anxious during more challenging cognitive tasks
5. Mania: N/A; she denies any history of mania, which is verified by her children and medical records
6. Depressed Mood: her children report that she has appeared increasingly depressed since her husband's death four years ago, as evidenced by loss of interest in usually pleasurable activities (grandchildren, playing cards), increased isolation, tearfulness, decreased appetite, and concentration problems. Mrs G was tearful when discussing her husband, and agreed that she has felt increasingly depressed. She feels the Effexor, which she started three years ago, has not been very helpful. She scored in the mildly depressed range on the Geriatric Depression Scale (GDS), which was consistent with her endorsement of symptoms on the GDS during her neuropsychological evaluation two years ago
7. Insight: insight appears intact upon interview; Mrs G reports that she needs some help accomplishing yardwork and some physical tasks around the home because of pain in her legs (which Dr B attributes to peripheral neuropathy and osteoarthritis), and she appears to have insight into her depressed mood over the past four years (she attributes this to her husband's death)
8. Impulsivity: N/A; she did not exhibit impulsivity during the interview or testing, her children deny that this is an issue, and there is no evidence of such in her medical records
9. Non-compliance: she has reportedly been non-compliant with her medications during times of intermittent confusion (which Dr B attributes to recurrent UTIs). Her non-compliance likely worsens when she does not take her Glyburide to manage her diabetes, and her blood sugar becomes labile
10. Other: relational stress and alleged financial exploitation related to her daughter Jane

Psychiatric/Emotional Factors (possible domains):	X Objective Assessment	X Clinical Interview

Values

What is the older adult's view of the situation? Mrs G feels that she is able to manage her home very well, though she does admit to having difficulty doing so during periods of confusion. She also feels she needs some assistance with physical tasks due to pain in her legs, but she is uncomfortable asking her family members for help ("I don't want to be a burden to them")

Preferences for how decisions made? And by whom? Mrs G would like to continue making her own decisions regarding management of her home and independent functioning ("I've always been independent. I don't want to go to a nursing home"). She indicates that she will draft advanced directives for the future, and would like her daughter, Mary, to be named as her Power of Attorney for Healthcare and Finance

Preferences for living setting? She would like to continue living in her own home in a rural area of Massachusetts

Goals including self assessment of quality of life? In regard to goals, she mentioned, "I want to take care of my dog and drive to the store whenever I want." Her quality of life appears impacted by her depression ("My life was much better when my husband was living. Sometimes I want to be with him")

Concerns, fears, preferences, religious views? She is afraid of being sent to a nursing home ("I'd rather die"). She is Catholic, and attends church regularly

Preferences for spending and saving? "I've always been a saver, and I like it that way"

Impact of culture, age, sexual orientation, diversity? She identifies herself as "an Irish woman who used to love to live like the Irish," clarifying that she used to love to attend parties and be social. She indicates that she has no interest in any future romantic relationships ("Bob was my one and only")

Views about guardianship (if applicable)? N/A

Risks

Is the risk new or old? New, within the past two years in the context of repeated UTIs and a diagnosis of mild mixed dementia

How serious is the risk? While there have been no serious issues yet, if repeated confusional episodes occur, her personal safety may be at risk due to medication non-compliance and decisions made in the context of impaired judgment

How imminent is the risk? Given her history of chronic UTIs for the past two years (Dr B estimates this has occurred about eight times), risk is likely imminent without oversight of this issue

What is the risk of harm to self? To others? Since her health has been previously compromised due to medication non-compliance in the context of confusion, she is likely to be at similar risk in the future. There are no indications of harm to others, but any instances of impaired judgment in the context of confusion may put others at risk if she were to make poor decisions (e.g., driving while confused)

Are there concrete instances of failure? There have been two hospital visits in the past two years to treat confusion related to chronic UTIs. She has also been treated as an outpatient for UTIs at least six times in the same period of time. According to her daughter, Jane, there may have been more instances of intermittent confusion, though this cannot be verified at this time

How objective is the assessment of risk? Risk assessment data was gathered through multiple methods (record review, informant interview, patient interview), with generally converging results, so assessment is deemed valid

H. Findings

Diagnoses and Prognoses

What diagnoses account for the deficits? Mild, mixed dementia

As compared to her low average to average estimated baseline intellectual functioning, she exhibits relative cognitive deficits in domains of working memory (moderately impaired), processing speed (mildly impaired), motor speed and dexterity (mildly impaired), verbal and non-verbal abstraction (low average), executive functioning (mildly impaired), complex verbal learning (low average), and verbal recall (mildly impaired, but with average performance under conditions of cueing/multiple choice). Cognitive functioning was within expected limits in domains of attention (average), new learning when provided with contextual cues (story learning = average), non-verbal recall, receptive language (intact), and visuospatial perception (average). Findings are generally consistent with previous neuropsychological test results, with the exception of slightly lower delayed list

(*Continued*)

Diagnoses and Prognoses
memory during current testing (mildly impaired versus borderline impaired previously). Given that the constellation of her cognitive strengths and weaknesses suggested a predominantly subcortical pattern of weakness, as well as a few cortical signs, etiology for these deficits is presumed to be mild mixed dementia. Mild deficits on functional measures of independent living skills (ILS—see results above) is likely related to dementia, given that deficits in abstract problem solving were noted (and likely relate to demonstrated executive functioning impairment). Although she endorses mild depression, this was not judged to account for her performance, given that she appeared engaged in testing, and given the consistency of her profile to previous testing **Can conditions be treated?** Regarding the dementia, she can continue to be treated with Aricept, which may delay future progression of her cognitive deficits. She will also need to maximize her treatment of her vascular risk factors—which put her at risk for future cognitive decline—by maximizing medication compliance, getting regular checkups, engaging in healthy behaviors that can lower the negative impact of vascular risk factors [healthy diet, exercise that is designed to work around her leg pain (e.g. swimming), and active cognitive engagement in novel tasks]. Regarding her intermittent confusion, continued exploration into the etiology and alternative treatments for her chronic UTIs should continue. Increased oversight of her mental status and education for Mrs G about early warning signs of UTIs may assist in early identification of future UTIs **Are deficits likely to get better, worse or stay the same?** Her dementia is likely to worsen over time, given that it has some features that are consistent with cortical/Alzheimer's pathology, though it is noted that she has exhibited only minimal worsening over the past two years (possibly because her predominant cognitive deficits are subcortical, and may not progress unless her underlying vascular health worsens), and her dementia is still classified as mild severity. Her mild depression may either stay stable or continue to worsen unless other treatment modalities are considered (e.g., bereavement-related psychotherapy in addition to existing medication regimen) **When should the older adult be re-evaluated?** Repeat neuropsychological evaluation is recommended in one year. Medical follow-up to continue exploration into etiology and different treatment approaches for UTIs will be necessary, but details are deferred to Dr B

Capacity Framework	Capacity Conclusions
1. The functional abilities constituent to the capacity; 2. Cognitive abilities, psychiatric/emotional functioning, and medical diagnoses and prognosis, *as they relate to the functional abilities*; 3. The individual's values, social network, and the specific risks of the capacity situation.	☐ Has capacity for decision/task in question ☐ Lacks capacity for decision/task in question X Has marginal capacity for decision/task in question. Mrs G has the capacity to be discharged to a home setting Nursing home placement is judged to be too restrictive in light of the mild nature of her dementia and given several areas of intact cognition and daily functioning. Guardianship is judged to be too restrictive for her retained strengths and her needs Specific recommendations are detailed below

Steps to Enhance Capacity	Would the Older Adult Benefit from:

Education, training, or rehabilitation?

- **Medical issues:** Teach warning signs of UTIs, so that she can contact Dr B for treatment
- **Family issues:** Reassure that she has the right to continue setting limits with her daughter, Jane, as she wishes.

Mental health treatment?

- **Psychotherapy:** Provide bereavement-related psychotherapy in conjunction with current regimen of Effexor. Consider involvement of family as appropriate. Discus with daughter Jane during feedback session, with Mrs G's permission. Inform Jane that Mrs G's diagnosis of dementia does not preclude her living on her own with some assistance. Invite both to consider how to make their relationship less stressful for Mrs G with family therapy

Occupational, physical, or other therapy?

- **Physical therapy:** Refer to physical therapy to learn exercises to increase her range of mobility in her legs in spite of her pain, which may allow her to accomplish more of the physical tasks around her home

Steps to Enhance Capacity	Would the Older Adult Benefit from:

Home and/or social services?

- **In-home services:** Refer for evaluation through the Aging Service Access Point to consider her need for home health aide, money management support, home chores, meals on wheels, in-home personal alarm, and her interest in senior center activities to decrease isolation. Given some of her difficulties with abstract daily problem solving, additional oversight should also include a focus on ensuring the safety of her home and assisting with complex tasks (e.g., determining whether to hire a repair person). This may be accomplished either through increased family support (e.g., family visiting a few times weekly) or through ongoing case management through her Aging Services case manager
- **Consider move to assisted living:** Moving to an assisted living community may also help to provide increased activities, and given that she was previously a social person, this may combat some of her loneliness and improve her depression and quality of life

Assistive devices or accommodations?

- **Pain referral:** Recommend an evaluation for management of leg pain that prevents her from carrying out some of the physical tasks in her home
- **Assistive walking referral:** Ask physical therapy to also determine if a cane or walker would be helpful

Medical treatment, operation or procedure?

- **Primary care:** Recommend continued regular medical checkups to ensure mental status and medication compliance are intact, and that vascular risk factors are well managed

Other?

- **Alzheimer's Association:** Provide family with contact information for the Alzheimer's Association (which provides resources for individuals with all types of dementia) so that they can learn communication strategies for individuals with memory problems, obtain information on support groups, and receive the contact information for the 24-hour hotline
- **Health care Proxy/Durable Power of Attorney.** Recommend that Mrs G proceed to complete health care proxy and durable power of attorney for health and finances to designate who she would like to be her agent in the event her capacity declines

FUTURE DIRECTIONS

Capacity assessment has recently emerged as a distinct field of legal, clinical, and behavioral research (Moye & Marson, 2007), built on the pioneering work of Grisso and Appelbaum (Appelbaum & Grisso, 1988; Grisso, 1986; Grisso & Appelbaum, 1995), followed by the seminal work by Marson (Marson, Chatterjee, Ingram, & Harrell, 1996; Marson, Ingram, Cody, & Harrell, 1995; Marson, McInturff et al., 1997), and others. The development of standardized capacity instruments has been central to the emergence of empirical capacity research. However, many of these instruments still need more normative data and empirical study, with special attention to issues of diversity. Given that so much rests on these assessments, the need for further normative research is imperative, as we need to be sure that observed "deficits" really represent deficits, rather than performance within the normal range for healthy adults on the task. Also, we need more reliability studies, so that we can be confident in interpreting potential decline via test—retest comparisons

Functional capacity measures are not intended to take the hard work out of professional clinical judgments of capacity, as no test will ever give a "score" for capacity (Grisso & Appelbaum, 1996). The case presented in this chapter clearly demonstrates the complexity of these evaluations, how factors that may affect the reliability and validity of standardized tests (e.g., sensory loss, cultural, and cohort differences) must be considered, and how conclusions rely on a synthesis of test and non-test data.

Despite the complexity of capacity assessment, new instruments that attempt to tailor the assessment to a particular competency issue can be very useful. However, some have expressed concern that instruments developed for competency issues might be over- or misused (Kapp & Mossman, 1996). As an analogy, although some are concerned about overreliance on the Mini-Mental State Exam (MMSE) in the diagnosis of dementia, few clinicians would make a diagnosis of dementia on the basis of an MMSE exam score alone. Rather, most clinicians make a diagnosis of dementia based on extensive evaluation of history, laboratory and other medical data, clinical interview, and testing. In the same way, overreliance or overinterpretation of capacity instrument scores is a risk, but is unlikely by most clinicians that appreciate the complexity of capacity assessments and the advantages and limitations of psychological assessment instruments. When used as part of a comprehensive multidisciplinary evaluation by a qualified user who is sensitive to issues in test administration and interpretation, capacity instruments are invaluable.

Research with capacity instruments has focused on five core issues in capacity: (1) nature of capacity impairment within different patient groups; (2) cognitive predictors of capacity performance within different patient groups; (3) reliability of capacity ratings across clinicians; (4) associations between different methods of capacity assessment (i.e., psychometric versus clinician-based approaches); and (5) longitudinal course of capacity change and decline (Moye & Marson, 2007). These studies have focused primarily on medical consent and financial capacity, and to a lesser extent on independent living and driving, with an emerging literature on research consent. More research is needed to clearly define the key domains essential for the capacity to live independently, as considered in guardianship and distinct from simple measurement of ADLs and IADLs. There is sparse research on testamentary capacity—a growing area of dispute in the context of aging, dementia, blended families and the tremendous intergenerational transfer of wealth in our society. The complex constructs of "self-neglect" and "undue influence" also await constructive definition and validation. Similarly, other capacities such as the capacity to accept/reject adult protective services and the capacity to complete an advance directive are in dire need of additional study and clinical commentary.

There is little research on the reliability of clinical judgments of capacity outside of Marson's work on consent capacity (Marson et al., 1997, 2000). Clinical judgments of capacity are human judgments, and as such are potentially influenced by personal, professional, and social contexts (Braun et al., in press). Empirical studies of cognitive decision-making outside of the capacity framework reveal that decision-making rarely conforms to the rational, logical models that are supposed to underlie them. Unfortunately, the bridge between the science of decision-making and clinical evaluation of capacity has not yet been built. Studies that consider how clinicians integrate multiple sources of capacity data with the elder's situation and values in the context of clinician factors are needed.

Capacity is a complex and enigmatic construct that must be studied, understood, and applied in practice. Its roots are in law rather than in a scientifically based theoretical framework. It has multiple components and determinants. Different clinicians arrive at different conclusions about capacity in similar cases. Unlike almost any other clinical assessment process, the outcome impacts not just the course of treatment, but an individual's ethically and legally sanctioned rights to self-determination. Therefore, the construct has immense personal and policy implications, but is challenging to study (and to obtain funding to study) precisely because of the intersections of law, ethics, clinical practice, and policy that are inherent and must be integrated. Although a clinician's opinion is currently the accepted standard for capacity determination—there is no "gold" standard—clinical opinion can be inaccurate, unreliable, and invalid. Thus, understanding capacity requires a construct validation approach, where multiple lines of reliability and validity data are interwoven to establish knowledge about the nature, workings, and measurement of the construct.

Spirited interdisciplinary collaboration between judges, lawyers, clinical professionals, and policy makers is critical to advancing capacity assessment and resolving issues of autonomy and protection for the growing population of older adults. At the same time, capacity assessment training should become part of the training for physicians, psychologists, and other clinicians who will work with older adults.

APPENDIX A: QUESTIONS TO ADD TO A CLINICAL INTERVIEW

Questions printed with permission from: *Assessment of Older Adults with Diminished Capacity: A Handbook for Psychologists.* © American Bar Association Commission on Law and Aging—American Psychological Association

Questions to add to a clinical interview for medical consent capacity evaluation

These questions are reprinted with permission from the Values Discussion Guide (Karel, Powell, & Cantor, 2004).

1. First, think about what is most important to you in your life. What makes life meaningful or good for you now?
2. Now, think about what is important to you in relation to your health. What, if any, religious or personal beliefs do you have about sickness, health care decision-making, or dying?
3. Have you or other people you know faced difficult medical treatment decisions during times of serious illness?
4. How did you feel about those situations and any choices that were made?
5. Some people feel a time might come when their life would no longer be worth living. Can you imagine any circumstances in which life would be so unbearable for you that you would not want medical treatments used to keep you alive?
6. If your spokesperson ever had to make a medical decision on your behalf, are there certain people you would want your spokesperson to talk to for advice or support (family members, friends, health care providers, clergy, other)?
7. Is there anyone you specifically would NOT want involved in helping to make health care decisions on your behalf?
8. How closely would you want your spokesperson to follow your instructions about care decisions, versus do what they think is best for you at the time decisions are made?
9. Should financial or other family concerns enter into decisions about your medical care? Please explain.
10. Are there other things you would like your spokesperson to know about you, if he or she were ever in a position to make medical treatment decisions on your behalf?

These questions are reprinted with permission from the *Assessment of Older Adults with Diminished Capacity: A Handbook for Psychologists.* © American Bar Association Commission on Law and Aging—American Psychological Association. This list of questions is based on those first developed for the first edition of this book. Additional questions were added by Dan Marson when this list was refined for, and subsequently published in, the ABA-APA Capacity Assessment series.

Questions to add to a clinical interview for financial capacity evaluation

1. What is your financial history? Are you in any debt? Do you live week to week? Are you able to plan ahead and save for the future?
2. Do you have enough money to provide for yourself in your retirement?
3. Have you made a will?
4. How knowledgeable are you about financial investments? What, if any, types of investments do you currently have?
5. What are the things you like to spend money on? In spending money, what are your highest priorities?
6. Are there people or organizations to whom you generally make gifts or contributions?
7. How would you like to invest and manage your money in the future? Do you want to stick with what you know, or are you open to new investment options?
8. Do you prefer higher-risk investments with a possibility of higher-return, or lower-risk investments with a smaller, guaranteed return?

9. If you needed help with your finances, who would you like to help you? Who can you trust to ensure your best interests?
10. How well does this person handle his or her own finances? Is he/she in debt? Does he/she have a good credit record? Is he/she knowledgeable about financial investments?
11. Do you currently have or would you like to obtain a financial advisor? Would this person be a more objective spokesperson than a relative or close friend?
12. Are there certain people with whom you would like your spokesperson to discuss financial decisions on your behalf (family, financial advisors, other)?
13. Is there anyone you specifically would not want to be involved in helping to make financial decisions on your behalf?
14. How closely would you want your spokesperson to follow your instructions about financial decisions, versus what he or she thinks is best for you at the time decisions are made? Are there other things you would like your spokesperson to know about you, if he or she were ever in a position to make financial decisions on your behalf?

Questions to add to a clinical interview for independent living capacity evaluation

1. Where are you living now? How long have you been there?
2. Does anyone live there with you? If not, do you have any fears or concerns about living alone?
3. Does anyone visit on a regular basis?
4. What family and/or friends live in your community who are important to you?
5. What is most important to you about where you live? What makes it "home"?
6. What kind of personal activities do you enjoy doing at home?
7. Are there community activities in which you enjoy participating?
8. What do you like about your house/apartment?
9. What do you not like about your house/apartment? What does not work well for you and why?
10. Do you feel that you can manage the house/apartment on your own? Have you noticed any changes in your abilities to manage?
11. Are there areas of your life that you feel you may need some assistance managing? For instance, do you have any trouble with housekeeping, yard work, preparing meals, shopping, driving, using the telephone, the mail, your health, taking medications, managing your money, or paying bills on your own?
12. Is there someone helping you with any of these things? If so, how long have they been assisting you?
13. If you needed help, who would you like to help you? Is there anyone that you would be wary of? Why?
14. Have you had any safety concerns at home? For instance, have you ever accidentally left the stove or oven on, fallen and been unable to get up by yourself, left your doors unlocked, or invited a stranger into your home?
15. Where would you like to live in the future? Have you ever considered moving to a place where there would be more help for you, such as senior housing, assisted living, or a nursing home? How do you feel about that? What fears or concerns do you have?

APPENDIX B: INTERVENTIONS TO ADDRESS DIMINISHED CAPACITY

This list is reprinted with permission from: *Assessment of Older Adults with Diminished Capacity: A Handbook for Psychologists.* © American Bar Association Commission on Law and Aging—American Psychological Association

The following list was based on a checklist of less restrictive alternatives to guardianship by Professor Joan O'Sullivan, University of Maryland School of Law, edited and refined by the ABA-APA Working Group on the Assessment of Capacity of Older Adults. This list details a wide range of legal and social interventions that can be used to assist someone with functional or decisional compromise instead of guardianship.

If the person needs medical treatment, but is not able to consent:

☐ ***Health Care Advance Directive***

Any written statement a competent individual has made concerning future health care decisions. The two typical forms of advance directive are the *living will* and the *health care power of attorney.*

☐ ***Surrogate decision making by an authorized legal representative, a relative, or a close friend***

In many states, the next of kin are authorized to make some or all medical treatment decisions in the absence of a health care advance directive or appointed guardian.

If the problem involves litigation against or by the disabled person:

☐ ***Appointment of guardian ad litem***

The court in which litigation is proceeding has authority to appoint a guardian ad litem solely for the purpose of representing the best interests of the individual in the litigation.

If the problem involves a family dispute:

☐ ***Mediation***

Referring a case to mediation before a hearing offers a personal, confidential, and less intimidating setting than the courtroom, as well as an opportunity for exploring underlying issues privately.

If the person needs help with financial issues:

☐ ***Bill paying services***

Also called *money management services*, these assist persons with diminished capacity through check depositing, check writing, checkbook balancing, bill paying, insurance claim preparation and filing, tax and public benefit preparation, and counseling.

☐ ***Utility company third party notification***

Most utility companies permit customers to designate a third party to be notified by the utility company if bills are not paid on time.

☐ ***Shared bank accounts (with family member)***

The use of joint bank accounts is a common strategy for providing assistance with financial management needs. However, if the joint ownership arrangement reaches most of the individual's income or assets, it also poses risk in its potential for theft, self-dealing, unintended survivorship, and exposure to the joint owner's creditors. A more secure arrangement is a multiple-party account with the family member or friend designated as agent for purposes of access to the account.

☐ ***Durable Power of Attorney for finances***

This legal tool enables a principal to give legal authority, as broadly or as narrowly as desired, to an agent or attorney in fact to act on behalf of the principal, commencing either upon incapacity or commencing immediately and continuing in the event of incapacity. Its creation requires sufficient capacity to understand and establish such an arrangement.

☐ ***Trusts***

Trusts can be established to serve many purposes, but an important one is the lifetime management of property of one who is or who may become incapacitated. They are especially useful where there is a substantial amount of property at stake and professional management is desired. Special or supplemental needs trusts and pooled income trusts are recognized under federal Medicaid and Social

Security laws as permissible vehicles for managing the funds of persons with disability who depend on government programs for their care needs.

☐ ***Representative payee***

A person or organization authorized to receive and manage public benefits on behalf of an individual. Social Security, Supplemental Security Income (SSI), veterans' benefits, civil service and railroad pensions, and some state programs provide for appointment of a "rep payee." Each program has its own statutory authorization and rules for eligibility, implementation, and monitoring.

☐ ***Adult protective services***

The term protective services encompasses a broad range of services. It includes various social services voluntarily received by seniors in need of support (e.g., homemaker or chore services, nutrition programs). It also includes interventions for persons who may be abused, neglected, or exploited, and which may lead to some form of guardianship.

If the person is living in an unsafe environment:

☐ ***Senior shared housing programs***

In shared housing programs, several people live together in a *group home* or apartment with shared common areas. *Congregate housing* refers to complexes with separate apartments (including kitchen), some housekeeping services, and some shared meals. Many congregate care facilities are subsidized under federal housing programs. Personal care and health oversight are usually not part of the facility's services, but they may be provided through other community social services.

☐ ***Adult foster care***

Adult foster care is a social service that places an older person, who is in need of a modest amount of daily assistance, into a family home. The program is similar to foster care programs for children. The cost varies and may be covered in part by the state social services program.

☐ ***Community residential care***

These are small supportive housing facilities that provide a room, meals, help with activities of daily living, and protective supervision to individuals who cannot live independently, but who do not need institutional care.

☐ ***Assisted living***

Assisted living facilities provide an apartment, meals, help with activities of daily living, and supervision to individuals who cannot live independently, but who do not need institutional care.

☐ ***Nursing home***

Nursing homes provide skilled nursing care and services for residents who require medical or nursing care; or rehabilitation services for injured, disabled, or sick persons.

☐ ***Continuing Care Retirement Communities (CCRCs)***

Continuing Care Retirement Communities, also called life care communities, usually require the payment of a large entry fee, plus monthly fees thereafter. The facility may be a single building or a campus with separate independent living, assisted living, and nursing care. Residents move from one housing choice to another as their needs change. While usually very expensive, many guarantee lifetime care with long-term contracts that detail the housing and care obligations, as well as its costs.

If the person needs help with activities of daily living or supervision:

☐ ***Care management***

This is provided by a social worker or health care professional, who evaluates, plans, locates, coordinates, and monitors services for an older person and the family.

☐ ***Home health services***

If the person needs medical care or professional therapy on a part-time or intermittent basis, a visiting nurse or home health aide from a home health agency may meet that need. Some services may be covered by Medicare or Medicaid, private insurance, or state programs

☐ ***Home care services***

Homemaker or chore services can provide help with housework, laundry, ironing, and cooking. Personal care attendants or personal assistants may assist an impaired person in performing activities of daily living (i.e., eating, dressing, bathing, toileting, and transferring), or with other activities instrumental to daily functioning.

☐ ***Adult day care services***

These are community-based group programs designed to meet the needs of functionally and/or cognitively impaired adults through an individual plan of care. Health, social, and other related support services are provided in a structured, protective setting, usually during normal business hours. Some programs may offer services in the evenings and on weekends.

☐ ***Respite care programs***

"Respite" refers to short-term, temporary care provided to people with disabilities in order that their families can take a break from the daily routine of caregiving. Services may involve overnight care for some period of time.

☐ ***Meals on Wheels***

Volunteers deliver nutritious lunchtime meals to the homes of people who can no longer prepare balanced meals for themselves. The volunteers also provide daily social contact with elders to ensure that everything is okay.

☐ ***Transportation services***

Because many elders cannot afford a special transit service, and are too frail to ride the bus, senior transportation services volunteers drive clients to and from medical, dental, or other necessary appointments, and remain with them throughout the visit.

☐ ***Food and prescription drug deliveries***

Either volunteer-based or commercially based delivery services for food or prescription drugs, may assist those who are unable to leave their home regularly.

☐ ***Medication reminder systems***

This may include a weekly pill organizer box, or another pill distribution system, or telephone reminder calls.

☐ ***Telephone reassurance programs***

These services use volunteers to provide a daily telephone call to older persons living alone.

☐ ***Emergency call system ("lifeline")***

Usually includes equipment added to the telephone line, plus a wireless signal button worn by the older adult. Trained responders provide emergency assistance in the event of a medical emergency in the home, such as a fall.

☐ ***Home visitors and pets on wheels***

Elder service agencies and other volunteer agencies may match elders with home visitors, including visiting pets, which provide social interaction and a form of monitoring.

☐ ***Daily checks on the person by mail carriers***

Many mail carriers, if notified that an elder at risk is living at an address, will monitor the home to ensure that mail has been picked up daily, and, if not, notify a designated individual.

☐ ***Housing modification***

A home may be modified or renovated to enhance safety and the use of technology in the home. For example, grab bars, ramps, night wandering alarms, medication prompt systems, and home-telehealth monitors may be added.

APPENDIX C: CAPACITY ASSESSMENT TOOLS

Instruments were selected for inclusion that:

1. Were developed to assess capacity (versus general functional assessment);
2. Have reliability and validity data.

The following instruments meet these criteria and are available for purchase through publishers.

Capacity to Consent to Treatment Instrument (CCTI) (Marson et al., 1995). The CCTI is based on two clinical vignettes, a neoplasm condition and a cardiac condition. Vignettes are presented orally and in writing; participants are then presented questions to assess their decisional abilities in terms of understanding, appreciation, reasoning, and expression of choice. Responses are subjected to detailed scoring criteria. To purchase, contact: Daniel Marson, JD, PhD

Sparks Center 650K
Department of Neurology
University of Alabama at Birmingham
1720 7th Avenue South
Birmingham, AL 35294-0017

The Financial Capacity Instrument (FCI) (Marson et al., 2000) was designed to assess everyday financial activities and abilities. The instrument assesses six domains of financial activity: basic monetary skills; financial conceptual knowledge; cash transactions; checkbook management; bank statement management; and financial judgment. The FCI is reported to require between 30 minutes and 50 minutes to administer, depending on the cognitive level of the examinee. The FCI uses an explicit protocol for administration and scoring. To purchase, contact: Daniel Marson, JD, PhD

Sparks Center 650K
Department of Neurology
University of Alabama at Birmingham
1720 7th Avenue South
Birmingham, AL 35294-0017

Independent Living Scales (ILS) (Loeb, 1996). The ILS is an individually administered instrument for adults over 65 that assesses the ability to care for oneself and/or property. The early version of the ILS, the Community Competence Scale (CCS), was constructed based on legal concepts, and to enhance expert testimony in guardianship cases. The ILS consists of 70 items in five subscales: Memory/Orientation; Managing Money; Managing Home and Transportation; Health and Safety; and Social Adjustment. An overall score reflects global independent functioning. The ILS has extensive information on norms, reliability, and validity. To purchase, contact: Psychological Corporation.

MacArthur Competence Assessment Tool-Treatment (MacCAT-T) (Grisso & Appelbaum, 1998). The MacCAT-T utilizes a semi-structured interview to guide the clinician through an assessment of understanding, appreciation, reasoning, and expressing a choice. Appreciation is assessed in two sections: whether there is "any reason to doubt" the diagnosis, and whether the treatment "might be of benefit to you." Reasoning is assessed through questions considering how patients compare treatment choices and consequences and apply treatment choices to everyday situations. To purchase, contact: Professional Resource Press.

APPENDIX D: CAPACITY WORKSHEET FOR PSYCHOLOGISTS

Reprinted with permission from: *Assessment of Older Adults with Diminished Capacity: A Handbook for Psychologists*by the ABA Commission on Law and Aging and the American Psychological Association (2008). Please read and review the handbook prior to using the worksheet.

Name: ______________________ Date(s) of Evaluation: ______________

Psychologist: ___________________ Place of Evaluation: ______________

A. Pre-Assessment Screening

Issue	Questions to consider
What functional and decisional capacities are in question:	What types of decisional or functional processes are in question? ***What data are needed?*** ***Am I appropriately qualified to assess these?***
Who is involved in this case:	Who is the client? Who are the interested parties? Who is requesting the evaluation? Who sees the report? Is the court or litigants involved?
Who is the older adult:	What is the person's history, age, cultural background, primary language, sensory functioning?
When does this evaluation need to be completed:	How urgent is the request? Is there a court date? What is the timeframe of interest?
Where and how will the evaluation take place:	In what setting does the evaluation take place? What accommodations are needed to maximize performance?
Why is this question being raised:	Why now? What is the history of the case? Will a capacity evaluation resolve the problem? Have all less restrictive alternatives and interventions been exhausted?
Is the patient medically stable:	Have all temporary and reversible causes of cognitive confusion been assessed and treated?

B. Informed Consent

Understanding	Issues to disclose
	Why is the evaluation requested?
	Procedures involved in evaluation?
	Potential risks?
	Potential benefits?
	Uses of the report?
	Limits on privacy and confidentiality?

☐ Understands and consents ☐ Questionable understanding but assents

☐ Understands and refuses ☐ Questionable understanding but refuses

C. Setting up the Assessment: Legal Standard and Functional Elements

What is the legal standard for the capacity in question?
What are the functional elements to consider?

D. Record Review

Medical records	Diagnoses
	Laboratory Tests
	Imaging
	Other Treatments
	Medications
Legal records	Documents filed in the court
	Financial statements
	HCP/POAHC documents
Other Records	

E. Collateral Interviews

Family
Staff/Professional Caregivers
Other

F. Accommodating and Enhancing Capacity during the Assessment

Assess recent events and losses, such as bereavement
Explore medical factors such as nutrition, medications, hydration
Select tests in consideration of cultural and language issues; administer tests in primary language
Select tests that are validated for the age of the person
Assess ability to read and accommodate reading difficulties
Adjust seating, lighting; use visual and hearing aids
Consider fatigue; take breaks; use multiple testing sessions

G. Assessment Data

Functional Elements	☐ **Objective Assessment**	☐ **Clinical Interview**
1. ____________ Level of impairment: Describe:		
2. ____________ Level of impairment: Describe:		
3. ____________ Level of impairment: Describe:		
4. ____________ Level of impairment: Describe:		
Cognitive Underpinnings (possible domains):	☐ **Objective Assessment**	☐ **Clinical Interview**
1. Sensory Acuity 2. Motor Activity and Speed of Processing 3. Attention and Concentration 4. Working Memory 5. Short-term/Recent Memory and Learning 6. Long-term Memory 7. Understanding or Receptive Language 8. Communication or Expressive Language 9. Arithmetic 10. Verbal Reasoning 11. Visual-Spatial and Visuo-Constructional Reasoning 12. Executive Functioning 13. Other		

(*Continued*)

Functional Elements	☐ Objective Assessment	☐ Clinical Interview
Psychiatric/Emotional Factors (possible domains):	☐ **Objective Assessment**	☐ **Clinical Interview**
1. Disorganized Thinking 2. Hallucinations 3. Delusions 4. Anxiety 5. Mania 6. Depressed Mood 7. Insight 8. Impulsivity 9. Non-compliance 10. Other		

Values	Possible Considerations
	What is the older adult's view of the situation? Preferences for how decisions made? And by whom? Preferences for living setting? Goals including self assessment of quality of life? Concerns, fears, preferences, religious views? Preferences for spending and saving? Impact of culture, age, sexual orientation, diversity? Views about guardianship (if applicable)?
Risks	**Possible Considerations**
	Is the risk new or old? How serious is the risk? How imminent is the risk? What is the risk of harm to self? To others? Are there concrete instances of failure? How objective is the assessment of risk?

H. Findings

Diagnoses and Prognoses	Possible Considerations
	What diagnoses account for the deficits? Can conditions be treated? Are deficits likely to get better, worse or stay the same? When should the older adult be re-evaluated?

Capacity Framework	Capacity Conclusions
1. The functional abilities constituent to the capacity; 2. Cognitive abilities, psychiatric/emotional functioning, and medical diagnoses and prognosis, *as they relate to the functional abilities*; 3. The individual's values, social network, and the specific risks of the capacity situation.	☐ Has capacity for decision/task in question ☐ Lacks capacity for decision/task in question ☐ Has marginal capacity for decision/task in question (if the case is not being adjudicated, recommended course of action)

Steps to Enhance Capacity	Would the Older Adult Benefit from:
	Education, training, or rehabilitation? Mental health treatment? Occupational, physical, or other therapy? Home and/or social services? Assistive devices or accommodations? Medical treatment, operation or procedure? Other?

ACKNOWLEDGMENTS

We thank Paul Anders, Michelle Mlinac, Kelly Trevino, Carolyn Stead, Brea Salib, and Becky Billings for their input on this chapter. We thank the ABA-APA Assessment of Capacity of Older Adults Workgroup for their ongoing dialog about capacity assessment.

REFERENCES

Allen-Burge, R., & Haley, W. E. (1997). Individual differences and surrogate medical decisions: Differing preferences for life-sustaining treatments. *Aging and Mental Health*, *1*, 121–131.

Alzheimer's Association (2006). Fact Sheets: Alzheimer's disease and other dementias; Growth of Alzheimer's disease through 2025; African Americans and Alzheimer's disease: The silent epidemic; Mild Cognitive Impairment; Early Onset Dementia: A National Challenge, a Future Crisis. Retrieved August 2, 2007. From http://www.alz.org

American Bar Association (2002). *Model Rules of Professional Conduct*. Washington, DC: Author.

American Bar Association and American Psychological Association Assessment of Capacity in Older Adults Project Working Group (2005). *Assessment of Older Adults with Diminished Capacity: A Handbook for Lawyers*. Washington DC: American Bar Association and American Psychological Association.

American Bar Association and American Psychological Association Assessment of Capacity in Older Adults Project Working Group (2006). *Judicial Determination of Capacity of Older Adults in Guardianship Proceedings: A Handbook for Judges. Washington, DC: American Bar Association and American Psychological Association.*

American Bar Association and American Psychological Association Assessment of Capacity in Older Adults Project Working Group (2008). *Assessment of Older Adults with Diminished Capacity: A Handbook for Psychologists*. Washington DC: American Bar Association and American Psychological Association.

American Psychological Association Multicultural Guidelines (2005). Retrieved 10/15/09 from: http://www.apa.org/pi/multiculturalguidelines/homepage.html

Anderer, S. J. (1997). *Development of an instrument to evaluate the capacity of elderly persons to make personal care and financial decisions. Unpublished Dissertation*. Allegheny University of the Health Sciences.

Appelbaum, P. S., & Grisso, T. (1988). Assessing patients' capacities to consent to treatment. *New England Journal of Medicine, 319*, 1635–1638.

Berg, J. W., Appelbaum, P. S., Lidz, C. W., & Parker, L. S. (2001). *Informed Consent: Legal Theory and Clinical Practice*. New York, NY : Oxford University Press.

Blackhall, L. J., Murphy, S. T., Frank, G., Michel, V., & Azen, S. (1995). Ethnicity and attitudes toward patient autonomy. *Journal of the American Medical Association, 274*, 820–825.

Blanchard-Fields, F. (1996). Emotion and everyday problem solving in adult development. In C. Magai, & S. H. McFadden (Eds.), *Handbook of emotion, adult development, and aging* (pp. 149–165). London, UK: Academic Press.

Braun, M. M. (2008). Neurological disorders. In D. Wedding, & M. Horton (Eds.), *Neuropsychological Assessment* (4th ed.) (pp. 31–67). New York, NY: Springer Publications.

Braun, M., Gurrera, R.J., Karel, M.J., Armesto, J.C., & Moye, J. (in press). Are clinician's ever biased in their judgments of the capacity of older adult's to make medical decisions? *Generations*

Busch, R. M., & Chapin, J. S. (2008). Review of normative data for common screening measures used to evaluate cognitive functioning in elderly individuals. *The Clinical Neuropsychologist, 22*, 620–650.

Bulcroft, K. A., Kielkopf, M. R., & Tripp, K. (1991). Elderly wards and their legal guardians: analysis of country probate records in Ohio and Washington. *Gerontologist, 31*(2), 156–164.

Cairns, R., Maddock, C., David, A. S., Hayward, P., Richardson, G., Szmukler, G., et al. (2005). Prevalence and predictors of mental incapacity in psychiatric inpatients. *British Journal of Psychiatry, 187*, 379–385.

Caralis, P. V., Davis, B., Wright, K., & Marcial, E. (1993). The influence of ethnicity and race on attitudes towards advance directives, life-prolonging treatments, and euthanasia. *The Journal of Clinical Ethics, 4*, 155–165.

Clemens, E., & Hayes, H. E. (1997). Assessing and balancing elderly risk, safety and autonomy: decision making practices of elder care workers. *Home Health Care Services Quarterly, 16*, 3–20.

Collopy, B. J. (1988). Autonomy in long term care: some crucial distinctions. *The Gerontologist, 28S*, 10–17.

Collopy, B. J. (1999). The moral underpinning of the proxy–provider relationship: Issues of trust and distrust. *Journal of Law, Medicine, and Ethics, 27*, 37–45.

Dudley, K. C., & Goins, R. T. (2003). Guardianship capacity evaluations of older adults: comparing current practice to legal standards in two states. *Journal of Aging and Social Policy, 15*, 97–115.

Edelstein, B. (1999). *Hopemont Capacity Assessment Interview Manual and Scoring Guide*. Morgantown, West Virginia: West Virginia University.

Eleazer, G. P., Honung, C. A., Egbert, C. B., Egbert, J. R., Eng, C., Hedgepeth, J., McCann, R., Strothers, H., et al. (1996). The relationship between ethnicity and advance directives in a frail older population. *Journal of the American Geriatrics Society, 44*, 938–943.

Finucane, M. L., Alhakami, A., Slovic, P., & Johnson, S. M. (2000). The affect heuristic in judgments of risks and benefits. *Journal of Behavioral Decision Making, 13*, 1–17.

Ganzini, L., Volicer, L., Nelson, W., & Derse, A. (2003). Pitfalls in the assessment of decision-making capacity. *Psychosomatics, 44*(3), 237–243.

Garrett, J. M., Harris, R. P., Norburn, J. K., Patrick, D. L., & Danis, M. (1993). Life-sustaining treatments during a terminal illness: Who wants what? *Journal of General Internal Medicine, 8*, 361–368.

Grisso, T. (1986). *Evaluating Competencies*. New York, NY: Plenum.

Grisso, T. (2003). *Evaluating Competencies: Forensic Assessments and Instruments* (2nd ed.). New York, NY: Kluwer Academic.

Grisso, T., & Appelbaum, P. S. (1995). Comparison of standards for assessing patient's capacities to make treatment decisions. *American Journal of Psychiatry, 152*, 1033–1037.

Grisso, T., & Appelbaum, P. S. (1996). Values and limits of the MacArthur treatment competence study. *Psychology, Public Policy, and Law, 2*, 167–181.

Grisso, T., & Appelbaum, P. S. (1998a). *MacArthur Competency Assessment Tool for Treatment (MacCAT-T)*. Sarasota, FL: Professional Resource Press.

Grisso, T., & Applebaum, P. S. (1998b). *Assessing Competence to Consent to Treatment*. New York, NY: Oxford.

Hopp, F. P., & Duffy, S. A. (2000). Racial variations in end-of-life care. *Journal of the American Geriatrics Society*, *48*, 658–663.

Hornung, C. A., Eleazer, G. P., Strothers, H. S., Wieland, G. D., Eng, C., McCann, R., et al. (1998). Ethnicity and decision-makers in a group of frail older people. *Journal of the American Geriatrics Society*, *46*, 280–286.

Horstman, P. (1975). Protective services for the elderly: the limits of parens patriae. *Missouri Law Review*, *40*, 215–236.

Hurme, S. B., & Appelbaum, P. S. (2007). Defining and assessing capacity to vote: the effect of mental impairment on the rights of voters. *McGeorge Law Review*, *38*, 931–1014.

Jefferson, A. L., Lambe, S., Moser, D. J., Byerly, L. K., Ozonoff, A., & Karlawish, J. T. (2008). Decisional capacity for research participation among individuals with mild cognitive impairment. *Journal of the American Geriatrics Society*, *292*, 1236–1243.

Johnson, M. M. S. (1990). Age differences in decision making: A process methodology for examining strategic information processing. *Journal of Gerontology*, *45*, 75–78.

Kahneman, D., Slovic, P., & Tversky, A. (1982). *Judgment under uncertainty: Heuristics and biases*. New York, NY: Cambridge University Press.

Kaplan, K. H., Strange, J. P., & Ahmed, I. (1988). Dementia, mental retardation, and competency to make decisions. *General Hospital Psychiatry*, *10*, 385–388.

Kapp, M. B., & Mossman, D. (1996). Measuring decisional capacity: cautions on the construction of a "capacimeter." *Psychology, Public Policy, and Law*, *2*, 73–95.

Karel, M. J. (2000). The assessment of values in medical decision making. *Journal of Aging Studies*, *14*, 403–422.

Karel, M. J., Powell, J., & Cantor, M. (2004). Using a values discussion guide to facilitate communication in advance care planning. *Patient Education and Counseling*, *55*, 22–31.

Keith, P. M., & Wacker, R. R. (1992). Guardianship reform: does revised legislation make a difference in outcomes for proposed wards. *Journal of Aging and Social Policy*, *4*, 139–155.

Kim, S. Y. H., Caine, E. D., Currier, G. W., Leibovici, A., & Ryan, J. M. (2001). Assessing the competence of persons with Alzheimer's disease in providing informed consent for participation in research. *American Journal of Psychiatry*, *158*, 712–717.

Kim, S. Y. H., Kim, H. M., Langa, K. M., Karlawish, J. H. T., Knopman, D. S., & Applebaum, P. S. (2009). Surrogate consent for dementia research. *Neurology*, *72*, 149–155.

Klessig, J. (1992). Cross-cultural medicine: A decate later—The effect of values and culture on life-support decisions. *Western Journal of Medicine*, *157*, 316–322.

Lai, J. M., & Karlawish, J. T. (2007). Assessing the capacity to make everyday decisions: a guide for clinicians and an agenda for future research. *American Journal of Geriatric Psychiatry*, *15*, 101–111.

Lawton, M. P., & Brody, E. M. (1969). Assessment of older people: self-maintaining and instrumental activities of daily living. *The Gerontologist*, *9*, 179–186.

Loeb, P. (1996). *Independent Living Scales*. San Antonio, TX: Psychological Corporation.

Markson, L. J., Kern, D. C., Annas, G. J., & Glantz, L. H. (1994). Physician assessment of patient competence. *Journal of American Geriatrics Society*, *42*, 1074–1080.

Marson, D. C., Chatterjee, A., Ingram, K. K., & Harrell, L. E. (1996). Toward a neurologic model of competency: cognitive predictors of capacity to consent in Alzheimer's disease using three different legal standards. *Neurology*, *46*, 666–672.

Marson, D. C., Earnst, K., Jamil, F., Bartolucci, A., & Harell, L. E. (2000). Consistency of physicians' legal standard and personal judgments of competency in patients with Alzheimer's disease. *Journal of the American Geriatrics Society*, *2000*(48), 911–918.

Marson, D. C., Hawkins, L., McInturff, B., & Harrell, L. E. (1997). Cognitive models that predict physician judgments of capacity to consent in mild Alzheimer's disease. *Journal of the American Geriatrics Society*, *45*, 458–464.

Marson, D. C., Ingram, K. K., Cody, H. A., & Harrell, L. E. (1995). Assessing the competency of patients with Alzheimer's disease under different legal standards. *Archives of Neurology, 52*, 949–954.

Marson, D. C., McInturff, B., Hawkins, L., Bartolucci, A., & Harrell, L. E. (1997). Consistency of physician judgments of capacity to consent in mild Alzheimer's disease. *The American Geriatrics Society, 45*, 453–457.

Marson, D. C., Sawrie, S., McInturff, B., Snyder, S., Chatterjee, A., Stalvey, T., et al. (2000). Assessing financial capacity in patients with Alzheimer's disease: a conceptual model and prototype instrument. *Archives of Neurology, 57*, 877–884.

Mitchell, A. (1978). Involuntary guardianship for incompetents: a strategy for legal services advocates. *Clearinghouse Review, 12*, 451–468.

Meyer, B. J. F., Russo, C., & Talbot, A. (1995). Discourse comprehension and problem solving: Decisions about the treatment of breast cancer by women across the lifespan. *Psychology and Aging, 10*, 84–103.

Moye, J., Gurrera, R. J., Karel, M. J., Edelstein, B., & O'Connell, C. (2006). Empirical advances in the assessment of the capacity to consent to medical treatment: clinical implications and research needs. *Clinical Psychology Review, 26*, 1054–1077.

Moye, J., Karel, M. J., Edelstein, B., Hicken, B., Armesto, J. C., & Gurrera, R. J. (2008). Assessment of capacity to consent to treatment: current research, the "ACCT" approach, future directions. *Clinical Gerontologist, 31*, 37–66.

Moye, J., & Marson, D. C. (2007). Assessment of decision making capacity in older adults: an emerging area of research and practice. *Journal of Gerontology, 62*, 3–11.

Moye, J., Wood, S., Edelstein, B., Armesto, J. C., Bower, E. H., Harrison, J. A., et al. (2007). Clinical evidence for guardianship of older adults is inadequate: findings from a tri-state study. *The Gerontologist, 47*, 604–612.

Ruchinskas, R. A. (2005). Risk assessment as an integral aspect of capacity evaluations. *Rehabilitation Psychology, 50*, 197–200.

Rutman, D., & Silberfeld, M. (1992). A preliminary report on the discrepancy between clinical and test evaluations of competency. *Canadian Journal of Psychiatry, 37*, 634–639.

Seckler, A. B., Meier, D. E., Mulvihill, M., & Cammer Paris, B. E. (1991). Substituted judgment: How accurate are proxy decisions? *Annals of Internal Medicine, 115*, 92–98.

Staats, N., & Edelstein, B. (1995). Cognitive changes associated with the declining competency of older adults. Los Angeles, CA: Paper presented at the Gerontological Society of America.

Starr, T. J., Pearlmann, R. A., & Uhlmann, R. F. (1986). Quality of life and resuscitation decisions in elderly patients. *Journal of General Internal Medicine, 1*, 373–379.

Streufert, S., Pogash, R., Piasecki, M., & Post, G. M. (1990). Age and management team performance. *Psychology and Aging, 5*, 551–559.

Titov, N., & Knight, R. G. (1997). Adult age differences in controlled and automatic memory processing. *Psychology and Aging, 12*, 565–573.

Uhlmann, R. F., & Pearlmann, R. A. (1991). Perceived quality of life and preferences for life-sustaining treatment in adults. *Archives of Internal Medicine, 151*, 495–497.

Virnig, B. A., & Morgon, R. O. (2002). *Assessing Capacity for Clinical Decisions and Research in Persons with Low English Proficiency: Ethical and Practical Challenges*. Netherlands: Springer.

Yates, J. F., & Patalano, A. L. (1999). Decision making and aging. In D. C. Park, R. W. Morrell, & K. Shifren (Eds.), *Processing of medical information in aging patients: Cognition and human factors perspective* (pp. 31–54). Mahwah, NJ: Lawrence Erlbaum.

CHAPTER

23 Household and Neighborhood Safety, Mobility

Catherine L. Lysack

Institute of Gerontology and Occupational Therapy & Gerontology, Wayne State University, Detroit, MI, USA

INTRODUCTION

Mobility and safety as a fundamental human concern

Living in a home and in a neighborhood where you feel safe, mobile, and independent is about as fundamental to daily living as one can get. For older adults this is no less true. How do you feel comfortable and secure in your daily activities if you have difficulty getting around your home and community and doing what you need to do? Yet, various health conditions and disabilities, as well as normal aging, bring changes to older bodies that challenge a person's physical abilities and participation in daily activities (Halter et al., 2009). For example, it is not unusual for older adults to have higher rates of heart disease, high blood pressure, and diabetes. Even normal age-related changes such as decreased muscle strength and range of joint motion, poorer vision, and more pain and inflammation are factors. These changes to the body, especially in the "oldest old" (i.e., adults over age 85 years), can negatively impact mobility and independence. Fortunately, there is specialized equipment, commonly called assistive devices and mobility aids, that help mitigate this. Walkers, canes, scooters, and wheelchairs provide mobility support in the home and neighborhood when ambulation is restricted or no longer possible. Home modifications also help. These include, for example, better lighting, removal of trip hazards, and installation of grab bars in the bathroom. Irrespective of the equipment or interventions undertaken, recommendations rely on timely and reliable mobility and safety assessment data. The data provided by evidence-based assessments focused on household and neighborhood safety and mobility help guide clinical decision-making with older adults. The data help identify functional impairments that put older adults at risk and highlight residual strengths and abilities that can be supported. These data are critical for treatment planning and service delivery.

ADL and IADL Assessment as a Starting Point

Any effort to find safety and mobility assessments will identify assessments of activities of daily living (ADL) and instrumental activities of daily living (IADL). Activities of daily living refer to the basic self-care tasks of everyday life. ADLs include dressing, bathing, and toileting, for example. Instrumental activities of daily life go beyond ADLs and include tasks necessary for an individual to live independently in the community. Examples of IADLs include using the telephone, managing money, and preparing meals. ADL and IADL assessments provide a general picture of a person's self-care abilities.

Handbook of Assessment in Clinical Gerontology. DOI: 10.1016/B978-0-12-374961-1.10023-5

There are a wide array of ADL and IADL assessments (Foti & Kanazawa, 2006; James, 2008). Two of the best known are the Katz ADL and the Barthel IADL Index. The "Occupational Therapy Practice Framework" published by the American Occupational Therapy Association (AOTA) provides a nomenclature and organizational scheme for occupational therapy practice in the United States which includes official definitions for 11 ADLs and 11 IADLs (AOTA, 2002). The definitions are consistent with the National Center for Health Statistics. Occupational therapists are the health care professionals who most often assess ADL and IADL in the hospital and community, but these assessments can be and are used by other professionals.

ADL and IADL assessment data, and more general assessments of function like the well-known Functional Independence Measure (FIM), are valuable tools because they are relatively quick and easy to use with solid predictive power. Data from ADL and IADL and FIM assessments can help predict who is at greatest risk for functional decline in the future. In research conducted with older adults in Michigan, FIM data collected in hospital helped predict which older adults would be discharged home alone, or not (Lysack, MacNeil, & Lichtenberg, 2001; Lysack, Neufeld, Mast, MacNeill, & Lichtenberg, 2003). The same studies showed that self-rated ADL and IADL status, perceptions shared by the older adults' themselves, added meaningful information. Results such as these underscore the value of simple ADL and IADL measures and general disability measures like the FIM in clinical gerontology. However, ADL and IADL assessments and general disability measures are not sufficient for understanding complex home safety and mobility issues, or for predicting, on a case-by-case basis, the underlying reason why one particular older adult is more vulnerable than another. To make these judgments more detailed assessments are required that measure the performance of each older adult within their particular home and neighborhood environment.

The Concepts "Person—Environment Fit" and "Aging in Place"

For those who assess the mobility and independence of older adults, two prominent ideas in gerontology are salient, the ideas of "person—environment fit" and "aging in place."

The idea of "person—environment fit" was first theorized by Powell Lawton nearly 30 years ago (Lawton, 1983). This concept suggests that it is the interaction between the abilities of an older adult and the particular environment in which they live that create the conditions for overall well-being. Thus, a "good fit" would imply a situation where the older adult was independent and safe because the environment did not "press" upon them, but rather supported them and accommodated their frailties. Think of the older adult wheelchair user who can be independent in a ranch-style home with specialized modifications, versus completely dependent in a traditional two-storey house lacking a wheelchair ramp outside and a stair glide to the second floor. In the neighborhood context, think about how much more secure that same older person would be if sidewalks were wide and well lit and pleasant surroundings attracted people of all ages to enjoy the events and activities found there, instead of being dimly lit, with empty and run-down buildings. As this chapter will show, the best assessments of household and neighborhood safety and mobility are those which measure functional performance at the intersection of the aging body and the social, natural, and "built" environments (Letts, Rigby, & Stewart, 2003).

The idea of "aging in place" is a newer concept but no less important. Aging in place refers to the preference that older adults show toward living in their own homes for as long as possible, rather than being forced to move because of their physical limitations or the limitations of their house (Gitlin, 2003; Rowles, 1983, 1993; Wahl & Gitlin, 2007). Surveys conducted by the American Association of Retired Persons (AARP) confirm that three-quarters of baby boomers want to live where they presently live until the end of life (AARP, 2000, 2003). Clinicians today are aware of these findings, and these findings shape practice and research. This is positive for older adults since research shows environmental modifications help reduce the risk of falls in older adults (Cumming, 2002; Mann,

Ottenbacher, Fraas, Tomita, & Granger, 1999), and improve functional ability (Freedman, Martin, & Schoeni, 2002; Murphy, Nyquist, Straburg, & Alexander, 2006; Stark, 2004; Wahl, Fänge, Oswald, Gitlin, & Iwarsson, 2009). Assessments provide the critical data necessary to identify exactly how and why a given older adult may be benefiting from environmental modifications or stressed by inadequate supports.

The Reality of Residential Transition in Late-Life

Although accurate and timely assessment of the mobility and safety of older adults is paramount at all times, it can be argued that it is of utmost importance when some critical event threatens the older adult's ability to remain at home independently. The moment of assessment may come slowly, as is the case when a patient has increasing dementia and management at home declines slowly over time. The critical moment of assessment may also come much more quickly, for the professional as well as the older adult and their family, as is the case with a pending discharge from hospital after a stroke or a hip fracture, for example. There is research to show that when an older adult who wants to remain at home can no longer do so, the psychological consequences can be devastating (Sherlock, 2005). Social isolation and depression are among the greatest immediate risks (Bruce et al., 2002). When the determination is that the older adult must move to a more supportive living situation like assisted living or a nursing home, there is also evidence that falls and other injuries increase immediately following the residential relocation (Gitlin, 2003). Most interesting is that this research shows that it is not only the frailty of the older adult that underlies the fall in the new environment, but also the delay in developing new habits and routines in the new environment (Gitlin, 2003). For these reasons, it is essential that the clinician identify the best assessment available and, together with interview data from the patient and family, formulate their recommendations carefully.

Another point about home and safety assessments is that an increasing number will focus on older women. Since women live longer than men, on average, and live more years with chronic health conditions and disabilities than their male counterparts, they will more often be the surviving spouse in a longstanding family home (National Center for Health Statistics, 2008). Among the population 75 years and over, nearly 50% of women are living alone, compared with 23% of men (NCHS, 2008; U.S. Census, 2003). Further, it is estimated that every woman over the age of 65 will make at least one residential move (Calvo, Haverstick & Zhivan, 2009; U.S. Census, 2003). Finally, Sergeant and Ekerdt (2008) have studied the motives for residential mobility in later life and the impact of downsizing on older adults. The authors conclude that residential mobility has numerous causes, but the ultimate decision to "downsize" is the culmination of many years of deliberation and "a constant process of evaluation and re-evaluation of the 'fit' between the home environment and its capability to support one's independence and quality of life" (Sergeant & Ekerdt, 2008, p.12). The reality of multiple residential moves in late-life reminds the clinician that home and safety assessment may need to be an ongoing one, as older adults move into different homes over time. The importance of careful reassessment is clearly important when the goal is to monitor changes in the older adults' abilities over time in the same environment, but also changes in functional ability when the older adult enters a new residential living situation.

The Purpose of the Chapter

The purpose of this chapter is to review home safety, community safety, and mobility assessments that recognize the capacities of the older adult within the context of their daily life. The chapter will take a practical approach, recognizing that busy clinicians need reliable screening tools and more comprehensive assessments.

The chapter organizes the extant literature into three major sections: (1) falls and balance assessments; (2) home safety assessments; and (3) assessments of neighborhood safety and mobility. It should be noted that while these assessments overlap to some degree with general assessments of an older adult's physical functioning, the assessments featured in this chapter are selected for their primary focus on safety and independence within the home and neighborhood environments. Each of the three sections describes the major clinical issues confronting the older adult in each area, including definitions of key terms, and then reviews the most useful evidence-based assessment instruments in that area. The goal of this chapter is to provide busy clinicians with up-to-date information about household and neighborhood safety and mobility, and describe a set of brief and practical assessment tools for use with older adults.

FALLS AND BALANCE ASSESSMENTS

Falls are a serious public health issue facing the elderly population. Approximately one-third of community-dwelling people over 65 years of age will experience one or more falls each year (CDC, 2008; Powell & Myers, 1995; Shumway-Cook, Baldwin, Polissar, & Gruber, 1997; Spirduso, 1995; Tinetti, Speechley & Ginter, 1988). For adults over age 80 years, the frequency of falls increases to nearly 40% (Nickens, 1985; Powell & Myers, 1995). Fall-related injuries are also the leading cause of all non-fatal injuries (CDC, 2008). Nearly 40% of falls occurring in the 65-years-of-age and over population are admitted to hospital for some type of treatment (Tideiksaar, 1997; Shumway-Cook et al., 1997). Common injuries include fractures, bruises, and soft tissue injuries. Serious injury occurs in 5—10% of individuals, including accidental death (Spirduso, 1995). Importantly, a serious fall can represent the end of independent living at home. Approximately 40—50% of fallers admitted to hospitals from their homes will not return home, but rather be admitted to nursing homes (Shumway-Cook et al., 1997; Tinetti et al., 1988).

Even if fallers do not suffer a serious injury, many experience significant restrictions in daily activities (Tinetti et al., 1988). Falling is associated with significant reduction in function and increased morbidity (CDC, 2008). In fact, older adults with impaired ADLs are 2.3 times more likely to sustain a fall when compared with older adults with no such impairment (American Geriatrics Society, British Geriatrics Society, American Academy of Orthopaedic Surgeons Panel on Falls Prevention, 2000; Rubenstein & Josephson, 2002). Older adults with balance and gait impairments are three times more likely to sustain a fall than older adults with no such impairments. It should not be surprising, then, that many older persons experience psychological difficulties directly related to the fall. Among these psychological consequences are fear of falling, loss of self-efficacy, activity avoidance, and loss of self-confidence.

Definitions

A fall is generally understood to mean an unexpected drop of mass from a higher point to a lower point, usually the floor or ground. Falls efficacy is defined as the level of perceived confidence an individual has about carrying out everyday activities without falling. Fear of falling is closely related to falls efficacy and is defined as a decrease in self-confidence to accomplish normal activities of daily living and adopt a lifestyle of inactivity resulting in significant muscular atrophy, most noticeable in lower extremity strength (Lachman et al., 1998; Maki et al., 1991; Tinetti, 1987; Wolfson, Judge, Whipple, & King 1995).

Clinical Considerations

Assessment of falling and balance and falls risk is more complex than it may appear at first. This is due to the complex relationships that exist between a person's basic physical abilities like trunk control and balance and lower extremity strength, for example, and falls risk. In addition to physical factors, there are important psychological variables that play a role. One's sense of confidence about doing things without falling may affect one's willingness to undertake certain activities in the home and wider community. The experience of having fallen and the development of a fear of falling are important factors implicated in activity restriction in older adults (Petersen, Murphy, & Hammel, 2003). Fear of falling is thought to increase the likelihood of future falls, at least for some older adults, through a negative cycle of fear and activity restriction. Research suggests the consequence of a fall is a fear of falling again, which causes restricted activity which in turn leads to diminished physical fitness and diminished confidence which further increases the likelihood of a fall (Scheffer, Schuurmans, Van Dijk, Van Der Hooft, & De Rooij, 2008). Not surprisingly, all of these physical and psychological dimensions of falling and falls risk have been the focus of instrument development. And while understanding is growing about the relationship between these various dimensions of falls and falls risk, it is still unclear how much constructs like fear of falling and falls efficacy, for example, overlap with one another, and the extent to which they predict future falls in populations of older adults. Thus, in selecting an assessment tool, gerontologists, researchers, health professionals, and other clinicians must be very attentive to the purpose to which they intend to put the tool. What dimension of falls risk is most important in each case? The choice of tool may also differ if the older adults are fit and active and independent community-dwelling persons or if they are frail and living in a nursing home or long-term care facility. Care must be taken to ensure the specific items on the assessment will provide the information necessary to meet their clinical objectives.

Methodological Considerations

Perrell and colleagues (2001) provide a very helpful review of falls risk assessment for use with elderly populations, including reliability and validity data about each tool and its sensitivity with different groups of older adults. Their review focuses on measures that objectively assess falls risk, that is, by measuring the actual performance of older adults doing common functional activities. These assessments are typically timed tests or measured in some other standardized way. While these assessments typically take longer to administer and require more equipment, they have the advantage of providing detailed data that may be useful if the goal is a more comprehensive assessment of an older adult's abilities or monitoring change or progress in an older adults' performance in specific tasks over time. In response to the growing demand for quicker assessments used for falls risk screening purposes, new tools have been developed that ask older adults themselves to rate their own perceptions and judgments related to falls risks. These tools are typically brief paper and pencil style questionnaires using Likert scales that are easy to complete and to score. Given specific clinical circumstances, more than one assessment may be indicated.

Both objective performance-based and self-rated measurement approaches are represented in the five assessments described below: the Berg Balance Scale (BBS); the Timed Up and Go (TUG) test; the Falls Efficacy Scale (FES); the Survey of Activities and Fear of Falling in the Elderly (SAFFE); the Fullerton Advanced Balance Scale (FABS); and the Activities-specific Balance Confidence Scale (ABC Scale) and the shorter version of the same scale called the ABC-6.

The Berg Balance Scale (BBS)

Description

The Berg Balance Scale (BBS; Berg, Wood-Dauphinee, Williams & Maki, 1992) is a 14-item scale designed to measure balance of the older adult in a clinical setting. The BBS is one of the earliest performance-based measures developed to assess balance status and falls risk in older adults

(Moreland et al., 2003). The original intent of the tool was to provide an objective measure that would be sensitive to the subtle changes in balance abilities and capable of identifying older adults at different levels of fall risk. The BBS has also been used to accurately distinguish older adults with a history of falls from those who have not fallen. Several studies have found the BBS to be a predictive measure of fall risk. Despite the fact that the BBS was originally validated using acute day-care patients, studies have used the BBS to study higher functioning older adults including active community-dwelling older adults. However, in these situations, the BSS appears to have a ceiling effect and is much less predictive (Boulgarides, McGinty, Willett, & Barnes, 2003; Brauer, Burns, & Galley, 2000). Critics also point out that the BBS does not include test items that evaluate impairments in the multiple sensory systems that contribute to balance and heightened fall risk among independently functioning older adults (Hernandez & Rose, 2008). Nonetheless, the BSS is likely the most widely used and well-known balance assessment (Moreland et al., 2003).

Equipment needed:	Ruler, 2 standard chairs (one with arm rests, one without), footstool or step, stopwatch or wristwatch, 15 ft walkway
Time needed:	15–20 minutes
Scoring:	A five-point ordinal scale, ranging from 0–4. "0" indicates the lowest level of function and "4" the highest level of function. Total score = 28
Interpretation:	41–56 = low fall risk 21–40 = medium fall risk 0–20 = high fall risk <36 fall risk close to 100%

Item description:	**SCORE (0–4)**
1. Sitting to standing	________
2. Standing unsupported	________
3. Sitting unsupported	________
4. Standing to sitting	________
5. Transfers	________
6. Standing with eyes closed	________
7. Standing with feet together	________
8. Reaching forward with outstretched arm	________
9. Retrieving object from floor	________
10. Turning to look behind	________
11. Turning 360 degrees	________
12. Placing alternate foot on stool	________
13. Standing with one foot in front	________
14. Standing on one foot	________
Total	________

Timed Up and Go (TUG) Test

Description

The Timed "Up and Go" Test (Podsiadlo & Richardson, 1991) measures, in seconds, the time taken by an individual to stand up from a standard arm chair (approximate seat height of 46 cm, arm height 65 cm), walk a distance of 3 meters (approximately 10 feet), turn, walk back to the chair, and sit down. This clinical test, developed in a medical setting, asks subjects to wear their regular footwear and use their customary walking aid (none, cane, walker). No physical assistance is given. They start with their back against the chair, their arms resting on the armrests, and their walking aid at hand. They are instructed that, on the word "go" they are to get up and walk at a comfortable and safe pace to a line on the floor 3 meters away, turn, return to the chair and sit down again. The subject walks through the test once before being timed in order to become familiar with the test. Either a stopwatch or a wristwatch with a second hand can be used to time the trial. Like the BSS, the TUG is well known and widely used where the clinical goal is to get an accurate objective assessment of balance. Also like the BSS, the scoring system is easy to use and provides a clinically useful indicator of falls risk for ambulatory older adults.

Equipment needed:	arm chair, tape measure, tape, stopwatch
Time needed:	10 minutes
Interpretation:	Normal healthy elderly usually complete the task in 10 seconds or less. Very frail or weak elderly with poor mobility may take 2 minutes or more.
Clinical guide:	<10 seconds = normal <20 seconds = good mobility, can go out alone, mobile without a gait aid <30 seconds = problems, cannot go outside alone, requires a gait aid A score of more than or equal to 14 seconds has been shown to indicate high risk of falls.

The Falls Efficacy Scale (FES)

Description

The Falls Efficacy Scale (FES; Tinetti, Richman, & Powell, 1990) and the Modified Falls Efficacy Scale (MFES; Hill, Schwarz, Kalogeropoulos, & Gibson, 1996) indicate the level of perceived confidence an individual has about carrying out everyday activities without falling. The FES scale was one of the first scales to assess the perceptions of older adults themselves. A well-known and widely used scale, the FES and now the MFES attend to the role of confidence and how confidence (or its opposite, fear) is implicated in falls. It should be noted that although the FES is often used to measure levels of fear of falling, it is thought that falls efficacy and fear of falling are related, but empirically and theoretically distinct, constructs (Tinetti et al., 1994; McAuley et al., 1997).

The FES differs from the BSS and the TUG in several major ways. First, it solicits the older adults' perceptions about falls risk; it does not measure their objective performance in any way. Second, the FES focuses on confidence; it does not measure objective balance or speed. Third, the FES assessment items are much more functional in orientation than either the BSS or the TUG. Thus, if the clinical concern is primarily with the psychological confidence of the older adult, or with assessment the older adult as they conduct "real" rather than "laboratory" activities, then the FES may be the assessment of choice. Note too that the modified FES expands the original set of items with four items related to the outdoor environment. Again, the functional nature of the MFES makes it a good choice for use with community-dwelling older adults.

Time needed:	5 minutes
Item description:	The FES is a 10-item test. The instruments are straightforward as follows: "On a scale from 1 to 10, with 1 being very confident and 10 being not confident at all, how confident are you that you do the following activities without falling?"

Take a bath or shower
Reach into cabinets or closets
Walk around the house
Prepare meals not requiring carrying heavy or hot objects
Get in and out of bed
Answer the telephone
Get in and out of a chair
Get dressed and undressed
Personal grooming (i.e., washing your face)
Get on and off the toilet

Interpretation:	A score of 70 or higher score indicates fear of falling
Modified FES:	The MFES includes four additional items related to the outdoor environment. These items are: using public transportation; crossing roads; light gardening or hanging out the wash; and using front or rear steps at home.

The Survey of Activities and Fear of Falling in the Elderly (SAFFE)

Description

The SAFFE (Lachman et al., 1998) is used to assess fear of falling and also the level of activity restriction related to fear of falling. The SAFFE contains 11 activities representing a variety of common ADLs and IADLs (e.g., taking a tub bath or shower), mobility (e.g., walking for exercise), and social activities (e.g., visiting friends or relatives). The SAFFE also has three subscales looking at levels of activity, worry about falling and restriction of activities within the last five years.

The SAFFE assessment is similar to the FES in that it assesses older adults' perceptions of their falls risk and the items assessed are very functional ADL and IADL tasks. The SAFFE goes further than the FES, however, in several important ways. First, the SAFFE includes an item related to going out to visit a friend or relative, a social activity, not included in the FES. It also includes "walking for exercise" and "going to a place with crowds." These items are broader than the more ADL focus of the FES. This makes it a better choice for active and independent community-dwelling older adults. Second, the SAFFE provides data on the relationship between feeling worried about doing an activity and not doing it which can be useful in the home health and community settings where research shows that a lack of confidence can lead older adults to significantly curtail their activities. The activity restriction dimension of the SAFFE can provide very useful data that may help to identify older adults who are intentionally limiting their participation in the community. This is very helpful information because research shows activity restriction has negative consequences for overall health and well-being (Li, Fisher, Harmer, McAuley, & Wilson, 2003). Loneliness and depression may be the longer-term consequence when older adults restrict their activities and social participation in the community due to fear of falls.

Items: The SAFFE is an 11-item test consisting of the following items:

Go to the store
Prepare simple meals
Take a tub bath
Get out of bed
Take a walk for exercise
Go out when it is slippery
Visit a friend or relative
Reach for something over your head
Go to a place with crowds
Walk several blocks outside
Bend down to get something

Instructions, Scoring and Interpretation

The SAFFE has three subscales, including fear of falling, activity restriction, and activity level. The fear-of-falling subscale reflects the extent to which participants are worried about the possibility of a fall while engaging in specific activities (e.g., going to a store; 1 = *very worried*, 2 = *a little worried*, 3 = *somewhat worried*, 4 = *not at all worried*). The score is calculated as an average because the number of items differs from participant to participant depending on the number of activities they engage in. Scores on the activity restriction subscale indicate the number of activities (e.g., social activities) that are avoided (compared to the past 5 years) to prevent falls (e.g., "Compared to 5 years ago, would you say that you engage in going to the store; 1 = *more often that you used to*, 2 = *about the same*, 3 = *less often that you used to*). Higher scores are indicative of high fear (fear-of-falling subscale) and high avoidance (activity restriction subscale). In contrast, higher scores on the activity level subscale (i.e., the number of activities that an individual engages in out of a list of 11) can be considered to be indicative of lower levels of avoidance. Lachman et al. (1998) have demonstrated that the SAFFE has satisfactory psychometric properties. Although the SAFFE may be less established than its predecessor the FES, the exercise and social items make it a better choice than the FES in certain situations, as does the emphasis on activity restriction.

Activities-Specific Balance Confidence Scale (ABC Scale)

Description

The ABC Scale (Powell & Myers, 1995) is test of balance confidence. It is also considered a test of fear of falling. The ABC Scale comes in a shorter six-item version called the ABC-6 (Peretz, Herman, Hausdorff, & Giladi, 2006). The 16-item version and the shorter ABC-6 are relatively new assessment tools. They were developed in response to research that showed how important balance and a sense of balance confidence are to predicting future falls. The ABC-6 is quickly becoming the assessment tool of choice for busy clinicians, given its brevity and ease of use and its predictive power that appears to be nearly as good as the full version (Lajoie & Gallagher, 2005). Both scales can be self-administered or administered via personal or telephone interview. A rating scale on an index card is used to facilitate in-person interviews. Participants' instructions are as follows: "For each of the following, please indicate your level of confidence in doing the activity without losing your balance or becoming unsteady by choosing one of the percentage points on the scale from 0% to 100%. If you do not currently do the activity in question, try and imagine how confident you would be if you had to do the activity. If you normally use a walking aid to do the activity or hold onto someone, rate your confidence as if you were using these supports. If you have any questions about answering any of these items, please ask the administrator." Scoring is summative, and divided by the number of items to yield a percentage score out of 100.

The Activities-specific Balance Confidence (ABC) Scale

For each of the following activities, please indicate your level of self-confidence by choosing a corresponding number from the following rating scale:

0%	10	20	30	40	50	60	70	80	90	100%
no confidence										completely confident

"How confident are you that you will not lose your balance or become unsteady when you...

1. ...walk around the house? ____%
2. ...walk up or down stairs? ____%
3. ...bend over and pick up a slipper from the front of a closet floor ____%
4. ...reach for a small can off a shelf at eye level? ____%
5. ...stand on your tiptoes and reach for something above your head? ____%
6. ...stand on a chair and reach for something? ____%
7. ...sweep the floor? ____%
8. ...walk outside the house to a car parked in the driveway? ____%
9. ...get into or out of a car? ____%
10. ...walk across a parking lot to the mall? ____%
11. ...walk up or down a ramp? ____%
12. ...walk in a crowded mall where people rapidly walk past you? ____%
13. ...are bumped into by people as you walk through the mall?____%
14. ... step onto or off an escalator while you are holding onto a railing? ____%
15. ... step onto or off an escalator while holding onto parcels such that you cannot hold onto the railing? ____%
16. ...walk outside on icy sidewalks? ____%"

The Fullerton Advanced Balance (FAB) scale

Description

The 10-item FAB scale (Rose, Lucchese, & Wiersma, 2006) is the newest performance-based measure reviewed in this chapter. The FAB was designed to comprehensively address the multiple dimensions of balance. The FAB scale includes static and dynamic balance activities performed in different sensory environments. This is one of the newest assessments in the area of falls and balance, and unlike many of the earlier assessments which were originally developed for more frail populations (although later widely used in more able-bodied populations), the FAB was specifically designed for use with independently functioning older adults. In recent testing (Hernandez & Rose, 2008), the FAB appears to be less prone to ceiling effects when used with independently functioning older adults. Following in the footsteps of the BBS and the FES, the FAB is a performance-based measure that focuses exclusively on balance-related static and dynamic tasks. The FAB appears quite sensitive to differences at the higher (more independent) end of the scale. The FAB scale is a predictive measure of faller status when used with independently functioning older adults. A practitioner can be confident in more than 7 out of 10 cases that an older adult who scores 25 or lower on the FAB scale is at high risk for falls and in need of immediate intervention. The authors state the FAB is also likely "to serve as a responsive outcome measure for showing change after a treatment intervention" (Hernandez & Rose, 2008, p. 2314).

Equipment needed:	stopwatch, pencil, 12-inch ruler, 6-inch-high bench [length, 18 in (45.6 cm); width, 14 in (35.6 cm); height, 6 in (15.2 cm)], masking tape, 2 foam pads [length, 18.5 in (47 cm); width, 15 in; height, 2.5 in (6.4 cm)], two 18 in lengths of non-slip material, a yardstick, and a metronome
Time needed:	10–12 minutes
Scoring:	Performance on each of the 10 individual test items is scored using a 5-point ordinal scale (0–4) with a maximum score of 40 points
Interpretation:	A practitioner can be confident in more than 7 out of 10 cases that an older adult who scores 25 or lower on the FAB scale is at high risk for falls and in need of immediate intervention

Individual FAB Items

The 10-item FAB scale involves the participant standing with feet together and eyes closed (item 1), reaching forward to retrieve an object (item 2), turning in a circle (item 3), stepping up and over a bench (item 4), tandem walking (item 5), standing on 1 leg (item 6), standing on foam with eyes closed (item 7), jumping for distance (item 8), walking with head turns (item 9), and recovering from an unexpected loss of balance (item 10).

Case Study 1—Falls assessment

Case description

Erma Oldfield is 78 years old and living alone in a two-bedroom bungalow with her two cats. She became a widow three years ago when her husband of 50+ years passed away. Erma is quite healthy for her age. She takes no prescription medications on a regular basis and she rides her bicycle for about an hour along a nearby neighborhood trail about three or four times a week, weather permitting. Erma takes care of all of her indoor housework and most of her outdoor yard work herself, although last year for the first time she hired someone to trim her trees and hedges, clear the leaves out of her gutters on her house, and wash all of her windows from the outside. Erma still drives, although she has had three minor car accidents in the last two years. No one was hurt in these collisions but they were all quite distressing to Erma when they happened. Erma herself feels she is doing "pretty well overall." Her biggest complaints are her declining vision and increased foot pain which seems to be getting worse every winter. Erma has a grown daughter Cindy who lives about one hour's drive away. Cindy is concerned that her mother is becoming less agile and fit, and worries that she might fall while riding her bicycle or while doing chores around the house. Cindy is also very worried that her mother is not a good driver and that a more significant car accident may be just around the corner. Erma has always been quite resistant to seek medical input and has not had a regular doctor for many years. She uses a walk-in clinic near her grocery store very occasionally for seasonal flu shots or a pain medication if her feet "flare up." Cindy has taken her mother to get new eye-glasses recently as well as new orthopedic shoes, but Erma feels that both were really not necessary and only helped "so-so." Cindy is urging her mother to make an appointment with a doctor now and stick with that doctor. She also wants her mother to be more forthcoming about her health concerns so together they can find better solutions to improve her function and safety at home.

Falls assessment procedures

Erma has not fallen yet, but she has two potential risk factors for a fall: declining vision and foot pain which can cause unsteadiness and loss of balance. On the positive side, she does not take multiple medications. Research shows that older adults taking more than four prescription medications have twice the falls risk as those who take no medications (Tinetti, 2003). To gain a quick sense of Erma's perceptions about her balance confidence, a clinician could administer the Activities Balance Confidence Scale which only requires about 10 minutes for Erma to answer the 16 questions. However, the downside of the ABC Scale is that Erma could report "high confidence," but may be overestimating her abilities, consciously or not. The use of the Fullerton Advanced Balance Scale is ideal in this case since it is the only objective measure to include multiple sensory systems. FAB items test for balance with eyes open and closed, and also under more demanding situations like "standing on foam with eyes closed" (item 7). FAB data can quickly identify areas of deficit and overall falls risk. If the results of the FAB put Erma at a mild or modest risk for falls, simple recommendations to improve home safety can be made. If risk is higher, further investigations or referral to a specialist may be warranted.

Issues of Diversity

There are no falls and balance assessments designed specifically for use with racial or ethnic minorities (Newton, 1997). On the face of it, there should be no reason for any minority older adult to be at higher risk for falls on the basis of their race or ethnicity *per se*. However, ethnic and racial minorities do have different rates of certain health conditions that increase their falls risk. For example, older African Americans have higher rates of hypertension and diabetes than their like-aged White peers. High blood pressure and diabetes, also more prevalent in African Americans, will increase falls risk too. Racial differences in the understanding of one's disease process can also be a factor in the assessment process, as Dilworth-Anderson and colleagues (2002, 2008) have shown in the context of dementia. There are other issues that increase falls risk of minorities, albeit less directly. The National Center for Health Statistics (2008) reports that 81% of White adults over age 65 in the United States have graduated from high school, but only 58% of older Blacks and 42% of older Hispanics. Lower educational attainment can negatively impact older adult's understanding of health information, but it also influences the kind of employment one has through one's working years, which in turn determines the type of health insurance and financial resources one has access to in later life. Since health care costs money, some older adults will be more disadvantaged. Clinicians need to be sensitive to these factors and work closely with their minority patients to be sure assessment data are interpreted with care, and recommendations for interventions are not only client centered, but culturally appropriate too.

HOME SAFETY ASSESSMENTS

Home safety assessments go a step beyond assessments of falls and balance. Home safety assessments are broader and include a wider array of factors in the home environment that can pose dangers and threats to functional performance in older adults. Many health conditions like arthritis, hip fracture, and a stroke, for example, limit an older adult's ability to climb stairs, carry out chores inside and outside of the home, and safely use the kitchen and bathroom, long known as the most dangerous rooms in a house from the point of view of home injuries. Home safety assessments also provide valuable information about the types of hazards in the home, as well as information about the ability of an older person to compensate for various bodily impairments through thoughtful adaptation of the environment. The contribution of home safety assessments is that they can identify modifiable risk factors. Falls among older adults can be reduced through evidence-based fall-prevention programs that address these modifiable risk factors. Most effective interventions focus on exercise alone or as part of a multifaceted approach that includes medication management, vision correction, and home modifications (Stevens & Sogolow, 2005). Since injuries in the home, most notably falls, are one of the most common reasons for admission to hospital and subsequent residential relocation in late life (CDC, 2008), it is an area demanding serious attention from clinicians.

Home safety assessments come in two main categories, checklists and "true assessments." Home safety checklists, while sometimes derived from home safety research, identify hazards in the home like improperly lit stairways and scatter rugs that pose a trip hazard. The use of these checklists is primarily educational. They are intended to raise awareness about the dangers in the home that can lead to injuries, falls and accidents. They are used by families and older adults themselves and health care professionals use them to encourage simple efforts that can be taken to remove these dangers in the home. The most common hazards are those that could potentially contribute to a fall, including trip hazards like electrical cords and small area rugs that are not secured, inadequate lighting, and poorly secured or absent handrails in stairways, for example. National organizations with rich educational resources related to home safety and home modifications to enhance safety and prevent falls in and around the home can be found on the internet, including: www.cdc.gov/injury; www.homesafetycouncil.org; www.rebuildingtogether.org; www.homemods.org. Most often home safety checklists do not calculate a score of any kind. They are simply indicators of the presence or absence of a potential problem. While visual inspection of checklist data in dramatic situations may point to home safety issues, more systematic assessment is needed to make a reliable determination about whether the older adult is "safe" or "at risk" at home.

"True" home safety assessments are those that include items that capture the phenomenon of home safety reasonably well and include a scoring system to guide clinical interpretation. Most home safety assessments available today have been developed by occupational therapists. For the most part they are interview-style assessments where "safety rating" is derived through professional evaluation of the physical environment itself in combination with the actual performance of the older adult doing a functional task in that home environment. Although standardized home safety assessments are not always used in clinical practice, oftentimes due to the time it takes to conduct these assessments, they provide significant advantages over home safety checklists. First, they are much more systematic and have been tested for their psychometric properties. Second, they provide a means of identifying at least the most "at risk" older adults. They also gather much more comprehensive data which is often required for justification of requests for home modifications and services, and for any effort to evaluate a fall prevention intervention. The biggest challenge confronting home safety assessment is the difficulty measuring the phenomenon of interest which is so much broader conceptually than, say, balance or even falls. How do instrument developers include sufficient items in their assessment to capture all of the dimensions of home safety? What follows is a review of the best known and most psychometrically sound home safety assessments.

Safety Assessment of Function and the Environment for Rehabilitation-Health Outcome Measurement and Evaluation (SAFER-Home) v.3

Description

The Safety Assessment of Function and the Environment for Rehabilitation-Health Outcome Measurement and Evaluation (SAFER-Home) v.3 is an occupational therapy assessment developed for use with the elderly and adults with disabilities living in the community. A group of experienced occupational therapists and researchers have developed the SAFER-Home v.3 after many years of clinical use and research studies in Toronto, Canada (Chui, Oliver, Marshall, & Letts, 2001). This tool has received the most psychometric testing of any home safety assessment and it is widely accepted to be the best clinical tool available (Chiu and Oliver, 2006; Letts, Scott, Burtney, Marshall, & McKean, 1998). It is also considered the "gold standard" for home safety research. It is available for purchase through COTA Health, Toronto (www.cotahealth.ca).

Items:	SAFER-Home v.3 consists of an easy-to-use checklist of 74 items grouped into 12 areas of concern: living situation; mobility; environmental hazards; kitchen; household; eating; bathroom and toilet; medication, addiction and abuse; leisure; communication and scheduling; wandering and personal care.
Time:	It takes about 45 minutes to an hour to complete the SAFER-Home v.3. The time taken depends on the size of the home and the complexity of the situation. The SAFER-Home v.3 can be used as a pre-discharge assessment. Inpatients can be assessed by an occupational therapist in their own home prior to hospital discharge. The assessment and intervention can ensure safety issues are addressed prior to discharge and facilitate the transition from hospital to home.
Scoring:	Safety is assessed based on the interaction of the person, occupation, and the environment. An occupational therapist uses interview, observation, and task performance to determine the rating. To rate an item, the occupational therapist considers the functional, social, environmental, and cultural aspects of the item.

The 100-page manual provides administrative instructions, detailed guidelines and seven case studies. It provides all the information needed to understand how the tool was developed and tested, whom it is designed for and how to use it. The guidelines and recommendations section provides extensive listings of questions and recommendations for therapists to conduct a comprehensive assessment and to make a wide range of suggestions on how to resolve the concerns identified. The manual also includes a set of case studies that walk the therapists through the process of doing an assessment and making appropriate recommendations.

Conceptually this is an ideal assessment since it is comprehensive and well tested in terms of its validity and reliability. However, its length (approximately 45 minutes) is an impediment to its use in practice settings. But it was not designed as a brief screening tool. Its value rests in its careful design and sensitivity in assessing older adults over time and when evaluation of the outcomes of environment modifications is the primary goal.

Westmead Home Safety Assessment

Occupational therapists in Australia developed two assessments of home safety in the mid to late 1990s, at the same time as the SAFER tool was being developed in Canada. These assessments were called the Westmead Home Safety Assessment (Clemson, Fitzgerald, & Heard, 1999) and the Home Falls and Accidents Screening Tool (Mackenzie, Byles, & Higginbotham, 2000) (see below). Both should be considered to be "home hazards checklists" rather than home safety assessments proper. They are briefly described here given their foundational place in the historical development of these assessments and despite their limitations, for their ongoing clinical use.

The Westmead Home Safety Assessment was developed to help therapists identify physical hazards in and around the home environments of elderly persons at risk of falls. The Westmead Assessment lists 72 possible home safety problems and therapists are asked to indicate "yes" or "no" to the presence of the problems. No score is calculated. The tool is simply used as a guide to therapist's recommendations to modify the home accordingly.

Home-Fast

The Home Falls and Accidents Screening Tool (Home-Fast) is a shorter 25-item tool. Like the Westmead Assessment, it is designed in a checklist format where a "no" response to any of the items indicates that no further therapist action is required. Although further psychometric testing is under way (Mackenzie, Byles, & Higginbotham, 2002) which may lead to a scoring system, at present the inability to calculate a risk score for individuals or to compare the scores of individuals to another are significant limitations of both the Westmead and Home-Fast assessments. The fact that both tools focus nearly exclusively on the physical attributes or hazards of the environment is also a significant drawback to using these tools, since it is now very well understood that the safety of an older adult is a function of their physical abilities and the environment in which they live. There is no such thing as a safe or even unsafe home in an absolute sense, it is only safe for a given person or not, given the specifics of their personal functioning and the type of environment they are in.

Cougar Home Safety Assessment (CHSA) v.4.0

Description

The Cougar Home Safety Assessment (CHSA) version 4.0 (Fisher, Baker, Koval, Lishok & Maisto, 1997; Fisher, Baker, Koval, Lishok & Stine, 2008) is relatively new assessment designed to be used by occupational therapists as part of an intervention effort to help people recognize and reduce safety hazards in their homes. Developed in the United States, it is a 78-item assessment that can be answered by observation, testing of certain home items, and questioning the resident. Items are organized into the following categories: fire hazards/carbon monoxide; emergency/medical; electrical/water temperature; flooring/hallways; kitchen; bedroom; bathroom(s); closets/storage areas; parking areas; entrances and disaster preparedness. In many respects, the CHSA is like the SAFER Tool in terms of types of items included. In other ways it is more like the Westmead and Home-Fast assessments developed before it. Like these older tools, the CHSA is basically a count of potential home hazards. Yet it has two small advantages: it has a scoring system and some of the items included in the assessment require objective performance by the older adult. Thus, the CHSA can be regarded as an assessment that attempts to quantify a specific older adult's safety within their particular home context.

Equipment: Thermometer, flashlight, reaching stick/yard stick to test smoke detector, pen

Scoring: The test administrator assesses the criteria using both observation and manual testing and is rated as safe or unsafe. The total number of items rated as safe is divided by the total number of items rated. This number is then multiplied by 100 to get a safety percentage.

Clinical Guidance

The focus of the CHSA is somewhat broader than the SAFER-Home. Propelled by the knowledge that the most vulnerable group of older adults are those who live alone (Lysack, MacNeill, & Lichtenberg, 2001), and that public health research points to hazards not traditionally assessed by occupational therapists, the CHSA includes items like the presence of carbon monoxide detectors and smoke detectors, for example, that are known to improve home safety in the population overall. The second difference between the two instruments is more conceptual: the CHSA provides a measure of home hazards (counting how many items in the environment are "safe" or not) versus the SAFER-Home which provides a measure of the "safety of the person" on each of the home safety items assessed. This is a key difference. Although the CHSA may identify the presence of many home hazards, this does not necessarily mean the older adult living in that home is "unsafe" or "at risk." Thus, it is suggested that the CHSA be used in conjunction with assessments of the older adult's performance and function to ensure that each individual's performance, environment, and occupation are assessed in home safety evaluation.

A major practical advantage of the CHSA is its availability. It can be downloaded and used with permission, at no charge from the developer's website at: http://www.misericordia.edu/misericordia_pg_sub.cfm?sub_page_id=935&subcat_id=108&page_id=338

Cougar Home Safety Assessment v.4.0

FIRE HAZARDS/CARBON MONOXIDE	Environment Safe	Environment Unsafe	Comments
1. There is a fire extinguisher present on every frequently used level of the house or apartment.			
2. There is a functional smoke detector on the ceiling in every level of the house or apartment (and near all bedrooms).			
3. Type and number of smoke detectors: Battery Electric Smoke detectors tested within last 6 months. Date tested:			
4. There is a functional carbon monoxide detector present on every level of the house or apartment.			

(Continued)

5. Type and number of carbon monoxide detectors:
   Battery
   Electric
   Carbon monoxide detectors tested within last 6 months.
   Date tested:
6. Portable heaters, ashtrays, candles, and other fire sources are located away from flammable objects.
7. Flammable objects are located away from stationary fire sources such as fireplaces, stoves, or radiators.
8. Flammable objects such as towels or curtains are located away from the stove area, and are at least 12″ from the baseboard or portable heater.
9. Chimney sweeps are conducted as follows: Every 3 months for wood; Bi-yearly for coal; Yearly for oil, gas, and any other fuel that does not produce smoke—if frequently used.

EMERGENCY/MEDICAL	Environment Safe	Environment Unsafe	Comments
10. At least one medical alert device is accessible at all times while in the house, and may be reached without significant risk of physical injury.			
11. At least one cordless or accessible telephone is on each level of the house.			
12. Emergency numbers are posted on or near the telephone, or are easily accessible without significant risk of physical injury (i.e., primary physician, pharmacy, closest family member, etc.).			
13. Flashlights are accessible and functional and may be reached without significant risk of physical injury.			
14. Assistive devices are in accessible areas (i.e., walkers, canes, low vision equipment, augmentative devices, long handled reacher, etc.).			
15. Medications are kept/stored in an accessible area and are no older than the expiration date.			
16. All areas of the home are well maintained and clean.			
17. A first aid kit, containing simple instructions, is easily accessible and may be reached without significant risk of physical injury.			

ELECTRICAL/WATER TEMPERATURE	Environment Safe	Environment Unsafe	Comments
18. Major appliances such as microwave oven, washer, dryer, and refrigerator may be accessed without significant risk of physical injury.			
19. All outlets and switches have plate covers, so that there is no exposed wiring and they are in easy reach.			
20. All cords are placed out of the flow of traffic or safely covered.			
21. Cords are not attached to walls or baseboards with nails or staples.			
22. Cords are in good condition (not frayed or cracked).			
23. Electrical cords and appliance cords are located away from the sink and stove areas.			

24. Ground fault switches are present in bathroom and kitchen outlets. *from* www.doityourself.com *"a ground fault interrupter, or ground fault circuit interrupter, is an electrical device that senses a fault in the electrical system and shuts down power to that device."*)			
25. Small electrical appliances (such as hairdryers, curling irons, toasters and electric shavers, etc.) are unplugged when not in use.			
26. Outlets do not appear to be overloaded.			
27. The water temperature is 120°F or lower as tested in a sink or tub.			
FLOORING/HALLWAYS	**Environment Safe**	**Environment Unsafe**	**Comments**
28. Floor surfaces are level with no more than 1/4 to 1/2 inch beveled transitions.			
29. Carpeting is secure and level.			
30. If throw rugs are present, they have a slip-resistant backing.			
31. Hallways, passageways, and stairways are free of clutter.			
32. Hallways, passageways, and stairways between rooms have lighting available.			
33. Night lights are available in all areas.			
34. Indoor stairways have a secure railing on at least one side.			
KITCHEN	**Environment Safe**	**Environment Unsafe**	**Comments**
35. Dials are labeled on stove.			
36. There is no excessive grease or clutter on or around the stove area.			
37. Commonly used items are stored in accessible locations and may be reached without significant risk of physical injury.			
38. Garbage cans, pet bowls, and other objects are not located in the walking path.			
39. There is a stable step stool or reaching stick to access items above arms' reach.			
40. The countertops are free of rough or sharp edges.			
41. There is adequate lighting over the stove and sink areas, where food is cut or sliced.			
42. Refrigerator and freezer are at an acceptable temperature and do not contain expired food.			
BATHROOM(S)	**Environment Safe**	**Environment Unsafe**	**Comments**
43. A slip-resistant mat or surface is outside all bathtubs or showers.			
44. A slip-resistant mat or abrasive strips are in all the bathtubs or showers.			
45. The following bathroom areas are accessible and may be reached without significant risk of physical injury.			
Tub:			
Sink:			
Toilet:			

(Continued)

46. A properly installed grab bar or other stable surface is available and secure near the tub and toilet.			
CLOSETS/STORAGE AREAS	**Environment Safe**	**Environment Unsafe**	**Comments**
47. Closets and/or storage areas have lighting available either inside or outside of the closet.			
48. Commonly used items within closets or storage are accessible and may be reached without significant risk of physical injury.			
49. Walk space near closets and storage areas are free of clutter.			
50. The garage, if used, is accessible and has adequate lighting.			
51. The attic, if used, is accessible and has adequate lighting.			
52. All chemical products are stored in a safe manner.			
53. Any weapons such as guns, knives, ammunition, etc., are out of the view of visitors and are in locked storage.			
PARKING AREA/ENTRANCES	**Environment Safe**	**Environment Unsafe**	**Comments**
54. Parking areas have lighting available and are operable.			
55. Parking areas are reasonably level.			
56. Walkways and sidewalks are clutter free and level.			
57. Walkways and sidewalks have lighting available and are operable.			
58. The doorbell and/or door knocker is/are functional.			
59. House numbers are visible on the home or mailbox.			
60. Outside stairways, if present, have a secure railing on at least one side.			
61. Entrances and doorways to home are free of clutter and hazards.			
62. Outside porches or exit areas have working lights available.			
63. Ramps, if present, are appropriately graded and have accessible handrails which may be reached without significant risk of physical injury.			
BEDROOM	**Environment Safe**	**Environment Unsafe**	**Comments**
64. The bed height allows for getting in and out safely.			
65. Pathways in the bedroom are clear.			
66. A phone is within reach of the bed.			
67. Lamps or light switches are within reach of each bed.			
68. Ash trays, smoking materials or other fire sources are located away from beds or bedding.			
DISASTER PREPAREDNESS	**Environment Safe**	**Environment Unsafe**	**Comments**
69. Disaster kit readily available. Includes: medication list, copy of medical records, extra food (non-perishable) and water, money, contact list, flashlight, Band-Aids, rope, extra clothes, and first aid kit.			

70. Copy of current medication list in a wallet/purse.
71. Copy of medication in a sealed plastic bag placed in disaster kit.
72. Extra month of medications available.
73. Copy of physician's name and contact information readily available.
74. Emergency escape route planned for evacuation.
75. Extra food (also non-perishable) and water in the house to last seven days.
76. Clothes and shoes available for immediate use during disaster or emergencies.
77. Emergency car kit is available for evacuation.
78. Plan for safe place in home in event of tornado/ hurricane/earthquake.

HOME SAFETY SUMMARY

Environment safe
Environment unsafe
Not rated

SAFETY SCORE

Percent safe = {# Safe} ÷ {78 minus # Not rated}
Date Hazards Found (include Item #)

Recommendations

Safety Assessment Scale (SAS)

The SAS (Poulin de Courval et al., 2006) is a very useful addition to the literature on home safety given its explicit focus on cognitive impairment and its role in home safety for older adults. The purpose of the SAS is to identify cognitively impaired clients at risk for accidents. The scale was developed in Canada and tested with 176 community-residing adults over age 65 diagnosed with dementia in Quebec, Alberta, and British Columbia. The SAS has excellent reliability as well as content, criterion, and construct validity.

There is a short and long version of the SAS. In both, there are items in seven sections: (1) caregiver and living environment; (2) smoking; (3) fire and burns; (4) nutrition; (5) food poisoning and toxic substances; (6) medication and health problems; and (7) wandering and adaptation to changing temperature. These areas of assessment are much broader than most other assessments of home safety and this makes it ideal for use by case managers, home health staff, and other health care professionals charged with making clinical decisions about an older adult's ability to remain safe at home. The short form consists of 19 items. It can be administered and scored in 5 minutes. The long form consists of 32 items and is recommended for use when a score of 15 or higher (indicating "at risk") on the short form is obtained. Scoring is straightforward, simple summing items. No specific equipment or training is needed to use the SAS.

Conveniently, the SAS can be downloaded at no charge on the Canadian Association of Occupational Therapists website http://www.caot.ca/pf/default.asp?pageid=1484. Although the developers of the SAS acknowledge that the SAFER Tool provides "a more exhaustive list for risk assessment in specific areas such as environmental hazards and functional limitations for falls or other safety issues" (p. 74), there is no doubt that for quick screening purposes in the home of older adults with dementia, their own instrument, the SAS, is the tool of choice.

Name

CLSC CÔTE-DES-NEIGES

S.A.S. SAFETY ASSESSMENT SCALE

CAREGIVER AND LIVING ENVIRONMENT (1)
a) This person lives on her own. Yes [1] No [0]
b) This person is alone at home.
Always [4] Most of the time [3] Occasionally [2] Never [1]

SMOKING (2)
This person leaves cigarette burn marks on the floor, furniture or clothing.
Yes [1] No [0]

FIRE AND BURNS (3)
a) The stove on/off buttons are located...
on the front of the stove [1] on the top of the stove [2]
behind the hotplates [3]
b) This person is capable of turning on the stove him/herself.
Yes [1] No [0] Doesn't know [1]
c) This person cooks his/her own food.
Always [4] Most of the time [3] Occasionally [2] Never [1]
d) This person forgets a pan on the stove.
Very often [4] Often [3] Sometimes [2] Never [1]
e) The heating system uses...
electricity [1] natural gas [2] wood [3]

NUTRITION (4)
a) This person receives meals-on-wheels or other prepared meals.
More than once a day [1] Once a day [2]
A few times a week (2 to 6 times a week) [3] Once a week or less [4]
b) This person's meals contain foods from different food groups
(dairy products, meat or fish, cereals, fruit and vegetables).
Always [1] Most of the time [2] Occasionally [3] Never [4]

FOOD POISONING AND TOXIC SUBSTANCES (5)
This person can tell the difference between food that is fresh and food
that is spoiled. Yes [0] No [1]

MEDICATION AND HEALTH PROBLEMS (6)
a) This person takes, on a regular basis...*
1 to 3 medications [2] 4 to 6 medications [3]
7 medications or more [4] Does not take any medication [1]
*prescribed medication only
b) This person takes medication to help him/her sleep or relax.
Yes [1] No [0]
c) Does this person suffer from any physical health problem?
None [1] Minor [2] Moderate [3] Severe [4]
d) This person accepts treatment for his/her physical health problems.
Yes [0] No [1] Does not apply [0]

WANDERING AND ADAPTATION TO CHANGING TEMPERATURE (7)
a) This person gets lost in familiar surroundings.
Very often [4] Often [3] Sometimes [2] Never [1]
b) Has this person ever gotten lost? Yes [1] No [0]
c) Can this person find his/her way home? Yes [0] No [1]
d) Does this person dress appropriately according
to the changing temperature, both indoors and outdoors?
Yes [0] No [1]

An Affiliated University Centre
Affiliated with McGill University

Assessed by SCORE ___ 47

The Limitations of Existing Home Safety Measures

Gitlin (2003) has written that the majority of home safety measures available assume that home environmental conditions pose the same level of risk to older people and do not account for the extent of exposure or the user interface. This is very fair criticism and it applies to all of the assessments reviewed above. Regarding Gitlin's point about the extent of exposure, these assessments do not take into account the amount of time an older adult is exposed to each "hazard." There is no weighting system designed into any of the assessments to control for this. Similarly, current assessments do not take into account what what Gitlin calls the "user interface" or what might be more simply described as the way an older adult chooses to perform a given task. Yet this might matter a great deal if the older adult is methodical rather than rushed; experienced in the task versus new to it. Perhaps doing a task in one way rather than another is what makes it safer, and not the task itself. According to Gitlin, measures of the home environment should but do not even begin to capture the more social (e.g., availability and participation of others, social roles) and cultural layers (e.g., beliefs and values that guide interactions within an environment) of the home environment, or what Lawton referred to as "higher order environmental attributes (e.g., engagement, stimulation, satisfaction, novelty, comfort, personal control, and personal continuity)" (p. 634). Gitlin (2003) further writes that although safety "is an environmental attribute that transcends user and place, the full range of items representing this domain may differ depending on person capabilities, contextual characteristics, and personal attributions and meanings." Instrument development, guided by theory, is urgently needed to reflect all of these significant shortfalls. Others have echoed these calls for instrument development (Vik, Nygård, & Lilja, 2007; Wahl, Fänge, Oswald, Gitlin, & Iwarsson, 2009), but the wait for better tools continues.

Case Study 2—Home safety assessment

Case description

Let's return to the case of Erma Oldfield, the 78-year-old woman we were introduced to in Case Study 1 earlier in this chapter. You will recall she had declining vision and foot pain which had been worsening with time. The results of the FABS assessment showed Erma had "moderate" falls risk. Additional neurological and visual perceptual tests identified no unusual findings, although her grip strength and a straight leg test showed her doctor that Erma was not quite as robust as she appeared. Laboratory tests also identified a chronic urinary tract infection and undiagnosed high blood pressure. Unfortunately, a week after receiving the test results and beginning new medications, Erma had her first fall, in the bathtub at home. She broke her wrist on her dominant right hand. About this time, Cindy began to see how many other things were problematic for her mother at home. There was a small flood in the house when, distracted by the phone, Erma forgot to turn off a kitchen tap. Erma also forgot a kettle on the stove when she left for church last Sunday. Fortunately, there was no major fire but the pot melted to the top of her stove. Both incidents were very upsetting to Erma and she has become more downhearted than usual. She is much less interested in having visitors and she tells Cindy she doesn't have the same energy to cook for herself as she used to. If you are the health care professional in charge of Erma's care, what would be your next step?

Home safety assessment procedures

The series of accidents in the home suggest doing a home safety screening assessment. Since there is evidence that cognition may be an issue and not only physical abilities, the Safety Assessment Scale would be the best choice from the assessments reviewed here. Although it is unclear if Erma's difficulties are related to cognitive decline it would take only 5 minutes to administer the SAS short form to get a baseline level of her abilities now. Erma Oldfield's safety at home may depend on it. If Erma's score on the SAS short form was greater than 15, it would be an indicator that she was "at risk." Review the case above and complete the SAS short form. You will see that Erma's score could be as high as 20 or 21. As a clinician you may decide that Erma's score is artificially raised by her recent fall and her adjustment to new medications. You may decide to wait and re-evaluate Erma Oldfield in 3 months after her cast is off, her blood pressure is well managed, and her infection has cleared. Part of your decision may involve more subtle psychosocial dimensions of the case, including how well Erma is adjusting to being a widow and what could be some diminishment in participation in her much-valued family life. Clinicians need to be aware that these less obvious psychosocial dimensions of older women's health require greater attention than they currently receive (Dillaway & Lysack, 2010). Another issue is limitations of the home safety assessments available. None of the instruments currently available can capture Erma's desired patterns of activity in the home, or her perceptions about how the home environment is influencing her activities and participation. A growing number of gerontologists are learning that older people want to participate more than they have the opportunity to. A number of studies state that participating in "meaningful doing" is important for staying healthy and for maintaining a higher level of quality of life for older adults (Vik, Nygård, & Lilja, 2007). These limitations in existing assessment tools must be addressed eventually through improved measurement tools, but until that time, careful clinical observation and interviewing remain crucial. An ongoing process of assessment and reassessment too will provide the data needed for home modifications and home-based tangible and personal social support services that will not only extend the amount of time that Erma can "age in place" but will enhance her quality of life at home as well.

Diversity issues

As you read Case Studies 1 and 2 which describe the falls risk and home safety situation of Mrs Erma Oldfield, do you imagine that she is White? Is this because she "seems" White from the case description, or is it because we are so used to seeing mostly images of White health care professionals and White patients in textbooks? Let's assume for a moment that "Mrs Oldfield" is a Middle Eastern woman named Mrs Fatima Youssef and she came to this country with her large extended family only 10 years ago speaking no English whatsoever. What would you do differently as the health care professional carrying out a falls risk assessment and a home safety assessment? Review the ABC Scale for balance confidence, the FABs screening tool for falls risk, and the SAS for home safety. Are there any items that could potentially cause difficulty? Are there any items that are not culturally relevant or require particular cultural sensitivity? It can be very useful to imagine how the people we encounter in the course of conducting clinical assessments and therapeutic interventions shape our interactions with them. A focus on optimal cultural competency must be the ethical clinician's constant concern.

NEIGHBORHOOD SAFETY AND MOBILITY ASSESSMENTS

For older adults and persons with disabilities, the safety of the neighborhood and one's ability to be mobile in the surrounding community are always major concerns. When the environment is lacking or inhospitable in some way, whether this is due to inaccessible buildings, fear of crime, or even unpleasant public spaces, older people will restrict their activities in these locales (Byrnes, Lichtenberg, & Lysack, 2006; Vik, Nygård, & Lilja, 2007). Activity restriction caused by problematic environments is itself a major risk factor for even further functional decline in older adults already vulnerable from age-related functional declines. From a public health perspective too, everything possible should be done to promote activity and mobility and remove barriers to activity and social participation (Tideiksaar, 2002; Tinetti, 2003; Wahl, Fänge, Oswald, Gitlin, & Iwarsson, 2009). The overall health and fitness of the population is at stake.

Unfortunately, and despite the established link between the quality of an environment and the health of people, the development of assessments to test neighborhood safety and mobility and its influence lag much further behind other areas. At least in part this is due to the complexity of environmental assessment. What factors should be included in a neighborhood assessment? What is the boundary of the neighborhood? What is the best way to measure barriers and facilitators in the environment? An additional problem is the overlap between safety and mobility assessments, as well as their overlap with so-called "participation" instruments based on the World Health Organization's International Classification of Functioning, Disability and Health (for a recent review of the latter see Noonan, Kopec, Noreau, Singer, & Dvorak, 2009). Participation assessments are certainly broader in nature and focus on the overall social engagement of the person in the environment. However, the concepts and their measurement continue to challenge the field. Practically speaking these impediments must be overcome, since it remains a major policy and perhaps even societal goal to provide the opportunities for older adults to "age in place." Aging in place is not possible if neighborhood conditions discourage people from remaining in their homes and neighborhoods as they grow older. It does not take very much for an older adult with some degree of frailty to have reduced mobility and thus activity restriction. For example, what happens when an older adult is too disabled to use existing public transportation services without assistance? If there is no viable alternative method of transportation then the older adult will not leave their home. Private transportation and family members may be available for doctor's appointments, but is it available on a regular basis to meet their IADL and social needs? Cost can be a barrier too. The consequences of restricted mobility (and thus activity restriction) are dire. It is not only that one's daily life activities are made more time consuming, unpleasant, and frustrating; restricted mobility for older adults can mark the beginning of a negative spiral of social isolation, loneliness, and depression (Li & Conwell, 2007). The inability to continue driving is associated with decreased activity and increased depression if satisfactory alternatives are not identified (Marottoli et al., 2000).

Depression in older adults is a significant threat to health and well-being. In 1999, a landmark U.S. Surgeon General's report on mental health found that 8–20% of older adults in the community, and up to 37% in primary care settings, suffer from depressive symptoms (U.S. Department of Health and Human Services, 1999). Recent research in a large sample ($n = 18{,}939$) of community-dwelling frail older adults admitted to long-term care in Michigan showed that 40.5% of the sample had recognized mental disorders, 39.6% used psychotropic medications, 24.5% had probable depression, and 1.4% had self-injury thoughts or attempts (Li & Conwell, 2007). Making treatment more challenging are other comorbid conditions. Impaired cognition, substance abuse, and medication misuse are all known to make depression worse, and complicate depression treatment (Bruce et al., 2002; Dalby et al., 2008). Yet this is the reality confronting many older adults.

Given the varied dimensions of the neighborhood that can impact safety, there are a very broad range of assessments in this realm. Generally speaking, these assessments are at an early phase of development. There are fewer assessments overall and the assessments that do exist tend to have been developed more for outcomes research purposes than for clinical screening purposes. As a result, the following section will be briefer than the falls assessment and home safety assessment sections above. The assessments reviewed below represent those which are best known in their class in the following areas: quality of the environment; environmental barriers; building accessibility; and safety of the neighborhood from a crime and personal security point of view.

Measure of the Quality of the Environment (MQE)

The best example of a subjective measure of the interaction of person and environment is the Measure of the Quality of the Environment (MQE; Fougeyrollas, Noreau, St Michel, & Boschen, 1999). The current version of the instrument (version 2.0) can be ordered online at: http://www.ripph.qc.ca/?rub3=&rub2=4&rub=18&lang=en&id_doc_sel=31.

A list of 109 environment features are scored on a 7-point scale ranging from major facilitators to major barriers to social participation. The environmental factors are classified into six categories: support and attitudes of family; income, job and income security; governmental and public services; physical environment and accessibility; technology; and equal opportunity and political orientations. The question used for each factor is "While taking into consideration your abilities and personal limits, indicate to what extent the situations or factors generally influence your daily life." The MQE is comprehensive and psychometrically strong, and includes many items related to employment, provision of government services, and equal opportunity. Recent research (Levasseur, Desrosiers, & St-Cyr Tribble, 2008) suggest the MQE is useful for older community-dwelling persons; however, its length and the recent finding that as many of half of the items are rated "not applicable" by older adults work against its use in this age group (Levasseur et al., 2008).

CRAIG Hospital Inventory of Environmental Factors (CHIEF and CHIEF-SF)

The CHIEF assessment was originally developed in the context of spinal cord injury (Whiteneck, et al., 2004). The CHIEF exists in two forms, the original 25-item assessment and the 12-item short form which are available with additional information online at: http://www.tbims.org/combi/chief/chiefrat.html. Both versions of the assessment have been used in other contexts, including with older adults. In both, items are scored for the frequency of encountering environmental barriers and the impact of the barrier on participation. The CHIEF includes five barrier factors: (1) attitude and support; (2) services and assistance; (3) physical and structural; (4) policy; and (5) work and school. The internal consistency and stability tests of both versions are similar and moderate to high. The CHIEF provides a measure of general environmental barriers that can be used for population surveys comparing people with and without disabilities. It is not sensitive to small changes, however, and therefore should not be used to measure changes in perceived environmental barriers over time.

The Community Health Environment Checklist (CHEC)

The CHEC is an objective assessment used to determine the accessibility of a building or site. The CHEC assessment comes out of the work of Stark and Gray at Washington University in St. Louis (Stark, Hollingsworth, Morgan, Chang, & Gray, 2008). The CHEC is informed by the ongoing theoretical work begun by the World Health Organization in its development of the International Classification of Functioning, Disability and Health. Thus, the CHEC is useful when the goal is to measure the extent to which factors in the environment can restrict mobility and participation in society.

The CHEC is composed of 65 questions that are divided into five sections: entering the building; using the building; restrooms; amenities; and usability of area of rescue assistance. A score of 100% indicates the highest level of accessibility that can be achieved. Scores for each feature are weighted and summed by subscale. Each subscale score is also summed to create a total receptivity score (maximum of 100). A receptivity score of 100 would indicate excellent receptivity and usability, with 75 suggesting moderate receptivity and 50 suggesting poor receptivity. Good internal consistency (Cronbach alpha, 0.95) has been reported for the Community Health Environment Checklist which can be administered in 10 to 90 minutes depending on building size and rater experience.

Neighborhood Environment Scale (NES)

The Neighborhood Environment Scale (NES) was developed for use in the context of children and families (Crum, Lillie-Blanton, & Anthony, 1996). Although the assessment targets young adolescents, nearly all of the items are relevant to older adults. The NES is an 18-item assessment containing items related to perceived personal safety (e.g., "I feel safe when I walk around my neighborhood by myself"), items focused on the physical appearance of the neighborhood (e.g., "In my neighborhood, many yards and alleys have broken bottles and trash lying around" and "There are abandoned or boarded-up buildings in my neighborhood") and appraisals of the dangers posed by others in the neighborhood (e.g., "The people who live in my neighborhood often damage or steal each other's property" and "Every few weeks, some adult gets beat up or mugged in my neighborhood"). Responses to items are assigned the code 1 = true or 0 = false. Scores range from 1 to 18 with higher scores indicating greater neighborhood disadvantage. Several items are reverse coded (see below). As with all the assessment in this category, there is very limited research on the reliability and validity of the tool and its clinical utility. However, given its brevity and apparent face validity, it may be useful in specific situations. Like many of the assessments reviewed in this chapter it is an easily administered assessment and it can be downloaded at no charge from the following website: http://chipts.ucla.edu/assessment/Assessment_Instruments/Assessment_files_new/assess_nes.htm.

Scoring Instructions for the NES

The NES uses the following response categories: 1 = true and 0 = false. Scores range from 1 to 18 with higher scores indicating greater neighborhood disadvantage. Items followed by an R should be reversed when scoring.

NES scale items

1. Within walking distance of my house there is a park or playground where I like to walk and enjoy myself, playing sports or games. **R**
2. There are plenty of safe places to walk or play outdoors in my neighborhood. **R**
3. Every few weeks, some kid in my neighborhood gets beat up or mugged.
4. Every few weeks, some adult gets beat up or mugged in my neighborhood.
5. In my neighborhood, I see signs of racism and prejudice at least once a week.
6. In my neighborhood, many yards and alleys have broken bottles and trash lying around.
7. I have seen people using or selling drugs in my neighborhood.
8. In the morning, or later in the day, I often see drunk people on the street in my neighborhood.
9. Most adults in my neighborhood respect the law. **R**
10. There are abandoned or boarded-up buildings in my neighborhood.
11. I feel safe when I walk around my neighborhood by myself. **R**
12. The people who live in my neighborhood often damage or steal each other's property.
13. The people who live in my neighborhood always take care of each other and protect each other from crime. **R**
14. Almost everyday I see homeless people walking or sitting around in my neighborhood.
15. In my neighborhood, the people with the most money are the drug dealers.
16. In my neighborhood, there are a lot of poor people who don't have enough money for food and basic needs.
17. For many people in my neighborhood, going to church on Sunday or religious days is a very important activity. **R**
18. The people in my neighborhood are the best people in the world. **R**

CONCLUSION

The population of older adults is growing and not surprisingly so is the demand for clinical tools to assess their function, mobility, falls risk, and home and neighborhood safety. This chapter focused on the home and neighborhood environment and reviewed assessments in three categories: (1) falls and balance assessments; (2) home safety assessments; and (3) assessments of neighborhood mobility and safety. Each of the sections reviewed the best known and most useful evidence-based instruments in that area, emphasizing their particular strengths and application. With these tools in hand clinicians have the resources to screen and identify older adults "at risk" for subsequent injury and functional decline. Assessments in this realm provide essential information to devise appropriate interventions.

REFERENCES

American Geriatrics Society, British Geriatrics Society, American Academy of Orthopaedic Surgeons Panel on Falls Prevention. (2000). Guideline for the prevention of falls in older persons. *J. Am. Geriatr. Soc.*, *49*, 664–672.

American Association of Retired Persons (AARP). (2000). *Fixing to stay.* Washington, DC: Author. Available online at: http://assets.aarp.org/rgcenter/il/home_mod.pdf Accessed: November 11, 2009.

American Association of Retired Persons (AARP). (2003). *These four walls.* Americans 45+ talk about home and community. Washington, DC: Author. Available online at: http://www.aarp.org/research/surveys/livcom/housing/design/articles/four_walls.html Accessed: November 11, 2009.

Berg, K., Wood-Dauphinee, S., Williams, J. I., & Maki, B. (1992). Measuring balance in the elderly: validation of an instrument. *Can. J. Public. Health*, *83*, S7–S11.

Boulgarides, L. K., McGinty, S. M., Willett, J. A., & Barnes, C. W. (2003). Use of clinical and impairment-based tests to predict falls by community dwelling older adults. *Phys. Ther*, *83*, 328–339.

Brauer, S. G., Burns, Y. R., & Galley, P. (2000). A prospective study of laboratory and clinical measures of postural stability to predict community dwelling fallers. *J. Gerontol*, *55*, M469–M476.

Bruce, M., McAvay, G., Raue, P., Brown, E., Meyers, B., Deohane, D., et al. (2002). Major depression in elderly home health care patients. *Am. J. Psych.*, *159*, 1367–1374.

Byrnes, M., Lichtenberg, P., & Lysack, C. (2006). Environmental press, aging in place, and residential satisfaction of urban older adults. *J. Appl. Soc.*, *23*, 50–77.

Calvo, E., Haverstick, K., & Zhivan, N. (2009). *Determinants and consequences of moving decisions for older Americans*. Center for Retirement Research. Working Paper 2009-16. Available online at: http://crr.bc.edu/images/stories/Working_Papers/wp_2009-16.pdf Accessed: November 11, 2009.

Centers for Disease Control and Prevention. (2008). Self-reported falls and fall-related injuries among persons aged >65 years—United States, 2006. *Morbidity and Mortality Weekly Reports*, *57*, 225–229.

Chiu, T., & Oliver, R. (2006). Factor analysis and construct validity of the SAFER-HOME. *OTJR: Occupation, Participation and Health*, *26*, 132–142.

Chui, T., Oliver, R., Marshall, L., & Letts, L. (2001). *Safety Assessment of Function and the Environment for Rehabilitation Tool (SAFER)*. Toronto, ON: Comprehensive Rehabilitation and Mental Health Services.

Clemson, L., Fitzgerald, M. H., & Heard, R. (1999). Content validity of an assessment tool to identify home fall hazards: the Westmead Home Safety Assessment. *Br. J. Occup. Ther.*, *62*, 171–179.

Crum, R., Lillie-Blanton, M., & Anthony, J. (1996). Neighborhood environment and opportunity to use cocaine and other drugs in late childhood and early adolescence. *Drug and Alcohol Dependence*, *43*, 155–161.

Cumming, R. G. (2002). Intervention strategies and risk-factor modification for falls prevention. A review of recent intervention studies. *Clinics in Geriatric Medicine*, *18*, 175–189.

Dalby, D., Hirdes, J., Hogan, D., Patten, S., Beck, C., Rabinowitz, T., & Maxwell, C. (2008). Potentially inappropriate management of depressive symptoms among Ontario home care clients. *Inter. J. Geriatric Psychiatry*, *23*, 650–659.

Dillaway, H., & Lysack, C. (2010). Psychosocial factors. In M. O'Connell (Ed.) (pp. 57-72) Women's Health Across the Lifespan. Bethesda, MD: American Society of Health-System Pharmacists.

Dilworth-Anderson, P., & Gibson, B. E. (2002). The cultural influence of values, norms, meanings, and perceptions in understanding dementia in ethnic minorities. *Alzheimer Disease & Associated Disorders*, *16* (Suppl. 2), S56–S63.

Dilworth-Anderson, P., Hendrie, H., Manly, J., Khachaturian, A., & Fazio, S. (2008). Diagnosis and assessment of Alzheimer's disease in diverse populations. *Alzheimer's & Dementia*, *4*, 305–309.

Fisher, G., Baker, A., Koval, D., Lishok, C., & Maisto, E. (1997). A field test of the Cougar Home Safety Assessment (version 2.0) in the homes of older persons living alone. *Austr. Occup. Ther. J*, *54*, 124–130.

Fisher, G., Kintner, L., Bradley, E., Costulas, D., Kozlevcar, J., Mahonski, K., et al. (2008). Home modification outcomes in the residences of older people as a result of Cougar Home Safety Assessment (Version 4.0) recommendations. *Californian Journal of Health Promotion*, *6*, 87–110.

Foti, D., & Kanazawa, L. (2006). Activities of daily living. In H. Pendleton, & W. Schultz-Krohnl (Eds.), *Pedretti's Occupational Therapy for Physical Dysfunction* (6th ed). Philadelphia, PA: Mosby-Elsevier.

Fougeyrollas, P., Noreau, L., St. Michel, G., & Boschen, K. (1999). *Measure of the Quality of Environment Version 2*. Lac St.-Charles, Quebec: INDCP.

Freedman, V. A., Martin, L. G., & Schoeni, R. F. (2002). Recent trends in disability and functioning among older adults in the United States. *J. Am. Med. Assoc.*, *288*, 3137–3146.

Gitlin, L. (2003). Conducting research on home environments: lessons learned and new directions. *The Gerontologist*, *43*, 628–637.

Halter, J., Ouslander, J., Tinetti, M., Studenski, S., High, K., Asthana, S., & Hazzard, W. (2009). *Hazzard's Principles of Geriatric Medicine and Gerontology*. Columbus, OH: McGraw-Hill.

Hernandez, D., & Rose, D. (2008). Predicting which older adults will or will not fall using the Fullerton Advanced Balance Scale. *Arch. Phys. Med Rehabil.*, *89*, 2309–2315.

Hill, K. D., Schwarz, J. A., Kalogeropoulos, A. J., & Gibson, S. J. (1996). Fear of falling revisited. *Arch. Phys. Med. Rehabil.*, *77*, 1025–1029.

James, A. B. (2008). Activities of daily living and instrumental activities of daily living. In E. Crepeau, E. Cohn, & B. Schell (Eds.), *Willard and Spackman's Occupational Therapy* (11th ed.). Philadelphia, PA: Lippincott, Williams & Wilkins.

Lachman, M. E., Howland, J., Tennstedt, S., Jette, A., Assmann, S., & Peterson, E. W. (1998). Fear of falling and activity restriction: the survey of activities and fear of falling in the elderly (SAFFE). *J. Gerontol. B. Psychol. Sci. Soc. Sci.*, *53*, 43–50.

Lajoie, Y., & Gallagher, S. P., (2004). Predicting falls within the Elderly Community: Comparison of postural sway, reaction time, the Berg balance scale and the Activity specific Balance Confidence (ABC) scale for comparing fallers and non-fallers. Archives of Gerontology and Geriatrics, 38, 11–26.

Letts, L., Rigby, P., & Stewart, D. (2003). *Using Environments to Enable Occupational Performance*. Thorofare, NJ: Slack.

Letts, L., Scott, S., Burtney, J., Marshall, L., & McKean, M. (1998). The reliability and validity of the safety assessment of function and the environment for rehabilitation (SAFER Tool). *Br. J. Occup. Ther.*, *61*, 127–132.

Levasseur, M., Desrosiers, J., & St.-Cyr Tribble, D. (2008). Do quality of life, participation and environment of older adults differ according to level of activity? *Health. Qual. Life. Outcomes*, *6*, 30, Published online April 29, 2008. doi: 10.1186/1477-7525-6-30.

Li, L., & Conwell, Y. (2007). Mental health care status of home care elders in Michigan. *The Gerontologist*, *47*, 528–534.

Li, F., Fisher, K. J., Harmer, P., McAuley, E., & Wilson, N. L. (2003). Fear of falling in elderly persons: association with falls, functional ability, and quality of life. *J. Geron.: Psych. Sci. and Soc. Sci.*, *58*, P283–P290.

Lysack, C., MacNeill, S., & Lichtenberg, P. (2001). The functional performance of elderly urban African-American women who return home alone after medical rehabilitation. *Am. J. Occ. Ther.*, *55*, 433–440.

Lysack, C., Neufeld, S., Mast, B., MacNeill, S., & Lichtenberg, P. (2003). After rehabilitation: an 18-month follow-up of elderly inner-city women. *Am. J. Occ. Ther.*, *57*, 298–306.

Mackenzie, L., Byles, J., & Higginbotham, N. (2000). Designing the home falls and accidents screening tool (HOME-FAST): selecting the items. *Br. J. Occup. Ther.*, *63*, 260–269.

Mackenzie, L., Byles, J., & Higginbotham, N. (2002). Reliability of the Home Falls and Accidents Screening Tool (HOME FAST) for measuring falls risk for older people. *Disabil. and Rehabil.*, *24*, 266–274.

Mann, W. C., Ottenbacher, K. J., Fraas, L., Tomita, M., & Granger, C. (1999). Effectiveness of assistive technology and environmental interventions in maintaining independence and reducing home care costs for the frail elderly. A randomized controlled trial. *Arch. Fam. Med.*, *8*, 210–217.

Marottoli, R., Mendes de Leon, C., Glass, T., Williams, C., Cooney, L., & Berkman, L. (2000). Consequences of driving cessation: decreased out-of-home activity levels. *J. Geron. Series B: Psych. Sci. and Soc. Sci.*, *55*, S334–S340.

Moreland, J., Richardson, J., Chan, D. H., O'Neill, J., Bellissimo, A., Grum, R. M., et al. (2003). Evidence-based guidelines for the secondary prevention of falls in older adults. *Gerontology*, *49*, 93–116.

Murphy, S. L., Nyquist, L. V., Straburg, D. M., & Alexander, N. B. (2006). Bath transfer in older adult congregate housing residents: assessing the person-environment interaction. *J. Am. Geriatrics Society*, *54*, 1265–1270.

National Center for Health Statistics (2008). Older Americans 2008: Key Indicators of Well-Being. Available online at: http://www.agingstats.gov/agingstatsdotnet/Main_Site/Data/Data_2008.aspx Accessed November 14, 2009.

Newton, R. A. (1997). Balance screening of an inner city older adult population. *Arch. Phys. Med. Rehabil.*, *78*, 587–591.

Nickens, H. (1985). Intrinsic factors in falling among the elderly. *Arch. Int. Med.*, *145*, 1089–1093.

Noonan, V., Kopec, J., Noreau, L., Singer, J., & Dvorak, M. (2009). A review of participation instruments based on the International Classification of Functioning, Disability and Health. *Disabil. and Rehabil.*, *31*, 1883–1901.

Perell, K., Nelson, A., Goldman, R. L., Luther, S. L., Prieto-Lewis, N., & Rubinstein, L. Z. (2001). Fall risk assessment measures: an analytic review. *J. Gerontol. A: Biol. Sci. Med. Sci.*, *56A*, M761–M766.

Peretz, C., Herman, T., Hausdorff, J. M., & Giladi, N. (2006). Assessing fear of falling can a short version of the Activities-specific Balance Confidence scale be useful? *Movement Disorders*, *21*, 2101–2105.

Peterson, E., Murphy, S., & Hammel, J. (2003). Resources for fall prevention and management of Fear of Falling. *J. Amer. Soc. Aging*, *XXVI*, 89–92.

Podsiadlo, D., & Richardson, S. (1991). The timed "up and go": a test of basic functional mobility for frail elderly persons. *J. Appl. Ger.*, *39*, 142–148.

Poulin de Courval, L., Gélinas, I., Gauthier, S., Gayton, D., Liu, L., Rossignol, M., et al. (2006). Reliability and validity of the Safety Assessment Scale for people with dementia living at home. *Can. J. Occ. Ther.*, *73*, 67–75.

Powell, L. E., & Myers, A. M. (1995). The Activities-specific Balance Confidence (ABC) scale. *J. Gerontol. A: Biol. Sci. Med. Sci.*, *50*, M28–M34.

Rose, D. J., Lucchese, M., & Wiersma, L. (2006). Development of a multidimensional balance scale for use with functionally independent older adults. *Arch. Phys. Med. Rehabil.*, *87*, 1478–1485.

Rowles, G. (1983). Place and personal identity in old age: observations from Appalachia. *J. of Environ. Psych.*, *3*, 299–313.

Rowles, G. (1993). Evolving images of place in aging and "aging in place." *Generations*, *17*, 65–70.

Rubenstein, L., & Josephson, K. (2002). The epidemiology of falls and syncope. *Clin. Geriatr. Med.*, *18*, 141–158.

Sergeant, J., & Ekerdt, D. (2008). Motives for residential mobility in later life. *Int. J. Aging Hum. Dev.*, *66*, 131–154.

Scheffer, A. C., Schuurmans, M. J., Van Dijk, N., Van Der Hooft, T., & De Rooij, S. E. (2008). Fear of falling: measurement strategy, prevalence, risk factors and consequences among older persons. *Age and Ageing*, *37*, 19–24.

Shumway-Cook, A., Baldwin, M., Polissar, N. L., & Gruber, W. (1997). Predicting the probability for falls in community-dwelling older adults. *Phys. Ther.*, *77*, 812–819.

Spirduso, W. W. (1995). Balance, posture and locomotion. In W. W. Spirduso (Ed.), *Physical Dimensions of Aging* (pp. 155–183). Chicago, IL: Human Kinetics Inc.

Stark, S. (2004). Removing environmental barriers in the homes of older adults with disabilities improves occupational performance. *Occup. Ther. J. Research: Occup. Particip. Health*, *24*, 32–39.

Stark., S., Hollingsworth, H., Morgan, K., Chang, M., & Gray, D. (2008). The inter-rater reliability of the Community Health Environment Checklist. *Arch. Phys. Med. Rehabil.*, *89*, 2218–2219.

Stevens, J. A., & Sogolow, E. D. (2005). Gender differences for non-fatal unintentional fall related injuries among older adults. *Inj. Prev.*, *11*, 115–119.

Tideiksaar, R. (1997). *Falling in Old Age: Its Prevention and Management*. New York, NY: Springer.

Tideiksaar, R. (2002). *Falls in Older People: Prevention and Management*. Baltimore, MD: Health Professions Press.

Tinetti, M. E. (2003). Clinical practice. Preventing falls in elderly persons. *N. Engl. J. Med.*, *348*, 42–49.

Tinetti, M. E. (1987). Factors associated with serious injury during falls by ambulatory nursing home residents. *J. Am. Geriatr. Soc.*, *35*, 644–648.

Tinetti, M. E., Speechley, M., & Ginter, S. F. (1988). Risk factors for falls among elderly persons living in the community. *N. Engl. J. Med.*, *319*, 1701–1707.

Tinetti, M. E., Richman, D., & Powell, L. (1990). Falls efficacy as a measure of fear of falling. *J. Gerontol. Psych. Sci.*, *45*, P239–P243.

US Department of Health and Human Services. (1999). *Mental health: a report of the Surgeon General*. Rockville, MD: National Institutes of Health, National Institute of Mental Health.

United States Census. America's families and living arrangements: 2003. Available at: http://www.census.gov/prod/2004pubs/p20-553.pdf. Accessed November 29, 2007.

Vik, K., Nygård, L., & Lilja, M. (2007). Perceived environmental influence on participation among older adults after home-based rehabilitation. *Phys. & Occup. Ther. Geriatrics*, *25*, 1–20.

Wahl, H.-W., & Gitlin, L. (2007). Environmental gerontology. In J. E. Birren (Ed.), *Encyclopedia of Gerontology. Age, Aging, and the Aged* (2nd ed.) (pp 494–501). Oxford, England: Elsevier.

Wahl, H.-W., Fänge, A., Oswald, F., Gitlin, L., & Iwarsson, S. (2009). The home environment and disability-related outcomes in aging individuals: what is the empirical evidence? *The Gerontologist*, *49*, 355–367.

Whiteneck, G., Harrison-Felix, C., Mellick, D., Brooks, C., Charlifue, S., & Gerhart, K. (2004). Quantifying environmental factors: a measure of physical, attitudinal, service, productivity, and policy barriers. *Arch. Phys. Med. Rehabil.*, *85*, 1324–1335.

Wolfson, L., Judge, J., Whipple, R., & King, M. (1995). Strength is a major factor in balance, gait and the occurrence of falls. *J. Gerontol. A: Biol. Sci. Med. Sci.*, *50A*(Special Issue), 64–67.

CHAPTER 24

Pain Assessment and Management in Older Adults

Theodore K. Malmstrom, Raymond C. Tait

Department of Neurology & Psychiatry, Saint Louis University School of Medicine, St Louis, MD, USA

INTRODUCTION

In the decade since the publication of the first edition of the *Handbook of Assessment in Clinical Gerontology*, interest in the topic of pain in older adults has mushroomed. A Medline search of publications with pain, geriatrics, aging, and older adults as keywords yielded 44,966 results, approximately 60% of which (26,744) dated to the past five years. Several converging lines of influence are likely to have contributed to this surge of interest. One line involves demographic trends: the proportion of the population aged 60 and over has increased steadily and will continue to do so in years to come (National Institute on Aging, 2007). Older adults also are more likely to develop health conditions with painful sequelae: up to 40% of older adults living independently experience pain at levels that can impact function (Thomas, Peat, Harris, Wilkie & Croft, 2004), and pain is estimated to impact up to 83% of older adults residing in alternative living facilities (Fox, Raina & Jadad, 1999). A second demographic consideration involves the projected growth in the population of older adults residing in alternative living facilities, particularly those with dementia. Pain management for older adults with severe dementia is very challenging, due in large part to the difficulties of assessment; thus, there is urgent need for the development of efficient assessment methodologies that facilitate effective treatment.

Aside from these demographic trends, a third line of influence reflects an increased awareness of the debilitating effects of diseases of later life and their often painful sequelae on quality of life, morbidity, and costs of care for the older adults who experience those diseases (Gagliese, 2009). Finally, the increased attention to the topic of pain management in older adults has served to highlight the problems and prospects in the area; as the literature has described the challenges of pain management among older adults more clearly, the range of researchable questions has expanded considerably. Nowhere have the challenges been outlined more clearly and has the research increased more dramatically than in the area of pain assessment. Indeed, a recent monograph that described the current status of that literature included over 400 references (Hadjistavropoulos et al., 2007a).

Why has there been such a surge in interest in pain assessment among older adults? Again, there are several factors that appear to be driving this line of study. First, there is an increased understanding of the neurocognitive processes associated with dementing conditions such as Alzheimer's disease. There is evidence that pain perception may remain intact, albeit with a decline in the communication abilities necessary to convey that experience to others (Benedetti et al., 2004). Second, despite increased attention to pain assessment in older adults with cognitive limitations, many questions still remain. The lack of a recognized, practical approach to pain assessment in older adults with cognitive incapacity underscores the need for continued work in the area. Thus, paralleling developments in the general

Handbook of Assessment in Clinical Gerontology. DOI: 10.1016/B978-0-12-374961-1.10024-7

field, gains in understanding have been limited, especially for patients with advanced dementia, and directions for future research remain largely defined by limitations in the studies undertaken to date.

Despite the halting nature of progress in the field, much has changed in our understanding of and approach to pain management in older adults with cognitive incapacity in the past decade. This chapter describes the current status of the field, with a heavy emphasis on pain assessment. The reasons for this emphasis are twofold. First, as noted above, pain assessment in dementia has been a particularly vigorous area of study. Second and, perhaps, more important, adequate assessment is needed both to identify persons for whom pain treatment is required and to evaluate the effectiveness of those treatments. Thus, effective assessment is also the backbone of effective treatment.

This chapter first examines our understanding of nociception among persons with neurocognitive deficits, as well as approaches to pain assessment in older adults with such deficits. The next section addresses the domains associated with the experience of pain, including sensory dimensions of the experience, psychological factors associated with it, and pain-related function. Throughout these sections we provide clinical vignettes to illustrate selected points. Another section provides an overview of current clinical practice guidelines for pain management that have been adopted by organizations most focused on the health of older adults, the American Geriatric Society (AGS), and the American Medical Directors' Association (AMDA). The final section discusses unresolved issues in the area, including issues related to both research and practice.

NEUROCOGNITION AND NOCICEPTION

The last decade has seen technological advances that have greatly furthered our ability to study neurocognitive processes associated with nociception, aging, dementia, and the intersection of the three areas. Because pain assessment historically has relied on self-report and because self-report is of limited value (at best) in patients with severely dementing conditions, this line of research is of particular importance to the assessment of pain. For example, if research were to document that dementing conditions consistently dull pain perception (i.e., dementia serves as an analgesic), treatment of pain could be titrated so as to be less aggressive. Other relationships between dementia and the experience of pain, of course, would point in other directions. In this section, we briefly review our current understanding of nociception in older adults, including the likely impact of dementing processes on the experience of pain.

Pain has long been recognized as an experience that involves sensory-discriminative, affective-motivational, and cognitive-evaluative dimensions (Melzack & Wall, 1965). Of the three, the cognitive-evaluative element of the experience, mediated by such mechanisms as beliefs and coping tactics (e.g., catastrophizing; Seminowicz & Davis, 2006), represents a particularly complex area for neurocognitive study as it involves multiple areas of the brain. Other aspects of the pain experience, however, have been linked to identifiable pathways. For example, the lateral pain system (spinothalamic tract, ventroposterior lateral thalamus, primary and secondary somatosensory cortices) subserves the sensory-discriminative elements of pain that are involved in coding the location, intensity, and quality of the sensation (Treede, Kenshalo, Gracely & Jones, 1999). The affective-motivational elements that are associated with emotion, arousal, and attention are linked to more medial structures (Price, 2000): the medial thalamus; hypothalamus; cingulate and insular cortex; prefrontal areas. Thus, disruptions in the functions of the lateral and medial structures are likely to directly impact related elements of the pain experience.

The relationship between aging and pain perception in cognitively intact older adults was highly uncertain at the time of the earlier chapter. More recent research has clarified the association to some degree. Evidence indicates that older adults generally detect nociceptive stimuli at levels comparable to those of younger adults (Gagliese & Melzack, 1997; Riley, Wade, Robinson & Price, 2000), but demonstrate pain thresholds that are higher (Gibson & Farrell, 2004). While the reasons for this difference remain speculative, there is increasing agreement that they relate to changes in the *quality* of the experience (i.e., its affective-emotional elements). That element, in turn, could be affected by changes in pain-related beliefs associated with aging (Harkins, 1996), by central nervous system changes (e.g., changes in white matter; Oosterman, van Harten, Weinstein, Scheltens & Scherder, 2006), or some combination of these and other factors (Gibson & Farrell, 2004).

The role of neurologic changes has been more clearly identified in patients with Alzheimer's disease (AD). Both histo-pathological and imaging studies of AD have shown changes that appear to target such medial structures as the hypothalamus, the cingulate and insular cortices, and the medial nuclei of the thalamus (Rub, Del Tredici, Del Turco & Braak, 2002; Thompson et al., 2003). Structures associated with the lateral pain pathway, however, are relatively well preserved, suggesting that Alzheimer's disease may preferentially spare the sensory-discriminative dimension. By comparison, transmission of neural impulses involving the affective-motivational dimension, at least theoretically, is likely to be disrupted. Secondary to the impact of Alzheimer's disease on memory and reasoning, appraisals of pain also are likely to be affected by disease processes (Cole et al., 2006).

The body of research that has studied dementia and dimensions of the pain experience largely supports the above relationships. With some consistency, that research has shown that pain detection and pain thresholds, both parameters related to the sensory-discriminative dimension, are relatively intact in patients with AD (Benedetti et al., 1999, 2004; Gibson, Voukelatos, Ames, Flicker & Helme, 2001). In contrast, evidence increasingly indicates that pain tolerance and pain reactivity are affected by the progression of AD. For example, pain intensity ratings are lower for AD patients than for patients without AD (Scherder & Bouma, 2000). Corresponding changes have been shown for pain tolerance: pain tolerance correlates with changes in Mini Mental State Examination (MMSE) scores, such that higher levels of tolerance are associated with lower MMSE levels (Benedetti et al., 1999). In turn, the tolerance appears to be related to reduced autonomic reactivity in AD patients (Rainero, Vighetti, Bergamasco, Pinessi & Benedetti, 2000), as well as a reduced capacity to anticipate noxious stimuli (Benedetti et al., 2004), both of which are likely to decrease motivational and affective components of the pain experience (Scherder, Sergeant & Swaab, 2003; Scherder, et al., 2005).

While there seems to be growing consensus on the neurophysiologic and neuroanatomic interactions of AD and pain perceptions, the implications of such research findings for assessment and treatment remain somewhat unclear. For patients with mild-to-moderate AD, there is evidence that valid and reliable self-report data can be used to assess pain intensity (Chibnall & Tait, 2001). The same cannot be said, of course, for patients with severe dementia. For the latter group, a host of observational approaches have been proposed (Hadjistavropoulos et al., 2007a), none of which have demonstrated clear superiority to the others. While an observational approach to pain assessment may be the only recourse for the latter group, questions have been raised as to whether this approach will yield data that are comparable to self-reports: arguments have been made that pain behaviors reflect the affective-motivational aspects of pain, rather than the sensory-discriminative dimension reflected in self-reports (Scherder et al., 2005). If so, a reasonable case could be made to incorporate observational approaches into assessment for patients across the dementia spectrum. Of course, such an approach would be potentially time consuming and costly, especially absent agreement regarding the observational system to be used.

THE PAIN EXPERIENCE

Since the publication of the *Gate Control Theory* (Melzack & Wall, 1965), pain has been recognized as modifiable not only by neuroanatomic and neurophysiologic factors such as those described above, but also by psychological, behavioral, and environmental factors. Figure 24.1 depicts the Glasgow Illness Model (Waddell, Newton, Henderson, Somerville & Main, 1993), a conceptual model that provides a visual representation of these factors. While the conceptual model described below is widely accepted, the importance of thorough pain assessment in older adults is borne out empirically as well. A recent study that compared adjustment status for cognitively intact older adults with and without chronic low back pain (CLBP) demonstrates widespread differences between the groups (Rudy, Weiner, Lieber, Slaboda & Boston, 2007). CLBP patients demonstrated greater dysfunction in multiple domains: (1) self-reported function; (2) performance-based function; (3) mood (depression); (4) CLBP-related diagnostic evidence (degenerative disc disease); and (5) the number of medical comorbidities that they demonstrated. Accordingly, assessment should encompass sensory, psychological, and functional dimensions of the pain experience. This section examines elements of each dimension with demonstrated importance to older adults and reviews instruments that have been used to assess those elements.

Pain Sensation

Pain Severity

Pain severity is the single feature of the pain experience that is most commonly assessed. As noted above, there is evidence that pain thresholds are somewhat higher for older than younger adults. Those differences, however, are of insufficient magnitude to generalize to individual cases (i.e., some older adults may magnify rather than minimize pain severity). Moreover, there are multiple possible reasons for the reported differences: (1) bona fide changes may exist in neurotransmission associated with aging (e.g., for visceral pain; Lasch, Castell & Castell, 1997); (2) older adults may cope with pain differently, perhaps, using different comparisons against which to evaluate pain (Riley et al., 2000); and (3) the differences may be related to the communication of discomfort rather than to the sensation itself (Benedetti et al., 2004). To complicate the picture further, tolerance for pain may actually *decrease* with age, especially when pain is severe or prolonged, secondary to pain summation

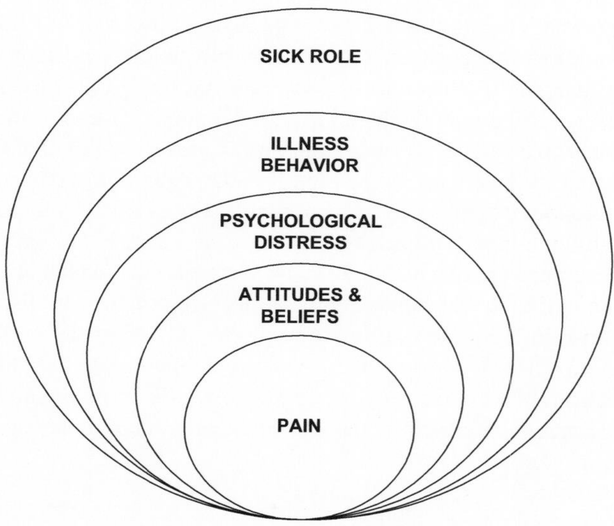

FIGURE 24.1

Glasgow Illness Model.

(adapted with permission from Waddell et al., 1993)

processes that are affected by age (Gibson & Farrell, 2004). Despite (or perhaps because of) the complexities of the above picture, it is reasonable to conclude at this time that the clinical assessment of sensory pain in older adults should be based on the assumption that the older adult experiences pain in a manner similar to the younger adult.

Case Study 1—Verbal descriptors

A 78-year-old White female was admitted to a subacute care facility following a fall in which she sustained a fracture of her right upper extremity. While she otherwise was medically stable, she also demonstrated widespread osteoarthritis and associated degenerative changes. She was approached shortly after her admission to assess whether she met inclusion criteria for a study. The study was designed to compare the measurement properties of several self-report instruments commonly used in the assessment of pain in older adults, and its primary inclusion criterion involved a patient report of some level of pain (in addition to several other criteria related to cognition). Because of the recent fracture, the patient was expected to qualify. When approached to estimate her current level of pain severity, however, the patient denied the presence of any pain, disqualifying her from study participation. In particular, when asked to describe the severity of her pain on a 1–100 scale, she responded: "I don't have any pain, so I guess I don't belong in your study. If you had asked me about stiffness, though, it's a different matter. I would rate my stiffness as 100 on your scale—it really gets in my way and probably is why I fell when I broke my arm."

Older adults are able to provide valid and reliable self-reports of pain severity using various measures. Self-report measures that have been tested in older adult samples include visual analog scales (VAS; e.g., Gagliese, Weizblit, Ellis & Chan, 2005), numeric rating scales (NRS; e.g., Chibnall & Tait, 2001), verbal descriptor scales (VDS; e.g., Herr, Spratt, Mobily & Richardson, 2004), and facial pain scales (FPS; e.g., Herr, Mobily, Kohout & Wagenaar, 1998). VAS are the least preferred self-report measures of those listed above due to consistently higher failure rates by older adults relative to other self-report measures (Herr, Spratt, Garand & Li, 2007). Error rates for NRS, VDS, and FPS are generally very low (Chibnall & Tait, 2001; Closs, Barr, Briggs, Cash & Seers, 2004; Herr et al., 2004; Peters, Patijn, & Lame, 2007). Studies that directly ask participants to rate scale preference show that older adults commonly select VDS and NRS as preferred scales (Herr et al., 2004, 2007; Peters et al., 2007). Similarly, studies demonstrate that the psychometric properties (reliability and validity) of NRS (Chibnall & Tait, 2001; Peters, Patijn & Lame, 2007) and VDS (Herr et al., 2007, 2004) are superior to other self-report measures. FPS, too, has acceptable reliability and validity among older adults (Herr et al., 1998). While there is no clear consensus on any individual class of pain intensity measures as the universal choice for use in older adults (Peters et al., 2007), a recent expert panel endorsed the use of NRS or VDS (Hadjistavropoulos et al., 2007a).

NRS scales require individuals to rate pain severity on a numeric scale (e.g., 0 "no pain" to 10 "worst possible pain"); there are several NRS variants with different anchor points or scale ranges. The 21-point Box Scale has a horizontal row of boxes labeled from 0 to 100 in five-point increments with the anchor points of 0 "no pain" and 100 "pain as bad as it could be" (Jensen, Miller & Fisher, 1998); it has performed well in comparison studies of self-report pain assessment measures with older adult populations (Chibnall & Tait, 2001; Peters et al., 2007). A typical VDS requires individuals to rate pain severity by selecting an adjective from several options that best characterize their pain (e.g., no pain, mild, moderate, severe, or very severe). VDS that use various descriptor terms (e.g., anchor point of "very severe pain" versus "excruciating") or numbers of descriptors (e.g., 5 versus 6) have been applied successfully in older adult populations (Hadjistavroloulos et al., 2007a). Preliminary data for a modified VDS, the Iowa Pain Thermometer (IPT), indicate the scale is acceptable and exhibits low error rates in older adults (Herr et al., 2007; Ware, Epps, Herr & Packard, 2006), but additional data are needed to fully evaluate the scale psychometrics.

Cognitive status is important to consider when choosing a self-report pain assessment measure. While self-report measures are generally not recommended among older adults with severe cognitive deficits (AGS Panel on Persistent Pain in Older Persons, 2002; American Medical Directors Association, 2009; Hadjistavropoulos et al., 2007a; Herr, Bjoro & Decker, 2006), older adults with mild to moderate cognitive impairment can provide valid self-reports of pain severity on both VDS and NRS scales (Chibnall & Tait, 2001; Ferrell, Ferrell & Rivera, 1995; Herr et al., 2004). A final consideration involves memory for pain in older adults. There is reasonable evidence that older adults with mild-to-moderate cognitive impairment can provide valid retrospective ratings of pain that they have experienced over a period of two weeks (Chibnall & Tait, 2001). The process by which to gauge actual levels of pain from retrospective ratings, however, differs between older adults with no cognitive impairment versus older adults with mild-to-moderate cognitive impairment. For older adults with no cognitive impairment, the best estimate of actual pain over a preceding two-week period is the average of the *usual* and *least* levels for that time period, reflecting a slight magnifying bias in such recollections. For older adults with mild-to-moderate impairment, however, the best pain estimate involves averaging *usual* and *worst* levels (Chibnall & Tait, 2001), an equation that reflects a tendency among older adults with mild-to-moderate impairment to discount pain. (A later section will review approaches to pain assessment for older adults with severe dementia.)

Pain Distribution

While pain severity is widely assessed and its importance long appreciated, pain distribution has received attention only recently in the literature on older adults. Typically, pain drawings are used to assess the distribution of pain; patients simply indicate the presence of pain on an outline of a human body. Not only can pain distribution be assessed reliably in younger adults (Margolis, Chibnall & Tait, 1988), but older adults, including nursing home residents, also are capable of completing pain drawings reliably (Gagliese, 2001). Among nursing home residents, however, the assessment is interview based and requires nursing staff participation.

Not only does the assessment of pain distribution orient staff to important elements of a resident's pain condition, there is considerable evidence that widespread pain is associated with other dimensions of adjustment. In particular, relative to a focal pain condition, multisite pain has been linked to higher levels of disability (Eggermont, Bean, Guralnik & Leveille, 2009; Kamaleri, Natvig, Ihlebaek & Bruusgaard, 2009; Mottram, Peat, Thomas, Wilkie & Croft, 2008; Soldato et al., 2007), higher levels of emotional distress (Wolfe & Michaud, 2009), and poorer levels of general health (Kamaleri, Natvig, Ihlebaek, Benth & Bruusgaard, 2008). Given the relative ease with which this important dimension of sensory pain can be assessed, as well as its clinical implications, it should be a routine part of clinical assessment.

Psychological Function

Psychological function subsumes two broad areas of importance in pain assessment: (1) the association between pain conditions and depression; and (2) the attitudes, beliefs, and coping responses that older adults employ in response to pain. The chapter will address the general literature regarding the former topic, but will put particular emphasis on several topics related to the latter: (1) efficacy expectations (both self efficacy and treatment efficacy); and (2) pain coping (with a particular focus on pain catastrophizing).

Pain and Depression

Of course, the association between pain and distress is well established and has long been recognized, particularly that between pain and depression (cf., Romano & Turner, 1985; Williamson & Schulz, 1992). While the association is well established, there is less agreement about the nature of the causal linkage between pain and depression. Some have argued that pain is often a manifestation of depression (Blumer & Heilbronn, 1982), such that pain complaints are primarily a psychosomatic phenomenon. Others have argued that the causal link is reversed: depression is primarily somatopsychic, i.e., secondary to pain and such pain-related sequelae as feelings of helplessness/hopelessness, decreased physical and social activities, reductions in income, etc. (Deshields, Jenkins & Tait, 1989). A third camp espouses an intermediate position: depression is most likely to be problematic and pain particularly disabling for people with limited resources, rendering them less resilient when confronted with the stresses endemic to the pain experience (Tait, 2004). Although a detailed discussion of this issue is beyond the scope of this chapter, the interested reader is referred to an excellent review of the topic (Gatchel & Dersh, 2002).

For the purposes of this chapter, we will assume that each of the three causal linkages described above applies to some segment of the broad population of older adults in pain. Certainly, the practitioner should be particularly attentive to the presence of pain in those patients with pre-existing major depressive disorder. Not only is pain a common complaint in that patient group, but the latter comorbidities potentiate the risk for functional decline (Reid, Williams, & Gill, 2003). The latter study involved baseline assessments of physical and emotional functioning with subsequent monthly interviews over a one-year follow-up for a cohort of 226 community-dwelling older adults (aged 70 and older). Over that year, baseline levels of depression strongly predicted functional decline, measured as the number of months that participants experienced disabling musculoskeletal pain. Moreover, functional decline undermined independence in such basic tasks as bathing, walking, dressing, and transferring. Such changes, if prolonged, can occasion substantial loss of independence and, potentially, the need for alternative living arrangements. Similarly, functional decline can lead to social isolation; older adults that lose access to a supporting social network are vulnerable to depression (or worsening depression in the case of patients with a pre-existing condition) and other comorbidities that can further undermine independence.

In the absence of a pre-existing depressive disorder, the patient with a chronic pain condition also merits careful attention. Particularly close attention should go to patients that describe severe levels of pain; as such patients are at risk for clinically significant distress (Gatchel & Dersh, 2002). Similarly, patients that describe widespread pain merit careful attention, as widely distributed pain also has been linked to high levels of depression (Tait, Chibnall & Margolis, 1990b). Possibly the most important element of the clinical assessment, however, involves attention to pain-related interference with basic life tasks: such interference has been shown to predict long-term distress and disability better than baseline measures of either pain or distress (Von Korff, Deyo, Cherkin & Barlow, 1993).

Case Study 2—Pain and depression

A 78-year-old white female lived independently despite chronic abdominal pain of a multi-year duration. Her independence was related, in part, to a successful analgesic regiment that her primary physician had instituted several years ago, involving QID administration of Darvocet. When her primary physician retired, he was replaced by a younger physician who was opposed to the long-term administration of opioid analgesics, despite their obvious long-term effectiveness for this patient. Instead, he tried a variety of anti-inflammatory, anti-depressant and anti-convulsant formulations, all without success. In despair, this patient shot herself in the stomach with a 22-caliber pistol. Initially, she was hospitalized on a general medical service to stabilize her, but then was transferred to a geriatric psychiatry service for treatment of depression. The service called in a pain consultant. Because the consultant attached great weight to the patient's history of adequate pain control prior to the medication changes, he recommended that the patient be placed back on QID Darvocet. The patient's emotional status improved rapidly, although her physical status remained somewhat impaired. She was transferred within days to a subacute facility where she underwent successful rehabilitation and then was discharged back home to live independently.

Efficacy Expectancy Beliefs

Efficacy expectancy beliefs are future-oriented beliefs regarding the likelihood that actions will yield desired outcomes. In the case of self efficacy, the beliefs reflect an individual's expectations that their actions will effect positive change (i.e., control beliefs), while outcome expectancies refer to beliefs that treatment and/or the actions of treatment providers will accomplish such change (i.e., outcome efficacy). A substantial literature documents association between self-efficacy, clinical adjustment, and response to treatment for older adult patients with chronic pain conditions (Resnick, 1998). Although a much smaller literature addresses outcome efficacy in older adults, the literature that exists has interesting implications, especially for those with cognitive limitations. Hence, both literatures merit attention.

Self-efficacy has been linked through an extensive literature with the three dimensions relevant to the general chronic pain population that are central to this chapter: pain; distress; and disability. For example, in a sample of older adults with osteoarthritis of the knee (mean age = 69.9 years), higher self-efficacy scores were associated with lower levels of reported pain, lower levels of depression, and greater exertion and speed on tests of walking (Marks, 2007). Similar results were reported with a sample with more widespread pain associated with rheumatoid arthritis, where higher self-efficacy was associated with less depression, less functional impairment, and more circumscribed pain (Rahman, Ambler, Underwood & Shipley, 2004).

A number of studies have focused on one of the dimensions described above. Those studies provide further support for the importance of self-efficacy as a mediating factor in clinical adjustment for older adults in pain. For example, self-efficacy beliefs were shown in one study to be a stronger predictor of depressive mood than levels of functional limitations (McIlvane, Schiaffino & Paget, 2007). Other studies speak to the central role of self-efficacy beliefs in disability status. Positive self-efficacy beliefs have been correlated with better functional status in older patients with prostate cancer (Perkins, Baum, Taylor, & Basen-Engquist, 2009), in older war veterans (Barry, Guo, Kerns, Duong & Reid, 2003), and in minorities from lower socioeconomic strata (Greene et al., 2006).

While there is strong support for self-efficacy as an important clinical variable in the assessment of older adults in pain, the above data do not speak clearly to the issue of causality—whether self-efficacy beliefs are a cause or an effect of the clinical parameters with which they have been associated. Obviously, this issue is important if the data are to be used to assist in the clinical management of this population (Clark & Nothwehr, 1999). If self-efficacy is a by-product of functional limitations, then the focus of clinical interventions should be on rehabilitation; if, instead, self-efficacy moderates response to treatment and/or long-term adjustment, it should be a treatment focus. Not surprisingly, the data on this topic are somewhat mixed. For example, a study that focused on physical predictors of self-efficacy among older patients with osteoarthritis pain found that stiffness, hamstring strength, and age were the strongest predictors of self-efficacy scores (Maly, Costigan & Olney, 2006). Similarly, there is evidence that an intervention that increases functional capacity also will boost participant perceptions of self-efficacy (Rejeski, Ettinger, Martin & Morgan, 1998).

The literature, however, provides stronger support for a central (causal) role for self-efficacy beliefs. Support for this is found in studies that controlled for self-efficacy beliefs statistically, longitudinal studies that examined self-efficacy and various other parameters of clinical status at baseline and at several time intervals thereafter, as well as treatment studies that assessed similar parameters before and after treatment. A study that used statistical controls examined older patients with and without chronic pain, examining their compliance with such physician-recommended self-management activities as regular exercise, eating well, and taking medications as prescribed (Krein, Heisler, Piette, Butchart & Kerr, 2007). The data showed that chronic pain negatively impacted each activity; after controlling for self-efficacy, however, the pernicious effects of pain were largely negated. Similarly, longitudinal research has shown that higher baseline levels of self-efficacy predict better clinical adjustment two or more years later, even after controlling for baseline differences in adjustment (Brekke, Hjortdahl, & Kvien, 2001). Moreover, longitudinal data suggest that self-efficacy is particularly important for individuals coping with baseline conditions that can impact function; those with lower levels of self-efficacy beliefs are more vulnerable to decline than are those with higher self-efficacy beliefs (Rejeski, Miller, Foy, Messier, & Rapp, 2001). Finally, a similar pattern emerges from treatment studies: interventions aimed at older adults with activity limitations most benefit participants with high levels of self-efficacy (Focht, Rejeski, Ambrosius, Katla, & Messier, 2005; Resnick, 1998).

Given the strength of the literature regarding self-efficacy, it is no surprise that several measures have been developed to assess this important construct. Two widely used measures are the Arthritis Self-Efficacy Scale (ASE; Lorig, Chastain, Ling, Shoor, & Holman, 1989) and the Pain Self-Efficacy Questionnaire (PSEQ; Nicholas, 2007). Because the PSEQ is more focused on pain and somewhat shorter than the ASE, it is shown in Appendix A.

Outcome efficacy beliefs have been much less studied among older adults, possibly because of the assumption that pain beliefs among older adults have many commonalities with those of younger adults. Accordingly, the literature regarding outcome efficacy beliefs is heavily weighted to younger adults, albeit with abundant evidence that expectancies for treatment significantly impact outcomes (DeGood & Tait, 2001).

Given the dearth of literature that explicitly references older adults, the implication is clear that the expectancy mechanisms that operate in younger adults apply *pari passu* to the older population. Recent research, however, raises questions about that assumption. An innovative approach to this topic examined the analgesic response to a topical anesthetic (lidocaine) among patients with Alzheimer's disease (Benedetti et al., 2006). Patients were either aware that an anesthetic was being applied (open approach) or unaware of the application (hidden). The direct analgesic effect, indicated by the response to the hidden application, was compared to the open effect in order to gauge the placebo response (i.e., the response that was mediated by outcome expectancies). AD patients with evidence of greater prefrontal impairment demonstrated a muted placebo response relative to those with less impairment. The results suggest that AD patients may have lower levels of outcome expectancy as prefrontal impairment progresses, a phenomenon that may deprive them of efficacy expectancy mechanisms that significantly enhance analgesic efficacy. If so, the implications of such findings are that such patients may require higher doses of analgesia in order to offset the expectancy decrement.

Pain Coping

As there is a huge volume of research regarding pain coping strategies that has emerged in recent years (cf., Degood & Tait, 2001), this chapter will address only that portion that specifically targets older adults. We provide a brief review of the range of coping strategies that have been studied vis-a-vis their relationship with pain adjustment. We then focus on pain catastrophizing, a construct that has been linked to multiple dimensions of clinical adjustment among patients with chronic pain conditions.

Pain coping responses differ significantly from the pain beliefs that were examined above. While pain beliefs refer to mental appraisals of a situation, coping involves the entire set of responses an individual produces in response to a stressor such as pain. Hence, a coping response may be a cognitive process (e.g., problem solving) or an overt behavior (e.g., stretching). Further, coping responses to pain can involve others; the patient that asks his spouse for assistance when facing a pain-related limitation demonstrates a form of coping. Finally, coping responses may be either adaptive or maladaptive, depending upon variables such as the internal and external resources available to the individual and the demands posed by the stressor (Lazarus & Folkman, 1984).

Case Study 3—Patient/Spouse coping

A 64-year-old White male had a 15-year history of low back pain. He underwent three surgeries in an effort to eliminate the pain, but ultimately was disabled by the condition and forced to retire from an engineering position that he held with a local aeronautics company. Following his forced retirement, he spent most of the next year at home, much of the time in bed with the blinds drawn and the lights out. His wife, a social worker, was concerned about his emotional and physical well-being and, over time, reduced her work hours and began to interact with him more as a social worker than as a spouse. Despite her efforts, he became depressed and was hospitalized for multidisciplinary treatment aimed at stabilizing medications, training in coping skills, and physical rehabilitation. He made good progress, and both he and his wife were brought into the treatment program prior to discharge for the purposes of discharge planning. When he returned for follow-up approximately a week later, his clinical condition had deteriorated markedly. Not only had he deteriorated, but his wife also had developed significant problems: she had begun brushing with such vigor that she broke several teeth. Detailed assessment of the home situation revealed that she had continued to treat him as she had grown accustomed to treating him, as a patient more than a spouse. Several sessions of joint psychotherapy were directed at re-establishing marital roles, giving the patient more responsibility for management of his health and for requesting help when he needed it. With the redefinition of roles, symptoms improved for both. Over the next month, the patient began to volunteer at a local hospital and the spouse had returned full-time to her work, roles that each had maintained successfully when further follow-up was determined to be unnecessary.

Although there is a potentially unlimited array of coping responses that could be studied, most research has focused on seven categories: diverting attention; coping self-statements; reinterpreting pain; ignoring sensations; hoping and praying; increasing behavior activities; and catastrophizing. Of these, the greatest attention has been directed at catastrophizing, which will be reviewed separately below. Of the other coping responses, most research has shown that older adults cope with pain in ways that are similar to younger adults. As might be expected, generally dysfunctional adaptation to pain (i.e., high levels of depression and/or disability) has been linked to passive coping strategies, such as prayer, ignoring pain, reinterpreting pain, and increased use of rest (Lopez-Lopez, Montorio, Izal, & Velasco, 2008; Rapp, Rejeski, & Miller, 2000; Sinclair, 2001). There are, however, several differences in coping patterns that have been identified for older adults. For example, fear of pain seems to play a larger role among older adults in explaining activity avoidance (Hadjistavropoulos et al., 2007b); conversely, the coping strategy of ignoring pain appears more adaptive in older than younger adults (Lopez-Lopez et al., 2008). Similarly, coping strategies characterized by praying and hoping appear to be more adaptive in older, minority patients than in non-minorities (Jones et al., 2008). While these data support the important role that coping responses play in the adjustment of older adults to chronically painful conditions, they also demonstrate important differences in successful coping that can characterize groups of older adults.

As noted earlier, coping responses may involve more than just the individual who is experiencing chronic pain—they also may involve a partner. Mounting evidence indicates that the nature of the communication between the person in pain and their partner may determine whether a positive adjustment to pain evolves. In particular, older adults in pain who are satisfied with the responses of their spouses are less likely to feel overwhelmed or depressed by pain than are counterparts who are not satisfied with spouse responses (Holtzman & Delongis, 2007). What are the qualities that seem to drive satisfaction? Several studies of patients with painful osteoarthritis suggest, not surprisingly, that they involve open communication (Porter, Keefe, Wellington, & de Williams, 2008) and accurate appraisals of the other's status (Cremeans-Smith et al., 2003). Moreover, there is evidence that training can positively impact spouse-assisted coping: patient/spouse dyads with osteoarthritis pain who underwent a 12-week training course showed significant increases in coping activities, perceived control over pain, and measures of physical fitness relative to dyads that did not receive such training (Keefe et al., 2004).

Catastrophizing, as noted above, is the coping response to pain that has seen the most focused attention (Chaves & Brown, 1987; Rosenstiel & Keefe, 1983; Sullivan, Bishop, & Pivik, 1995). It has been described as a significant cognitive component of the pain experience involving an exaggerated negative orientation to aversive stimuli (Sullivan et al., 1995). Catastrophizing is comprised of three elements that include ruminating about pain (e.g., "When I am in pain, I keep thinking about how badly I want the pain to stop"), appraising pain in a manner that magnifies its threat value (e.g., "When I am in pain, I become afraid that the pain will get worse"), and devaluing resources available to cope with pain (e.g., "When I am in pain, I feel I can't go on"). The primary measure currently used to assess the construct is the Pain Catastrophizing Scale (PCS; see Appendix B), a 13-item self-report inventory that was developed to measure the extent to which people catastrophize in response to pain (Sullivan et al., 1995). In a large literature, catastrophic thinking has been shown to correlate positively with many aspects of the pain experience, including pain intensity, emotional distress, pain-related disability, health services use, pain behavior, and reliance on medication (Goubert, Crombez, & Van Damme, 2004; Linton, Buer, Vlaeyen, & Hellsing, 2000; Sullivan, Stanish, Waite, Sullivan, & Tripp, 1998; Sullivan, Rodgers, & Kirsch, 2001; Sullivan & Neish, 1999).

Catastrophizing has been studied heavily in younger adults and to a lesser degree in older adults. Results of the latter studies are largely consistent with those of the former: in older adults with chronic pain, higher levels of catastrophizing are associated with higher levels of depression (Lopez-Lopez et al., 2008), higher levels of disability (Rapp et al., 2000; Shelby et al., 2008), and higher levels of reported pain (Shelby et al., 2008). Pain catastrophizing and self-efficacy appear to overlap: the latter study found levels of self-efficacy mediated relationships between catastrophizing and multiple clinical domains. Such results suggest that interventions aimed at improving pain management skills should address both catastrophizing and self efficacy.

Although the above discussion addresses catastrophizing as a cognitive coping skill, there is debate as to whether it should be treated as a skill or, instead, as a more enduring attribute or trait (Keefe, Lefebvre, & Smith, 1999). While the preponderance of opinion falls on the side of catastrophizing as a dysfunctional coping strategy, the debate is far from resolved, as the strategy has proved quite refractory to change. Indeed, some of the more effective treatment approaches have involved highly individualized exposure treatments, modeled after therapies successful in the treatment of anxiety disorders (Vlaeyan, de Jong, Sieben, & Crombez, 2002).

Whether catastrophizing is a particularly intractable coping strategy or a relatively stable attribute, there is evidence that the structure and content of pain catastrophizing cognitions may vary in association with demographic and situational factors. As noted above, catastrophizing subsumes three distinct elements for the general chronic pain population: rumination; magnified threat appraisal; and helplessness. The structure of catastrophizing for Black minorities in pain, however, may involve only two dimensions: rumination and powerlessness (Chibnall & Tait, 2005). Moreover, for patients coping with cancer pain, the content of catastrophizing cognitions appears to differ from that of patients with chronic non-malignant pain: cancer patients who catastrophize may view pain increases as signifying disease progression, impending death, etc. (Deshields et al., in press).

Aside from the predictably strong correspondence between catastrophizing and clinical adjustment, there is some research on catastrophizing and cognition that may have implications for older adults. Neurophysiologic research has shown that people that demonstrate high levels of catastrophizing also exhibit enhanced activity in brain regions associated with emotional distress when exposed to experimental pain inductions (Seminowicz & Davis, 2006). Those emotional responses may serve to enhance recall for pain: among patients experiencing arthritis pain, those who report high levels of catastrophizing demonstrate superior memory for pain, relative to low catastrophizing patients (Lefebvre & Keefe, 2002). If emotional reactivity associated with catastrophizing mediates memory, then patients with demonstrated tendencies to catastrophize, whose pain-related memories may fade less rapidly, may remain reactive to pain even as cognitive capacities wane.

Pain and Function

An increasing literature documents strong associations between chronic pain and dysfunction in older adults. As was noted previously, loss of function is an issue of particular significance in the older adult population. Functional decline (especially in mobility) has been shown to occasion depression (Chou, 2007; Gayman, Turner, & Cui, 2008), to inhibit recovery from depression (Mavandadi et al., 2007), to be associated with multiple other comorbidities (Juhakoski, Tenhonen, Anttonen, Kauppinen, & Arokoski, 2008; Leong, Farrell, Helme, & Gibson, 2007), and to predict mortality (Malmstrom et al., 2007). Further, the loss of function can have grave implications for independent living, especially when the mobility needed to carry out the basic activities of daily living is threatened (Bryant, Grigsby, Swenson, Scarbro, & Baxter, 2007). Finally, once functional capacity is compromised in an older adult, functional restoration can be a complex and challenging task that may require attention to a range of psychological factors, as well as rehabilitation of physical capacity (Weiner & Herr, 2002). For all of these reasons, the assessment of pain-related function (and/or its obverse, disability) is of crucial importance among older adults.

In this section we will briefly review several approaches to the assessment of pain-related function in older adults. Those approaches fall generally into one of three categories: self-report measures; observational measures; and performance measures. This chapter will not review of any one of these areas exhaustively, as the burgeoning literature on assessment renders that impractical. Instead, among self-report and performance measures, we examine those that are commonly used and that are relatively straightforward to administer. For observational measures, many of which have been employed among patients with cognitive impairments, we provide a somewhat more extensive review.

Self-Report Measures

Several brief measures that have been used to evaluate disability related to non-specific pain in older adults include the SF-36 (Ware & Sherbourne, 1992), the Brief Pain Inventory (BPI; Cleeland & Ryan, 1994), and the Pain Disability Index (PDI; Pollard, 1984; Tait, Chibnall, & Krause, 1990a). Each measure has good psychometric properties and is easily administered and scored. The SF-36, however, assesses health-related functional interference, rather than interference related to pain, so that a patient's general health status should be considered when interpreting the instrument. The BPI and the PDI both are pain specific, reliable, and with good evidence supporting their validity. The BPI is a 9-item instrument (although one item has seven sub-parts) that assesses pain distribution, severity, treatment effectiveness, and pain-related interference. Although initially developed to assess pain associated with cancer, it now is widely used to assess various pain conditions and has been translated into multiple languages. The PDI is a 7-item scale comprised of two subscales: one subscale measures pain-related interference with voluntary activities (e.g., household chores, socializing); and the other measures interference with obligatory activities (e.g., sleeping, bathing). Because the briefest of these measures is the PDI, it is included in Appendix C. As with the other measures noted above, it has been used successfully in research with older adults (Ruger et al., 2008; Fuentes, Hart-Johnson, & Green, et al., 2007).

Aside from these general measures of pain-related disability, several measures of condition-specific pain have been used with older adults. For example, the Western Ontario McMaster Universities Osteoarthritis Index (WOMAC; Bellamy, Buchanan, Goldsmith, Campbell, & Stitt, 1988) has been widely used to assess dysfunction associated with osteoarthritis, the most common painful condition among older adults (Jones et al., 2008; Juhakoski et al., 2008; Merle-Vincent et al., 2007). The

WOMAC is a 24-item self-report instrument used to assess pain, disability, and joint stiffness in patients with osteoarthritis. As with the BPI, the WOMAC has been widely used and translated into multiple languages. Similarly, several brief measures have been used to assess disability specific to low back pain, the Oswestry Disability Questionnaire (ODQ; Fisher, 2008) and the Roland-Morris Questionnaire (RMQ; Ersek, Turner, Cain, & Kemp, 2008). Both of these measures have been used extensively and are appropriate for clinical and research purposes when used with cognitively intact older adults.

Observational measures

In response to the challenges of pain assessment in patients with cognitive impairment such as dementia, much research in the past decade has focused on the use of behavioral observation measures to assess pain in older adults with dementia. While evidence has shown that older adults with mild to moderate cognitive impairment can provide valid self-reports of pain (Chibnall & Tait, 2001; Closs et al., 2004), the same cannot be said of older adults with advanced dementia, necessitating the use of alternative strategies in the latter group. While the latter point is not controversial, several important issues remain in regard to its implications: (1) at what point on the dementia spectrum should self-report assessment methods give way to behavioral observation methods; and (2) which neurocognitive functions (e.g., working memory, semantic memory, episodic memory, frontal/executive function) are most closely linked to the capacity of older adults with dementia to provide accurate self-report? These issues notwithstanding, studies of patients with cognitive compromise have shown that pain does affect behavior and that pain treatment impacts behavior in measurable ways (Chibnall, Tait, Harman, & Luebbert, 2005; Feldt, 2000; Fuchs-Lacelle & Hadjistavropoulos, 2004; Kovach, Noonan, Griffie, Muchka, & Weissman, 2002). We will briefly review that literature and then discuss an observational measure that has received considerable recent attention: the Pain Assessment Checklist for Seniors with Limited Ability to Communicate (PACSLAC; Fuchs-Lacelle & Hadjistavropoulos, 2004; Zwakhalen, Hamers, & Bergers 2007).

Presently, there are no fewer than 20 observational pain assessment tools that appear in recently published review papers on this subject (see Bjoro & Herr, 2008; Hadjistavropoulos et al., 2007a; Herr et al., 2006; Herr, Bursch, & Black, 2008; Zwakhalen, Hamers, Abu-Saad, & Berger, 2006). These tools differ along several dimensions: (1) the types of behaviors that are observed (e.g., facial expressions, verbalizations, body movements, social interactions); (2) the number of items rated (e.g., 10 or fewer, more than 10); (3) the time period required for observation (e.g., 1 minute, 5 minutes, etc.); and (4) the methods used to elicit behaviors (e.g., prescribed activities, usual daily activities). The sheer number of instruments that have been developed to assess pain using behavioral observation precludes an exhaustive overview here; the interested reader is referred to several excellent, recent reviews (cited below) for further details of available observational measures. Instead, we briefly review the psychometric properties of behavioral observation pain assessment tools.

Research establishing the measurement properties of observational pain assessment measures is still in its early stages. Consequently, no specific tool is recommended for wide adoption in clinical practice (Bjoro & Herr, 2008). Instead, recent reviews emphasize the overall need for further study into the reliability, validity, and clinical applicability of observational measures (Bjoro & Herr, 2008; Hadjistavropoulos et al., 2007a; Herr et al., 2006, 2008; Zwakhalen et al., 2006). One recent review (Herr et al., 2008) presented a systematic evaluation of empirical evidence on 17 observational tools, summarized in Table 24.1. Measures were evaluated along five dimensions, each on a 4-point scale (3 = evidence is strong, 2 = evidence supports need for further testing, 1 = evidence is insufficient and/or tool revisions are needed, and 0 = evidence is absent): conceptualization; subjects and setting; administration, scoring and feasibility; reliability; validity. As shown in Table 24.1, most measures received scores of 1 or 2 across categories, and only one measure (PAINAD) received any category

Table 24.1 2008 Evaluation of Observational Pain Assessment Measures*

	Conceptualization	Subjects & Setting	Administration, Scoring, & Feasibility	Reliability	Validity	Sum of Score
Abbey	1	1	1	1	1	5
ADD Protocol	2	2	2	1	2	9
CNPI	2	2	2	2	2	10
CPAT	1	1	1	0	1	4
DBS/MDS	2	2	0	1	2	7
Dis DAT	1	1	1	0	1	4
DS-DAT	2	2	1	2	2	9
Doloplus 2	2	2	2	2	2	10
EPCA-2	2	2	1	2	2	9
FLACC	0	1	0	1	1	3
MOBID	2	1	1	1	1	6
NOPPAIN	2	2	2	2	2	10
PACSLAC	2	2	2	2	2	10
PADE	1	2	2	1	2	8
PAINAD	2	3	3	3	2	13
PAINE	2	2	1	2	1	8
PBOICIE	1	1	0	1	1	4

**Used with permission of Keela Herr, PhD, RN, AGSF, FAAN, College of Nursing, The University of Iowa, copyright 2008*
*** ADD Protocol is not included as an assessment tool, but as a protocol for validation of presence of pain*
**** Ratings: 0 = Evidence is absent; 1 = Available evidence is insufficient and/or tool revisions are needed; 2 = Available evidence supports need for further testing; 3 = Available evidence is strong*
***** Tools: Abbey = Abbey Pain Scale (Abbey et al., 2004); ADD = Assessment of Discomfort in Dementia Protocol (Kovach et al., 1999); CNPI (Checklist of Nonverbal Pain Indicators (Feldt, 2000); CPAT = Certified Nurse Assistant Pain Assessment Tool (Cervo et al., 2007); DBS/MDS = Discomfort Behavior Scale (Stevenson et al., 2006); Dis DAT = Disability Distress Assessment Tool (Regnard et al., 2007); DS-DAT = Discomfort Scale-Dementia of the Alzheimer's Type (Hurley et al., 1992); Doloplus 2 = Doloplus 2 (Wary & Doloplus, 1999); FLACC = Faces, Legs, Activity, Cry and Consolability Pain Assessment Tool (Merkel et al., 1997); EPCA-2 = Elderly Pain Caring Assessment 2 (Morello et al., 2007); MOBID = Mobilization-Observation-Behavior-Intensity-Dementia Pain Scale (Husebo et al., 2007); NOPPAIN = Nursing Assistant-Administered Instrument to Assess Pain in Demented Individuals (Snow et al., 2004); PACSLAC = Pain Assessment Checklist for Seniors with Limited Ability to Communicate (Fuchs-Lacelle, & Hadjistavropoulos, 2004); PADE = Pain Assessment for the Dementing Elderly (Villaneuva et al., 2003); PAINAD = Pain Assessment in Advanced Dementia Scale (Warden et al., 2003); PAINE = Pain Assessment in Noncommunicative Elderly Persons (Cohen-Mansfield, 2006); PBOICE = Pain Behaviors for Osteoarthritis Instrument for Cognitively Impaired Elders (Tsai et al., 2008)*

rating of 3. We briefly discuss one instrument, the PACSLAC, to illustrate the points from this discussion.

The PACSLAC (Fuchs-Lacelle & Hadjistavropoulos, 2004) rates the presence/absence of 60 pain-related behaviors in four categories following a period of activity: (1) facial expressions (13 items); (2) activity/body movement (20 items); (3) social/personality/mood (12 items); and (4) other (physiologic indicators, eating, sleeping, vocal behaviors; 15 items). The total scale score ranges from 0 to 60, with 60 representing the presence of 60 pain behaviors. Evidence regarding the reliability of the instrument is good: Fuchs-Lacelle and Hadjistavropoulos (2004) report good internal reliability (Chronbach's alpha = 0.85), and good inter-rater reliability ($r = 0.89$) has been found between researcher and care-giver ratings of patients in dementia care facilities (Cheung & Choi, 2008). Evidence regarding validity is less strong: moderate support was found for the PACSLAC to differentiate between painful, distressing, or calm events (based on retrospective ratings), and guidelines to facilitate interpretation of PACSLAC scores are lacking (Zwakhalen et al., 2006). Nonetheless, there is evidence that routine use of the PACSLAC by nurses over a 3 month period improved pain management (increased PRN use of analgesic medications) in a long-term care unit (Fuchs-Lacelle, Hadjistavropoulos, & Lix, 2008), although it is not clear whether that change reflects properties of the instrument or simply increased attention to behavioral indicators of distress over that time period. Obviously, at 60 items the PACSLAC is somewhat cumbersome to administer, and several studies have described shortened versions of the instrument (van Nispen tot Pannerden et al., 2009; Zwakhalen et al., 2007;). In sum, like many of the other instruments studied, the PACSLAC demonstrates promise, but still requires considerable work.

An unresolved, substantive issue that remains regarding the use of behavioral observation to assess pain is when to apply this approach in a clinical setting. Prevailing opinion is that observations should be initiated upon noticeable change in behavior (e.g., Kovach et al., 1999, 2006). While this recommendation makes conceptual sense, nursing home staff, burdened by competing demands, may have difficulty identifying changes in behavior (Chibnall et al., 2005). Hence, cognitively impaired patients needing treatment for pain may not be readily identified in a long-term care setting.

Case Study 4—Pain and mobility

A 95-year-old White female with severe osteoarthritis had lived in a nursing home for four years secondary to functional limitations related to pain and to dementia of the Alzheimer's type (DAT). In the nursing home, she demonstrated very limited mobility and typically could be found sitting on a couch beside the nursing station. In her time in the nursing home, she developed affection for an 82-year-old male resident. She demonstrated her affection physically, reaching out to him whenever he walked by the couch in an attempt to grab his crotch. Her guardian enrolled her into a pain assessment study in which behavioral observation was built around an analgesic trial. Patients enrolled in the trial were randomly assigned to a protocol where they received either an active analgesic (acetaminophen) or a placebo for four weeks; after four weeks, they were moved into the other condition. During the time that the patient was in the placebo phase of the trial, there was no observable change in her behavior. During the analgesic phase, however, she demonstrated a marked increase in her levels of activity. This activity increase was viewed with annoyance by the nursing staff: because of her increased mobility, she was able to demonstrate her affection repeatedly and at multiple locations around the nursing unit. Hence, despite the obvious increase in mobility associated with the analgesic phase of the trial, the staff physician decided against instituting routine acetaminophen administration following her trial participation.

Performance Measures

Functional performance measures include objective tests of prescribed tasks, such as standing, balancing, lifting, or walking. Many of these tests measure timed performance on a given task administered by a trained observer. For example, a performance test may require an individual to walk 4 meters at their usual pace (e.g., Miller, Wolinsky, Andresen, Malmstrom, & Miller, 2008b) or at a rapid walking pace (e.g., Reid, Williams, & Gill, 2005), or to walk up and down a flight of stairs as quickly as possible (e.g., Miller, Nicklas, & Loeser, 2008a). Functional performance tests also may include measures of strength (e.g., handgrip, knee), using a dynamometer, or endurance (e.g., total distance achieved in a six minute walk; e.g., Leveille et al., 1999). Among older adult populations, studies have demonstrated that functional performance measures are robust at differentiating between individuals with differing pain levels (Reid et al., 2005; Eggermont et al., 2009; Leveille et al., 1999; Miller, 2008a; Onder et al., 2006; Weaver et al., 2009). Physical performance measures also are valid alternative methods of collecting functional data in older adults with impaired cognitive function that precludes use of self-report measures (Guralnik, Branch, Cummings, & Curb, 1989).

One functional performance measure, in particular, that has been used widely in gerontology over the last decade and, more recently, in pain studies (e.g., Eggermont et al., 2009; Onder et al., 2006;

Weaver et al., 2009) is the Short Physical Performance Battery (SPPB; Guralnik, Ferrucci, Simonsick, Salive, & Wallace, 1995; Guralnik et al., 1994). The SPPB is a standardized battery with three components: walking speed; chair stands; and standing balance. It has established predictive validity for various behavioral outcomes, including disability (Guralnik et al., 1989; Onder et al., 2005), health services utilization (Penninx et al., 2000), and mortality (Perera, Studenski, Chandler, & Guralnik, 2005). The SPPB also is sensitive to change in physical status over time (Miller et al., 2008b) and to interventions in randomized controlled trials (Pahor et al., 2006).

The administration of the SPPB is straightforward. Walking speed is measured (meter/second) over a 4-meter course on which participants walk at their usual pace. The chair stand component requires a sturdy chair without arms at an appropriate height for participants. Participants cross their arms over their chests and complete five rises and returns as quickly as possible. Chair stand is scored as time to complete the task (or a maximum of 60 seconds). Balance is measured using a hierarchical set of tasks, including side-by-side stand, semi-tandem stand, and tandem stand. Established scoring rules are used to quantify balance across tasks (Guralnik et al., 1995, 1994). Raw scores on each SPPB component (walking speed, chair stands, balance) are converted to a 0–4 scale (0 = inability to complete the test; 4 = highest level of performance). The sum of the 0–4 scales (0–12) is used as a composite measure of physical performance (Guralnik et al., 1995, 1994; Ostir, Volpato, Fried, Chaves, & Guralnik, 2002).

CLINICAL PRACTICE GUIDELINES

Interdisciplinary clinical practice guidelines for managing pain in older adults are available from the American Geriatrics Society (AGS) (AGS Panel on Persistent Pain in Older Persons, 2002; AGS Panel on the Pharmacological Management of Persistent Pain in Older Persons, 2009) and the American Medical Directors Association (AMDA) (2009). The AGS and AMDA guidelines represent evidence-based and expert recommendations for pain management, and provide a framework that addresses key considerations for health professionals in the care of older adults with pain. While the general principles put forth by AGS and AMDA overlap considerably, the AMDA guidelines target professionals working in the long-term care (LTC) setting. AGS (AGS Panel on Persistent Pain in Older Persons, 2002; AGS Panel on the Pharmacological Management of Persistent Pain in Older Persons, 2009) and AMDA (2009) also provide comprehensive guidelines on the pharmacologic treatment of pain in older adults. Here we provide an overview of the AGS and AMDA clinical practice guidelines with an emphasis on the central role of assessment in pain management.

American Geriatrics Society (AGS)

The AGS guidelines focus on the management of chronic pain in older adults aged 75 and above because of the high levels of frailty, disability, comorbid conditions, sensory deficits, and dementia which complicate pain assessment and management and assessment of pain in this group (AGS Panel on Persistent Pain in Older Persons, 2002). Relative to pain assessment, the following emphases shape the five primary guidelines: (1) the necessity of undertaking appropriate diagnostic testing in order to understand the underlying cause(s) of pain; (2) the value of an interdisciplinary approach; (3) that self-report of pain remains the gold standard for older adults, including those with mild-to-moderate cognitive impairment; (4) that older adults may be reluctant to admit pain; and (5) that information from ancillary sources (families and caregivers) can be valuable.

Of the five primary AGS (AGS Panel on Persistent Pain in Older Persons, 2002) guidelines, the first two are straightforward: (1) health professionals should assess older adults for persistent pain when care begins (e.g., admission, new provider, etc.); and (2) health professionals should recognize that persistent pain is a significant problem if it impacts an older adult's physical or psychosocial function. In the latter case, the third guideline advises a comprehensive assessment that should include a thorough history and physical examination. The history should document: (1) pain characteristics (i.e., pain intensity, duration, location, etc.); (2) how pain impacts quality of life (i.e., physical and/or psychosocial function); (3) patients' understanding both of pain and pain management; (4) patients' previous use of analgesics, including effectiveness and side effects; (5) previous treatments and their efficacy; and (6) identification and discussion of patients' concern(s) regarding past or current pain treatments. The physical examination should include: (1) evaluation of area of pain origin; (2) musculoskeletal exam; (3) neurological exam; and (4) observed tests of physical performance (e.g., usual activities, physical performance, etc.). Of course, appropriate diagnostic and laboratory tests should be done when questions arise from the history and physical exam.

Recommendations for pain assessment are consistent with materials discussed earlier in this chapter. Self-report measures are recommended for older adults with normal cognitive function or with mild-to-moderate dementia, using a standardized, validated pain assessment scale (no specific scale is recommended). As noted earlier, older adults may use a range of descriptors for pain (e.g., aching, soreness, burning, etc.), so health professionals should consider such terminology when screening for pain. Pain-related functional interference should be ascertained by direct questions, supplemented when appropriate with standardized instruments such as the Pain Disability Index. Patients with mild-to-moderate cognitive impairment may require extra time, repeat instructions, or assistance from family members. The guidelines recommend against reliance on only clinician or informant ratings to assess pain intensity, however, unless a patient is unable to provide such information.

A fourth AGS (AGS Panel on Persistent Pain in Older Persons, 2002) guideline applies to patients with advanced dementia and recommends behavioral observation to assess pain-related behaviors, including verbalizations (e.g., moaning, groaning) and body movements (e.g., guarding, tensing). While AGS does not recommend a specific behavioral observation instrument, the guidelines underscore the importance of differentiating between pain behaviors that occur during movement (e.g., walking, transfers) versus pain behaviors that occur in the absence of movement. When pain behaviors are observed during movement, the guidelines suggest the use of analgesic medication prior to the initiation of activities (e.g., bathing, transfers), as well as non-pharmacologic approaches (e.g., physical therapy) to minimize activity-related pain. When pain behaviors are independent of movement, the guidelines suggest the investigation of a specific cause of pain behavior (e.g., infection, constipation) and/or whether basic needs (e.g., thirst, hunger) are being met. Finally, should no curable cause of pain be identified, AGS suggests that an analgesic trial may be used as a means to reduce non-movement pain behaviors.

The final AGS (AGS Panel on Persistent Pain in Older Persons, 2002) guideline emphasizes the importance of reassessment for persistent pain at regular intervals following the initial assessment. Further, the guideline recommends that the same instrument(s) be used for reassessment as for the initial assessment. The efficacy and potential side effects of any treatments also should be monitored as part of reassessment.

American Medical Directors Association (AMDA)

As noted earlier, while compatible with guidelines issued by AGS, the AMDA (2009) clinical practice guidelines provide recommendations for acute and persistent pain management specific to long-term care (LTC). The AMDA guiding principles emphasize that the core of pain management in LTC involves individually tailored care plans. AMDA emphasizes the need for interdisciplinary care (i.e., input from patient, caregivers, physicians, nurses, therapists, etc.) and recognizes the importance of institutional commitment to effective pain management in LTC settings. In particular, the guidelines emphasize the importance of communication, consistency in language, documentation, and education.

The specific AMDA pain management guidelines are organized in four categories: recognition; assessment; treatment; and monitoring.

Pain recognition includes an evaluation of the presence (or absence) of pain, identification of pain characteristics, diagnosis of possible source(s) of pain, and provision of interim treatment (as necessary). The recognition of pain begins with routine assessment upon admission and at least quarterly thereafter; assessment should occur daily for LTC residents with conditions known to cause pain. Evaluation of pain characteristics should include a pain intensity rating on an appropriate scale, description of pain characteristics, identification of known activities/circumstances that improve or worsen pain, and determination of impact of pain on function (e.g., sleep, activities of daily living, quality of life). Observation of patient behaviors and function also is encouraged, especially at times of activity (e.g., bathing, therapy, activities). Interim treatment should be provided if existing treatment is inadequate.

Pain recognition activities in LTC settings begin with a medical history and physical examination. The history should include: relevant diagnoses and conditions; solicitation of information from family regarding diagnoses and conditions; medication use along with known adverse events associated with medication use; and information regarding previous clinical care (assessments and treatments) for pain. Consistent with AGS guidelines, AMDA advises further diagnostic tests, evaluations, and consultations (as needed) to determine the cause of pain, if unknown, following a medical history and physical examination. A thorough assessment also should investigate the effect of pain on function and quality of life.

The development and implementation of interdisciplinary, individualized care plans is recommended to treat pain in LTC patients. The care plan should identify an assessment measure and frequency of repeat assessments to monitor pain, and also monitor functional outcomes, especially those important to an individual patient (e.g., ambulation, social activity, etc.). A treatment plan should establish goals for pain reduction and improvements in relevant functional outcomes with input from patients and caregivers. Finally, the AMDA guidelines emphasize the importance of routine pain monitoring, including both the assessment of pain intensity and the impact of pain on function, quality of life, sleep, mood, etc. Such monitoring is critical to the evaluation of treatment efficacy; if monitoring shows treatment to be ineffective, treatment should be adjusted as necessary or referral to specialists initiated.

CONCLUDING REMARKS

There has been enormous progress in the past decade in the assessment and treatment of pain in older adults. Ten years ago, relatively few recognized the prevalence of pain in the older age group, much less the complexities of assessment and the importance of effective treatment. Presently, updated guidelines exist for the treatment of pain in older adults who reside in the community and in alternative living arrangements. Moreover, new technologies have enabled research into anatomic and physiologic substrates that modulate neurocognitive processes associated with the experience of pain. Some of that work translates directly into clinical applications (e.g., Bennedetti et al., 2006; Seminowicz, Mikulis, & Davis, 2004).

Progress in the assessment realm, however, has been more mixed. We now know that older adults detect painful stimuli at levels that are similar to younger adults, but appear to have higher pain thresholds, possibly secondary to changes in their affective/motivational response to pain (Scherder et al., 2005). We now realize that older adults with mild-to-moderate dementia can provide valid self-reports and that selected self-report scales are superior to others in assessing pain in that subgroup. On the other hand, although there are many investigators attempting to address the issue, we have yet to identify a practical and widely accepted method of assessing pain in older adults with advanced dementia. This shortcoming represents a major clinical and ethical problem, inasmuch as pain appears to be widespread in this large and increasing subgroup of older adults.

Similar problems exist in relation to the treatment of pain in this age group. In general, pain continues to be undertreated, both in the community and in alternative living settings (Pahor et al., 1999). Moreover, many of the medications commonly used to treat pain are associated with medical complications when used in older adults, including non-steroidal medications (MacLean, 2001), central nervous system medications (Hanlon et al., 2009), and opioids (Fine, 2004). While these complications can be managed in many cases with appropriate medical oversight, such oversight often requires both special expertise and time commitment, commodities that can be scarce in current health care. Treatment difficulties also can be magnified by regulatory complications. For example, the Food and Drug Administration (FDA) issued a strong safety warning in June 2009 against the use of acetaminophen-containing analgesic compounds (with further restrictions likely to follow), secondary to the large number of those compounds and the potential for consumers to consume them in quantities that can cause liver damage. While that alert clearly was based on empirical data, other data have shown that acetaminophen is a safe analgesic for many older adults relative to other analgesic treatments (Bannwarth et al., 2001). Further, some of the most commonly used (and safe) analgesics in nursing homes, where considerable medical and nursing oversight exist, involve compounds that contain acetaminophen (Guay, Lackner, & Hanlon, 2002). Hence, the FDA safety warning and any subsequent proscriptions against the use of acetaminophen-containing compounds are likely to further complicate the treatment of pain in a population where pain management already is problematic.

In light of both the progress and problems highlighted above (and throughout this chapter), there has been a recent call to establish a subfield of pain research that focuses on pain and aging (Gagliese, 2009). To a large degree, this research subfield already has emerged, impelled forward by discoveries such as those described in preceding pages and by the need for further discovery. The clinical picture described above, however, justifies a call that extends beyond the realm of research to further clinical and programmatic activities designed to better the quality of care rendered to this vulnerable population.

APPENDIX A: PAIN SELF-EFFICACY QUESTIONNAIRE (PSEQ)*

Please rate how confident you are that you can do the following things at present, despite the pain. To indicate your answer circle one of the numbers on the scale under each item, where 0 = not at all confident and 6 = completely confident.

1. I can enjoy things, despite the pain.

1______	2______	3______	4______	5______	6______
Not at all Confident					Completely Confident

2. I can do most of the household chores (e.g., tidying-up, washing dishes, etc.), despite the pain.

1______	2______	3______	4______	5______	6______
Not at all Confident					Completely Confident

3. I can socialize with my friends or family members as often as I used to do, despite the pain.

(continued on next page)

* Used with the permission of M. K. Nicholas. (Nicholas, M. K. Self-efficacy and chronic pain. In a paper presented at the annual conference of the British Psychological Society, St. Andrews, Scotland, 1989.)

1______ 2______ 3______ 4______ 5______ 6______

Not at all Confident ... Completely Confident

4. I can cope with my pain in most situations.

1______ 2______ 3______ 4______ 5______ 6______

Not at all Confident ... Completely Confident

5. I can do some form of work, despite the pain ("work" includes housework, paid and unpaid work).

1______ 2______ 3______ 4______ 5______ 6______

Not at all Confident ... Completely Confident

6. I can still do many of the things I enjoy doing, such as hobbies or leisure activity, despite pain.

1______ 2______ 3______ 4______ 5______ 6______

Not at all Confident ... Completely Confident

7. I can cope with my pain without medication.

1______ 2______ 3______ 4______ 5______ 6______

Not at all Confident ... Completely Confident

8. I can still accomplish most of my goals in life, despite the pain.

1______ 2______ 3______ 4______ 5______ 6______

Not at all Confident ... Completely Confident

9. I can live a normal lifestyle, despite the pain.

1______ 2______ 3______ 4______ 5______ 6______

Not at all Confident ... Completely Confident

10. I can gradually become more active, despite the pain.

1______ 2______ 3______ 4______ 5______ 6______

Not at all Confident ... Completely Confident

APPENDIX B: PAIN CATASTROPHIZING SCALE*

Below are statements that describe different thoughts and feelings about pain. Circle the number on the scale (0 = Not at all to 4 = All the time) that best describes the way *you* feel when you experience pain.

1. "When I'm in pain, I worry all the time about whether the pain will end." Do you do this not at all, to a slight degree, to a moderate degree, to a great degree, or all the time?
   0 = NOT AT ALL
   1 = TO A SLIGHT DEGREE
   2 = TO A MODERATE DEGREE
   3 = TO A GREAT DEGREE
   4 = ALL THE TIME

* Used with the permission of Michael J. L. Sullivan, Copyright 1995.

2. "When I'm in pain, I feel I can't go on." Do you feel this way not at all, to a slight degree, to a moderate degree, to a great degree, or all the time?
   0 = NOT AT ALL
   1 = TO A SLIGHT DEGREE
   2 = TO A MODERATE DEGREE
   3 = TO A GREAT DEGREE
   4 = ALL THE TIME
3. "When I'm in pain, it's terrible and I think it's never going to get any better." Do you think this way not at all, to a slight degree, to a moderate degree, to a great degree, or all the time?
   0 = NOT AT ALL
   1 = TO A SLIGHT DEGREE
   2 = TO A MODERATE DEGREE
   3 = TO A GREAT DEGREE
   4 = ALL THE TIME
4. "When I'm in pain, it's awful and I feel that it overwhelms me." Do you feel this way not at all, to a slight degree, to a moderate degree, to a great degree, or all the time?
   0 = NOT AT ALL
   1 = TO A SLIGHT DEGREE
   2 = TO A MODERATE DEGREE
   3 = TO A GREAT DEGREE
   4 = ALL THE TIME
5. "When I'm in pain, I feel I can't stand it anymore." Do you feel this way not at all, to a slight degree, to a moderate degree, to a great degree, or all the time?
   0 = NOT AT ALL
   1 = TO A SLIGHT DEGREE
   2 = TO A MODERATE DEGREE
   3 = TO A GREAT DEGREE
   4 = ALL THE TIME
6. "When I'm in pain, I become afraid that the pain will get worse." Do you think this way not at all, to a slight degree, to a moderate degree, to a great degree, or all the time?
   0 = NOT AT ALL
   1 = TO A SLIGHT DEGREE
   2 = TO A MODERATE DEGREE
   3 = TO A GREAT DEGREE
   4 = ALL THE TIME
7. "When I'm in pain, I keep thinking of other painful events." Do you think this way not at all, to a slight degree, to a moderate degree, to a great degree, or all the time?
   0 = NOT AT ALL
   1 = TO A SLIGHT DEGREE
   2 = TO A MODERATE DEGREE
   3 = TO A GREAT DEGREE
   4 = ALL THE TIME
8. "When I'm in pain, I anxiously want the pain to go away." Do you do this not at all, to a slight degree, to a moderate degree, to a great degree, or all the time?
   0 = NOT AT ALL
   1 = TO A SLIGHT DEGREE
   2 = TO A MODERATE DEGREE
   3 = TO A GREAT DEGREE
   4 = ALL THE TIME
9. "When I'm in pain, I can't seem to keep it out of my mind." Do you do this not at all, to a slight degree, to a moderate degree, to a great degree, or all the time?
   0 = NOT AT ALL

1 = TO A SLIGHT DEGREE
2 = TO A MODERATE DEGREE
3 = TO A GREAT DEGREE
4 = ALL THE TIME

10. "When I'm in pain, I keep thinking about how much it hurts." Do you think this way not at all, to a slight degree, to a moderate degree, to a great degree, or all the time?
0 = NOT AT ALL
1 = TO A SLIGHT DEGREE
2 = TO A MODERATE DEGREE
3 = TO A GREAT DEGREE
4 = ALL THE TIME

11. "When I'm in pain, I keep thinking about how badly I want the pain to stop." Do you think this way not at all, to a slight degree, to a moderate degree, to a great degree, or all the time?
0 = NOT AT ALL
1 = TO A SLIGHT DEGREE
2 = TO A MODERATE DEGREE
3 = TO A GREAT DEGREE
4 = ALL THE TIME

12. "When I'm in pain, there's nothing I can do to reduce the intensity of the pain." Do you feel this way not at all, to a slight degree, to a moderate degree, to a great degree, or all the time?
0 = NOT AT ALL
1 = TO A SLIGHT DEGREE
2 = TO A MODERATE DEGREE
3 = TO A GREAT DEGREE
4 = ALL THE TIME

13. "When I'm in pain, I wonder whether something serious may happen." Do you think this way not at all, to a slight degree, to a moderate degree, to a great degree, or all the time?
0 = NOT AT ALL
1 = TO A SLIGHT DEGREE
2 = TO A MODERATE DEGREE
3 = TO A GREAT DEGREE
4 = ALL THE TIME

APPENDIX C: PAIN DISABILITY INDEX*

The rating scales below measure the impact of pain in your everyday life. We want to know how much your pain is preventing you from doing your normal activities. For each of the 7 categories of life activity listed, *circle* the *one* number that best reflects the level of disability you typically experience. A score of 0 means no disability at all. A score of 10 means that all the activities which you would normally do have been disrupted or prevented by your pain. Your rating should reflect the *overall* impact of pain in your life, not just when the pain is at its worst. Make a rating for every category. If you think a category does not apply to you, circle "0."

1. Family/Home Responsibilities. This category refers to activities related to the home or family. It includes chores and duties performed around the house (e.g., yard work) and errands or favors for other family members (e.g., driving the children to school).

0 1 2 3 4 5 6 7 8 9 10
no disability mild moderate severe total disability

2. Recreation. This category includes hobbies, sports, and other leisure-time activities.

0 1 2 3 4 5 6 7 8 9 10
no disability mild moderate severe total disability

3. Social Activity. This category includes parties, theater, concerts, dining out, and other social activities that are attended with family and friends.

0 1 2 3 4 5 6 7 8 9 10
no disability mild moderate severe total disability

4. Occupation. This category refers to activities that are directly related to one's job. This includes nonpaying jobs as well, such as that of a homemaker or volunteer worker.

0 1 2 3 4 5 6 7 8 9 10
no disability mild moderate severe total disability

5. Sexual Behavior. This category refers to the frequency and quality of one's sex life.

0 1 2 3 4 5 6 7 8 9 10
no disability mild moderate severe total disability

6. Self-Care. This category includes personal maintenance and independent daily living activities (e.g., taking a shower, driving, getting dressed, etc.).

0 1 2 3 4 5 6 7 8 9 10
no disability mild moderate severe total disability

7. Life-Support Activity. This category refers to basic life-supporting behaviors such as eating, sleeping, and breathing.

0 1 2 3 4 5 6 7 8 9 10
no disability mild moderate severe total disability

* Reprinted from *Pain 40*, Tait, R. C., Chibnall, J.T. & Krause, S. The pain disability index; psychometric properties, 171–182, 1990, with permission from Elsevier.

REFERENCES

Abbey, J., Piller, N., De Bellis, A., Esterman, A., Parker, D., Giler, L., & Lowcay, B. (2004). The abbey pain scale: a 1-minute numerical indicator for people with end-stage dementia. *International Journal of Palliative Nursing*, *10*, 6–13.

AGS Panel on Persistent Pain in Older Persons. (2002). The management of persistent pain in older persons. *J. Am. Geriatr. Soc.*, *50*, S205–S224.

AGS Panel on the Pharmacological Management of Persistent Pain in Older Persons. (2009). Pharmacological management of persistent pain in older persons. *J. Am. Geriatr. Soc.*, *57*, 1331–1346.

American Medical Directors Association. (2009). *Pain Management Clinical Practice Guideline*. Columbia, MD: AMDA.

Bannwarth, B., Pehourcq, F., Lagrange, F., Matoga, M., Maury, S., Palisson, M., & Le Bars, M. (2001). Single and multiple dose pharmacokinetics of acetaminophen (Paracetamol) in polymedicated very old patients with rheumatic pain. *J. Rheumatol.*, *28*, 182–184.

Barry, L. C., Guo, Z., Kerns, R. D., Duong, B. D., & Reid, M. C. (2003). Functional self-efficacy and pain-related disability among older veterans with chronic pain in a primary care setting. *Pain*, *104*, 131–137.

Bellamy, N., Buchanan, W. W., Goldsmith, C. H., Campbell, J., & Stitt, L. W. (1988). Validation study of WOMAC: a health status instrument for measuring clinically important patient relevant outcomes to antirheumatic drug therapy in patients with osteoarthritis of the hip or knee. *J. Rheumatol.*, *15*, 1833–1840.

Benedetti, F., Arduino, C., Costa, S., Vighetti, S., Tarenzi, L., Rainero, I., & Asteggiano, G. (2006). Loss of expectation-related mechanisms in Alzheimer's disease makes analgesic therapies less effective. *Pain, 121*, 133–144.

Benedetti, F., Arduino, C., Vighetti, S., Asteggiano, G., Tarenzi, L., & Rainero, I. (2004). Pain reactivity in Alzheimer patients with different degrees of cognitive impairment and brain activity deterioration. *Pain, 111*, 22–29.

Benedetti, F., Vighetti, S., Ricco, C., Lagna, E., Bergamasco, B., Pinessi, L., & Rainero, I. (1999). Pain threshold and tolerance in Alzheimer's disease. *Pain, 80*, 377–382.

Bjoro, K., & Herr, K. (2008). Assessment of pain in the nonverbal or cognitively impaired older adult. *Clinics in Geriatric Medicine, 24*, 237–262.

Blumer, D., & Heilbronn, M. (1982). Chronic pain as a variant of depressive disease: the pain-prone disorder. *J. Nerv. Ment. Dis., 170*, 381–406.

Brekke, M., Hjortdahl, P., & Kvien, T. K. (2001). Self-efficacy and health status in rheumatoid arthritis: a two-year longitudinal observational study. *Rheumatology, 40*, 387–392.

Bryant, L. L., Grigsby, J., Swenson, C., Scarbro, S., & Baxter, J. (2007). Chronic pain increases the risk of decreasing physical performance in older adults: the San Luis Valley Health and Aging Study. *J. Gerontol., Ser. A, 62*, 989–996.

Cervo, F. A., Raggi, R. P., Bright-Long, L. E., Wright, W. K., Rows, G., Torres, A. E., Levy, R. B., & Komaroff, E. (2007). Use of the certified nursing assistant pain assessment tool (CPAT) in nursing home residents with dementia. *American Journal of Alzheimer's Disease & Other Dementias, 22*, 112–119.

Chaves, J. F., & Brown, J. M. (1987). Spontaneous cognitive strategies for the control of clinical pain and stress. *Journal of Behavioral Medicine, 10*, 263–276.

Chibnall, J. T., & Tait, R. C. (2001). Pain assessment in cognitively impaired and unimpaired older adults: a comparison of four scales. *Pain, 92*, 173–186.

Chibnall, J. T., & Tait, R. C. (2005). Confirmatory factor analysis of the Pain Catastrophizing Scale in African American and Caucasian Workers' Compensation claimants with low back injuries. *Pain, 113*, 369–375.

Chibnall, J. T., Tait, R. C., Harman, B., & Luebbert, R. A. (2005). Effect of acetaminophen on behavior, well-being, and psychotropic medication use in nursing home residents with moderate-to-severe dementia. *J. Am. Geriatr. Soc., 53*, 1921–1929.

Cheung, G., & Choi, P. (2008). The use of the Pain Assessment Checklist for Seniors with Limited Ability to Communicate (PACSLAC) by caregivers in dementia care. *N. Z. Med. J., 121*, 21–29.

Chou, K. L. (2007). Reciprocal relationship between pain and depression in older adults: evidence from the English Longitudinal Study of Ageing. *J. Affective Disord., 102*, 115–123.

Clark, D. O., & Nothwehr, F. (1999). Exercise self-efficacy and its correlates among socioeconomically disadvantaged older adults. *Health Education & Behavior, 26*, 535–546.

Cleeland, C. S., & Ryan, K. M. (1994). Pain assessment: global use of the Brief Pain Inventory. *Annals of the Academy of Medicine, Singapore, 23*, 129–138.

Closs, S. J., Barr, B., Briggs, M., Cash, K., & Seers, K. (2004). A comparison of five pain assessment scales for nursing home residents with varying degrees of cognitive impairment. *J. Pain Symptom Manag., 27*, 196–205.

Cohen-Mansfield, J. (2006). Pain Assessment in Noncommunicative Elderly persons—PAINE. *Clinical Journal of Pain, 22*, 569–575.

Cole, L. J., Farrell, M. J., Duff, E. P., Barber, J. B., Egan, G. F., & Gibson, S. J. (2006). Pain sensitivity and fMRI pain-related brain activity in Alzheimer's disease. *Brain, 129*, 2957–2965.

Cremeans-Smith, J. K., Stephens, M. A., Franks, M. M., Martire, L. M., Druley, J. A., & Wojno, W. C. (2003). Spouses' and physicians' perceptions of pain severity in older women with osteoarthritis: dyadic agreement and patients' well-being. *Pain, 106*, 27–34.

DeGood, D. E., & Tait, R. C. (2001). Assessment of pain beliefs and pain coping. In D. C. Turk, & R. Melzack (Eds.), *Handbook of Pain Assessment—Second Edition* (pp. 320–345). New York, NY: The Guilford Press.

Deshields, T. L., Jenkins, J. O., & Tait, R. C. (1989). The experience of anger in chronic illness: a preliminary investigation. *International Journal of Psychiatry in Medicine, 19*, 299–309.

Deshields, T. L., Tait, R. C., Manwaring, J., Trinkaus, K. M., Naughton M., Hawkins J., & Jeffe, D. B. (in press). The Cancer Pain Inventory: Preliminary development and validation. *Psycho-Oncology.*

Eggermont, L. H., Bean, J. F., Guralnik, J. M., & Leveille, S. G. (2009). Comparing pain severity versus pain location in the MOBILIZE Boston study: chronic pain and lower extremity function. *J. Gerontol., Ser. A*, *64*, 763–770.

Ersek, M., Turner, J. A., Cain, K. C., & Kemp, C. A. (2008). Results of a randomized controlled trial to examine the efficacy of a chronic pain self-management for older adults. *Pain*, *138*, 29–40.

Feldt, K. S. (2000). The checklist of nonverbal pain indicators (CNPI). *Pain Management Nursing*, *1*, 13–21.

Ferrell, B. A., Ferrell, B. R., & Rivera, L. (1995). Pain in cognitively impaired nursing home patients. *J. Pain Symptom Manag.*, *10*, 591–598.

Fine, P. G. (2004). Pharmacological management of persistent pain in older patients. *Clinical Journal of Pain*, *20*, 220–226.

Fisher, K. (2008). Assessing clinically meaningful change following a programme for managing chronic pain. *Clinical Rehabilitation*, *22*, 252–259.

Focht, B. C., Rejeski, W. J., Ambrosius, W. T., Katula, J. A., & Messier, S. P. (2005). Exercise, self-efficacy, and mobility performance in overweight and obese adults with knee osteoarthritis. *Arthritis & Rheumatism*, *53*, 659–665.

Fox, P. L., Raina, P., & Jadad, A. R. (1999). Prevalence and treatment of pain in older adults in nursing homes and other long-term care institutions: a systematic review. *Can. Med. Assoc. J.*, *160*, 329–333.

Fuchs-Lacelle, S., & Hadjistavropoulos, T. (2004). Development and preliminary validation of the pain assessment checklist for seniors with limited ability to communicate (PACSLAC). *Pain Management Nursing*, *5*, 37–49.

Fuchs-Lacelle, S., Hadjistavropoulos, T., & Lix, L. (2008). Pain assessment as intervention: a study of older adults with severe dementia. *Clinical Journal of Pain*, *24*, 697–707.

Fuentes, M., Hart-Johnson, T., & Green, C. R. (2007). The association among neighborhood socioeconomic status, race and chronic pain in black and white older adults. *J. Natl. Med. Assoc.*, *99*, 1160–1169.

Gagliese, L. (2001). Assessment of pain in elderly people. In D. C. Turk, & R. Melzack (Eds.), *Handbook of Pain Assessment—Second Edition* (pp. 119–133). New York, NY: The Guilford Press.

Gagliese, L. (2009). Pain and aging: the emergence of a new subfield of pain research. *J. Pain*, *10*, 343–353.

Gagliese, L., & Melzack, R. (1997). Age differences in the quality of chronic pain: a preliminary study. *Pain Research and Management*, *2*, 157–162.

Gagliese, L., Weizblit, N., Ellis, W., & Chan, V. W. (2005). The measurement of postoperative pain: a comparison of intensity scales in younger and older surgical patients. *Pain*, *117*, 412–420.

Gatchel, R. J., & Dersh, J. (2002). Psychological disorders and chronic pain: are there cause-and-effect relationships? In D. C. Turk, & R. J. Gatchel (Eds.), *Psychological Approaches to Pain Management: A Practitioner's Handbook—Second Edition* (pp. 30–51). New York, NY: The Guilford Press.

Gayman, M. D., Turner, R. J., & Cui, M. (2008). Physical limitations and depressive symptoms: exploring the nature of the association. *Journals of Gerontology Series B—Psychological Sciences & Social Sciences*, *63*, S219–S228.

Gibson, S. J., & Farrell, M. (2004). A review of age differences in the neurophysiology of nociception and the perceptual experience of pain. *Clinical Journal of Pain*, *20*, 227–239.

Gibson, S. J., Voukelatos, X., Ames, D., Flicker, L., & Helme, R. D. (2001). An examination of pain perception and cerebral event-related potentials following carbon dioxide laser stimulation in patients with Alzheimer's disease and age-matched control volunteers. *Pain Research & Management*, *6*, 126–132.

Goubert, L., Crombez, G., & Van Damme, S. (2004). The role of neuroticism, pain catastrophizing and pain-related fear in vigilance to pain: a structural equations approach. *Pain*, *107*, 234–241.

Greene, B. L., Haldeman, G. F., Kaminski, A., Neal, K., Lim, S. S., & Conn, D. L. (2006). Factors affecting physical activity behavior in urban adults with arthritis who are predominatly African-American and female. *Physical Therapy*, *86*, 510–519.

Guay, D. R., Lackner, T. E., & Hanlon, J. T. (2002). Pharmacologic management: noninvasive modalities. In D. K. Weiner, K. Herr, & T. E. Rudy (Eds.), *Persistent Pain in Older Adults: An Interdisciplinary Guide for Treatment* (pp. 160–187). New York, NY: Springer Publishing Company.

Guralnik, J. M., Branch, L. G., Cummings, S. R., & Curb, J. D. (1989). Physical performance measures in aging research. *J. Gerontol., Ser. A*, *44*, M141–M146.

Guralnik, J. M., Ferrucci, L., Simonsick, E. M., Salive, M. E., & Wallace, R. B. (1995). Lower-extremity function in persons over the age of 70 years as a predictor of subsequent disability. *N. Engl. J. Med.*, *332*, 556–561.

Guralnik, J. M., Simonsick, E. M., Ferrucci, L., Glynn, R. J., Berkman, L. F., Blazer, D. G., et al. (1994). A short physical performance battery assessing lower extremity function: association with self-reported disability and prediction of mortality and nursing home admission. *J. Gerontol.*, *49*, M85–M94.

Hadjistavropoulos, T., Herr, K., Turk, D. C., Fine, P. G., Dworkin, R. H., Helme, R., et al. (2007a). An interdisciplinary expert consensus statement on assessment of pain in older persons. *Clinical Journal of Pain*, *23*, S1–S43.

Hadjistavropoulos, T., Martin, R. R., Sharpe, D., Lints, A. C., McCreary, D. R., & Asmundson, G. J. (2007b). A longitudinal investigation of fear of falling, fear of pain, and activity avoidance in community-dwelling older adults. *Journal of Aging & Health*, *19*, 965–984.

Hanlon, J. T., Boudreau, R. M., Roumani, Y. F., Newman, A. B., Ruby, C. M., Wright, R. M., et al. (2009). Number and dosage of central nervous system medications on recurrent falls in community elders: the Health, Aging, and Body Composition study. *J. Gerontol., Ser. A*, *64*, 492–498.

Harkins, S. W. (1996). Geriatric pain: pain perceptions in the old. *Clinics in Geriatric Medicine*, *12*, 435–459.

Herr, K., Bjoro, K., & Decker, S. (2006). Tools for assessment of pain in nonverbal older adults with dementia: a state-of-the-science review. *J. Pain Symptom Manag.*, *31*, 170–192.

Herr, K., Bursch, H., & Black, B. (2008). State of the art review of tools for assessment of pain in nonverbal older adults. City of Hope Pain & Palliative Resource Center (http://prc.coh.org/PAIN-NOA.htm).

Herr, K. A., Mobily, P. R., Kohout, F. J., & Wagenaar, D. (1998). Evaluation of the faces pain scale for use with the elderly. *Clinical Journal of Pain*, *14*, 29–38.

Herr, K., Spratt, K. F., Garand, L., & Li, L. (2007). Evaluation of the Iowa pain thermometer and other selected pain intensity scales in younger and older adult cohorts using controlled clinical pain: a preliminary study. *Pain Medicine*, *8*, 585–600.

Herr, K. A., Spratt, K., Mobily, P. R., & Richardson, G. (2004). Pain intensity assessment in older adults: use of experimental pain to compare psychometric properties and usability of selected pain scales with younger adults. *Clinical Journal of Pain*, *4*, 207–219.

Holtzman, S., & Delongis, A. (2007). One day at a time: the impact of daily satisfaction with spouse responses on pain, negative affect and catastrophizing among individuals with rheumatoid arthritis. *Pain*, *131*, 202–213.

Husebo, B. S., Strand, L. I., Moe-Nilssen, R., Husebo, S. B., Snow, A. L., & Ljunggren, A. E. (2007). Mobilization-Observation-Behavior-Intensity-Dementia pain scale (MOBID): development and validation of a nurse-administered pain assessment tool for use in dementia. *J. Pain Symptom Manag.*, *34*, 67–80.

Hurley, A. C., Volicer, B. J., Hanrahan, P. A., Houde, S., & Volicer, L. (1992). Assessment of discomfort in advanced Alzheimer patients. *Research in Nursing & Health*, *15*, 369–377.

Jensen, M. P., Miller, L., & Fisher, L. D. (1998). Assessment of pain during medical procedures: a comparison of three scales. *Clinical Journal of Pain*, *14*, 343–349.

Jones, A. C., Kwoh, C. K., Groeneveld, P. W., Mor, M., Geng, M., & Ibrahim, S. A. (2008). Investigating racial differences in coping with chronic osteoarthritis pain. *Journal of Cross-Cultural Gerontology*, *23*, 339–347.

Juhakoski, R., Tenhonen, S., Anttonen, T., Kauppinen, T., & Arokoski, J. P. (2008). Factors affecting self-reported pain and physical function in patients with hip osteoarthritis. *Arch. Phys. Med. Rehabil.*, *89*, 1066–1073.

Kamaleri, Y., Natvig, B., Ihlebaek, C. M., Benth, J. S., & Bruusgaard, D. (2008). Number of pain sites is associated with demographic, lifestyle, and health-related factors in the general population. *Eur. J. Pain*, *12*, 742–748.

Kamaleri, Y., Natvig, B., Ihlebaek, C. M., & Bruusgaard, D. (2009). Does the number of musculoskeletal pain sites predict work disability? A 14-year prospective study. *Eur. J. Pain*, *13*, 426–430.

Keefe, F. J., Blumenthal, J., Baucom, D., Affleck, G., Waugh, R., Caldwell, D. S., et al. (2004). Effects of spouse-assisted coping skills training and exercise training in patients with osteoarthritic knee pain: a randomized controlled study. *Pain*, *110*, 539–549.

Keefe, F. J., Lefebvre, J. C., & Smith, S. J. (1999). Catastrophizing research: avoiding conceptual errors and maintaining a balanced perspective. *Pain Forum*, *8*, 176–180.

Kovach, C. R., Logan, B. R., Noonan, P. E., Schlidt, A. M., Smerz, J., Simpson, M., & Wells, T. (2006). Effects of the Serial Trial Intervention on discomfort and behavior of nursing home residents with dementia. *American Journal of Alzheimer's Disease & Other Dementias*, *21*, 147–155.

Kovach, C. R., Noonan, P. E., Griffie, J., Muchka, S., & Weissman, D. E. (2002). The assessment of discomfort in dementia protocol. *Pain Management Nursing*, *3*, 16–27.

Kovach, C. R., Weissman, D. E., Griffie, J., Matson, S., & Muchka, S. (1999). Assessment and treatment of discomfort for people with late-stage dementia. *J. Pain Symptom Manag.*, *18*, 412–419.

Krein, S. L., Heisler, M., Piette, J. D., Butchart, A., & Kerr, E. A. (2007). Overcoming the influence of chronic pain on older patients' difficulty with recommended self-management activities. *Gerontologist*, *47*, 61–68.

Lasch, H., Castell, D. O., & Castell, J. A. (1997). Evidence for diminished visceral pain with aging: studies using graded intraesophageal balloon distension. *Am. J. Physiol.*, *272*, G1–G3.

Lazarus, R. S., & Folkman, S. (1984). *Stress, Appraisal, and Coping*. New York, NY: Springer Publishing Company.

Lefebvre, J. C., & Keefe, F. J. (2002). Memory for pain: the relationship of pain catastrophizing to the recall of daily rheumatoid arthritis pain. *Clinical Journal of Pain*, *18*, 56–63.

Leong, I. Y., Farrell, M. J., Helme, R. D., & Gibson, S. J. (2007). The relationship between medical comorbidity and self-rated pain, mood disturbance, and function in older people with chronic pain. *J. Gerontol., Ser. A*, *62*, 550–555.

Leveille, S. G., Guralnik, J. M., Hochberg, M., Hirsch, R., Ferrucci, L., Langlois, J., et al. (1999). Low back pain and disability in older women: independent association with difficulty but not inability to perform daily activities. *J. Gerontol., Ser. A*, *54*, M487–M493.

Linton, S. J., Buer, N., Vlaeyen, J., & Hellsing, A. (2000). Are fear-avoidance beliefs related to the inception of an episode of back pain? A prospective study. *Psychology & Health*, *14*, 1051–1059.

Lopez-Lopez, A., Montorio, I., Izal, M., & Velasco, L. (2008). The role of psychological variables in explaining depression in older people with chronic pain. *Aging & Mental Health*, *12*, 735–745.

Lorig, K., Chastain, R. L., Ung, E., Shoor, S., & Holman, H. R. (1989). Development and evaluation of a scale to measure perceived self-efficacy in people with arthritis. *Arthritis & Rheumatism*, *32*, 37–44.

MacLean, C. H. (2001). Quality indicators for the management of osteoarthritis in vulnerable elders. *Ann. Intern. Med.*, *135*, 711–721.

Malmstrom, T. K., Andresen, E. M., Wolinsky, F. D., Miller, J. P., Stamps, K., & Miller, D. K. (2007). Mortality risk in older inner-city African Americans. *J. Am. Geriatr. Soc.*, *55*, 1049–1055.

Maly, M. R., Costigan, P. A., & Olney, S. J. (2006). Determinants of self efficacy for physical tasks in people with knee osteoarthritis. *Arthritis & Rheumatism*, *55*, 94–101.

Margolis, R. B., Chibnall, J. T., & Tait, R. C. (1988). Test-retest reliability of the pain drawing instrument. *Pain*, *33*, 49–51.

Marks, R. (2007). Physical and psychological correlates of disability among a cohort of individuals with knee osteoarthritis. *Canadian Journal on Aging*, *26*, 367–377.

Mavandadi, S., Ten Have, T. R., Katz, I. R., Durai, U. N., Krahn, D. D., Llorente, M. D., et al. (2007). Effect of depression treatment on depressive symptoms in older adulthood: the moderating role of pain. *J. Am. Geriatr. Soc.*, *55*, 202–211.

McIlvane, J. M., Schiaffino, K. M., & Paget, S. A. (2007). Age differences in the pain-depression link for women with osteoarthritis. Functional impairment and personal control as mediators. *Women's Health Issues*, *17*, 44–51.

Melzack, R., & Wall, P. D. (1965). Pain mechanisms: a new theory. *Science*, *150*, 971–979.

Merkel, S. I., Voepel-Lewis, T., Shayevitz, J. R., & Malviya, S. (1997). The FLACC: a behavioral scale for scoring postoperative pain in young children. *Pediatric Nursing*, *23*, 293–297.

Merle-Vincent, F., Couris, C. M., Schott, A. M., Perier, M., Conrozier, S., Conrozier, T., et al. (2007). Cross-sectional study of pain and disability at knee replacement surgery for osteoarthritis in 299 patients. *Jt., Bone, Spine*, *74*, 612–616.

Miller, G. D., Nicklas, B. J., & Loeser, R. F. (2008a). Inflammatory biomarkers and physical function in older, obese adults with knee pain and self-reported osteoarthritis after intensive weight-loss therapy. *J. Am. Geriatr. Soc.*, *56*, 644–651.

Miller, D. K., Wolinsky, F. D., Andresen, E. M., Malmstrom, T. K., & Miller, J. P. (2008b). Adverse outcomes and correlates of change in the short physical performance battery over 36 months in the African American Health Project. *J. Gerontol., Ser. A*, *63*, 487–494.

Morello, R., Jean, A., Alix, M., Sellin-Peres, D., & Fermanian, J. (2007). A scale to measure pain in non-verbally communicating older patients: the EPCA-2 study of its psychometric properties. *Pain*, *133*, 87–98.

Mottram, S., Peat, G., Thomas, E., Wilkie, R., & Croft, P. (2008). Patterns of pain and mobility limitation in older people: cross-sectional findings from a population survey of 18,497 adults aged 50 years and over. *Quality of Life Research*, *17*, 529–539.

National Institute on Aging. (2007). *Why population aging matters. A global perspective*. Department of Health and Human Services. Publication No. 07–6134.

Nicholas, M. K. (2007). The pain self-efficacy questionnaire: taking pain into account. *Eur. J. Pain*, *11*, 153–163.

Onder, G., Cesari, M., Russo, A., Zamboni, V., Bernabei, R., & Landi, F. (2006). Association between daily pain and physical function among old-old adults living in the community: results from the ilSIRENTE study. *Pain*, *121*, 53–59.

Onder, G., Penninx, B. W., Ferrucci, L., Fried, L. P., Guralnik, J. M., & Pahor, M. (2005). Measures of physical performance and risk for progressive and catastrophic disability: results from the Women's Health and Aging Study. *J. Gerontol., Ser. A*, *60*, 74–79.

Oosterman, J. M., van Harten, B., Weinstein, H. C., Scheltens, P., & Scherder, E. J. (2006). Pain intensity and pain affect in relation to white matter changes. *Pain*, *125*, 74–81.

Ostir, G. V., Volpato, S., Fried, L. P., Chaves, P., & Guralnik, J. M. (2002). Reliability and sensitivity to change assessed for a summary measure of lower body function: results from the Women's Health and Aging Study. *Journal of Clinical Epidemiology*, *55*, 916–921.

Pahor, M., Blair, S. N., Espeland, M., Fielding, R., Gill, T. M., Guralnik, J. M., et al. (2006). Effects of a physical activity intervention on measures of physical performance: results of the lifestyle interventions and independence for elders pilot (LIFE-P) study. *J. Gerontol., Ser. A*, *61*, 1157–1165.

Pahor, M., Guralnik, J. M., Wan, J. Y., Ferrucci, L., Penninx, B. W., Lyles, A., Ling, S., & Fried, L. P. (1999). Lower body osteoarticular pain and dose of analgesic medications in older disabled women: the Women's Health and Aging Study. *Am. J. Public Health*, *89*, 930–934.

Penninx, B. W., Ferrucci, L., Leveille, S. G., Rantanen, T., Pahor, M., & Guralnik, J. M. (2000). Lower extremity performance in nondisabled older persons as a predictor of subsequent hospitalization. *J. Gerontol., Ser. A*, *55*, M691–M697.

Perera, S., Studenski, S., Chandler, J. M., & Guralnik, J. M. (2005). Magnitude and patterns of decline in health and function in 1 year affect subsequent 5-year survival. *J. Gerontol., Ser. A*, *60*, 894–900.

Perkins, H. Y., Baum, G. P., Taylor, C. L., & Basen-Engquist, K. M. (2009). Effects of treatment factors, comorbidities and health-related quality of life on self-efficacy for physical activity in cancer survivors. *Psycho-Oncology*, *18*, 405–411.

Peters, M. L., Patijn, J., & Lame, I. (2007). Pain assessment in younger and older patients: psychometric properties and patient preference of five commonly used measures of pain intensity. *Pain Medicine*, *8*, 601–610.

Pollard, C. A. (1984). Preliminary validity study of the pain disability index. *Perceptual & Motor Skills*, *59*, 974.

Porter, L. S., Keefe, F. J., Wellington, C., & de Williams, A. (2008). Pain communication in the context of osteoarthritis: patient and partner self-efficacy for pain communication and holding back from discussion of pain and arthritis-related concerns. *Clinical Journal of Pain*, *24*, 662–668.

Price, D. D. (2000). Psychological and neural mechanisms of the affective dimension of pain. *Science*, *288*, 1769–1772.

Rahman, A., Ambler, G., Underwood, M. R., & Shipley, M. E. (2004). Important determinants of self-efficacy in patients with chronic musculoskeletal pain. *J. Rheumatol.*, *31*, 1187–1192.

Rainero, I., Vighetti, S., Bergamasco, B., Pinessi, L., & Benedetti, F. (2000). Autonomic responses and pain perception in Alzheimer's disease. *Eur. J. Pain*, *4*, 267–274.

Rapp, S. R., Rejeski, W. J., & Miller, M. E. (2000). Physical function among older adults with knee pain: the role of pain coping skills. *Arthritis Care & Research*, *13*, 270–279.

Regnard, C., Reynolds, J., Watson, B., Matthews, D., Gibson, L., & Clarke, C. (2007). Understanding distress in people with severe communication difficulties: developing and assessing the Disability Distress Assessment Tool (DisDAT). *Journal of Intellectual Disability Research*, *51*, 277–292.

Reid, M. C., Williams, C. S., & Gill, T. M. (2003). The relationship between psychological factors and disabling musculoskeletal pain in community-dwelling older persons. *J. Am. Geriatr. Soc.*, *51*, 1092–1098.

Reid, M. C., Williams, C. S., & Gill, T. M. (2005). Back pain and decline in lower physical function among community-dwelling older person. *J. Gerontol., Ser. A*, *60*, 793–797.

Rejeski, W. J., Ettinger, W. H., Martin, K., & Morgan, T. (1998). Treating disability in knee osteoarthritis with exercise therapy: a central role for self-efficacy and pain. *Arthritis Care & Research*, *11*, 94–101.

Rejeski, W. J., Miller, M. E., Foy, C., Messier, S., & Rapp, S. (2001). Self-efficacy and the progression of functional limitations and self-reported disability in older adults with knee pain. *Journals of Gerontology Series B-Psychological Sciences & Social Sciences*, *56*, S261–S265.

Resnick, B. (1998). Efficacy beliefs in geriatric rehabilitation. *Journal of Gerontological Nursing*, *24*, 34–44.

Riley, J. L., Wade, J. B., Robinson, M. E., & Price, D. D. (2000). The stages of pain processing across the adult lifespan. *Journal of Pain*, *1*, 162–170.

Romano, J. M., & Turner, J. A. (1985). Chronic pain and depression: does the evidence support a relationship? *Psychological Bulletin*, *97*, 18–34.

Rosenstiel, A. K., & Keefe, F. J. (1983). The use of cognitive strategies in chronic low back pain patients: relationship to patient characteristics and current adjustment. *Pain*, *17*, 33–44.

Rub, U., Del Tredici, K., Del Turco, D., & Braak, H. (2002). The intralaminar nuclei assigned to the medial pain system and other components of this system are early and progressively affected by the Alzheimer's disease-related cytoskeletal pathology. *Journal of Chemistry and Neuroanatomy*, *23*, 279–290.

Rudy, T. E., Weiner, D. K., Lieber, S. J., Slaboda, J., & Boston, J. R. (2007). The impact of chronic low back pain on older adults: a comparative study of patients and controls. *Pain*, *131*, 293–301.

Ruger, L. J., Irnich, D., Abahji, T. N., Crispin, A., Hoffmann, U., & Lang, P. M. (2008). Characteristics of chronic ischemic pain in patients with peripheral arterial disease. *Pain*, *139*, 201–208.

Scherder, E., Oosterman, J., Swaab, D., Herr, K., Ooms, M., Ribbe, M., et al. (2005). Recent developments in pain in dementia. *BMJ*, *330*, 461–464.

Scherder, E. J., & Bouma, A. (2000). Visual analogue scales for pain assessment in Alzheimer's disease. *Gerontology*, *46*, 47–53.

Scherder, E. J., Sergeant, J. A., & Swaab, D. F. (2003). Pain processing in dementia and its relation to neuropathology. *Lancet Neurol.*, *2*, 677–686.

Seminowicz, D. A., & Davis, K. D. (2006). Cortical responses to pain in healthy individuals depends on pain catastrophizing. *Pain*, *120*, 297–306.

Seminowicz, D. A., Mikulis, D. J., & Davis, K. D. (2004). Cognitive modulation of pain-related brain responses depends on behavioral strategy. *Pain*, *112*, 48–58.

Shelby, R. A., Somers, T. J., Keefe, F. J., Pells, J. J., Dixon, K. E., & Blumenthal, J. A. (2008). Domain specific self-efficacy mediates the impact of pain catastrophizing on pain and disability in overweight and obese osteoarthritis patients. *J. Pain*, *9*, 912–919.

Sinclair, V. G. (2001). Predictors of pain catastrophizing in women with rheumatoid arthritis. *Archives of Psychiatric Nursing*, *15*, 279–288.

Snow, A. L., Weber, J. B., O'Malley, K. J., Cody, M., Beck, C., Bruera, E., et al. (2004). NOPAIN: a nursing assistant-administered pain assessment instrument for use in dementia. *Dementia Geriatr. Cognitive Disorders*, *17*, 240–246.

Soldato, M., Liperoti, R., Landi, F., Finne-Sovery, H., Carpenter, I., Fialova, D., et al. (2007). Non malignant daily pain and risk of disability among older adults in home care in Europe. *Pain*, *129*, 304–310.

Stevenson, K. M., Brown, R. L., Dahl, J. L., Ward, S. E., & Brown, M. S. (2006). The Discomfort Behavior Scale: a measure of discomfort in the cognitively impaired based on the Minimum Data Set 2.0. *Research in Nursing & Health*, *29*, 576–587.

Sullivan, M. J., Bishop, S. R., & Pivik, J. (1995). The Pain Catastrophizing Scale: development and validation. *Psychological Assessment*, *7*, 524–532.

Sullivan, M. J., & Neish, N. (1999). The effects of disclosure on pain during dental hygiene treatment: the moderating role of catastrophizing. *Pain*, *79*, 155–163.

Sullivan, M. J., Rodgers, W. M., & Kirsch, I. (2001). Catastrophizing, depression and expectancies for pain and emotional distress. *Pain*, *91*, 147–154.

Sullivan, M. J., Stanish, W., Waite, H., Sullivan, M., & Tripp, D. A. (1998). Catastrophizing, pain, and disability following soft tissue injuries. *Pain*, *77*, 253–260.

Tait, R. C. (2004). Compensation claims for chronic pain: effects on evaluation and treatment. In R. H. Dworkin, & W. S. Breitbart (Eds.), *Psychosocial Aspects of Pain: A Handbook for Health Care Providers* (pp. 547–570). Seattle, WA: IASP Press.

Tait, R. C., Chibnall, J. T., & Krause, S. J. (1990a). The Pain Disability Index: psychometric properties. *Pain*, *40*, 171–182.

Tait, R. C., Chibnall, J. T., & Margolis, R. B. (1990b). Pain extent: relations with psychological state, pain severity, pain history, and disability. *Pain*, *41*, 295–301.

Thomas, E., Peat, G., Harris, L., Wilkie, R., & Croft, P. R. (2004). The prevalence of pain and pain interference in a general population of older adults: cross-sectional findings from the North Staffordshire Osteoarthritis Project (NorStOP). *Pain*, *110*, 361–368.

Thompson, P. M., Hayashi, K. M., de Zubicaray, G., Janke, A. L., Rose, S. E., Semple, J., et al. (2003). Dynamics of gray matter loss in Alzheimer's disease. *J. Neurosci.*, *23*, 994–1005.

Treede, R. D., Kenshalo, D. R., Gracely, R. H., & Jones, A. K. (1999). The cortical representation of pain. *Pain*, *79*, 105–111.

Tsai, P. F., Beck, C., Richards, K. C., Phillips, L., Roberson, P. K., & Evans, J. (2008). The Pain Behaviors for Osteoarthritis Instrument for Cognitively Impaired Elders (PBOICIE). *Research in Gerontological Nursing*, *1*, 116–122.

van Nispen tot Pannerden, S. C., Candel, M. J., Zwakhalen, S. M., Hamers, J. P., Curfs, L. M., & Berger, M. P. (2009). An item response theory-based assessment of the pain assessment checklist for seniors with limited ability to communicate (PACSLAC). *J. Pain*, *10*, 844–853.

Villanueva, M. R., Smith, T. L., Erikson, J. S., Lee, A. C., & Singer, C. M. (2003). Pain Assessment for the Dementing Elderly (PADE): reliability and validity of a new measure. *Journal of the American Medical Directors Association*, *4*, 1–8.

Vlaeyan, J. W., de Jong, J., Sieben, J., & Crombez, G. (2002). Graded exposure in vivo for pain-related fear. In D. C. Turk, & R. J. Gatchel (Eds.), *Psychological Approaches to Pain Management: A Practitioner's Handbook—Second Edition* (pp. 210–233). New York, NY: The Guilford Press.

Von Korff, M., Deyo, R. A., Cherkin, D., & Barlow, W. (1993). Back pain in primary care. Outcomes at 1 year. *Spine*, *18*, 855–862.

Waddell, G., Newton, M., Henderson, I., Somerville, D., & Main, C. J. (1993). A Fear-Avoidance Beliefs Questionnaire (FABQ) and the role of fear-avoidance beliefs in chronic low back pain and disability. *Pain*, *52*, 157–168.

Warden, V., Hurley, A. C., & Volicer, L. (2003). Development and psychometric evaluation of the Pain Assessment in Advanced Dementia (PAINAD) scale. *Journal of the American Medical Directors Association*, *4*, 9–15.

Ware, J. E., Jr., & Sherbourne, C. D. (1992). The MOS 36-item short-form health survey (SF-36). I. Conceptual framework and item selection. *Medical Care*, *30*, 473–483.

Ware, L. J., Epps, C. D., Herr, K., & Packard, A. (2006). Evaluation of the Revised Faces Pain Scale, Verbal Descriptor Scale, Numeric Rating Scale, and Iowa Pain Thermometer in older minority adults. *Pain Management Nursing*, *7*, 117–125.

Wary, B., & Doloplus, C. (1999). Doloplus-2, a scale for pain measurement. *Soins. Gerontologie*, *19*, 25–27.

Weaver, G. D., Kuo, Y. F., Raji, M. A., Al Snih, S., Ray, L., Torres, E., & Ottenbacher, K. J. (2009). Pain and disability in older Mexican-American adults. *J. Am. Geriatr. Soc.*, *57*, 992–999.

Weiner, D. K., & Herr, K. (2002). Comprehensive interdisciplinary assessment and treatment planning: an integrative overview. In D. K. Weiner, & K. Herr (Eds.), *Persistent Pain in Older Adults: An Interdisciplinary Guide for Treatment* (pp. 18–57). New York, NY: Springer Publishing Company.

Williamson, G. M., & Schulz, R. (1992). Pain, activity restriction, and symptoms of depression among community-residing elderly adults. *J. Gerontol.*, *47*, P367–P372.

Wolfe, F., & Michaud, K. (2009). Predicting depression in rheumatoid arthritis: the signal importance of pain extent and fatigue, and comorbidity. *Arthritis & Rheumatism*, *61*, 667–673.

Zwakhalen, S. M., Hamers, J. P., Abu-Saad, H. H., & Berger, M. P. (2006). Pain in elderly people with severe dementia: a systematic review of behavioural pain assessment tools. *BMC Geriatr.*, *6*, 3.

Zwakhalen, S. M., Hamers, J. P., & Berger, M. P. (2007). Improving the clinical usefulness of a behavioural pain scale for older people with dementia. *Journal of Advanced Nursing*, *58*, 493–502.

CHAPTER

Assessments in Driver Rehabilitation

25

Joseph M. Pellerito Jr.

Department of Occupational Therapy, College of Health and Human Services, Western Michigan University, Kalamazoo, MI, USA

INTRODUCTION

Driving a motor vehicle is an indispensable method of transportation and a personal and meaningful symbol of what it means to participate fully in mainstream American life. (Pellerito, 2006)

One of the most important rites of passage for people of all ages is earning a driver's license. People living in both urban and rural areas are highly dependent on the automobile to meet their travel and community mobility needs (Hensher & Alsnih, 2003; Molnar, Eby & Miller, 2003; U.S. Department of Transportation, 2003). Driving is an important symbol of adult autonomy and independence. It provides a sense of personal competence, enables access to essential services and meaningful social interactions, and can support the ability of older people to age in place in familiar surroundings (U.S. Department of Transportation, 2003). The independent community mobility afforded by driving also influences the roles people assume, the formation and maintenance of primary (e.g., family and extended family) and secondary (e.g., friends, clubs, religious affiliations) group ties, the daily operation of households and businesses, the pursuit of meaningful activities in a variety of social settings (Carr, 1993; Johnson, 1995; Victor, 1994), and a positive self-concept and high self-esteem (Carr, 1993; Galski, Bruno & Ehle, 1992; Gillins, 1990; Kalz et al., 1990; Stubbins, 1977). Overall, driving and its associated car culture, especially in developed countries, influence the ways in which individuals interact with others, perceive the world and themselves, and imagine how others perceive them (Lyman & Vidich, 2000).

OLDER DRIVERS AS A GROUP

The proportion and number of older drivers in the United States has increased dramatically over the past two decades (Lundberg, Hakamies-Blomqvist, Almkvist & Johansson, 1998) and it is anticipated that this trend will continue (Freund & Szinovacz, 2002). There are 35 million Americans 65 years of age or older, which is approximately 13% of the total U.S. population; the number of older drivers is expected to double and reach 70 million by the year 2030 (U.S. Department of Transportation, 2003). Drivers age 55 and older comprised 28% of the driving population in 2000 and that number is expected to increase to 39% by the year 2050 (Cushman, 1996; Marottoli & Drickamer 1993).

Older Americans resemble the broader population when it comes to their dependence on privately owned automobiles (U.S. Department of Transportation, 2003). More than four out of five trips undertaken by people over the age of 65 in the United States are in passenger vehicles that are usually

Handbook of Assessment in Clinical Gerontology. DOI: 10.1016/B978-0-12-374961-1.10025-9

their own (National Research Council, 1988). It is understandable that older Americans continue to drive even after experiencing the cumulative effects of aging and chronic disease, and the disabling effects of traumatic injuries, chronic disabilities, and the aging process (Molnar et al., 2003). There is significant variation in the functional abilities of older drivers as well. Although it has been estimated that about one-third of the population over age 65 have limitations that render them unable to perform a significant number of activities of daily living (ADL), more than two-thirds of these people continue to drive (Rosenbloom, 1993).

The effects of aging and the concomitant challenges associated with disabling health conditions can work in tandem to reduce the functioning, safety, independence, and well-being of older Americans. Lysack et al. (2003) posited that when a person is hospitalized after experiencing the effects of a traumatic or chronic health condition, current medical rehabilitation is considered complete after an individual: (1) survives an initial or recurring disabling event; (2) reaches an optimal level of functioning that is primarily measured in physical terms; and (3) returns home or to an alternative destination to resume as many routines and meaningful activities as possible (which may or may not include driving). Community and public policy perspectives take into consideration the long-term consequences of aging and disabilities. They assert that social outcomes of rehabilitation should be measured by the extent to which a person can reconstruct a positive self-image, resume key life roles, re-engage with primary and secondary group members, return to meaningful work and leisure activities, and participate in the community (Lysack et al. (2003); Pellerito, 2009).

There is growing concern among some health care professionals and the general public that there is mounting evidence that older driver subgroups account for a disproportionate number of traffic accidents and morbidity and mortality. The oldest drivers, that is, individuals who are 75 years of age or older, experience traffic accidents at a rate second only to the youngest drivers between 15 and 24 years of age (O'Neill, 1992; Williams & Carsten, 1989). More than 7000 elderly drivers die in automobile accidents on U.S. highways and roads annually (Kulash, 2000); the number of older drivers 70 years of age and older killed in vehicular accidents nationwide has increased 39% over a 10-year period (Aging News Alert, 2000). Florida had the most elderly auto fatalities in 1999, followed by Texas, California, Pennsylvania, and Michigan (Aging News Alert, 2000). Motor vehicle accidents are the leading cause of accidental deaths for people age 65–74 and second leading cause (after falls) for older people in general (U.S. Department of Health and Human Services, 1991). By age group, drivers 80 years of age or older have the highest fatality rate, drivers 65–79 the third highest, and drivers 16–24 the second highest (U.S. Department of Commerce, 1995). Physiologic changes, concomitant medical conditions, and medications associated with aging can impair driving ability (Molnar et al., 2003). Thus, as the number of older drivers increases, their competence to drive has become a growing concern for themselves and their families, professional caregivers, and the public. Medical doctors possess an added responsibility because they have the legal authority and ethical responsibility to report individuals (i.e., to their state's department of motor vehicles or DMV) they deem unsafe to drive (Underwood, 1992). Other health care team members and family caregivers also share the ethical responsibility and burden of helping to facilitate driving retirement (i.e., planned and a participatory and willful decision on the part of the elder to stop driving for his or her sake and for the well-being of other road users) or driving discontinuance (i.e., unplanned and without consent) when necessary. Safe driving is similarly the concern of the general public, the automobile manufacturing industry, researchers and teachers, and the insurance industry.

Driving: A Rite (of Passage) or a Right?

In contemporary industrialized societies in the United States and abroad driving is not considered an inalienable right, but a privilege that is granted by the government and defined in legal terms; however, for many people, driving is much more than a privilege, luxury, or instrumental activity of daily living

(IADL) as some would suggest; it is an activity of daily living (ADL) (Pellerito, 2006) that is necessary for a full and productive social life in urban and rural areas around the world. Many people equate the possession of a driver's license with choice, freedom, and self-identity (Pellerito, 2009). Drivers with functional impairments, whether due to accidental injury, illness, aging-related changes, or some other cause or combination of causes, have the same needs to drive or access the community as passengers or both. However, persons experiencing difficulties driving and accessing alternatives to driving that enable community mobility are often either unaware that there are driving specialists who could help them or are uncertain about the steps necessary to engage professionals equipped to address their concerns.

Health care professionals should explore the ways in which an impairment or disability may be impacting their clients' driving and community mobility during their initial evaluations, and subsequent goal-setting should reflect their clients' needs irrespective of the setting where health care (e.g., occupational therapy, psychology, neuropsychology) services are rendered. In other words, professional caregivers should not wait for their clients (or their clients' caregivers) to broach this topic but should address it during their initial evaluations.

When physical or cognitive limitations or both impair safe driving, screening driver readiness and conducting comprehensive driver rehabilitation evaluations may become necessary, which can result in driving discontinuance. Despite an increased interest in people with disabilities as a group and what it means to age successfully, many health care professionals are unaware of the field of driver rehabilitation and the tools available to assist clients receive a comprehensive driving evaluation or assistance with transitioning from driver to non-driver status. They are unaware of the professionals who comprise a driver rehabilitation evaluation team, simple self-assessments that can help to screen driver fitness (e.g., following a stroke or brain injury), and some of the tools designed to facilitate discussions between practitioners and clients about strategies that can help to ensure that the transition from driver to non-driver status is successful. Next we will examine the composition of the driver rehabilitation team and the key services it provides to clients and patients and their family caregivers.

DRIVER REHABILITATION TEAM AND KEY SERVICES

The services that are offered by a driver rehabilitation program are usually a good indicator of the professionals who comprise a particular program's team structure. Every driver rehabilitation program employs primary team members to provide key driver rehabilitation services irrespective of the program's service delivery model, team structure, or service offerings. Among the driver rehabilitation team members is the driver rehabilitation specialist (DRS); the DRS plays the central role in providing efficacious driver rehabilitation and, more recently, community mobility services to clients and their caregivers. DRSs conduct comprehensive driver rehabilitation evaluations with the aim of determining their clients' driver readiness. DRSs work with other health care professionals, including ancillary team members, to help ensure that clients achieve their driver rehabilitation goals, community mobility goals, or both. Table 25.1 lists primary and ancillary driver rehabilitation team members and Table 25.2 presents key driver rehabilitation services, as well as the professionals responsible for the services rendered.

SELF-ASSESSMENTS THAT CAN HELP TO SCREEN DRIVER READINESS

Introduction

Some older drivers grapple to answer the question, "Am I fit to continue driving a motor vehicle?" while others do not. Professional caregivers should be prepared to encourage their clients to engage in what can be a complex decision-making process. Eby et al. (2009) have published an excellent

Table 25.1 Primary and Ancillary Driver Rehabilitation Team Members

Primary Team Members	Ancillary Team Members
• Client • Client's chief caregivers • Primary DRS assigned to the client's case, such as an occupational therapist who has specialized in driver rehabilitation • Neuropsychologists • Vehicle modifier (also known as the mobility equipment dealer) • Physician(s), such as the client's physiatrist or general practitioner • Case manager	• Client's friends and extended family members • Occupational therapy generalists • Occupational therapy assistants • Other allied health professionals, such as speech-language pathologists, audiologists, physical therapists, therapeutic recreation specialists, social workers, nurses, physicians, psychologists, orthotists, and prosthetists • Other allied health professionals working as specialists in driving related interventions, such as occupational or physical therapy wheeled mobility and seating specialists, occupational therapy low-vision specialists, surgeons, ophthalmologists, geriatricians, etc. • Occupational therapists or other allied health professionals specializing in driver rehabilitation who are not assigned to a particular client's case but are consulted for input by the primary DRS • State motor vehicle department staff responsible for licensing and re-licensing driver applicants

Table 25.2 Key Driver Rehabilitation and Community Mobility Services

Services	Person(s) Responsible forService Delivery
• Self-screening tools	Client or client's caregiver or both with or without the assistance of a health care professional
• Clinical screening or assessment	OT generalists during an ADL or IADL evaluation or DRS
• Clinical evaluations of physical, sensory, and cognitive abilities	OT generalists during an ADL or IADL evaluation or DRS
• In-vehicle pre-driving assessments help determine the best vehicle type, adapted driving aids, and structural modifications before taking a client on the road	OT DRS
• On-road evaluations examine the client's ability to access a vehicle, stow and secure an ambulation aid as necessary, and drive a vehicle with or without structural modifications, adaptive driving equipment, or both	OT DRS
• Off-street training (i.e., closed-circuit course) can be conducted on a driving range or in an isolated parking lot, which enables clients to learn and practice driving skills in a protected physical environment • Driving simulators can be used to assess driver readiness or for driver remediation and training in a protected virtual environment	OT DRS

Table 25.2 Key Driver Rehabilitation and Community Mobility Services *(Continued)*

Services	Person(s) Responsible forService Delivery
• On-road training while using a specific vehicle with or without modifications, adapted driving controls, or both	OT DRS
• Recommendations for adapted driving aids	OT DRS
• Recommendations for vehicle modifications	OT DRS
• Client–vehicle fittings	OT DRS
• Developing and implementing driving retirement plans and providing counseling that includes exploring strategies to facilitate alternative community mobility	OT DRSs, OT generalists, driver educators, and other health science professionals such as physicians, neuropsychologists, psychologists, social workers, and others
• Identifying and using alternatives to driving for community mobility	OT DRSs, OT generalists, driver educators, and other health science professionals
• Exploring funding options for driver rehabilitation and community mobility services and equipment	OT DRSs, OT generalists, driver educators, and other health science professionals
• Utilize education and training resources	Client or client's caregiver or both

resource for professionals, older drivers, elders currently receiving health care services, and caregivers titled "Promising approaches for promoting lifelong community mobility." Molnar and her colleagues, with the support of the AARP, have succinctly reviewed many of the challenges associated with elder community mobility and offer "promising approaches" that address specific mobility-related concerns. This resource is currently available in PDF format and an updated web-based version that can be updated with greater regularity will be available online.

Eby et al. (2003) posited that "making informed decisions about driving fitness requires meaningful information about the changes in driving-related abilities drivers may experience and how these changes affect driving" (p. 6). The ability for elders to engage in activities that are meaningful to them can be impacted by health-related challenges associated with specific diagnoses. The effects of these conditions impact individuals differently due to many factors such as access to health care (e.g., physical medicine and rehabilitation), drug therapy regimens, lifestyle choices, and environmental factors; therefore, self-screening tools tend to focus on functional declines that can affect driving, rather than on the medical conditions that lead to these declines. Self-screening tools vary in complexity in terms of both usage protocols and where they are utilized. Screening can be a first step in identifying at-risk drivers and is intended to identify functional impairments that can result in a decline of driving abilities. Screening may prompt and/or inform the need for a comprehensive driver rehabilitation evaluation and should not be used by itself to determine driving fitness. A comprehensive evaluation including both a clinical and on-road assessment should be completed to determine whether an elder should continue driving and under what conditions. "Collectively, screening and assessment contribute to a comprehensive, multifaceted approach for identifying older drivers who may be at risk" (Molnar et al., 2003, p. 6).

The Roles of the Health Care Professional

Physicians and other health care professionals, family and friends, and even older drivers themselves can also play an important role in the screening process. Physicians are uniquely positioned to identify functional impairments that can affect driver fitness and lead to driving-related problems. Early detection of declining health and associated functional abilities among elders can result in opportunities to refer clients for physical medicine and rehabilitation services such as occupational, physical, and speech and hearing therapy. Other specialists (e.g., low vision, hand therapy, cognitive, and assistive technology specialists, to name a few) may also become engaged in the clients' care to assist them with identifying and implementing rehabilitation intervention plans that include remediation or compensation strategies (or both).

It is interesting to note that when the ability to drive a motor vehicle is compromised, evidence suggests that older drivers will stop driving voluntarily, if advised to do so by their personal physician or rehabilitation specialist or both (Pellerito, 2006). Unfortunately, many physicians report that they are uncomfortable with making fitness-to-drive decisions or lack the necessary information to do so. In such cases, patients can be referred to occupational therapists certified as driving rehabilitation specialists for a comprehensive driver rehabilitation evaluation (i.e., clinical and on-road driving assessments). As described in the recently published *Occupational Therapy Practice Guidelines for Driving and Community Mobility for Older Adults*, occupational therapists consider driving an occupation, and the overarching goal of occupational therapy for individuals is continued engagement in meaningful occupations (Molnar et al., 2007).

> *Evaluation of driving by an occupational therapist generally includes an initial interview to obtain medical and driving history, a clinical assessment of visual, cognitive, and psychomotor abilities, and an on-road driving assessment. Once declines in functional abilities have been identified, driver rehabilitation specialists can determine whether a return to driving is possible through training and rehabilitation, and what specific remedial activities should be undertaken.*
>
> **(Molnar et al., 2007, pp. 11–12)**

HOME-BASED DRIVING SELF-ASSESSMENT TOOLS

Molnar et al. (2007) also identified home-based self-screening tools that are appealing because elders can use them within the comfort and privacy of their home environments. "Because self-screening can be done privately with the results remaining confidential, it may be less threatening than other types of screening and something older drivers would be willing to do earlier in the aging process and to repeat over time" (Molnar et al., 2007, p. 14). Home-based tools are especially useful for older drivers who are cognitively intact because they impart information about factors that can lead to driving-related declines over time. Awareness of these factors serves as a means for elders and their caregivers to recognize some of the warning signs or "red flags" that reflect declining health and functional abilities.

Having access to this information also can assist elders in making informed decisions about driving, as well as facilitate discussions between older drivers and their families about driver fitness and related concerns. "Older drivers must be free of serious cognitive impairment and must be honest in their responses and willing to follow through on suggested courses of action for the process to be of real benefit. Thus, older adults with dementia, who lack insight into their impairments in driving-related abilities, are not good candidates for self-screening and may be resistant to other screening and assessment efforts" (Molnar et al., 2007).

Driving Decisions Workbook

Molar et al. (2007) developed an excellent self-screening resource for clients, their caregivers, and professionals titled the *Driving Decisions Workbook*, a paper and pencil instrument developed by the

University of Michigan Transportation Research Institute (UMTRI). The workbook is designed to increase older drivers' self-awareness and general knowledge about driving-related declines in abilities, and to make recommendations about driving compensation and remediation strategies that could extend safe driving, as well as further evaluation that might be needed. Development of the self-screening instrument was based on review of the literature, focus groups with older drivers and the adult children of older drivers, and a panel of experts on older driver abilities and evaluation. Based on findings from these activities, a model of the influences on driving decisions was developed with three domains for screening potential problems with driving—health (medical conditions and medication use), driving abilities (vision, cognition, and psychomotor), and experiences, attitudes, and behavior. Preliminary testing of the workbook indicated that it correlated with an on-road driving test, as well as several clinical tests of functional abilities, most of which are part of the test battery from the Model Driver Screening and Evaluation Program. Older drivers considered the workbook to be useful and reported their intent to make changes in their driving or seek further evaluation as a result of completing it.

SAFER Driving Enhanced Driving Decisions Workbook

In follow-up work to the *Driving Decisions Workbook*, Molnar et al. (2009) created a web-based self-screening instrument that is based on "health concerns" that affect driving—that is, the symptoms that people experience due to medical conditions, medications used to treat them, and the general aging process—rather than the medical conditions or medications themselves. The *SAFER Driving: Enhanced Driving Decisions Workbook* simplifies the self-screening process based on the premise that health conditions and medications produce a relatively small number driving related concerns. Molnar et al. (2009) reported that preliminary testing of the instrument shows that it correlated with a clinical evaluation and on-road assessment administered through an established driving assessment program, and that study participants reported planning to make changes in their driving or seek further evaluation after using the tool.

The AAA Roadwise Review

Another self-screening tool is the AAA Roadwise Review, a CD-Rom-based tool that allows elders to address their functional performance on assessments that are reported to predict safe driving abilities. The design of the tool was influenced by elders who participated in numerous focus groups. The tool enables older adults to assess their safe driving abilities and offers links to feedback tailored to individual performance on each of the performance measures. Feedback on their test outcomes can assist them in deciding how to use the performance information to keep driving safely (e.g., seek a DRS for a formal driving assessment). There are no published evaluation results available for AAA Roadwise Review, but AAA reports that users enjoy the program and report that they follow the recommendations provided.

These self-screening tools are only a representative sample of numerous tools available to clients, caregivers, and professionals. Their effectiveness in terms of validity and reliability requires continued scrutiny. Molnar et al. (2007) asserted the following: "While early self-screening results are encouraging, there is clearly a need for further research to evaluate the effects of self-screening on driver behavior. In particular, objective data are needed about the actual changes in behavior made by drivers as a result of self-screening (e.g., seeking out further assessment and evaluation, participating in driver education/training activities, and modifying and/or reducing actual driving), and ultimately whether self-screening leads to reductions in crash involvement" (p. 17). It is clear, however, that self-screening tools can be added to any practitioner's cadre of assessment strategies meant to be efficacious for their clients and their clients' caregivers alike.

BOX 25.1 LOCATING A DRIVER REHABILITATION SERVICE PROVIDER

Clients or caregivers wishing to locate a comprehensive driver rehabilitation program often begin their search by speaking with their family physicians. The physician is usually aware of the local or regional driver rehabilitation programs and can write a prescription requesting a formal driving evaluation for their client as necessary. The referral is often as succinct as a phrase (or even a word or two) that simply requests that a "driver evaluation" be completed; the physician usually does not specify the need for a clinical versus an on-road evaluation that is followed by on-road training using appropriate adaptive driving equipment or exploration of alternatives to driving to enable community mobility.

Another way clients and caregivers seek out driver rehabilitation services is by either directly calling or stopping by a facility where a driver rehabilitation program is offered or where a mobility equipment dealer's (i.e., vehicle modifier) shop is located. In the latter case the mobility equipment dealer should encourage the client to seek out a driver rehabilitation specialist (DRS) who can provide a comprehensive driver evaluation. If the client or caregiver is unclear about what kinds of services should be offered, the dealer should refer them to Table 25.2 that presents a succinct listing of driver rehabilitation and community mobility key services and the professionals who provide them.

Clients undergoing rehabilitation as inpatients or outpatients to address an injury or illness may also be referred by the occupational therapist working in the capacity as a generalist or by any one of the other driver rehabilitation team members (e.g., physiatrist, physical therapist, speech-language pathologist, nurse, social worker, neuropsychologist, or therapeutic recreation specialist) for a comprehensive driver evaluation. Many community-based organizations (e.g., religious organizations, centers for independent living, and assisted living centers) also search for driver rehabilitation programs suitable to address their clients driving needs, community mobility needs, or both. In any case prospective clients and caregivers can be referred to the ADED's or AOTA's websites for a state-by-state listing of driver rehabilitation service providers. Finally it is crucial that professionals also assist prospective clients to explore funding options to help ensure they get the services they need to achieve their driver rehabilitation and community mobility goals related to being a driver, passenger, or both.

Professionals who comprise the driver rehabilitation team enable driver rehabilitation programs to operate. Each member of the driver rehabilitation team performs a vital role during comprehensive driver rehabilitation evaluations (i.e., clinical and on-road assessments). The primary team members include the client, DRS, neuropsychologist, vehicle modifier, and funding source agent. Ancillary services also support the primary team by providing complementary evaluation and interventions that enable driving or community mobility goals or both to be achieved. Driver rehabilitation specialists work to continuously improve the standards of driver rehabilitation practice to effectively address the complex issues and challenges that preclude clients' from driving or accessing dependable alternative transportation or both. See Box 25.1 for information on locating a driver rehabilitation service provider. Finally, self-screening tools that can be used by clients (and their caregivers) to periodically assess their driver fitness help identify functional deficits, and prompt an individual or professional to seek out the services of a driver rehabilitation specialist (e.g., a comprehensive driver evaluation) were presented.

CLINICAL-BASED SCREENING TOOLS FOR DRIVING FITNESS

In some settings, such as an outpatient OT clinic, a client may be referred specifically for an assessment to determine their readiness to participate in a comprehensive driver rehabilitation evaluation. Two options are listed below for rehabilitation specialists (e.g., physicians) which can be used in the predriving screening process.

Gross Impairments Screening (GRIMPS)

A Gross Impairments Screening (GRIMPS) battery has been developed as a tool for driver licensing agency staff to provide early detection of driving impairments in the well-elderly population (NHTSA, 2003). The battery consists of tests in two domains:

- Physical measures: Rapid pace walk, foot tap, head-neck rotation, and arm reach
- Perceptual-cognitive measures: Motor-Free Visual Perception Test (visual closure subtest; MVPT), Trail Making Test Part B, cued/delayed recall, scan test, dynamic trails, computer-based test, and Useful Field of Vision (UFOV) test-subtest 2 (processing speed and divided attention) (NHTSA, 2003).

The Assessment of Driving-Related Skills (ADReS)

ADReS is designed for use by physicians. It is comprised of brief assessments designed to target essential functions that are required for safe driving including: vision; cognition; and motor skills. Any impairment in these functions may increase the client's risk for crashes (NHTSA, 2003); however, the ADReS does not claim to predict crash risk. The ADReS uses the Snellen chart to test visual acuity, confrontation testing to evaluate visual field of view, Trail Making Test Part B, Clock Drawing Test (CDT), rapid pace walk, manual range of motion (ROM) testing, and manual muscle strength testing. The test is fully described and a score sheet is provided in the *Physicians Guide to Assessing and Counseling Older Drivers*.[5]

Some OT clinics coordinate efforts with their local driver rehabilitation service providers to develop a screening instrument for their settings. The battery of tests covers the essential skill areas of physical abilities, attention, visual perception, and cognition, but uses different testing instruments to avoid a practice effect with evaluations conducted by the DRS.

For the active driver and caregivers there are many resources, driving self-screens, and impairment indicators. One example is the Association for Driver Rehabilitation Specialists (ADED), which has published warning signs listed by disability on its website. The Safe Mobility for Life project also has the "How Is Your Driving Health" brochure, Self-Awareness checklist, and Tips to Help You Drive Safely Longer, to name a few. These valuable resources are available at no cost to OT generalists, neuropsychologists DRSs, clients, caregivers, and others.

THE DRIVER REHABILITATION CLINICAL EVALUATION

The driver rehabilitation clinical evaluation entails assessing clients' discrete fundamental performance areas that are considered to be critical to the task of operating a motor vehicle. The word "clinical" refers to the frequent practice of administering driver rehabilitation tests or assessments in an occupational therapy clinic and has been used to differentiate this portion of the comprehensive driver rehabilitation evaluation from the on-road (i.e., behind-the-wheel) evaluation. The clinical evaluation can be conducted in a variety of bricks and mortar locations (i.e., both hospital- and community-based locations) and can serve a variety of purposes, including helping the driver rehabilitation specialist (DRS) to do the following:

- Establish the client's ability to meet basic criteria (e.g., visual acuity) set by the driver licensing agency for securing or maintaining a driver's license;
- Develop a client profile that highlights existing strengths and weaknesses related to pre-driving activities (e.g., transferring into the vehicle and stowing a mobility aid) and basic driving skills;

- Identify the need for initiating referrals to other specialists (e.g., neuropsychologists, wheeled mobility and seating specialists, low vision specialists);
- Prepare to conduct an individualized on-road evaluation;
- Determine the client's potential to learn new skills and benefit from adaptive driving equipment options;
- Develop compensatory strategies for driving or alternatives to driving that enable community mobility; and
- Develop a customized driver training plan that is tailored to meet the unique needs of the client.

The predictive value of the clinical evaluation has not been well established in the professional literature; however, researchers and practitioners are collaborating to develop evaluation protocols that are both reliable and valid. There is no consensus among DRSs as to which clinical tests can most effectively predict driver readiness; however, there are numerous assessments that are used by DRSs. See Appendix A for a comprehensive list of frequently used tests by DRSs while conducting clinical evaluations.

Data collected during the clinical evaluation is almost never sufficient to provide a definitive recommendation that a client is safe or unsafe to drive, with a few exceptions to be discussed later in this chapter. Rather the clinical evaluation is most beneficial in helping the DRS to predict and understand the client's on-road driving performance; therefore, a comprehensive driver rehabilitation evaluation must include both the clinical evaluation and the on-road evaluation. This section will focus on the component tests that comprise the clinical evaluation that provides the foundation upon which the on-road evaluation of a client's driving performance can be conducted.

Clinical evaluations are conducted by DRSs such as occupational therapists specializing in driver rehabilitation and community mobility services. The clinical evaluation is comprised of a series of tests that are by and large accepted by the professional community within the United States. As previously mentioned, the clinical evaluation is the first of two components that make up the comprehensive driver rehabilitation evaluation and must be completed before an on-road evaluation can be initiated. DRSs use the clinical evaluation to analyze client factors (i.e., strengths and limitations) in a variety of performance or skill areas. The on-road evaluations of actual driving performance require clients to integrate these skills in a smooth, coordinated manner to ensure successful outcomes. It also is important that the DRS be aware of the state statutes regarding driving, procedures for reporting individuals (who are not safe to drive) to their respective state department of motor vehicles, and the expected level of expertise for each DRS practicing in their respective states.

Test selection

The battery of tests that comprise the clinical evaluation can be expanded and abbreviated based on the issues that are specific to the client; for example, a client with an incomplete spinal cord injury (SCI) would require a detailed assessment of their physical capacities and deficits, and the long-term potential for further recovery. By contrast a physical assessment may not be needed for an individual with a diagnosis of attention deficit disorder (ADD), who has not reported having had a history of sensorimotor limitations. Using these examples, a brief screening of cognitive skills (versus a full cognitive evaluation) may be all that is required for the individual diagnosed with an SCI, as opposed to the need to provide a far more thorough assessment of visual perception, cognition, and academic skills for the client diagnosed with ADD and associated learning disabilities.

McKenna (1998) offered the following suggestions for preferred characteristics of tests if they are to be included in the battery of driver rehabilitation clinical assessments. The assessment tools should require basic skills, could be easily passed by the majority of the population, and should not depend on intelligence level. Each of the tests should have a direct functional correlate to the driving task and, most importantly, should be validated by the on-road evaluation.

ADED (2004) published the *Best Practices for the Delivery of Driver Rehabilitation Services* and lists the following components as core parts of the driver rehabilitation clinical evaluation:

- Interview and medical history;
- Physical assessments;
- Visual assessments; and
- Cognitive assessments.

Interview and Medical History

The DRS begins the interview by reviewing what to expect during each stage of the comprehensive driver rehabilitation evaluation and training (i.e., clinical evaluation, on-road evaluation, and on-road training). The current status of the client's driver's license must be determined by the DRS and discussed with the client, as this may determine possible limits to the behind-the-wheel assessment. The DRS must be familiar with the licensing requirements in their state; for example, an on-road evaluation may not be conducted if the individual's driving privilege has been revoked by the licensing agency. A state may require the readministration of the law test if the client's license has been expired beyond a specified length of time. This would indicate the need to include an assessment of the client's ability to demonstrate their knowledge of the rules of the road by passing a paper and pencil test that includes questions usually presented in a multiple-choice format. If the client has been deemed unsafe to drive, the DRS can play an important role in assisting them with resources about driving discontinuance and alternatives to driving for community mobility that are affordable, accessible, and reliable.

The state's licensing and medical reporting regulations should be discussed with the individual. See Appendix E for a listing of licensing laws and reporting requirements by state. Many clients who have been referred for a driver rehabilitation evaluation may be unaware of the specific laws pertaining to driving with a disability, aging-related health concerns, or both. A release of information form may be completed by the DRS and delivered to the licensing agency, the physician, and other relevant parties. The possible outcomes of the driver evaluation should be clearly defined in advance, as well as the policy of the driver rehabilitation program regarding reporting drivers who may present a danger to themselves and the public.

In addition to assessing driving performance, the DRS reviews the client's driving habits and patterns. Several questionnaires are available to elicit this information and include questions that address items such as typical distances traveled by motor vehicle, times of the day when the client is most often behind the wheel, the kinds of traffic environments they are accustomed to driving in, and motor vehicle crash history (Stav, 2004; Owsley et al., 1999). Questions can be included to address the client's ability to analyze their strengths and weaknesses, as well as any tendency to self-limit driving, such as avoiding high-volume traffic or not driving at night. If a cross-check of the client's insight and awareness of deficits is needed, the questionnaire can also be given to a family member to complete.

PHYSICAL ASSESSMENT

An assessment of the client's physical skills enables the DRS to anticipate potential challenges the client may face with vehicle control and helps guide the decision-making process for selecting adapted driving equipment, vehicle modifications, and driver training strategies. The information acquired during the clinical evaluation can be used to determine the preferred vehicle type and adaptive driving aids for the on-road assessment.

Height and Limb Length

For clients of short stature or who have limbs that are shorter than the normal range, the DRS should consider the implications for vehicle modifications. A seating system may be needed to position the individual for enhanced line of sight to help ensure correct viewing of the traffic environment. Modifications may be needed to resize or reposition the steering wheel or to add an on/off switch to the driver's front airbag. A vehicle with power adjustable brake and accelerator pedals, after-market extensions, or the use of hand controls may be viable adapted driving options. A client of above average height may need to make careful choices as to the type of vehicle [e.g., van, sport utility vehicle (SUV), truck] for ease of entering and exiting the vehicle and for proper positioning and line of sight once inside of the vehicle. Measurements of the length of the client's limbs and trunk and taking digital photographs of the client seated in the mocked-up vehicle are valuable for design purposes and to establish a visual baseline measurement, formulate recommendations, and to illustrate and support the client's need for third-party reimbursement.

Range of Motion and Strength

The client's ability to turn their head from side to side is important for visual scanning, tracking, and searching techniques, especially while in traffic, stopped or yielding at an intersection, or both. Neck ROM tends to decrease as people age (Isler, Parsonson & Hansson, 1997). The DRS should ask the client to look to the right and left, measure the client's ROM using a goniometer, and document any limitations. If limitations in the client's neck ROM are not likely to improve, the DRS should consider recommending an adapted mirror system in the vehicle. Barry et al. (2003) found that the use of a cervical brace had a negative impact on driving performance primarily due to decreased head ROM and exaggerated blind spots. Moreover, drivers were observed to compensate for decreases in neck ROM by decreasing their speeds and slowing their acceleration when executing lane changes, which increased the likelihood of traffic accidents.

The DRS should measure any limitations in the client's upper extremity joint ROM. Limitations in ROM may indicate the need to elevate the client's seat height in the vehicle or to modify the size or position of the steering wheel. Limited reach may also affect the client's ability to access secondary controls, such as lights, turn signals, windshield wipers, and heating and air-conditioning controls.

A manual muscle test (MMT) of the client's arm strength also may be warranted. Because operation of a motor vehicle's controls involves a coordination of movements, the action of steering or of hand control use can be imitated and the degree of strength and ability noted. A dynamometer and pinch gauge can be used to assess hand grip and pinch strength. Reduced effort steering or electronic gas and brake pedals may be appropriate for clients with decreased upper and lower extremity strength. Various steering devices may be considered for individuals with decreased grip/grasp and pinch (e.g., lateral, three-jaw chuck, and tip) strength.

Joint ROM and strength of the lower extremities (especially the right leg) should also be assessed. Limitations in hip, knee, and ankle motion may affect the client's ability to enter and exit the vehicle and may influence the type of vehicle that is recommended. Limitations in lower extremity ROM also may affect proper positioning necessary for reaching the brake and accelerator pedals and sitting at a proper viewing height. The client's ability to move their foot from the gas pedal to the brake pedal can be further assessed during brake reaction testing.

Range of motion restrictions are common after a total hip replacement, which may make it difficult for the client to transfer into and out of a motor vehicle safely and efficiently. The client may be at risk for falling when walking to and from the vehicle and when entering or exiting the vehicle. If surgery was performed on a client's right hip, there may be interference with accelerator-to-brake reaction time. Ambulation aids, such as a walker or cane, would require the client to safely stow and retrieve the device. The technique employed to perform these tasks must preclude hip external rotation and hip flexion greater than 90 degrees. The client may need to explore adapted driving controls (e.g., left foot gas pedal with a right accelerator pedal block). Limitations in right ankle ROM (e.g., due to an ankle fracture or the use of a right ankle-foot orthosis following a stroke), would hinder a client's ability to apply the correct amount of pressure on the accelerator and brake pedals. The client may intend to compensate by lifting their leg from the hip; however, this technique is fatiguing and negatively affects brake reaction time and accelerator pedal control. If both legs are affected, hand controls may be a consideration.

Sensation

Proprioception and kinesthetic awareness, or the knowledge of the position of the extremity and its movement through space, respectively, also are important to driving. Clients with decreased position sense and kinesthetic awareness may have difficulty with accurate foot placement on the pedals and coordination of foot movement on and between the accelerator and brake pedals. Other important sensory input required to drive a motor vehicle includes the ability to sense light and deep pressure, which allows drivers to judge the amount of force they are exerting on the accelerator pedal and brake pedal.

Sensation of the upper and lower extremities also should be considered; for example, a client diagnosed with right hemiplegia after a cerebrovascular accident (CVA) might have good recovery of arm motion, but may also have decreased sensation in the involved extremities. Consequently steering may be more accurate employing the left arm only with a steering (i.e., spinner) knob.

Another consideration is whether the client's health condition is progressive or static; for example, consider a person with diabetes mellitus (DM) who underwent a right leg amputation because of circulatory problems. Although they may demonstrate satisfactory sensation in the left lower extremity, adequate brake reaction speed, and good driving performance using a left foot accelerator, the DRS, after consultation with the physician, may proactively recommend hand controls in anticipation of further (i.e., progressive) sensory loss in the left leg.

Coordination

Coordination of arm and leg motion is critical to safely control a motor vehicle. Because the vehicle becomes an extension of the driver, the vehicle amplifies coordination deficits; for example, a client with Parkinson's disease (PD) may only be exerting slight tremulous motion on the steering wheel; however, the vehicle may be moving from side to side resulting in poor lane keeping and increasing the likelihood of a traffic accident. Another example presents an individual with cerebral palsy (CP) exerting excess force on the brake, resulting in a harder stop than is desired, and increasing the risk of a rear end collision.

Muscle Tone

An assessment of muscle tone will help the DRS understand the degree of the individual's motor control for handling the vehicle. An example would be an individual diagnosed with a traumatic brain injury (TBI) that resulted in a mild left hemiparesis who wishes to steer the vehicle using both hands. However, as the client drives and muscle tone increases, the left hand begins pulling the steering wheel to the left, causing the vehicle to cross the centerline of the road. In this example the client may be able to better control their steering using a right spinner knob. The DRS can then assess the client's ability to use their left hand for operation of the secondary controls, such as the lights, wipers, and turn signals.

Intermittent spasm activity can be a problem for individuals with SCI. Sudden severe spasms affecting the client's legs, trunk stability, and arm motion can seriously impact vehicle control. Typically an individual with an SCI learns to avoid the motions that can trigger a spasm, but sometimes hitting a speed bump while driving or riding as a passenger in a vehicle, for example, can facilitate increased spasm activity. A referral to a physician for medication management may be indicated.

Clients with CP may experience the effect of primitive reflexes impacting their voluntary motion; for example, head turning to the right or left may elicit arm extension to that side, resulting in a tendency to steer in that direction. There may be associated reactions from one extremity to another. A client using hand controls may notice that steering to the left results in a similar motion in the left arm, thereby increasing acceleration via the hand controls while turning. One extreme example is illustrated by the client who was unable to apply the brake without eliciting a startle reaction that caused him to release his grasp on the steering wheel. Typically an extended in-vehicle evaluation period is needed to determine whether the individual can develop the ability to inhibit these reflexive motions to maintain control over the vehicle. Another consideration would be the client's ability to access the secondary controls of the vehicle, such as the turn signals, lights, and the heating and air-conditioning system. An alternate access method may need to be considered.

Apraxia, or deficits in motor planning, can be a factor in clients with TBI, stroke, or dementia, to name a few. Individuals with autism spectrum disorders also can have deficits in motor coordination (Capo, 2001). These deficits can have serious implications for the client's ability to control the motor vehicle, depending on the severity of the apraxia noted.

Endurance

The DRS can observe the client's endurance for activity during the span of the clinical evaluation and interview the client about their awareness of their stamina and the changes in their movement capacity when fatigued. Motor and cognitive fatigue can be a particular problem for individuals with multiple sclerosis (MS). It may be advisable to schedule the assessment to be completed over several sessions with at least one appointment in the afternoon, so that the client's limitations that are exacerbated by the time of day can be noted and compensation strategies considered. This factor can be further assessed during the on-road evaluation. For example, an individual may be able to drive satisfactorily with standard controls during the morning hours but may experience a decrease in vehicle handling abilities later in the day, indicating the need to assess the use of adapted driving equipment on an as-needed basis. Clients' awareness of their endurance limitations is important because they will need to self-limit their driving to shorter trips, specific times of the day, and have a back-up plan for support and an alternative to driving themselves.

Reaction Speed

The time required to identify and respond to a stimulus can be critical to safe driving in a dynamic, complex traffic environment. A decrease in response time has been documented in clients diagnosed with acquired brain injury (Brower, Withaar, Tant, & van Zomeren, 2002; Groeger, 2000), stroke (Klavora et al., 1995), MS (Schultheis, Garay, & DeLuca, 2001; Shawaryn, Schultheis, Garay, & DeLuca, 2002;), and in the elderly population (Korteling, 1990; Marottoli & Drickamer, 1993). Some state licensing agencies have set criteria for acceptable brake reaction speed. In Maryland, for example, the Motor Vehicle Administration (MVA) requires a minimum reaction speed of 0.5 second (0.5/sec), tested on the American Automobile Association (AAA) Brake Reaction Timer. The AAA instruction manual indicates that a reaction time of 0.39 second falls at the 50th percentile for men and women, with ages ranging from 21 to 80 years (AAA, undated). Unfortunately the AAA no longer distributes this equipment; therefore, alternative reaction speed testing equipment must be used.

Porto Clinic

The Porto Clinic assessment tool provides an assessment of simple and complex reaction time and near-versus far-point vision and depth perception. The client is instructed to apply pressure to the accelerator in response to a green light on the control panel. When the light changes to yellow, the client should reduce pressure on the accelerator and apply the brake in response to the red light. The instrument then measures the speed of the client's response, which is judged against the norms provided. It is worthwhile to note that brake reaction testing does not assess the client's ability to control the amount of pressure placed on the accelerator or brake pedals. These skills would be further assessed in the vehicle.

Vericom Braking Reaction Timer

The Vericom braking reaction timer (Vericom Computers, Inc., Rogers, MN) is an in-vehicle assessment tool. The Vericom braking reaction timer draws power from the vehicle's battery via the accessory power outlet. It has a suction-mounted control panel just above the center dashboard, which is used by the DRS. A small display is mounted within the view of the driver but without blocking visibility of either the road environment or the vehicle's dashboard gauges.

This test is conducted in a large, vacant parking lot or a designated driving range. Driving practice is provided to allow the driver to become familiar with the handling of the vehicle and to demonstrate sufficient vehicle control skills. The driver is instructed to accelerate beyond a minimum of 25 mph, and at random intervals the DRS activates a red light, indicating the need for a hard brake. The Vericom braking reaction timer will measure reaction time, stopping time, brake speed, reaction distance, stopping distance, and peak *G* (i.e., the maximum *G* or gravity force generated). Vericom suggests that the average reaction time is normally considered to be 0.75 second (Vericom, 2004).

It has been noted that reaction time in the vehicle is generally slower than the rate measured during the clinical evaluation. Response time is also likely to be slowed when the driver is surprised or the driving situation is stressful, or both (Sanders & McCormick, 2003).

Several visual perceptual/cognitive tests also provide a means to rate visual processing speed, notably the MVPT-3 and the Trail Making Test. These provide a useful comparison with the client's performance on the brake reaction speed tests and may indicate a client's potential to improve. For example, an individual who has an average response time on the MVPT-3 but fails the brake reaction test may have a specific impairment of lower extremity functioning and may respond well to treatment. By comparison a client who scores low on both measures is demonstrating a more global deficit in processing and response rate, and remediation may not be as successful.

Balance

A client's balance affects their ability to travel to and from the vehicle and to safely enter or exit the vehicle. The client's sitting balance can be a factor when making turns, particularly for individuals with SCIs and other diagnoses that impact sitting balance. Decreased sitting balance may be compensated for by seating systems, additional seat belts, or both. A preliminary assessment of balance can be done during the clinical evaluation by interviewing the client and by pushing slightly (i.e., perturbations) on their shoulder from the right or left and then observing their ability to maintain an erect sitting posture or their need to compensate (e.g., initiating arm or leg motion or both). The

DRS is advised to provide clients with close supervision and use a transfer belt during these assessment procedures to minimize the risk of a client falling.

Considerations Regarding Wheelchairs

The client's skill in transferring from a wheelchair to and from a vehicle would be more specifically assessed in the vehicle, but an initial discussion of techniques, adaptive equipment, and endurance could be held during the clinical evaluation. The DRS should note that the act of transferring to the driver's side of the vehicle presents different challenges than transferring to the passenger's side. Many clients who have been passengers since the onset of their injuries may not have as much experience in transferring on the driver's side of the vehicle.

It is also important to note the make and model of the wheelchair or scooter and to discuss plans for storage of the equipment in the vehicle. Another significant issue is the individual's indication of their need and intention to acquire a new wheelchair or scooter, which will influence current and future vehicle modification recommendations. An OT or PT wheeled mobility and seating specialist consultation may be needed to fully address this issue.

Visual Assessment

The driver rehabilitation specialists (DRS) see clients of driving age for many reasons. Any illness or injury that affects the body's ability to function physically and/or cognitively may have an effect on the ability to drive or access alternative transportation. Many individuals seek rehabilitation specifically for "low vision" driving. Some require bioptic lenses as driving aides. It is more common, however, that the DRS encounters vision-related driving issues through routine screening and testing of clients who are referred to them for a variety of reasons; for example, clients that are contending with impairments due to illness, injury, and/or aging-related concerns. Clients seeking assistance due to a particular primary diagnosis may also have underlying symptoms of macular degeneration, cataracts, glaucoma, visual field loss and other eye conditions that may or may not be related to the primary condition, and may or may not have even been diagnosed and treated in the past. Because vision plays an enormous role in enabling clients to safely operate a vehicle, it is the responsibility of the DRS to carefully evaluate the client's functional visual ability as a key assessment component that is a part of the comprehensive driver rehabilitation evaluation. For example, the DRS needs to be able to distinguish whether a person's driving difficulty comes not from an issue related to turning the wheel physically, but is related to not being able to perceive the lane markers. An evaluation of visual acuity, contrast, and visual fields will assist the DRS in isolating the cause of the difficulty. It is also important to note that the DRS is unqualified for and should not attempt to make diagnoses of the cause of visual impairments.

The vision screening process enables the DRS to identify and describe observed symptoms that should cue them to generate recommendations and/or referrals to a qualified ophthalmologist, optometrist, or other medical professionals for in-depth evaluation, intervention, and follow-up. While symptoms of vision loss may be observed and reported by many health care professionals, formal diagnosis and medical treatment must be left to those professionals that are fully qualified to do so.

THE ROLE OF VISION IN THE OPERATION OF A MOTOR VEHICLE

Visual function is an essential component of driving. Up to 95% of all information absorbed by the driver while operating a motor vehicle is obtained through the visual sense (Shiner & Schieber, 1991). Visual function includes acuity, visual field of view (central and peripheral), contrast sensitivity and glare recovery, scanning and tracking, and visual perceptual skills. The successful driver must be able to integrate all of these components in order to comprehend fully the ever-changing environment through which they are moving.

Parameters for Licensure by the Bureau of Motor Vehicles

Visual acuity and peripheral visual field are the primary factors used by state governments to determine whether a person has the visual skills necessary to operate a motor vehicle with competence. The law governing the operation of a motor vehicle in the United States is prescribed by each state and varies somewhat between states. Generally, some degree of acuity between 20/20 and 20/200 is required. Some states also require a minimal peripheral field of view in one or both eyes of between 70 degrees (monocular) to 140 degrees with bi-ocular vision. Acuity of 20/40 or poorer may require corrective lenses, while acuity of less than 20/100 may require specialized aides and training (Colenbrander et al., 1999). Some states have a minimum peripheral field of view requirement and some do not. Many states have conditional or restricted licensing for a variety of issues including visual impairments. The most common is the need for corrective lenses while driving, but some states restrict drivers to driving during daylight hours only and several states allow biotic driving. A policy statement by the American Academy of Ophthalmology suggests that visual acuity may not be the most reliable indicator of driving ability (American Academy of Ophthalmology, 2001). There is ongoing research exploring the best methods of assessing a client's visual ability to drive, and tests such as the Useful Field of View (UFOV) may provide a more thorough assessment of visual function relative to the operation of a motor vehicle. Please refer to Appendix E for a state-by-state review as prepared by the National Transportation Safety Board (NTSB, Vol. III, Appendix III). Currently, detailed information regarding state driving vision requirements should be obtained from the Bureau of Motor Vehicles or Department of Public Safety for the particular state in question.

Visual Skills

Visual acuity is the ability of the visual system to recognize detail at various distances. Sufficient acuity is needed to read text, recognize faces, and identify objects both near and far. Some degree of visual acuity is required to read signs and dashboard instruments, as well as recognize objects such as other vehicles and pedestrians while driving. The most common tests of visual acuity are given by a range of professionals using eye charts. The most frequently used charts are the Snellen Eye Chart, Colenbrander 1-m Chart, ETDRS (Early Treatment of Diabetic Retinopathy Study), Bailey-Lovie, and LEA charts.

The client is asked to read a series of letters of known height at a prescribed distance, with the smallest legible letters read indicating the degree of near or far acuity. Snellen described the "standard eye" as being able to read letters subtending five degrees of arc, and developed his chart to test acuity. Used as the standard for years, the Snellen chart has several flaws, such as lack of geometric progression, a variable number of letters per line, and lack of proportional spacing to letter size. Current charts, such as the ETDRS, employ a geometric progression of the symbols used on the chart, called a logarithmic Minimum Angle of Resolution (logMAR). Each line contains the same number of symbols, with each line value equaling 0.1 log unit, or 25%, smaller than the preceding line (when starting at the top of the chart). This standardization allows for consistency in evaluation of acuity levels. Charts are designed for assessing near and far distance acuity. The terms "20/20," 20/40," and so forth, are the notations derived from the Snellen chart and are the most commonly recognized visual acuity "values." Most of the other eye charts provide a "Snellen equivalent," which is a conversion of the metric measurement of acuity into the more familiar Snellen terminology.

Field of view is the portion of the viewing area that can be perceived by the client without turning their head irrespective of visual acuity. Field of view has natural limitations defined by a client's eyebrows and cheekbone structure and the shape and size of their nose. Other natural limitations depend upon the shape and structure of the eye itself, particularly as it relates to visual images entering the eye from the periphery, and subsequently where the image falls on the outer edge of the retina. Due to these natural limitations, the normal field of view is approximately 90 degrees temporally or towards the ear, 60 degrees nasally or towards the nose, 70 degrees below the horizontal plane, and 45 degrees above the horizontal plane. Part of the total field of view is "binocular" accounting for approximately 120 degrees in the middle of the field of view because the visual fields of both eyes overlap. Because the visual fields overlap, each of the eyes views an object from a slightly different angle providing stereoscopic or binocular vision, a key component of depth perception.

Peripheral vision is that portion of the field of view along the outer limits of the entire field, and is the second aspect of vision that is most frequently tested by state licensing bureaus. Though commonly referring to the field of view in a horizontal plane at an angle of approximately 90 degrees, temporally, from each eye, the peripheral field also includes the vertical plane above and below the visual center. Peripheral vision is important in order to recognize movements approaching from the far left or right, such as a vehicle at an intersection or a vehicle passing from behind in another lane. It is also important in the detection of street signs and traffic lights above the center of vision, as well as responding to the instruments on the dash, such as a flashing warning light that is located below the center of view. Peripheral vision is not used to identify objects so much as it is used as a cue to shift central vision from one object to one coming into the field of view in order to identify it and initiate a process of assessing potential responses to the visual stimuli.

Another important aspect of the field of view is that portion of the visual field seen by the macula, the central field of view. This portion of the retina, with a radius of approximately 30 degrees, is used for detail and color and is responsible for visual acuity. The retina is a specialized layer of photoreceptor cells on the posterior portion of the eye which converts light into nerve impulses that are sent to the occipital lobes of the brain for processing and interpretation. The retina, made up of two types of receptors called "rods," detects light and dark shades and movements while the "cones" detect color and detail. Rods are found more predominantly around the outer portion of the retina and are useful for night vision and detecting objects along the periphery of the field of view. The cones are found in the central "macula" area of the retina, culminating at the fovea. Reading and recognition of object detail including the color and texture of objects is dependent upon the function of the cones in the macula. Diseases such as macular degeneration damage areas of the macula, leaving crucial areas of the most important part of the central field of view distorted, hazy, or blank. These damaged areas are called scotomas. Imagine trying to read this sentence, or the instrumentation on the dashboard of your motor vehicle, when the word or number you look at is missing because of macular damage.

Contrast sensitivity, scanning, and glare recovery are other aspects of visual function that are vital to driving skill but which are not evaluated by state licensing bureaus. Contrast sensitivity describes the ability of the eye to detect various shades of gray or color shades. The ability to differentiate subtle shadings or detect details in poor lighting conditions greatly impacts acuity. Contrast is the measure of visual perception between light and dark, whether that is black and white, various shades of gray, or various shades of color. The black print on the white page you are reading is a very distinct contrast, but most of our visual images are composed of less sharply defined tones and shades. Indeed, the beauty we find in many things such as a rose petal comes from the delicate and subtle shades of coloring inherent in its features. Contrast sensitivity within the context of the visual aspects of driving skill is important for object recognition, reading of road signage, location of the curb, and dividing lanes and recognition of lights, such as brake and traffic lights. Persons demonstrating difficulty with contrast, such as those with cataracts, have increased difficulty with these and other driving tasks. This can be compounded when driving in less than optimum lighting conditions. Even though the client may have adequate acuity in the clinical or community setting where the pre-driving assessment has taken place, the DRS must ask how acuity is affected by glare, rain, cloudy or foggy days, or driving at dusk or at night. Early morning and at dusk are the two most difficult times of the day to perceive objects, because there is often insufficient light for the cones to see color and detail, but too much light to benefit from the rods that are designed for night vision.

Glare is a common distraction for all drivers. Sunlight reflecting from another vehicle, from a wet or icy pavement, and headlights or even the sun itself can momentarily affect anyone's ability to see. When the driver has cataracts or perhaps some type of retinal disease, recovering visual function after encountering a glare situation can take many seconds or even minutes! Visual acuity can be greatly reduced under these circumstances and can lead to loss of control of the vehicle and worse.

Several screening tools are available and if the DRS identifies deficits in a client's visual skills, a referral to a vision specialist should be initiated. There are some useful tools for assessing vision skills and a brief description of them follows.

Optec 5000

The Optec 5000 is a vision screening tool (Stereo Optical Co., 2009). The slide package designed for driving includes an assessment of near-point vision (to assess acuity for the dashboard controls of a vehicle or to adequately view the clinical evaluation tests), distance vision, peripheral vision, color discrimination, depth perception, and sign recognition. The Optec also has tumbling E slides, which can be useful to assess far-point acuity for clients with aphasia. A recommended addition, because of its importance to driving, is the contrast package (Stereo Optical Co., 2009).

This measures an individual's contrast sensitivity, which would indicate their vision during poor lighting conditions (e.g., at night, at dusk, on a cloudy day, on a rainy day).

Titmus Vision Screener

The Titmus Vision Screener, like the Optec, provides assessment of near and distance acuity, traffic color recognition, depth perception, and peripheral vision. For clients with language impairment, visual acuity slides using number stimuli or tumbling Es are available. Slides also are provided for traffic sign recognition set at 20/40 or 20/70 visual acuity. The ability to recognize common traffic signs can be one pertinent indicator of driver readiness for clients with dementia. Note that the Porto Clinic also provides a means to assess acuity and depth perception as previously stated.

COGNITIVE SKILLS

There are six categories of cognitive skills that influence driving performance: (1) attention; (2) processing speed; (3) language functions; (4) memory functioning; (5) visuospatial and visuomotor functioning; and (6) executive functioning (Coleman Bryer et al., 2006).

Attention

Simple or sustained attention includes being able to focus on a single stimulus for various periods of time. Focusing on multiple pieces of information simultaneously is known as complex or divided attention (i.e., multitasking). Working memory is considered the most complex aspect of attention and involves complex attentional processes that depend on executive functioning. Impairment in visuospatial attention, such as visual neglect or field loss, can result from damage to the right parietal lobe of the brain. Driving performance may be negatively affected by attention deficits; for example, a driver may not see obstacles on or near the road or comprehend important events on the road as they are unfolding. They also may become easily distracted by non-essential stimuli (e.g., radio, conversation, billboard, cell phone) or be unable to process several events simultaneously. Attentional abilities have been recognized as predictive of driving fitness (Engum et al., 1988).

Processing Speed

The time it takes to verbally or physically respond to a stimulus is referred to as processing speed. Deficits in attention often accompany impairments in processing speed; however, even in cases where this is not demonstrated, a deficit in either one of these areas increases the likelihood of driving cessation following a TBI or stroke, for example. Although a client who demonstrates processing speed deficits may be able to adequately focus on a specific stimulus or event while driving (e.g., a specific hazard), they may not be able to process the stimulus in sufficient time to plan and implement an appropriate response, such as demonstrating an avoidance maneuver to avert a potential crash. Processing speed deficits are a common manifestation of TBIs and dementia, and other aging-related health challenges.

Language Functioning

The ability to communicate by comprehending information by hearing (auditory) or seeing (written) and respond appropriately via verbal or non-verbal communication is known as language functioning. Although the relationship between driving and language disruption is not immediately apparent, alexia (the inability to read) or aphasia (the inability to understand or express language or both) may impact driving performance (Golper, Rau & Marshall, 1980; Mackenzie & Paton, 2003). For example, an individual with alexia may be unable to interpret road signs, particularly those that cannot be immediately identified by shape, and an individual with aphasia may be unable to ask for or respond to directions or assistance. Language functioning deficits are often overlooked when making decisions about a client's driving fitness; however, studies have revealed that left hemisphere damage with symptoms such as aphasia is sufficient to substantially compromise driving performance.

25.9.4 Memory

Driving performance also can be substantially affected by memory functioning. Memory occurs in three stages: (1) encoding or the ability to acquire new information; (2) consolidation or the transformation of new information to permanent storage (i.e., long-term memory); and (3) retrieval or the ability to recall (i.e., remember) learned material. Memory deficits can be manifested when a client is unable to learn new driving routes or to recall those routes without extensive rehearsal, or both. Among individuals with Alzheimer's disease (AD), as dementia advances from a severity level of "very mild" to "mild," driving impairment becomes a significant traffic safety problem (Dubinsky, Stein & Lyons, 2000). Although memory problems are most commonly associated with dementia, deficits in memory also are common after TBI, stroke, multiple sclerosis (MS), and aging-related health conditions. Decreased memory functioning, which is a part of normal aging, is not a concern unless there is a diagnosis of dementia (Coleman Bryer et al., 2006).

Memory Assessments

The Trail Making Test has been highly correlated with driving performance (Hopewell, 2002). The Trail Making Test was initially designed as part of the U.S. Army Individual Test Battery (1944) and is now in the public domain. The administration instructions are provided in detail in *A Compendium of Neuropsychological Tests: Administration, Norms and Commentary* (Spreen & Strauss, 1998); they are reproduced in Appendix B.

Norms are available for persons aged 18 to 89 years, and it has been noted that scores decrease for individuals with advanced age or lower education levels (Tombaugh, 2004). A government study (NHTSA, 2003) suggested that a timed score of 100 seconds on the Trails B subtest would indicate a need for further testing of driving performance because it correlated with increased crash risk.

CLOX is a clock drawing test that is designed to differentiate executive function and visual-spatial praxis (Royall, Cordes, & Polk, 1998). In CLOX 1 the client is requested to draw a clock, and in CLOX 2 the client copies a clock drawn by the evaluator. Standardized instructions are provided: "Draw me a clock that says 1:45. Set the hands and numbers on the face so that a child could read them" (Royall et al., 1998, p. 589). For CLOX 2 the evaluator draws a clock in a circle printed on the scoring sheet, following a specific sequence. The client is then asked to copy the evaluator's drawing. The two drawings are then scored, and the client's performance for the two testing conditions is compared. The test is particularly valuable for clients with dementia and Alzheimer's disease.

The Rivermead Behavioral Memory Test is a test of everyday memory skills, including the ability to remember names, faces, pictures, appointments, a brief story, a short route within the room, and the location of a personal object hidden in the room. Normal performance would result in one or two errors on the 12-test items (Wilson, Cockburn, & Baddeley, 1985).

Visuospatial Functioning and Visuomotor Functioning

Visuospatial and visuomotor functioning are required to help ensure optimal driving performance (Galski et al., 1992). There are five categories of visuospatial disorders (Benton et al., 1993): deficiencies in localizing particular points in space; challenges with judging direction; problems with perceiving the distance between oneself and another object (e.g., depth perception); impaired topographical orientation (i.e., knowing one's location in a particular geographic area or region); and unilateral visual neglect. Deficits in visuospatial functioning can affect a client's ability to pinpoint the locations of various visual stimuli while behind the wheel of a motor vehicle (e.g., other road users and the surrounding physical environment). A sense of being disoriented or becoming lost can be manifestations of visuospacial deficits as well.

Visuomotor deficits affect one's ability to plan and initiate movements in response to what is seen (i.e., visual stimuli). The most notable aspect of visuomotor functioning within the context of driving is visual scanning. Visual scanning is the ability to search within one's field of view to locate an object or series of objects. Functional scanning requires coordinated movement of the eyes (and head) horizontally, vertically, and diagonally to locate a particular object. Maintaining one's gaze upon a selected object enables a client to focus their lens to maximize visual acuity for optimal object recognition (e.g., rapidly braking in response to seeing a child in the street). Tracking combines both scanning and motion. In other words, the client finds and fixates on an object and, if it is moving, such as a vehicle or pedestrian, tracks (i.e., follow) the movement of the object. Another example of visual tracking is the necessity of a driver to identify and follow the dividing lines on a highway. In a cognitively intact individual visual scanning occurs in an organized fashion and the systematic approach to examining the visual environment plays an important role in how the environment is perceived. Many persons with brain disorders have abnormal eye movements that result in an inaccurate comprehension of the world as it is seen and perceived. Risk for motor vehicle crashes while driving increases substantially when abnormal eye movements are detected (Webster, Rapport, Godlewski, & Abadee, 1994; Webster et al., 1995).

Executive Functioning

This and the following section are taken from Pellerito (2006).

Executive functioning represents the highest level of cognitive functioning and is especially susceptible to impairment after brain damage. There is growing recognition that this domain of cognition has a tremendous impact on functional outcomes such as driving. Executive functioning includes a broad spectrum of abilities, including anticipatory behavior, problem solving, self-monitoring, and self-assessment, all of which are critical aspects of risk and fitness to drive. The term can also encompass other high-level aspects of cognitive functioning that sometimes overlap with the domain of attention, including multitasking, mental flexibility, inhibitory ability, and attentional vigilance functions. Other aspects of executive functioning include abstract thinking, insight, and preserved personality functioning. Often neuropsychological test batteries for driving assessment have been brief, largely neglecting important domains such as executive functioning (Gouvier et al., 1989; Korteling & Kaptein, 1996; Rothke, 1989; Sivak, Olson, Kewman, Won, & Henson 1981). Although the ability to drive a motor vehicle relies heavily on perception, motor skills, and information processing speed, numerous investigators have emphasized the special importance of executive functions in making determinations about an individual's driving ability.

The Role of Executive Functioning in Driving

Various studies indicate that risk for accidents is moderated by higher-order cognitive abilities (Coleman et al., 2002; Daigneault, Joly & Frigon, 2002; Hopewell, 2002; Mazer, Korner-Bitensky, & Sofer, 1998; Schank & Sundet, 2000) and that performance on tasks of executive functioning is predictive of on-road driving ability. Coleman et al. (2002) reported that performance on tasks of executive functioning, combined with years post injury and disability at discharge from a rehabilitation hospital, predicted post-discharge traffic accidents and violations after TBI. Similarly Daigneault et al. (2002) reported that older drivers with a history of accidents performed more poorly than control subjects on tasks of executive functioning. The standard versions of the *Trails B* (Reitan & Davison, 1974) and the *Stroop* (Trenerry et al., 1989) tests, both commonly used neuropsychological tasks evaluating executive function, have shown strong correlations with driving ability (Hopewell, 2002; Schanke & Sundet, 2000). Other commonly used tests of executive functioning that have shown strong predictive utility include the *Matrix Reasoning* and *Letter–Number Sequencing* subtests of the Wechsler Adult Intelligence Scale (WAIS)-III (Wechsler, 1997), the *Colored Trails Test* (D'Elia et al., 1996), the *Tower of London* (Culbertson & Zillmer, 2001), and the *Wisconsin Card Sorting Test* (Heaton, 1981).

Executive functions also play a major role in the functional capacity of other cognitive and motor functions. Perceptual and motor skills may be intact but functionally hindered by the complexity of the stimulus challenge. The *Useful Field of Vision* (UFOV; Ball & Owsley, 1992) test illustrates this point by combining assessment of simple peripheral vision with assessment of functional visual capacity during conditions of increased cognitive load. Selective and divided attention tasks are included to mimic real world conditions in which stimulus fields may be complex and cluttered. Research using the UFOV test generally has demonstrated that the functional range of peripheral vision is inversely related to cognitive load (Fisk, Novack, Mennemeier, & Roenker, 2002). The UFOV test has shown strong predictive validity for crashes and driving evaluations and 86% accuracy predicting the outcome of driving evaluations (Ball, Owsley, Sloane, Roenker, & Bruni, 1993; Goode et al., 1998; Mazer et al., 2003; Myers, Ball, Kalina, Roth, & Goode, 2000; Owsley et al., 1998) among older adults. The test is gaining popularity in the driving evaluation process; however, generalizability of UFOV validity research to persons with acquired brain disorders, such as stroke and TBI, has been limited.

Two studies indicated that the UFOV test might be useful in assessing driving readiness in TBI survivors (Calvanio et al., 2004; Fisk et al., 2002). TBI survivors performed more poorly on the UFOV test than did college students, and the authors interpreted this finding as possibly indicative of a higher risk for crashes (Fisk et al., 2002); however, no actual assessment of driving safety was conducted. In fact only 9% of the TBI survivors scored above the UFOV test cutoff associated with increased risk of crash among healthy older adults. Considering that TBI survivors fail driving evaluations at rates of 30–60%, it may not have good predictive validity in this population. Fisk et al. (2002) and Calvanio et al. (2004) found that the UFOV test correlated strongly with several standard visual attention tests, including *Trails A* and *B*, but neither study directly examined the relationship of performance on the UFOV test and actual driving ability. Although these findings provide some support for generalizing crash-risk research on the UFOV test to persons with TBI, a high correlation between the UFOV test and *Trails B*, an inexpensive paper-and-pencil test, highlights the importance of simultaneously examining the unique predictive powers of measures used to assess fitness to drive.

Visual Perception Tests

The MVPT was designed and standardized for adults for the normal population and the brain-injured population (Bouska & Kwatny, 1983). It has norms for people aged 18 to 80 years and is a motor-free test of visual perceptual abilities, including spatial relationships, visual discrimination, figure-ground, visual closure, and visual memory (Colarusso & Hammill, 1972). This test provides a profile of basic visual perceptual skills needed to drive, as well as an indication of a client's speed in processing visual information, and has been correlated to driving performance (Korner-Bitensky et al., 2000).

MVPT-3 (Colarusso & Hammill, 2003) is the version of the test that is available at the time of this writing. The test has been expanded to 65 items. Several subsections have been added (e.g., spatial orientation and figure-ground, as well as more difficult items requiring visual closure and visual short-term memory). The test norms now extend to ages ≥94 years. A means to record and judge response speed has also been included, which is critical for responding to the rapid processing of traffic interaction (McKenna, 1998). This version of the test was recently introduced and is markedly more difficult. Test norms also do not exist as of yet to correlate test performance with the determination of driving risk.

The (TVPS-R) is similar in format to the MVPT but provides a consistent number of test items for each of its seven subtests: visual discrimination; visual memory; visual-spatial relationships; visual form constancy; visual sequential memory; visual figure ground; and visual closure. The test offers an upper level (UL) version that provides norms for young people aged 12 to 18 years. The test has recently been revised to add less difficult items and to refine the norms (Gardner, 1996).

The Hooper Visual Organization Test provides 30 drawings of common objects that have been cut apart and rearranged. The client is asked to name the object and so must mentally rotate the parts into a recognizable whole. The test was normed on subjects ranging in ages from 13 to 80 years (Hooper, 1979).

In the UFOV test, the concept of "useful field of view" refers to the brain's ability to comprehend visual information with the head and eyes in a stationary position (Mestre, 2004).

The UFOV test is administered on a computer using a touch screen. The test involves a series of slides and objects the client must remember amid background visual distractions. It tests visual memory, visual attention, and divided attention with structured and unstructured components. The test differs substantially from standard eye examinations that measure visual acuity or visual function and the ability to see an object at a given distance (National Institute on Aging, 1998). The UFOV has been shown to be a strong predictor of crash risk in older drivers (Owsley et al., 1998).

Inclusion of a visual-motor test to the clinical evaluation is advisable because driving is not a motor-free task. The test also should be used for the population for which it has been designed. For example, a test that assesses the developmental level of a skill, such as visual-motor coordination, is valuable for use with individuals with developmental disabilities such as CP, mental retardation (MR), and spina bifida (SB). By contrast a test such as the Benton Test of Visual Retention has been designed for individuals with acquired deficits such as TBI and CVA. This test does not provide developmental norms; however, it does provide an indication of memory for visual stimuli and a measure of visual inattention. In contrast, unilateral neglect would not be a likely deficit noted with a client with CP, for example.

The Beery-Buktenica Developmental Test of Visual-Motor Integration (VMI) consists of 27 geometric forms of increasing complexity. The client is required to copy each form without erasing. The results are analyzed by specific criteria, and norms are provided for young people aged 3 to 18 years (Beery, 1997).

The Benton Visual Retention Test provides three sets of 10 geometric designs and allows for four methods of administration. It assesses the client's ability to copy the designs and demonstrate recall in one of three different conditions. The versatility of the test allows for repeated administration while minimizing the practice effect. The test is also sensitive to inattention, demonstrated by an increased number of errors for designs on the right or left of the page. The norms can be adjusted for age and education level; norms are provided for those aged 8 to 89 years (Sivan, 1992).

The Dynavision has a series of lights arranged in a large circle on a metal board. The board is adjustable so that a client can be tested at different heights or from a seated position. The large size helps to ensure that a significant portion of the client's visual field is stimulated. The lights are illuminated in a random pattern, and the client is required to touch each light to turn it off or to cause another light to activate. There are several modes of increasing complexity that require various response patterns by the client. There has been some evidence that visual-motor training using this tool can result in improvement of a client's on-road driving performance (Klavora, Gaskovski & Forsyth, 1995).

DRIVING KNOWLEDGE

Tests of driving knowledge are informal tests that demonstrate the client's knowledge of the rules of driving. They test the client's ability to recognize road signs, familiarity with vehicle laws, and practical applications of the rules of the road. A familiar example would be the law test provided by many driver-licensing agencies to qualify an individual for a learner's permit. Similar tests are also available from driver education courses. For experienced drivers tests of defensive driving techniques are available. Although these tests provide an indication of the client's knowledge of information pertinent to driving, they do not assess or predict the client's functional driving skills or ability to integrate knowledge and performance skills when on the road.

A Driver Performance Test (DPT) consists of 40 brief videotaped driving scenes, each taken from the perspective of the driver in the vehicle. Each video is followed by a multiple-choice question. The test items are given point scores for the best to the least acceptable answer. The scores can be compared with those of experienced drivers of automobiles and light trucks, and can be analyzed for strengths and weaknesses in the skills of Search, Identify, Predict, Decide, and Execute, which are the critical skills for safe operation of a motor vehicle (Safe Performance Associates, undated).

Interpretation of the Test Results

As previously stated the primary value of the clinical evaluation is to prepare the DRS for on-road testing and to provide a possible explanation of the client's on-road performance. It has also been stressed throughout this chapter that a decision to "pass" or "fail" a client should not be based on the clinical evaluation alone. However, there are a few exceptions to this rule. A recommendation against driving that is based on clinical evaluation results is appropriate in the following situations:

- The client does not meet the standards set by the driver-licensing agency. If the client does not meet the vision criteria, brake reaction speed, if applicable, or various medical qualifications (e.g., a seizure disorder that is controlled by medication for a specified time period), a referral to a specialist (e.g., vision care or neurologist) or for further therapy may be considered.
- The client scores in the severely deficient ranges on all or most of the tests included in the clinical evaluation. This situation may occur with clients who have severe deficits from such diagnoses as TBI or stroke or from progressive diseases such as dementia, PD, MS, and amyotrophic lateral sclerosis (ALS), to name a few. In the cases of such conditions as head trauma or stroke, consideration may be given to a recommendation for further therapy if the onset is relatively recent or if therapeutic efforts have been minimal in the client's past. The potential for improvement may be limited in those with progressive disorders. It is also advisable to discuss the recommendations with the physician to gather additional understanding of the client's prognosis.

The DRS may choose to perform the on-road evaluation to provide additional concrete feedback to the client who is disputing the recommendations of the clinical evaluation. It would be advisable that the on-road evaluation be carried out in an off-street, protected environment before moving to evaluate the client's on-road driving performance. A driving simulator may also provide the client with an opportunity to practice driving in a protected virtual environment.

Coordination With the On-Road Evaluation

In some settings the DRS may perform both the clinical evaluation and the on-road evaluation. In other models of driver rehabilitation service provision, different individuals handle the two phases of the comprehensive evaluation. If there are two DRSs involved in the evaluation, an open line of communication between the two practitioners is essential. The information learned from the clinical tests needs to be conveyed to the on-road evaluator so that he or she can be prepared to observe the client performing certain aspects of the driving task that are expected to be challenging and to be ready for possible problems that may arise. The clinical evaluation is not necessarily predictive of on-road performance; therefore, the practitioner who conducts only the clinical evaluation needs to be mindful of a possible discrepancy between clinical and on-road performance. Conversely the practitioner who only observes a client's on-road driving performance needs to appreciate the value of standardized testing of abstract measures, such as subtle visual perceptual and cognitive functions. There needs to be mutual respect between each of the respective DRSs and an acknowledgment that every client must receive both components of the comprehensive driver rehabilitation evaluation. It is only by joining efforts that a meaningful analysis can be completed, producing the best possible recommendations for the client being served.

APPENDIX A: ASSESSMENTS THAT COMPRISE THE DRIVER REHABILITATION CLINICAL ASSESSMENT

Clinical Evaluation Components	Client Factors Assessed	Assessments
		Note: Asterisks denote optional assessments that can be completed by the DRS or data can be provided to the DRS by a therapist generalist. Formal assessments versus observations and interviews are conducted depending on the client's or patient's functional status and diagnosis or diagnoses. Check marks indicate routine or customary assessments conducted by the DRS as part of the clinical driver rehabilitation evaluation.
• Initial interview with client (may include caregiver)	• Client's medical and social history	• Interview guide that is program specific
• Physical assessments	• Height and limb length • ROM • Strength • Fine motor coordination • Muscle tone	• Consultation with the primary OT and PT generalists as needed or observation and assessment or both • Goniometric ROM measurements* (procedure and norms available in Pendleton, H. M., & Schultz-Krohn, W. (Eds.) (2006). *Pedretti's Occupational Therapy Practice Skills for Physical Dysfunction.* (6th ed.). St. Louis, MS: Mosby Elsevier. Manual Muscle Testing (MMT)* (procedure and norms available in Pendleton, H. M., & Schultz-Krohn, W. (Eds.) (2006). *Pedretti's Occupational Therapy Practice Skills for Physical Dysfunction* (6th ed.). St. Louis, MS: Mosby Elsevier • Hand-held dynamometry* (norms available in Mathiowetz et al., 1985; positioning available in Pendleton, H. M., & Schultz-Krohn, W. (Eds.). (2006). *Pedretti's Occupational Therapy Practice Skills for Physical Dysfunction.* (6th ed.). St. Louis, MS: Mosby Elsevier. Hand-held pinch gauge* (procedure available in Pedretti, 2009); (adult Norms available from Mathiowetz et al. 1985) • Nine Hole Peg test* (tool available from Sammons Preston Rolyan, P.O. Box 5071, Bolingbrook, IL 60440 (1-800-547-4333); (adult norms available from Oxford et al., 2003)

Clinical Evaluation Components	Client Factors Assessed	Assessments
	• Proprioception	Examination and observation* (procedure and norms in Pendleton, H. M., & Schultz-Krohn, W. (Eds.) (2006). *Pedretti's Occupational Therapy Practice Skills for Physical Dysfunction* (6th ed.). St. Louis, MS: Mosby Elsevier
	• Kinesthesia	• Examination and observation* (procedure and norms available in Pendleton, H. M., & Schultz-Krohn, W. (Eds.) (2006). *Pedretti's Occupational Therapy Practice Skills for Physical Dysfunction* (6th ed.). St. Louis, MS: Mosby Elsevier
	• Endurance	• Examination and Observation* (procedure and norms available in Pendleton, H. M., & Schultz-Krohn, W. (Eds.) (2006). *Pedretti's Occupational Therapy Practice Skills for Physical Dysfunction* (6th ed.). St. Louis, MS: Mosby Elsevier
	• Sitting balance (static and dynamic) • Standing balance	• Berg Balance Scale* (available at www.chcr.brown.edu/Balance.html) • Tinetti Assessment Tool* (including balance test and gait test) (available at http://www.anodynetherapy.com/PDF%20Files/Tinetti.pdf
	• Ambulation status	• Dynamic Gait Index* (available at http://r-sports.hp.infoseek.co.jp/siryou/balance/dgi.doc
	• Primary ambulation aid used	• Consultation with the primary OT and PT generalists as needed or interview and observation or both
	• Wheeled mobility and seating	• Consultation with the primary OT and PT generalists as needed or interview and observation or both
	• Tactile sensation • Light and deep pressure • Stereognosis	• Sensation* (procedure and norms available in Pendleton, H. M., & Schultz-Krohn, W. (Eds.) (2006). *Pedretti's Occupational Therapy Practice Skills for Physical Dysfunction* (6th ed.). St. Louis, MS: Mosby Elsevier
	• Brake reaction speed	• The Vericom braking reaction timer (Vericom Computers, Inc., Rogers, MN)
Visual assessments	• Visual acuity • Peripheral vision • Depth perception • Color perception • Road sign recognition • Binocular glare testing • Contrast sensitivity • Stereopsis • Contrast sensitivity • Peripheral vision • Tracking • Convergence • Saccades • Pursuits	• Snellen Chart* (available at www.mdsupport.org/snellen.html) • Optec 5000 Vision Tester (see http://www.stereooptical.com/html/optec-5000.html)

(*Continued*)

Clinical Evaluation Components	Client Factors Assessed	Assessments
Cognitive and visual perceptual assessments	• Form constancy • Visual memory • Visual closure • Visual discrimination	• Motor-Free Visual Perceptual Test-3* (MVPT-3) • TVPS-R* • Hooper Visual Organization Test • Trail Making Test (Part A) • Useful Field Of View (UFOV) • The Beery-Buktenica Developmental Test of Visual-Motor Integration* (VMI) • The Benton Visual Retention Test
	• Search, identify, predict, decide, and execute	• Driver Performance Test* (DPT)
General knowledge	• Tests of driving knowledge	• Informal tests that demonstrate the client's knowledge of the rules of driving.

DRS, *Driver rehabilitation specialist;* ROM, *range of motion;* MMT, *manual muscle testing;* PT, *physical therapist.*

APPENDIX B: INSTRUCTIONS FOR THE TRAIL MAKING TEST PARTS A AND B

Administration—Part A

Sample A. When ready to begin the test, place the Part A test sheet in front of the subject. Give the subject a pencil, and say: *"On this page* (point) *are some numbers. Begin at number 1* (point to '1') *and draw a line from one to two* (point to '2'), *two to three* (point to '3'), *three to four* (point to '4'), *and so on, in order, until you reach the end* (pointing to the circle marked 'END'). *Draw the lines as fast as you can. Do not lift the pencil from the paper. Ready! Begin!"*

If the subject makes a mistake on Sample A, point it out, and explain it. The following explanations of mistakes are acceptable:

1. "You started with the wrong circle. This is where you start (point to '1')."
2. "You skipped this circle (point to the one omitted). You should go from number one (point) to two (point), two to three (point) and so on, until you reach the circle marked 'END' (point)."
3. "Please keep the pencil on the paper, and continue right onto the next circle."

After the mistake has been explained, the examiner marks out the wrong part and says: *"Go on from here"* (point to the last circle completed correctly in the sequence).

If the subject still cannot complete Sample A, take the subject's hand and guide the pencil (eraser end down) through the trail. Then say: *"Now you try it. Put your pencil, point down. Remember, begin at number one* (point) *and draw a line from one to two* (point to '2'), *two to three* (point to '3'), *three to four* (point to '4'), *and so on, in order until you reach the circle marked 'END'* (point). *Do not skip around but go from one number to the next in the proper order. If you make a mistake, mark it out. Remember, work as fast as you can. Ready! Begin!"*

If the subject succeeds this time, go on to Part A of the test. If not, repeat the procedure until the subject does succeed, or it becomes evident that he or she cannot do it.

If the subject completes the sample item correctly and in a manner that he or she knows what to do, say: *"Good! Let's try the next one."* Turn the page, and give Part A of the test.

Test. Say, "On this page are numbers from 1 to 25. Do this the same way. Begin at number one (point) and draw a line from one to two (point to '2'), two to three (point to '3'), three to four (point to

'4'), and so on, in order until you reach the end (point). Remember, work as fast as you can. Ready! Begin!"

Start timing. If the subject makes an error, call it to his or her attention immediately, and have the subject proceed from the point where the mistake occurred. Do not stop timing.

If the examinee completes Part A without error, remove the test sheet. Record the time in seconds. Errors count only in the increased time of performance. Then say: *"That's fine. Now we'll try another one."* Proceed immediately to Part B, sample.

Administration—Part B

Sample. Place the test sheet for Part B, sample side up, flat on the table in front of the examinee, in the same position as the sheet for Part A was placed. Point with the right hand to the sample and say: *"On this page are some numbers and letters. Begin at number one* (point) *and draw a line from one to* A (point to 'A'), *A to two* (point to '2'), *two to B* (point to 'B'), *B to three* (point to '3'), *three to C* (point to 'C'), *and so on, in order until you reach the end* (point to circle marked 'END'). *Remember, first you have a number* (point to '1'), *then a letter* (point to 'A'), *then a number* (point to '2'), *then a letter* (point to 'B'), *and so on. Draw the lines as fast as you can. Ready! Begin!"*

If the subject makes a mistake on Sample B, point it out, and explain it. The following explanations of mistakes are acceptable:

1. "You started with the wrong circle. This is where you start (point to '1')."
2. "You skipped this circle (point to the one omitted). You should go from one (point) to A (point), A to two (point), two to B (point), B to three (point), and so on, until you reach the circle marked 'END' (point)." If it is clear that the subject intended to touch the circle but missed it, do not count it as an omission, but caution him or her to touch the circle.
3. "You only went as far as this circle (point). You should have gone to the circle marked 'END' (point)."
4. "Please keep the pencil on the paper, and go right onto the next circle."

After the mistake has been explained, the examiner marks out the wrong part and says: *"Go on from here"* (point to the last circle completed correctly in the sequence).

If the subject still cannot complete Sample B, take the subject's hand and guide the pencil (eraser end down) through the circles. Then say: *"Now you try it. Remember you begin at number one* (point) *and draw a line from one to* A (point to 'A'), *A to two* (point to '2'), *two to B* (point to 'B'), *B to three* (point to '3'), *and so on until you reach the circle marked 'END'* (point). *Ready! Begin!"*

Test. If the subject completes the sample item correctly, say: *"Good. Let's try the next one."* Turn the page over and proceed immediately to Part B, and say: *"On this page are some numbers and letters. Begin at number one* (point) *and draw a line from one to* A (point to 'A'), *A to two* (point to '2'), *two to B* (point to 'B'), *B to three* (point to '3'), *three to C* (point to 'C'), *and so on, in order until you reach the end* (point to circle marked 'END'). *Remember, first you have a number* (point to '1'), *then a letter* (point to 'B'), *and so on. Do not skip around, but go from one circle to the next in the proper order. Draw the lines as fast as you can. Ready! Begin!"*

Start timing. If the subject makes an error immediately, call it to his or her attention and have the subject proceed from the point where the mistake occurred. Do not stop timing.

If the subject completes Part B without error, remove the test sheet. Record the time in seconds. Errors count only in the increased time of performance.

From Spreen, O. & Strauss, E. *A Compendium of Neuropsychological Tests*, New York, 1991, Oxford University Press.

APPENDIX C: GUIDELINES FOR MOTOR VEHICLE ADMINISTRATORS: LICENSE RENEWAL REQUIREMENTS

State/Province	2001 Licensing Renewal Requirements and Distinctions for Older Drivers*
Alabama	4-year renewal cycle (in person). No tests for renewal. Minimum acuity 20/60 in one eye with/without corrective lenses. May *not* use bioptic telescopic lens to meet acuity standard. *No special requirements for older drivers.*
Alaska	5-year renewal cycle (mail in every other cycle). No renewal by mail for drivers aged 69+ and for drivers whose previous renewal was by mail. Vision test required at in-person renewal. Minimum 20/40 in one eye for unrestricted license. 20/40 to 20/100 needs report from eye specialist; license request determined by discretion. May use bioptic telescopic lens in certain conditions.
Arizona	12-year renewal cycle. At age 65, reduction of interval to 5 years. New photograph and vision test at renewal; no renewal by mail after age 70 (available to active duty veterans and dependents only). Minimum acuity 20/40 in one eye required; acuity of 20/60 restricted to daytime only. May *not* use bioptic telescopic lens to meet acuity standard.
Arkansas	4-year renewal cycle. Vision test required at renewal, with minimum 20/40 required for unrestricted license. Acuity of 20/60 restricted to daytime only. Bioptic telescopes permitted in certain circumstances. *No special requirements for older drivers.*
California	5-year renewal cycle (may be mail in for no more than two sequential cycles) with vision test and written knowledge test required. No renewal by mail at age 70. Minimum visual acuity is 20/200 (best corrected) in at least one eye as verified by an optometrist or ophthalmologist. Bioptic lenses are permitted for driving but may not be used to meet 20/200 acuity standard.
Colorado	10-year renewal cycle (mail in every other cycle). At age 61, reduction in renewal to 5 years. No renewal by mail at age 66. Vision test required at renewal. Written test required only if point accumulations result in suspension (12 points in 12 months, or 18 points in 24 months, for nonminor and noncommercial drivers). Minimum acuity must be 20/70 in the better eye if worse eye is 20/200 or better, 20/40 if worse eye is worse than 20/200. Bioptic telescopes are permitted to meet acuity standard.
Connecticut	4-year renewal cycle (in person). Vision test required at in person. 20/40 required in better eye for unrestricted license; 20/50 to 20/70 restricted license; in some circumstances, a license may be issued when acuity is 20/200. No license may be issued to drivers using telescopic aids. Reduction of interval to 2 years may be requested by drivers aged 65+.
Delaware	5-year renewal cycle (in person). No tests required for renewal. Minimum acuity 20/40 for unrestricted license, restricted license at 20/50; beyond 20/50 driving privileges denied. Bioptic telescopes treated on case-by-case basis. *No special requirements for older drivers.*

State/Province	2001 Licensing Renewal Requirements and Distinctions for Older Drivers*
District of Columbia	4-year renewal cycle (in person). Unrestricted license for 20/40 acuity; 20/70 in better eye requires 140E visual field for restricted license. At age 70, vision test required and physician signature attesting to physical and mental capability to drive; a medical report plus reaction test may also be required. At age 75 written knowledge and road tests may be required.
Florida	6-year renewal cycle for clean driving record; 4-year renewal cycle for unclean record. In-person renewal required every third cycle. Vision test at in-person renewal. Must have 20/70 in either eye with or without corrective lenses. Monocular people need 20/40 in fellow eye. Bioptic telescopes are *not* recognized to meet acuity standard. *No special requirements for older drivers.*
Georgia	4-year renewal cycle (in person). Vision test required for renewal (within previous 6-month period). Acuity 20/60 in either eye with or without corrective lenses. Bioptic telescopes permitted for best acuity as low as 20/200, with restrictions. *No special requirements for older drivers.*
Hawaii	6-year renewal cycle for drivers ages 18 to 71 (in person). Vision test required, with 20/40 standard for better eye. Bioptic telescopes permitted for driving but not for passing vision test. Reduction of interval to 2 years for drivers aged 72+.
Idaho	4-year renewal cycle (mail in every other renewal). Vision test required: 20/40 in better eye for no restrictions; 20/50–20/60 requires annual testing; 20/70 denied license. Use of bioptic telescopes is acceptable, but acuity must reach 20/40. Driving test may be required if examiner thinks it is needed. No renewal by mail after age 69.
Illinois	4-year renewal cycle for ages 21 to 80 (mail in every other cycle for drivers with clean records and no medical report review requirements). Vision test at in-person renewal: 20/40 in better eye for no restrictions, 20/70 in better eye results in daylight-only restriction. May have 20/100 in better eye and 20/40 through bioptic telescope. Written test every 8 years unless clean driving record. From ages 81 to 86 reduction of interval to 2 years. At age 87 reduction of interval to 1 year. No renewal by mail, vision test required, and on-road driving test required at age 75+.
Indiana	4-year renewal cycle (in person). Vision screening at renewal, including acuity and peripheral vision. 20/40 in better eye for no restriction; restricted license for 20/50. Bioptic telescope lenses permitted for best acuity as low as 20/200, with some restrictions, if 20/40 achieved with telescope. At age 75 renewal cycles are reduced to 3 years. (Mandatory drive test for people age 75+ eliminated 1/19/00.) Drive test required for people with 14 points or 3 convictions in 12-month period.
Iowa	Renewal cycle of 2 years or 4 years at driver's option. Vision screening at renewal: 20/40 in better eye with or without corrective lenses; 20/50 in better eye results in restricted license for daylight only; 20/70 in better eye results in restricted license for daylight only up to 35 mph. Bioptic telescopes are not permitted to meet acuity requirement. At age 70 renewal cycle is 2 years.

(*Continued*)

State/Province	2001 Licensing Renewal Requirements and Distinctions for Older Drivers*
Kansas	6-year renewal cycle for ages 16–64 (in person). Vision and knowledge test at renewal. Minimum acuity: 20/40 better eye; 20/60 better eye with doctor report; worse than 20/60 must demonstrate ability to operate vehicle safely and have safe record for 3 years. At age 65 renewals every 4 years.
Kentucky	4-year renewal cycle (in person). No tests required for renewal. Minimum visual acuity 20/200 or better with corrective lenses in better eye; 20/60 or better using a bioptic telescopic device. *No special requirements for older drivers.*
Louisiana	4-year renewal cycle (mail in every other cycle). Vision test at renewal. Minimum acuity 20/40 in better eye for unrestricted; 20/50–20/70 with restrictions; 20/70–20/100 possible restricted license; less than 20/100 in better eye, referred to Medical Advisory Board (MAB). No renewal by mail to drivers age 70+ or those with a conviction of moving violation in 2-year period before renewal.
Maine	6-year renewal cycle. At age 65 renew every 4 years. Vision screening test at renewal for age 40, 52, and 65; every 4 years after age 65. Minimum acuity 20/40 better eye without restrictions; 20/70 better eye with restrictions.
Maryland	5-year renewal cycle. Vision tests required for renewal (binocular, acuity, peripheral). Minimum acuity of at least 20/40 plus continuous field of vision at least 140E in each eye for unrestricted license; at least 20/70 in one or both eyes for restricted but requires continuous field of view of at least 110E with at least 35E lateral to the midline of each side; 20/70–20/100 requires special permission from MAB. Medical report required for new drivers age 70+. (Maryland law specifies that age alone is not grounds for re-examination of older drivers.)
Massachusetts	5-year renewal cycle (in person). Vision screening at renewal: 20/40 better eye for unrestricted; 20/70 better eye for restricted; 20/40 through telescope, 20/100 through carrier. *No special requirements for older drivers.* (Massachusetts law prohibits discrimination by reason of age for licensing issues.)
Michigan	4-year renewal cycle (mail in every other cycle if free of convictions). Vision and knowledge test at renewal. Minimum acuity 20/40 better eye for unrestricted; 20/70 better eye with daylight only restriction; 20/60 if progressive abnormalities or diseases of the eye. *No special requirements for older drivers.*
Minnesota	4-year renewal cycle. Vision test at renewal: 20/40 in better eye for no restrictions; 20/70 in better eye for speed limit restrictions; 20/100 better eye referred to driver evaluation unit. *No special requirements for older drivers.* (Minnesota law specifies that age alone is not justification for re-examination.)
Mississippi	4-year renewal cycle (in person). Vision test at renewal: 20/200 best corrected without telescope; 20/70 with telescope. *No special requirements for older drivers.*
Missouri	6-year renewal cycle (in person). At age 70, reduction in renewal cycle to 3 years. Vision test and traffic sign recognition test required at renewal. Minimum acuity: 20/40 in better eye for unrestricted; up to 20/160 for restricted.

State/Province	2001 Licensing Renewal Requirements and Distinctions for Older Drivers*
Montana	8-year renewal cycle for ages 21–67. Vision test at renewal: 20/40 in better eye for no restrictions; 20/70 in better eye with restrictions on daylight and speed; 20/100 in better eye possible restricted license if need is shown. For ages 68–74, renewal cycle reduced to 1–6 years. At age 75 renewal cycles reduced to 4 years.
Nebraska	5-year renewal cycle. Vision test at renewal: Knowledge test if violations on record. Acuity 20/40 required in better eye, but 17 restrictions are used, depending on vision in each eye. *No special requirements for older drivers.*
Nevada	4-year renewal cycle (mail in every other cycle if qualified). Minimum acuity 20/40 in better eye. Bioptic telescopes permitted to meet acuity standard: 20/40 through telescope, 20/120 through carrier, 130E visual field. Vision test and medical report required to renew by mail at age 70.
New Hampshire	4-year renewal cycle (in person). Vision test at renewal: 20/40 better eye for unrestricted; 20/70 in better eye with restrictions. At age 75 road test required at renewal.
New Jersey	4-year renewal cycle (10-year in-person digitized photo licenses implemented in 2003). Periodic vision retest: 20/50 better eye; 20/70 in better eye with restrictions. Bioptic telescope permitted to meet acuity standard. *No special requirements for older drivers.*
New Mexico	4- or 8-year renewal cycle. Drivers may not apply for 8-year license if they will reach the age of 75 during the last 4 years of the 8-year period. Vision test required for renewal; knowledge and driving test may be required Minimum acuity: 20/40 better eye; 20/80 better eye with restrictions.
New York	5-year renewal cycle. No tests for renewal. Minimum best corrected acuity 20/40 in one eye; 20/40–20/70 best-corrected one eye requires minimum 140E horizontal visual field; 20/80–20/100 best corrected in one eye requires minimum 140E horizontal visual field plus 20/40 through bioptic telescopic lens. *No special requirements for older drivers.*
North Carolina	5-year renewal cycle (in person). Vision and traffic sign recognition tests required for renewal. Acuity 20/40 in better eye required for unrestricted; 20/70 better eye with restrictions. Bioptic telescopes are *not* permitted for meeting acuity standard but are permitted for driving. *No special requirements for older drivers, except that people age 60+ are not required to parallel park in the road test.*
North Dakota	4-year renewal cycle. Vision test required for renewal: 20/40 better eye for unrestricted; 20/70 in better eye with restrictions. Bioptic telescopes permitted to meet acuity standard: 20/130 in carrier, 20/40 in telescope, full peripheral field. *No special requirements for older drivers.*
Ohio	4-year renewal cycle. Vision test required for renewal: 20/40 better eye for unrestricted; 20/70 better eye with restrictions; bioptic telescopes permitted to meet acuity standards. *No special requirements for older drivers.*
Oklahoma	4-year renewal cycle (in person). No tests for renewal. Minimum acuity: 20/40 better eye for unrestricted; 20/100 better eye with restrictions. Bioptic telescopes *not* permitted to meet acuity standard

(*Continued*)

State/Province	2001 Licensing Renewal Requirements and Distinctions for Older Drivers*
	but may be used for driving. *No special requirements for older drivers.*
Oregon	8-year renewal cycle (mail in every other cycle). Vision screening test once every 8 years at age 50+. Minimum acuity: 20/40 better eye for unrestricted; 20/70 better eye with restrictions. Bioptic telescopes *not* permitted to meet acuity standard but may be used for driving.
Pennsylvania	4-year renewal cycle. Drivers age 65+ may renew every 2 years. Random physical examinations for all drivers age 45+; most selected are age 65+. Minimum acuity: 20/40 better eye for unrestricted; up to 20/100 combined vision with restrictions. Bioptic telescopes *not* permitted to meet acuity standards but may be used for driving.
Rhode Island	5-year renewal cycle. Vision test required for renewal: 20/40 better eye. At age 70 renewal cycles reduced to 2 years.
South Carolina	5-year renewal cycle (in person). Renewal by mail if no violations in past 2 years and if license is not suspended, revoked, or canceled. Vision test and knowledge test required if >5 points on record. Minimum acuity: 20/40 better eye for unrestricted; 20/70 in better eye if worse eye is 20/200 or better; 20/40 if worse eye is worse than 20/200. Bioptic telescopes *not* permitted to meet acuity standard but may be used for driving. *No special requirements for older drivers.*
South Dakota	5-year renewal cycle. Vision test required for renewal: 20/40 better eye for unrestricted; 20/60 better eye with restrictions. *No special requirements for older drivers.*
Tennessee	5-year renewal cycle (mail in every other cycle). Minimum acuity: 20/30 better eye; 20/70 better eye with restrictions; 20/200 better eye requires bioptic telescopes with 20/60 through the telescope. Bioptic telescopes are permitted to meet standard. No tests required for renewal. *No special requirements for older drivers.*
Texas	6-year renewal cycle (effective 01/01/02; staggered 4–6 years until 2002). Vision test required for renewal: 20/40 better eye; 20/70 better eye with restrictions. Bioptic telescopes are permitted to meet acuity standard, and driver must pass a road test. *No special requirements for older drivers.*
Utah	5-year renewal cycle (mail in every other cycle if no suspensions, no revocations, no convictions for reckless driving, and no more than 4 reportable violations). Vision test required for drivers age 65+ every renewal. Minimum acuity: 20/40 for unrestricted; 20/100 in better eye with restrictions. Bioptic telescopes are *not* permitted to meet acuity standard.
Vermont	2- or 4-year renewal cycle. Minimum acuity: 20/40 in better eye; bioptic telescopes are permitted to meet visual acuity standard, and driver must pass road test. No tests for renewal. *No special requirements for older drivers.*
Virginia	5-year renewal cycle (mail in every other cycle unless suspended or revoked, 2+ violations, seizures/blackouts, DMV medical review indicator on license, failed vision test). Vision test required for renewal. Minimum acuity: 20/40 better eye for unrestricted; 20/200 with restrictions; bioptic telescopes are permitted with 20/200 through carrier, 20/70 through telescope. Knowledge and road test

State/Province	2001 Licensing Renewal Requirements and Distinctions for Older Drivers*
	required if 2+ violations in 5 years. *No special requirements for older drivers.*
Washington	5-year renewal cycle (in person). Vision test required for renewal. Minimum acuity 20/40 better eye; 20/70 better eye with restrictions. Bioptic telescopes are permitted to meet acuity standards. Other tests may be required if License Service Representative deems it necessary. *No special requirements for older drivers.*
West Virginia	5-year renewal cycle. Minimum acuity: 20/60 better eye; if worse than 20/60, optometrist or ophthalmologist must declare ability to be safe. Bioptic telescopes are *not* permitted to meet acuity standard but may be used for driving. No tests required for renewal. *No special requirements for older drivers.*
Wisconsin	8-year renewal cycle (in person). Minimum acuity: 20/40 better eye; 20/100 better eye with restrictions. Bioptic telescopes are *not* permitted to meet acuity standards but may be used for driving. Vision test required for renewal. *No special requirements for older drivers.*
Wyoming	4-year renewal cycle (mail in every other cycle). Vision test required for renewal (for mail in and in person). Minimum acuity; 20/40 better eye; 20/100 better eye with restrictions. Bioptic telescopes are permitted to meet acuity standard. *No special requirements for older drivers.*
Alberta	No mandatory retesting; medical review and vision test at ages 75, 80, and every 2 years thereafter.
British Columbia	No mandatory retesting; medical review at age 80 and every 2 years thereafter.
Manitoba	Annual license renewal. No mandatory retesting; no periodic medical review. Minimum acuity of 6/12 (20/40) −2 in the better eye with or without correction. May drive with restrictions with acuity of 6/12 (20/40) −3, to 6/18 (20/60) −2 in the better eye. Telescopic lenses not eligible for any class of license. Minimum horizontal field requirement of 120° with both eyes tested together or tested separately and results superimposed. Visual fields to be measured at or 10° above or below fixation. Standards exist for hemianopsia and quadratic field defects, color perception, and diplopia. Drivers with depth perception and diabetic retinopathy impairments must meet visual acuity and field standards. On recommendation from a physician, mature drivers can be requested to complete medical, vision, or oral test.
New Brunswick	4-year renewal for passenger vehicle license (may be renewed by mail). No tests required for renewal. Minimum visual acuity (corrected) must be at least 20/40 in at least one eye. *No special requirements for older drivers.*
Newfoundland and Labrador	5-year renewal cycle (may be by mail if current photo is on file). No tests required for renewal. Drivers age 75 must present a medical exam form from their physician to renew their licenses. Drivers age 80 must provide a medical report every 2 years.
Northwest Territories	No mandatory retesting; medical review at ages 75, 80, and every 2 years thereafter.

(*Continued*)

State/Province	2001 Licensing Renewal Requirements and Distinctions for Older Drivers*
Nova Scotia	No mandatory retesting; no periodic medical review; drivers 65+ involved in a collision must take a written and on-road test.
Nunavut	5-year renewal cycle (in person). No tests required for renewal unless medical concerns have been identified. *No special requirements for older drivers.*
Ontario	5-year renewal cycle (in person). At age 80, renewal every 2 years. Mail-in renewal is an option for drivers with no testing requirements who have had photo taken within past 2 years. Mandatory written knowledge test, vision test, and participation in a 90-minute group education session on safe driving at age 80 and every 2 years thereafter; includes driver record review. Senior drivers may be required to pass a road test before being relicensed if they have an excessive number of demerit points showing on their record. Some drivers may be required to pass a road test before being relicensed if, in the opinion of the instructor, they may represent a safety risk. Collision-involved drivers aged 70+ who are convicted of a collision-related offense must take mandatory vision, knowledge, and road tests. Vision requirements include 20/40 acuity in better eye, with or without corrective lenses, and 120°. No periodic medical review requirement under Section 203 of Highway Traffic Act; physicians required to report any patient aged 16+ with a medical condition that may make driving dangerous. Medical report may be required on a cyclical basis if there is evidence of a medical condition that may eventually interfere with safe operation of motor vehicle.
Prince Edward Island	3-year renewal cycle (may be renewed by mail, but regular renewal is in person). No tests required for renewal. Minimum acuity for original license 20/40 in better eye. *No special requirements for older drivers.* On recommendation from the police, physician, or family member, mature drivers can be requested to complete medical, vision, or oral test.
Quebec	2-year renewal cycle (may be renewed by mail, but driver must come to a service center every 4 years to have a picture taken). At ages 75, 80, and every 2 years thereafter, drivers must present a medical examination and optometric report (with acceptable exam results) when renewing. No tests required for renewal, but a declaration of illness or impairment that has not been previously reported must be reported upon renewal. Visual requirements for licensing include 20/40 vision with or without glasses in at least one eye, and minimum field of vision of 120 degrees.
Saskatchewan	Annual renewals required for all drivers (may be renewed by mail). No tests required for renewal unless driver's license indicates that an annual vision, road, or medical exam is required. When a license is issued or renewed, any medical condition that may affect a driver's ability to drive must be reported to SGI. If the license indicated that an annual medical exam report is required, then a medical report must be presented at the time of renewal. Minimum visual requirements for passenger vehicle driver license: 20/50 with both eyes examined together (aided or unaided); field of vision must measure a minimum of 120 degrees (both eyes measured together). *No special requirements for older drivers.* On recommendation from the police,

State/Province	2001 Licensing Renewal Requirements and Distinctions for Older Drivers*
	physician, or family member, mature drivers can be requested to complete medical, vision, or oral test.
Yukon	No mandatory retesting; medical review and vision test at age 70, every 2 years to age 80, annually thereafter.

**Information about each jurisdiction was obtained from one or more of the following sources: DMV licensing official, DMV website, DMV Driver's Manual, research report, Insurance Institute for Highway Safety.*
Staplin, L., Lococo, K. H., Gish, K. W. et al. Model driver screening and evaluation program final technical report: DOT HS 809 581. Guidelines for motor vehicle administrators, Washington, DC, 2003, National Highway Traffic Safety Administration. Available at: http://www.nhtsa.dot.gov/people/injury/olderdrive/modeldriver/. Accessed January 5, 2004.

APPENDIX D: STATE OF MICHIGAN'S DRIVER LICENSING REQUIREMENTS AND REPORTING LAWS

This section has been reprinted with permission from the AMA

Each state has its own licensing and license renewal criteria for drivers of private motor vehicles. In addition, certain states require physicians to report unsafe drivers or drivers with specific medical conditions to the driver licensing agency. This chapter contains licensing agency contact information, license requirements and renewal criteria, reporting procedures, and Medical Advisory Board information listed by state. These materials are provided to physicians as a reference to aid them in discharging their legal responsibilities. The information in this chapter should not be construed as legal advice nor used to resolve legal problems. If legal advice is required, physicians should consult an attorney who is licensed to practice in their state. Information for this chapter was primarily obtained from each state's driver licensing agency and reflects the most current information at the time of publication. Please note that this information is subject to change. When information for this chapter was not available from an individual state's driver licensing agency, the following references were used:

(1) Coley, M. J. & Coughlin, J. F. State driving regulations. Adapted from: National Academy on an Aging Society. *The Public Policy and Aging Report.* 2001, 11(4). Epilepsy Foundation. Driver information by state. Available at: http://www.efa.org/answerplace/drivelaw/searchform.cfm. Accessed January 10, 2003.

(2) Insurance Institute for Highway Safety. U.S. driver licensing renewal procedures for older drivers. Available at: http://www.hwysafety.org/safety_facts/state_laws/older_drivers.htm. Accessed May 12, 2003. Massachusetts Medical Society. *Medical Perspectives on Impaired Driving* (1st ed.). Available at: www.massmed.org/pages/impaireddrivers.asp. Accessed May 12, 2003.

(3) National Highway Traffic Safety Administration. State reporting practices. Available at: http://www.nhtsa.gov/people/injury/olddrive/FamilynFriends/state.htm. Accessed May 12, 2003.

(4) Peli, E. & Peli, D. *Driving with Confidence: A Practical Guide to Driving with Low Vision.* Singapore: World Scientific Publishing Co. Pte. Ltd. 2002. *State and Provincial Licensing Systems: Comparative Data.* Arlington, VA: American Association of Motor Vehicle Administrators. 1999.

(5) Supplemental Technical Notes. In: Staplin, L., Lococo, K., Byington, S., & Harkey, D. *Guidelines and Recommendations to Accommodate Older Drivers and Pedestrians.* Washington, DC: Federal Highway Administration. 2001.

(6) Michigan Driver Licensing Agency Michigan Department of State 517 322-1460 contact information: 7707 Rickle Road, Lansing, MI 48918. www.michigan.gov/sos

APPENDIX E: LICENSING REQUIREMENTS

Visual acuity: Each eye with/without correction........................20/40

Both eyes with/without correction ....20/40 to and including 20/50

If one eye blind—other with/without correction........................20/50

Absolute visual acuity minimum ....Minimum of 20/70 in better eye with daylight-only restriction; minimum of 20/60 if progressive abnormalities or disease of the eye exist.

Are bioptic telescopes allowed? ....Yes. A road test is required.

Visual fields: Minimum field requirement ....110°−140° in both eyes; if less than 110° to/including 90°, there are additional conditions and requirements.

Visual field testing device ....Not specified

Color vision requirement: None

Type of road test: Standardized course and requirements

Restricted licenses: Restrictions are based on review of medical input and re-examination testing. Examples include radius limitations, daylight-only driving, and no expressway driving.

License renewal procedures

Standard: Length of license validation ....4 years

Renewal options and conditions ....Mail-in every other cycle, if free of convictions.

Vision testing required at time of renewal?..................................Yes

Written test required?...Yes

Road test required?...Yes, if license has been expired more than 4 years.

Age-based renewal procedures: No

Reporting procedures

Physician/medical reporting: Physicians are encouraged to report unsafe drivers. They may do so by completing a "Request for Driver Evaluation" form (OC-88). This form can be downloaded from the Michigan Department of State website.

Immunity: None

Legal protection: None

DMV follow-up: The driver is notified in writing of the referral. The notification includes a notice of date, time, and location of driver re-examination as well as any medical statements to be completed by the driver's doctor.

Other reporting: The Department accepts referrals for re-examination from family, police, public officials, and others who have knowledge of a driver's inability to drive safely or health concerns that may affect his/her driving ability.

Anonymity: Reporting is not anonymous. However, the Department will release the name of the reporter only if he/she is a public official (e.g., police, judge, state employee). The names of non-public official reporters will be released only under court order.

Medical Advisory Board (MAB)

Role of the MAB: The MAB advises the Department of State on medical issues regarding individual drivers. Actions are based on the recommendation of specialists.

MAB contact information: For additional information, contact the Driver Assessment Office at 517 241-6840.

REFERENCES

Aging News Alert (October 24, 2000). Fatalities rise among older drivers.

American Academy of Ophthalmology (2001). Policy statement: vision requirements for driving, Approved by the Board of Trustees, October 2001. Available at: http://www.aao.org/aao/member/policy/driving.cfm. Accessed January 14, 2004.

American Automobile Association (AAA): Automatic brake reaction timer: instructions for use. Heathrow, FL, undated, American Automobile Association.

Army Individual Test Battery: Manual of directions and scoring, Washington, DC, 1944, War Department, Adjutant General's Office. Cited in Lezak, M.D. (1995). *Neuropsychological Assessment*. New York, NY: Oxford University Press, pp. 381–384.

Association for Driver Rehabilitation Specialists. (2004). *Best practices for the delivery of driver rehabilitation services*. Ruston, LA: Association for Driver Rehabilitation Specialists.

Ball, K., Owsley, C., Sloane, M. E., Roenker, D. L., & Bruni, J. R. (1993). Visual attention problems as a predictor of vehicle crashes in older drivers. *Invest Ophthalmol. Vis. Sci.*, *34*, 3110–3123.

Ball, K., & Owsley, C. (1992). The useful field of view test: a new technique for evaluating age-related declines in visual function. *J. Am. Optom. Assoc.*, *63*, 71–79.

Barry, C. J., Smith, D., Lennarson, P., Jermeland, J., Darling, W., Stierman, L., & et al. (2003). The effect of wearing a restrictive neck brace on driver performance. *Neurosurg.*, *53*, 98–102.

Beery, K. E. (1997). *The Beery-Buktenica Developmental Test of Visual-motor Integration Manual* (rev. ed) Parsippany, NJ: Modern Curriculum Press.

Benton, A. L., Hamsher, K. S., Varney, N. R., et al. (1983). *Contributions to Neuropsychological Assessment*. New York, NY: Oxford University Press.

Blumer: *A Public Philosophy for Mass Society*. Champaign, IL: University of Illinois Press.

Brower, W. H., Withaar, F. K., Tant, M. L., & Van Zomeren, A. H. (2002). Attention and driving in traumatic brain injury: a question of coping with time-pressure. *J. Head Trauma. Rehabil.*, *17*, 1–15.

Calvanio, R., Williams, R., Burke, D. T., Mello, J., Lepak, P., Al-Adawi, S., et al. (2004). Acquired brain injury, visual attention, and the Useful Field of View Test: a pilot study. *Arch. Phys. Med. Rehabil.*, *85*, 474–478.

Capo, L. C. (2001). Autism, employment, and the role of occupational therapy. *Work*, *16*, 201–207.

Carr, D. (1993). Assessing older drivers for physical and cognitive impairment. *Geriatrics*, *48* 46–51

Colarusso, R. P., & Hammill, D. D. (1972). *Motor-free Visual Perception Test Manual* (1st ed.) Novato, CA: Academic Therapy Publications.

Colarusso, R. P., & Hammill, D. D. (2003). *Motor-free Visual Perception Test Manual* (3rd ed.) Novato, CA: Academic Therapy Publications.

Coleman, R. D., Rapport, L. J., Ergh, T. C., Hanks, R. A., Ricker, J. H., & Millis, S. R. (2002). Predictors of driving outcome after traumatic brain injury. *Arch. Phys. Med. Rehabil.*, *83*, 1415–1422.

Coleman Bryer, R., Rapport, L. J., & Hanks, R. A. (2009). Determining fitness to drive: Neurophysical Considerations. In J. M. Pellerito, Jr. (Ed.), *Driving retirement*. Munich, Germany: VDM Publishing House, Ltd.

Colenbrander, A., Goodwin, L., & Fletcher, D. (2007). Vision Rehabilitation and AMD. *International Ophthalmology Clinics*, *47*(1), 139–148.

Culbertson, W. C., & Zillmer, E. A. (2001). Tower of London. *Drexel University.* Odessa, FL: Psychological Assessment Resources.

Cushman, L. A., & Cogliandro, F. C. (1999). On-road driving post-stroke: cognitive and other factors. *Arch. Clin. Neuropsychol.*, *14*, 799.

Cushman, L. A. (1996). Cognitive capacity and concurrent driving performance in older drivers. *IATTS Research*, *20*(1), 38–45.

D'Elia, L., Satz, P., Uchiyama, C., et al. (1996). *Color Trails Test*. Odessa, FL: Psychological Assessment Resources.

Daigneault, G., Joly, P., & Frigon, J. Y. (2002). Executive functions in the evaluation of accident risk of older drivers. *J. Clin. Exp. Neuropsychol.*, *24*, 221–238.

Dubinsky, R. M., Stein, A. C., & Lyons, K. (2000). Practice parameter: risk of driving and Alzheimer's disease (an evidence-based review). *Neurology*, *54*, 2205–2211.

Eby, D. W., Molnar, L. J., Shope, J. T., et al. (2003). Improving older driver knowledge and awareness through self-assessment: The Driving Decisions Workbook. *Journal of Safety Research*, *34*, 371–381.

Eby, D. W. (2009). SAFER driving: The enhanced driving decisions workbook. *Annual Lifesavers Conference*. Nashville, TN.

Engum, E., Cron, L., Hulse, C., et al. (1988). Cognitive behavioral driver's inventory. *Cogn. Rehabil.*, 34–50, September/October.

Fisk, G. D., Novack, T., Mennemeier, M., & Roenker, D. (2002). Useful field of view after traumatic brain injury. *J. Head Trauma Rehabil.*, *17*, 16–25.

Fisk, G. D., Owsley, C., & Mennemeier, M. (2002). Vision, attention, and self-reported driving behaviors in community-dwelling stroke survivors. *Arch. Phys. Med. Rehabil.*, *83*, 469–477.

Freund, B., & Szinovacz, M. (2002). Effects of cognition on driving involvement among the oldest old: variations by gender and alternative transportation opportunities. *The Gerontologist*, *42*(5), 621–633.

Galski, T., Bruno, R. L., & Ehle, H. T. (1992). Driving after cerebral damage: a model with implications for evaluation. *American Journal of Occupational Therapy*, *46*(4), 324–332.

Gardner, M. F. (1996). *Test of visual perceptual skills manual* (rev. ed). Hydesville, CA: Psychological and Educational Publications.

Gillins, L. (1990). Yielding to age: when the elderly can no longer drive. *Journal of Gerontological Nursing*, *16*, 12–15.

Golper, L. A., Rau, M. T., & Marshall, R. C. (1980). Aphasic adults and their decisions on driving: an evaluation. *Arch. Phys. Med. Rehabil.*, *61*, 34–40.

Goode, K., Ball, K., Sloane, M., et al. (1998). Useful field of view and other neurocognitive indicators of crash risk in older adults. *J. Clin. Psychol. Med. Settings*, *5*, 425–440.

Gouvier, W. D., Maxfield, M. W., Schweitzer, J. R., Horton, C. R., Shipp, M., Nelson, K., & Hale, P. N. (1989). Psychometric prediction of driving performance among the disabled. *Arch. Phys. Med. Rehabil.*, *70*, 745–750.

Groeger, J. A. (2000). *Understanding Driving: Applying Cognitive Psychology to a Complex Everyday Task*. East Sussex, UK: Psychology Press.

Heaton, R. K. (1981). *Wisconsin Card Sorting Test Manual*. Odessa, FL: Psychological Assessment Resources.

Hooper, H. E. (1979). *The Hooper Visual Organization Test Manual*. Los Angeles, CA: Western Psychological Services.

Hopewell, C. A. (2002). Driving assessment issues for practicing clinicians. *J. Head Trauma Rehabil*, *17*, 48–61.

Isler, R. B., Parsonson, B. S., & Hansson, G. J. (1997). Age related effects of restricted head movements on the useful field of view of drivers. *Accid. Anal. Prevent.*, *29*, 793–801.

Johnson, J. E. (1995). Rural elders and the decision to stop driving. *Journal of Community Health Nursing*, *12*(3), 131–138.

Kalz, R. T., Golden, R. S., Butler, J., Tepper, D., Rothke, S., Holmes, J., et al. (1990). Driving safely after brain damage: follow up of 22 patients with matched controls. *Archives of Physical Medicine and Rehabilitation*, *71*, 133–137.

Klavora, P., Gaskovski, P., & Forsyth, R. (1995). Test-retest reliability of three Dynavision tasks. *Perceptual Motor Skills*, *80*, 607–610.

Klavora, P., Gaskovski, P., Martin, K., Forsyth, R., Heslegrave, R. J., Young, M., & Quinn, R. P. (1995). The effects of Dynavision rehabilitation on behind the wheel driving ability and selected psychomotor abilities of persons after stroke. *Am. J. Occup. Ther.*, *49*, 534–542.

Korner-Bitensky, N., Mazur, B. L., Sofer, S., Gelina, L., Meyer, M. B., & Morrison, C. (2000). Visual testing for readiness to drive after stroke: a multicenter study. *Am. J. Phys. Med. Rehabil.*, *79*, 253–259.

Korteling, J. E., & Kaptein, N. A. (1996). Neuropsychological driving fitness tests for brain-damaged subjects. *Arch. Phys. Med. Rehabil.*, *77*, 138–145.

Korteling, J. E. (1990). Perception-response speed and driving capabilities of brain-damaged and older drivers. *Hum. Factors*, *32*, 95–108.

Kulash, D. (2000). Safe mobility for a maturing society: a strategic plan and national agenda. *Transportation in an Aging Society: A Decade of Experience*. Originally presented as proceedings from the International Conference November 1999.

Lundberg, C., Hakamies-Blomqvist, L., Almkvist, O., & Johansson, K. (1998). Impairments of some cognitive functions are common in crash-involved older drivers. *Accident Analysis and Prevention*, *30*(3), 371–377.

Lyman, L.M., & Vidich, A.J. (Eds.) (2000). *Selected Works of Herbert*

Lysack, C., Neufeld, S., Mast, B., McNeil, S., & Lichtenberg, P. (2003). After rehabilitation: an 18-month follow-up of elderly inner-city women. *American Journal of Occupational Therapy*, *57*(3), 298–306.

Mackenzie, C., & Paton, G. (2003). Resumption of driving with aphasia following stroke. *Aphasiology*, *17*, 107–122.

Marottoli, R. A., & Drickamer, M. A. (1993). Psychomotor mobility and the elderly driver. *Clin. Geriatr. Med.*, *9*, 403–411.

Mazer, B. L., Korner-Bitensky, N. A., & Sofer, S. (1998). Predicting ability to drive after stroke. *Arch. Phys. Med. Rehabil.*, *79*, 743–750.

Mazer, B. L., Sofer, S., Korner-Bitensky, N., Gelinas, I., Hanley, J., & Wood-Dauphinee, S. (2003). Effectiveness of a visual attention retraining program on the driving performance of clients with stroke. *Arch. Phys. Med. Rehabil.*, *84*, 541–550.

McKenna, P. (1998). Fitness to drive: a neuropsychological perspective. *J. Mental Health*, *7*, 9–18.

Mestre, D. R. (2004). *Dynamic Evaluation of the Useful Field of View in Driving*. Marseilles, France: Cognitive Neurosciences Centre.

Molnar, L. J., Eby, D. W., & Miller, L. L. (2003). *Promising Approaches for Enhancing Elderly Mobility.* Ann Arbor, MI: University of Michigan Transportation Research Institute.

Molnar, L. J., Eby, D. W., St. Louis, R. M., & Neumeyer., A. (2007). *Promising Approaches for Promoting Lifelong Community Mobility.* Ann Arbor, MI: University of Michigan, Transport Institute.

Molnar, L. J., & Eby, D. W. (2009). Getting around: Meeting the boomers' mobility needs. In R. Houston (Ed.), *Boomer bust? economic and political issues of the graying society., vol. 2*. Praeger Publishing.

Myers, R. S., Ball, K. K., Kalina, T. D., Roth, D. L., & Goode, K. T. (2000). Relation of useful field of view and other screening tests to on-road driving performance. *Percept. Mot. Skills*, *91*, 279–290.

National Highway Traffic Safety Administration (NHTSA). (2003). *Project Summary and Model Program Recommendations (DOT HS 809 582).* Model driver screening and evaluation program: final technical report. Volume 1. Washington, DC: US Department of Transportation.

National Institute on Aging (1998). New test predicts crash risk of older drivers. Science Blog.

National Research Council. (1988). *Transportation in an ageing society: improving mobility and safety for older persons.* Special Report 218, vol. 1. Washington, DC: Transportation Research Board.

O'Neill, D. (1992). Physicians, elderly drivers, and dementia. *Lancet*, *2*, 99–104.

Owsley, C., Ball, K., McGwin, G., Jr., Sloane, M. E., Roenker, D. L., White, M. F., et al. (1998). Visual processing impairment and risk of motor vehicle crash among older adults. *JAMA*, *279*, 1083–1088.

Owsley, C., Stalvey, B., Wells, J., & Sloane, M. E. (1999). Older drivers and cataract: driving habits and crash risk. *J. Gerontol. Med. Sci*, *54A*, M203–M211.

Pellerito, J. M. (Ed.). (2006). *Driver Rehabilitation and Community Mobility: Principles and Practice*. St. Louis, MO: Elsevier Mosby.

Pellerito, J.M. (2009).

Posse, C., McCarthy, D. P., & Mann, W. C. (2006). A pilot study of interrater reliability of the assessment of driving-related skills older driving screening tool. *Topics in Geriatric Rehabilitation*, *22*(2), 113–120.

Radford, K. A., & Lincoln, N. B. (2004). Concurrent validity of the stroke drivers screening assessment. *Arch. Phys. Med. Rehabil.*, *85*, 324–328.

Reitan, R. M., & Davison, L. A. (1974). *Clinical Neuropsychology: Current Status and Applications*. New York, NY: Halstead Press.

Rosenbloom, S. (1993). Transportation needs of the elderly population. *Clinics in Geriatric Medicine*, *9*, 297–310.

Rothke, S. (1989). The relationship between neuropsychological test scores and performance on driving evaluation. *Int. J. Clin. Neuropsychol.*, *11*, 134–136.

Royall, D. R., Cordes, J. A., & Polk, M. (1998). CLOX: an executive clock drawing task. *J. Neurosurg. Psychiatr.*, *64*, 588–594.

Safe Performance Associates (Undated). *Driver Performance Test Manual*. Clearwater, FL: Safe Performance Associates

Sanders, M. S., & McCormick, E. J. (2003). Human factors and the automobile. In M. S. Sanders, & E. J. McCormick (Eds.), *Human Factors in Engineering and Design*. New York, NY: McGraw-Hill, Inc.

Schanke, A., & Sundet, K. (2000). Comprehensive driving assessment: neuropsychological testing and on-road evaluation of brain injured patients. *Scand. J. Psychol.*, *41*, 113–121.

Schultheis, M. T., Garay, E., & DeLuca, J. (2001). The influence of cognitive impairment on driving performance in multiple sclerosis. *Neurology*, *56*, 1089–1094.

Shawaryn, M. A., Schultheis, M. T., Garay, E., & Deluca, J. (2002). Assessing functional status: exploring the relationship between the multiple sclerosis functional composite and driving. *Arch. Phys. Med. Rehabil.*, *83*, 1123–1129.

Shiner, D., & Schieber, F. (1991). *Visual requirements for safety and mobility of older drivers. Hum. Factors*, *33*. Silver Spring, MD: CD Publications.

Sivak, M., Olson, P., Kewman, D., Won, H., & Henson, D. L. (1981). Driving and perceptual/cognitive skills: behavioral consequences of brain damage. *Arch. Phys. Med. Rehabil.*, *62*, 476–483.

Sivan, A. B. (1992). *Benton Visual Retention Test Manual* (5th ed.) San Antonio, TX: The Psychological Corporation.

Spreen, O., & Strauss, E. (1998). *A Compendium of Neuropsychological Tests: Administration, Norms and Commentary*. New York, NY: Oxford University Press.

Stav, W. B. (2004). *Driving Rehabilitation: A Guide for Assessment and Intervention*. San Antonio, TX: The Psychological Corporation.

Stereo Optical Co., Inc. (2009). *Vision Tester Slide Packages and Instructions*. Stereo Optical Co., Inc.

Stubbins, J. (1977). *Social and Psychological Aspects of Disability: What about Leisure?* Baltimore, MD: University Park Press.

Tombaugh, T. T. (2004). Trail Making Test A and B: normative data stratified by age and education. *Arch. Clin. Neuropsychol.*, *19*, 203–214.

Trenerry, M. R., Crosson, B., Deboe, J., et al. (1989). *Stroop Neuropsychological Screening Test*. Psychological Assessment Resources.

U.S. Department of Commerce, Economics and Statistics Administration. (1995). *Statistical Abstract of the U.S.* (115th ed.) Washington, DC: Bureau of Census.

U.S. Department of Health and Human Services. (1991). *Bound for Good Health: A Collection of Age Pages*. Bethesda, MD: National Institute on Aging.

U.S. Department of Transportation. (2003). *Safe Mobility for a Maturing Society: Challenges and Opportunities*. Washington, DC: Government Printing Office.

Underwood, M. (1992). The older driver: clinical assessment and injury prevention. *Archives of Internal Medicine*, *152*(4), 735–740.

Vericom (2004). *Vericom Manual VC3000*, Version 3.2.5.

Victor, C. (1994). *Old Age in Modern Society* (2nd ed.) London, UK: Chapman and Hall.

Wang, C. C., Kosinski, C. J., Schwartzberg, J. G., et al. (2003). *Physician's Guide to Assessing and Counseling Older Drivers*. Washington, DC: National Highway Traffic Safety Administration.

Webster, J. S., Rapport, L. J., Godlewski, M. C., & Abadee, P. S. (1994). Effect of attentional bias to right space on wheelchair mobility. *J. Clin. Exp. Neuropsychol.*, *16*, 129–137.

Webster, J. S., Rhoades, L. A., Morrill, B., Rapport, L. J., Abadee, P. S., Sowa, M. V., et al. (1995). Rightward orienting bias, wheelchair maneuvering, and fall risk. *Arch. Phys. Med. Rehabil.*, *76*, 924–928.

Wechsler, D. (1997). *Wechsler Adult Intelligence Scale* (3rd ed.) San Antonio, TX: Psychological Assessment Corp.

Williams, A. F., & Carsten, O. (1989). Driver age and crash involvement. *Am. J. Public Health*, *79*, 326–327.

Wilson, B., Cockburn, J., & Baddeley, A. (1985). *The Rivermead Behavioral Memory Test Manual*. Reading, UK: The Thames Valley Test Company.

Index

Printed and bound by CPI Group (UK) Ltd, Croydon, CR0 4YY

11/06/2025

01899189-0017